Procedural Dermatosurgery

A Step by Step Approach

Procedural Dermatosurgery
A Step by Step Approach

Editors

Biju Vasudevan
MD FRGUHS (Dermatosurgery)
Professor (Derm & Ven)
Base Hospital Lucknow
Lucknow, Uttar Pradesh, India

Manas Chatterjee MD
Professor and Head
Department of Dermatology
INHS Asvini
Mumbai, Maharashtra, India

Shilpa K MD FRGUHS (Dermatosurgery)
Assistant Professor
Bangalore Medical College and Research Institute
Bengaluru, Karnataka, India

Assistant Editors

Divya Gorur MD FRGUHS
Senior Resident
Department of Dermatology
Bangalore Medical College and Research Institute
Bengaluru, Karnataka, India

Madura C MD FRGUHS (Dermatosurgery)
Consultant Dermatologist, Dermatosurgeon and
Hair Transplantation Surgeon
Cutis Academy of Cutaneous Sciences
Bengaluru, Karnataka, India

Harish Prasad MD FRGUHS
Consultant Dermatologist
Apollo and HCG Cancer Hospital
VITALS Klinic
Bengaluru, Karnataka, India

Savitha AS MD
Assistant Professor
Department of Dermatology
Sapthagiri Institute of Medical Sciences
Bengaluru, Karnataka, India

Shekhar Neema MD
Assistant Professor
Department of Dermatology
Command Hospital
Kolkata, West Bengal, India

Sujala S Aradhya
MD (DVL) FRGUHS (Dermatosurgery)
Consultant Dermatologist and Dermatosurgery
Sujala Polyclinic and Laboratory
Bengaluru, Karnataka, India

Foreword
Dr (Col) Manas Chatterjee MD

ASSOCIATION OF CUTANEOUS SURGEONS (I)
1995

JAYPEE *The Health Sciences Publisher*
New Delhi | London | Panama

Jaypee Brothers Medical Publishers (P) Ltd

Headquarters

Jaypee Brothers Medical Publishers (P) Ltd
4838/24, Ansari Road, Daryaganj
New Delhi 110 002, India
Phone: +91-11-43574357
Fax: +91-11-43574314
E-mail: jaypee@jaypeebrothers.com

Overseas Offices

JP Medical Ltd
83 Victoria Street, London
SW1H 0HW (UK)
Phone: +44 20 3170 8910
Fax: +44 (0)20 3008 6180
E-mail: info@jpmedpub.com

Jaypee-Highlights Medical Publishers Inc
City of Knowledge, Bld. 235, 2nd Floor, Clayton
Panama City, Panama
Phone: +1 507-301-0496
Fax: +1 507-301-0499
E-mail: cservice@jphmedical.com

Jaypee Brothers Medical Publishers (P) Ltd
17/1-B, Babar Road, Block-B, Shyamoli
Mohammadpur, Dhaka-1207
Bangladesh
Mobile: +08801912003485
E-mail: jaypeedhaka@gmail.com

Jaypee Brothers Medical Publishers (P) Ltd
Bhotahity, Kathmandu, Nepal
Phone: +977-9741283608
E-mail: kathmandu@jaypeebrothers.com

Website: www.jaypeebrothers.com
Website: www.jaypeedigital.com

Inquiries for bulk sales may be solicited at: jaypee@jaypeebrothers.com

Procedural Dermatosurgery: A Step by Step Approach

First Edition: **2018**

ISBN: 978-93-5270-212-1

Printed at Sanat Printers

Dedicated to

Our families, teachers, students and patients

Editorial Advisory Committee

Contributors

Aarti Sarda MD
Senior Resident
KPC Medical College
Kolkata, West Bengal, India

Abhilasha MD MD
Junior Resident
Rajarajeshwari Medical College and Hospital
Bengaluru, Karnataka, India

Abhishek De MD FAGE
Associate Professor
Calcutta National Medical College
Kolkata, West Bengal, India

Akshi Bansal MD
Department of Dermatology
Bangalore Medical College and Research Institute
Bengaluru, Karnataka, India

Aman Dua MD
Consultant Dermatologist and
Hair Transplant Surgeon
AK Clinics Pvt Ltd
Ludhiana, Punjab, India

Amit Kerure
Consultant Dermatologist
Mumbai, Maharashtra, India

Anagha Ramesh MD
Consultant Dermatologist
Bengaluru, Karnataka, India

Aneesh KP MBBS
Senior Resident
Department of Dermatology
Base Hospital Lucknow
Lucknow, Uttar Pradesh, India

Ankan Gupta MD DNB
Assistant Professor
Department of Dermatology
Christian Medical College
Vellore, Tamil Nadu, India

Anupam Das MD
Assistant Professor
KPC Medical College and Hospital
Kolkata, West Bengal, India

Avitus John Prasad DDVL
Managing Director
SP Derma Center
Madurai, Tamil Nadu, India

Biju Vasudevan MD FRGUHS (Dermatosurgery)
Professor (Derm & Ven)
Base Hospital Lucknow
Lucknow, Uttar Pradesh, India

Bipin Deshpande DVD FAAD (USA)
Chaitanya Clinic
Dahanukar Colony and Head
Department of Cosmetology
Noble Hospital
Pune, Maharashtra, India

BM Shashikumar MD FIADVL (Dermatopath)
Associate Professor
Department of Dermatology
Mandya Institute of Medical Sciences
Mandya, Karnataka, India

BS Chandrashekar
Chief Dermatologist and Medical Director
Cutis Academy of Cutaneous Sciences
Bengaluru, Karnataka, India

Chaithra Shenoy
Consultant Dermatologist and Cosmetologist
Cutis Academy of
Cutaneous Sciences
Bengaluru, Karnataka, India

Chander Grover MD DBM MNAMS
Professor
Dermatology and STD
University College of Medical Sciences and
Guru Teg Bahadur Hospital
New Delhi, India

Debdeep Mitra MD DNB
Graded Specialist
Department of Dermatology, Base Hospital
New Delhi, India

Debjit Kar MD DVL FIADVL
Consultant Dermatologist and Dermatosurgeon
Assistant Professor
Department of Dermatology
Hi-Tech Medical College and Hospital
Rourkela, Odisha, India

Dhanashree Bhide MD
Consultant Dermatologist
Dhadphale Nursing Home
Pune, Maharashtra, India

Divya Gorur MD FRGUHS
Senior Resident
Department of Dermatology
Bangalore Medical College and Research Institute
Bengaluru, Karnataka, India

Eswari L MD FRGUHS (Dermatosurgery)
Assistant Professor
Bangalore Medical College and Research Institute
Bengaluru, Karnataka, India

Gautam Kumar Singh MD
Cl Spl (Dermatology)
Military Hospital Kirkee
Pune, Maharashtra, India

Govind Mittal MD FRGUHS (Dermatosurgery)
Consultant Dermatologist, Dermatosurgeon and Dermatotrichologist, Excel Care Hospital
Bengaluru, Karnataka, India

Harish Prasad MD FRGUHS
Consultant Dermatologist
Apollo and HCG Cancer Hospital
VITALS Klinic
Bengaluru, Karnataka, India

Imran Majid MD
Associate Professor
Cutis Institute of Dermatology
Srinagar, Jammu and Kashmir, India

Koushik Lahiri DVD(CAL) FIAD FFAADV MRCPS(Glasgow) FRCP(Edin) FRCP(London)
Consultant Dermatologist
Wizderm Speciality Hair and Skin Clinic
Kolkata, West Bengal, India

Kumaresan M MD Diplomate ABHRS
Professor
PSG Hospitals
Coimbatore, Tamil Nadu, India

Lakshmi DV MD FRGUHS
Senior Resident
Department of Dermatology
Bangalore Medical College and Research Institute
Bengaluru, Karnataka, India

Leelavathy B MD
Professor and Head
Department of Dermatology
Bangalore Medical College and Research Institute
Bengaluru, Karnataka, India

Madhulika Mhatre
Consultant Dermatologist
Mumbai, Maharashtra, India

Madura C MD FRGUHS (Dermatosurgery)
Consultant Dermatologist, Dermatosurgeon and Hair Transplantation Surgeon
Cutis Academy of Cutaneous Sciences
Bengaluru, Karnataka, India

Manas Chatterjee MD
Professor and Head
Department of Dermatology
INHS Asvini
Mumbai, Maharashtra, India

Meenaz Khoja DDV
Consultant Dermatologist
GMF Ruby Hall Clinic and MMF Joshi Hospital
Pune, Maharashtra, India

Munish Paul MD Dermatology
Consultant Dermatologist
Skin Laser Centre
New Delhi, India

Nagesh TS MD DNB
Associate Professor
Department of Dermatology
Sapthagiri Institute of Medical Sciences
Bengaluru, Karnataka, India

Narendra Patwardhan MD DDV
Consultant Dermatologist
Shriyash Clinic
Deccan Gymkhana
Pune, Maharashtra, India

Nilesh Goyal MRCP DNB DVD SCS Dip
Leslie Baumann International Cosmetic Dermatology Fellow and Consultant Cosmetic Dermatologist
Juvenis Clinic, Lilavati Hospital and Bombay Hospital
Mumbai, Maharashtra, India

Nirav V Desai DNB
Dermatologist and Hair Transplant Surgeon
AK Clinics, Ludhiana, Punjab and
New Delhi, India

Nirmal B Krishna MD FRGUHS (Dermatosurgery)
Assistant Professor and Consultant
Department of Dermatology
Velammal Medical College and
Research Institute
Madurai, Tamil Nadu, India

Niti Khunger MD DDV DNB
Professor and Consultant Dermatologist
VM Medical College and Safdarjang Hospital
New Delhi, India

Nitin Barde MD FRGUHS (Dermatosurgery)
Assistant Professor
Indira Gandhi Government Medical College
Nagpur, Maharashtra, India

Pavan Raj R MD FRGUHS (Dermatosurgery)
Consultant Dermatologist and Dermatosurgeon
Cutis Academy of Cutaneous Sciences
Bengaluru, Karnataka, India

Pradeep Kumari DNB MNAMS FCPS DVD
Chief Dermatologist
Skin and Surgery International and
Asia Institute of Hair Trnasplant
Pune, Maharashtra, India

Pradyumna Vaidya DVD DNB
Consultant Dermatologist
Dr Vaidya's Skin and Laser Clinic
Pune, Maharashtra, India

Priyanka Agarwal MD
Senior Resident
Rajarajeshwari Medical College and Hospital
Bengaluru, Karnataka, India

Pushpa KR MD FRGUHS
Dermatologist and Dermatosurgeon
Epitome Skin and Laser Centre
Bengaluru, Karnataka, India

Raghunatha Reddy MD DNB FRGUHS
Professor and Head
Department of Dermatology
MVJMC&RC
Consultant Dermatologist and Dermatosurgeon
Dr Raghu's Mathapitha Skin Clinic
Bengaluru, Karnataka, India

Rajesh Verma MD
Professor and Head
Department of Dermatology
Base Hospital Lucknow
Lucknow, Uttar Pradesh, India

Rasya Dixit
Consultant Dermatologist
Dr Dixit Cosmetic Dermatology Clinic
Bengaluru, Karnataka, India

Revathi TN
Professor
Department of Dermatology
Bangalore Medical College and Research Institute
Bengaluru, Karnataka, India

Satish Udare
Consultant Dermatologist
Navi Mumbai, Maharashtra, India

Savita Yadav MD
Assistant Professor
Department of Dermatology and Venereology
All India Institutes of Medical Sciences
New Delhi, India

Savitha AS MD
Assistant Professor
Department of Dermatology
Sapthagiri Institute of Medical Sciences
Bengaluru, Karnataka, India

Sharad Mutalik DVD
Consultant Dermatologist
Cutaneous and Laser Surgeon
Maharashtra Medical Foundation
Pune, Maharashtra, India

S Sacchidanand MD DVD DHA FRCP (Glasgow)
Director of Medical Education
Government of Karnataka
Dean cum Director
Department of Health and Education
Bangalore Medical College and Research Center
Bengaluru, Karnataka, India

Salim T MD
Medical Director and Clinical Head
Cutis Institute
Kozhikode, Kerala, India

Shehnaz Arsiwala MD DDV
Renewderm Centre, Saifee Hospital and
Prince Aly Khan Hospital
Mumbai, Maharashtra, India

Shekhar Neema MD
Assistant Professor
Department of Dermatology
Command Hospital
Kolkata, West Bengal, India

Shilpa K MD FRGUHS (Dermatosurgery)
Assistant Professor
Bangalore Medical College and Research Institute
Bengaluru, Karnataka, India

Shruthi C MD
Department of Dermatosurgery
Bangalore Medical College and
Research Institute
Bengaluru, Karnataka, India

Shyamanta Barua MD
Assistant Professor
Department of Dermatology
Assam Medical College and Hospital
Dibrugarh, Assam, India

Somesh Gupta MD
Additional Professor
Department of Dermatology
All India Institutes of Medical Sciences
New Delhi, India

Soumya Jagadeesan MD
Associate Professor
Department of Dermatology
Amrita Institute of Medical Sciences
Kochi, Kerala, India

Sujala S Aradhya MD (DVL) FRGUHS (Dermatosurgery)
Consultant Dermatologist and Dermatosurgery
Sujala Polyclinic and Laboratory
Bengaluru, Karnataka, India

Sukesh Mathapathi MS MD DNB FIADVL
Consultant Dermatotrichologist
People Tree - CITI - Fortis Hospitals
Bengaluru, Karnataka, India

Suman Patra MD
Senior Resident
All India Institutes of Medical Sciences
New Delhi, India

Surajit Gorai MD DNB MNAMS
Consultant Dermatologist
Apollo Gleneagles Hospitals
Kolkata, West Bengal, India

Sushil Tahiliani MD DV&D
Hinduja Hospital and Research Center
Bharatiya Arogya Nidhi Hospital
Asian Heart Institute
Mumbai, Maharashtra, India

Sushmitha Jayaprasad
MD FRGUHS (Aesthetic Dermatology)
Junior Consultant
Cutis Academy of Cutaneous Sciences
Bengaluru, Karnataka, India

Swapnil Shah MD
Associate Professor
Ashwini Rural Medical College
Solapur, Maharashtra, India

Syed Mubashir MD FRGUHS (Dermatosurgery)
Department of Dermatology
Government Medical College
Srinagar, Jammu and Kashmir, India

Teena Ramesh MD FRUGHS (Aesthetic Dermatology)
Consultant
Cutis Academy of Cutaneous Sciences
Bengaluru, Karnataka, India

Tolong K MD
Consultant Dermatologist
Shija Hospitals and Research Institute
Imphal, Manipur, India

Umashankar Nagaraju MD
Professor
Rajarajeshwari Medical College and Hospital
Bengaluru, Karnataka, India

Vaishalee Kirane DVD DNB
Dermatologist and Trichologist
Ruby Hall Clinic
Aditya Birla Memorial Hospital and
Joshi Hospital
Pune, Maharashtra, India

Vandana Chatrath MD
Dermatologist and Dermatological Surgeon
Delhi Dermatology Group
New Delhi, India

Varsha DV DVD FRGUHS Dermatosurgery (Madrid)
Consultant Dermatologist
BOSS Hospital
Bengaluru, Karnataka, India

Venkataram Mysore
MD DNB DipRC Path (LOND) FRCP (GLASGOW) FISHRS
Venkat Charmalaya, Bengaluru, Karnataka, India

Vinay Saraf MD DVD
Senior Consulting Dermatologist
Nanavati Superspeciality Hospital
Mumbai Skin and Laser Clinic
Mumbai, Maharashtra, India

Message

Message from President of ACS(I)

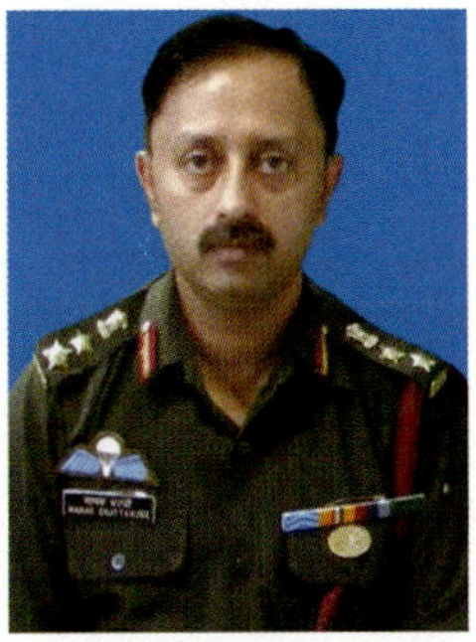

The step by step book to Dermatosurgical Procedures, a proposal of the fledgling Association of Cutaneous Surgeons (India)[ACS(I)] Academy as it gains wings, has been a project close to my heart as ACS(I) President as well as to all members of the ACS(I) executive. At the ACS(I), it has been our endeavor to throw open our gates to a more universal acceptance of dermatosurgery as a potent therapeutic tool in the hands of the dermatologist. We have tried to ensure that the skill and practice of dermatosurgery are acquired by those at the furthest reaches of our great nation. Toward this end, this book is meant to act as the carrier of the knowledge of basic and advanced skill in this growing branch of dermatology to every corner of our country. Being as it is a developing field, new skills and specialists are being added to the expanding fold of the specialty. This book will address the needs of those who join the dermatosurgery bandwagon.

This being a first-time effort, there are improvements that would be needed as we go along. I am sure that future editions would improve on this concept that the editors have so lucidly espoused in the form of this book. Being a sister text of our highly successful Textbook of Dermatosurgery, it would be a worthy companion next to the operating table for those of us who need to be in constant touch with a quick guide as we perform the procedures that characterize our branch.

I wish this effort the very best and am sure of its acceptance by the rank and file of dermatosurgeons in India and abroad.

Jai Hind

Dr (Col) Manas Chatterjee MD
President, ACS(I), 2015–17
Professor and Head
Department of Dermatology
INHS Asvini
Mumbai, Maharashtra, India

Foreword

It is indeed a privilege for me to write this foreword for a singularly unique endeavor of the Association of Cutaneous Surgeons (India) which has been executed with great aplomb by Dr (Lt Col) Biju Vasudevan and his team. This illustrated step by step book to the performance of various procedures would be a welcome addition to the desk of the budding dermatosurgeon who is all set to explore the world of procedural dermatology.

Dermatosurgery has gained a strong foothold in the practice of dermatology with procedural management being required by almost a third of all patients being seen in our OPDs and clinics. There is a felt need for a book that succinctly details the steps of the various procedures without going into details of the theoretical basis of these therapeutic modalities. This would enable an enthusiast to start with the procedures, get the desired results which would enhance his interest in the details of these modalities. It is in this niche that this book would find a place in the young practitioner's mindset. In addition, established seniors, sometimes need to revisit what they have been doing to enhance their skills and find new ways of enhancing their outcomes.

The step by step book is embellished with images detailing the key steps of the various procedures which would make it easier for the dermatosurgeon to understand and emulate the said steps and thus would increase his confidence in these mostly simple but effective modalities of surgical dermatotherapeutics. The short descriptions are meant to enhance understanding without it being an encroachment on the limited time available when the dermatosurgeon is just about to embark on a procedure. In this respect, this short companion is meant to be on the side of the specialist in his hour of need.

It is hereby hoped that this short treatise be a stepping stone to betterment of dermatosurgical care of our patients.

Dr (Col) Manas Chatterjee MD
President, ACS(I), 2015–17
Professor and Head
Department of Dermatology
INHS Asvini
Mumbai, Maharashtra, India

Preface

This book *Procedural Dermatosurgery: A Step by Step Approach* is a dream project of the Association of Cutaneous Surgeons (India)[ACS(I)] Academy and involves the description of various surgical procedures in a stepwise manner. It contains the detailed steps involved in doing various dermatosurgical procedures accompanied by figures for each of the steps. This would help all budding and practicing dermatosurgeons to easily carry out these procedures just by reading and having a visual outlook of the respective surgeries.

The chapters are contributed by eminent dermatosurgeons who are experts in their respective fields from all over the country. The book will be a ready reference for dermatologists, dermatosurgeons, dermatology residents and will also be a guide for other specialties when they encounter a dermatosurgery case.

Tips and tricks, modifications, complications and recent advances are highlighted for each procedure. The chapters are concise and have been made crisper by addition of tables, flowcharts and algorithms.

We are sure this book will be a welcome addition to all concerned.

Regards

Biju Vasudevan
Manas Chatterjee
Shilpa K

Acknowledgment

We are very thankful to all faculty and residents of Bangalore Medical College, Bengaluru, Karnataka, India.

Contents

CHAPTER 1

Essential Dermatosurgical Instruments

Rajesh Verma, Aneesh KP, Ankan Gupta

INTRODUCTION

A surgical instrument is a designed tool or device used for carrying out desired actions during a surgery, e.g. cutting a biological tissue, holding it or to provide access for viewing a deeper lying structure. Some surgical instruments are designed for general use in surgery, while there are some which are tailor-made for a specific role in a specific procedure, e.g. instruments for nail procedures, implanters in hair transplantation, dermatomes for taking a skin graft, etc. (Table 1.1).

Surgical equipment is as important to the procedure as to the doctor. Faulty and ineffective instruments can do just as much damage as an unqualified doctor could. High quality precision equipment can considerably influence the outcome of any procedure, more so in case of cosmetic procedures involving face and exposed parts of the body. Utmost care must be taken in selecting the correct instrument for a particular step; however, the surgeon must not be obstinate and learn to improvise with instruments like using a chalazion clamp in oral mucosal procedures.

GENERAL INSTRUMENTS

Forceps

This is a handheld, hinged instrument used for grasping and holding objects. The arms of the forceps are used as extensions of thumb and index finger in stabilizing or holding the tissue, sutures or dressings. The free tips of the forceps are modified for various uses. There are two basic type of forceps—the nonlocking type and locking type which are also known as clamps.

Table 1.1: Classification of dermatosurgical instruments.

General instruments	1. Graspers/Forceps 2. Cutters (Scalpel, scissors, cutters, trocars, splitters) 3. Retractors/Distractors 4. Clamps/Occluders 5. Sealers (Staples, sutures) 6. Scopes and probes 7. Measuring devices (Rulers and calipers) 8. Markers (Skin marking pens)
Special instruments	1. Vitiligo surgery instruments 2. Hair transplant instruments 3. Nail surgery instruments

Adson's Tissue Forceps

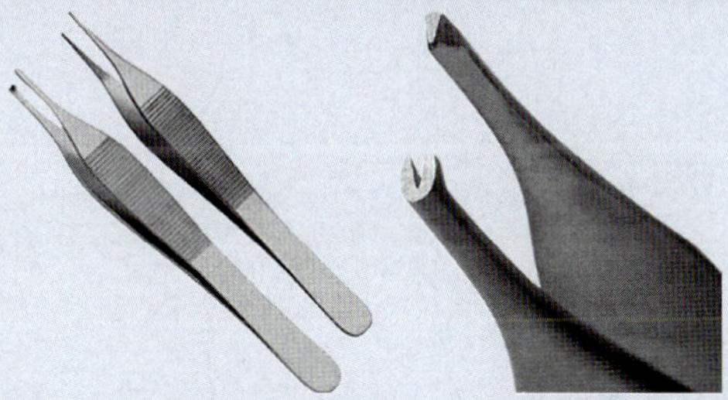

Description	A type of dissecting forceps with wider blade and better grip.
Uses	Hold wound edges during exploration and suturing. Removing recipient plugs in hair transplant.
Remarks	Easy to control as the blades provide better grip.

Allis Forceps

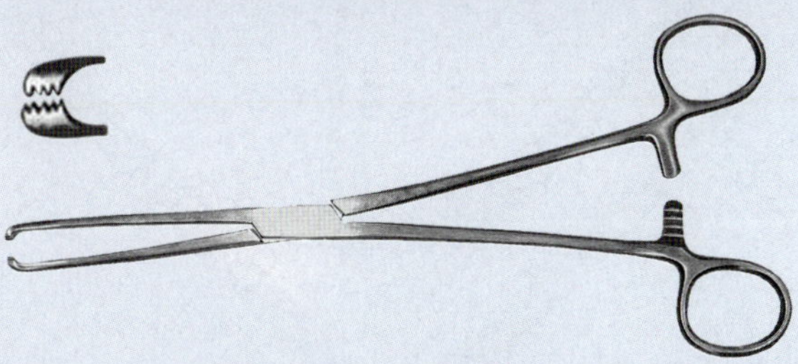

Description	A surgical instrument with sharp teeth, used to hold or grasp heavy tissue. Two straight blades with interdigitating teeth at the tip. Handle has a ratchet with 3 catches.
Uses	Corn enucleation surgery.
Remarks	Can damage tissues, if used inappropriately, hence it is used to hold the tissue which has to be removed.

Cheatle Forceps

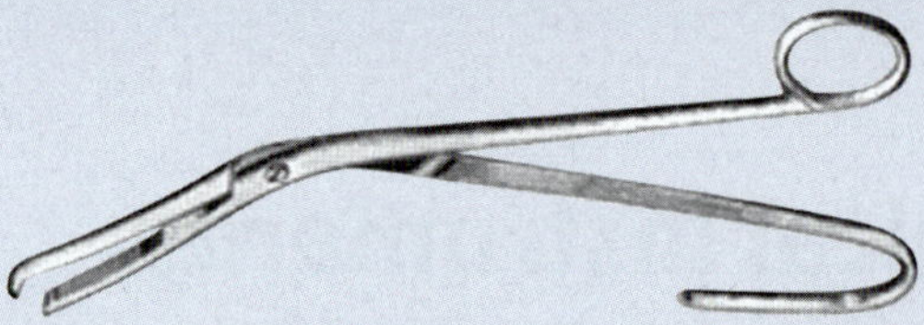

Description	Forceps with long handles with complete ring at one end and partial at other.
Uses	To pick up sterilized articles/gauze pieces from tray.
Remarks	The tips are kept dipped in antiseptic solution.

Epilation Forceps

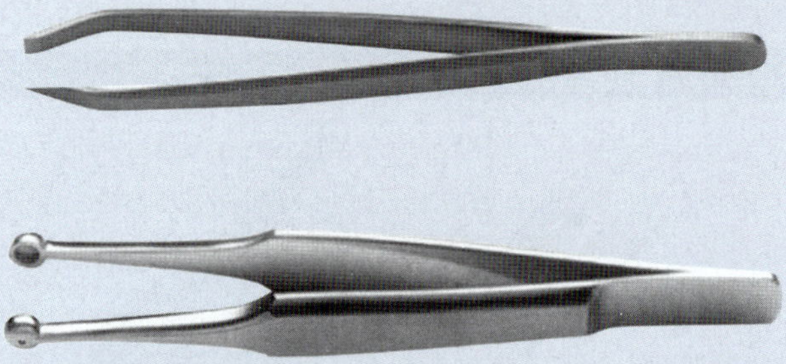

Description	A kind of small spring forceps, used for removing unwanted hair.
Uses	In electroepilation to pull out destroyed hair.
Remarks	Various types are available. For example, Beer epilation forceps, Douglas forceps.

Dissecting Forceps (Toothed/Plain)

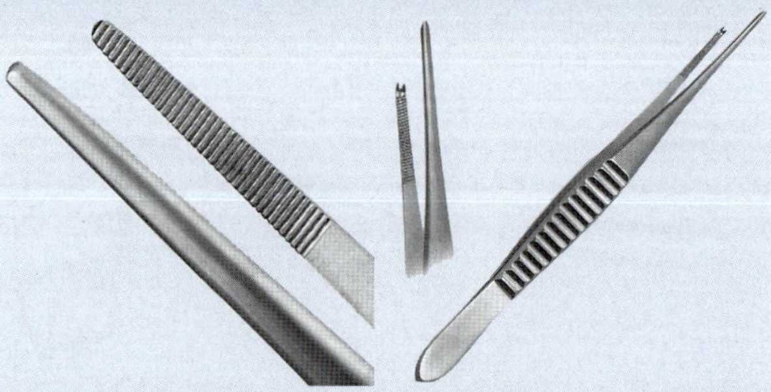

Description	Forceps with toothed or plain tips and variable types of grip. Plain forceps have horizontal serrations at the tip and toothed ones have two teeth on one jaw and interdigitating tooth on the other. Spring tension at one end holds the grasping ends apart until pressure is applied. This allows one to quickly and easily grasp small objects or tissue to move and release it, or to grasp and hold tissue with easily variable pressure.
Uses	Plain dissecting forceps are used for holding delicate structures like blood vessels, nerves, etc. Toothed dissecting forceps are used for holding tough tissues like skin, fascia, tendon, etc.
Remarks	Various types of dissecting forceps have been designed according to the use For example, Plane dressing forceps, Adson forceps, Bonney's forceps, Gillie's forceps, Lane's forceps, Mc'Indoe's forceps, DeBakey's forceps, Gerald's forceps, Bayonet's forceps, etc.

Sponge Holding Forceps

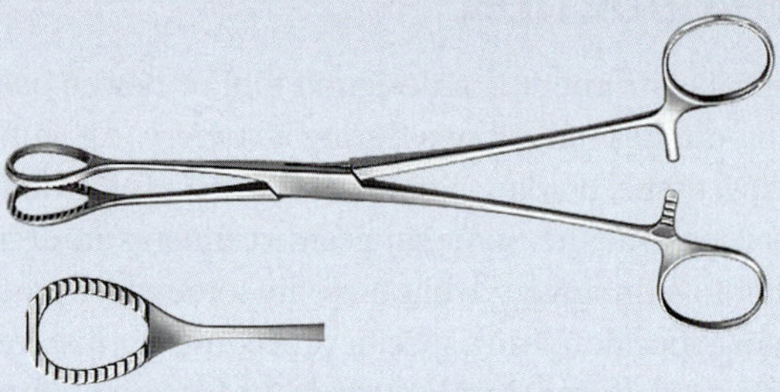

Description	Large size hinge forceps with fenestrations/hole at the tip of the blades. The handles are ratcheted as well as looped. Sponge holding forceps can either be curved or they may be straight. Transverse inner surface is serrated to provide better grip.
Uses	Hold sponges and/or cotton wool swabs in preparing the surgical site.

Hemostatic Forceps/Artery Forceps

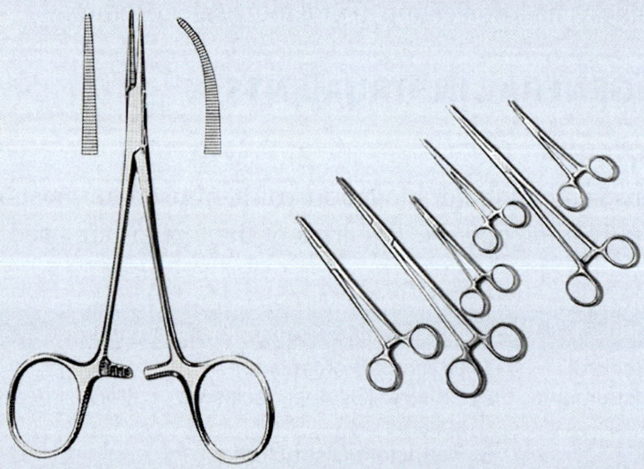

Description	Forceps with gradually tapering blades towards the tip with serrations at the tip. Commonly referred to as "Artery forceps". The tip may be either straight or curved. They are available in three different sizes; large, medium and small. The small size artery forceps is also referred to as "Mosquito artery forceps".

Uses	Catch cut end of blood vessels. Blunt dissection in lipoma and sebaceous cyst excision. Crushing pedicles of skin tag and DPN. To hold the free ends of suture in ear lobe repair and nerve biopsy. Three point traction in circumcision.
Remarks	Medium and small sizes are commonly used in dermatosurgery.

Iris Forceps

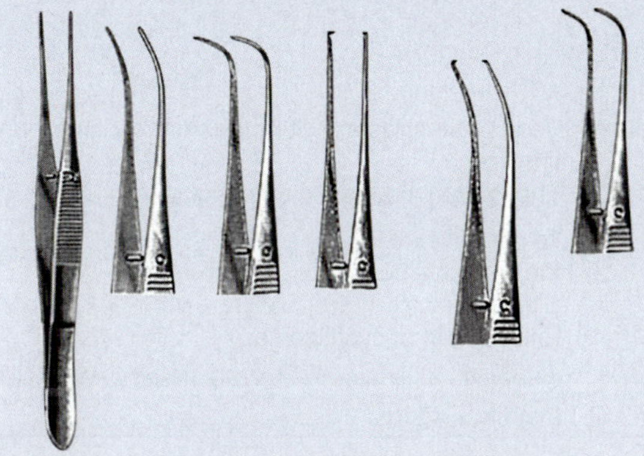

Description	A kind of fine spring forceps originally used in ophthalmic surgery to hold iris tissue. But it also finds application in fine surgeries like skin grafting, hair transplant, etc. The tip may be straight/curved or plane/toothed.
Uses	Miniature punch grafting. Split thickness skin grafting. Blister grafting.
Remarks	Various designs are available with different names. Common ones used in dermatosurgery are illustrated.

Iris forceps—Graefe

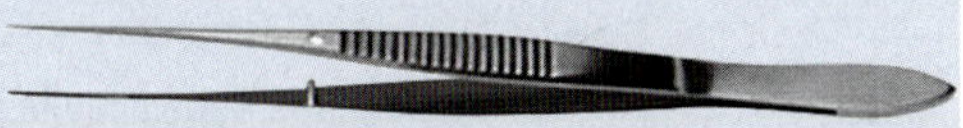

Iris forceps—Stevens

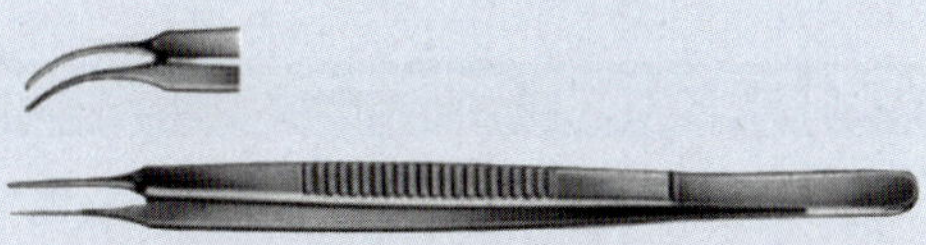

Iris forceps—Bishop Harman

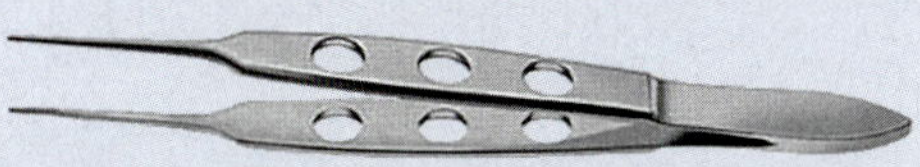

Iris forceps—Forester

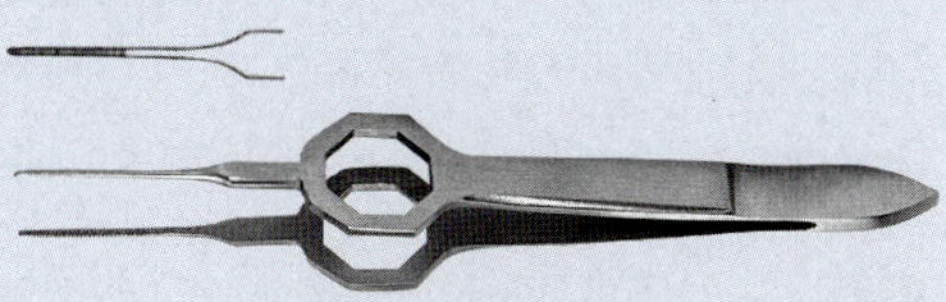

Iris forceps—Gill

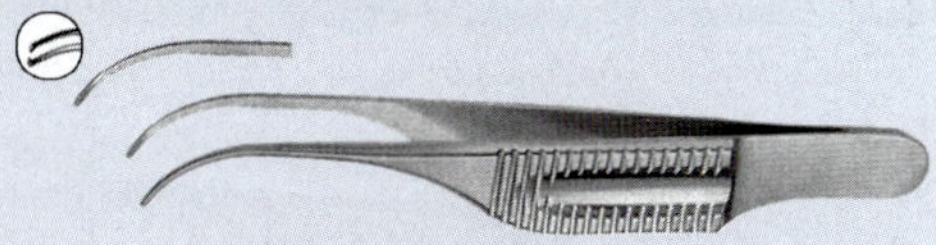

Iris forceps—Mod-Tuebingen

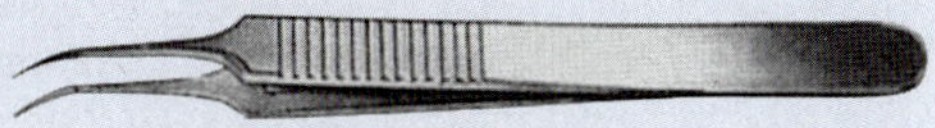

Jeweler Forceps

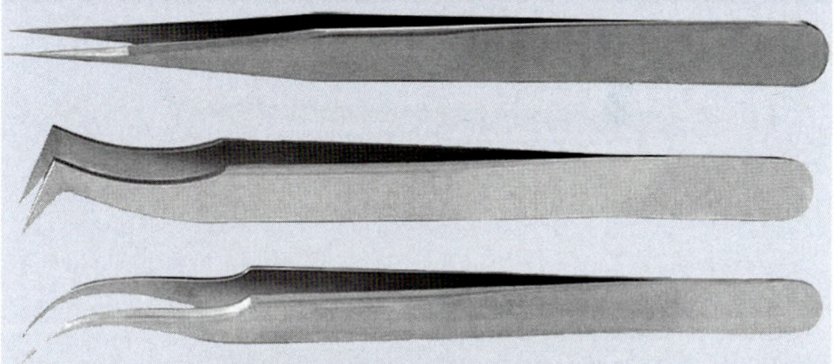

Description	A small thumb forceps with very fine pointed blades, used to grasp tissues in microsurgical procedures.
Uses	Miniature punch grafting. Punch biopsy. Implantation of follicular units in hair transplantation.
Remarks	The tip may be straight, bent or curved.

Scissors

Scissors are cutting instruments with two blades hinged together at a fulcrum. These are available in various sizes and types. Scissors can be classified as having sharp or blunt edges and as straight and curved.

Dressing Scissors/Nurses Scissors

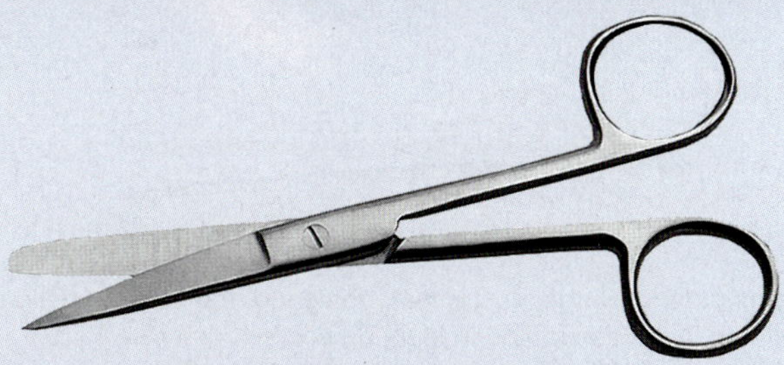

Description	The lower blade is blunted and the upper blade is sharp.
Uses	To cut the dressing without injuring the skin.

Lister Bandage Scissors

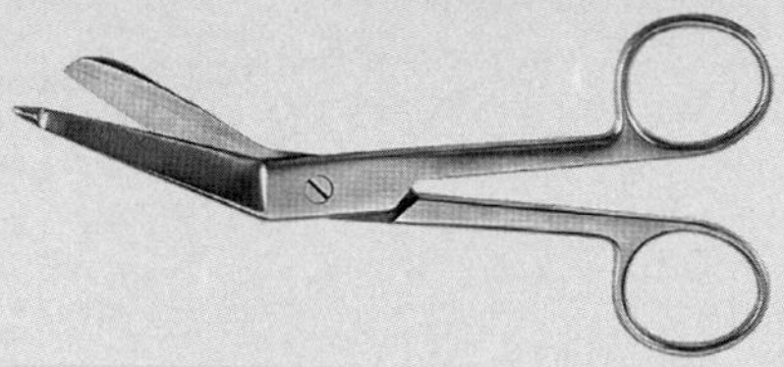

Description Thick blunt plate at the tip of the lower blade to avoid injury.
The blades are curved to an angle for ease of use.

Uses To cut the dressing without injuring the skin.

Mayo Scissors

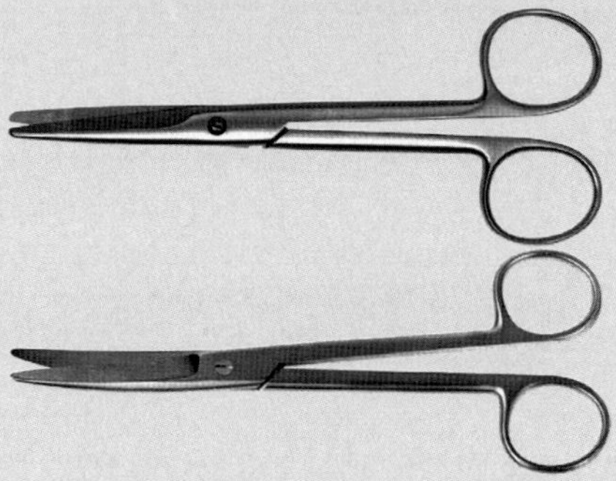

Description A type of surgical scissor with flattened blades.
Blades may be straight or curved.

Uses *Straight*: Cutting dressing, Vaseline impregnated gauze, suture materials, dressing pads, etc.
Curved: Removal of warts after electrocautery, cutting skin tags, sample taking out the biopsy from tough areas.

Remarks Was developed by Mayo Clinic.
Most often used to cut fascia in general surgery.

Metzenbaum Scissors

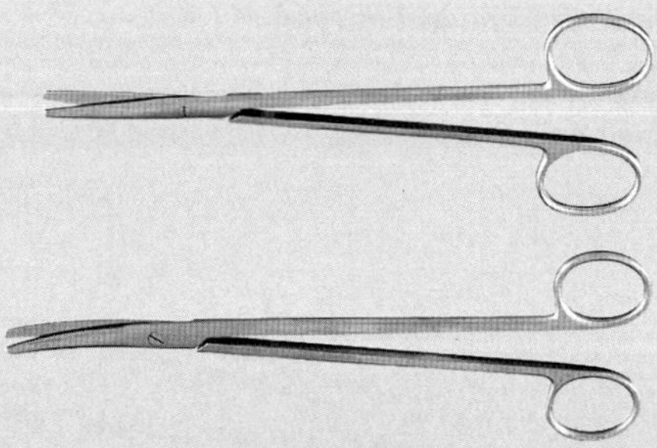

Description Surgical scissors designed for cutting delicate tissue and in blunt dissection.
Have a relatively long shank-to-blade ratio.

Uses Cutting skin tags.
Skin biopsy.
Split thickness skin grafting.

Iris Scissors

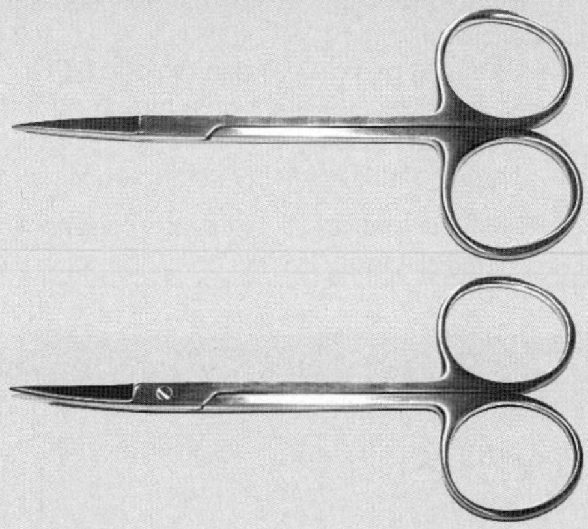

Description Very small scissors with an extremely sharp and fine tip.
The tip may be curved or straight.

Uses To cut delicate tissue.
Ideal for cutting mucous membranes.
Skin biopsy.
Enucleation of cyst/lipoma.

Remarks Originally designed for the fine detail work of ophthalmic surgery.

Gradle Scissors

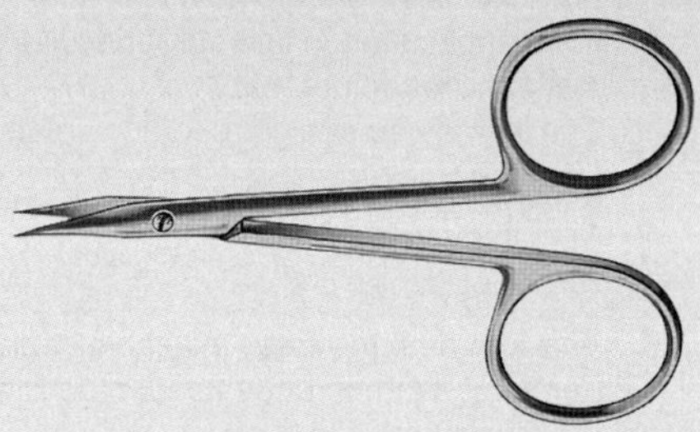

Description Short blades with thin pointed ends.
May be curved or straight.

Uses Cut delicate tissues especially in periorbital area.
Cut skin tags.

O'Brien Scissors

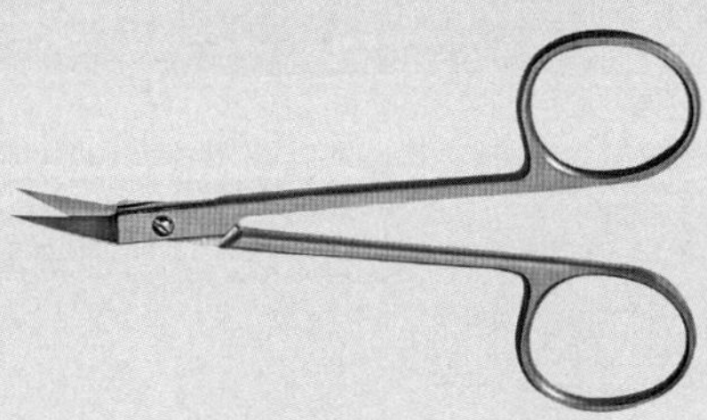

Description Small scissors with angled short blades with pointed edges.

Uses Cut suture in delicate or tight areas.

Spencer Scissors

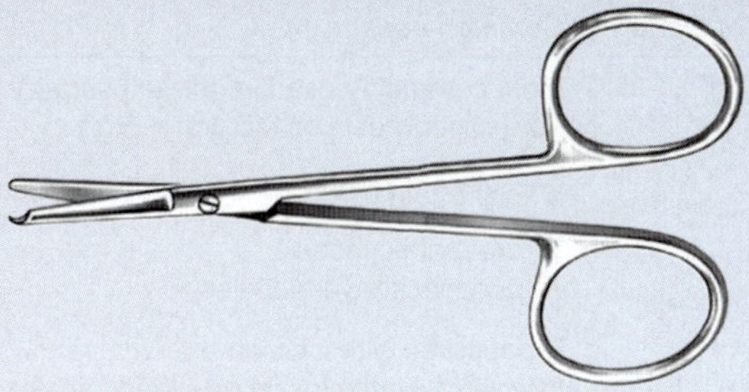

Description Small scissors with a small hook shaped tip on one blade.

Uses Suture removal.

Remarks The small hook shaped tip on one blade slides under sutures to slightly lift them before cutting for removal. This hook also holds the suture, so it does not slip off the blade of the scissors prior to cutting.

Double S-Shaped Curved Scissors

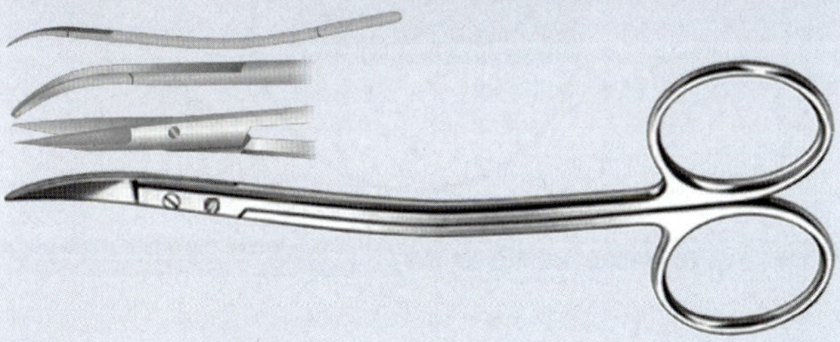

Description Small scissors with two curves which form the alphabet "S".

Uses Useful to operate at a depth.
Miniature punch grafting at recipient site.
Hair transplantation surgery to cut deeper donor grafts.

Undermining Scissors

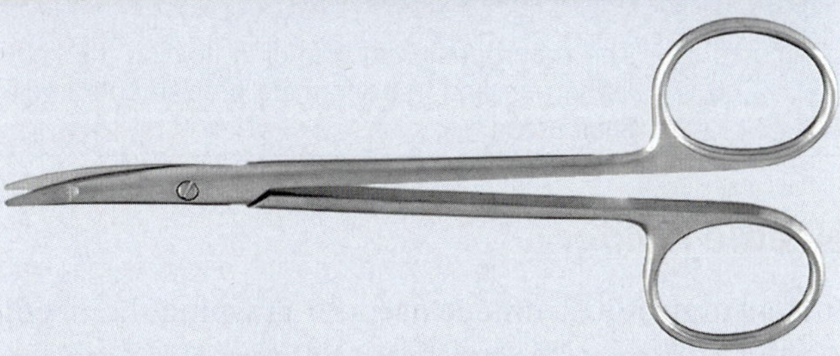

Description Small scissors with longer shanks.
Distal part is flattened to provide thinner operating edge.

Uses In surgeries where considerable undermining is required.

Remarks For example, Ragnell dissecting scissors.

Castroviejo Spring Scissors

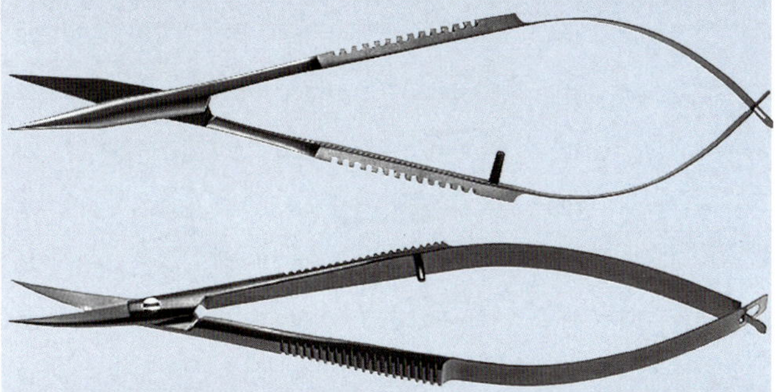

Description Small scissors with thin short blades and spring action.
The tip may be curved or straight.

Uses For fine work involving delicate tissue like face.
To cut the graft in blister grafting and split thickness skin grafting.

Remarks The unique design features allow extremely smooth cutting of fine and coarse tissue with reduced trauma.

Scalpels

Consists of disposable steel blades which can be fitted on to reusable stainless steel handles. Some handles are designed to fit a specific hand hold. For example, Beaver style handle is shaped like a pen and is suited for close, precise cuts; other handles, such as Bard-Parker style are flatter. A particularly common type of handle, called the No. 3 Bard-Parker style, has a metric ruler to measure precise cuts. Another common type of handle is the rounded Siegel style, designed for curved incisions. The Bard-Parker handle (BP handle) is the commonly used handle in dermatosurgery.

The sizes of surgical blades which fit into various sizes of BP handle is given in Table 1.2. Various sizes and shapes of blades available are listed in Figure 1.1. Commonly used blades in dermatology and their uses are enumerated in Table 1.3.

Table 1.2: Bard-Parker handle and surgical blades.

Size of BP handle	*Size of blade*
Handle #3	10, 11, 12, 13, 14, 15, 15B, 15C, 16, 17
Handle #4	20, 21, 22, 22A, 23, 24, 25, and 36
Handle #7	10, 11, 12 and 15
Handle #9	6, 9, 10, 11, 12, 15 and 16
Handle #B3	6, 9, 10, 11, 12, 12D, 13, 14, 15

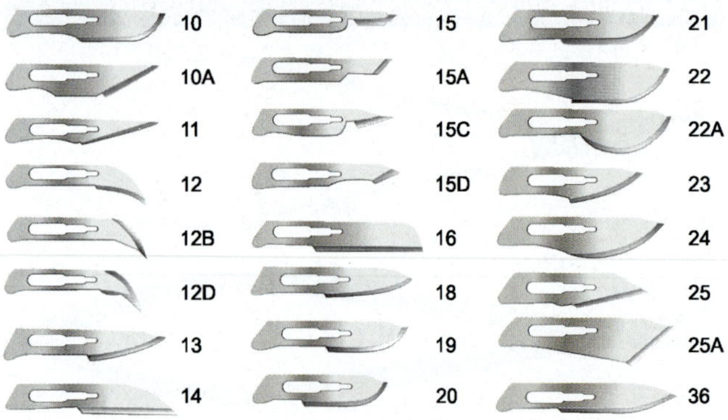

Fig. 1.1: Sizes of surgical blades.

Bard-Parker Handle

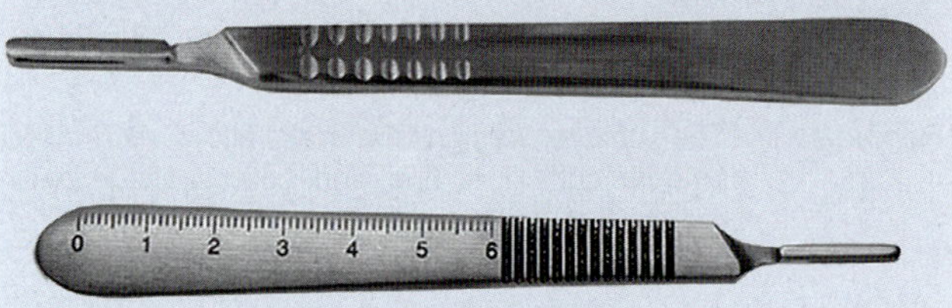

Description	Flat blade holders of various sizes. Different sizes are suited for particular blade sizes. Handle #3 has a metric ruler to measure the size of the incision.
Uses	For handling the surgical blade safely and precisely during procedures like skin biopsy, enucleation/excision of cyst, etc.
Remarks	The flat design is helpful to have a better grip of the knife. Longer handles are denoted by the letter L after the size of the handle. For example, 3L, 4L, etc.

Siegel Handle

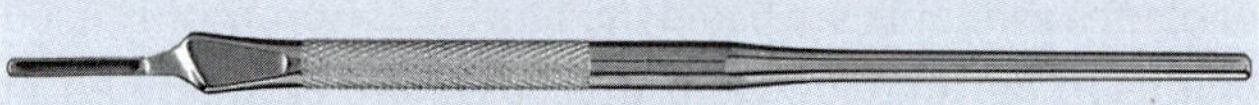

Description	Round bodied blade handle designed to hold standard surgical blades. The distal end has a prominence similar to that of Bard-Parker handle. Also referred to as handle #7.
Uses	To hold the knife like a pen.
Remarks	The round design is helpful in holding the knife like a pen and in performing precise cuts in difficult areas.

Table 1.3: Commonly used blades in dermatosurgery.

Size of blade	*Common uses*
15	Most commonly used in dermatosurgery. For procedures with incision < 5 cm.
15D	Incision < 5 cm in delicate areas like face.
11	To drain abscesses. To perform shave biopsies.
10, 21	Procedures with incision > 5 cm. In areas with thick skin (trunk and scalp). For excision of large lesions, wound debridement.

Beaver Handle

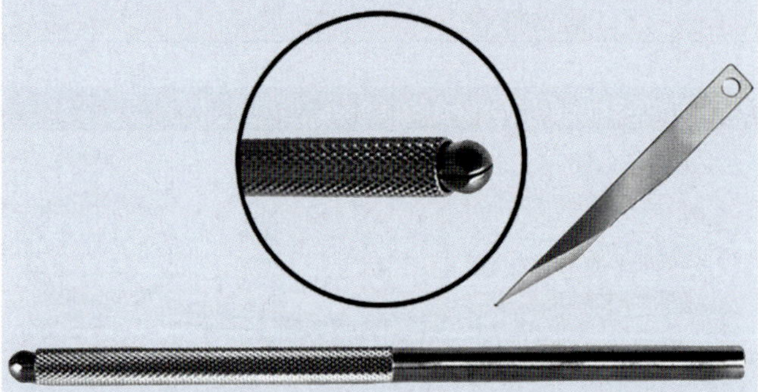

Description	Round bodied blade handle shaped like a pen. The distal end has a slit into which the blade can be placed and fixed. Specific set of blades referred to as "Beaver mini blades" are available for use with this type of handle.
Uses	To hold the knife like a pen. For close and precise cuts.
Remarks	The round design is helpful in holding the knife like a pen and in performing precise cuts in difficult areas.

Needle Holder

It is a surgical instrument used for grasping the needle during suturing. Most needle holders have a clamp mechanism to lock the needle in place. The size of the needle holder to be used should be determined by the size of the needle and the anatomical site of the surgery. The jaws of a needle holder are textured and short to maintain a firm grip on the needle.

Mayo-Hegar Needle Holder

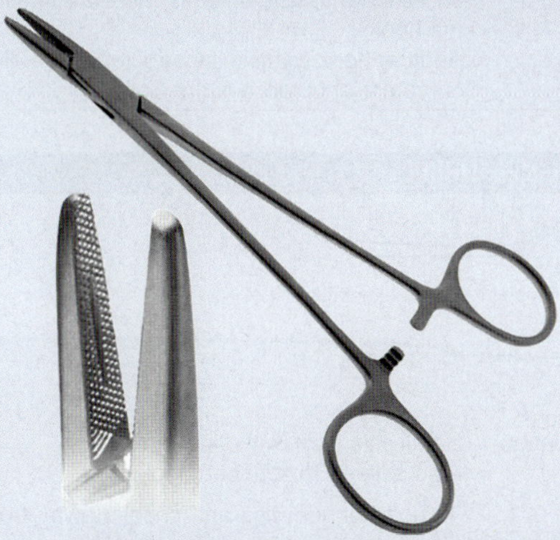

Description	Larger size needle holder with long shanks. Serrated tips with central longitudinal depression.
Uses	For holding larger size needles—3.0 and 2.0 suture needles. For performing sutures involving larger areas like trunk, limbs, etc.
Remarks	The cross serrations help to provide better hold on the needle used.

Ryder Needle Holder

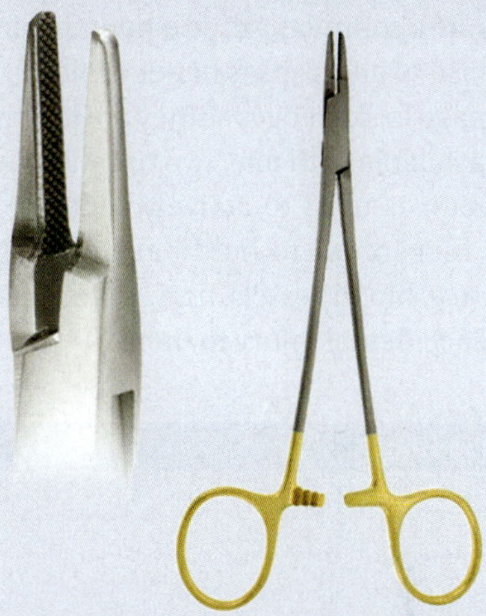

Description	Smaller size needle holder with long shanks. Tips are thinner with cross-serrations.
Uses	For holding smaller size needles—4.0 and 5.0 suture needles. For performing sutures involving delicate skin like face, earlobe, periorbital area, etc.
Remarks	The thin short blades help to provide better grip to small sized needles.

Crile-Wood Needle Holder

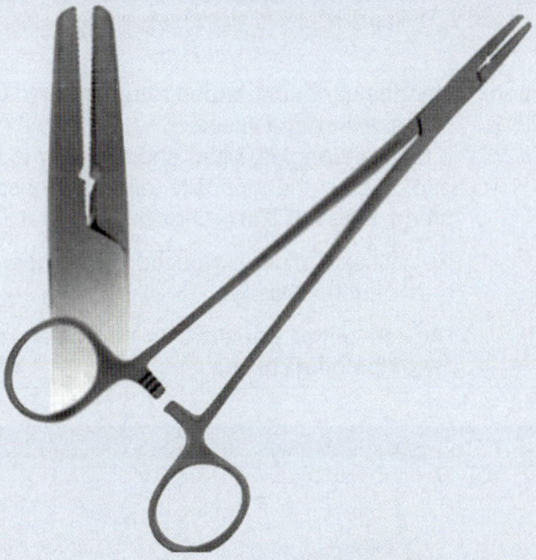

Description	Smaller size needle holder than Mayo-Hegar with long shanks. Serrated tips with transverse groove to accommodate the needle.
Uses	For holding larger size needles. For performing sutures involving larger areas like trunk, limbs, etc.
Remarks	The transverse groove helps in achieving a good perpendicular grip of the needle.

Castroviejo's Needle Holder

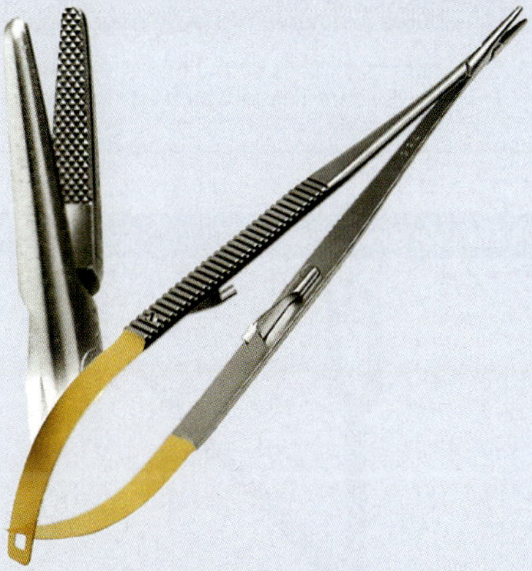

Description	Small size needle holder with spring action. Very thin tips for fine work.
Uses	For holding smaller size needles—4.0 and 5.0 suture needles. For performing sutures involving delicate skin like periorbital area. Used in delicate cosmetic surgeries.
Remarks	The thin short blades help to provide better grip to small sized needles.

Skin Hooks and Retractors

Skin hooks are a commonly used equipment in dermatology where the use of a forceps is better avoided. It can reduce undue damage to skin edges as they are less traumatic. Skin hooks are available with one, two or multiple teeth.

A retractor is used to actively separate the edges of a surgical incision or to hold back underlying organs/structures (e.g. blood vessels, nerves, deeper cysts, etc.), so as to avoid accidental injury to them.

Guthrie Skin Hook

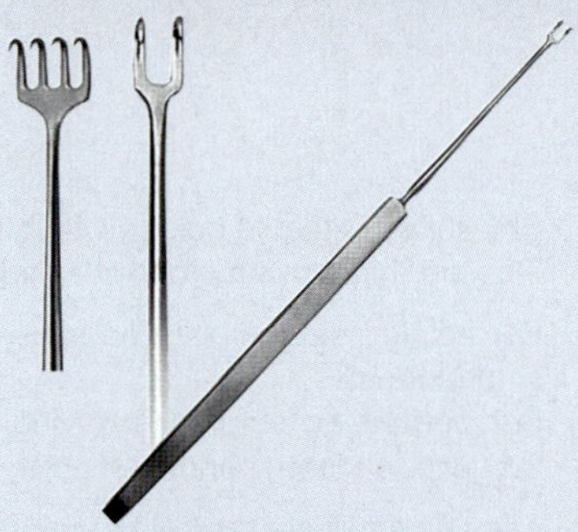

Description	Small skin hook with two, three or four prongs. The tip is flattened. The prongs may be sharp or blunt.
Uses	To retract skin while performing deep procedures like nerve biopsy, tendon repair, etc.
Remarks	Skin hooks are useful in avoiding use of forceps on delicate tissue which is more traumatic than the hooks.

Joseph's Double Skin Hook

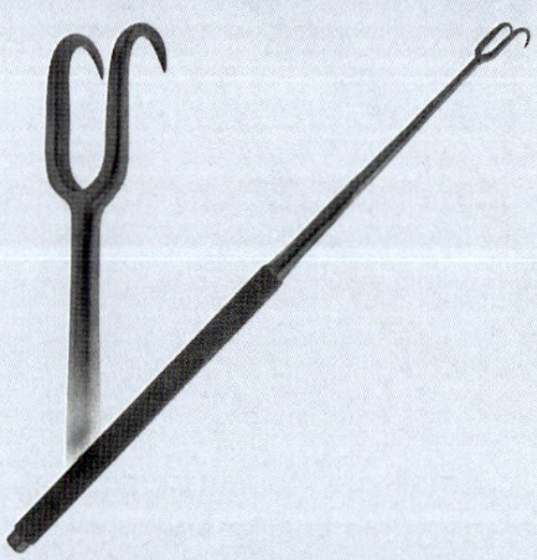

Description	Small skin hook with two prongs. The tip is "U" shaped. The tip is not flattened when compared to Freer skin hook.
Uses	To retract skin while performing deep procedures like nerve biopsy, tendon repair, etc. Provides better field of vision when compared to Freer skin hook.
Remarks	Skin hooks are useful in avoiding use of forceps on delicate tissue which is more traumatic than the hooks. Another hook with similar structure but a different curvature angulation is the Cottle's hook.

Frazier Skin Hook

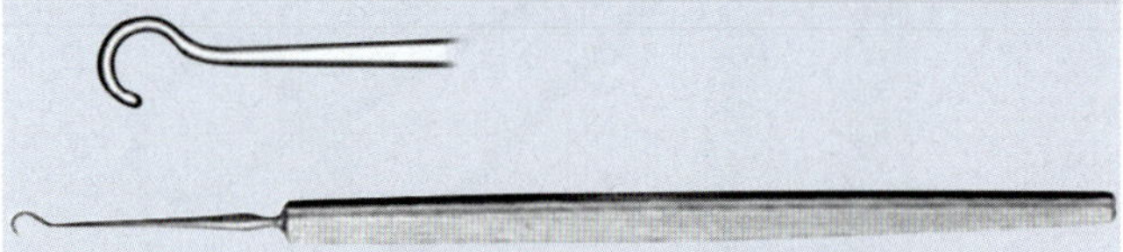

Description	Small skin hook with single prong. Also called Frazier Dura hook.
Uses	To hold tongue, lips and cheeks away from the surgical area.
Remarks	Provide better visualization and easy accessibility of the surgical site.

Senn Retractor

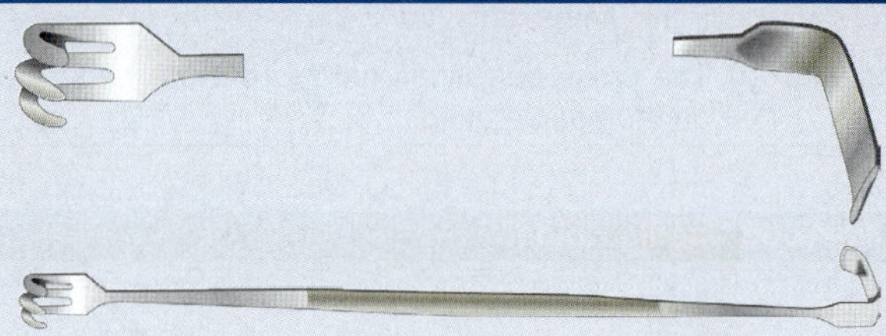

Description	Handheld, double-ended retractor used to retract primarily surface tissue. It has one angled, blunt end and, at the opposite end, facing the opposite direction has a three prong, rake tip. The prongs may be sharp or blunt.
Uses	Retract skin in deep procedures like nerve biopsy and tendon surgeries.
Remarks	Provide better visualization and easy accessibility of the surgical site.

Haber Spreader

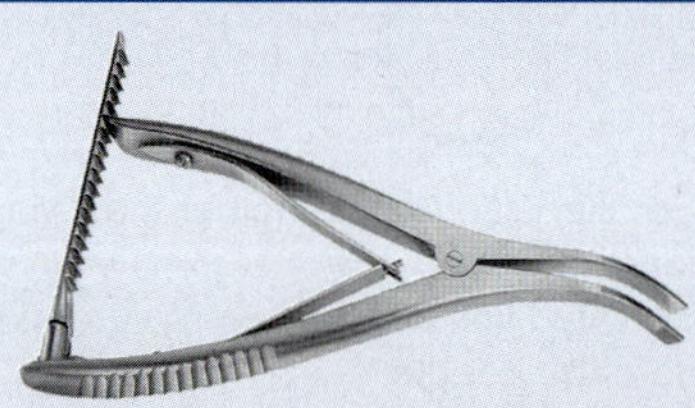

Description	A set of straight handles connected to a set of curved front arms, and culminating in a set of jaws with four sharp staggered prongs.
Uses	It is used separate a superficial incision along a natural tissue dissection plane.

Other General Instruments

Curette	
Description	Sharpened scrapping instrument. Loop shaped cutting edge at both edges.
Uses	Curettage of various benign and malignant cutaneous growth.
Remarks	Different types are in use.
Fox Dermal curette	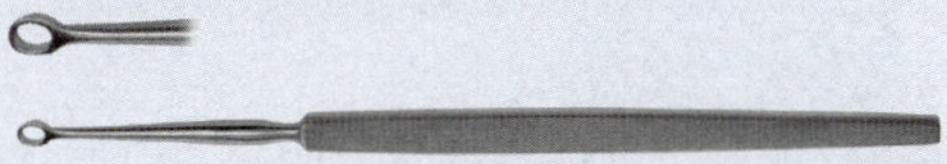
Piffard Dermal curette	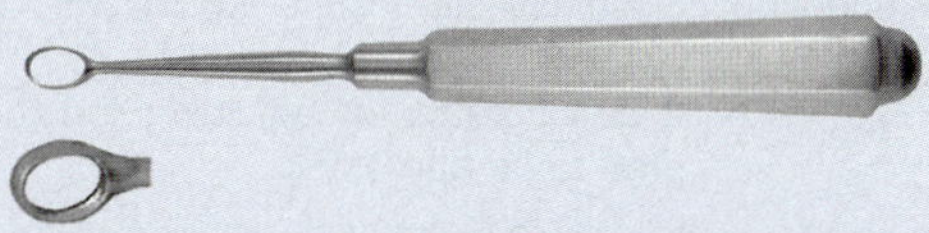
Rein Round curette	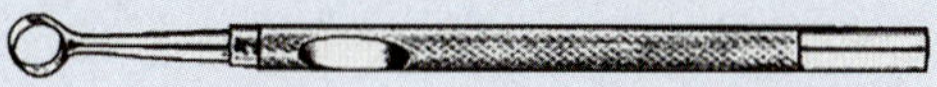

Volkmann Double Ended Scoop

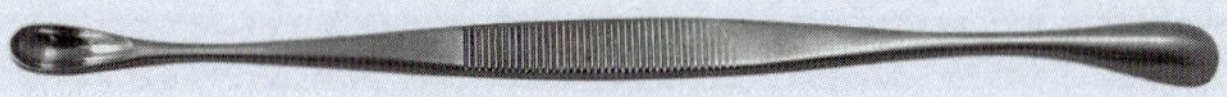

Description	A modification of curette. Stout handle with spoon shaped extension at the ends. Extensions maybe round or oval with sharp edges.
Uses	Scooping abscess cavities. Nail surgeries. Corn enucleation. Ulcer debridement. Application of pellet in cell based vitiligo surgeries.

Maneksha's Manual Dermabrader

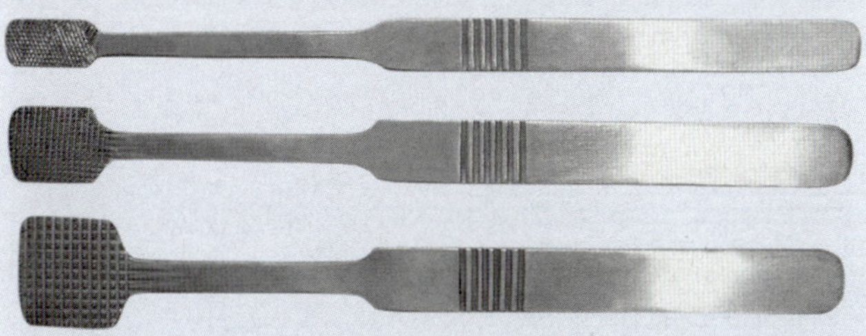

Description	It has a handle with thumb rest and a rectangular plate at the distal end. The plate has horizontal and vertical sharp teeth. Various sizes of 3 to 25 mm are available.
Uses	Recipient area preparation in STSG, SBEG, and NCES. Dermabrasion of acne scars. Tattoo removal. Debridement of wound/ulcer.

Comedone Extractor

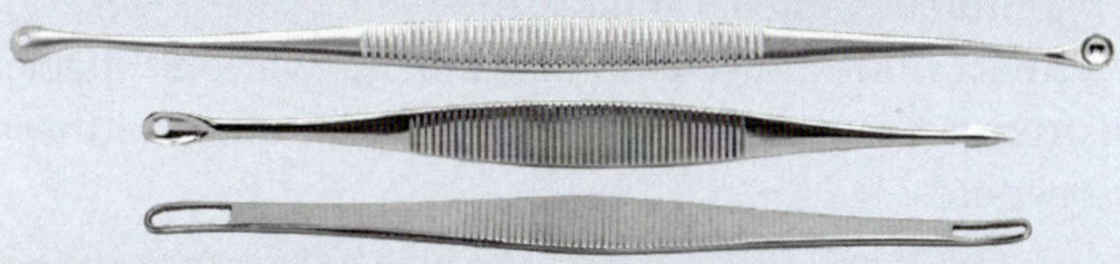

Description	Central handle with two perforated cups at the ends.
Uses	Expression of comedones.
Remarks	Used keeping the convexity of the cup held against the comedones. For example, Saalfield comedone extractor, Schaumberg comedone extractor.

Chalazion Clamp

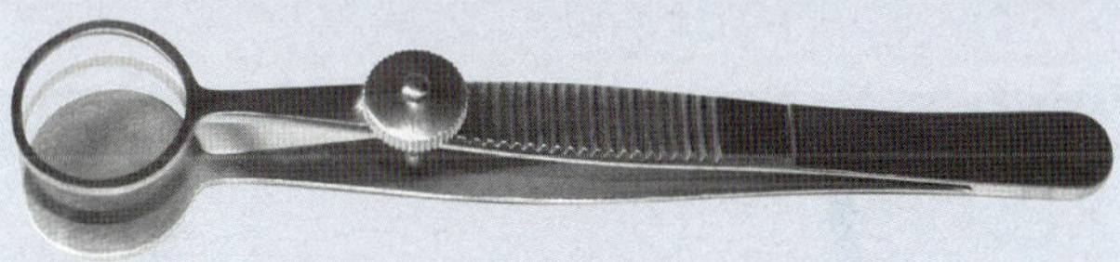

Description	It has a forceps-like handle with one distal tip with a flat solid oval plate and another distal tip with a ring-like aperture. The shaft has a thumbscrew.
Uses	Oral mucosal biopsy. Deroofing of mucocele. Minor salivary gland biopsy. Ear lobe repair. Scrotal surgery. Nasal lesions on ala nasi.
Remarks	Various types are available. For example, Braid chalazion clamp, Desmarres Chalazion clamp, Weis Chalazion clamp, etc.

Instruments for Specific Procedures

Vitiligo Surgery

The following transplantation procedures are employed for hypopigmentation disorders.

Tissue Grafts

- Thin and ultra-thin split-thickness skin grafts (STSG)
- Suction blister epidermal grafts (SBEG)

- Mini-punch grafts (MPG)
- Hair follicular grafts (HFG)

Cellular Grafts

- Noncultured epidermal cell suspension (NCES)
- Cultured "pure" melanocytes (CM)
- Cultured epithelial grafts (CE)

Apart from the general instruments, various special instruments are also required to perform many of these procedures.

Razor Blade Holder

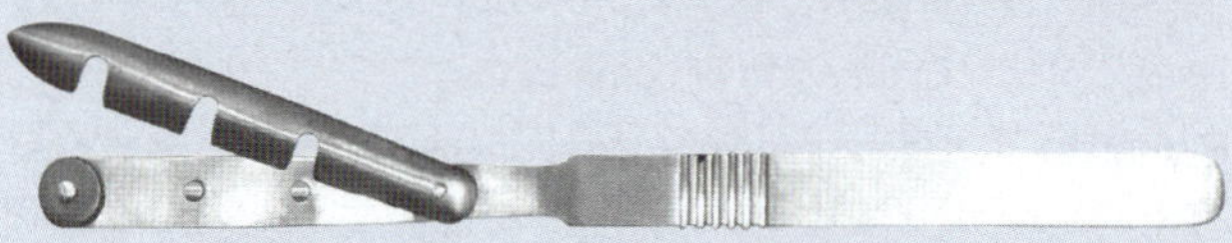

Description	Stainless steel holder which can fit in standard razor blades. The blade is fixed by thumbscrew.
Uses	To obtain split thickness skin grafts from the donor site.
Remarks	Ideal for harvesting small grafts. Both the sides of the blade are exposed and can be used conveniently.

Silver Knife

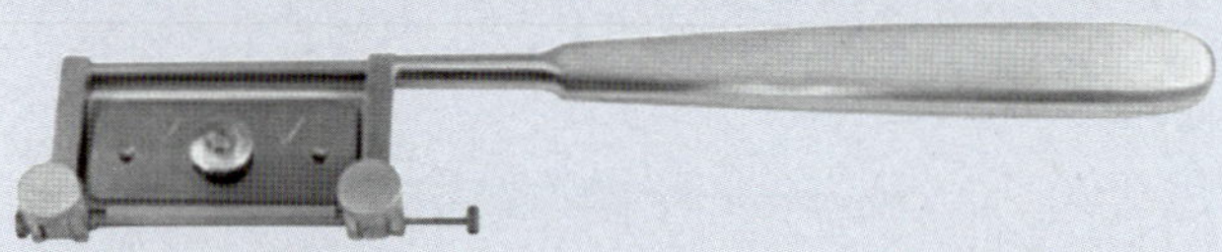

Description	Stainless steel knife which can fit regular razor blades. It has screws for adjusting the thickness of the graft to be harvested.
Uses	To obtain split thickness skin grafts from the donor site.
Remarks	Ideal for harvesting small intricate grafts from areas which would not be accessible with the larger standard knives, such as the ear, dorsa of the hands or scalp.

Humby Knife

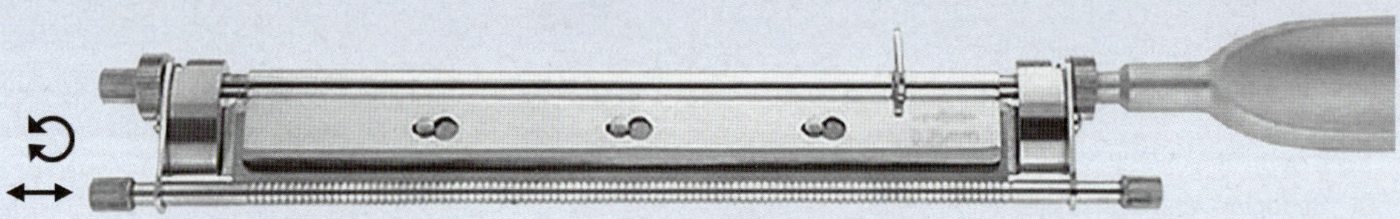

Description	A long knife (12 inch long) with disposable blade (6¼ inch long). It has a handle and a plate where the blade is attached. The design of the plate is slightly different in different modifications of the knife available. These knives have an in-built adjustable guard which can limit the maximal thickness of the graft harvested. A thumbscrew is used to adjust the thickness of the graft.
Uses	To obtain split thickness skin grafts from the donor site.
Remarks	Watson modification is the most commonly used modification of Humby knife.
Braithwaite modification (1955 Fenton Braithwaite)	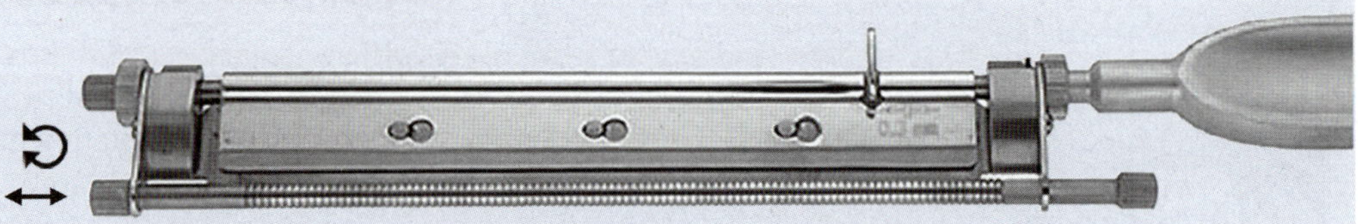 First modification of Humby knife which can be sterilized without dismantling. The guard oscillates and rotates when the knife is used. Thickness of the graft harvested can vary because of the "play" of the guard.

Watson modification
(1960 John Watson)

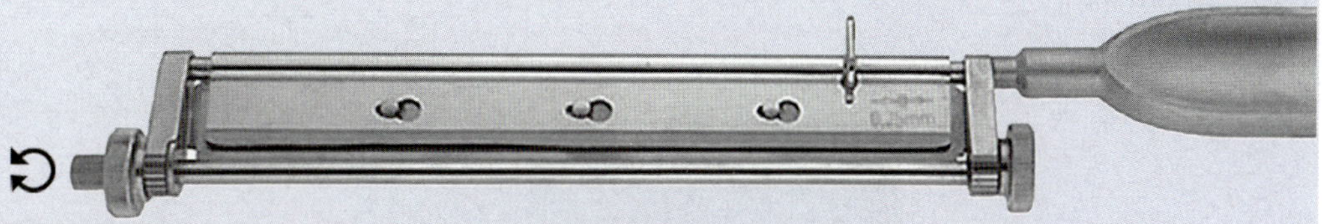

Modified Braithwaite design with a fine, smooth guard with no movement.
The guard passes eccentrically through the bushes at both ends enabling control of thickness of graft with adjustment of a single knob.
It eliminates "play" of the guard but can cause considerable "drag" on the skin as the guard is fixed.

Cobbett modification
(1968 J Cobbett)

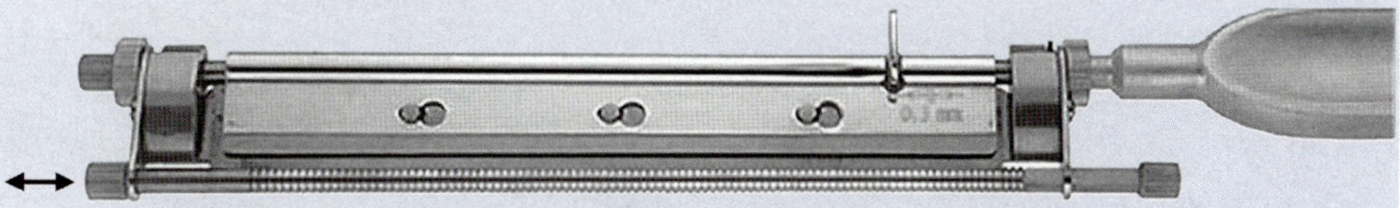

Another modified Braithwaite design with oscillating guard to eliminate "drag".
The guard is fixed to a "D" shaped hole to avoid rolling up of the graft harvested on to the guard.

Powered Dermatomes

Description	These are mechanical dermatomes which use either compressed air/water, DC current or AC current. Different types are available.
Uses	To obtain split thickness skin grafts from the donor site. Rapidly remove long strips of skin.
Remarks	Operation is simple. Procedure can be performed with least number of assistants.

Brown's dermatome

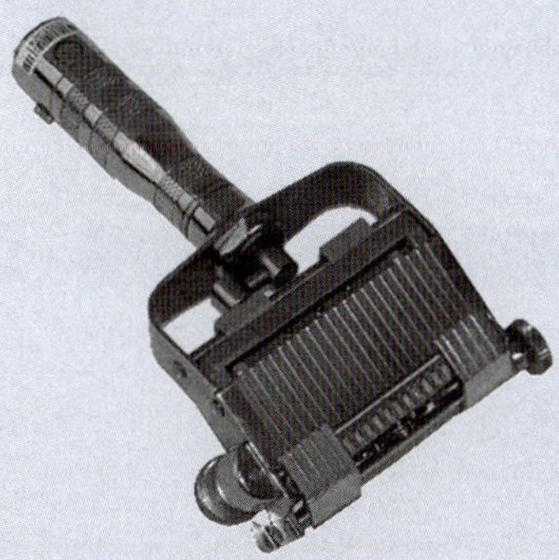

Zimmer dermatome

First mechanical dermatome to be introduced.
Works with compressed air/water.

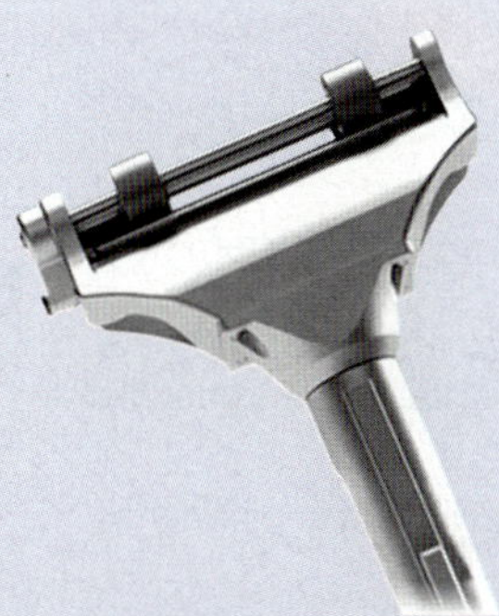

Both electric operated and nitrogen gas propelled versions are available.

Davol Dermatome

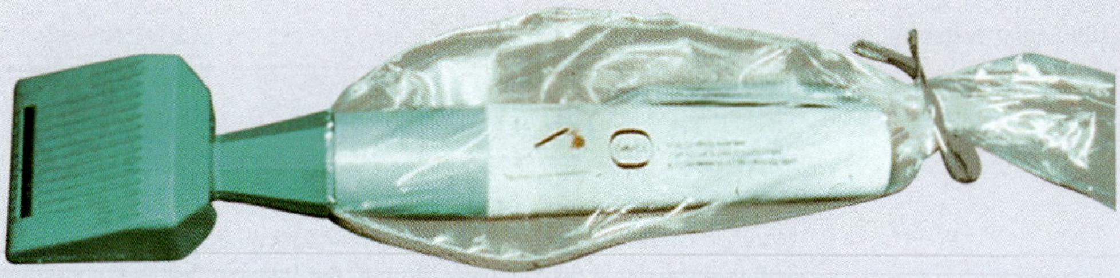

Cordless, battery operated dermatome. Ideal for harvesting small grafts.

Padgett Dermatome

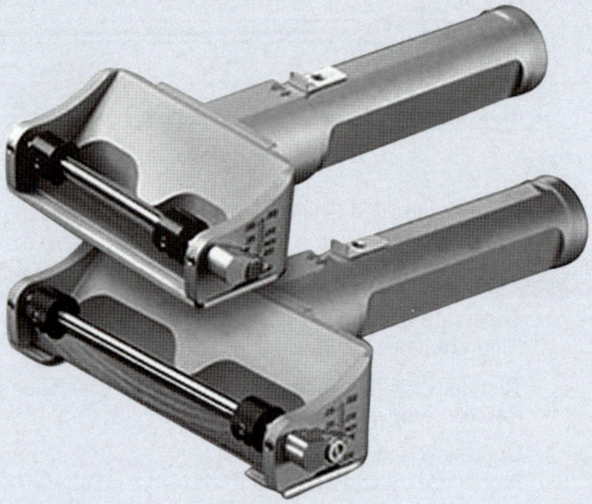

AC current operated dermatome.

Nail Surgery

Nail Splitter

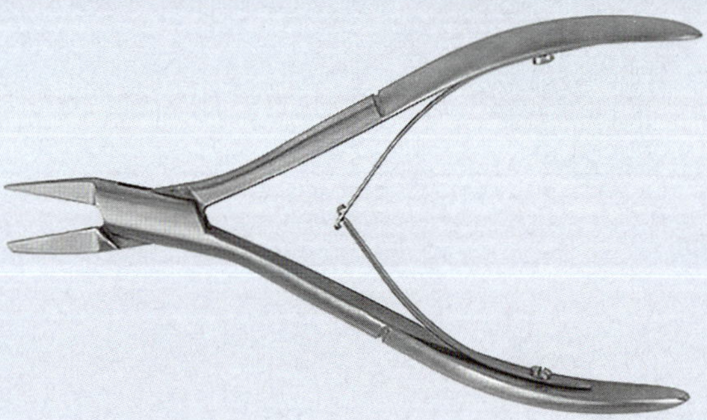

Description	Also referred to as English anvil pattern nail splitter. Has sharp triangular shaped anvil opposed by a sharp and flat edge at the distal end and double spring at the handle.
Uses	To cut longitudinal strip of nail plate in partial nail avulsion.
Remarks	The nail plate is split from the distal to the proximal end.

Nail Spatula

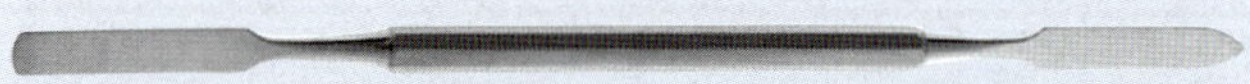

Description	Rod shaped/ flattened equipment with flat edges. The tip of the flat edges may be modified into different shapes.
Uses	Proximal and lateral nail fold separation in nail avulsion, nail matrix biopsy, etc.
Remarks	Spatula is inserted between the proximal/lateral nail fold and nail plate and gently separated by lateral movements.

Freer Septum Elevator

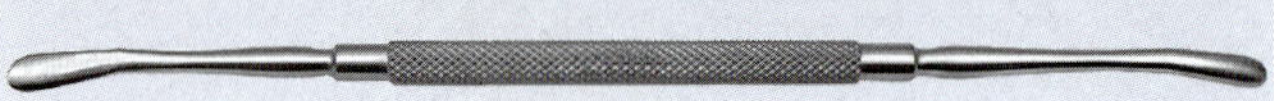

Description	Rod shaped equipment with thin curved blades.
Uses	To loosen distal nail plate from hyponychium, proximal nail fold and lateral nail folds.

Skin Biopsy

Punches

Description	Circular blade ranging in size from 1 to 8 mm which is attached to a pencil-like handle. May be provided with corresponding size plungers.
Uses	Skin biopsy involving delicate areas, cosmetically important areas, etc. Proximal and distal nail matrix biopsies, nail bed biopsy. Mini punch grafting in vitiligo surgery.
Remarks	The common punch size used to diagnose most inflammatory skin conditions is the 3.5 or 4 mm punch.

Reusable metallic punches with plungers

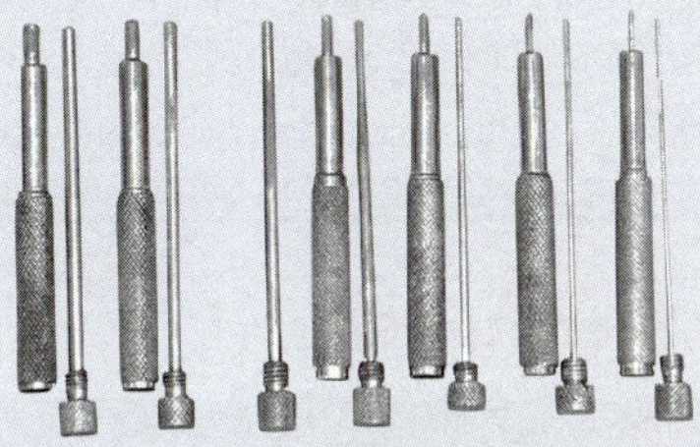

Disposable punches

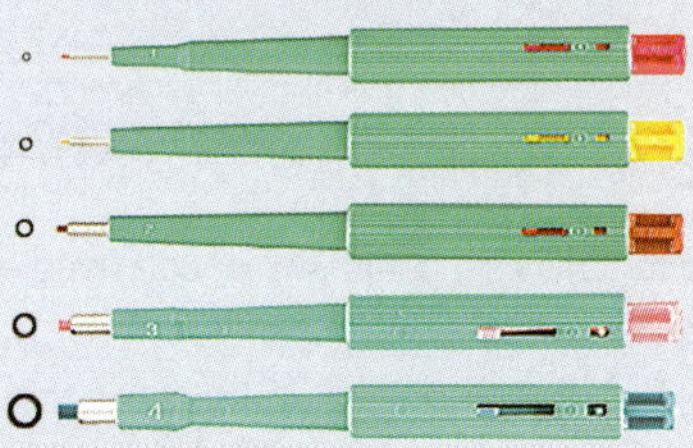

Disposable punches with stainless steel blades of sizes varying from 1 to 8 mm.
Punches with or without and inbuilt plungers are available.

Disposable elliptical punches

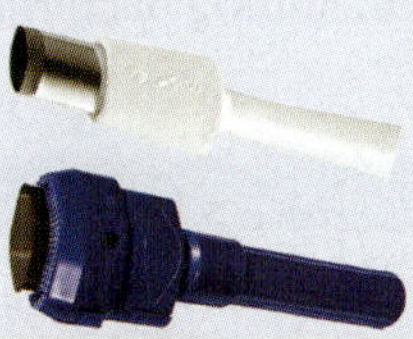

Disposable elliptical punches with fixed and moveable blades are available.
Used for better closure of the wound and for better comsetic results especially on the face and exposed parts.

Dermablade/BiopBlade

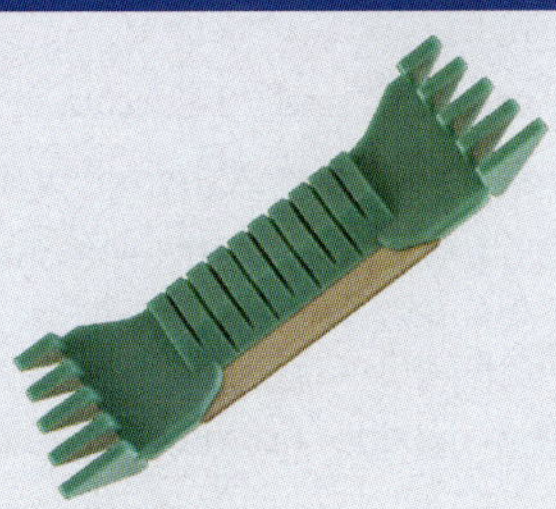

Description	Small, flexible, sterile blade with plastic side grips.
Uses	Shave biopsy.
Remarks	Can also be used for harvesting small STSG in vitiligo surgery.

Hair Transplantation

Implanters

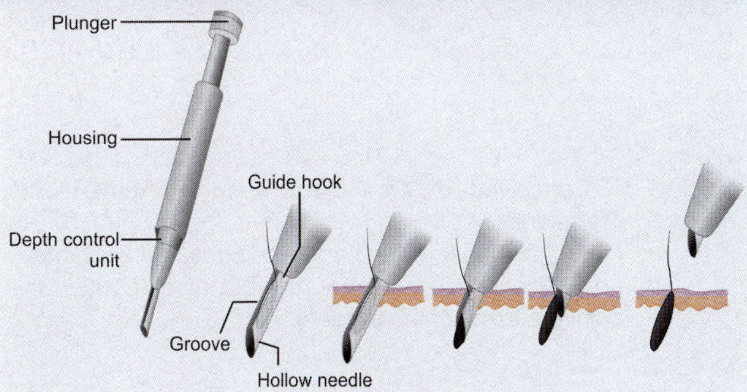

Description	An attempt to automate and quicken the process of implantation of hair.
Uses	In hair implantation of scalp, eyebrow and other parts of body.
Remarks	In a single move a slit is created and without removing the implanter the graft can be placed.

Choi implanter (Korea)

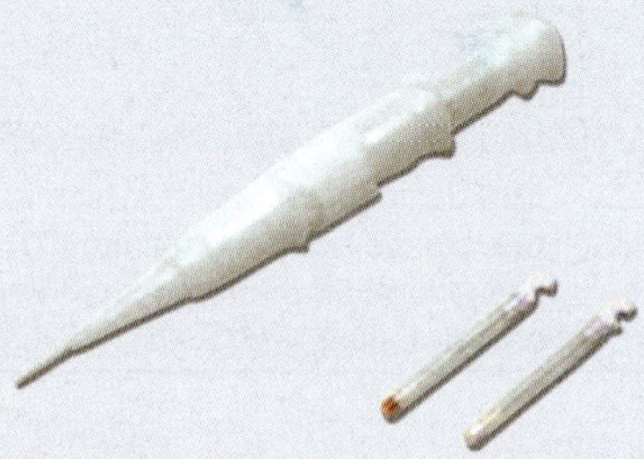

Originated at the Kyungpook National University (KNU) in Korea

Atlanta implanter (USA)

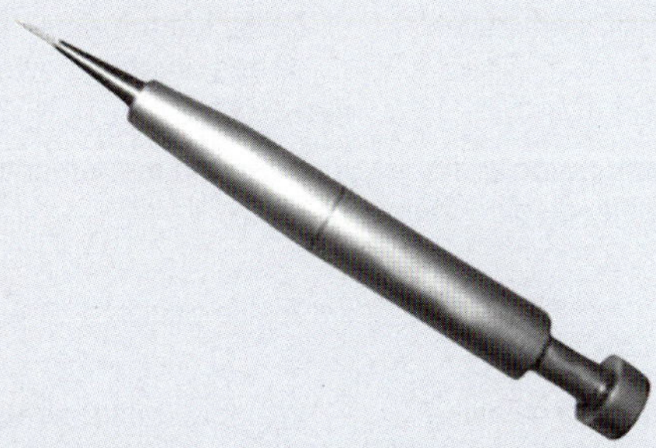

Suited for large or super mega sessions, up to 4000 plus grafts as well as smaller sessions for eye lashes, eye brows, cut scars and corrective surgery procedures with great convenience and speed.

SAVA Implanter (India)

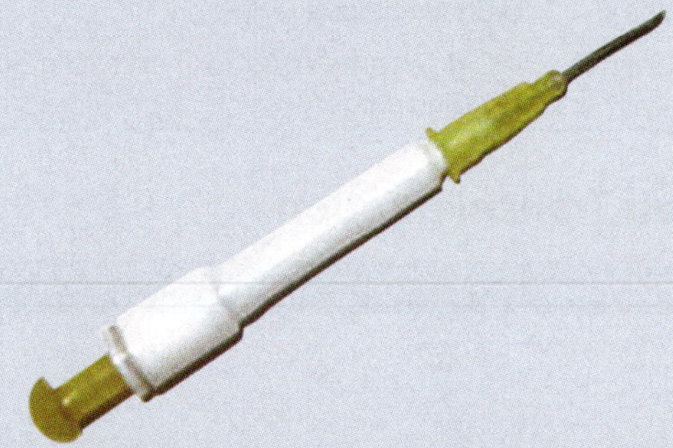

Conceived by Dr Sajeev Vasa of Ahmedabad, Gujarat.
An inexpensive, high quality disposable implanter.
Minimises the graft trauma, but also reduces the overall cost of the surgery.

Lion Implanter (Spain)

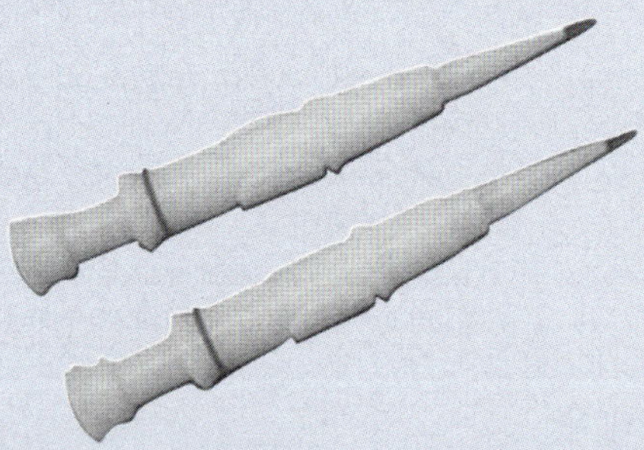

The device uses a clip, which is not found in previously used hair transplanters. This clip reduces the procedural time and makes the replacement of the needle easier.

Circumcision Instruments

Plastibell Clamp

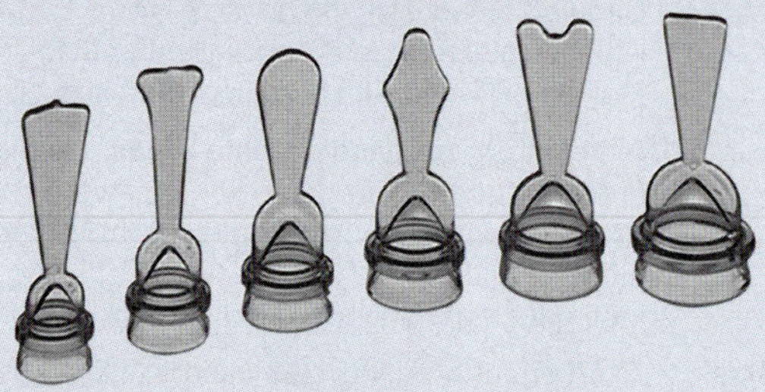

Description	It is a plastic device designed for circumcising infant males.
Uses	Circumcision.
Remarks	Other popular available clamps include Gomco clamp and the Mogen clamp.

Acne Scar Surgeries

Nokor Needle

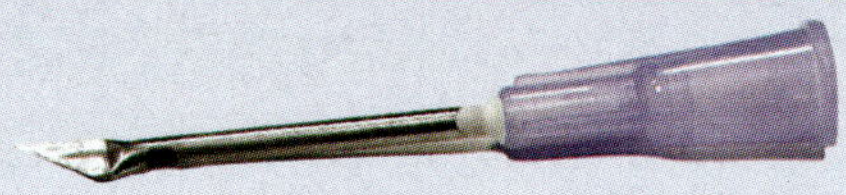

Description	It is a 1.5 inch, 18-gauge needle with a flat pointed end.
Uses	Subcision.
Remarks	For treatment in boxcar acne scars.

Sterilization of Instruments

Defined as a process that destroys or eliminates all forms of microbial life including bacterial endospores.

Sterilization Methods

Method	*Suitable for*	*Remarks*
Hot air sterilization	Glass instruments, forceps, scissors, scalpels, swabs, dusting powder	1 hour at 160°C ½ hour at 180°C 10 min at 200°C
Steam autoclaving (Gravity displacement)	Wrapped instruments/utensils	Most widely used method 30 min at 121°C or 15 min at 132°C and drying time of 15–30 min.
	Textile packs	30 min at 121°C or 25 min at 132°C and drying time of 15 min.
Steam autoclaving (Dynamic air removal)	Wrapped instruments/utensils	4 min at 132°C and 20–30 min of drying time
	Textile packs	4 min at 132°C and 20 min of drying time
Cold sterilization or Chemical sterilization	Sharp metallic instruments	2% Glutaraldehyde, 70% Alcohol, Carbolic acid, Lysol, etc. can be used Instrument immersed for at least 30 min
Gas sterilization	Glass, Rubber articles Fumigating OTs, hand pieces of hand machine.	Ethylene dioxide, Formaldehyde used

Sterilization of Dermatological Equipment		
Skin grafting for vitiligo	Stainless punches	Autoclaving
	Disposable punches	Not to be reused
	Artery forceps	ETO sterilization
	Blades, forceps, scissors	Autoclaving
Hair transplant	Needles, Forceps, Cutting boards, Blades, BP handle, Artery forceps, Adson's forceps, Needle holder	Autoclaving
	Plastic blade holders, Plastic bottles for spraying saline	ETO sterilization or prolonged exposure to chemical disinfectant like Glutaraldehyde
Chemical peels	Brushes to apply chemicals on face	ETO sterilization
Laser	Metal spacers, Interchangeable metal hand pieces	Autoclaving
	Interchangeable plastic hand pieces, Goggles	ETO sterilization or prolonged exposure to chemical disinfectant like Glutaraldehyde

CHAPTER 2

Local Anesthesia for Dermatosurgical Procedures

Sushil Tahiliani, Savitha AS

INTRODUCTION

Dermatologists routinely perform procedures, which may either be diagnostic or therapeutic. Most of these procedures are performed under local anesthesia in an outpatient setting. According to workforce guideline: "Office-based dermatologic surgery is defined as surgery performed by a licensed physician to diagnose and treat certain skin conditions using topical, local, infiltrative, or tumescent anesthesia in an office or facility outside of ambulatory surgical centers and hospital settings."[1] As most of the procedures performed are elective procedures, the overall comfort of the patient is also important.

ANESTHETIC AGENTS

The structure of local anesthetics can be divided into three distinct parts: an aromatic portion (lipophilic), intermediate chain (composed of either ester or amide linkage), and amine group (hydrophilic). This is the basis of local anesthetic classification as either esters or amides. Ester anesthetics are metabolized via the plasma enzyme and pseudocholinesterase. Hydrolysis is rapid and the by-products are excreted in the urine. Amide anesthetics are metabolized primarily by the liver. They should be used with caution in patients with liver disease (Table 2.1).

COMBINATION OF LOCAL ANESTHETICS WITH ADRENALINE

This combination offers following advantages:

- Decreases anesthetic absorption and systemic toxicity with improved efficacy; thus smaller amounts required.
- Prolonged duration of action (almost doubled); especially with lignocaine and procaine.
- Less bleeding at operative site; especially useful on vascular areas with better visualization of operative field.

Adrenaline may potentially induce adverse effects. Therefore, its use must be carefully considered in patients with heart disease and those patients concomitantly taking β-blockers.

DIFFERENT TYPES OF ADMINISTRATION OF LOCAL ANESTHESIA

- Surface anesthesia
- Infiltrative anesthesia
- Tumescent anesthesia
- Nerve blocks

Topical Anesthesia/Surface Anesthesia

Topical anesthesia causes superficial loss of pain sensation after direct application of local anesthetic solutions,

Table 2.1: Pharmacological properties of commonly used local anesthetics.

Agent	*Procaine*	*Prilocaine*	*Lidocaine*	*Bupivacaine*
Onset of action (min)	2–5	>2	<2	5
Duration of action (min)	20–30	30–90	30–60	120–240
Duration of action with adrenaline	30–45	120	120	180–240
Elimination half life (hrs)	0.66	1.5	1.6	3.5
Max dose	500 mg or 7 mg/kg	350 mg	300 mg 4.5 mg/kg	175 mg or 2 mg/kg
Max dose with adrenaline	600 mg	550 mg	500 mg or 7 mg/kg	200 mg

ointments, gels or sprays. They reversibly block nerve conduction near their site of administration by targeting free nerve endings in the dermis or mucosa, thereby producing temporary loss of sensation in a limited area.

Factors Affecting the Action of Topical Anesthesia[2]

- *Drug form*: Free bases are lipophilic and can penetrate the stratum corneum on their own, whereas the salt forms require special delivery systems to do so.
- *Melting point and eutectic mixtures*: The lower the melting point, the better the penetration is. Eutectic mixtures have a lower melting point, thus better penetration than either component by itself.
- *Concentration of drug in vehicle*: Higher the concentration of drug in the vehicle, higher the rate of penetration.

Skin Permeation Enhancers

These compounds, promote skin permeability by increasing the permeability of the stratum corneum temporarily and reversibly. They can be:

- Solvents, e.g. water, alcohols, glycerol, low molecular weight ethers, sucrose esters, silicone fluids, etc.
- Surfactants, e.g. ionic and nonionic bile salts
- Miscellaneous chemicals, e.g. urea, anticholinergic drugs.

Physical Means of Enhancing Permeation

Skin penetration of topically applied anesthetics can be enhanced by following physical measures:

- Exfoliation of the skin.
- Degreasing by alcohol.
- By covering the application area with a dressing or patch of nonporous material such as micropore and tegaderm.
- *Iontophoresis*: Lignocaine HCl 10%/adrenaline 0.1% topical iontophoretic patch (LidoSite) is the first Food and Drug Administration (FDA) approved prefilled active anesthetic patch.

  Disadvantages of iontophoresis technique are:
  - Can cause skin irritation at higher current densities or upon longer application.[3]
  - Prolonged application can also cause electrochemical polarization in the skin, which decreases the magnitude of current flow through the skin.

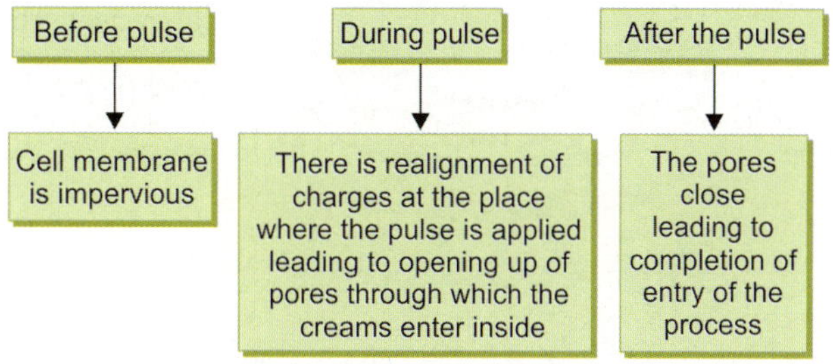

Fig. 2.1: Schematic diagram of electroporation.

  - The mild electrical sensation can be uncomfortable for some patients.
  - It cannot be used over large surface areas of the body.
- Electroporation (uses short electrical impulses of high voltage to create transient pores in the skin) (Fig. 2.1).[4]
- Sonophoresis or phonophoresis (low frequency, ultrasonic energy to disrupt stratum corneum): The ultrasound enhances drug delivery by cavitation, micro steaming and heating (Fig. 2.2).
- Magnetophoresis/magnetokinesis (application of magnetic field to enhance permeation).[5]
- Thermal energy (heat increases skin permeability).
- Erbium:YAG laser pretreatment.[6] Reapplication of topical anesthetic after first pass of ablative lasers produces quicker and deeper anesthesia.
- Skin pretreatment with a hand-applied, plastic microneedle array.[7]

Eutectic Mixture of Local Anesthetics

Eutectic mixtures are compounds, which melt at lower temperatures than any of their components, permitting higher concentrations of anesthetics for use. It is 5% oil in water emulsion cream with a melting point of 18°C and consists of 25 mg/mL of lignocaine, 25 mg/mL of prilocaine, a thickener, an emulsifier, and distilled water adjusted to a pH level of 9.4. EMLA can be used safely on mucosa also.

Commonly Used Method of Application

Topical anesthesia is applied in a thick layer (1–2 g/10 cm^2, up to a maximal dose of 20 g/200 cm^2) to intact skin. After application, the area is covered with a patch of tegaderm or clear plastic wrap to facilitate penetration through the stratum corneum (Fig. 2.3). Depth of anesthesia depends on the contact time with Eutectic Mixture of Local Anesthetics (EMLA).

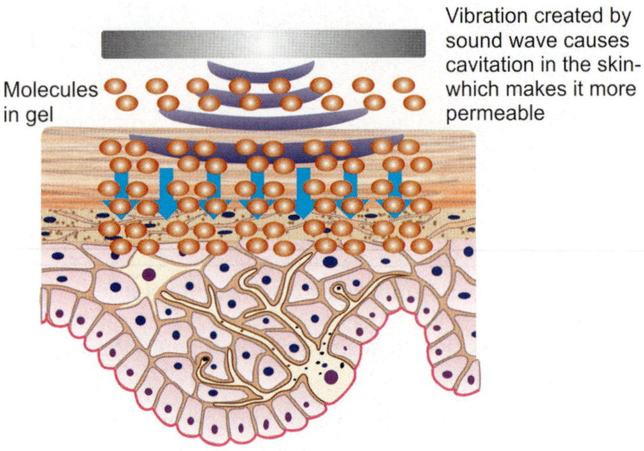

Fig. 2.2: Schematic diagram of sonophoresis.

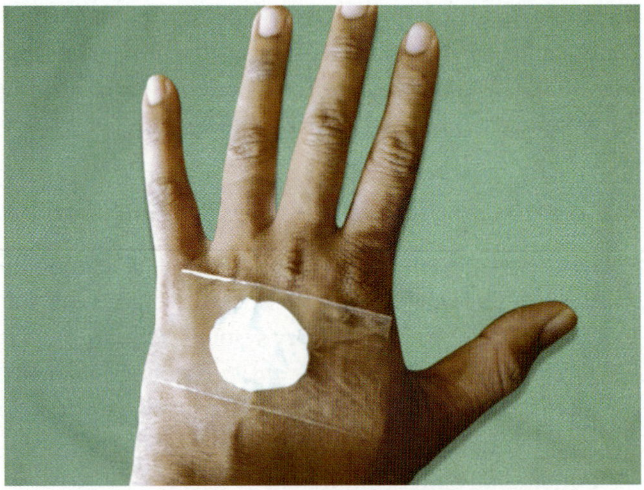

Fig. 2.3: Topical anesthesia applied under occlusion.

Anesthetic effect has been shown to reach a maximal depth of 3 mm after a 60-min application, and 5 mm after a 120-min application. Dermal analgesia can be expected to increase for up to 3 hours under occlusive dressing and persist for 1–2 hours after removal of the cream. Eutectic mixture of local anesthetics are not reliably effective on the palms and soles because of variable penetration.[2]

Advantages of Topical Anesthesia

- Painless as compared to infiltrative anesthesia
- Safely used in patients with needle anxiety
- No tissue edema which can distort surgical site.

Disadvantages of Topical Anesthesia

- Expensive
- Onset time: 30–45 minutes
- Allergic reactions in sensitive patients
- EMLA is a pregnancy category B agent, should be used cautiously in nursing mother, because lignocaine is excreted through breast milk
- With 60 minutes application, the depth of anesthesia obtained is only 3 mm. More invasive procedures are less tolerable under topical anesthesia.

Indications of Topical Anesthesia

- Nonablative laser treatments
- Skin biopsy, Botulinum toxin and filler injections
- To lessen the pain of infiltrative anesthesia
- Pregnant women and nursing women.

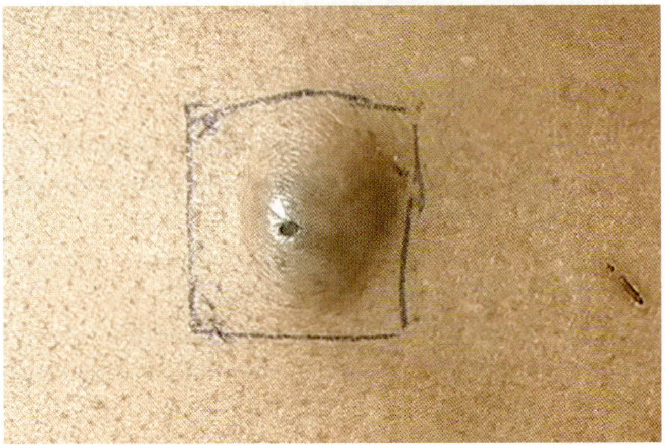

Fig. 2.4: Marking the borders of the lesion prior to infiltration.

Infiltrative Anesthesia

This is the most commonly used technique of anesthesia. Here the anesthetic agent is directly injected into the site of lesion either intradermally or subcutaneously. 1% lignocaine is the most commonly used anesthetic agent.

Tip: Direct infiltration to the surgical site causes distortion of landmarks, so marking the area is important prior to infiltration (Fig. 2.4).

Procedure (Fig. 2.5)

- Skin is held taut.
- Bevel of the needle inserted, preferably into follicular opening as this reduces the pain.
- Infiltrate the area adequately at the level of deep dermis.
- Appearance of peau d' orange indicates the level is in upper dermis, which causes discomfort to the patient (Fig. 2.6).

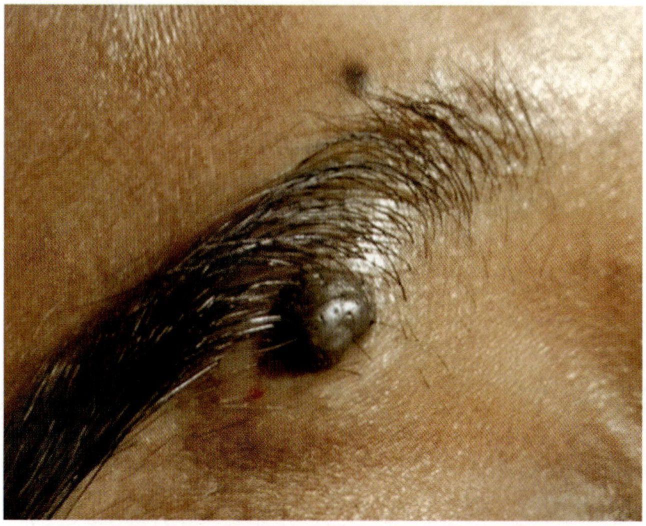

Fig. 2.5: Direct infiltration of anesthesia beneath the lesion.

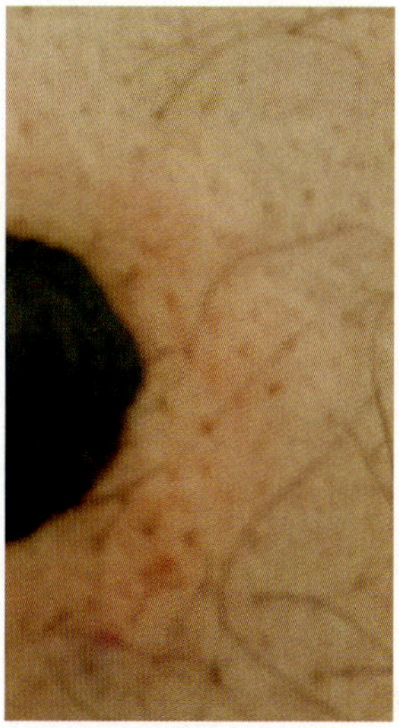

Fig. 2.6: Peau d' orange when infiltration is in upper dermis.

- Additional needle pricks when required are to be placed in previously anesthetized adjacent areas and then proceed to nonanesthetized area to reduce the pain due to needle prick (refer to images of ring block).

Ring Block/field Block (Figs. 2.7A to E)

Ring block is a type of infiltration anesthesia. The anesthetic agent is infiltrated circumferentially around the surgical site, without direct injection in the operative field.

A ring block is useful when the distortion of a surgical site due to the infiltration of anesthesia is not desired. Injection should be into both superficial and deep planes to be effective.[8]

Advantages: Ring blocks allow a decreased volume of anesthetic to be used to anesthetize a larger area.

Steps: Steps for ring block/field block are shown in Figures 2.7A to E.

Needleless Dermajet

This is a needleless pressure injection syringe, used for the intradermal infiltration of drugs in a soluble state. This technique achieves almost painless tissue infiltration with a high velocity microspray in single or multiple doses of 0.1 cc to a depth of 2 to 5 mm, without actual contact with the site of injection. A fine jet emitted under great pressure punctures the tissue without scoring, with a minimum amount of trauma, raising instantaneously a well-defined pinpoint wheal (Figs. 2.8A to D).[9]

Tumescent Anesthesia[10]

This term is used to describe injection of high volume, low concentration lidocaine/epinephrine solution used by dermatologic surgeons for liposuction, hair transplantation, laser resurfacing, flaps and grafts, etc. The solution provides anesthesia safely, is practically painless to inject, and markedly decreases bleeding. Epinephrine (1:1,000,000) is added for hemostasis, and the solution is buffered with sodium bicarbonate to decrease injection discomfort. Concentrations as high as 55 mg/kg have been used safely with the tumescent technique. The absorption kinetics of lidocaine change when high-volume, low-concentration solutions are used. Decreased concentrations of lidocaine also result in slower plasma absorption with decreased peak plasma levels.[8] The tumescent technique for local anesthesia permits regional local anesthesia of the skin and subcutaneous tissues by using direct infiltration rather than a proximal nerve block. By using large volumes of a dilute anesthetic solution consisting of lidocaine (0.1% or 0.05%) and epinephrine (1:1,000,000) in physiologic saline, the tumescent technique produces swelling and firmness, or tumescence, of targeted fatty areas. Recent clinical studies of the absorption pharmacokinetics of lidocaine with the tumescent technique have shown that peak plasma lidocaine levels occur approximately 12 to 15 hours after beginning the infiltration.

Clinical local anesthesia persists for up to 18 hours, obviating the need for postoperative analgesia.

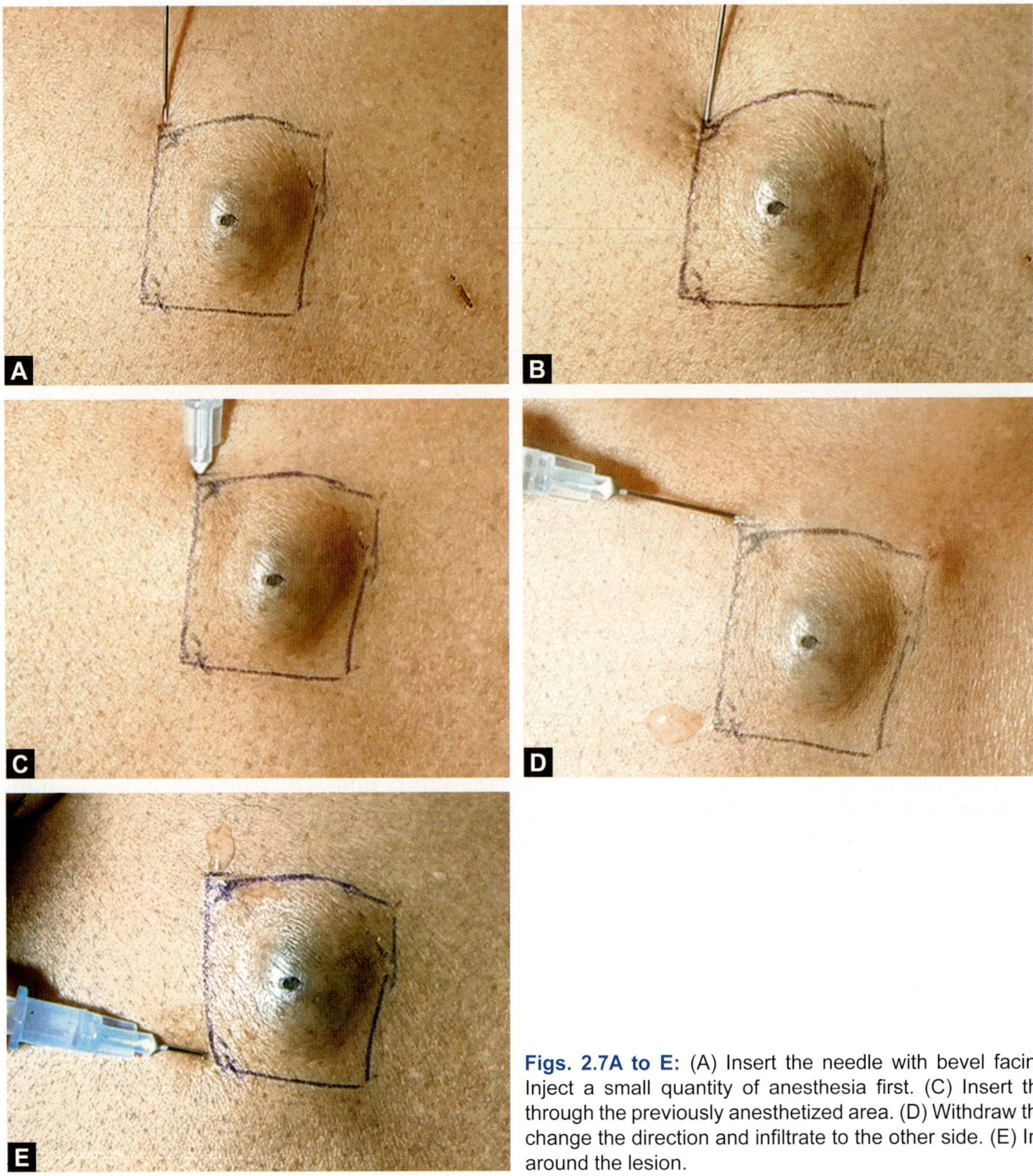

Figs. 2.7A to E: (A) Insert the needle with bevel facing up. (B) Inject a small quantity of anesthesia first. (C) Insert the needle through the previously anesthetized area. (D) Withdraw the needle, change the direction and infiltrate to the other side. (E) Infiltrate all around the lesion.

Complications of Infiltrative and Tumescent Anesthesia

Local: The local effects are summarized in Table 2.2.

Systemic effects[11]: Systemic effects are most often encountered after the unintentional intravenous injection or administration of an excessive dose of an anesthetic. Adding a vasoconstrictor (e.g. epinephrine) can reduce the systemic absorption of an anesthetic. When using topical anesthetics, strict adherence to the maximal dose and area recommended is advised. Great caution must be exercised when using topical anesthetics on mucosal surfaces because of the much greater absorption. Allergic reactions, although systemic, are not related to serum levels of the anesthetic, but rather, they are considered idiosyncratic and can occur at any dose.

Maximum safe doses of lidocaine, and lidocaine with epinephrine is 4.5 mg/kg body weight and 7 mg/kg respectively. The CNS is affected in a predictable and dose-dependent fashion. As serum levels of lidocaine increase,

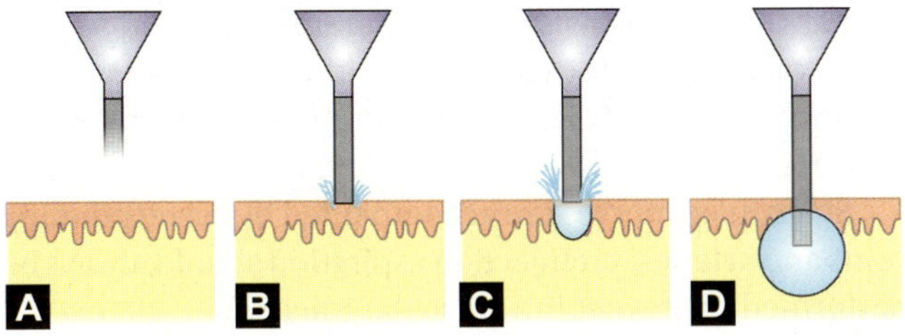

Figs. 2.8A to D: (A) A fine jet is emitted from the nozzle at high velocity (> 100 m per second). (B and C) Impact of the jet on the skin surface punctures the tissue. (D) As the hole in the skin becomes deeper, the liquid that has accumulated in the hole slows down the incoming jet, and the progression of the hole in the skin is stopped.

effects on the CNS become more severe. At serum lidocaine levels in the range of 1–5 μg/mL, patients may complain of tinnitus, light headedness, circumoral numbness, diplopia, or a metallic taste in the mouth. In addition, they may complain of nausea and/or vomiting, or they may become more talkative. As serum levels increase to 5–8 μg/mL, nystagmus, slurred speech, localized muscle twitching, or fine tremors may be noticed. Patients also have been noted to have hallucinations at these levels. If blood lidocaine levels reach 8–12 μg/mL, focal seizure activity occurs; this can progress to generalized tonic-clonic seizures. Respiratory depression occurs at extremely high blood levels (20–25 μg/mL) and can progress to coma. If signs of CNS toxicity are noted, steps must be taken to reduce hypoxia and acidosis, because these states increase the toxicity of local anesthetics. The patient's airway should be maintained, and supplemental oxygen provided. If blood levels of carbon dioxide increase, protein binding of lidocaine decreases and this results in higher levels of free lidocaine in the blood. Increased respiration and respiratory alkalosis increase the seizure threshold and decrease the uptake of the local anesthetic into the CNS.

Compared with the CNS, the cardiovascular system is less susceptible to the effects of local anesthetics. Most adverse effects of the cardiovascular system that occur with the administration of local anesthetics are a result of the addition of epinephrine rather than direct effects of the anesthetic. However, high blood levels of local anesthetics directly reduce cardiac contractility. In addition to the direct vasodilatory effects of most local anesthetics, the decrease in cardiac function can cause hypotension. Atrioventricular blocks, bradycardia, and ventricular arrhythmias also are reported; these are more common in patients with known conduction disturbances and those requiring antiarrhythmic medications.

Table 2.2: Local effects.

Complications	*Cause*	*Prevention and treatment*
Pain	• Due to needle puncture of the skin • Acidic pH 3.5-4.5 due to epinephrine • Tissue irritation from the anesthetic • Distention of tissues	• Slow administration • Add sodium bicarbonate
Ecchymosis	• Perforation of cutaneous blood vessels (Common in mucous membranes, head, and genitalia) • Patient has a bleeding diathesis • Aspirin or other anti-coagulants like green tea, vitamin C, vitamin E, gingko biloba	• Reassurance. Will disappear over time. The fresh hematoma may require drainage with an 18-gauge needle, followed by the application of a pressure dressing.
Infection	• Proper sterile technique is not used	• Use proper sterile techniques

Allergic reactions: Allergic reactions to local anesthetics are extremely rare, especially with amide local anesthetics, and account for less than 1% of the reactions caused by local anesthetics. Reactions can be type I (i.e. anaphylactic) or type IV (i.e. delayed-type hypersensitivity) reactions. These reactions are idiosyncratic and not dose dependent. Skin prick and intradermal test results are negative in the vast majority of patients, but some authors recommend testing with the most commonly used amide local anesthetic (lidocaine). Clinical signs of type I reactions include pruritus, urticaria, facial swelling, wheezing, dyspnea, cyanosis, laryngeal edema, nausea, vomiting, and abdominal cramping. Epinephrine with a concentration of 1:1000 should be administered subcutaneously in a dose of 0.3–0.5 mL. This dose can be repeated every 20–30 minutes to a maximum of 3 doses. If anaphylaxis ensues, a 5 mL dose of epinephrine 1:10,000 should be administered intravenously. Type IV (i.e. delayed-type hypersensitivity) reactions account for 80% of allergic reactions to local anesthetics. They are more common with the use of topical anesthetics and may occur with anesthetics of both amide and ester subtypes. Clinical manifestations are similar to those of allergic contact dermatitis and include erythema, plaques, and pruritus. Patients with a history of type IV reactions are not at an increased risk of type I reactions due to amide type anesthetics. Contact dermatitis caused by topical anesthetics should be treated with topical steroid preparations.

Nerve Blocks

A nerve block involves placing the local anesthetic solution in a specific location at or around the main nerve trunk that will effectively depolarize that nerve and obtund sensation in the area of sensory distribution of that particular nerve.

Advantages

Single accurately placed injection can obtund large areas of sensation without tissue distortion at operative site.

Disadvantages

- Sensation of numbness in areas other than the operative site
- Lack of hemostasis at the operative site due to lack of vasoconstrictor component of the local anesthetic injection, which is obtained in injection form at site directly.

Since many nerves are accompanied by corresponding veins and arteries, preinjection aspiration should always be performed to prevent intravascular injection.

Commonly Used Nerve Blocks

Supraorbital nerve block (Figs. 2.9A to D): Supraorbital nerve exits the supraorbital foramen, and divides into medial and lateral branches, each branch accompanied by its artery.

Supratrochlear nerve block (Figs. 2.10A and B): The supratrochlear nerve block is often performed in

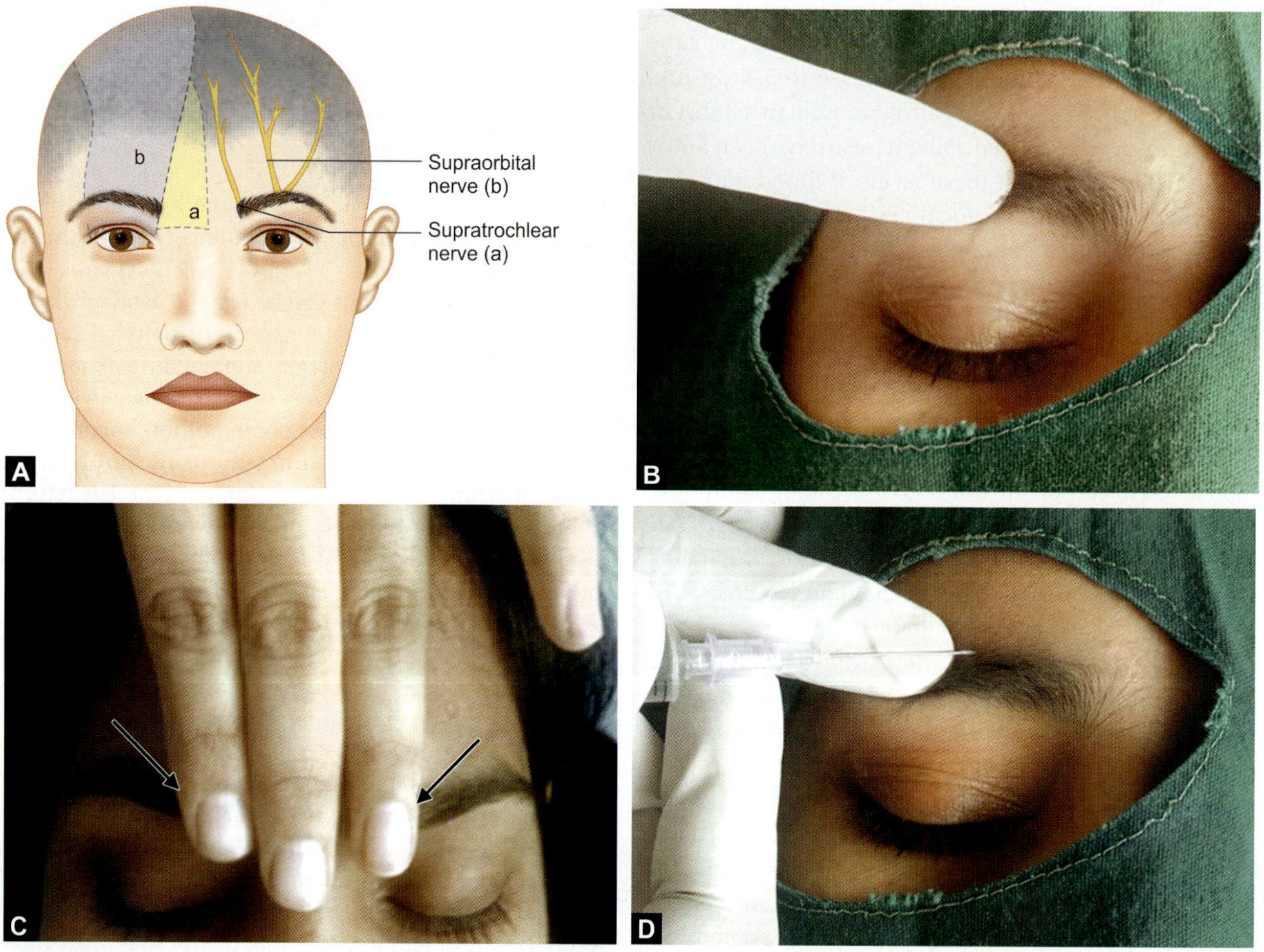

Figs. 2.9A to D: (A) Supraorbital and supratrochlear nerve and areas supplied by them. (B) The supraorbital foramen is located with the pulp of the index finger of nondominant hand along the supraorbital ridge until a subtle notch is felt. (C) Another method is to place three fingers centered vertically over glabella, the major branches of supraorbital nerve emerge just lateral to the fingers. (D) Insert the needle just lateral to the foramen, it will seek the bone contact (with less than 10 mm generally) at the edge of the foramen. Inject very slowly 1.5–2 mL of anesthetic solution with the needle facing medially.

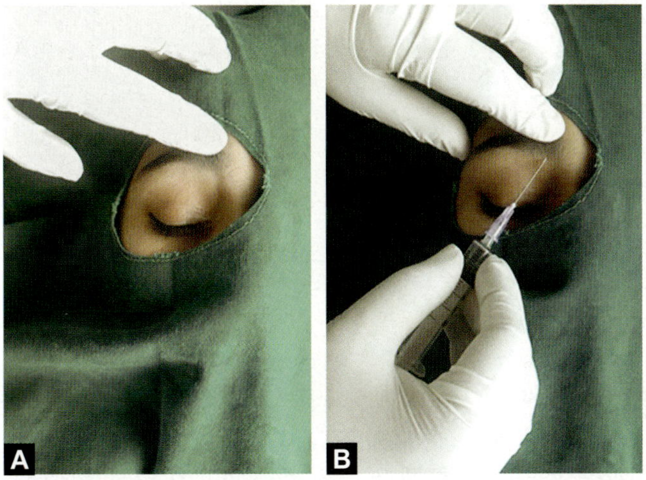

Figs. 2.10A and B: Supratrochlear nerve block: Insertion is on the supraorbital ridge approximately 1 cm medial to the supraorbital notch between the notch and the bridge of the nose.

conjunction with the supraorbital nerve block to achieve regional anesthesia over the ipsilateral forehead.

Infraorbital nerve block (Figs. 2.11A to C): The infraorbital nerve leaves by the infraorbital foramen located at 4–7 mm below the infraorbital bone edge.

Extraoral technique: The extraoral technique of infraorbital nerve block is shown in Figures 2.11A and B.

Endo-oral method: The endo-oral method of infraorbital nerve block is shown in Figure 2.11C.

Mental nerve (Figs. 2.12A and B): The mental nerve is the terminal branch of the inferior alveolar nerve. It enters the face through the mental foramen and supplies the inferior lip and the chin.

1. *Intraoral approach (Fig. 2.12A)*
2. *Transcutaneous route (Fig. 2.12B)*

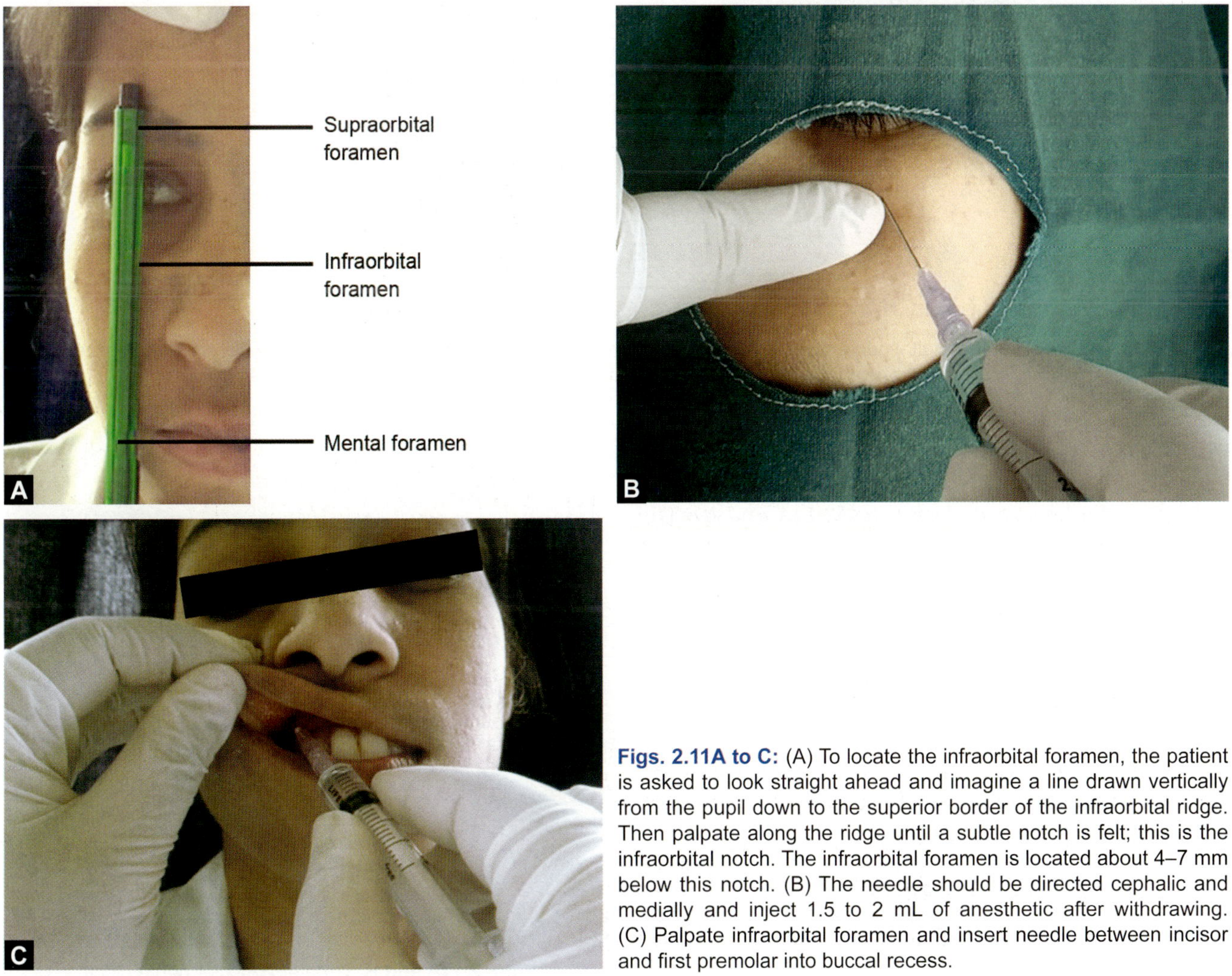

Figs. 2.11A to C: (A) To locate the infraorbital foramen, the patient is asked to look straight ahead and imagine a line drawn vertically from the pupil down to the superior border of the infraorbital ridge. Then palpate along the ridge until a subtle notch is felt; this is the infraorbital notch. The infraorbital foramen is located about 4–7 mm below this notch. (B) The needle should be directed cephalic and medially and inject 1.5 to 2 mL of anesthetic after withdrawing. (C) Palpate infraorbital foramen and insert needle between incisor and first premolar into buccal recess.

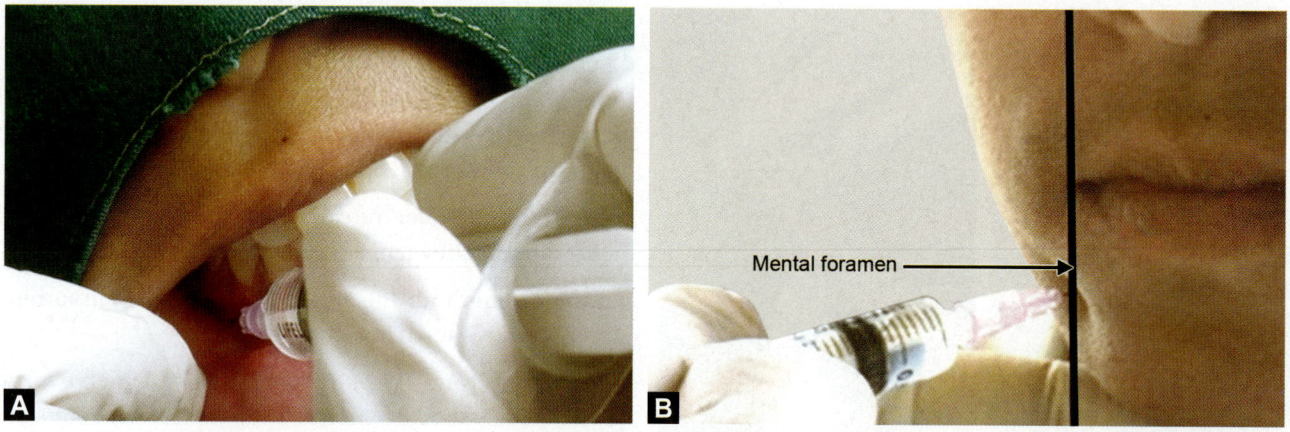

Figs. 2.12A and B: (A) The mental foramen is palpable between the 2 lower premolar teeth. Insert the needle along the lower gum line into the buccal fold between the premolar teeth near the foramen. (B) Insert needle at mental foramen, advance needle perpendicular to bone until periosteum is reached, withdraw the needle and inject 2–3 mL of anesthetic near the mental foramen, but not straight into it.

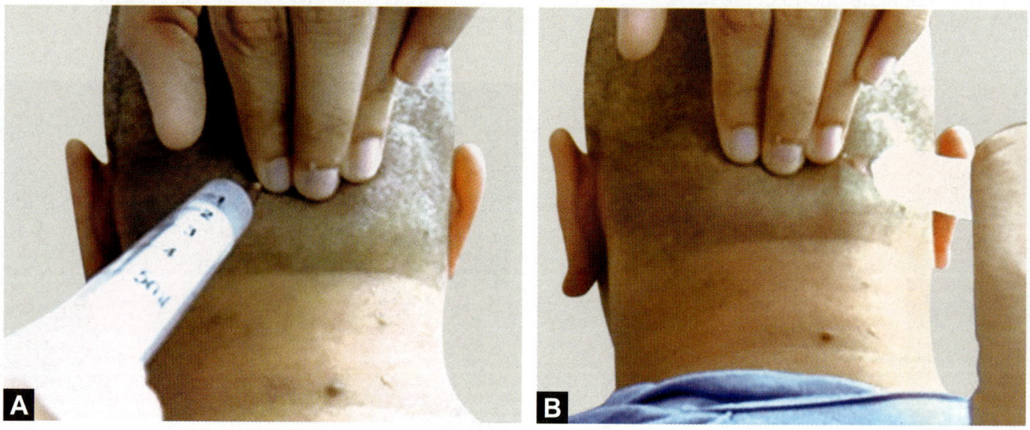

Figs. 2.13A and B: Greater occipital nerve block: Place three fingers on superior nuchal line with middle finger on the external occipital protuberance, point of injection is just lateral to the lateral fingers on either side.

Greater occipital nerve block: The greater occipital nerve block is shown in Figures 2.13A and B.

Greater auricular nerve block (Figs. 2.14A and B): The greater auricular nerve numbs the lower third of the ear and the lower postauricular skin. Locate the mastoid tip and inject local anesthetic both anterior and posterior to the mastoid.

Digital nerve blocks (Figs. 2.15A to C): Each digit is innervated by 4 digital nerves. The 2 palmar digital nerves innervate the palmar aspect of the digit and the nail bed, whereas the dorsal nerves innervate the dorsum of the digit.

a. *Proximal digital nerve block* (Fig. 2.15B)
b. *Transthecal block (Fig. 2.15C)*

Distal Digital Block (Wing Block)[12]

The procedure for distal digital block is shown in Figures 2.16A to C.

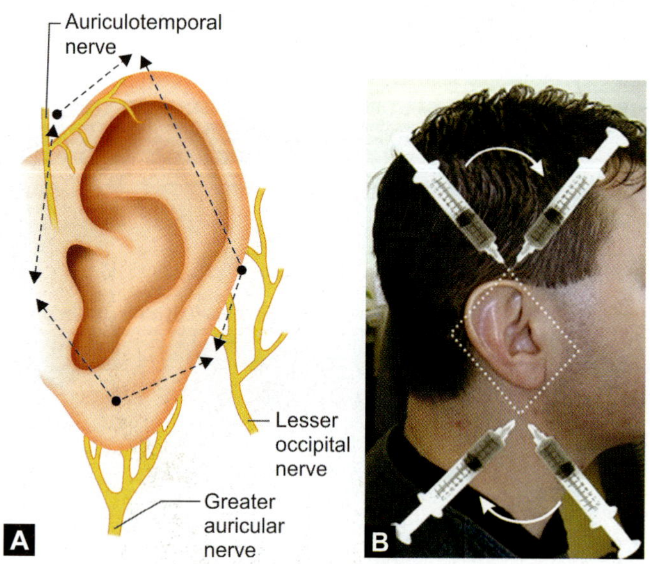

Figs. 2.14A and B: Greater auricular nerve block.

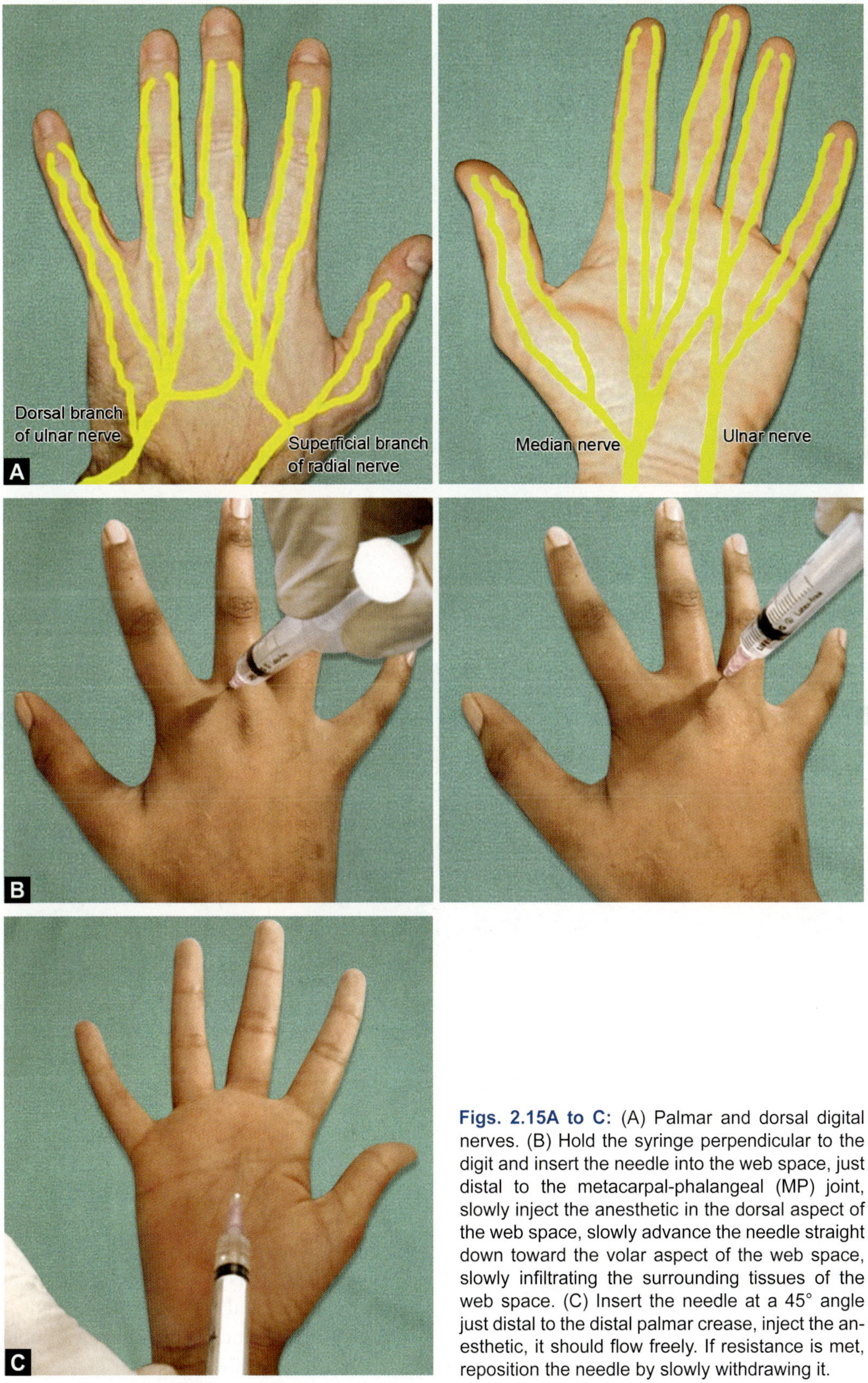

Figs. 2.15A to C: (A) Palmar and dorsal digital nerves. (B) Hold the syringe perpendicular to the digit and insert the needle into the web space, just distal to the metacarpal-phalangeal (MP) joint, slowly inject the anesthetic in the dorsal aspect of the web space, slowly advance the needle straight down toward the volar aspect of the web space, slowly infiltrating the surrounding tissues of the web space. (C) Insert the needle at a 45° angle just distal to the distal palmar crease, inject the anesthetic, it should flow freely. If resistance is met, reposition the needle by slowly withdrawing it.

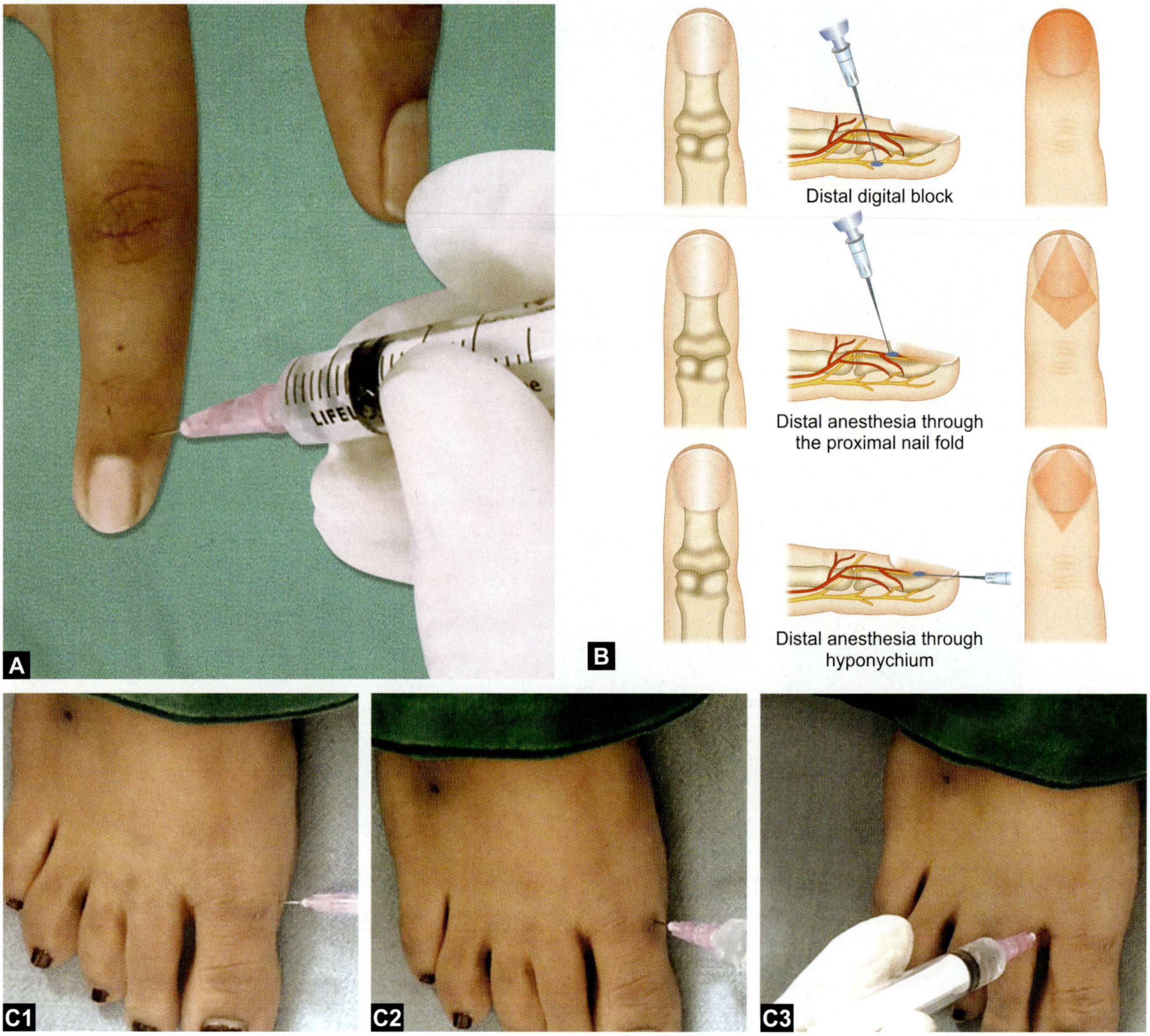

Figs. 2.16A to C: (A) Needle is inserted 2–3 mm proximal to the junction of proximal and lateral nail fold. Insert the needle vertically and advance towards ventral aspect, inject about 0.5 to 1 mL of anesthetic agent. (B) Three types of distal digital blocks with areas covered (C1) Insert the needle at a 90° angle at the medial aspect of the digit, just distal to the metatarsal-phalangeal joint. (C2) Slowly inject the anesthetic as the needle is advanced toward the volar/plantar side, without piercing the volar skin. (C3) Make another injection over the already anesthetized skin at the lateral aspect of the digit, with the needle at 90°, advancing it from the dorsal to ventral aspect, as was done medially.

Three-sided digital block: Figure 2.16C shows the three-sided distal digital block technique.

TIPS FOR REDUCING PAIN DURING ANESTHESIA

- Topical anesthesia prior to needle puncture
- Smaller size needles, 30 gauge needles
- Injection through cutaneous pores
- Slow infiltration; infiltrate as one advances the needle slowly.
- Distraction: Massage or vibration; an assistant who "hand holds" and chats with the patient.
- Buffered lidocaine with sodium bicarbonate and freshly mixed epinephrine.
- Re-inject in anesthetized areas; minimize sticks.

Absorbable Sutures (*see* Box 3.2)

Absorbable sutures loose most of their tensile strength within 60 days by proteolysis or hydrolysis (Fig. 3.1). These sutures provide support to the tissues till healing occurs. Natural absorbable sutures are digested by proteolytic enzymatic digestion while synthetic sutures undergo hydrolysis in tissue. These sutures are placed deep into wound in the subcutaneous and deeper dermis layer to eliminate dead space and approximate the wound edges, and provide strength till healing occurs.

These sutures should not be placed very superficially as otherwise it may result in splitting of suture or epithelialization of suture tunnels.

Important properties of absorbable sutures are presented in Table 3.1.

Nonabsorbable Sutures (Box 3.3)

Nonabsorbable sutures (Box 3.3) retain most of their strength 60 days after placement and most elicit little inflammatory response (Fig. 3.2). These sutures are generally used for epidermal closure and require manual removal.

Important properties of some of the non absorbable sutures are presented in Table 3.2.

Polybutester suture characteristics are similar to polypropylene suture, but offers better handling including lower memory, increased flexibility, higher elasticity and better knot security. But this suture has not been widely used in dermatologic surgery still.

Besides the absorbability, the other important consideration when making a choice of suture is whether the suture is monofilament and multifilament. Monofilament suture is made up of single strand and requires careful handling. While multifilament sutures are made from

Box 3.3: Nonabsorbable suture.

Monofilament

- Polypropylene (Prolene)
- Nylone (Ethilon)
- Polybutester (Novafil)
- Hexafluoropropylene

Multifilament

- Surgical silk
- Cotton
- Polyester (Dacron)
- Polyamide braided

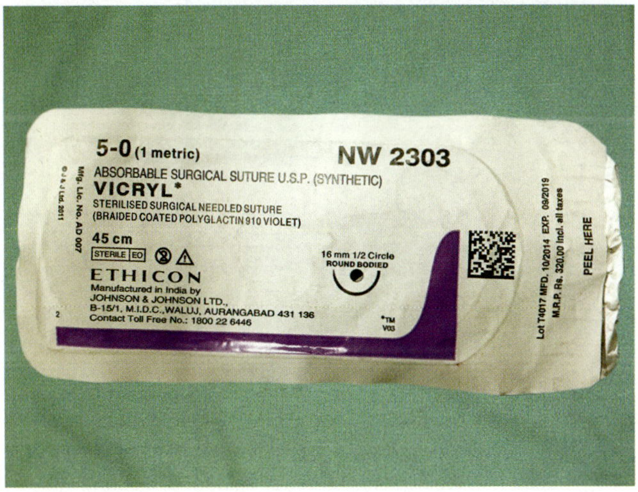

Fig. 3.1: Most commonly used absorbable suture—'Vicryl'. Note that suture and needle characteristics are mentioned on the package.

Table 3.1: Important properties of absorbable sutures.

Properties	*Handling*	*Knot security*	*Tissue reactivity*	*Time to lose strength*	*Use*	*Other comments*
Catgut	Fair	Poor	High	Proteolysis by 60 days	Mucosa	—
Polyglycolic acid	Fair to good	Fair to good	Low to moderate	Hydrolysis by 90–120 days	As buried suture	Available in beige, violet and green color
Polydioxanone (PDS)	Poor	Poor	Low	Hydrolysis by 180–210 days	Resorbed slowly; suited for wounds requiring support for long term	Violet or clear color
Poliglecaprone 25 (Monocryl)	Excellent	Good	Low	Hydrolysis by 9–120 days	As buried suture in wound requiring long term support	Clear
Polyglactin 910 (Vicryl)	Good	Fair	Low-moderate	Hydrolysis by 60–90 days	As buried suture in wound requiring short-term dermal support	Violet or clear; one study reported higher risk of hypertrophic scar

Table 3.2: Properties of nonabsorbable sutures.

Properties	*Handling*	*Knot security*	*Tissue reactivity*	*Tensile strength*	*Use*	*Other comments*
Polypropylene	Poor	Poor	Low	Moderate	Widely used for epidermal closure; also for invisible suture as very-low friction coefficient	Blue or clear
Nylon monofilament	Poor	Poor	Low	High	Percutaneous closure; widely used	Green, black or clear; Pre-moistened monofilament has better handling
Surgical silk	Excellent	Excellent	High	Low	Mucosa, flexures as very soft suture	Black
Polyester	Good	Good	Low-moderate	Very-high	Not much used in dermatology; costly	Green or clear. Coated suture has lesser tissue drag

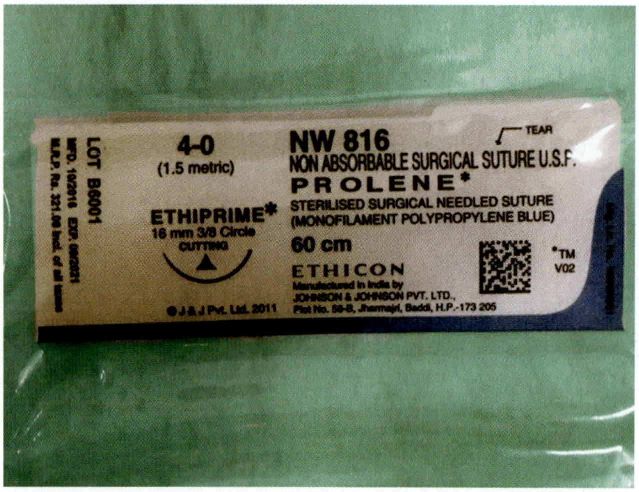

Fig. 3.2: Polypropylene suture (Prolene) is the most commonly used nonabsorbable suture for epidermal closure.

twisting or braiding of several thin filaments together. Difference in the characteristics of these two suture types have been enumerated in Table 3.3.

Table 3.3: Properties of monofilament and multifilament sutures.

Monofilament	*Multifilament*
• Lesser strength	• Greater tensile strength
• Less pliability	• More pliability
• Difficult handling	• Handling easy
• Knots slip	• Knots well
• Stiff	• Less stiff
• Infection risk low	• Risk of infection
• Friction low	• Coefficient of friction high

Local wound factors like tension in the wound, risk of infection, site, depth of placement of suture determines the kind of suture we need to close the wound edges. General tips for making a choice are enumerated in Box 3.4.

Box 3.4: General tips for making suturing material choice.

1. Smallest suture which provides adequate strength is preferred
2. Multifilament sutures have greater capillarity—avoided in contaminated wounds
3. Monofilament sutures can easily slide through tissue, therefore good for tough tissues.
4. Knot strength is directly proportional to friction coefficient of the suture material, thus when suturing with Prolene, extra knots are required
   - Simple interrupted without tension—Prolene, Polybutester
   - Mucosa, intertriginous area–Silk, polyester
   - Invisible suture—Vicryl
   - Non absorbable long term tensile strength—Nylon
   - Buried suture:
     - Low tension—Vicryl/Monocryl
     - Tension high/prolonged period—PDS
     - Contaminated wound—PDS
     - Subcuticular—Monocryl (good knot security)

We have to decide the size of the suture also. Sutures are available in sizes varying from 11-0 to 5. Greater the number of zeroes lesser is the diameter of the suture. Table 3.4 provides the approximate guide for suture size to be used for different body parts.

NEEDLES

Surgical needles are made up of high quality stainless steel which is very resistant to corrosion. Surgical needle parts comprise of point, body and swage (Fig. 3.3). Point is that part of needle which extends from tip of needle to the point of maximum cross-sectional area of needle. Swage is that part of needle to which the suture material is attached. Body of the needle is the main bulk which lies between point and swage.

Table 3.4: Guide to suture size.

Site	*Size of suture*
Scalp	3–0/4–0
Face	5–0
Eyelid	6–0
Ear lobe	6–0
Trunk and limbs	4–0

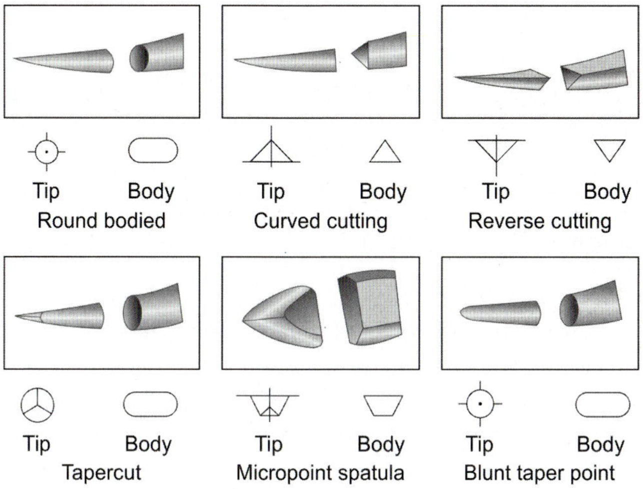

Fig. 3.4: Different types of cross-section of the body of the needle.

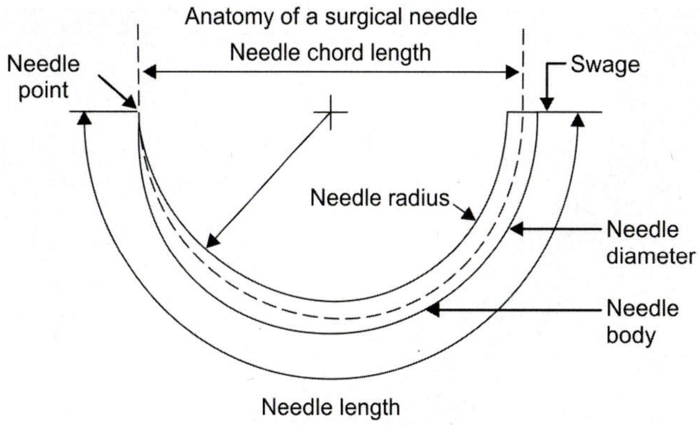

Fig. 3.3: Parts of the needle.

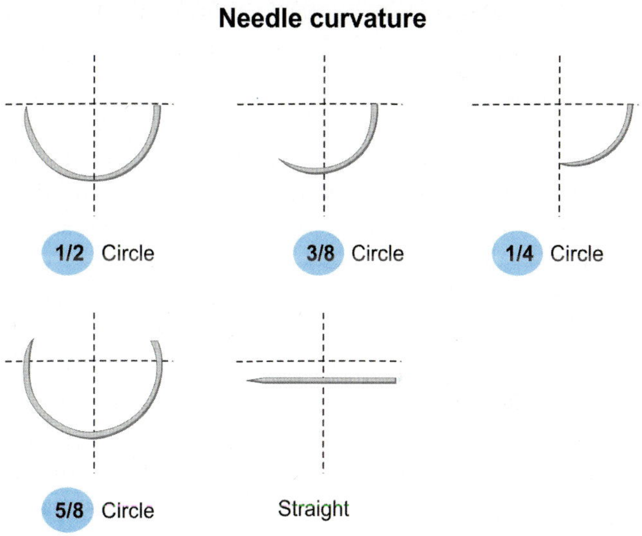

Fig. 3.5: Different shapes of the curvature of the needle.

Needles are classified based on:

- Attachment of suture—traumatic needles are needles with eye and without attached suture, while atraumatic needles do not have eye and the suture material is directly attached to one end of the needle. Dermatologists mainly use atraumatic needles as they are less traumatic to tissue, handling is easy, saves time and there is no risk of unthreading of the suture.
- Based on cross-section of body of the needle (Fig. 3.4), they are classified into round body needle and cutting needle. Cutting needles have triangular cross-section. Conventional cutting needle has sharp inner margin pointing towards the wound edge while reverse cutting needle has the sharp margin pointing outwards from the wound margin. Reverse cutting needle are most suited for cosmetic surgery as they cause little trauma while making the maneuvering of the needle through the tissue easier. Round body needle cause least tearing of tissue, therefore more suitable for delicate areas.
- Based on shape of the body—classified into straight and curved needles. In dermatosurgery, primarily curved needles are used. Length of curvature of the needle can be 1/4th, 3/8th, ½, or 5/8th of circle (Fig. 3.5). Most commonly 3/8th of a circle needle is used in dermatosurgery.
- Based on size of needle—needle length is the distance measured along the needle from the point to the swage. Different needle lengths are available for each suture size.

SUTURING TECHNIQUES

In order to have good approximation of wound edges with minimal tension, we have to do multilayer closing of the wound. Appositional sutures are buried sutures placed in subcutaneous and deeper dermis for approximation of wound margins, eliminating the dead space, redistributing the tension away from the wound edges and evert the

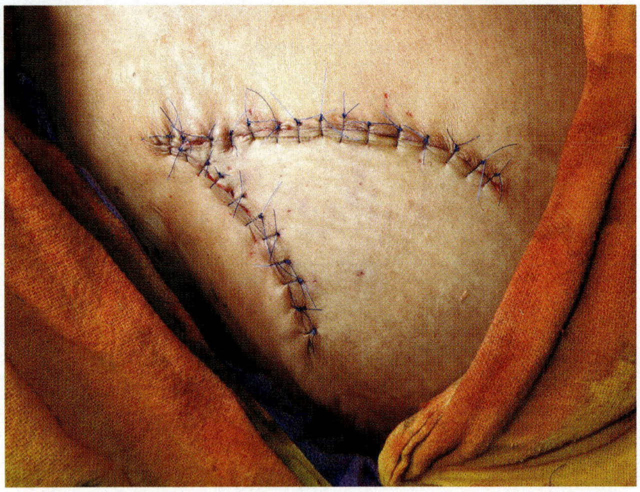

Fig. 3.6: Simple interrupted sutures with good wound margin eversion.

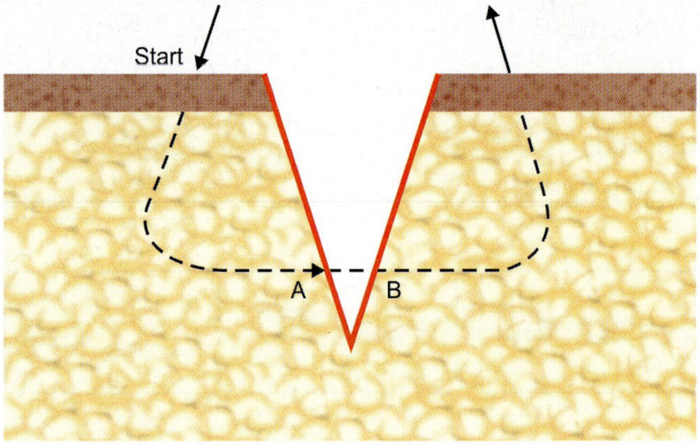

Fig. 3.7: When placing interrupted suture final configuration should be pear shaped in order to have good eversion of wound margins.

wound margins. Buried sutures should be placed at even level across the wound to prevent step off deformity and too superficial placement should be avoided as it can result in spitting of suture from the surface.

Epidermal sutures are placed on skin surface to provide precise epidermal wound edge approximation. Toothed forceps should be used for grasping, stabilizing and elevating the wound margins when passing the needle through the tissue.

Depending upon the technique, different suturing methods can be categorized into interrupted sutures, continuous/running sutures and other special sutures. Proper suturing technique will result in well-approximated and everted wound margins. Buried suture is generally one size larger than the epidermal suture.

Interrupted Sutures

1. ***Simple interrupted sutures***: It is the most basic and commonly performed suturing technique (Fig. 3.6).

Steps

- Insert the needle perpendicular to the skin surface 3–5 mm away from the wound margin.
- Traverse the epidermis and full thickness of dermis and exit into the wound.
- Enter the needle into the opposite wound margin.
- Traverse the dermis and exit the needle perpendicular to the epidermis.
- Then tie the knot.

Tips (Figs. 3.7 and 3.8)

- Entry and exit point of the needle should be equidistant from the wound edges.
- The final configuration of stitch should be pear shaped as it results in good wound eversion.
- Depth of tissue bite should be equal on two sides, so as to avoid mismatched wound edge heights.
- Distance between two sutures depends upon the site and tension in the wound. Generally over face, the gap kept is 3–5 mm.
- Suture should be just tight enough for epidermal apposition; very tight sutures can result in tissue strangulation and scarring.

Advantages

- It is very simple technique and can be easily mastered.
- If the wound edges are of different thickness, then by altering the depth of tissue bite on two sides, leveled approximation can be achieved.
- Do not impair cutaneous circulation when compared to running sutures.

Disadvantages

- Takes more time compared to running sutures.
- Can leave cross-hatched linear scars.

2. ***Horizontal mattress suture:*** It helps to reduce tension, evert wound edges and close the dead space (Figs. 3.9A and B).

Steps

- Enter the needle perpendicularly at a gap of 5–7 mm from wound edge.
- Traverse the epidermis, dermis and may be subcutaneous layer.

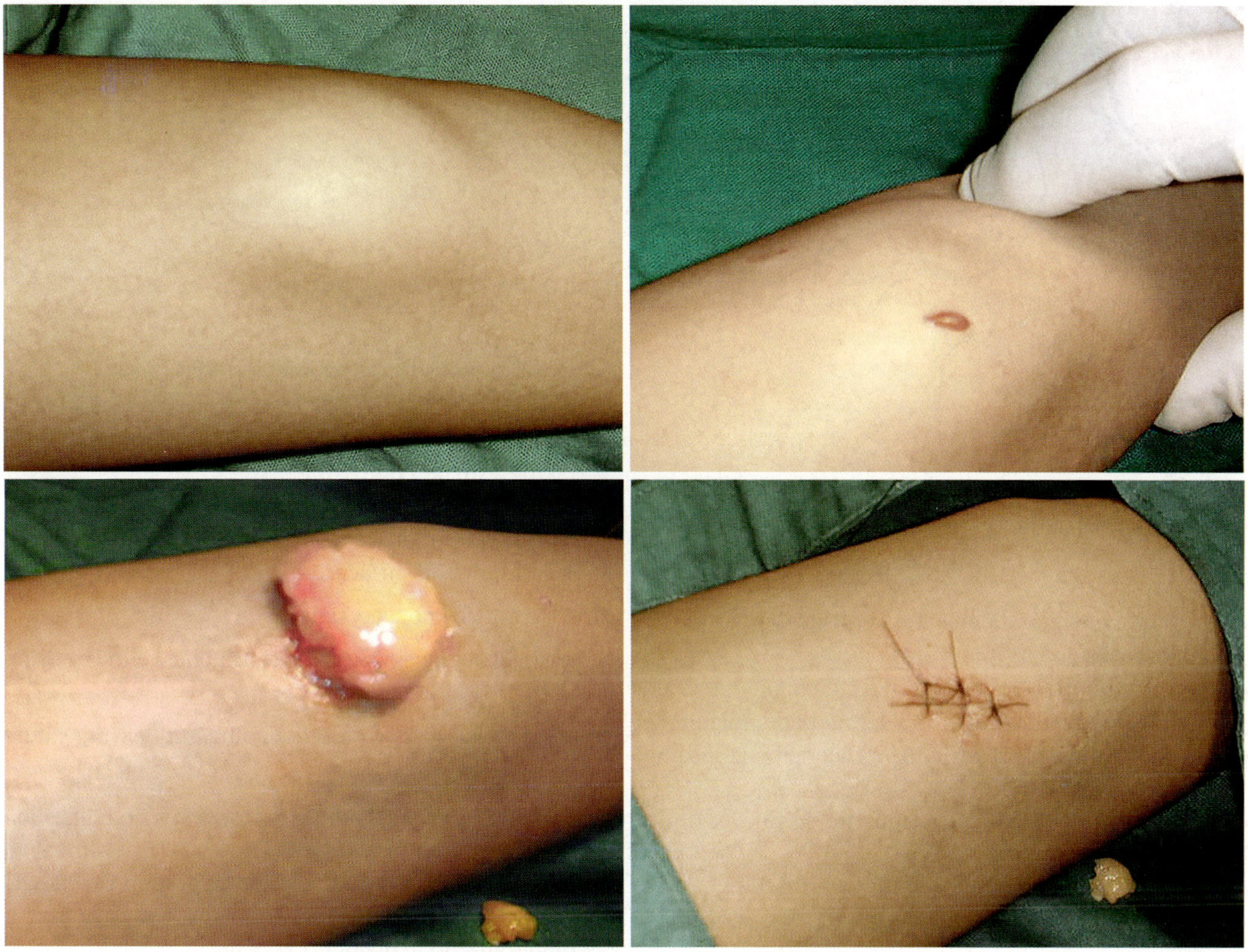

Fig. 3.8: Simple interrupted epidermal closure after lipoma excision.

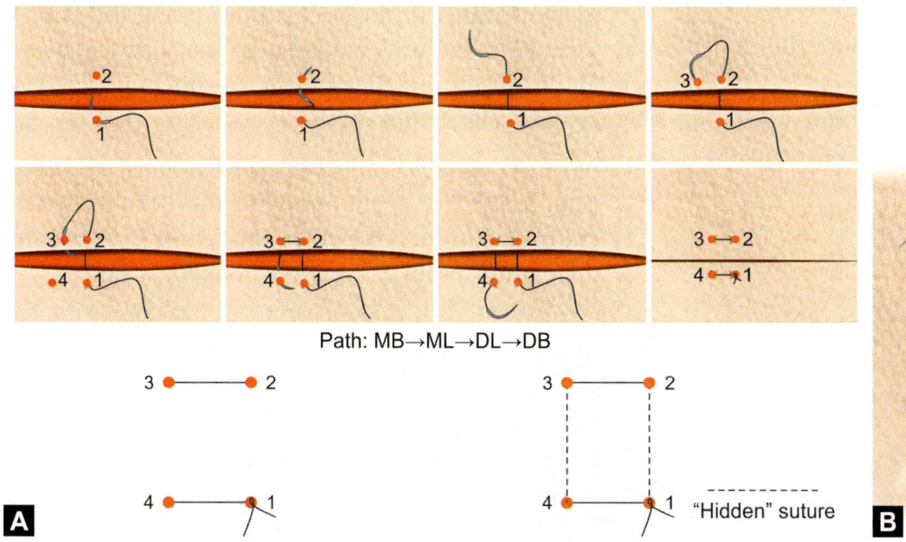

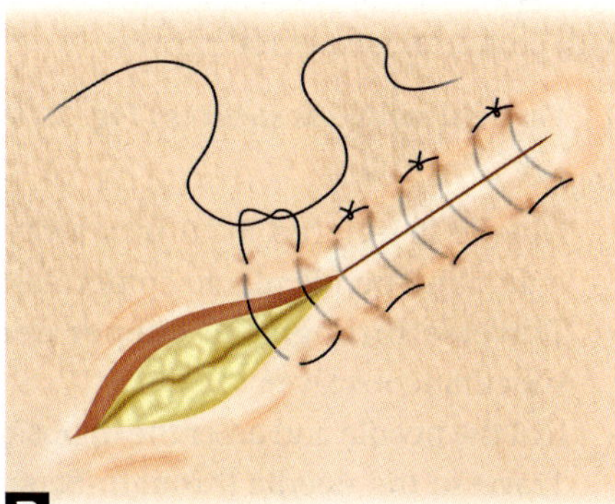

Figs. 3.9A and B: Horizontal mattress suture.

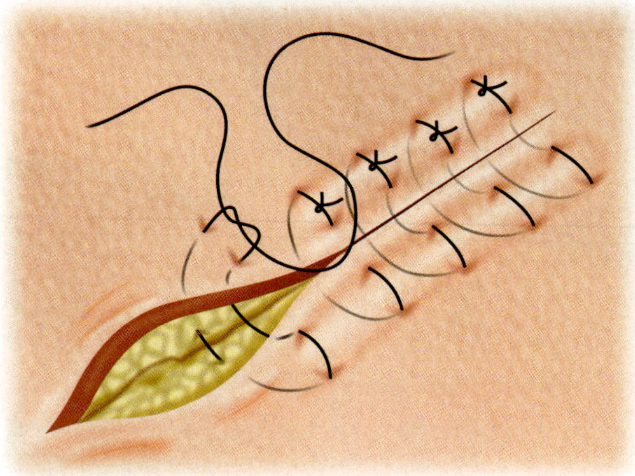

Fig. 3.10: Vertical mattress suture.

- Exit the needle and enter the opposite wound at the same level.
- Traverse the needle through the subcutaneous layer, dermis and exit through the epidermis perpendicularly.
- Re-enter the needle again 5–10 mm laterally on the same side of the suture line.
- Traverse the needle through the tissue as done previously.
- Finally needle exits from the original entry side.
- Tie the knot on the surface.

Tips

- Tie knot just tightly enough to approximate the edges.
- Remove the sutures early to avoid edge necrosis.

Advantages: Wound eversion better, and reduces dead space.

Disadvantages: Takes more time, risk of wound edge necrosis high if suture tied tightly, therefore avoid in tissues with compromised blood supply.

3. ***Vertical mattress sutures (Fig. 3.10)***

Steps

- Needle is entered 5–10 mm away from the wound margin perpendicular to epidermal surface.
- Traverse through the deeper dermis and may be subcutaneous layer.
- Exit the needle and enter the opposite wound edge.
- Traverse the needle through the subcutaneous layer, dermis and exit the needle on surface.
- Reverse the needle on the needle holder.

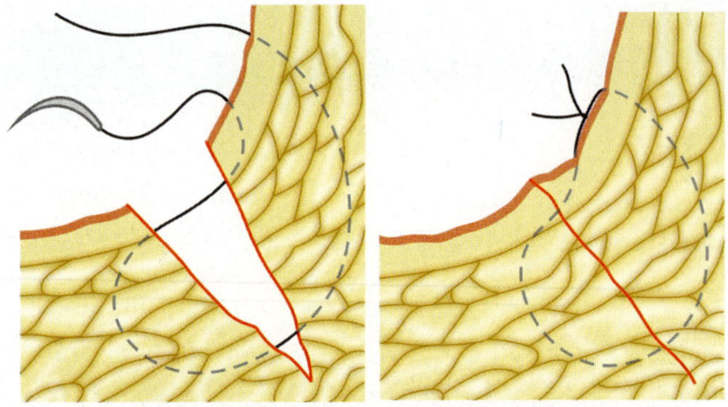

Fig. 3.11: Half buried vertical mattress suture.

- Re-enter the needle 1–3 mm away from the wound edge taking a smaller bite of the tissue.
- Take similar small bite and exit the needle on the first side of the wound.
- Tie the knot on surface.

Tips: Do not tie knot very tightly.

Advantages: Reduces wound tension, good wound eversion and closes dead space.

Disadvantages: Risk of cross-hatching and leaving suture marks more.

4. ***Half buried vertical mattress suture*:** It is a modification of vertical mattress suture (Fig. 3.11). It is similar to vertical mattress suture, except that when the needle is traversing through the opposite wound edge, it penetrates up to deeper part of dermis without exiting the skin surface and then needle exits through the original wound margin 2–3 mm away from the wound margin in line with the original entry point. Then knot is secured. In this way we have only two entry exit points for the needle and therefore this technique is good for cosmetically significant sites.

5. ***Far near near far modified vertical mattress suture (Fig. 3.12)*:** It is again a modification of the vertical mattress suture. It provides very good strength and therefore is useful in wounds with high tension.

Steps

- Enter the needle 5–10 mm away from the wound margin.
- Traverse the needle to the opposite side and exit around 2–3 mm away from wound edge.
- Reenter the needle 2–3 mm away from the wound margin on the original entry side.
- Again traverse the tissue through the wound margin.

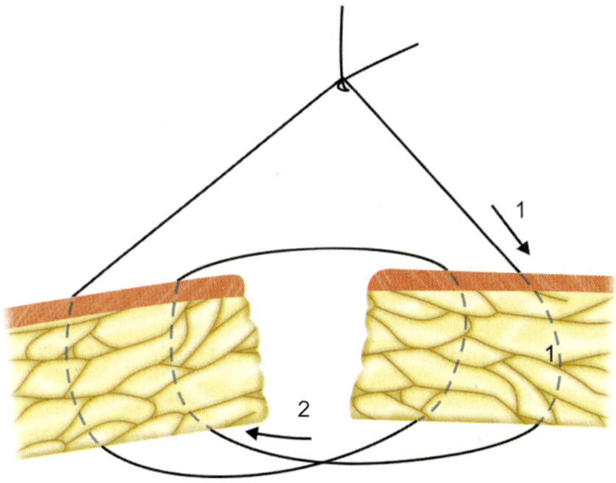

Fig. 3.12: Far near near far modified vertical mattress suture.

- Enter the opposite wound edge and exit 5–10 mm away from the wound margin.
- Tie the knot.

Tips: Depth of tissue bites should be symmetric on two sides for good alignment of wound edges.

Advantages: Very good for high tension wounds and provides good wound eversion.

Disadvantages: Chances of misalignment high, if symmetric tissue bites are not taken.

6. ***Pulley sutures***: It is a minor modification of vertical mattress sutures. In this, we place the vertical mattress sutures as described before but before tying the knot the thread is traversed through the loop on the opposite side of the wound edge. After that the knot is tied. It provides additional wound closure strength.

Continuous/Running sutures

Running stitches should not be used in wounds with moderate to severe tension in wound margins as they can strangulate the vascular plexus and damage the tissue. Their main advantage is ease and speed of application.

1. ***Simple running suture***: It is also called as continuous over and over suture (Fig. 3.13).

Steps

- Simple interrupted stitch is placed, tied but not cut.
- Then a series of simple interrupted stitches are placed without tying or cutting the suture.
- The whole length of wound is traversed like this.
- Knot is tied at the end of suture line between loop of last pass and the tail end of the suture.

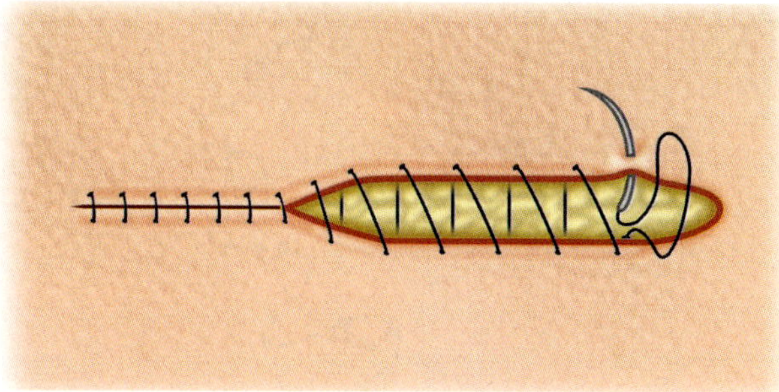

Fig. 3.13: Simple running suture.

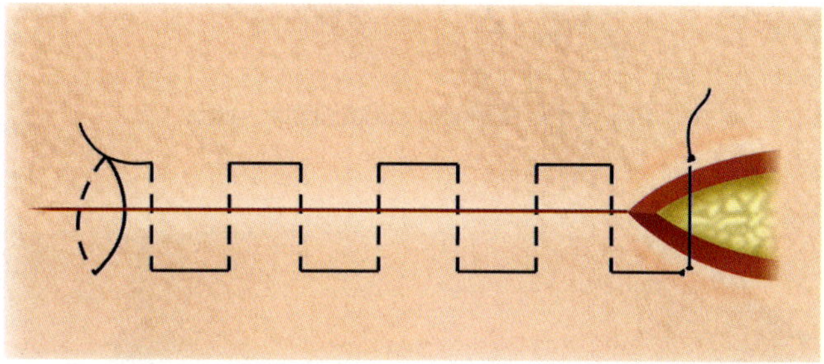

Fig. 3.14: Running horizontal mattress suture.

Advantages: Useful for long wounds as suture placement is very quick.

Disadvantages: Strength poor and risk of wound dehiscence high, if suture breaks at one point.

2. ***Running horizontal mattress suture (Fig. 3.14)***

Steps

- Place a interrupted suture and do not cut the thread.
- On the same side laterally enter the needle and exit on the other side.
- Then enter the needle laterally on the exit side itself.
- Keep on doing the same steps on the two sides, i.e exit and entry on the same side of wound margin.
- Final knot placed between last loop and the suture end.

Advantages: Provides very good wound eversion.

Disadvantages: More time consuming compared to simple running suture.

3. ***Running subcuticular suture (Fig. 3.15)***: It is placed when there is no tension in wound edges and site is cosmetically significant as with this technique there will not be any suture marks.

Steps

- Needle is introduced into skin 4–6 mm distal from one end of wound.
- It traverses through the tissue and enters the wound at the apex.

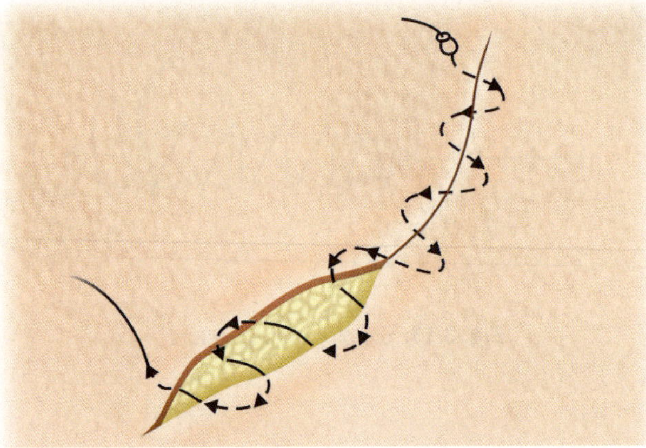

Fig. 3.15: Running subcuticular stitch.

- Free end of the suture is tied on itself.
- Then horizontal tissue bites are taken in the dermis alternately from both wound edges.
- The length of wound is traversed and when the other apex is reached needle is taken out by puncturing 4–6 mm distal to the apex of the wound.
- Then knot is tied on the suture itself.

Tips

- Both absorbable and non absorbable sutures can be used. Prolene is the preferred non absorbable suture as it is monofilament and its coefficient of friction is very low (Fig. 3.16). If absorbable sutures are used then the knots are buried at the time of placing the sutures (Fig. 3.17).

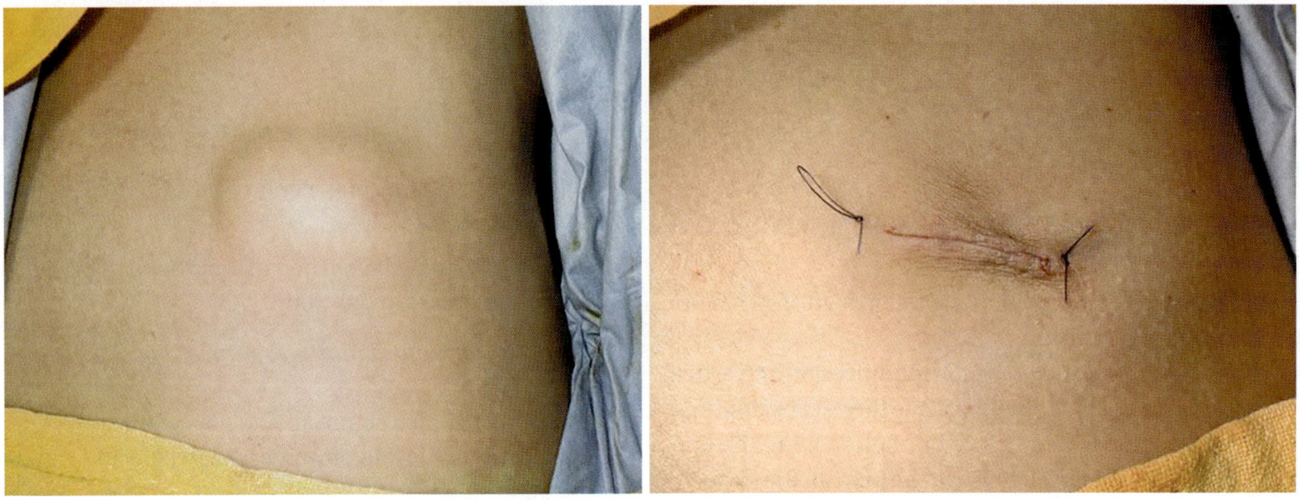

Fig. 3.16: Running subcuticular stitch with knots on surface after excision of lipoma over back.

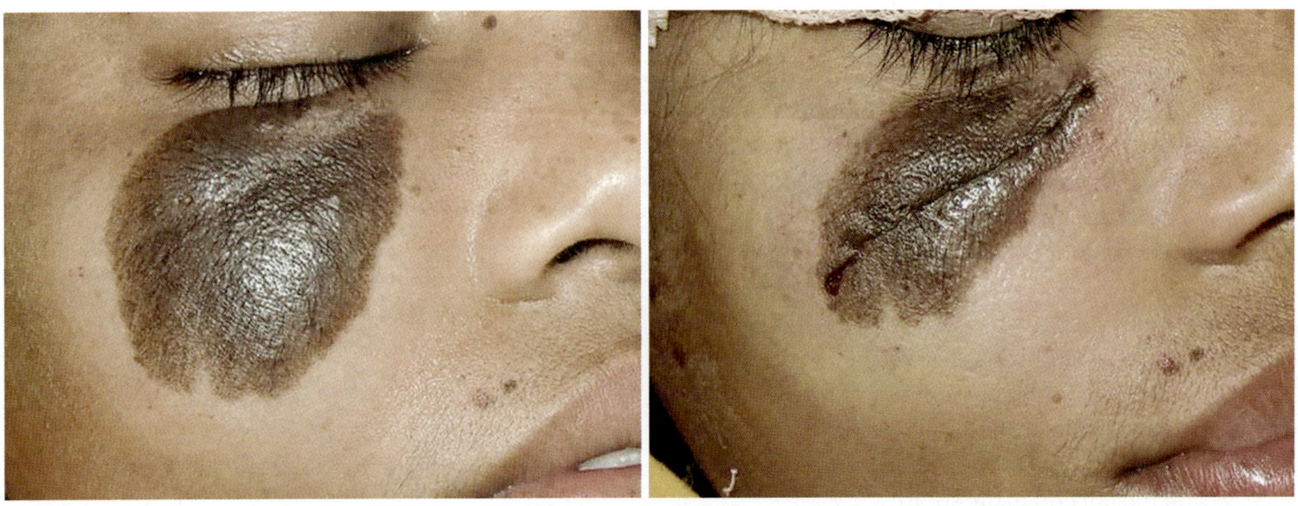

Fig. 3.17: Running subcuticular stitch with buried knots after partial elliptical excision of congenital melanocytic nevi over the face.

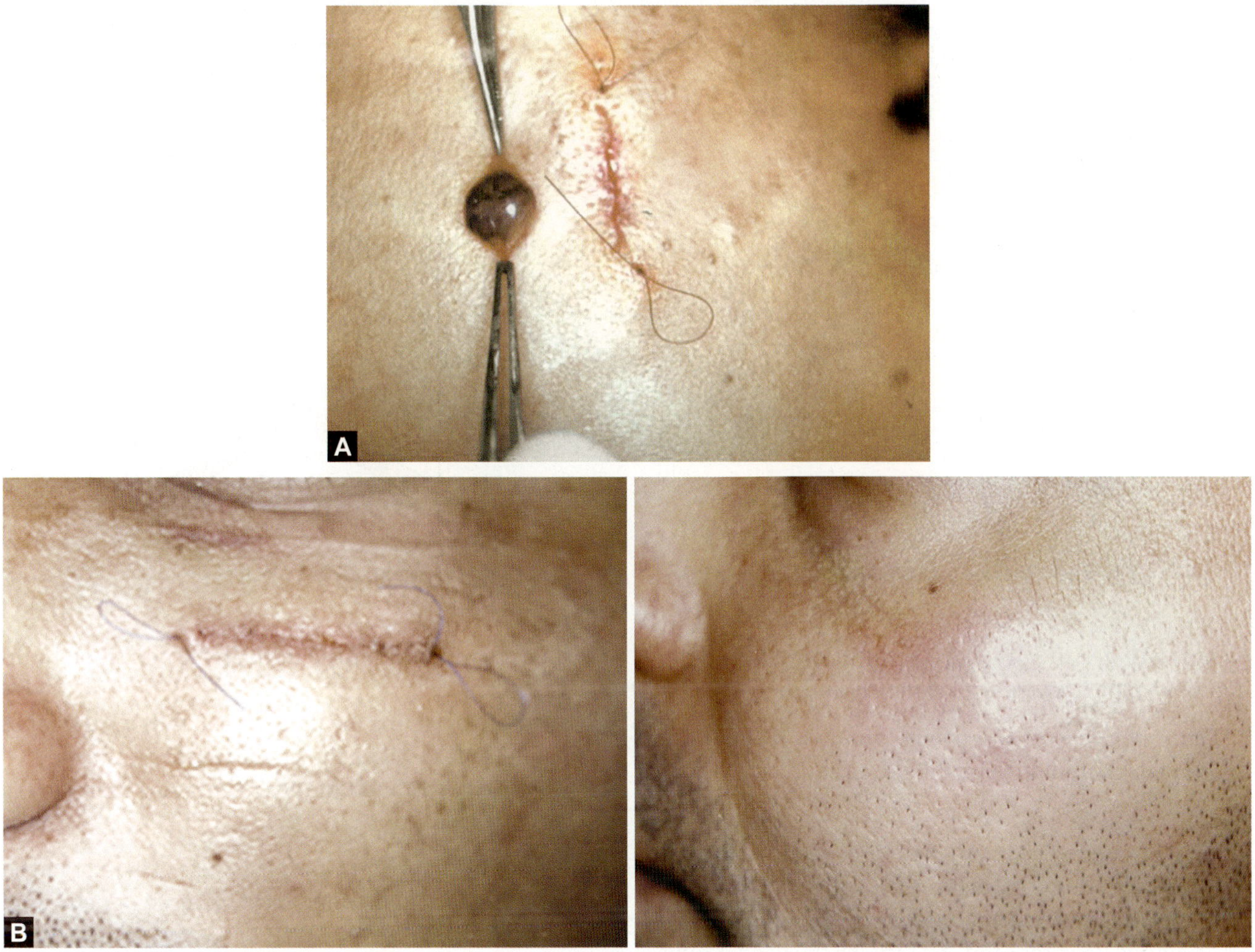

Figs. 3.18A and B: Running subcuticular suture gives very good esthetic scar.

- Horizontal bites should be taken at same level on both the sides.
- The bites should be parallel to the skin surface.
- Steristrips can be applied as a support for better approximation of skin edges.
- If approximation not good at some points along the length of wound then 1–2 simple interrupted stitches can be placed at those particular points.

Advantages
- Cosmetically very good results as there are no suture marks and cross-hatching (Figs. 3.18A and B).
- Quicker to perform.
- Avoids suture removal when absorbable suture is being used. So useful in children.

Disadvantages
- It is suitable only for wounds with no tension as it does not provide much strength.
- Also suitable for closing wounds with equal thickness of wound margins.
- Very long wound should not be closed using this technique.

4. ***Running subcutaneous suture (Fig. 3.19):*** It is placed in subcutaneous layer to close the dead space.

Steps
- Simple interrupted stitch is placed in subcutaneous layer at one end of wound without cutting the suture.
- Running suture is placed by taking horizontal bites alternately from the two wound margins.
- Then knot is tied at the end to the loop of last pass.

Tips: Take deep bites into the fat.

Advantages: The suture can be placed quickly, eliminates dead space and provides good wound eversion.

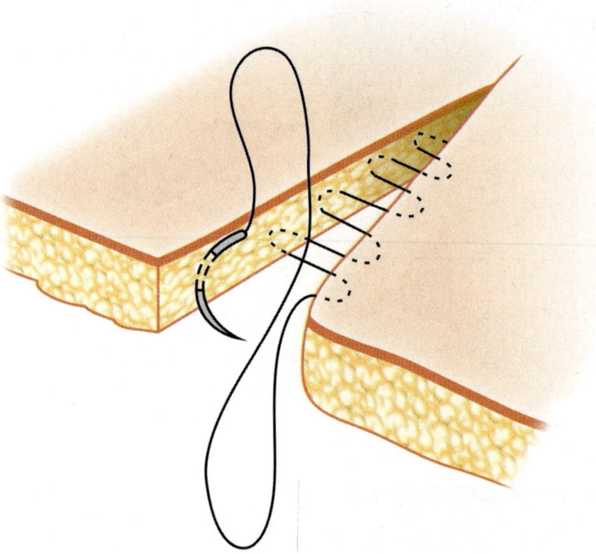

Fig. 3.19: Running subcutaneous suture.

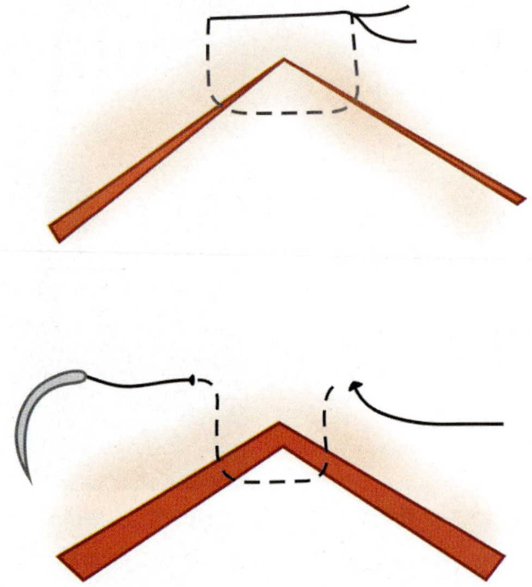

Fig. 3.20: Tip suture.

Disadvantages: If thread gets cut at one point, then approximation is affected all along the length of wound.

5. ***Running dermal subdermal sutures*:** It is good for wound under mild to moderate tension.

Steps

- First place a buried interrupted vertical stitch at one end of the wound, and cut only the free suture tail.
- Now insert the needle into the subcutaneous layer (pointing upwards) and exit through the deep dermis.
- Enter the needle (pointing downwards) into the dermis of opposite side and exit through the subcutaneous layer.
- Place running sutures by traversing the needle as described above and without tying knots.
- Place knot when the other end of wound is reached. Then cut.

Advantages: Suture can be placed quickly, eliminates dead space well.

Disadvantages: Low suture strength.

Other Special Suturing Techniques

1. ***Tip sutures (Fig. 3.20)*:** Half buried horizontal mattress sutures. These sutures are used while doing flap surgery or scar revision surgeries (W-plasty).

Steps

- Suture is first passed though the one wound edge to which the flap tip is going to be attached.
- Then the needle is passed through the dermis of the tip of the flap.
- Needle after exiting the tip is passed through the other wound edge to which the tip is going to be attached
- Needle exits through the epidermis and then knot is being tied.

Tips: Tissue bite taken into the tip or angle of flap should be at appropriate depth in order to avoid raised or depressed flap.

Advantages: Very useful for aligning the tips and angles of the flap and minimizes suture marks.

Disadvantages: Difficulty in placing this stitch, if wound tension high while doing the closure.

2. ***Purse string sutures*:** It is basically a buried horizontal mattress suture placed in deeper dermis, all around the circumference of the wound edge to close the dead space.

Advantages: It distributes the tension all around the wound edges, good hemostasis.

Disadvantages: Can strangulate the tissue, if tied too tightly.

SUTURE REMOVAL

Appropriate timing and technique of suture removal is important to avoid suture marks, infection and wound gaping. Sutures should not be removed too early as it might result in wound dehiscence and also delayed removal is not preferred as that might result in suture marks.

Table 3.5: Suture removal time.

Anatomic site	*Timing of suture removal (days)*
Scalp	7–10
Eyelids	4–6
Face	5–7
Ears	5
Trunk	7–12
Upper limbs	10–14
Lower limbs	10–14

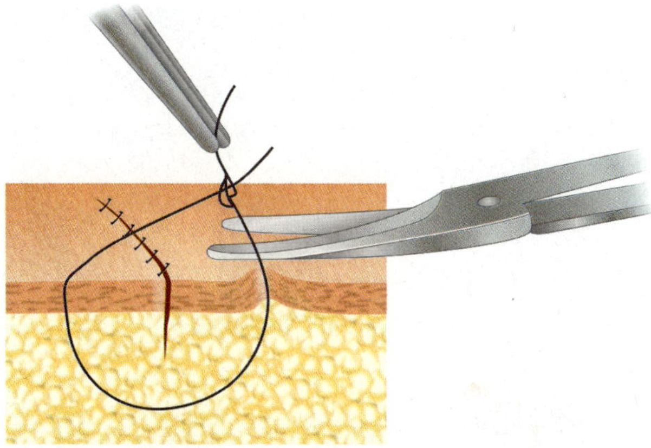

Fig. 3.21: Suture removal technique.

The time of suture removal depends upon the site and tension in wound. In general sutures are removed between 5 to 15 days after suture placement. Table 3.5 provides a general guide regarding the time of suture removal according to the site. Staged removal of sutures should be done when significant tension is present in wound or in high movement areas.

Consider early removal of sutures in case of: secondary infection, none to minimal tension in wound margins, cosmetically significant sites, and do delayed removal in case there is tension in the wound edges and healing is delayed.

Figure 3.21 depicts the technique of removal of interrupted sutures. First clean the suture area with antiseptic solution, then grasp the suture with forceps and pull towards the opposite side, so that the knot gets lifted. Cut the suture immediately beneath the knot using the suture cutting forceps. Then grasp the suture by its knot and pull it towards the wound or suture line as pulling in the opposite direction can lead to wound dehiscence. Look for the four limbs of suture radiating out from the knot that was removed and examine the wound for any residual suture bits. Steristrips can be applied after suture removal in order to provide support to the wound margins for additional time period.

For removal of running sutures, cut alternating loops and then pull the intervening loop. In case of running subcuticular sutures, the technique of suture removal will depend upon the type of sutures used. In case of absorbable sutures, we need to pull the knot, cut beneath the knot at both the ends and leave the suture buried inside. While in case of nonabsorbable sutures cut beneath the knot on one side and then pull the suture slowly from the opposite end.

COMPLICATIONS AND THEIR MANAGEMENT

In this last section of the chapter we are presenting a brief discussion on the immediate complications which arise after the suturing of wound edges:

- Wound dehiscence occurs when sutures are removed before complete epithelialization and healing up of the wound. This occurs when there is secondary infection or excessive tension in wound edges. Sometimes it follows inadvertent suture removal following knot slippage. If the wound margins are healthy, then resuturing can be done or otherwise tissue can be allowed to heal with secondary intention.
- Secondary infection can be easily prevented by taking good postoperative care of wound and prescribing prophylactic oral antibiotics in case of risk of infection.
- Hematoma (Fig. 3.22) formation occurs due to bleeder or excessive ooze in the wound. Early hematoma is due to bleeder and requires opening up of the wound and treating the bleeder. Delayed hematoma is usually the result of incomplete closure of cavity and collecting up of the ooze. In this case the decision to open up the wound and draining up of the hematoma will depend upon the size of hematoma and its progression. Small hematoma which is not progressing further can be just observed and allowed to undergo fibrosis, while a bigger hematoma which is likely to compromise the final result needs to be drained.
- Retained suture material can occur when we are not careful while removing the sutures. This increases the chances of infection, reactions and later spitting of the suture. A close watch for these side effects should be done.

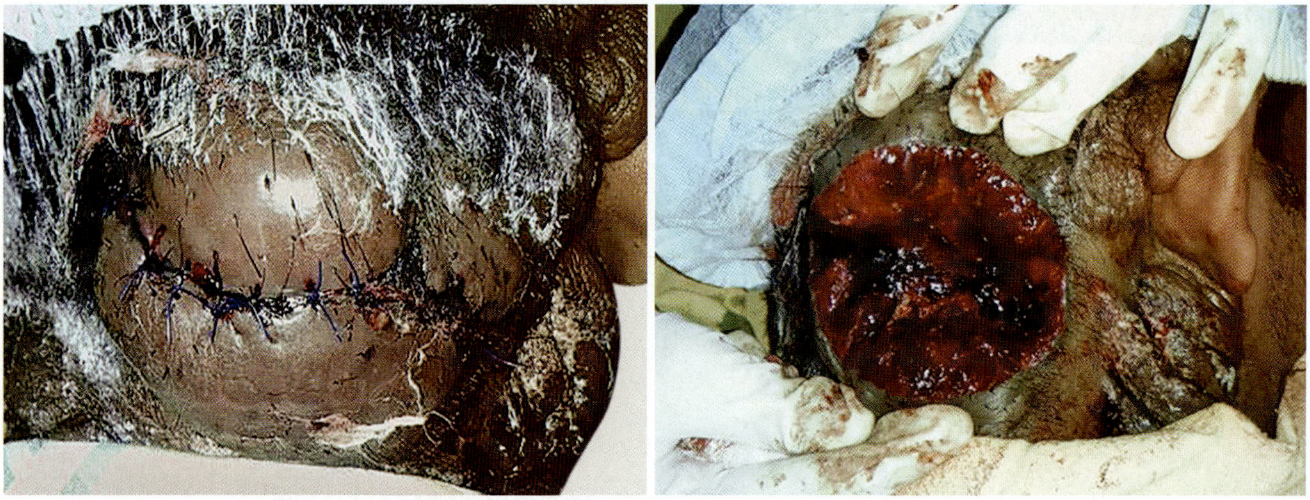

Fig. 3.22: Acute hematoma formed after partial plexiform neurofibroma excision has to be reopened, hemostasis achieved and sutured again in layers.

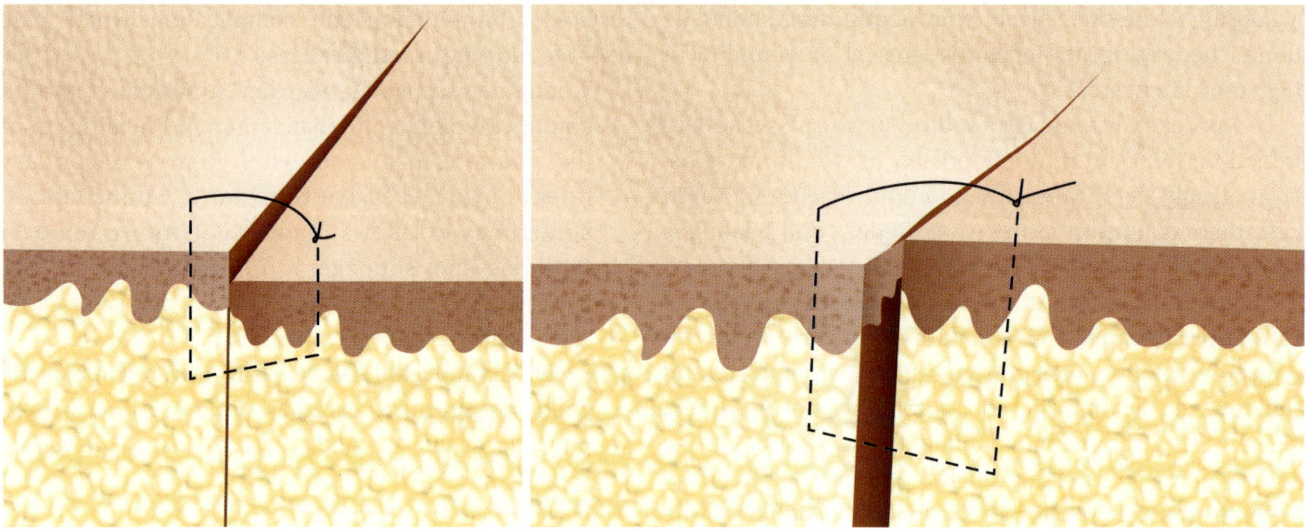

Fig. 3.23: Step off deformity.

- Spitting of suture occurs when the suture knot is placed too superficial in the wound. The suture end protrudes out through the scar line.
- Step off deformity (Fig. 3.23) is when the wound edges are not at same level. This results when buried sutures cross the two wound margins at unequal levels (*see* Figs. 3.18A and B). It can be corrected by removing and reapplying the buried sutures or by taking unequal tissue bites when placing the epidermal sutures.
- Suture tracks (Fig. 3.24) occur when the sutures are left for long periods, or larger caliber sutures are applied or the sutures are tied too tightly.

Tips for getting a good suture line are provided in Table 3.6.

OTHER MEANS OF WOUND CLOSURE

Include skin tapes, surgical adhesive and staples.

Skin Tapes

Skin tapes are wound closure tapes made up of microporous nonocclusive material with a thin film of acrylic polymer adhesive on one side. Steristrips and cover strips are examples of two commercially available wound closure tapes. They are available in different widths. Most commonly they are used to support sutured wounds. They can be used alone in wounds with very little tension

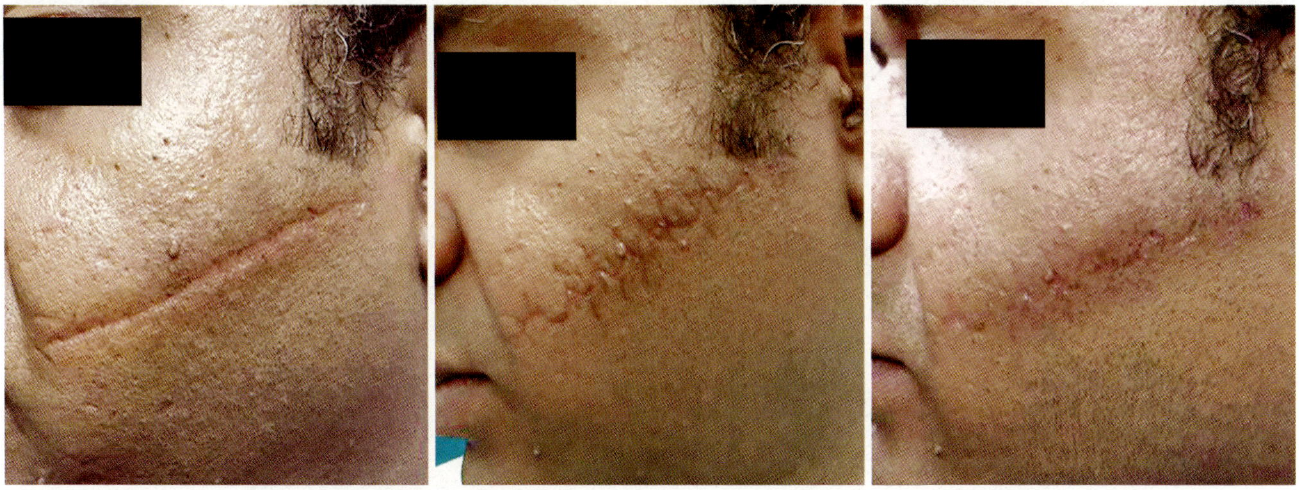

Fig. 3.24: Suture tracks due to tight suture placement after scar revision surgery were managed with fractional ablative CO_2 laser.

Table 3.6: Tips and tricks for good suture line.

S no	*Problem*	*Comment*
1.	Complete understanding of available different suture materials	Helps in making appropriate choice
2.	Imperfection detected when closing wound	Take corrective measures then itself as it is difficult to do scar revision at later date
3.	Knot slippage occurs due to high tension in wound or because of low coefficient of friction of suture material	Increase the initial number of throws of knot, take help of assistant to hold the wound edges together when placing knot
4.	Breakage of suture during tying	Low tensile strength or caliber of suture material, excessive tension in wound margins
5.	Breakage or bending of needle can be avoided	Use appropriate size needle and corresponding size needle holder and move the needle in arc motion when passing through the tissue
6.	Wound margins should be well-approximated and everted at the end of surgery	Vertical mattress epidermal suture, running subcuticular suture help in everting wound margins. Arc needle away from wound margins when placing epidermal suture
7.	Two wound margins should be at same level as otherwise it results in step off deformity; common when uneven wound margin thickness on two sides or wrong placement of buried sutures	If step off deformity severe, then replace and remove incorrect sutures. If mild, then take different thickness tissue bites on two sides (deeper bite on lower side) when placing epidermal sutures
8.	Suture tracks occur due to delayed removal of sutures, and or higher caliber of suture material and or when sutures are tied too tightly	Remove sutures at the earliest possible, use sutures of thinner caliber, and do not tie sutures too tightly
9.	When excising lipoma, give incision smaller then the lipoma as they slip out easily through a smaller incision line.	

(Fig. 3.25), to close superficial lacerations. They are not useful for hairy area and highly mobile areas.

Area should be dry and wound margins well-approximated before applying the wound tapes. Tapes are placed perpendicularly across the wound without overlapping one another. Patient is instructed to keep the area clean and dry. Tapes become loose and can be removed in around one week time.

Their main advantage is speed and ease of application, lower infection risk and no second visit for suture removal is required. For good adherence of tape, degrease with alcohol and apply tincture benzoin around the wound margins.

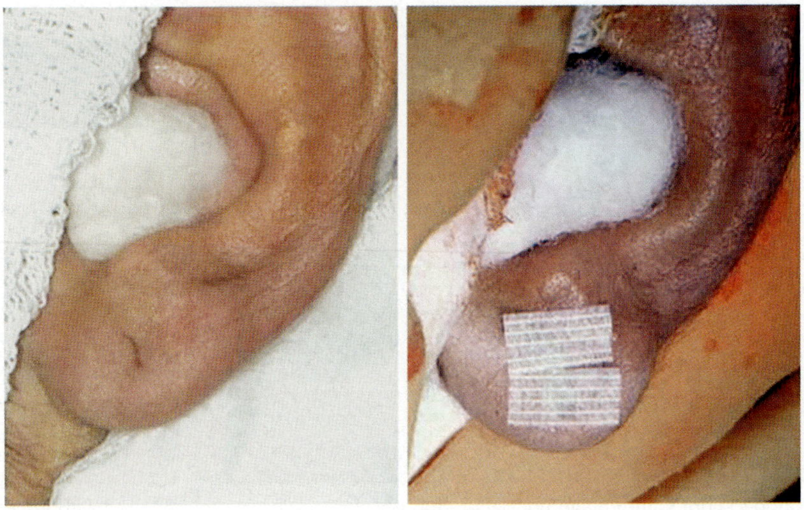

Fig. 3.25: Adhesive tapes alone were used for closure of wound margins when doing split ear lobe repair as there is no tension in wound edges.

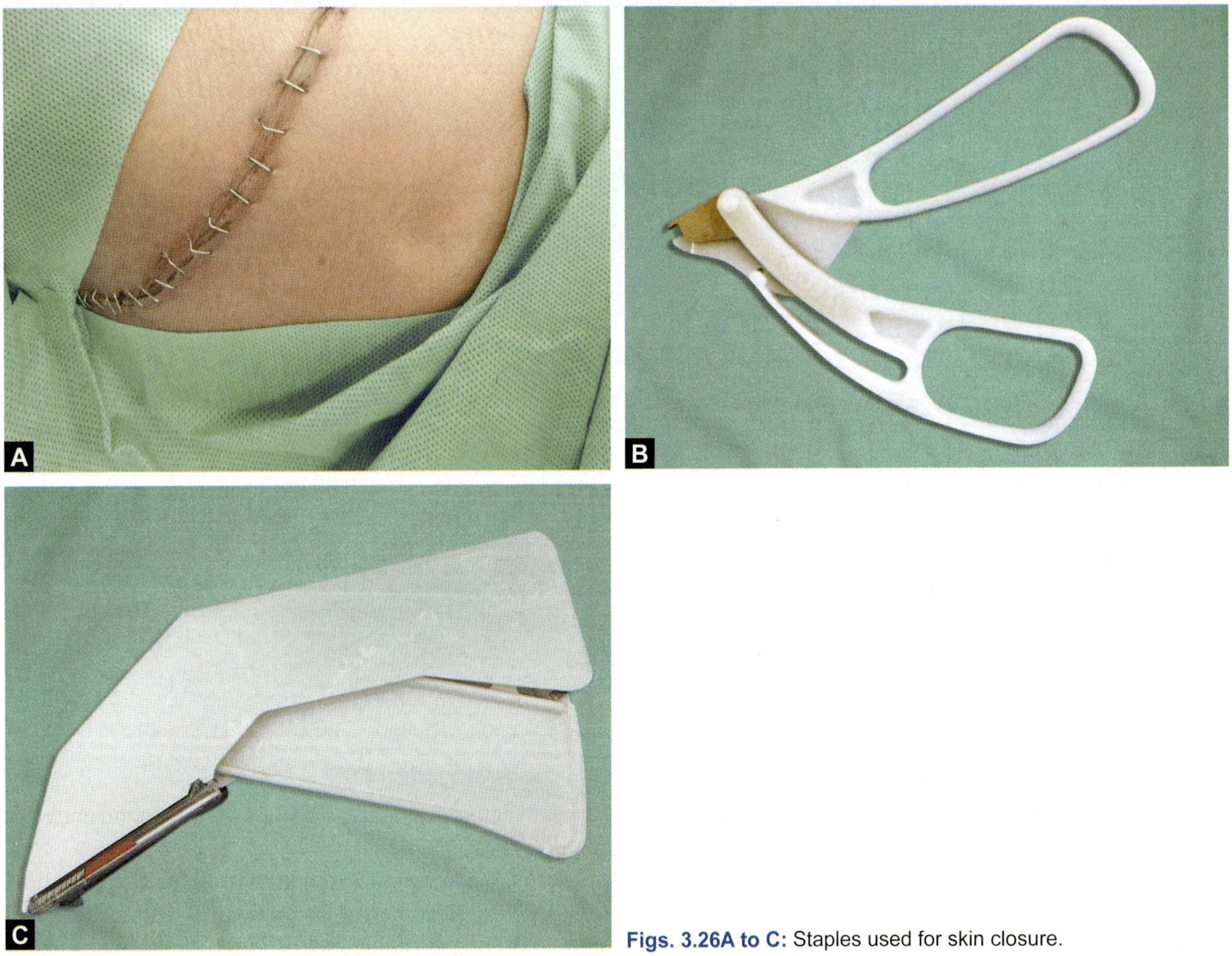

Figs. 3.26A to C: Staples used for skin closure.

Surgical Adhesives

They can be used when there is no tension in wound edges.

Material: Chemically tissue adhesives are all cyanoacrylate compounds. Two commercially available chemicals are octyl-2-cyanoacrylate (Dermabond and Ethicon) and N-butyl-2-cyanoacrylate (Indermil, Syneture). It is available as single use prefilled vials with different applicator tips. It is in liquid form and polymerizes when comes in contact with water or water containing tissue forming a flexible film that bonds to the underlying surface. Polymerization occurs through an exothermic reaction in which a small amount of heat is generated. Octyly-2-cyanoacrylate has more bonding strength, flexibility and less tissue toxicity compared to the N-butyl-2-cyanoacrylate.

How to use?

- Clean the closure site with alcohol or acetone.
- Tissue edges should be completely approximated before applying the tissue glue.
- Thin layer of tissue glue is applied all over the wound edges extending 5–10 mm beyond the wound edges.
- Two to three layers are applied for octyl-2-cyanoacrylate while single layer is enough for N-2-butyl cyanoacrylate.
- Patient is instructed to avoid any shearing forces over wound edges and also not to perform any wound care at home.

Adhesive comes out in 7–14 days with epidermal turn over. Patient should not apply any ointment or cream over the adhesive.

Advantages

- Very quick to use
- No need for suture removal
- Adhesive forms a film that has antibacterial activity and is impermeable to water as well
- No formal training required
- Especially useful in children and uncooperative patient
- No suture marks.

Disadvantages

- They do not evert the wound edges
- Do not use adhesive in areas subject to repeated trauma or highly mobile area otherwise
- Do not use near eyes and in infected wounds
- Contraindicated in those allergic to cyanoacrylate
- Expensive.

Staples

Staples are rarely used by dermatologist. Surgeons use them for closing wound over body (Figs. 3.26A to C) and limbs and under high tension. Staples are made from high quality stainless steel and have to be removed in 1–2 weeks time. Their main advantage is that they are quick to apply, there is decreased risk of infection as well as reactivity, and they provide good wound eversion. Their main disadvantage is their cost, cannot be used over highly mobile areas, and leave cross hatch skin marks.

CHAPTER 4

Dressings in Dermatosurgery

Salim T, Soumya Jagadeesan, Surajit Gorai

INTRODUCTION

Dressings are an important part of the therapeutic armamentarium of any dermatologist. In addition to the care of surgical sites, the dermatologists are also involved in the treatment of acute and chronic wounds. With the advances in the last few decades, we are faced with an increasing variety of dressing materials to choose from. The selection of the dressing is often crucial and depends on the practitioner's skilled assessment of the wound and the knowledge of how to provide an optimum wound healing environment through the use of the available appropriate dressings.

PRINCIPLES OF WOUND DRESSINGS

The principles of wound dressings have changed dramatically in the recent years with the changing social needs and the new insights into the pathophysiologic mechanisms of wound healing. Previously, it was not uncommon for a patient to be admitted for a prolonged period in the hospital for the management of a nonhealing ulcer, with frequent and often painful change of dressings. Currently, with the inadequate resources to provide in-patient treatment to all chronic wounds and with the reduced acceptance of prolonged morbidity, new parameters of dressings have emerged. A dressing is no longer a passive covering for wounds; it performs a rather active role in promoting wound healing and repair. The wound being recognized as a synthetic environment where numerous complex cellular processes are interlinked in the process of repair, the modern dressings are designed to nurture the cellular environment of the wound.[1]

Moist Healing Environment

One of the most important observations in the last several decades is that, the wound that is kept adequately moist heals faster. The evidence for this is more in acute wounds. However, even in chronic wounds, moisture-retentive dressings have been found to lead to a number of desirable outcomes such as pain control, painless autolytic debridement and stimulation of granulation tissue. Also, occlusion of the wound is contraindicated in the presence of infection. The principle behind moisture allowing greater re-epithelialization is not fully known. The proposed mechanisms include: (1) dry wound surface and scab inhibiting keratinocyte migration; (2) a favorable electrical gradient in moist wounds; (3) retention of cytokines and other growth factors in the wounds occluded with moisture-retentive dressings.[2-4]

The Role of Oxygen

For a long time, it was believed that the availability of oxygen was critical in wound healing. The subsequent studies have shown that hypoxia in fact triggers keratinocyte migration, promotes angiogenesis and stimulates the secretion of growth factors by the dermal fibroblasts.[5] The use of a semipermeable dressing can provide adequate oxygen tension required for the wound to heal properly.

The characteristics of an ideal dressing are listed in Table 4.1.[6]

Table 4.1: Characteristics of an ideal dressing.

- Absorbs extra exudates
- Allows gaseous exchange
- Barely need changing
- Comfortable and conformable
- Cost effective
- Damage protector (prevent further trauma)
- Long shelf life
- Noncytotoxic, nonsensitizing
- Provide sterile environment
- Provide thermal insulation

Table 4.2: Advantages and disadvantages of the conventional dressings.

Advantages	*Disadvantages*
Inexpensive, readily available	Require frequent replacement, hence time-consuming
Less chance of adherence to the wound	Can cause maceration of the wound and the surrounding skin, if left in situ for a long time
Can be molded into deeper wounds, will fill the dead space and absorb exudates	Lack specialized properties

TYPES OF DRESSINGS

Conventional Dressings

The conventional dressings that are still being used widely are made of materials like cotton, silk, linen, cellulose, etc. and have been tried and tested since historical times. Other materials like white petrolatum, antibacterial agents like povidone-iodine, chlorhexidine or balsam of Peru may be impregnated in the conventional dressings, depending on the indication. It is important to know about the conventional dressings before we move to modern dressings.

The conventional dressing is usually a 'layered' or composite dressing which is either a 'pressure' or 'nonpressure' dressing.

The 3 layers commonly seen are:

1. A contact interface layer
2. The absorbent layer
3. The outer 'wrap'.

The contact layer is the one that is directly in contact with the wound and is usually permeable to fluids and is nonadherent. A layer of antibiotic ointment or a contact layer of nonadhesive material, such as paraffin gauze or antibiotic impregnated tulle, serves this purpose. The middle absorbent layer is usually composed of materials like cotton pads or gauze and helps to absorb the exudates and to mold to the shape of the wound. The outer layer (like a tape or a roller bandage) helps to secure the dressing in place. Each layer should be in close contact with the adjacent layer with no gaps or air pockets.

In a pressure dressing, the key difference is that more bulk is added to the absorbent layer with the aim of creating hemostasis. The usual sites of pressure dressings include the scalp and digits. It is commonly applied immediately after a surgical procedure and changed in 24 hours. Care should be taken that the pressure created does not become excessive, where it can result in ischemia and tissue necrosis.[7]

The advantages and disadvantages of the conventional dressings are listed in Table 4.2.[8]

Modern Dressings

Occlusive dressings: These are of 6 categories—alginates, hydrogels, hydrocolloids, films, foams and hydrofibers. Their properties are listed in Table 4.3.[7] **Absorbent dressings** include *alginates* (Figs. 4.1A to F), *hydrofiber, foam dressings* and the more sophisticated super-absorbent dressings containing polyacrylate polymers. They handle fluid in different ways. Foams simply soak up fluid, alginates change in structure from a dry product to a gel and hydrofibers draw and lock the fluid away from the wound bed. **Moist dressings** work by either preventing the skin surrounding a wound from losing moisture or by actively donating moisture to the wound area. Examples are either *hydrocolloids* or *hydrogels*, both working by either adding or helping to maintain moisture by promoting autolytic debridement. **Surgical dressings** are used to cover the incision wounds postoperatively and generally, low adherent transparent polyurethane dressings like *films* (Figs. 4.2A and B) or island dressings are used for this purpose.

Antimicrobial Dressings

In the modern times, sophisticated dressings have emerged which provide adequate bacterial control over the wound site. They are impregnated with antimicrobial substances like silver and iodine and reduce the need for frequent topical application and dressing change.[7] Recent advances in antiseptic technology have resulted in the development of products that are less harmful to healthy tissue while being highly effective in destroying pathogens; some examples are honey, silver, iodine, cadexomer iodine and polyhexamethylene-biguanide (PHMB).

In older silver-containing dressings, the silver ions were present in the form of silver nitrate ($AgNO_3$) and silver sulfadiazine. However, newer formulations consist of high-density polyethylene mesh impregnated with

Table 4.3: Properties of occlusive dressings.[7]

Type	*Properties*	*Indications*	*Advantages*	*Disadvantages*	*Trade names available*	*Tips*
Alginates	1. Derived from brown seaweeds (phaeophyceae) 2. Forms a gel when in contact with the wound surface, which can be lifted off at dressing removal or rinsed away with sterile saline	Infected wounds and highly exudative wounds Full-thickness burns Particularly useful in postoperative packing	Highly absorbent with spontaneous sucking ability The ion-exchange properties of some alginates make them hemostatic agents Nonadherent Conforms to wound shape No reports of toxicity Useful in infected wounds	Requires secondary dressing to absorb the exudates and these need to be changed regularly Possess an unpleasant appearance and odor; the yellowish color of the gel may be mistaken for pus	KALTOSTAT	May be used in dry wounds also, but after moistening with saline and daily dressing change to prevent dessication
Hydrocolloids	Usually composed of a hydrocolloid matrix bonded onto a vapor-permeable film or foam backing; forms a gel that provides a moist environment when in contact with the wound surface	Moderately exudative wounds Chronic ulcers Burns Surgical and traumatic wounds	Adhere to wound edges and therefore, allows the patient to bathe and shower. Capillary action facilitates debris removal Thermal insulation	Opaque Risk of maceration of surrounding skin Possible wound trauma with dressing change Gel has unpleasant appearance and odor; like alginates, may be mistaken for pus Caution in infected wounds	DUODERM TEGASORB	Can be cut according to size in the sheet form. When it absorbs the exudates- causes autolytic debridement and improves angiogenesis waterproof
Hydrogels	Consist of cross-linked insoluble polymers and up to 96% water	Mildly exudative wounds Lasers, superficial burns Chemical peels burn Graft donor sites	Donates fluid to necrotic tissue Soothing, cushioning and cooling effect (reduces temperature by about 5°C) Reduction of postoperative pain Semitransparent	Absorption is slow Requires secondary dressing Maceration can occur Caution in infected wounds	HI-ZEL	The cooling effect of the dressing can be augmented by prior refrigeration Topical antibiotic may be applied to prevent bacterial colonization, especially gramnegative bacteriae
Films	Thin, elastic, transparent sheets of polyurethane or other synthetic semipermeable, self-adhesive, polymer dressing	Intravenous catheter sites Skin tears Split-thickness graft donor sites Laser resurfacing	Translucent, can inspect the wound without removing the dressing Permeable to water vapor Can be left on the wound for days Tends to reduce postoperative pain Creates bacterial barrier	Difficult to position properly May adhere to wound as it dries No mechanical protection for the wound Possible exudate accumulation; not suitable for exudative wounds Nonabsorbent	TEGADERM	Can be used as a 'splint' to hold a thin split-thickness graft stiff as it is being harvested from the donor site
Foams	Normally contain hydrophilic polyurethane or silicone foam	Highly exudative wounds Dermabrasion Burns Laser resurfacing	Absorbent Permeable to water vapor Conforms to wound shape Thermally insulates Increases comfort	Opaque Cannot be used on dry wounds Possible undesirable drying effect on inadequately exudative wounds Needs to be frequently changed, almost daily	MEPILEX, ALLEWYN	Silicone-based rubber foams, known as silastic foams can be used for packing cavities or deep ulcers, such as pilonidal sinuses
Hydrofiber	Resemble alginates, are not occlusive and are more absorbent than standard hydrocolloid dressings	Highly exudative wounds Diabetic leg ulcers Burns Surgical wounds cavities Graft donor sites	Highly absorbent, 3 times more than alginates Anti-inflammatory properties Antimicrobial properties Reduces odor formation Reduced wear and tear	Requires secondary dressings Can cause maceration	ACQUACEL	Need secondary dressing

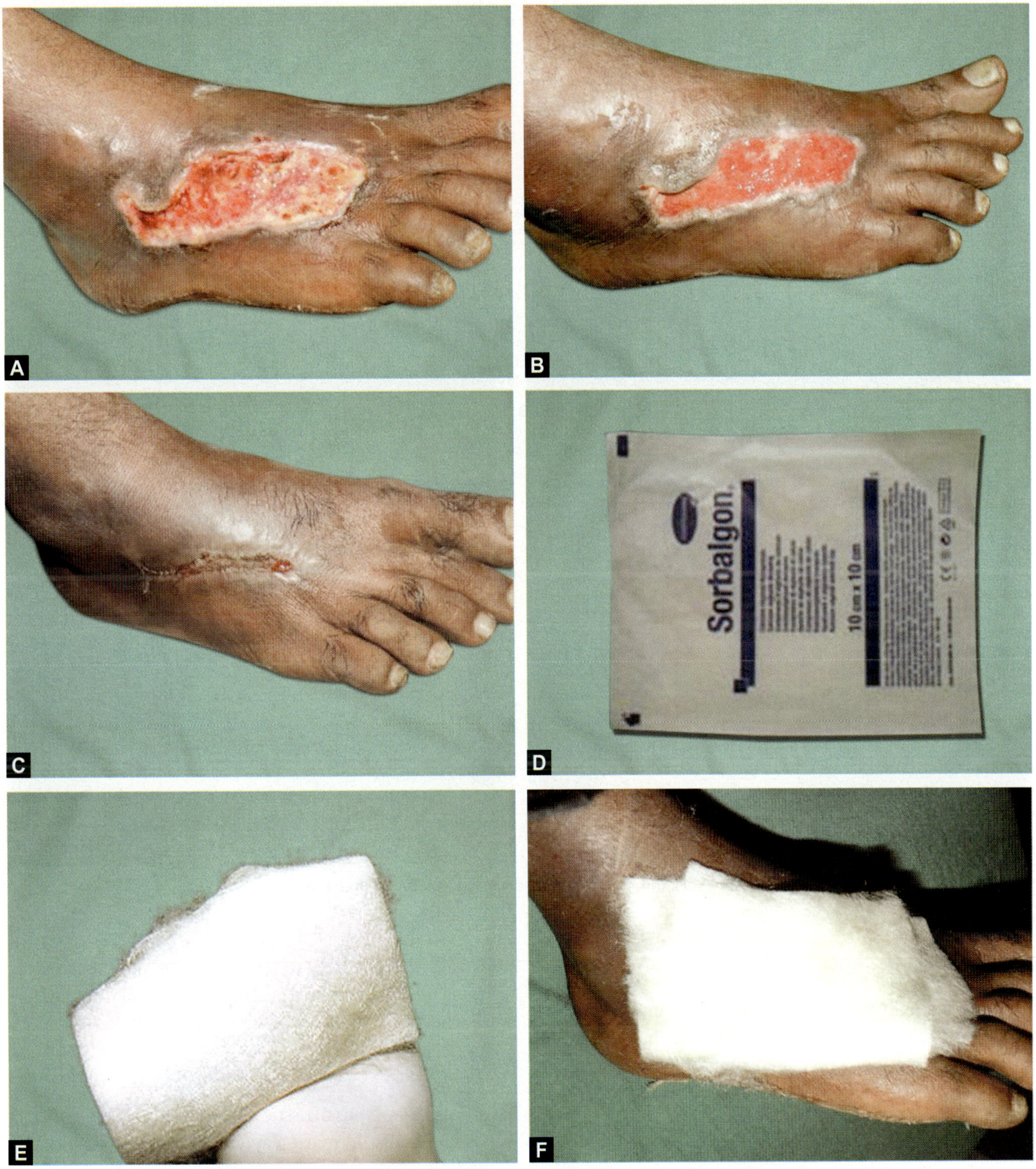

Figs. 4.1A to F: Alginate dressings used effectively in nonhealing leg ulcers.

nanocrystalline silver. Examples of nanocrystalline silver dressings include Acticoat™, Actisorb®, etc. Similarly povidone-iodine which has been used as an antiseptic, has been shown to inhibit wound healing, but the newer formulations release iodine at such low rates that it has not been found to be cytotoxic on the keratinocytes.[7,9-11]

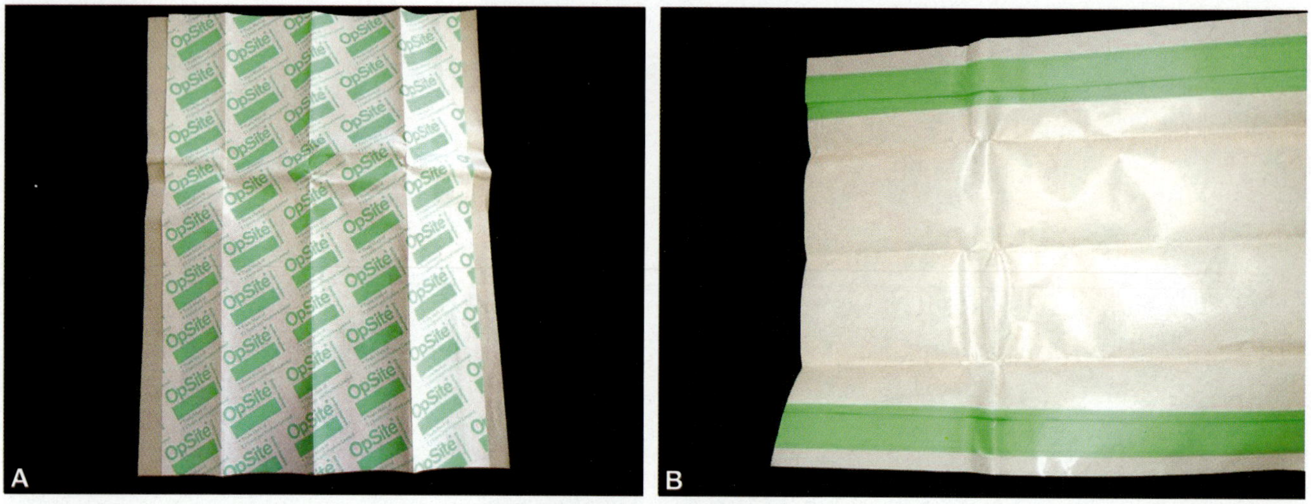

Figs. 4.2A and B: Film dressings.

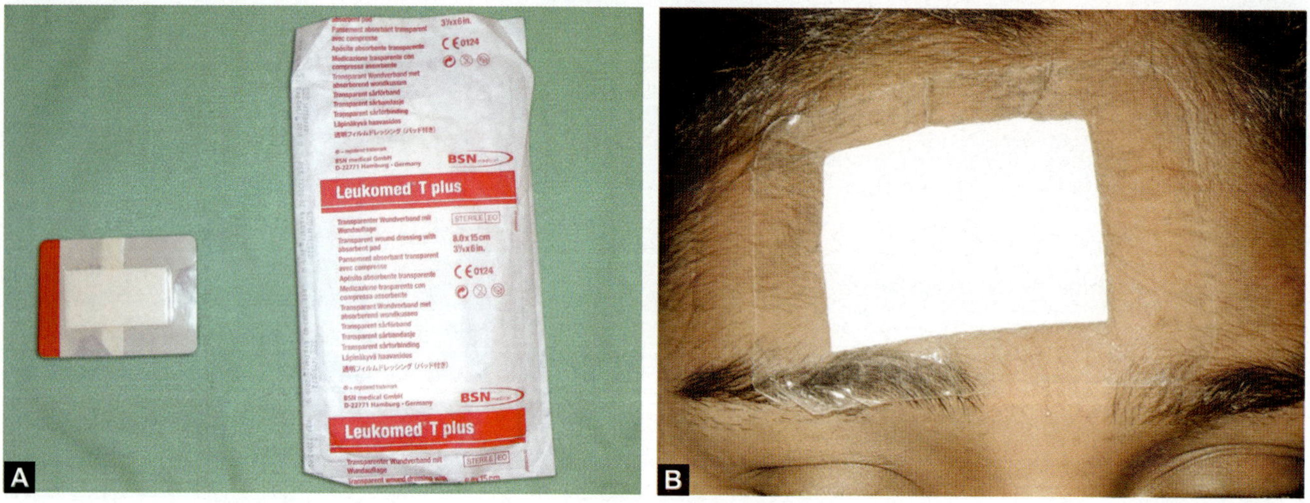

Figs. 4.3A and B: Composite dressing with a pad and a film.

Composite Dressings

With the changing times and increasing demands, newer designs of occlusive/semiocclusive dressings have emerged. Composite dressings which incorporate 2 or more types of occlusive dressings are now in vogue; they typically have three layers. These are:

- A contact layer that is semi or nonadherent (hydrogel/hydrocolloid/alginate/foam)
- An absorptive layer
- An outer layer with an adhesive border like a film. (e.g. Lukomed Tplus®, Figs. 4.3A and B).

They are more waterproof and eliminate the need for a secondary retention dressing. There are also composite dressings which combine the advantage of an occlusive/semiocclusive dressing and an antimicrobial dressing like silver- based dressings (e.g. ACQUACEL Ag).

Tissue Engineered Skin–Equivalents

There are three types of tissue engineered skin -equivalents: epidermal grafts, dermal replacements, and composite grafts (with both epidermal and dermal component).

Epidermal grafts: Autologous keratinocytes obtained from the skin biopsy specimen of the patients are co-cultured with irradiated murine fibroblasts that serve as a feeder layer. A sheet of keratinocytes that is two to eight cells thick is formed and is attached to petroleum gauze. The graft must be sutured into place and the gauze backing is removed after 1 week, when the keratinocytes have attached to the wound. The commercially available product in the United States of America is Epicel®. There are additional epidermal grafts available outside of the US, such as Laserskin® and Celaderm™.[12,13]

Dermal replacements: Major component is collagen; occasionally, extracellular matrix, fibroblasts and basement membrane material are added. Can be xenogenic or allogenic. The goal is to provide a temporary biologic dressing to stimulate the process of healing.[14-16]

Composite grafts: Apligraf is a bi-layered human skin equivalent that is derived from the neonatal foreskin. Consists of keratinocytes with epidermal and dermal skin equivalents. The graft can repair itself, if wounded.[7,14]

CHOOSING A SUITABLE DRESSING[17]

Dressings in Dermatosurgery (How are they Used and Applied?)

General Measures while Applying/ Changing Dressings

- Hand hygiene must be practised before and after the dressing change.
- The tape or adhesive portion of the previous dressing if present is removed by pulling it parallel to the skin surface and in the direction of hair growth. Alcohol wipes or nonirritating solvents help in removing the adhesive quickly and painlessly.
- The old dressing is removed and placed in the appropriate biomedical waste disposal bin. A dressing should never be handled by an ungloved hand for the risk of transmitting pathogenic organisms.
- Clean the wound area with saline or antimicrobial solution; look for any signs of infection. Should keep in mind that with occlusive dressings like hydrocolloids or alginates, a brownish material may be seen on the wound surface, which is not pus.
- Apply the dressing; in case of modern dressings, keep in such a way that the sticky side of the dressing which adheres to the paper sticks to the wound.
- If a tape is used to secure the dressing, the correct way to use it is by placing the tape at the center of the dressing and pressing the tape down on both sides, applying tension evenly away from midline.
- An elastic adhesive bandage may be used to hold the dressings in place on mobile areas, or where pressure is required.

Dressings for Surgical Incision Wounds

Following a wound created by a surgical procedure, like an excision biopsy, sutures are usually placed to achieve hemostasis, better cosmesis, reduce risk of infection and better healing. In such a case, the wound heals by first intention. However, on some occasions, it may not be advantageous to close the wound in this way owing to the presence of a persistent source of infection, or if the wound is too small or some other reason. In these situations, the wound will be being encouraged to heal from the base upwards by the use of appropriate dressings that promote healing by secondary intention.

- An antibiotic ointment may be applied over the suture site, which will prevent infection and prevent the contact layer of the dressing from sticking to the sutures or the wound.
- It is generally considered best practice to cover all surgical incisions postprocedure and, when practical, this should involve low adherence, transparent polyurethane dressings, which protect the wound and give the opportunity to check the surgical incision site for any signs of wound infection without having to disturb the dressing itself. These dressings can be left in place for between 3 to 5 days, during which time the epithelialization process may be completed. If the procedure is a minor one such as a skin biopsy, the dressing may be dispensed with after a day or two; thereafter, the layer of antibiotic may be sufficient.
- If oozing of fluid (blood or exudate) from the incision site is anticipated in the immediate postoperative phase, dressings should incorporate an integral central pad of absorbent material (island dressings). These island dressings combine the advantages of transparent low-adherent polyurethane film dressings while also having the ability to absorb small amounts of exudate, aiding the normal debridement process in the wound and help to prevent any adverse effect on healing.
- After suture removal, tapes may be used as external splints; e.g. Steri-strips-(Figs. 4.4A to D) as they support the tissue, enable collagen remodelling and minimize the risk of hypertrophic scar formation.
- Conventional dressings (pressure or nonpressure dressings) may also be considered in surgical wounds that heal by first intention.

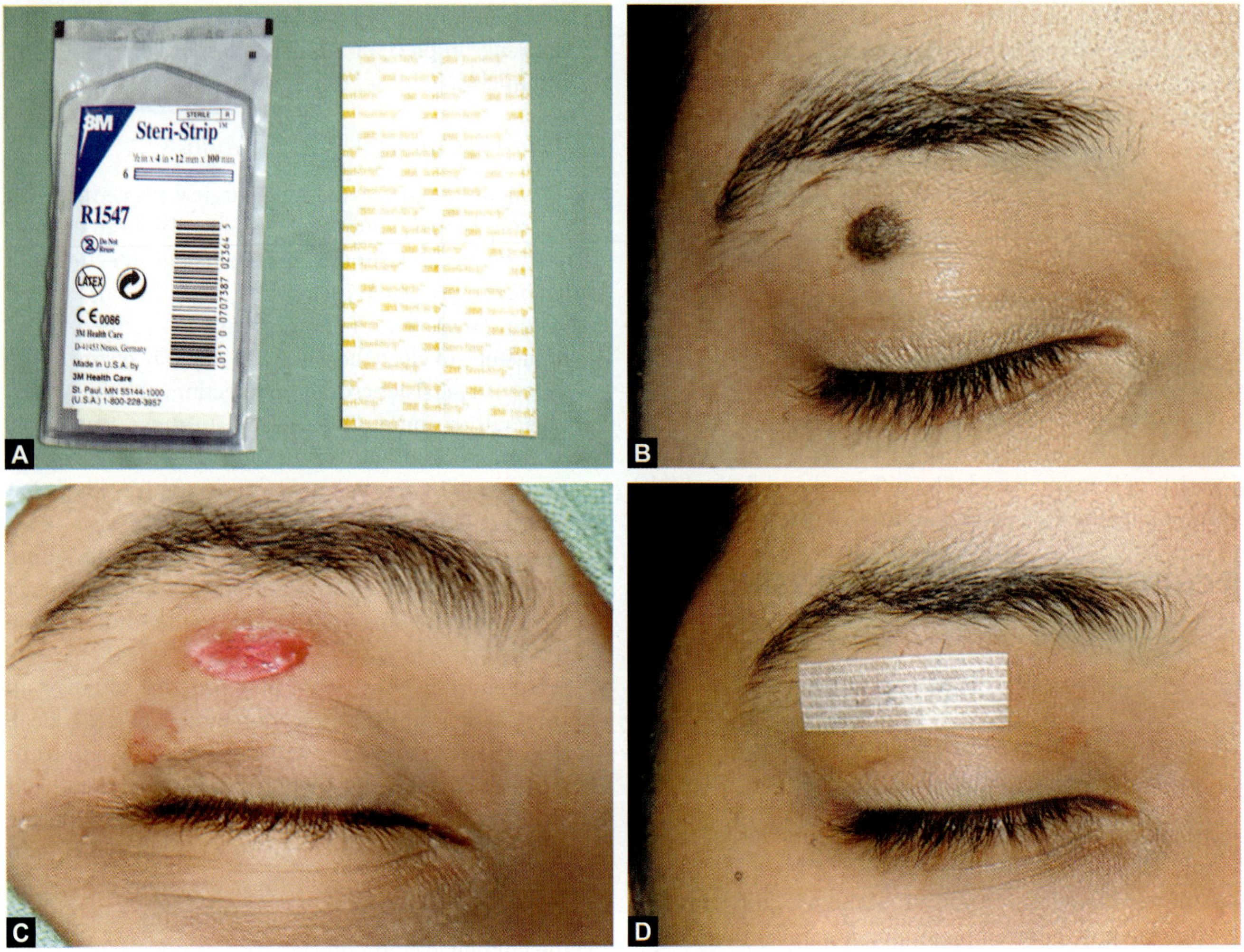

Figs. 4.4A to D: Steristrips, illustrated as dressing following excision of a mole.

Leg Ulcers

In more than 80% cases of leg ulcers, the etiology is venous insufficiency. In venous ulcers, moisture retention can be best achieved by occlusive dressings; but studies have not demonstrated the superiority of one category over the other. Therefore, the choice of the occlusive dressing depends on the practitioner's and the patient's preference. However, simple nonadherent dressings are generally recommended in the management of venous leg ulcers. Honey dressings, silver dressings or the routine use of topical antiseptics or antimicrobials are not recommended in the routine treatment of patients with venous leg ulcers.[18-20]

Compression is thought to be of utmost importance in the management of venous ulcers. Patients should be offered the strongest compression that maintains patient concordance. An ankle pressure of 30 to 40 mm Hg should be achieved to reduce edema, prevent capillary leakage and thereby improve healing rates of ulcers. At initiation of compression, patients should be assessed for skin complications within 24 to 48 hours. In patients with an ABPI < 0.8, and in patients with diabetes, compression should only be used under specialist advice and with close monitoring.[18-20]

Compression can be achieved by dressings, usually layered pressure dressings. With graduated compression stockings, the patient can independently wear it, provided they are able and healthy. Besides compression stockings, single layer and multilayered compression bandages are also available. Combining compression with occlusive dressings has been found to augment the healing rates of venous ulcers.

The Unna boot is a type of compression bandage which has been used for many years in the treatment of stasis ulcers. It was originally a cotton bandage

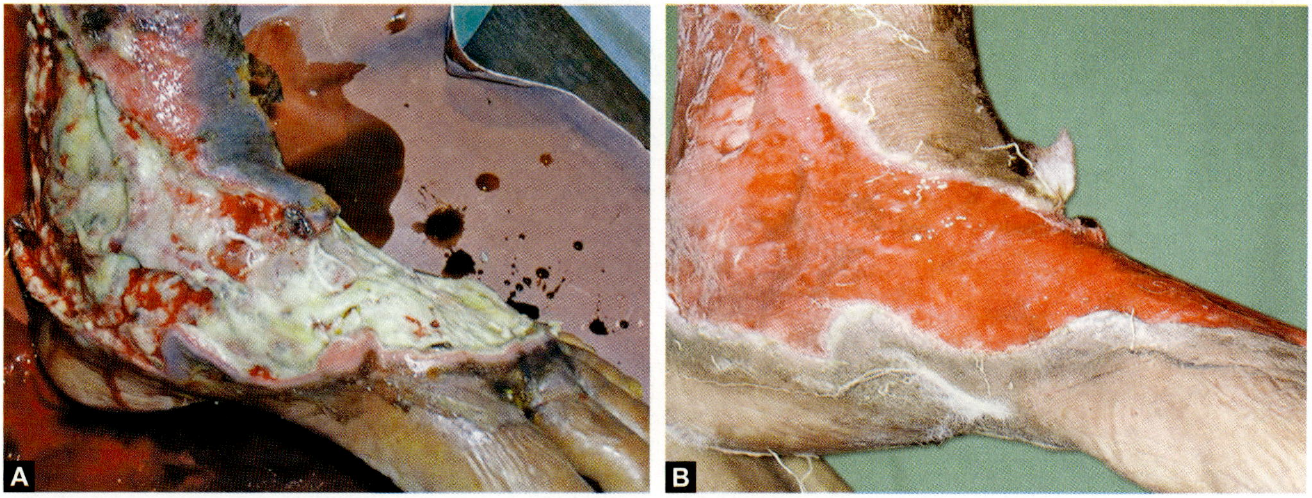

Figs. 4.5A and B: Enzymatic debridement using Papain, collagenase dressings. The photograph is before and after 10 days of papain dressing.

impregnated with zinc oxide, gelatin and glycerin paste. Applied in a semirigid state, Unna boot confers the dual advantage of compression along with the moisture retentive properties of an occlusive dressing. It should be applied by qualified medical personnel and changed at least weekly. Nowadays, flexible compression bandages are more preferred (when compared to the rigid nature of Unna's boot). They come in different varieties—elastic/inelastic, single/multilayered, long- or short-stretch compression, etc. The major concern is in identifying how much tension is needed while prescribing elastic compression bandages.[7]

The authors have used papain dressings and amniotic membrane dressings to good effect in leg ulcers (Figs. 4.5 and 4.6).

Pressure Sores

Overall, the quality of clinical evidence for wound dressings was found to be low to very low in most of the meta-analyses. No recommendations could be made about using specific types of dressings, except that gauze dressings should not be used for pressure ulcers. The NICE guideline development group emphasized that the effectiveness of each dressing would depend on the type of pressure ulcer and, therefore, chose to recommend a dressing that promotes the optimum healing environment, rather than a specific type of dressing. NICE advises that clinicians should discuss the type of dressing with the person with the pressure ulcer and, if appropriate, their family or caretakers, taking into account the person's pain and tolerance, the position of the ulcer, the amount of exudate and the frequency of dressing change. A dressing that promotes a warm, moist wound healing environment should be considered for grade 2, 3 and 4 pressure ulcers.[18]

A Cochrane data analysis found that hydrocolloid, film and foam dressings were found to prevent pressure ulcers compared with standard care. However, the authors also noted that dressings do not replace best practices, such as turning and repositioning, skin care, good nutrition and continence management.[21]

Vitiligo Surgery

Surgeries have become an indispensible tool in the current management of vitiligo. Procedures ranging from tissue grafts to cellular techniques have revolutionized the therapeutic options. Cosmetic outcome can be greatly improved if the right dressing can be applied in the right method during the surgery.

It is important to secure the grafts on the recipient area while carrying out miniature punch grafting. Dressings do have a significant role in proper immobilization and in securing the grafts. Various surgical adhesives like octyl cyanoacrylate, flexible collodion, etc., have been used in miniature punch grafting.

Cyanoacrylate tissue glue (Fig. 4.7) is helpful in providing quick and effective immobilization of donor grafts and securing grafts over areas that are difficult to treat, like the genitalia, groin, eyelids, palms, and fingertips.[22] The tiny droplets of octyl cyanoacrylate are expressed from

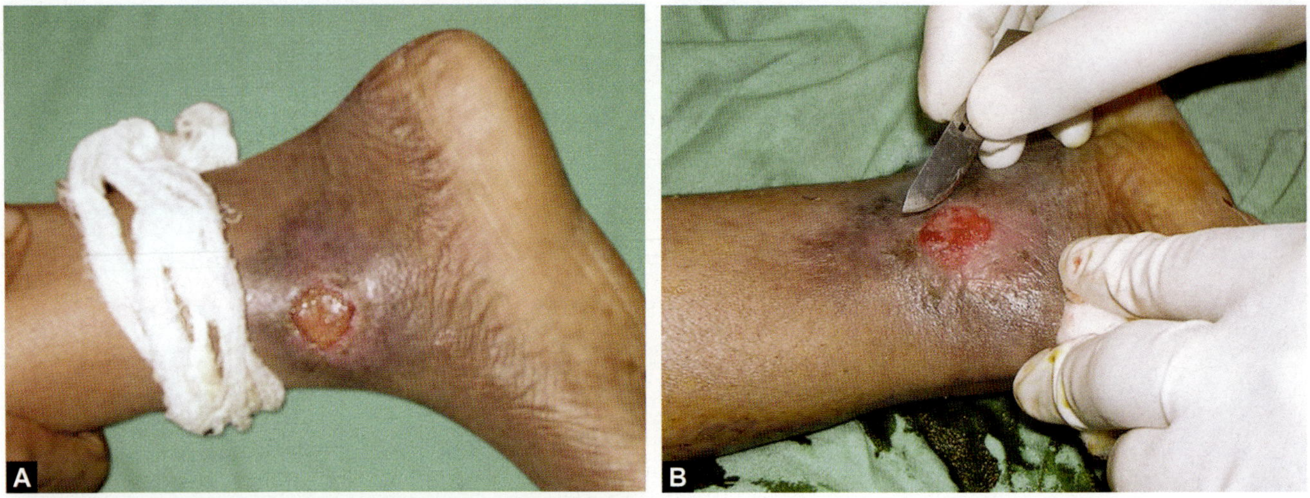

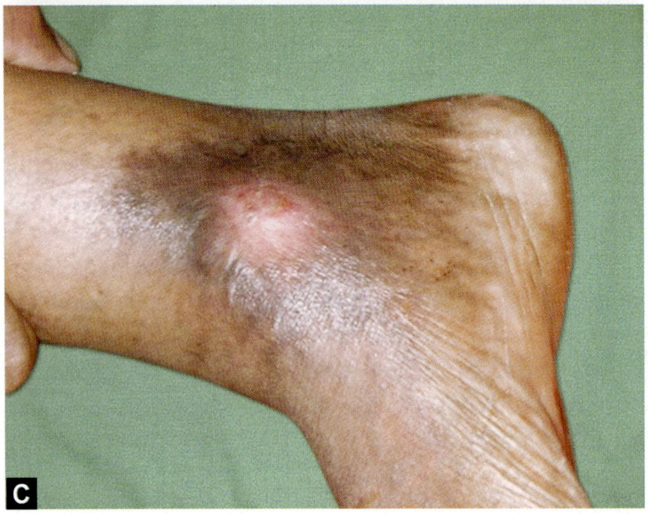

Figs. 4.6A to C: Amniotic membrane in ulcer treatment as dressings.

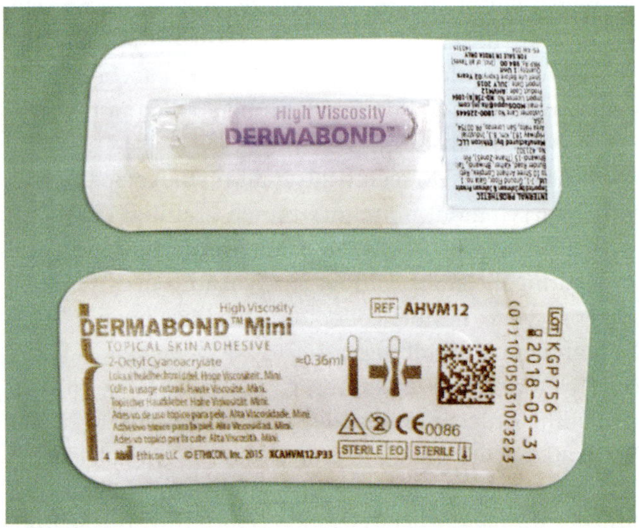

Fig. 4.7: Cyanoacrylate tissue glue.

the needle tip; broken further into even smaller droplets by taking it on another sterile needle tip, and applied only at four points, at 12, 3, 6 and 9 o'clock positions between the edges of the donor grafts and the recipient wells. The adhesion between the graft and the recipient wells start within 10 seconds and is complete within 1 minute of application. No dressing or immobilization is required in any patients. Apart from the adhesive property, octyl cyanoacrylate also exhibits antimicrobial properties against staphylococci, *Pseudomonas*, and *E. coli*.[23]

Alternatively, paraffin embedded nonadherent sterile gauze (Jelonet®) can be applied as a primary dressing followed by surgical pad and elastic adhesive dressings to immobilize the area (Fig. 4.8).

In split thickness grafting and suction blister grafting, octyl cyanoacrylate gel can be used to secure the graft in position in place of sutures (Figs. 4.9A and B). Adhesive film dressings like Opsite® can be used as secondary dressings over the recipient site. Opsite is a transparent, adhesive film. The film is moisture vapor permeable, conformable and extensible which is widely used to provide a moist wound environment for superficial wounds. Opsite provides moisture vapor permeability, allowing the excess exudate to evaporate, helping to prevent skin maceration. The grafts can also be placed in position using sutures or without sutures and further dressed with absorbent pads and hydrofilm dressings. Lukomed T plus® is a film dressing with absorbent pad which can be directly applied over a grafted site.

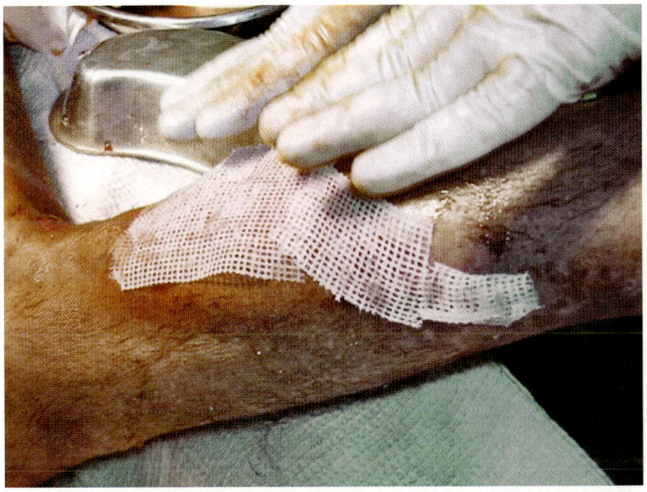

Fig. 4.8: Paraffin embedded nonadherent sterile gauze (Jelonet®) can be applied as a primary dressing in miniature punch grafting.

In cellular grafting techniques, primary dressing is done using collagen dressings. After applying the basal layer cell suspension, collagen sheets are used as primary covers to create a biological environment (Fig. 4.10). Alternatively, amniotic membrane can also be used (Figs. 4.11A and B). Mepitel dressing is also used in places where collagen sheets are not available (Figs. 4.12A and B). This is then covered with a sterile pad and finally with Tegaderm (3M) dressing.

Nail Surgeries

In nail surgery, the postoperative dressings must have these properties: nonadherent, absorbent, perfectly fixed and with adequate pressure to prevent bleeding.

Application of an antiseptic ointment covered with a paraffin embedded nonadherent sterile gauze (Jelonet®, Bactigrass®, Sofratulle®) as a first layer will protect the wound from drying and will allow easy and painless removal. Mepitel® is another nonabsorbent, porous, semitransparent flexible poyamide net, silicon- coated dressing useful as a primary dressing in nail surgeries and cellular grafting surgeries in vitiligo.

Second layer of dressing is made of 3 or 4 layers of absorbent mesh gauze that will absorb exudates and bleed and provide protection against trauma. Secure final layer of dressing can be made of elastic adherent plasters such as elastoplast, which will keep the surgical area secure and exert sufficient pressure so as postoperative bleeding can be prevented. Care should be taken to leave the tip of the toes and fingers uncovered so as to inspect for cyanosis if the dressing is too tight.

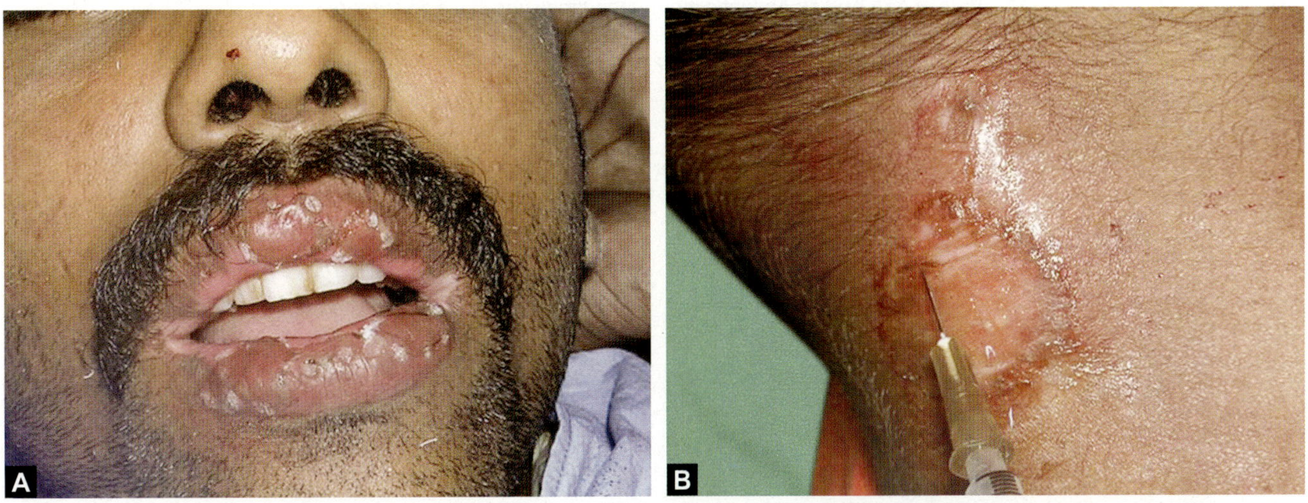

Figs. 4.9A and B: Tissue glue for securing grafts in SBEG, ultrathin epidermal grafting—applied over the periphery of grafts to secure them in place.

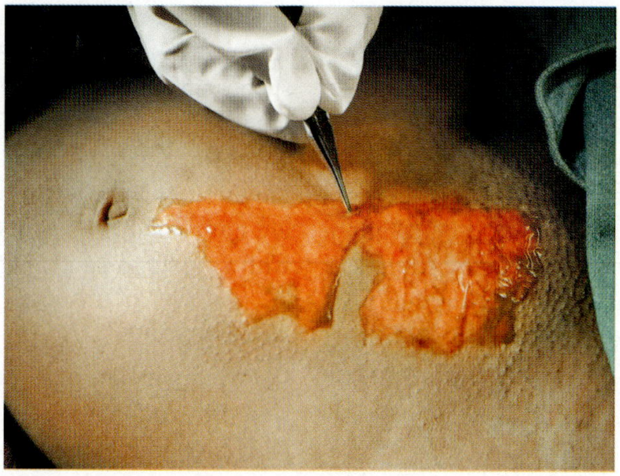

Fig. 4.10: Collagen dressings used as primary dressings in cellular grafts in vitiligo surgery.

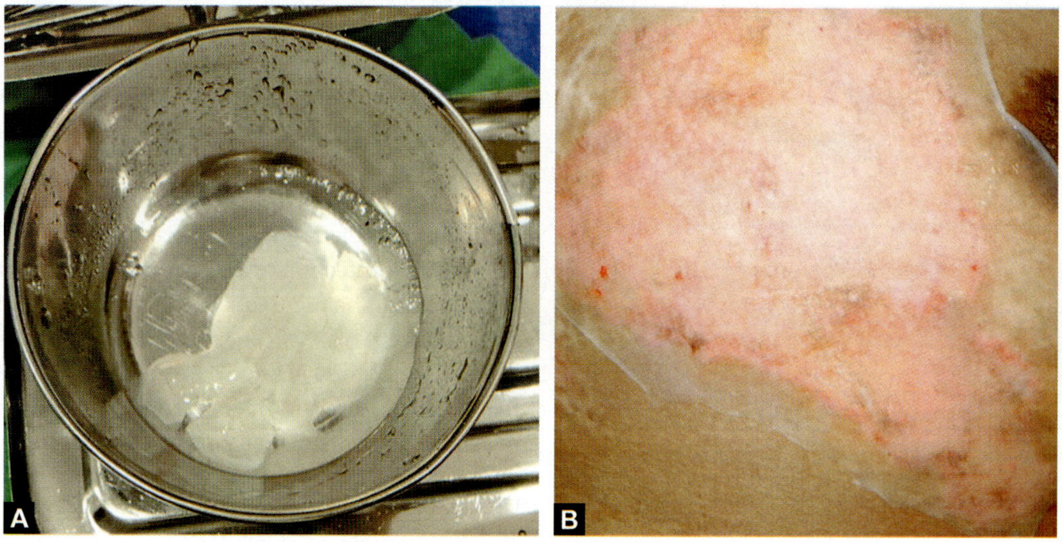

Figs. 4.11A and B: Amniotic membrane dressings in vitligo surgery.

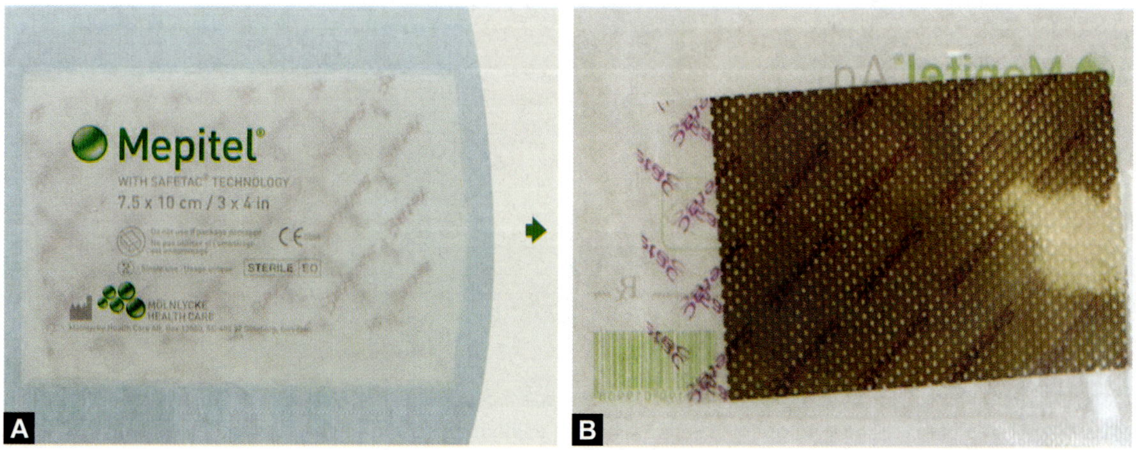

Figs. 4.12A and B: Mepitel dressings.

Recently, authors have found a new self-adhesive bandage without any chemical adhesive namely Coban® to be very effective in nail surgeries. The advantage being nonallergic and can be easily reapplied if the patient feels the dressing too tight without disturbing the inner layers of the dressing. It is a stretchable and self-adhesive dressing suitable for pressure dressings and also provides effective hemostasis (Figs. 4.13A to D).

Dressing Removal and Replacement in Nail Surgery

If the wound is clean and there is no bleeding on the first inspection, pressure dressings are not required further. Bertrand Richert suggested a simple dressing which provides protection to the toes and the surgical wound.[24] We found this method useful in our practice. This will also cover the tip of the toe and protect. A large porous plaster, half split into four on its length will cover easily a great toe or a finger (Figs. 4.14A to E).

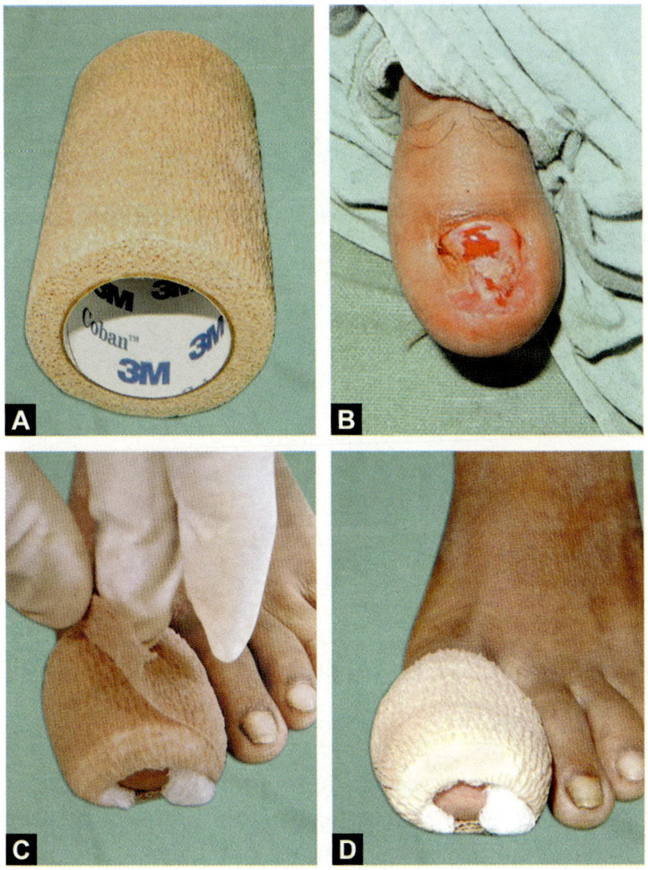

Figs. 4.13 A to D: Coban® dressings in nail surgeries.

Hair Transplant

A pressure dressing may be given on the donor area after a hair transplant surgery. The recipient area is generally left uncovered with the newer techniques, but sometimes a nonadherent dressing may be given depending on the preference of the surgeon. The patient is called back the next day for inspection of the surgical site.

Liposuction

Absorbent dressings are generally given on the incision sites to facilitate drainage. Patients are also required to wear compression garments in the postoperative period.

Laser Surgery

The primary goal after laser resurfacing is total and uniform re-epithelialization. In the absence of infection and with the use of occlusive dressings, this is possible within 5 to 7 days. Delay in re-epithelialization has been attributed to crust formation, to which the wound is most prone during the first 2 to 3 postoperative days. The dressings may be open or closed. By open, we mean that the wound is left alone after applying a cream or ointment without covering it. The application is repeated in frequent intervals. Whereas by closed dressings, any of the 4 categories of occlusive dressings (except alginates and hydrofibers) may be used. Studies have shown that postlaser procedure, closed/occlusive dressings fared better in terms of re-epithelialization and patient comfort, when compared to open dressings. Foam dressings and hydrogel/hydrocolloid dressings are widely used postprocedure. In significant postlaser resurfacing wounds, the protocol recommended is— the dressing is placed immediately after the procedure and then the patient is called for review on postoperative day 1 and 2, when the wound is cleansed and the dressing is changed. The replacement dressing remains in place till day 5, when the dressing is changed to an open dressing.[7,25] But in most cases especially for laser done over face, e.g. acne scars, closed dressing is cosmetically less acceptable.

COMPLICATIONS OF WOUND DRESSINGS

- Maceration of the skin surrounding a wound may occur, if a dressing with a low absorptive capacity is used on a heavily exuding wound.

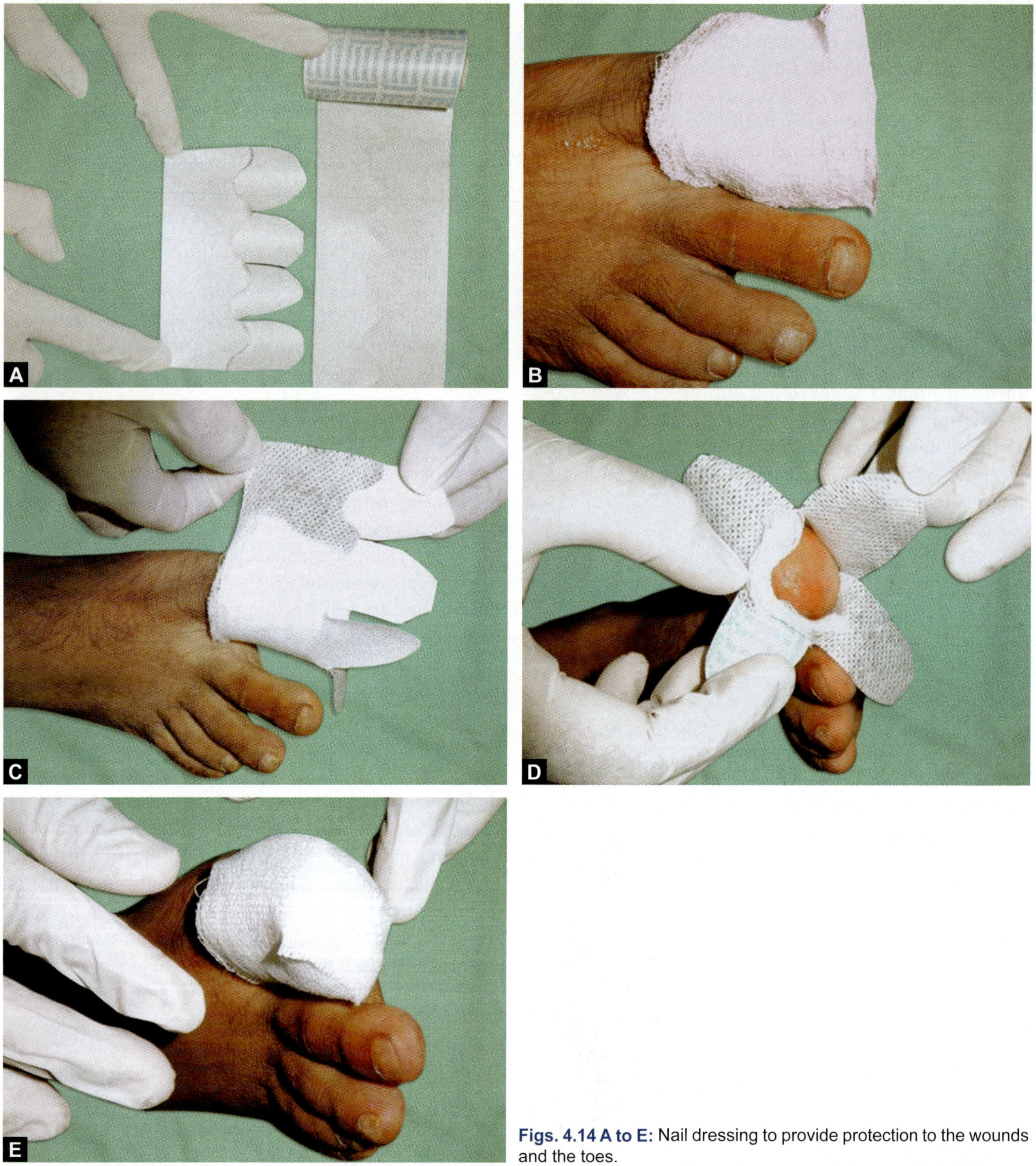

Figs. 4.14 A to E: Nail dressing to provide protection to the wounds and the toes.

- If the dressing is highly absorptive, then more frequent dressing changes may be needed, in addition to investigation and management of the cause of the exudate (such as infection).
- Conversely, use of a highly absorptive dressing on a dry wound may lead to disruption of healthy tissue on the wound surface and cause pain when removed.

- Iodine containing dressings should not be used in young children, pregnant or lactating women, or patients with known or suspected iodine sensitivity. As iodine is absorbed, caution must be taken when using these dressings in large wounds, wound with cavities, patients with a history of thyroid disease.
- Gauze dressings should not be used on pressure sores.

TIPS AND TRICKS

- To avoid the formation of bubbles/air pockets while applying dressings like films; the caregiver may use the proximal end of the thumb forceps and move it from one side to the other end of the dressing (like applying butter with a knife).
- The skin surrounding a highly exuding wound may be further protected through the use of emollients (such as 50:50 mix of white soft paraffin and liquid paraffin) or the application of barrier films.
- Hydrogel dressings have two removable thin sheets of polyethylene film, with some types containing a supportive inner gel mesh. For application to the wound, the film on the contact side is removed, leaving the outer film in place. With this mode of application, the dressing is semipermeable to gases and water vapor. If the outer film is also removed, then the dressing becomes permeable to fluid too; exudate can pass to a secondary gauze dressing. They are particularly useful in cosmetic procedures like chemical peels, laser resurfacing, dermabrasion, etc.

REFERENCES

1. Hayward PG, Morrison WA. Current concepts in wound dressings. Aust Prescr. 1996;19:11-3.
2. Gilje O. On taping (adhesive tape treatment) of leg ulcers. Acta Derm Venereol. 1948;28:454-67.
3. Winter GD. Formation of the scab and the rate of epithelialization of superficial wounds in the skin of the young domestic pig. Nature. 1962;193:293-4.
4. Eaglstein WH, Davis SC, Mehle AL, Mertz PM. Optimal use of an occlusive dressing to enhance healing. Effect of delayed application and early removal on wound healing. Arch Dermatol. 1988;124:392-5.
5. Li W, Dasgeb B, Phillips T, et al. Wound-healing perspectives. Dermatol Clin. 2005;23:181-92.
6. Jones V, Grey JE, and Harding KG. Wound dressings. BMJ 2006;332:777-80.
7. Menaker GM, Mehlis SL, Kasprowicz S. Dressings. In: Bolognia J, Jorizzo JL, Schaffer, JV (Eds). Dermatology. Philadelphia: Elsevier Saunders. 2012.
8. Matthews DN. Dressing of open wounds and burns with tulle gras. Lancet. 1941;237(6124):43–4.
9. Carter MJ, Tingley-Kelley K, Warriner RA 3rd. Silver treatments and silver-impregnated dressings for the healing of leg wounds and ulcers: a systematic review and meta-analysis. J Am Acad Dermatol. 2010;63:668-79.
10. Cooper RA. Iodine revisited. Int Wound J. 2007;4:124-37.
11. Hansson C. The effects of cadexomer iodine paste in the treatment of venous leg ulcers compared with hydrocolloid dressing and paraffin gauze dressing. Cadexomer Iodine Study Group. Int J Dermatol.1998;37:390-6.
12. Carsin H, Ainaud P, Le Bever H, et al. Cultured epithelial autografts in extensive burn coverage of severely traumatized patients: a five year single center experience with 30 patients. Burns. 2000;26:379-87.
13. Lobmann R, Pittasch D, Muhlen I, Lehnert H. Autologous human keratinocytes cultured on membranes composed of benzyl ester of hyaluronic acid for grafting in nonhealing diabetic foot lesions: a pilot study. J Diabetes Complications. 2003;17:199-204.
14. Bello YM, Falabella AF. Use of skin substitutes in dermatology. Dermatol Clin. 2001;19:555-61.
15. Smith DJ. Use of Biobrane in wound management. J Burn Care Rehabil. 1995;16(3 Pt 1):317-20.
16. Davis DA, Arpey CJ. Porcine heterografts in dermatologic surgery and reconstruction. Dermatol Surg. 2000;26:76-80.
17. British National Formulary (2015) BNF 70 September 2015-March 2016. Appendix 4; 1294-1319. BNF Group, London.
18. Chronic wounds: advanced wound dressings and antimicrobial dressings. NICE Guidelines. March 2016.
19. Agency for Healthcare Research and Quality (2014) Chronic venous ulcers: a comparative effectiveness review of treatment modalities. Comparative Effectiveness Review 127.
20. Scottish Intercollegiate Guidelines Network (2010) Management of chronic venous leg ulcers. SIGN Guideline 120.
21. Huang L, Woo KY, Liu LB, et al. Dressings for preventing pressure ulcers: a meta-analysis. Adv Skin Wound Care. 2015; 28:267-73.
22. Ghorpade A. Use of tissue glue for punch grafting in vitiligo—A preliminary report. Indian J Dermatol Venereol Leprol 2004;70:159-61.
23. Toriumi DM, O'Grady K, Desai D, Bagal A. Use of octyl-2-cyanoacrylate for skin closure in facial plastic surgery. Plast Reconstr Surg. 1998;102:2209-19.
24. Richert B,Di Chiacchio N, Haneke E. Nail Surgery ed 2011. 16-21, Informa healthcare UK.
25. Weinstein C, Ramirez O, Pozner J. Postoperative care following carbon dioxide laser resurfacing. Avoiding pitfalls. Dermatol Surg. 1998;24:51-6.

CHAPTER 5

Skin Biopsy Techniques

Shyamanta Barua, Anupam Das, BM Shashikumar

INTRODUCTION

"Bio" means life and "opsia" means to view. Therefore, biopsy means to view life. The term "biopsy" was coined by Ernest Besnier in 1879. Skin biopsy is a very commonly performed procedure in dermatology. It not only helps in confirming the diagnosis, but also it has become an important tool to document evidences in this world of litigations and consumer activism.[1-4] Therefore, the knowledge of the details of this procedure cannot be overemphasized. In this chapter, we have briefly reviewed the various techniques of skin biopsy. Table 5.1 highlights the advantages and disadvantages of different biopsy techniques.

Table 5.1: Advantages and disadvantages of different biopsy techniques.

Techniques	*Advantages*	*Disadvantages*
Shave biopsy	Performed quickly Require little training Do not require sutures for closure Excellent hemostasis achieved in patients with bleeding disorders or in those taking warfarin or aspirin	Does not include deeper tissue Avoided in pigmented lesions (nevi)
Punch biopsy	Can be easily performed Can be used both for diagnostic as well as therapeutic purposes Areas with good vasculature heal rapidly without scarring Low incidence of infection and bleeding	Pain and discomfort, if periosteum is hit accidentally Material obtained may not be adequate Biopsy may not include deeper tissue
Excision biopsy	Serves both diagnostic and therapeutic purpose Allows for multiple studies (culture, histology, immunofluorescence, electron microscopy) from a single biopsy site	Require the greatest amount of expertise and time Always require sutures Better performed with an assistant Complications may occur

INDICATIONS[2-4]

- *Diagnostic*: Confirmation of clinical diagnosis or cases where clinical diagnosis is not possible (neoplastic conditions, bullous dermatoses, appendageal tumors, etc.). Besides, special investigations like immunofluorescence also rely on the basic skin biopsy as the first step.
- *Prognostic*: Helpful in assessing the effectiveness of a therapeutic intervention on a previously diagnosed disease. Done mainly in autoimmune blistering dermatoses, leprosy and connective tissue diseases.
- *Therapeutic*: Helpful in situations like pyogenic granuloma, small nevi, cysts where biopsy will serve as the treatment modality as well.

CONTRAINDICATIONS[2-4]

- Infection at site of biopsy
- Previous allergies to topical medications like antibiotics and anesthetics
- Factors interfering with hemostasis like drugs (warfarin) and disorders associated with bleeding
- Uncontrolled diabetes mellitus
- Patients with a tendency to develop keloids.

SELECTION OF SITE OF BIOPSY[2-4]

The indications of biopsy are numerous and the selection of the site is extremely important. The site is decided on the basis of differential diagnosis, size of the lesion, special investigations which have been planned, etc.[4,5]

- *Inflammatory conditions*: Lesions with most advanced stages of inflammation must be chosen, with the inclusion of the adjacent normal skin as well.[6-9]
- *Blistering dermatoses*: Earliest lesions, preferably less than 48 hours lesions must be chosen.[10]
- *Vasculitic conditions*: Lesions which are earliest to appear are preferably chosen for biopsy, in order to identify the predominant type of infiltrating cells.[10]

- *Neoplastic conditions*: Attempts should be made to excise the entire lesion. Small lesions may be removed entirely and in case of large lesions, it is prudent to choose the center of the lesion.
- *Immunofluorescence studies*: In blistering dermatoses, perilesional skin is chosen for samples which are to be sent for immunofluorescence studies.
- If possible, areas like face (cosmetically important), tibia (poor healing characteristics) axilla, groin (chances of secondary infection), deltoid and chest wall (tendency of hypertrophic scarring), etc. must be avoided.[5,6,10]

ANESTHESIA BEFORE SKIN BIOPSY[2-4]

The commonest local anesthetic which is used before doing a skin biopsy is Lignocaine 1%/2%. Local anesthesia can be achieved either by infiltrating in the surrounding area, in a ring or field form around the lesion or into the nerve and also by applying it locally as EMLA (eutectic mixture of local anesthetics).[4,11]

By combining adrenaline with lignocaine, the duration of the anesthesia can be increased and blood loss can be minimized. Precaution has to be taken while injecting the combination in certain areas like the nasal tip, other acral areas and in certain associated conditions like connective tissue disorders, peripheral vascular disorders, etc.[12-14]

Prior to performing a skin biopsy, proper documentation with clinical photographs is done. This is followed by taking written informed consent, following universal precautions, cleaning the area using isopropyl alcohol, povidone-iodine, or chlorhexidine gluconate and infiltration of local anesthesia.

TECHNIQUES OF SKIN BIOPSY[2-4,15,16]

Shave Biopsy (Figs. 5.1A to C)

Shave biopsy is ideal for superficial skin lesions like actinic keratoses, seborrheic keratosis, acrochordon, planar warts, and squamous cell or superficial basal carcinomas. But it

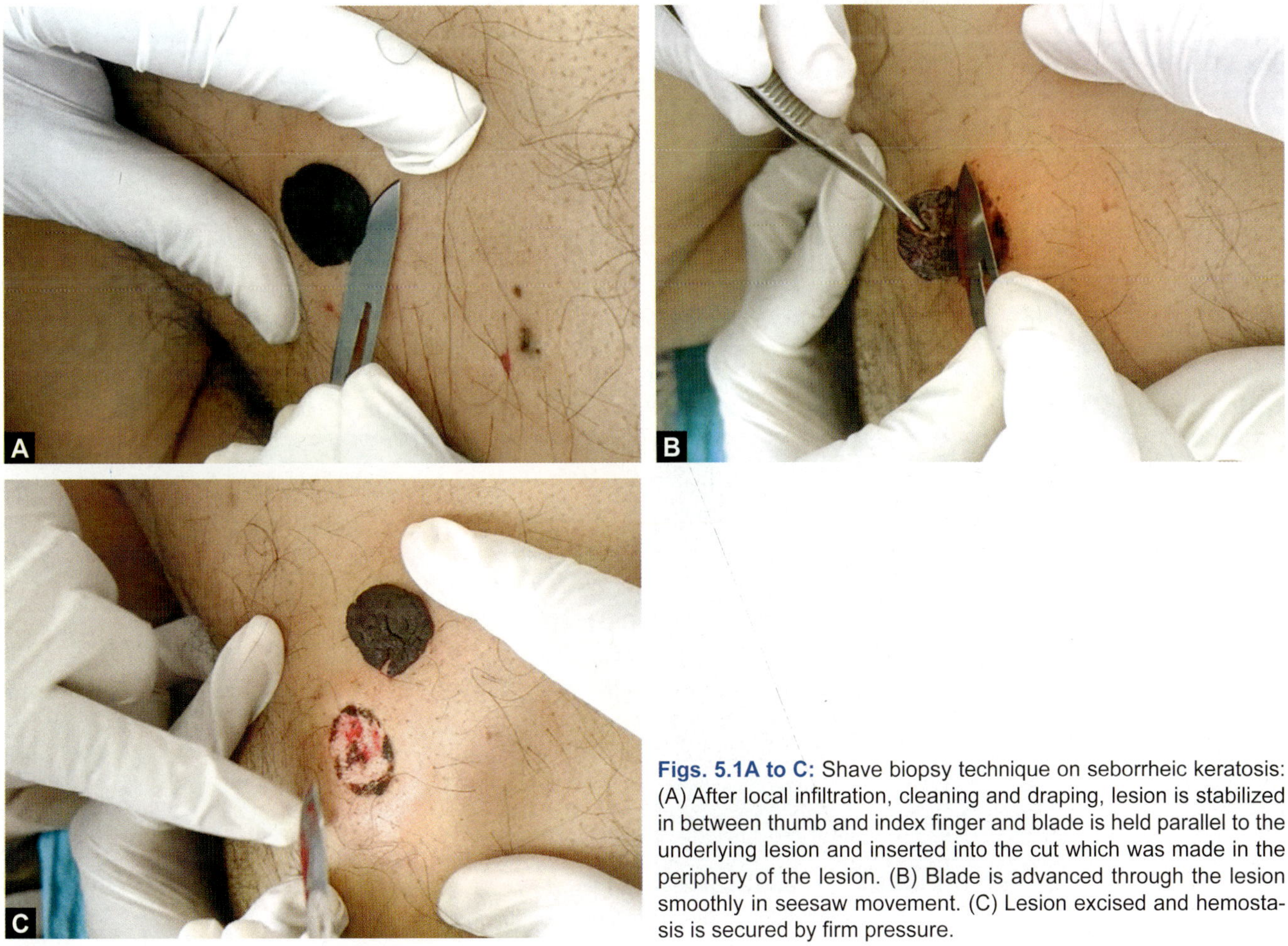

Figs. 5.1A to C: Shave biopsy technique on seborrheic keratosis: (A) After local infiltration, cleaning and draping, lesion is stabilized in between thumb and index finger and blade is held parallel to the underlying lesion and inserted into the cut which was made in the periphery of the lesion. (B) Blade is advanced through the lesion smoothly in seesaw movement. (C) Lesion excised and hemostasis is secured by firm pressure.

is contraindicated for pigmented lesions like melanoma. It can be superficial which involves removal of epidermis only or epidermis along with limited superficial dermis or deep shave biopsy (saucerization biopsy). A double-edge razor blade, curved scissor or No. 15 blade can be used for superficial shave biopsy whereas deeper shave biopsy is done with No. 15 blade. Relaxed skin tension lines (RSTLs) are observed carefully and a direction perpendicular to these lines is chosen. The lesion is stabilized in between thumb and index finger, following which a scoring incision is made in the periphery of the lesion.

- The blade is held parallel to the underlying lesion and inserted into the cut which was made in the periphery of the lesion and the blade is advanced through the lesion smoothly.
- Hemostasis is secured by firm pressure or chemical hemostatic agents (20% aluminum chloride in absolute alcohol, trichloroacetic acid or silver nitrate).
- For pedunculated lesions, shave biopsy using scissors is the preferred technique.
- Superficial lesions are preferably removed using a razor blade.
- Antibiotic cream and pressure gauze dressing is applied over the area.

Tips: Shave Biopsy[1]

- By raising a wheal by injecting the local anesthetic below the lesion to be biopsied, the shave can be facilitated. This makes the lesion rise up and it can be held between thumb and forefinger to stabilise it before shave.
- Manipulation of the angle of the blade can lead to ideal depths. Keeping the blade always parallel to skin surface helps in avoiding deep penetration (Figs. 5.2A to D). Use of hemostatic agents helps in reduced bleeding and to keep a dry wound.

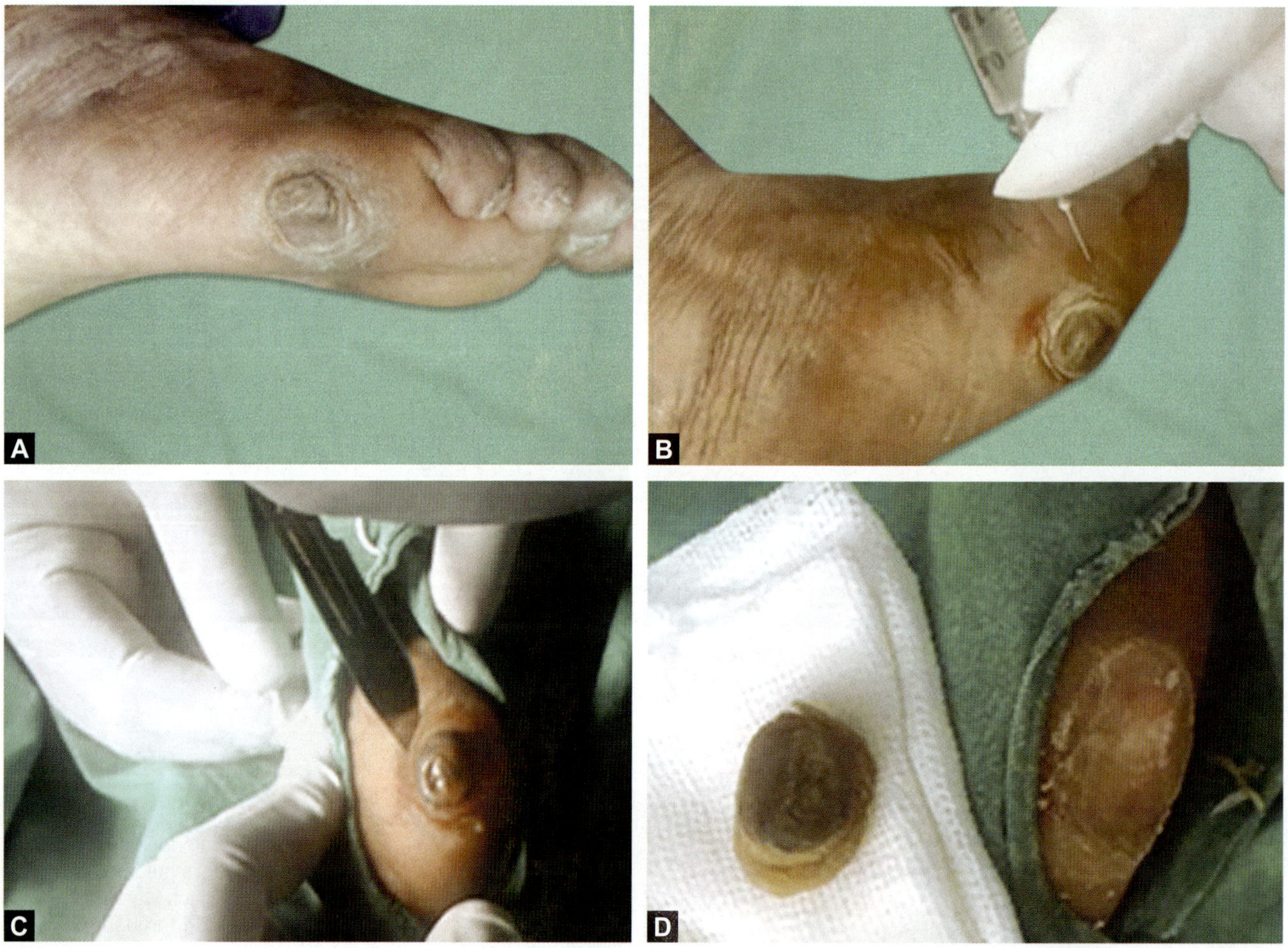

Figs. 5.2A to D: Shave biopsy on the foot.

Punch Biopsy

It is proably one of the most common surgeries done by a dermatologist. It is ideal for diagnostic purposes in a biopsy and also helps in removing small lesions entirely. It has the advantage of better cosmesis compared to a shave biopsy. Though a range of 2–10 mm can be chosen, ideally biopsies should at least be of 3 mm diameter (Fig. 5.3). The best choice is 4 mm, though in certain vital areas 3 mm is acceptable. In case, more than 3 mm punches are used, it is preferable to place one or two sutures to minimize the scarring. Figure 5.4 shows the instruments used for punch biopsy and Figures 5.5A to H show the steps of punch biopsy.

- RSTLs are identified and the punch is held perpendicular to these lines (Figs. 5.6A to D).
- Vertical steady pressure is applied over the lesion and the punch is rotated in a clockwise direction and slowly progressed towards the interior of the lesion. Once, the subcutaneous tissue is reached, the punch is withdrawn when a "give away" feel is perceived.
- The tissue is held carefully with forceps and thereafter, it is cut at the base using a scissor or blade. This ensures that the tissue is not crushed or damaged. Instead of forceps same needle used for local anesthesia can be used to hold the tissue (Fig. 5.7).
- Hemostasis is secured and the wound is sutured by prolene preferably. Sutures are removed after 1 week.

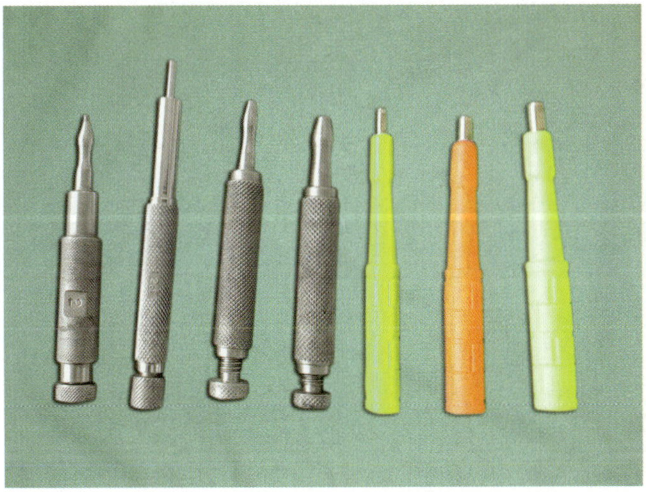

Fig. 5.3: Various types and sizes of punches. Both disposable and reusable punches are available.

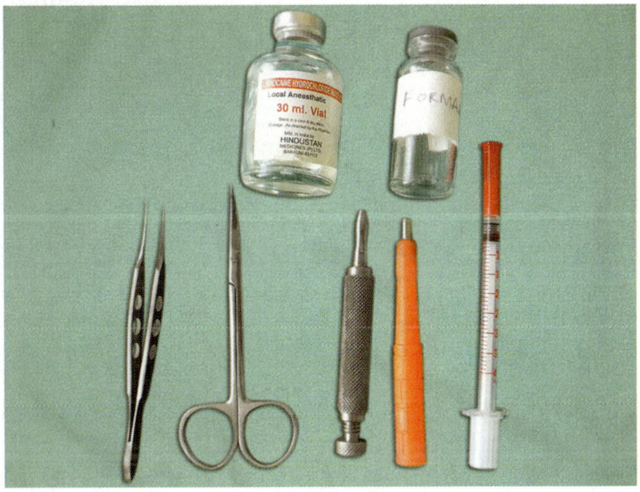

Fig. 5.4: Various instruments used for punch biopsy.

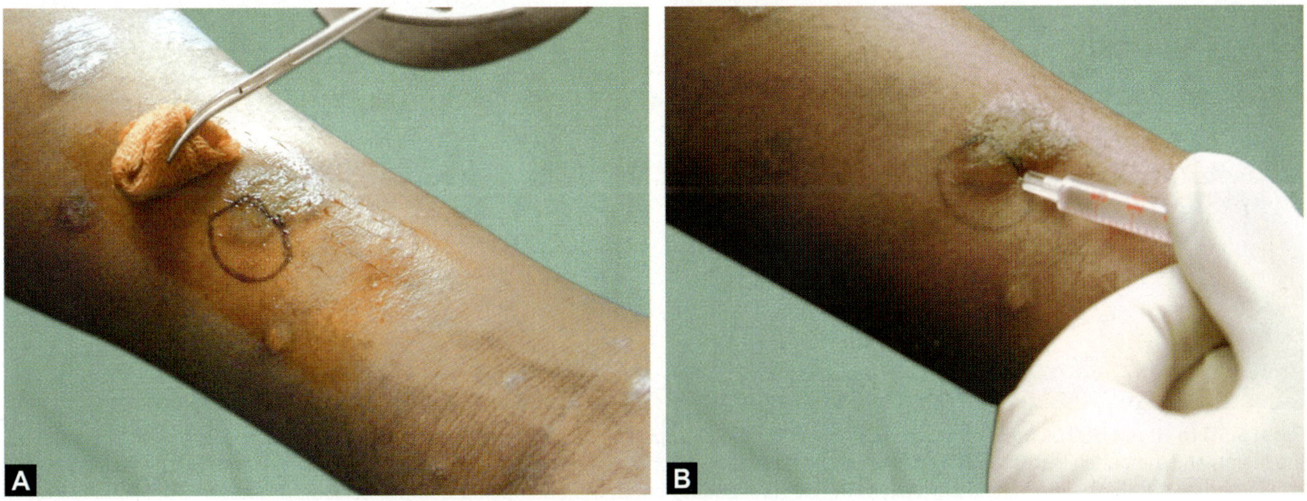

Figs. 5.5A and B: Punch biopsy technique: (A) Cleaning and draping. (B) Local infiltration with lignocaine.

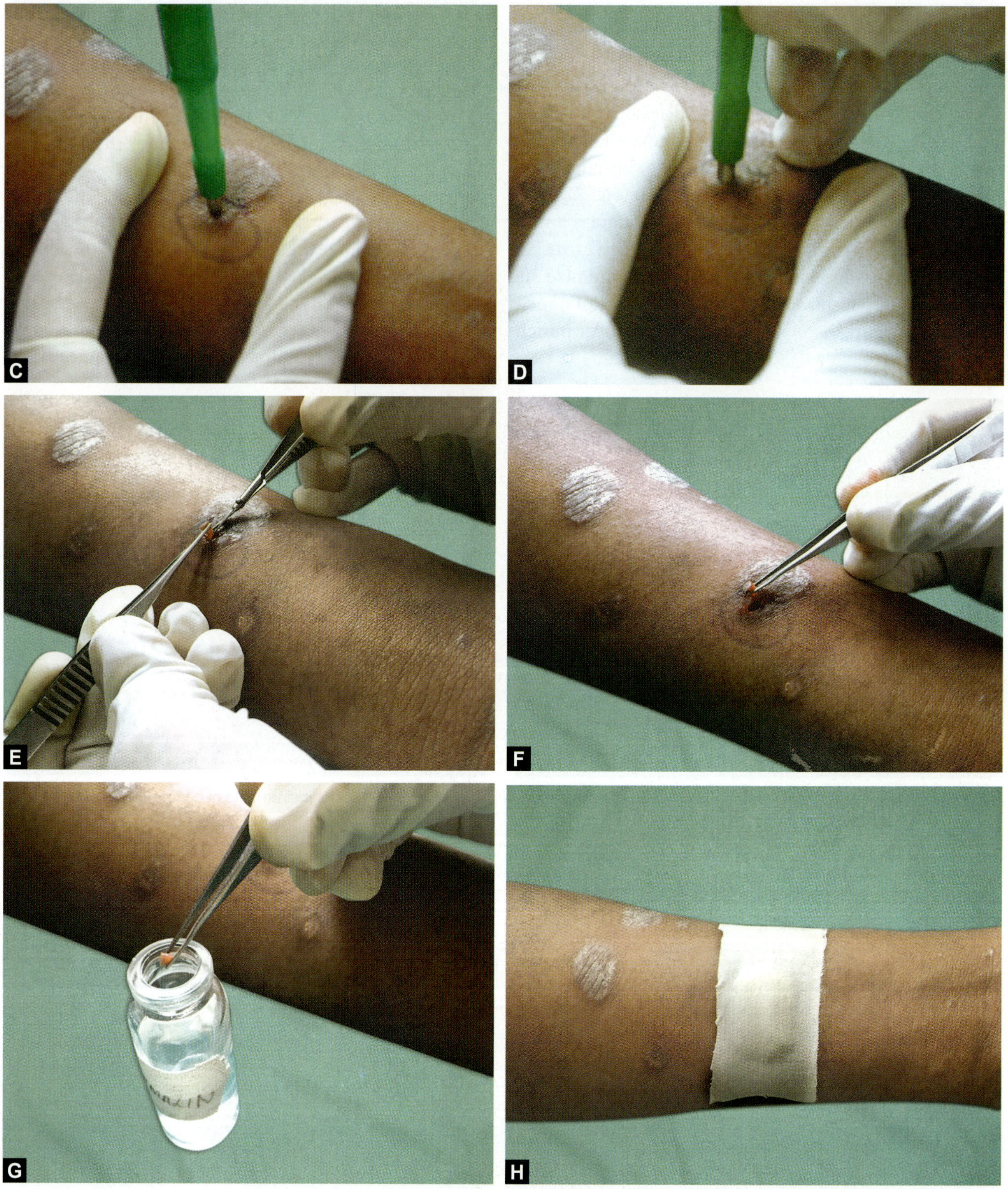

Figs. 5.5C to H: (C) RSTLs are identified and the punch is held perpendicular to these lines and vertical steady pressure is applied over the lesion and the punch is rotated in a clockwise direction. (D) Punch is rotated till subcutaneous tissue is reached, that is till "give away" feel is perceived. (E) Tissue is held carefully with fine forceps and cut at the base using a sharp scissor. (F and G) Cut tissue is gently transferred to 10% buffered formalin. (H) Wound is dressed with antiseptic cream. (RSTL: Relaxed skin tension line).

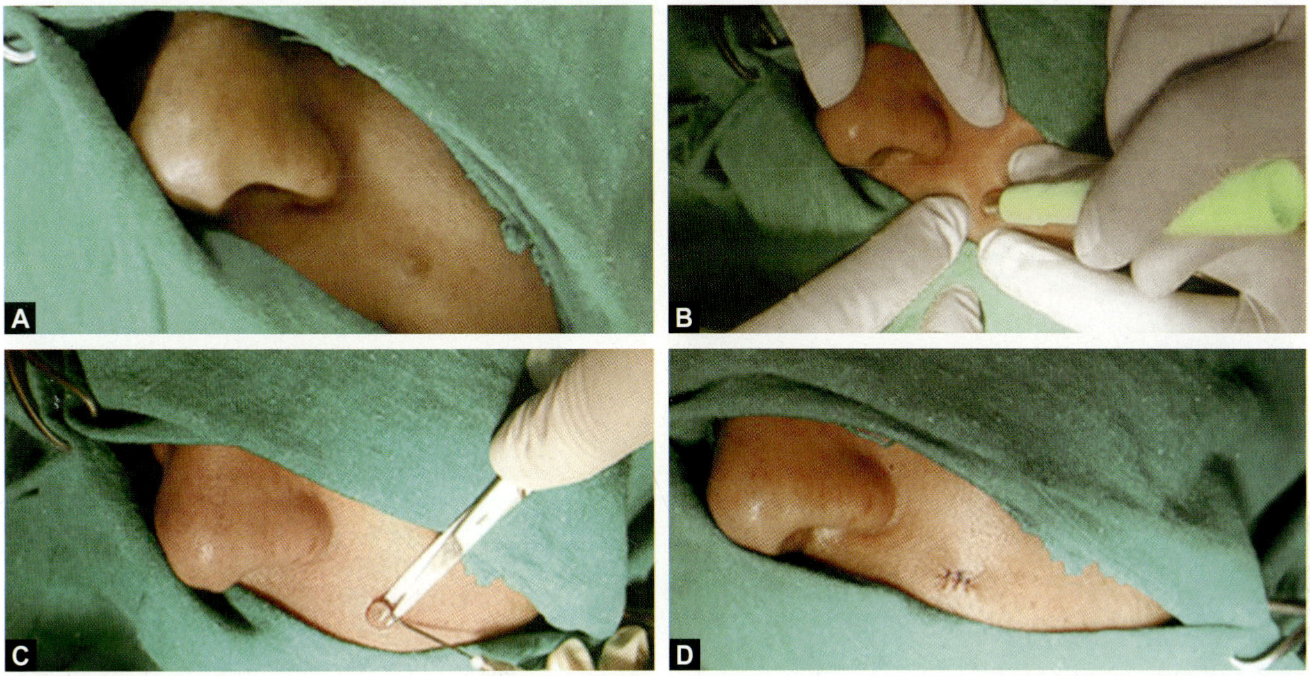

Figs. 5.6A to D: Punch biopsy on the face with pressure applied perpendicular to RSTL. (RSTL: Relaxed skin tension line).

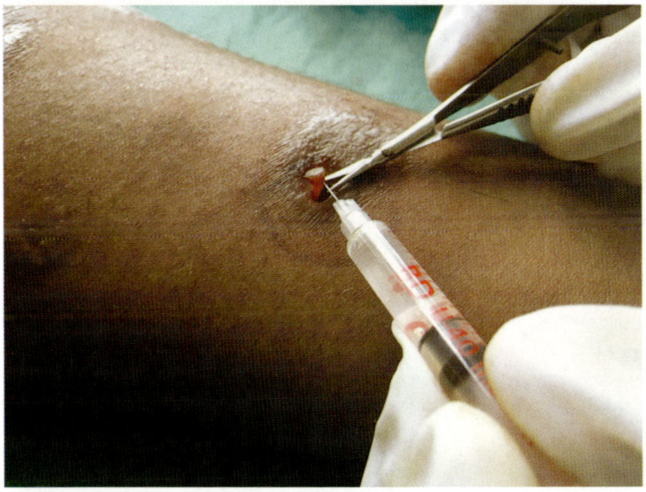

Fig. 5.7: Insulin syringe can be used to handle the tissue.

Tips: Punch Biopsy

- While using punch, do not continuously try to remove punch and check the progressive depth of penetration. This results in ragged edges and biopsy tissue may shred.
- While punching, application of pressure by fingers in a downward direction may help the tissue to pop out in an easy fashion. Gentle handling of popped tissue with fine forceps or a needle tip is pivotal in preventing crush artifact.

Excision Biopsy (Figs. 5.8A to D)

- The method of local anesthesia is preferably a ring block.
- A surgical marker is chosen and the area to be excised is marked in the shape of an ellipse, whose apex has an angle of 30 degrees and the length thrice that of the breadth. Besides, 3–5 mm of the normal skin should be included.
- Scalpel with No. 15 blade is taken and the area is stretched carefully, following which an incision is given at the apex of the ellipse. The incision is gradually progressed towards the length of the ellipse. Similarly, incision is given on the other side.
- The ellipse of tissue is separated from the underlying subcutaneous tissue using forceps.
- Hemostasis is secured, wound is sutured, antibiotic cream applied and dressing is done. Sutures are removed after 1 week.

Incision Biopsy

The basic procedure is similar to excision biopsy. However, unlike excision biopsy, only a part of the lesion is removed in incision biopsy.

Curette Biopsy (Figs. 5.9 and 5.10)

A sharp curette is used to scrape off the friable part of the lesion, even without using local anesthesia.

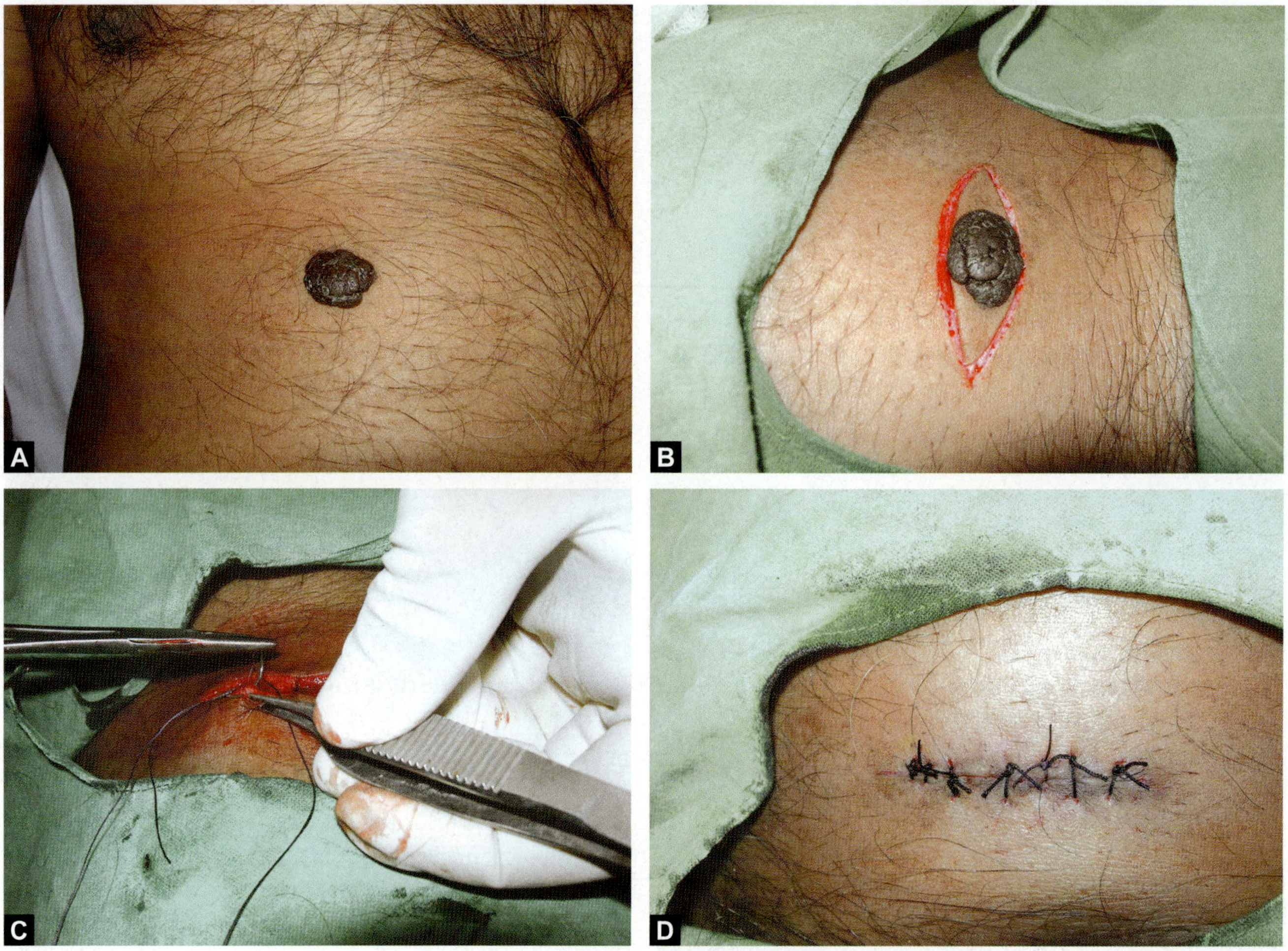

Figs. 5.8A to D: Excision biopsy: (A) After local infiltration, cleaning, draping and marking of lesion done. (B) Elliptical incision is placed with vertex angle of 30° and length to width ration of 3:1. (C) Tissue is excised and sent for histopathology and wound is sutured. (D) Interrupted suture or subcuticular sutures are placed.

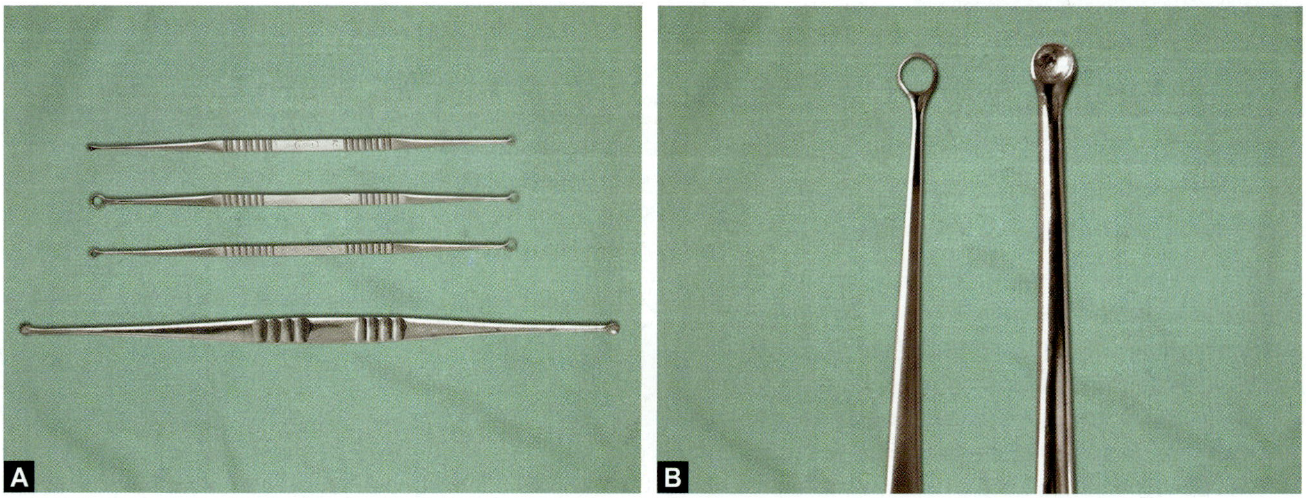

Figs. 5.9A and B: (A) Different sizes and varieties of curette. (B) Scoop and ring variety.

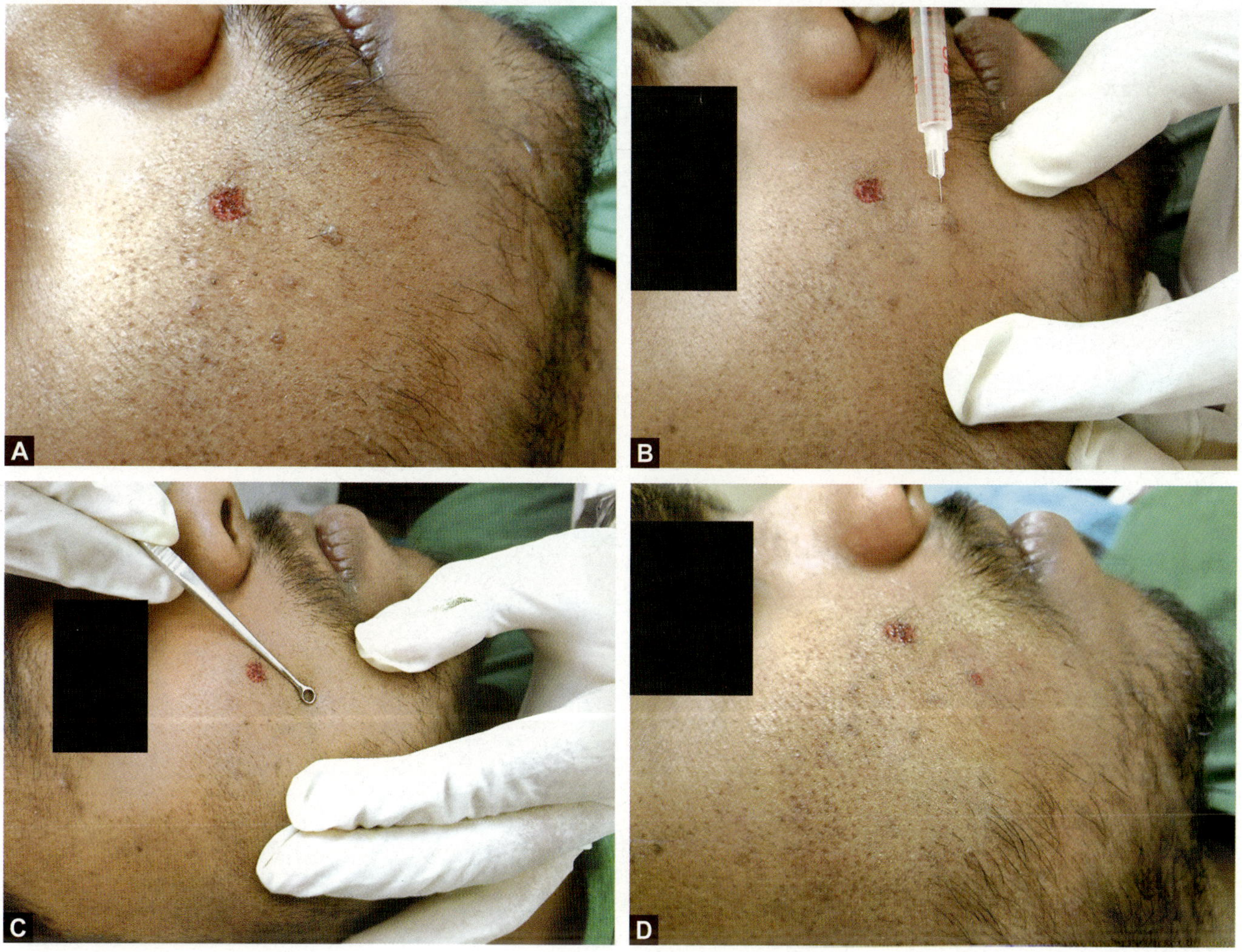

Figs. 5.10A to D: Curettage technique: (A) Plane wart which is cleaned. (B) Local anesthesia is infiltrated. (C) Curettage is done. (D) Resultant wound is left open.

Skin Surface Biopsy[17]

This is the best technique for diagnosing demodicidosis and for evaluation of mite density in such cases. The skin surface is smeared with the gel of Cyanoacrylate and a glass slide is used to press the area down. When the slide is taken off from the surface of skin, it is stained and the examined under the microscope (Figs. 5.11A to D).

Snip Biopsy

This is used in cases of pedunculated or really superficial lesions like acrochordons, seborrheic keratosis and filiform warts. The peduncle is first held with the forceps and it is used to give mild upward traction so that the lesion's base is exposed for the snip to be carried out (Fig. 5.12).

POST-BIOPSY CONSIDERATIONS:[2-4,18]

- The biopsy specimen is to be placed in 10% formalin which is buffered and then seen under light microscopy.
- For immunofluorescence studies, sample is placed in Michel's solution or phosphate buffered saline.
- Wound dressings should be preferably occlusive or semiocclusive, to ensure better and faster healing.
- The dressing must be removed in 24–36 hours and thereafter cleaned with soap and water twice daily followed by application of topical antibiotics.
- Sutures can be removed in 7 to 10 days and the site checked for any post-procedural complications.

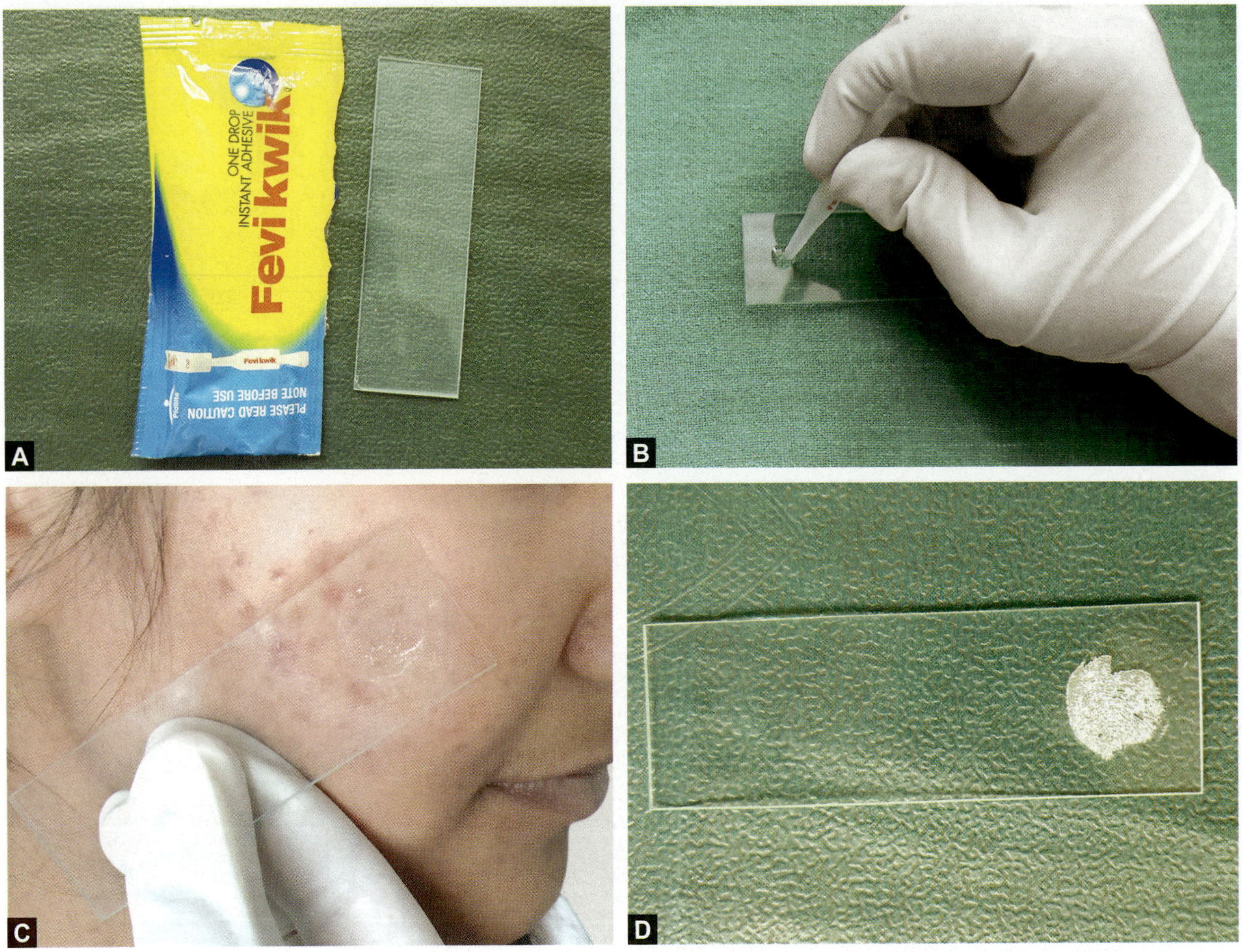

Figs. 5.11A to D: Skin surface biopsy: (A) Instruments require for skin care biopsy—Cyanoacrylate gel or Fevikwik and clean glass slide. (B) A drop of Fevikwik is applied to an area of 1 × 1 cm over the edge of the slide. (C) Slide is pressed over the area and left for 5 min. (D) Slowly removed and slide is stained with KOH. (KOH: Potassium hydroxide).

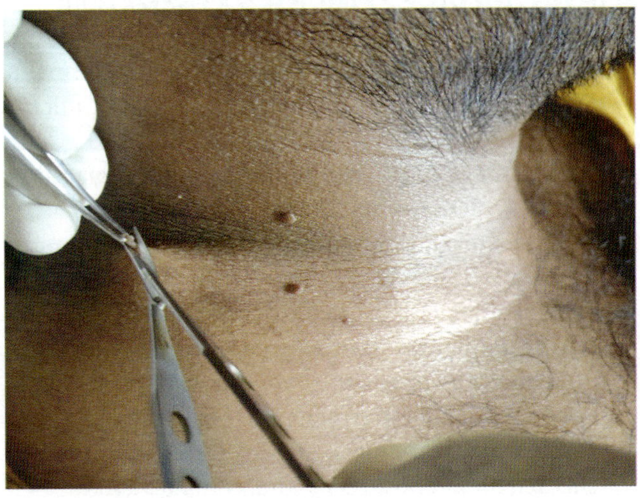

Fig. 5.12: Snip biopsy.

COMPLICATIONS

- Hypersensitivity to local anesthetics[19]
- Discomfort associated with administration of local anesthetics (pain, stinging, burning, etc.)[19]
- Bleeding and hematoma formation (more common in scalp, face, genitals and in elderly patients with atrophic skin)
- Infection (*Staphylococcus*, *Streptococcus*, or *Candida*)
- Allergic reactions to topical antibiotics
- Irritant reactions to tape
- Keloids or hypertrophic scars.

BIOPSY AT SPECIAL SITES

- **Scalp biopsy:** Scalp is a very vascular structure. So, lignocaine with adrenaline is preferred over plain

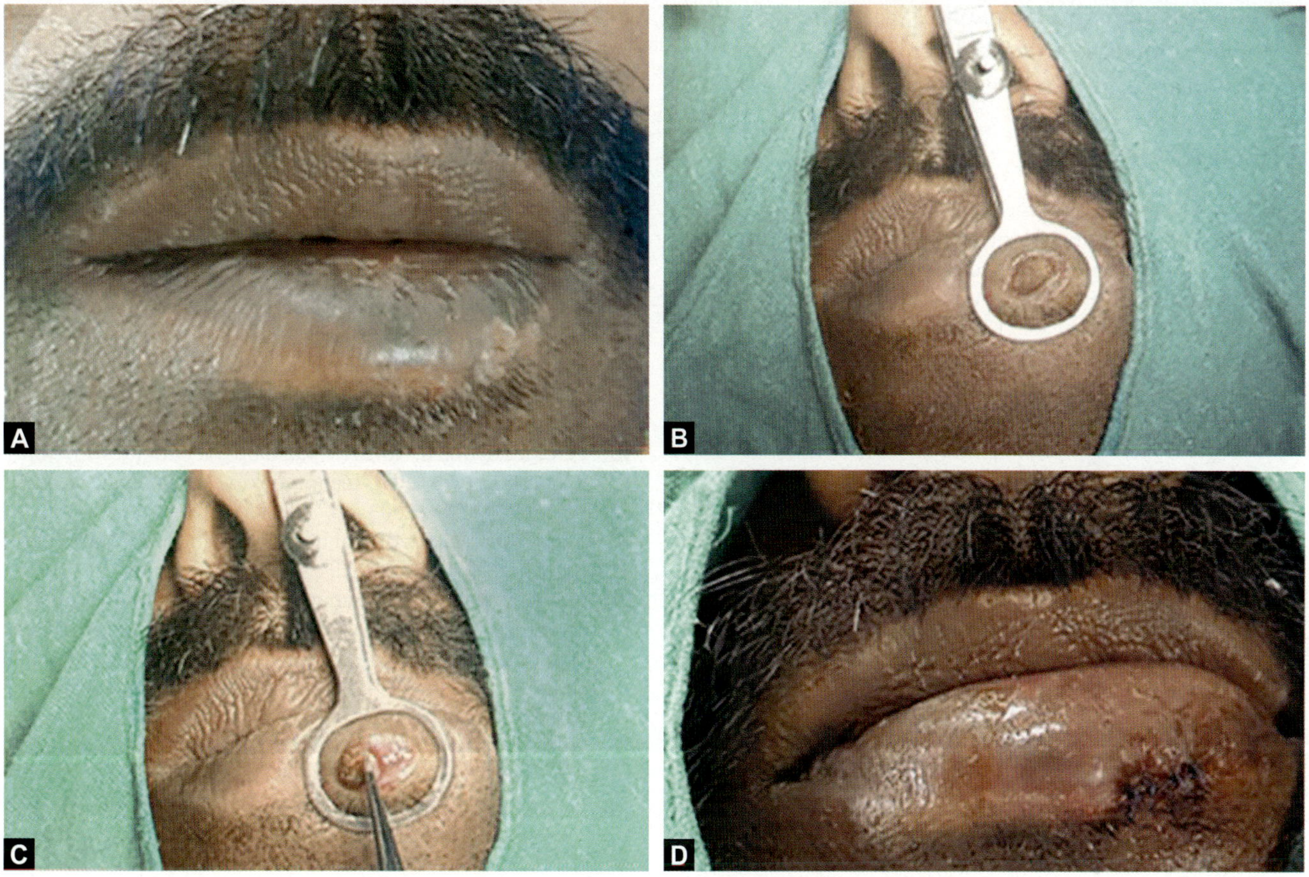

Figs. 5.13A to D: Excision biopsy using chalazion clamp.

lignocaine for local anesthesia. While performing biopsy circumferential pressure can be giving through ring of the artery forceps to obtain hemostasis. Punch should be advanced parallel to the direction of hair in order to avoid transaction of follicle. Two punches of 4/5 mm taken is always better and depth aimed should be subcutaneous tissue. One of the punch biopsy specimens will have to be cut horizontally for getting tangential sections and the other vertically for longitudinal ones. Sutures are placed which can be removed after 7–12 days.

- **Oral biopsy:** Oral biopsy can be done with same technique as skin biopsy. Oral mucosa being more vascular, chalazion clamp can be used to achieve hemostasis over lip, anterior buccal mucosa and tongue (Figs. 5.13A to D). Care should be taken while taking biopsy near second upper molar, as it's floor is adjacent to sublingual salivary glands.
- **Nail biopsy:** Biopsy of various structures of the nail unit is performed for both diagnostic and therapeutic purposes. Nail biopsies can either be by excision, punch or longitudinal sections. The excision or punch biopsies can be carried out in all parts of nail like nail plate, nail matrix, nail bed or nail fold. Details can be found in nail chapter.
- **Biopsy of the face:** Facial biopsy is avoided unless it is absolute necessary to prevent cosmetic disfigurement. Incision biopsy is better avoided and punch biopsy with 3 mm punch is preferred if necessary. While doing a biopsy on face, the excision long axis should always be parallel to the RSTL. This will result in a better scar. 5.0 and 6.0 sutures are to be used for better cosmetic outcome.
- **Penile biopsy:** It should always be borne in mind that injecting epinephrine is better avoided under the lesions on penile shaft and a ring block is better for glans lesions.
- **Biopsy of the breast:** Punch biopsy is done in similar fashion as with other areas. Fusiform biopsy is done for Paget's disease of breast with semilunar shape incision taken near or directly on the areola edge.

- **Biopsy of palms and soles:** The incision is made along the flexion crease or it should cross at 45° across high tension areas while taking biopsy of palms and soles.

REFERENCES

1. Seia Z, Musso L, Palazzini S, et al. Skin Biopsy Procedures: How and Where to Perform a Proper Biopsy. In: Khopkar U (Ed.). Skin Biopsy—Perspectives. Intech, Rijeka, Croatia; 2011. pp. 3–18.
2. Nischal U, Nischal KC, Khopkar U. Techniques of skin biopsy and practical considerations. J Cutan Aesthet Surg. 2008;1:107-11.
3. Alguire PC, Mathes BM. Skin biopsy techniques for the internist. J Gen Intern Med. 1998;13:46-54.
4. Mutalik S. How to make local anesthesia less painful? J Cutan Aesthet Surg. 2008;1:37-8.
5. Harrison PV. A guide to skin biopsies and excisions. Clin Exp Dermatol. 1980;5:235-43.
6. Pinkus H. Skin biopsy: a field of interaction between clinician and pathologist. Cutis. 1977;20:609-14.
7. Arca MJ, Bierman JS, Johnson TM, et al. Biopsy techniques for skin, soft-tissue, and bone neoplasms. Surg Oncol Clin North Am. 1995;4:157-74.
8. Bart RS, Kopf AW. Techniques of biopsy of cutaneous neoplasms. J Dermatol Surg Oncol.1979;5:979-87.
9. Peters MS, Winkelman RK. The biopsy. Dermatol Clin. 1984;2:209-17.
10. Pariser RJ. Skin biopsy: lesion selection and optimal technique. Mod Med. 1989;57:82-90.
11. Bjerring P, Arendt-Nielsen L. Depth and duration of skin analgesia to needle insertion after topical application of EMLA. Br J Anaesth. 1990;64:173-7.
12. Krunic AL, Wang LC, Soltani K, et al. Digital anesthesia with epinephrine: an old myth revisited. J Am Acad Dermatol. 2004;51:755-9.
13. Lalonde D, Bell M, Benoit P, et al. A multicenter prospective study of 3,110 consecutive cases of elective epinephrine use in the fingers and hand: the Dalhousie Project clinical phase. J Hand Surg Am. 2005;30:1061-7.
14. Thomson CJ, Lalonde DH, Denkler KA, et al. A critical look at the evidence for and against elective epinephrine use in the finger. Plast Reconstr Surg. 2007;119:260-6.
15. Perez M, Lodha R, Nouri K. Skin biopsy techniques. In: Nouri K, Leal-Khouri S (Eds). Techniques in Dermatologic Surgery. St. Louis: Mosby; 2003. pp. 75-80.
16. Achar S. Principles of skin biopsies for the family physician. Am Fam Physician. 1996;54:2411-8.
17. Bunyaratavej S, Rujitharanawong C, Kasemsarn P, et al. Skin scrapings versus standardized skin surface biopsy to detect Demodex mites in patients with facial erythema of uncertain cause—a comparative study. Indian J Dermatol Venereol Leprol. 2016;82:519-22.
18. Telfer NR, Moy RL. Wound care after office procedures. J Dermatol Surg Oncol.1993;19:722-31.
19. Fisher MM, Pennington JC. Allergy to local anaesthesia. Br J Anaesth. 1982;54:893-4.

CHAPTER 6

Excisions of Cysts and Small Tumors

Dhanashree Bhide, Harish Prasad

INTRODUCTION

In dermatology practice we come across variety of cysts and tumors requiring excision for cosmetic as well as medical reasons, and also for correct histopathological diagnosis.

As trained dermatosurgeons we can carry out excision of smaller lesions with good cosmetic outcome if proper techniques are mastered. In this chapter we will highlight simple and easy to perform procedures, with tips and tricks for each method.

The classification of tumors and cysts is very exhaustive and beyond the scope of this chapter. However, the broad classification of tumors, which needs to be remembered, includes:

- Keratinocytic tumors—Basal cell carcinoma (BCC), squamous cell carcinoma (SCC), Bowen's disease, actinic keratoses, acanthomas and verrucae
- Melanocytic tumors
- Appendageal tumors
- Hematolymphoid tumors
- Soft tissue tumors
- Neural tumors
- Inherited tumor syndromes.[1,2]

As far as tumors are concerned, keratinocytic tumors are most frequently encountered in practice. We will be mentioning common conditions and their method of excision in the following chapter.

SMALL TUMORS AND CYSTS

Junctional nevi, pyogenic granulomas, milia, sebaceous cysts, lipomas and a variety of smaller benign tumors and cysts can be removed by simple elliptical excision. Modified techniques can be employed in certain special situations.

Sometimes there is diagnostic dilemma and preservation of tissue architecture is essential for histopathological examination. In such situations, simple excision can be preferred over radiofrequency or laser.

Simple Elliptical Excision

Principles of Procedure

Before planning the ellipse one must consider the local anatomy, likely nature of the tumor whether benign or malignant, cosmetic units when operating on face, RSTL lines and the functional outcome of the procedure.

Steps (Figs. 6.1 and 6.2)[3]

- Written consent and xylocaine skin test
- Pretreatment photograph
- Standard aseptic precautions
- Marking of the margins before infiltration
- Local anesthesia infiltration
- Incision line parallel to lines of closure, i.e. relaxed skin tension lines (RSTL) and minimum skin tension lines (MSTL)
- Length to width ratio is 3:1 or 4:1
- Tips of ellipse should meet at an angle of 30°
- On face, try to give scar in single cosmetic unit
- Scalpel held perpendicular to the skin at the beginning of incision and then moved at an angle of 45° (Fig. 6.2F)
- Edges undermined before suturing.

Modifications

- While excising epidermal raised lesions, instead of elliptical incision, the lesion can be shave excised and feathering of base with coagulation can be done using radiofrequency (Figs. 6.3A to D)
- Base can be coagulated using radiofrequency. Appropriate sized punch can be used and 1 to 2 stay sutures can be taken to facilitate healing by primary intention and give a cosmetically better acceptable scar.

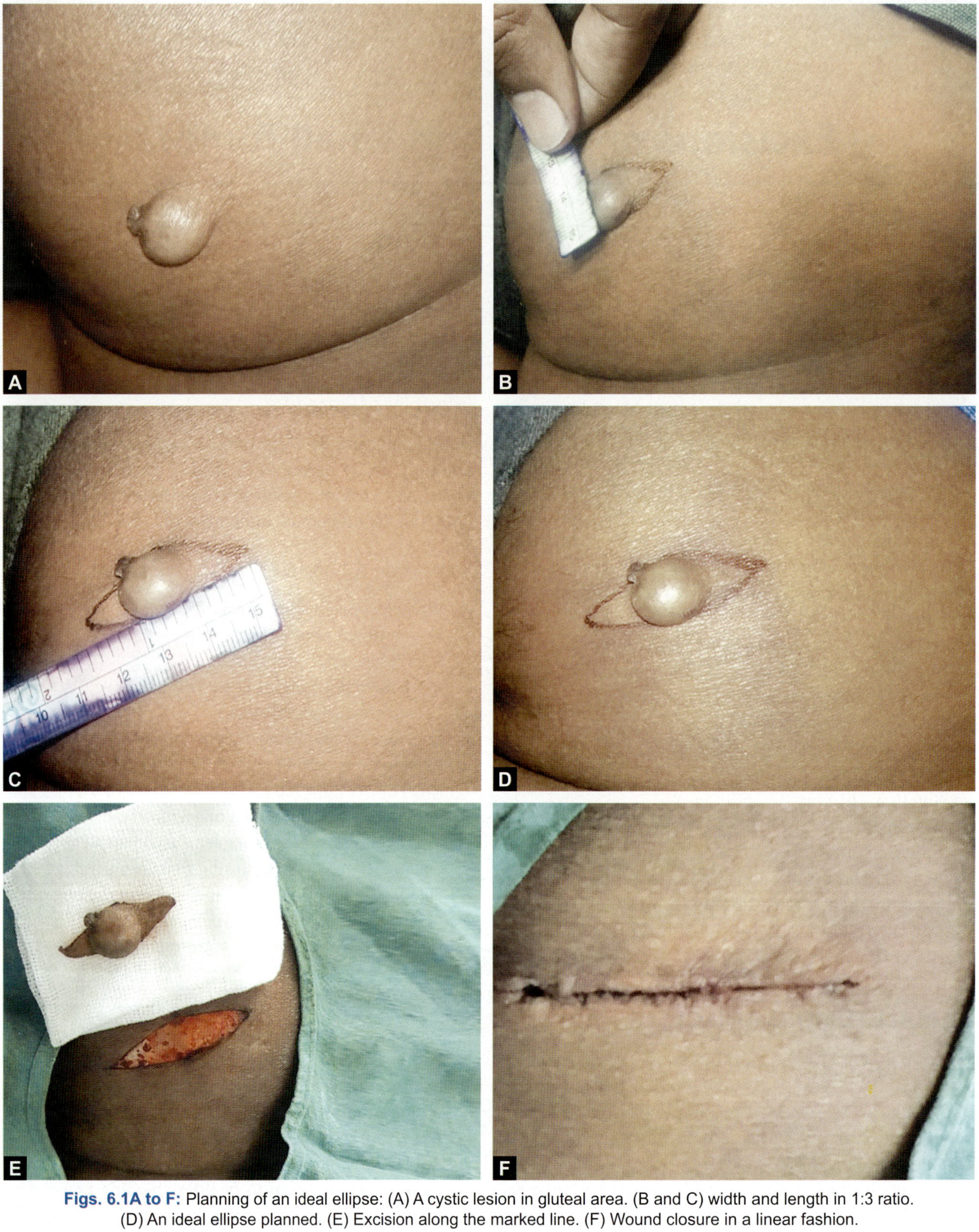

Figs. 6.1A to F: Planning of an ideal ellipse: (A) A cystic lesion in gluteal area. (B and C) width and length in 1:3 ratio. (D) An ideal ellipse planned. (E) Excision along the marked line. (F) Wound closure in a linear fashion.

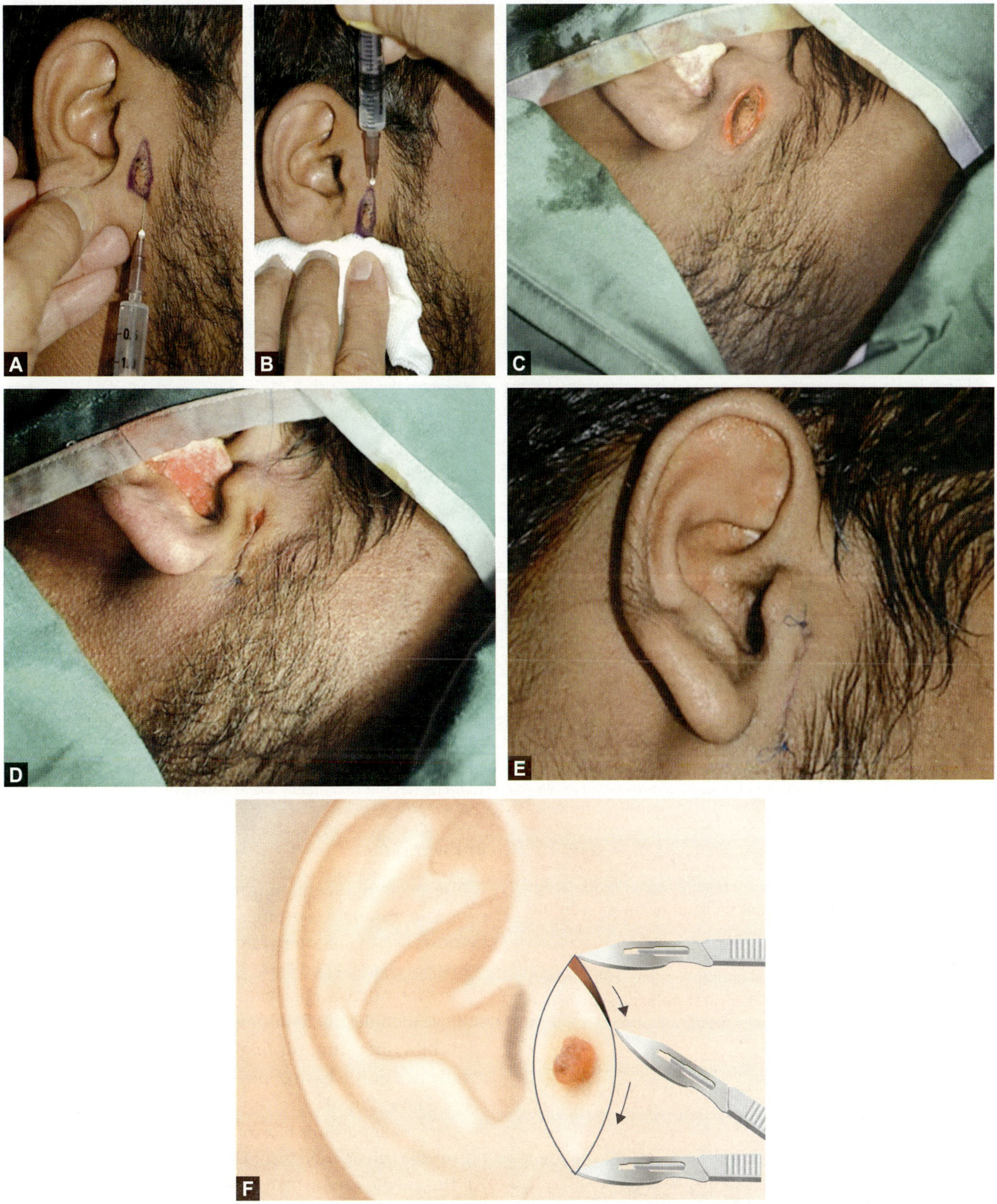

Figs. 6.2A to F: Elliptical excision: (A and B) Injection of local anesthesia after planning an ellipse. (C) Ellipse being excised. (D and E) Wound closure in straight line. (F) Diagrammatic representation.

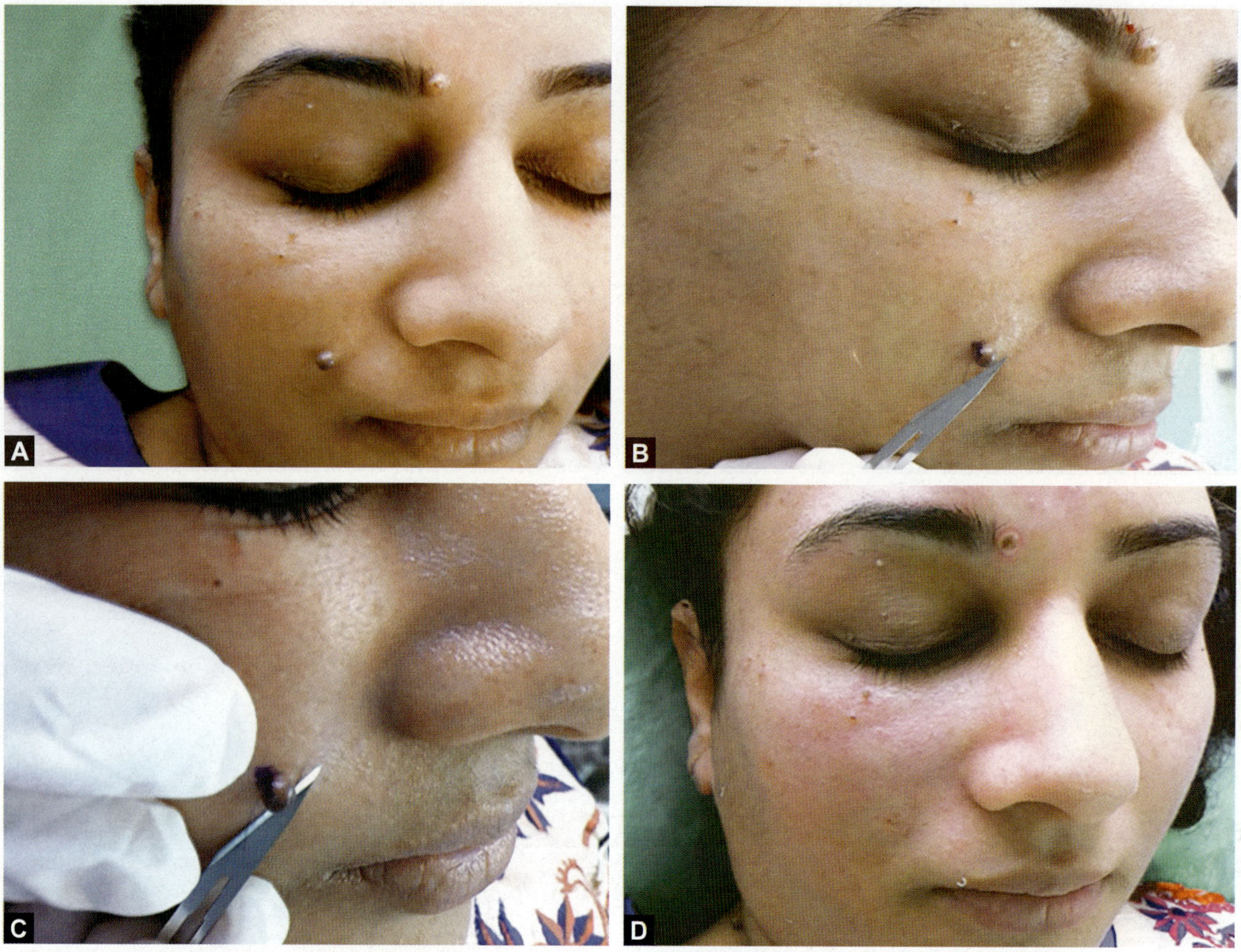

Figs. 6.3A to D: Shave excision of benign raised lesion: (A) Benign raised lesion on right cheek. (B) Blade introduced at 45° angle to base. (C) Blade being held parallel to base. (D) After complete shave excision.

TIPS AND TRICKS[4]

- Incision should be vertical along the Langer's line except in scalp where horizontal incision or incision in the direction of hair may be taken.
- On back, avoid giving scar in bra strap area.
- It has been observed that simple looking scalp tumors can give surprises on histological examination and hence proper excision techniques should be observed in this very vascular area.
- While performing surgeries in certain locations especially periorbital and neck region, one must know the anatomical details as important vessels pass very superficially in these sites.
- For smaller lesions, sharp 15 no. blade may be used and for larger lesions, 10 no. blade may be used.
- Finest possible suture according to the area should be chosen: face 6/0 and other areas 4/0.
- Preferably use monofilament sutures over braided ones.

Innovations

While excising scalp tumors or vascular lesions like pyogenic granulomas in other locations, in order to achieve hemostasis, ring of artery forceps can be used to give firm pressure (Figs. 6.4 and 6.5).

In oral mucosa, chalazion clamp can be very useful to achieve bloodless field during surgery.

While operating on fingers and toes, rubber band can be tied at the base of finger to achieve bloodless field (Figs. 6.6A to C).

For smaller lesions like milia or small cysts, bevel of 21 no. needle can be used to make fine incision (Figs. 6.7A and B). The needle can be bent at 90° and the bent corner used to extract milia.

While operating on pedunculated lesions, sharp scissors can be used after infiltration anesthesia.

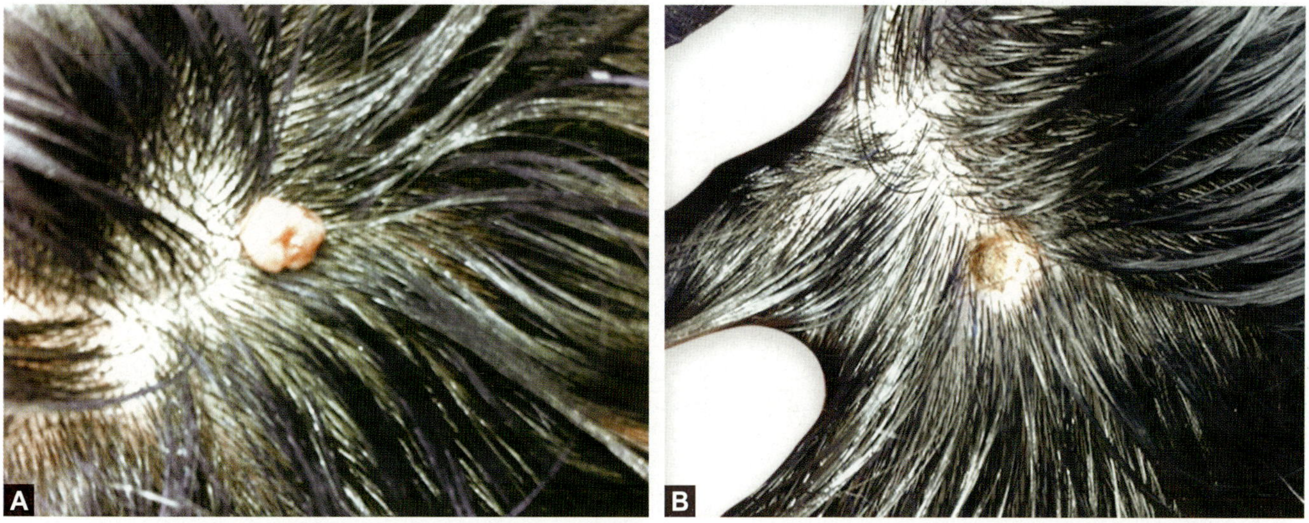

Figs. 6.4A and B: (A) Scalp tumor. (B) Scalp tumor after bloodless excision due to compression with scissor handle.

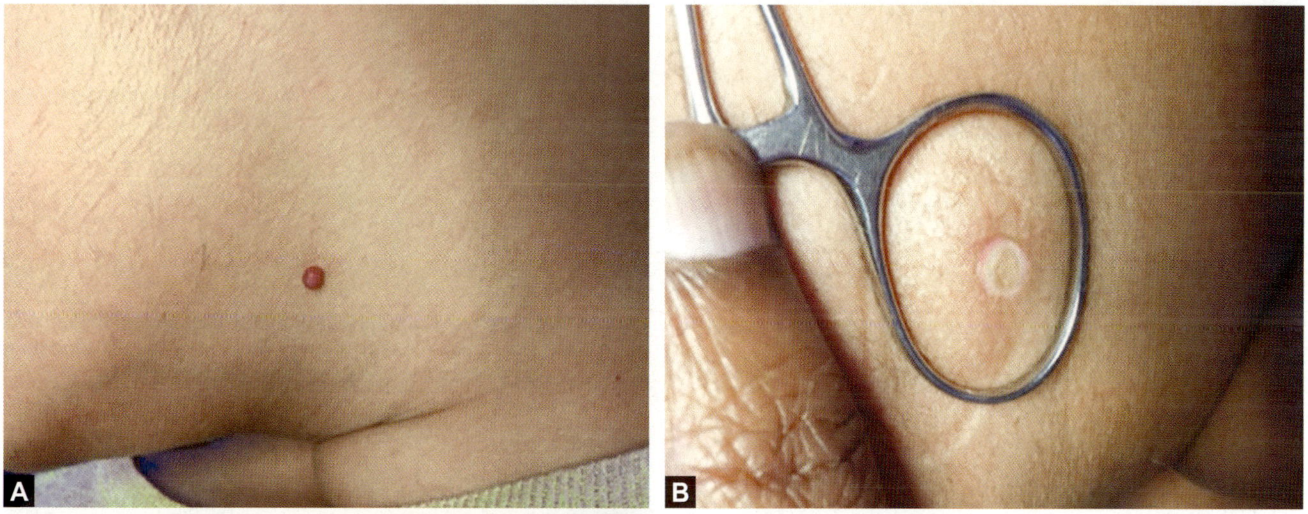

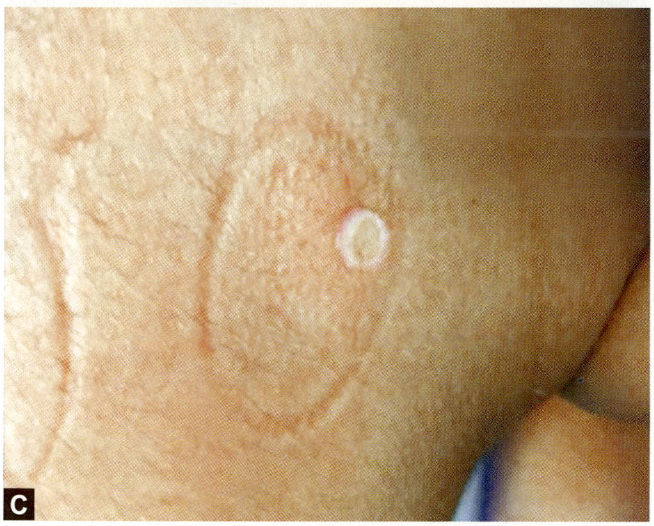

Figs. 6.5A to C: (A) Pyogenic granuloma. (B) Pressure with artery with minimal bleeding. (C) Bloodless field.

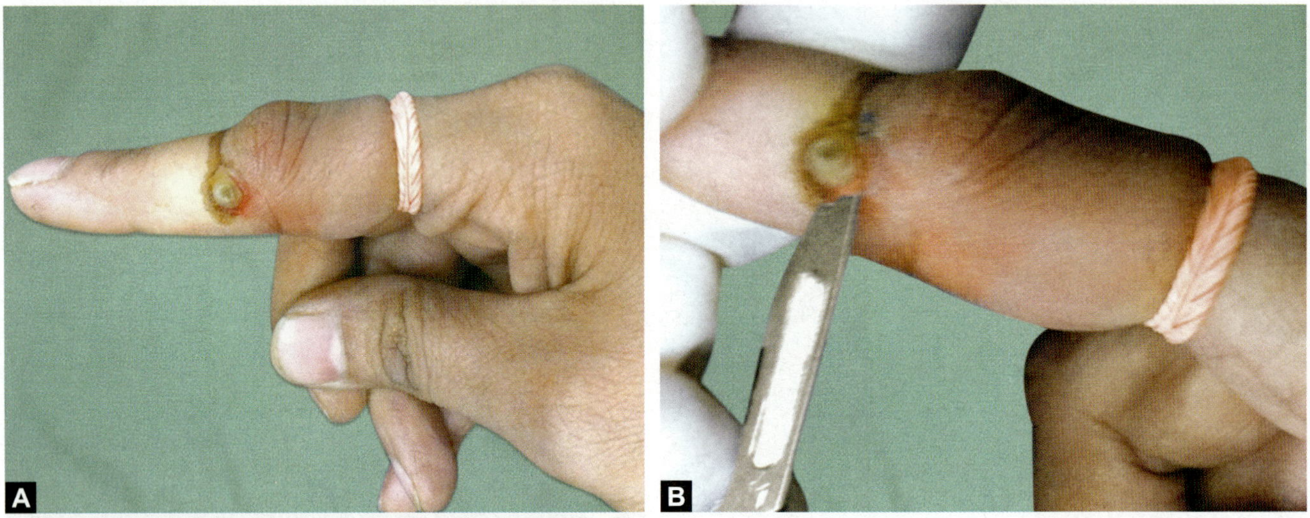

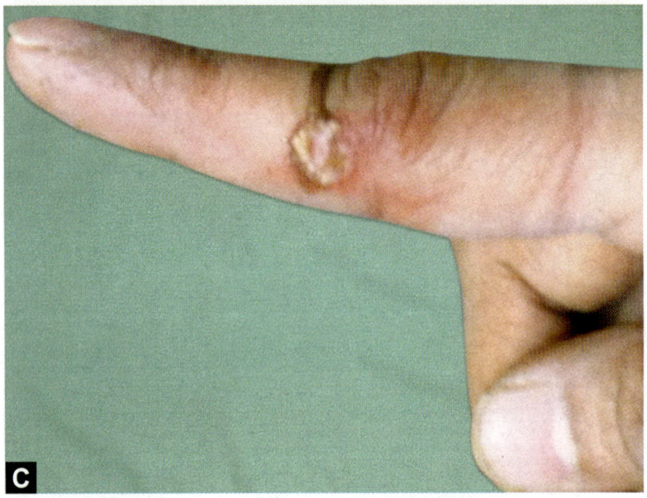

Figs. 6.6A to C: (A) Digital fibrokeratoma of index finger with tourniquet tied. (B) Lesion being excised without bleeding. (C) A bloodless field after tourniquet removal.

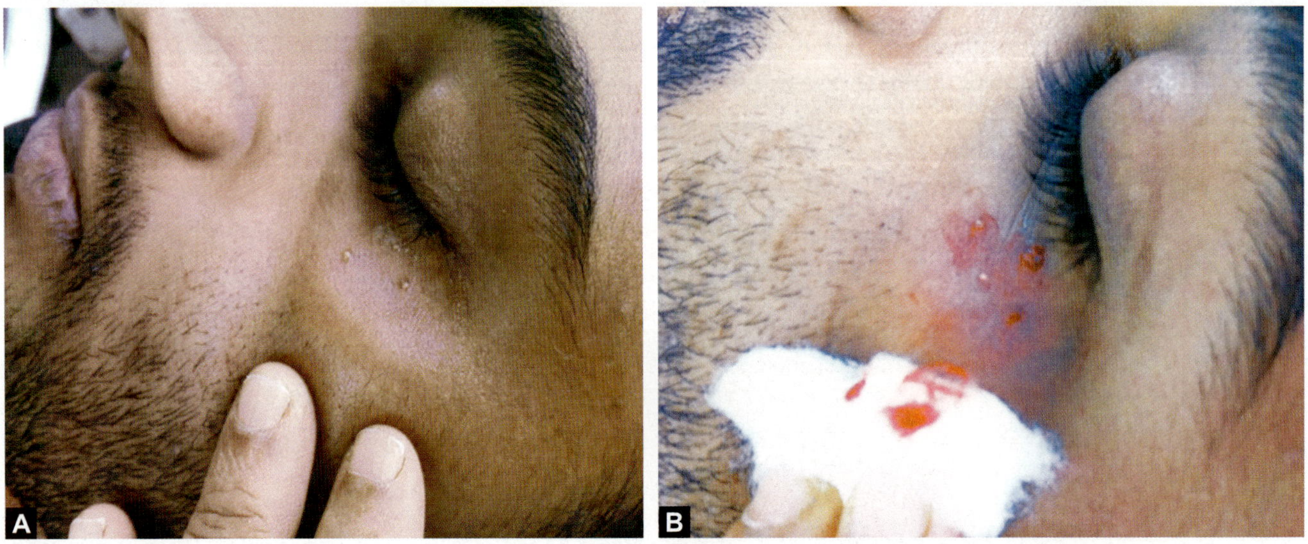

Figs. 6.7A and B: (A) Intraepidermal inclusion cyst of milia. (B) Needling out of milia.

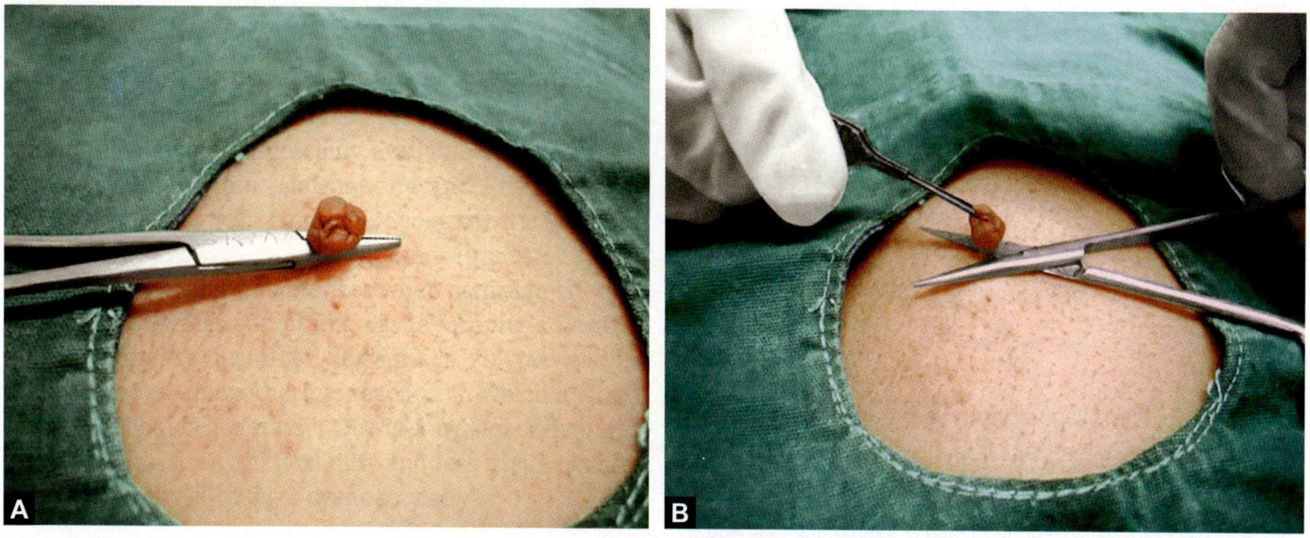

Figs. 6.8A and B: (A) Pedunculated lesion being compressed at the base with artery forceps. (B) Pedunculated lesion being cut with absolutely no bleeding.

Before excising, crushing of base with straight artery forceps significantly reduces the chances of bleeding (Figs. 6.8A and B).

Complications[5-8]

If done properly, complications are rare. Rarely following complications may be seen:

- Hematoma formation
- Infection
- Dehiscence
- Necrosis
- Dog ear formation.

Dog Ear Deformity

Dog ears are the standing cone deformities or one sided extra mound of redundant tissue, which is seen after the excision and repair of certain skin lesions (seen at the edge of incision).

Causes of Dog Ear

- When simple elliptical excisions are planned and the angle of excision is more than 30°.
- In flap surgeries when defects of unequal sides are formed
- In plastic surgery procedures like abdominoplasty surgery, or tummy-tuck surgery, breast lift where skin tightening can result in redundant skin.

Prevention of Formation of Dog Ear

- Anticipation of dog ear formation is very important to prevent its formation. Well planned elliptical excision with appropriate width and length ratio and angle will prevent coning in simple excisions.
- However, if unequal sides of wound are formed due to some anatomical variation, the following techniques can be followed to prevent dog ear formation:
  - Rule of halves (Fig. 6.9). In this technique first stitch is placed at the center of the defect. Then the remaining halves on either side are sutured. This will spread excess tissue on both sides equally over the entire length of the wound.
  - Another way of preventing dog ear formation is through formation of Burow's triangle (Fig. 6.10).

A triangular tissue on longer side of the wound is excised and closed thus decreasing the length. Burow's triangle can be drawn anywhere along the length, so that the line of closure merges with RSTL, junction of anatomical unit or hairline.

Correction of Dog Ears

Dog ear once formed can be repaired in number of ways.

- Apex of the dog ear is divided using a scalpel, thus creating two smaller triangles which are then cut at the base and wound closed in linear fashion (Figs. 6.11 and 6.12).

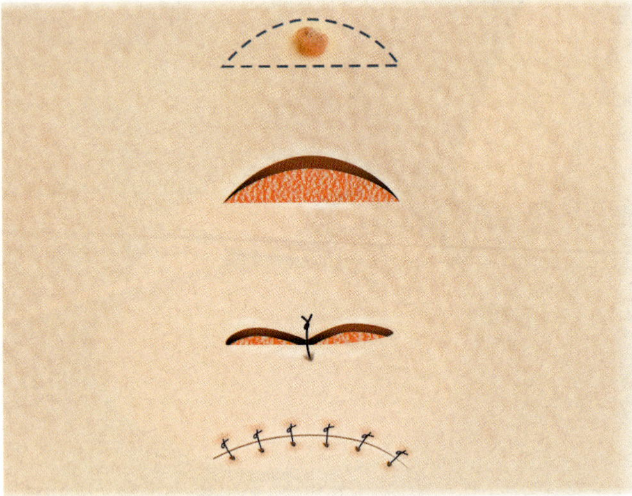

Fig. 6.9: Rule of halves. A center stitch is placed first followed by on stitches on either side.

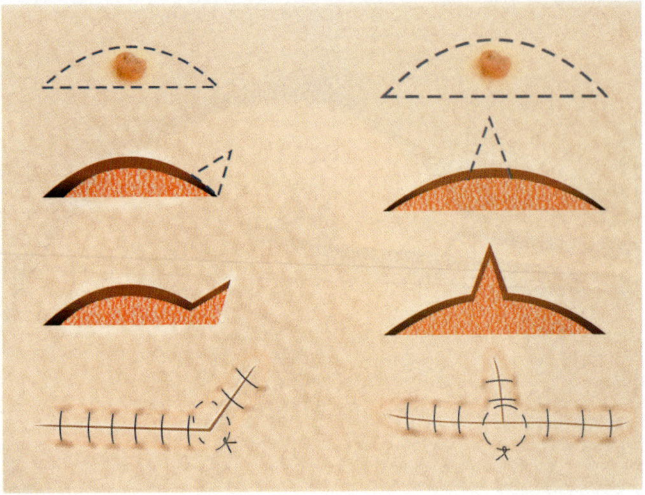

Fig. 6.10: Burow's triangle to reduce the length on longer side of wound.

- Place a skin hook in the tip of the dog ear, pull the tissue to one side and incise one triangle on this side and same thing repeated on the other side. A single large triangular tissue is discarded and wound closed in a linear fashion (Fig. 6.13).
- Dog ear can also be repaired by simply excising extra cone of skin as a new ellipse, thus extending the line of closure but maintain the direction same as original wound (Fig. 6.14).
- In another technique, linear incisions are made on either side of redundant tissue. Later this tissue is unfolded and made to lie flat on the wound. Excess triangular tissue on either side is excised and wound is closed in the shape of M at the end (Fig. 6.15).

Pseudo Dog Ear Formation

Removal of less tissue at the edges than in the center as in the figure can result in pseudo dog ears (Figs. 6.16A and B).

Conclusion

For smaller benign cysts and tumors, simple excision with specific modifications is a very useful tool for both diagnostic as well as cosmetic indications.

BASAL CELL CARCINOMA

All basal cell carcinomas need excision.

Principle of Excision

- To achieve complete excision to avoid recurrence
- As most lesions occur on face and neck area, good cosmetic as well as functional outcome is necessary
- On nose, it is difficult to identify peripheral and deep margins. Hence there is almost 2.5 times higher incidence of recurrence. It is mandatory to carefully examine 100% of the margin on histology to achieve satisfactory results.

Types of Excision

- Wide local excision
- Mohs micrographic surgery.

Wide Local Excision

Indications:

- Primary BCC
- Lesions on trunk, neck and extremities
- Nodular superficial type
- Size less than or equal to 0.5 cm on face and less than or equal to 2 cm on body areas other than face.

Principle of excision and modifications: The size of the tumor, anatomical location, ulceration and apparent depth of penetration determine the clinical excision margin. Histological subtype is also important in determining the management in BCC.[9] While treating the primary lesions, goal should be to remove the lesion totally at first surgical intervention because primary lesions have higher cure rates and recurrent lesions are known to be more aggressive. Smaller primary BCC can be excised with 3 mm margin.[10-12] Use of 4 mm margin is satisfactory for primary well-defined BCC which is <2 cm in diameter. Occasionally 3 and 2 mm margins may give similar cure rates.[13,14] It is found that about 5% of

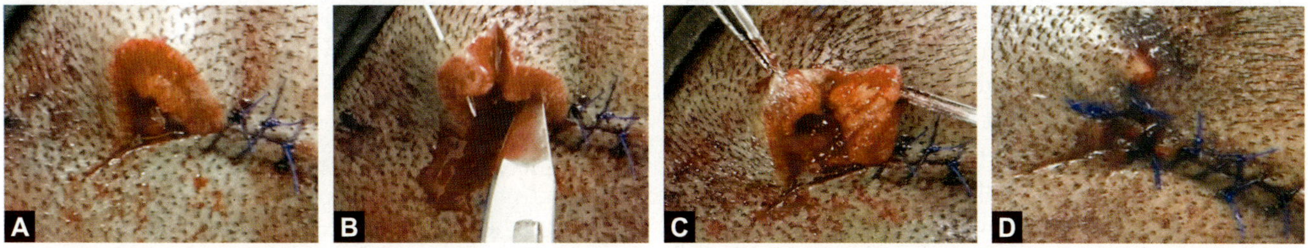

Figs. 6.11A to D: (A) A large standing cone deformity formed at the edge in a flap surgery. (B) Incised at the apex of cone with scalpel. (C) Two triangles cut from the base. (D) Wound closed in linear fashion.

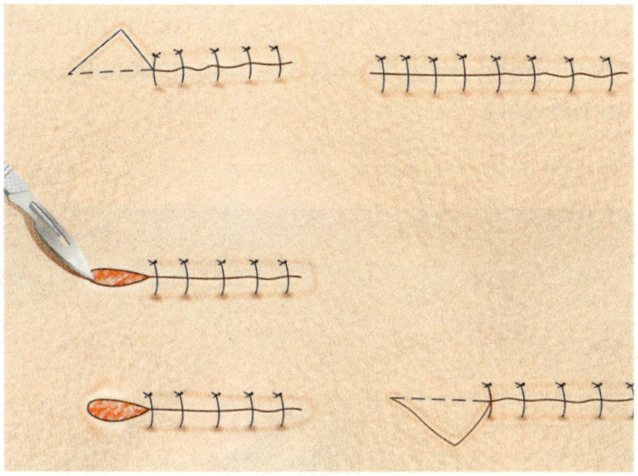

Fig. 6.12: Dog ear correction with creation of two triangles with incision at the apex of cone.

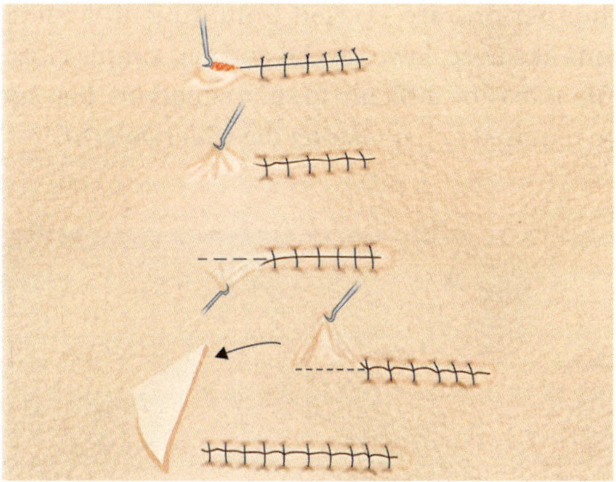

Fig. 6.13: Single triangle technique for dog ear correction.

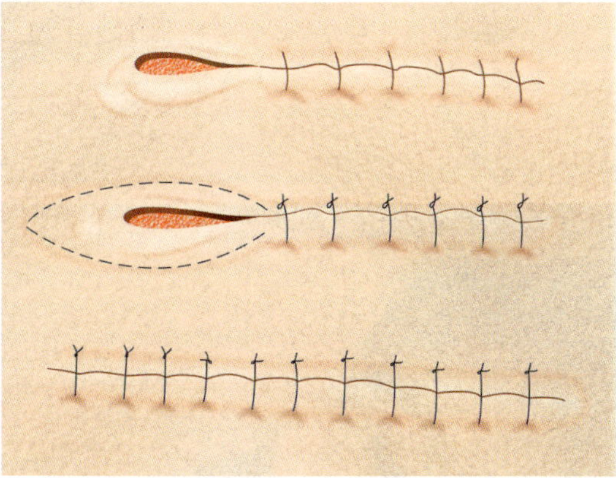

Fig. 6.14: Dog ear correction with simple elliptical excision.

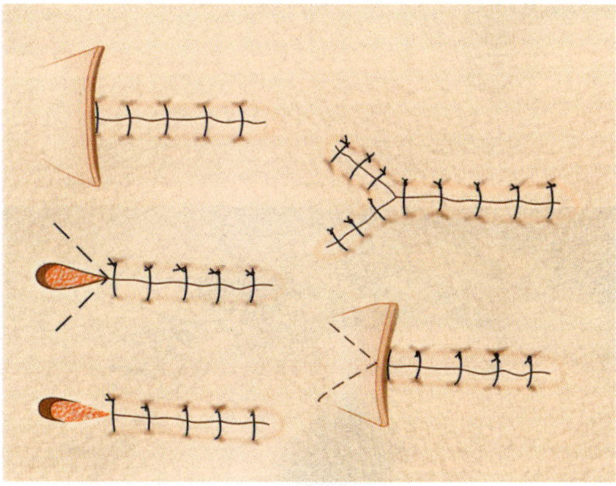

Fig. 6.15: Dog ear correction with M plasty.

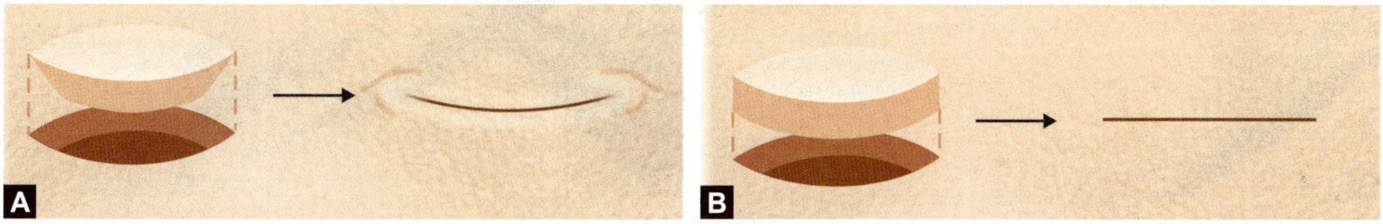

Figs. 6.16A and B: Removal of less tissue at the tips of excision results in pseudo dog ear as in (A) as compared to (B) which results in uniform flat closure.

small well-defined BCCS extend 4 mm beyond the clinical margin. Hence, 4 to 5 mm peripheral margin will increase the peripheral clearance rate to almost 95%.[15-18] Hence, it is the preferred margin for primary BCC with indolent histology. However, studies by Lalloo and Sood support margin of 2 mm for treatment of simple well-demarcated, nonrecurrent lesions in head and neck area. Ideally for recurrent high-risk BCC, Mohs surgery is a preferred option. But, if Mohs surgery is not preferred by the patient, then 5 to 6 mm margin of excision should be taken.[10]

When lesions are excised from difficult anatomical locations like nose, lower eyelid and ear: simple closure of the wound may be difficult. In such situations, flap surgery may be required to reconstruct the wider defects.

Steps (Figs. 6.17 and 6.18)

Similar to simple excision.

> **TIPS AND TRICKS**
>
> Correct orientation of specimen is necessary so that histopathologist will be able to comment on the margins on all sides.

Preoperative use of dermoscopy or loupe magnification helps in recognizing clinical margins and favors complete excision. This helps in minimizing the recurrence rate. Positive dermoscopic features are ulceration, multiple blue gray globules, leaf-like areas, telangiectasia and absent pigment network.[19]

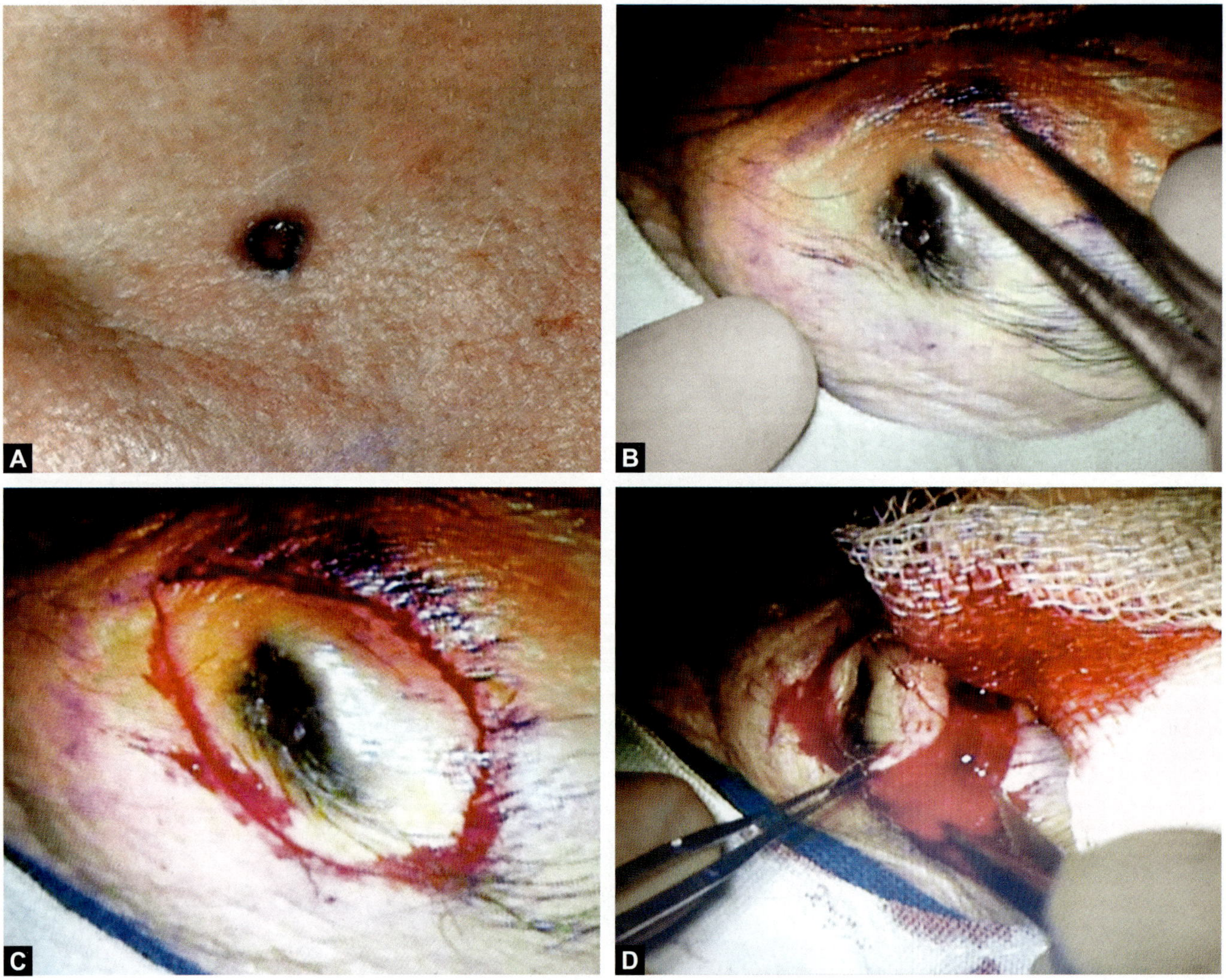

Figs. 6.17A to D

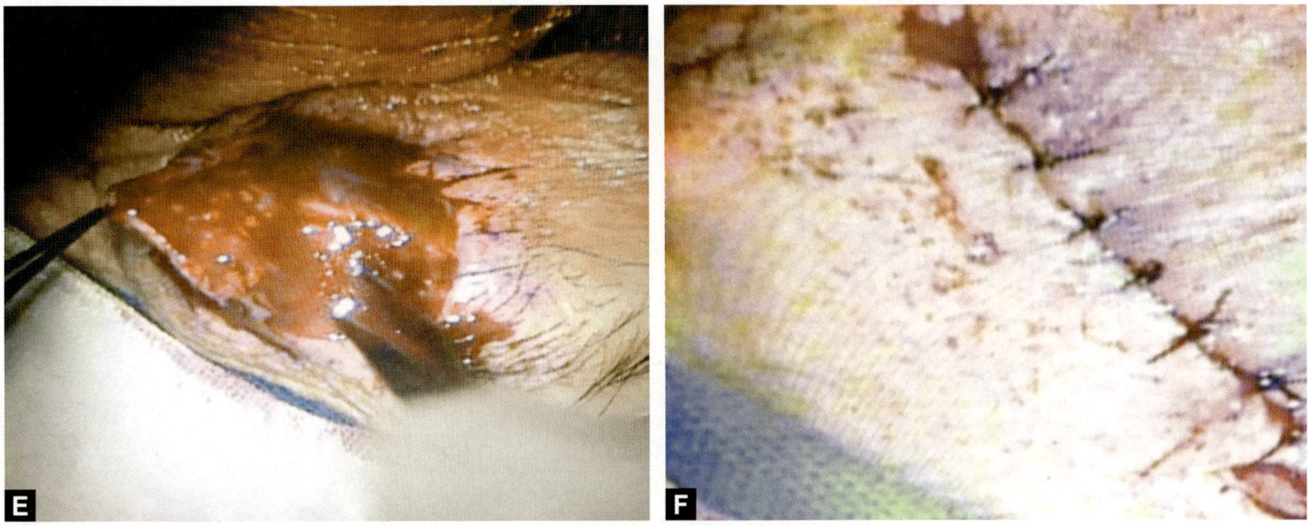

Figs. 6.17A to F: (A) Suspected pigmented BCC. (B) Ellipse planned with wide margin. (C to E) intraoperative images of elliptical excision. (F) Final linear closure of the wound.

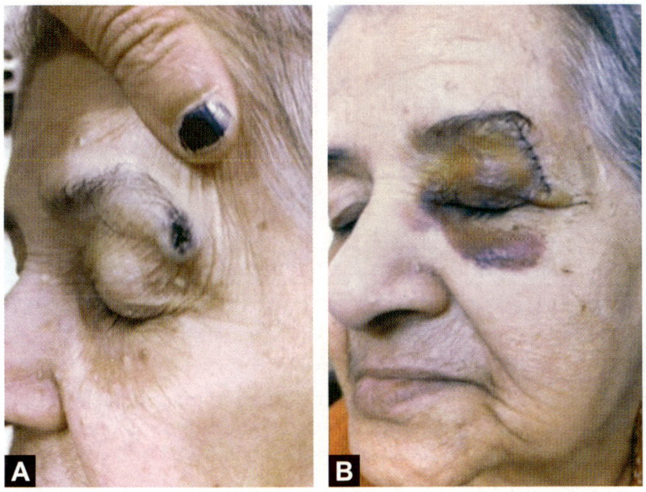

Figs. 6.18A and B: Simple excision and closure of suspected BCC. With (A) before and (B) immediately after excision.

Use of curettage prior to excision may increase cure rate by accurately defining true borders.

Preoperative biopsy to determine aggressiveness of the disease is necessary to determine the excision margin.[20,21]

Complications

- Incomplete excision and recurrence
- Disfigurement.

Conclusion

Wide local excision is a good treatment option for primary lesions, if adequate margin of excision is taken. It is necessary to take wider margin in high-risk areas like face. The resultant defect in such case is difficult to close by direct closure and to give good functional and cosmetic result, grafts and flaps may be necessary.[22]

Mohs Micrographic Surgery (Figs. 6.19A to D)

Indications[23-25]

- Recurrent lesions
- H-zone of face—ear, nose, eyelid and lips
- Aggressive growth
- More than or equal to 0.5 cm on face, more than or equal to 2 cm on areas other than face. Size more than 2 cm, unclear borders, aggressive histology
- Ill-defined borders, incomplete excision, multicentric, radiation, neurotropism, genetic syndromes with multiple tumors
- Useful for other nonmelanoma skin cancers.[26]

Principles of excision

- Examination of 100% tissue margins
- Achieve high cure rates
- Conserve the tissue.

Modifications

As against simple excision it is done in stages. Excised tumor is mapped, frozen sections are examined for tumor extent and then according to the extent, excision is performed in second stage to achieve complete excision.

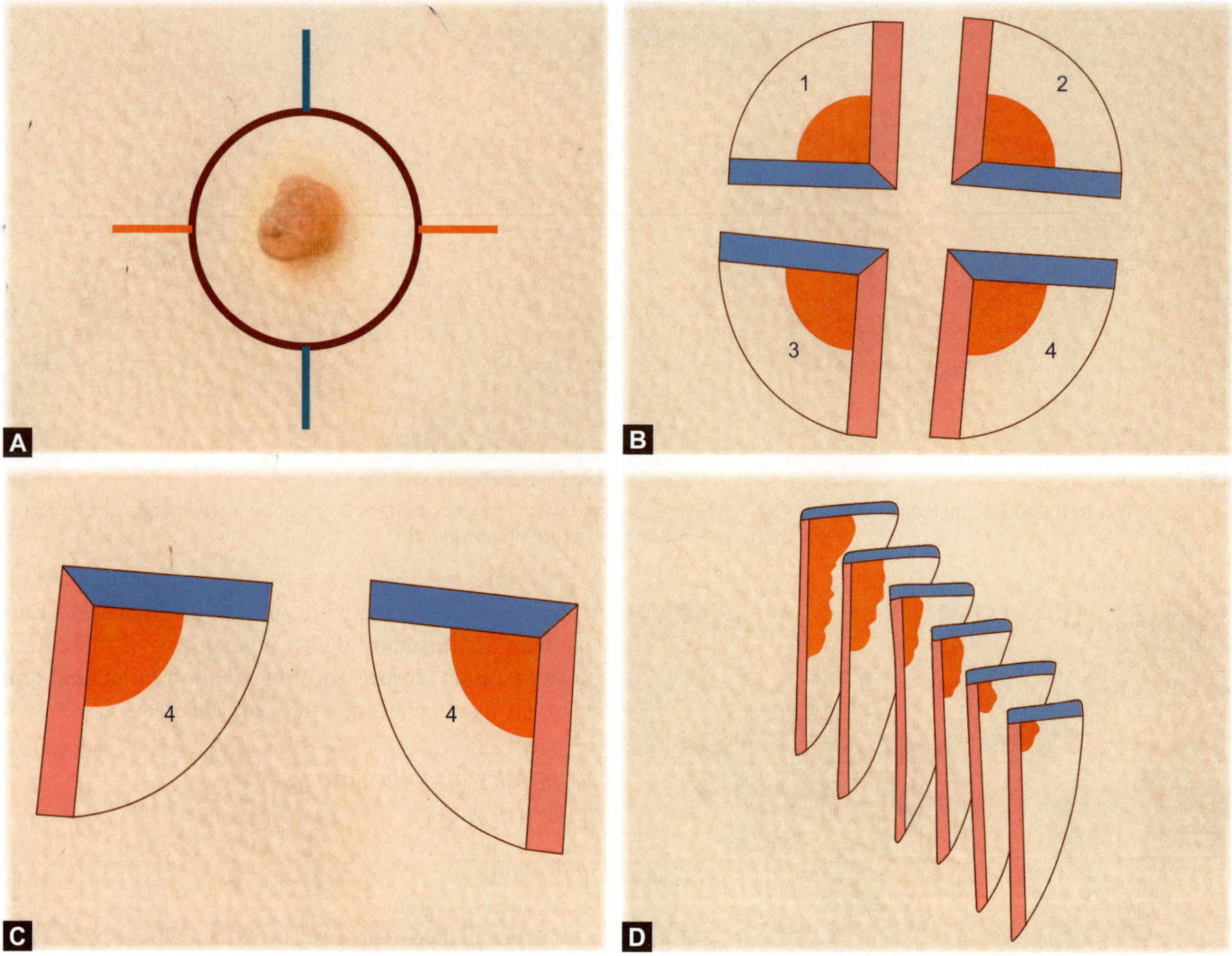

Figs. 6.19A to D: (A) Tumor marked, debulked with curette and excision done 2 to 3 mm beyond the curetted margin. (B) Marking done to preserve anatomical orientation cut into 4 pieces. (C) Specimen turned over and put in cryostat, so that epidermis and deepest margins are in one plane. (D) Frozen section is prepared, horizontal sections taken and examined after H and E staining.

Steps

- Identification of tumor, marking the margins, infiltration of local anesthesia
- Debulking with curette
- Excision is done 2 to 3 mm beyond the curetted margin with scalpel angle of 45° involving entire depth of dermis. Saucer-shaped piece of tissue is obtained. Anatomical orientation is preserved by marking with different colors. Dressing is given and patient waits for about 45 minutes
- Sectioning is done along the scored lines. Specimen is turned over and mapped to maintain the anatomical orientation
- Horizontal sections are taken, put into cryostat and examined under microscope after staining with H and E stain. The sections are prepared in such a way that epidermal and dermal margins are in the same plane.

Color Key

- Red—tumor
- Pink—vertical margin
- Blue—horizontal margin.

TIPS AND TRICKS

Use of curettage prior to excision of BCC may increase cure rate by accurately defining true borders.[15,20,21]

Complications

- Infection
- Scarring.

Conclusion

Mohs micrographic surgery allows examination of 100% of tumor margin and hence chances of recurrence are minimal. In high-risk areas where wider margins are taken it is essential to use flaps and grafts to give good cosmetic and functional results. However, for primary lesions, which are smaller in size, this technique can be labor intensive and costly. Hence, in these circumstances wide local excision can be performed after prior dermoscopic examination and prior skin biopsy to determine the extent of tumor.

Alternative Methods

Curettage and cautery, cryotherapy, radiation, photodynamic therapy, and topical imiquimod.[27]

SEBACEOUS CYST/EPIDERMOID CYST

Introduction

Sebaceous cyst or epidermoid cyst is a benign swelling with punctum on the surface occurring because of rupture of the pilosebaceous follicle. Excision is indicated, if the lesion becomes secondarily infected causing pain, or if it is of a large size in cosmetically important location, e.g face or in a location where normal body function is affected, e.g. lesion on back can be uncomfortable while sleeping. If any inflammation is noticed it is advisable to wait till it settles, as the cyst wall is friable and likely to rupture leading to incomplete excision.

Principles of Excision

- It is mandatory to completely excise the capsule to prevent recurrence
- Dead space should be properly obliterated
- Infiltration of anesthesia should be in a field block manner to avoid rupture of cyst wall while injecting
- The aim of treatment should be to give minimal scar and rapid recovery.

Types of Excision

- Traditional wide excision
- Mini hole technique.

Traditional Wide Excision

Traditional wide excision follows the principles of basic elliptical surgery. The advantage of these techniques are that they ensure complete removal of cyst wall thus preventing recurrence. However, they result in longer scar as compared to mini hole techniques (Figs. 6.20A to D).

Indications

- Cysts on face
- Large cysts which have never been infected or ruptured.

Advantages

- Entire capsule can be removed through a smaller hole facilitating faster healing
- Minimum scar
- No sutures required
- Less surgical time
- Minimum bleeding.

Disadvantages

Accidental rupture of cyst wall may lead to incomplete removal and increase chances of recurrence.

Steps (Figs. 6.21A to J)

- Field block is given using xylocaine 2% with adrenaline after taking all aseptic precautions
- Always mark lesion before infiltration, as small lesions can be obliterated after injection
- Gentle massage to facilitate diffusion of anesthetic
- Wait for 10 mins to achieve effect of adrenaline
- Small 1 to 2 mm hole is created on the surface of the cyst
- The hole is widened with artery forceps
- All the contents are expressed out giving gentle pressure
- The empty cyst wall is slowly pulled out through the hole
- The dead space is flushed with betadine and then normal saline
- Dressing is applied.

Modifications

- Use of scoop to express the contents. During accidental rupture of cyst wall, this can be a useful method

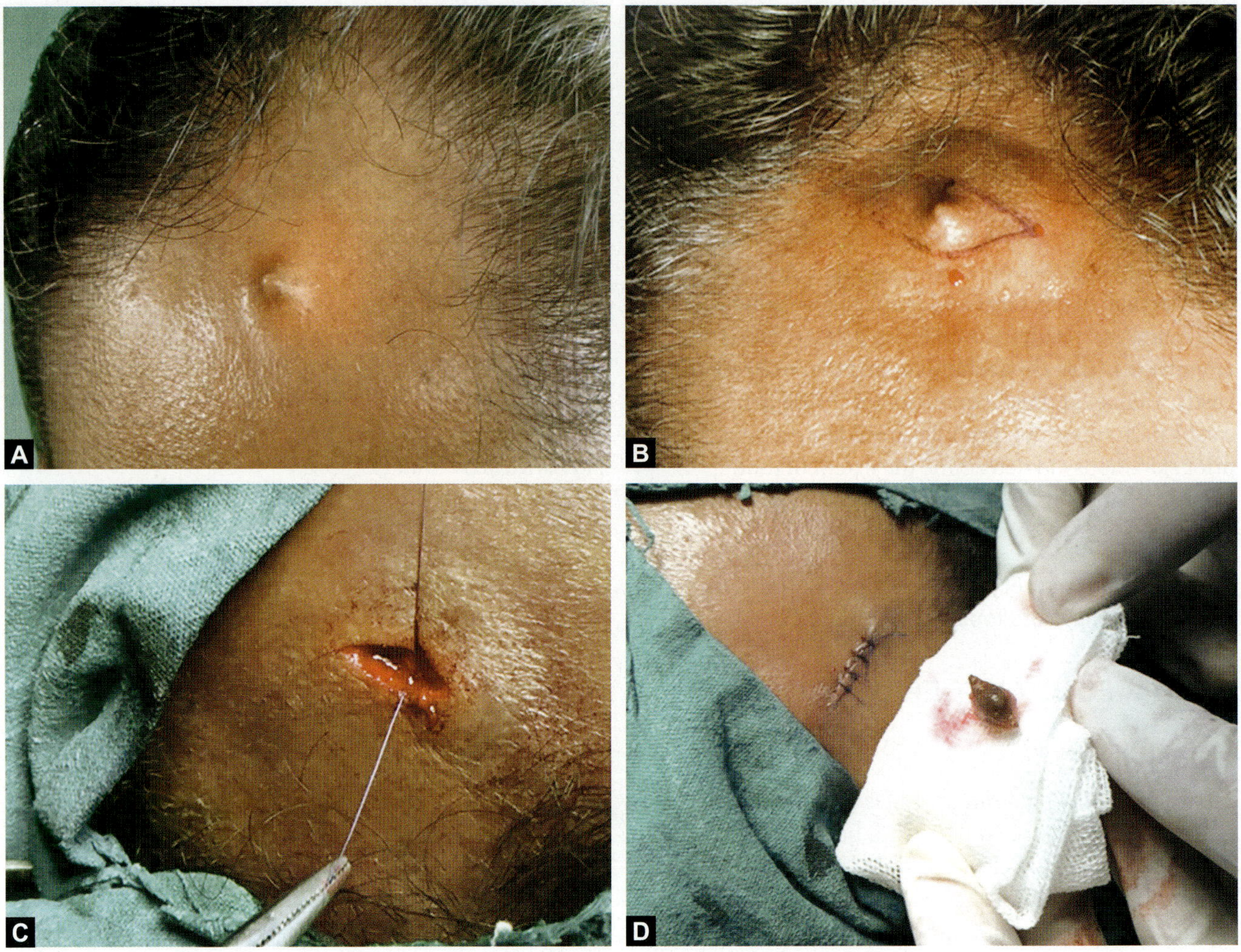

Figs. 6.20A to D: Traditional wide excision. (A) Sebaceous cyst over forehead showing punctum. (B) An ellipse planned around the punctum. (C) Excision of cyst. (D) Linear closure of wound mini hole technique.[27-30]

- Application of lateral pressure instead of vertical pressure to squeeze the contents. This can minimize the chances of wall rupture.
- Use of 2 to 3 mm punch instead of scalpel to make mini hole.
- Using the bevel of 20 gauge needle to widen the punctum
- Waiting till the inflammation subsides as the inflamed tissue is friable.[29]
- Hydrodissection (Figs. 6.22A to K) A small wedge incision is made on the top of the cyst taking care not to stab the cyst wall. The wedge is then cut away from the rest of the skin but left on the dermis intact. Using skin hook and scissors/scalpel, hydrodissection is done carefully between the cyst wall and the skin cover using the wedge as a support. The corners of the wedge can be released and the dissection continued till the cyst is delivered in toto. Advantage is that of a small scar.
- Removal by using 2 step technique.[30] This method is used as an alternative for treating uninfected cysts especially larger cysts and cysts in areas where the skin is thick. In first step the cyst contents are removed after making mini hole by using CO_2 laser. After a gap of 1 month the cyst wall is removed by minimum incision technique. The logic of removing the capsule after 1 month is that after expulsing the contents the capsule crumples and becomes small in size. This facilitates complete removal of the cyst wall, causes minimal handling and produces inconspicuous scar. Other advantages of using CO_2 laser are less bleeding, almost no chances of infection and easy manipulation during procedure.

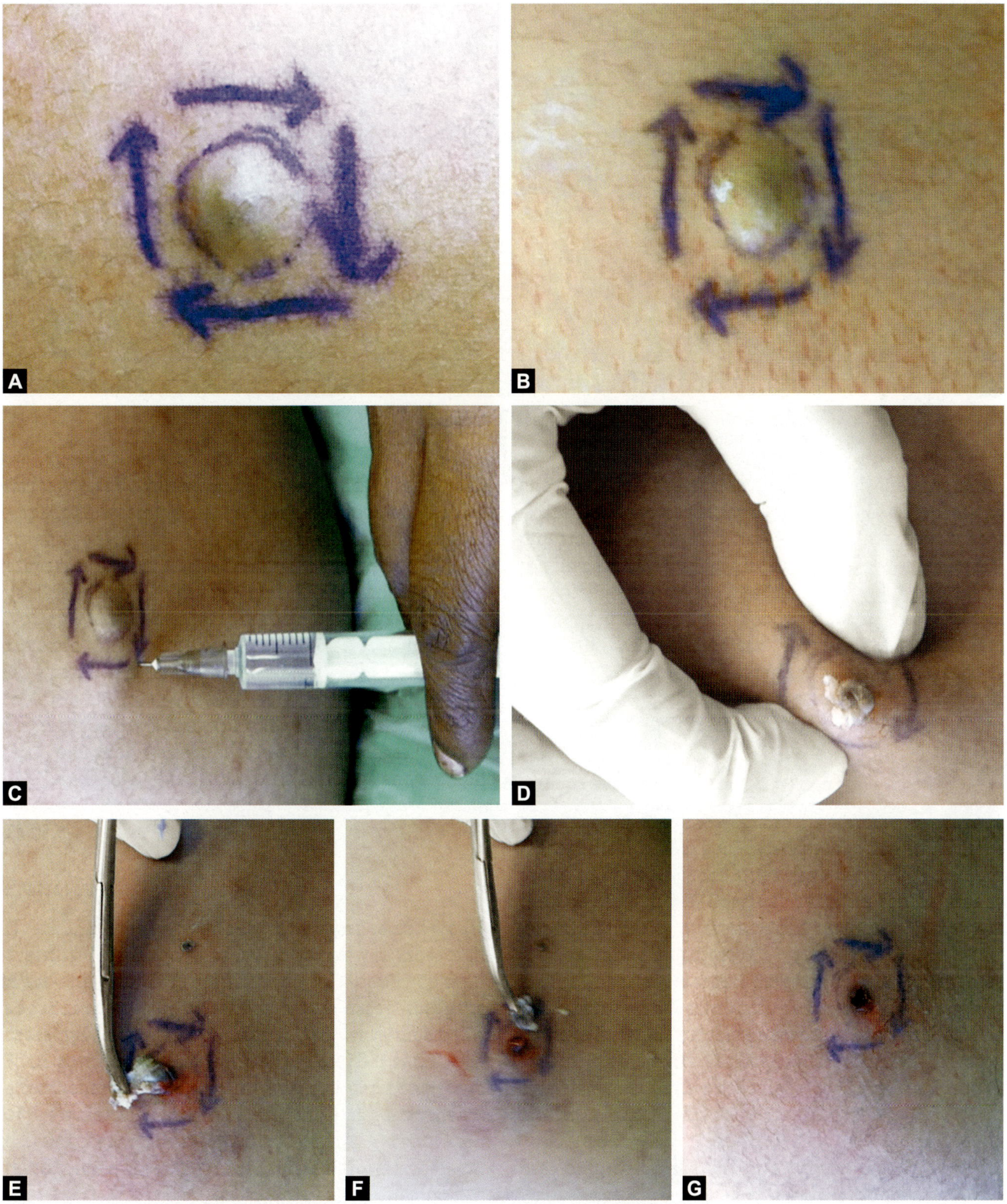

Figs. 6.21A to G: (A and B) The lesion to be excised marked and painted (C) Field block anesthesia being given. (D) Contents being expressed through the narrow hole. (E) Cyst wall held with artery and being pulled out with gentle pull. (F) Complete removal of cyst wall. (G) Minimal defect can be closed with single suture.

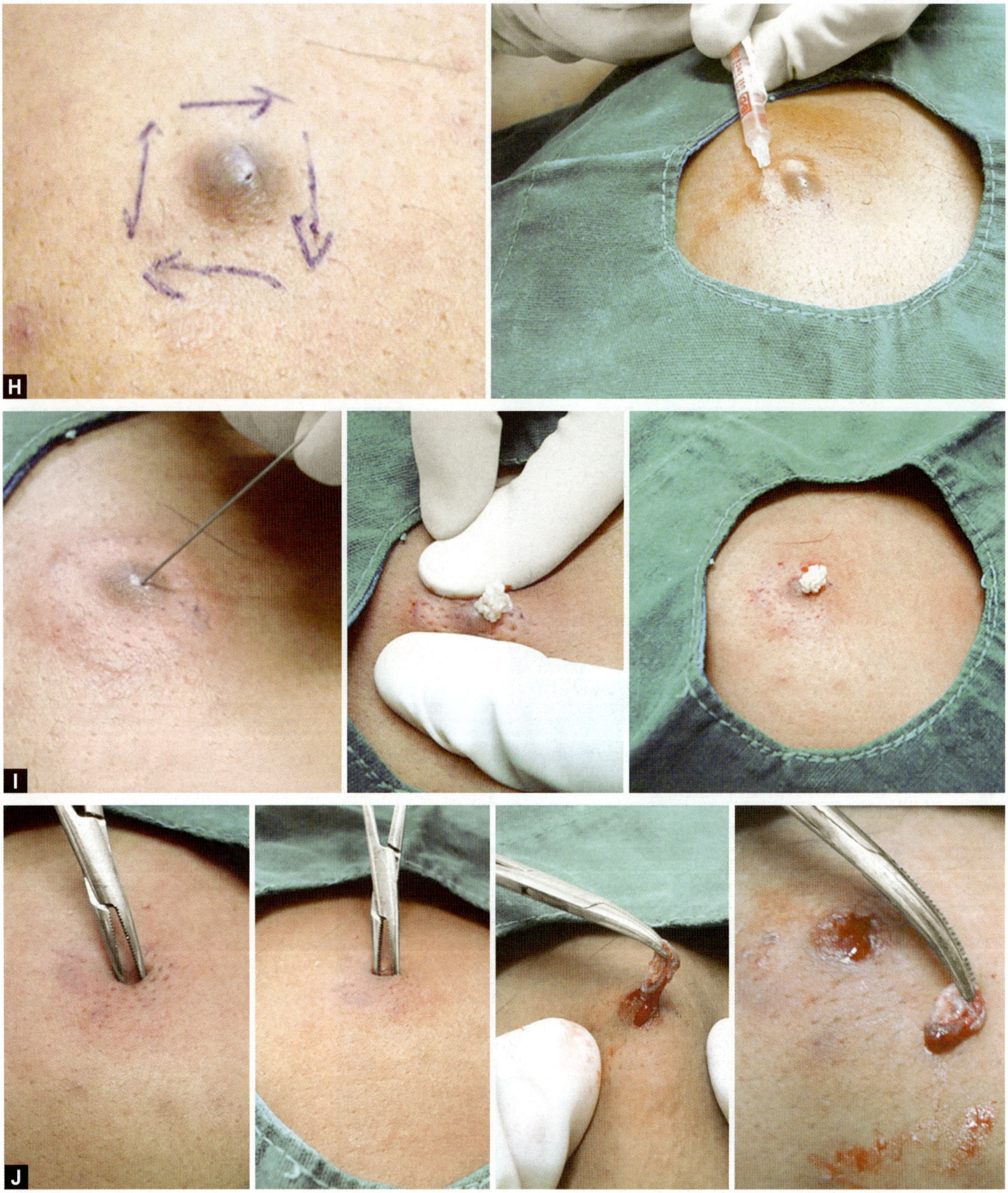

Figs. 6.21H to J: (H) Cyst margin marked and field block being given. (I) Bevel of 20G needle used to make a hole and express the contents. (J) Cyst wall being removed with artery forceps.

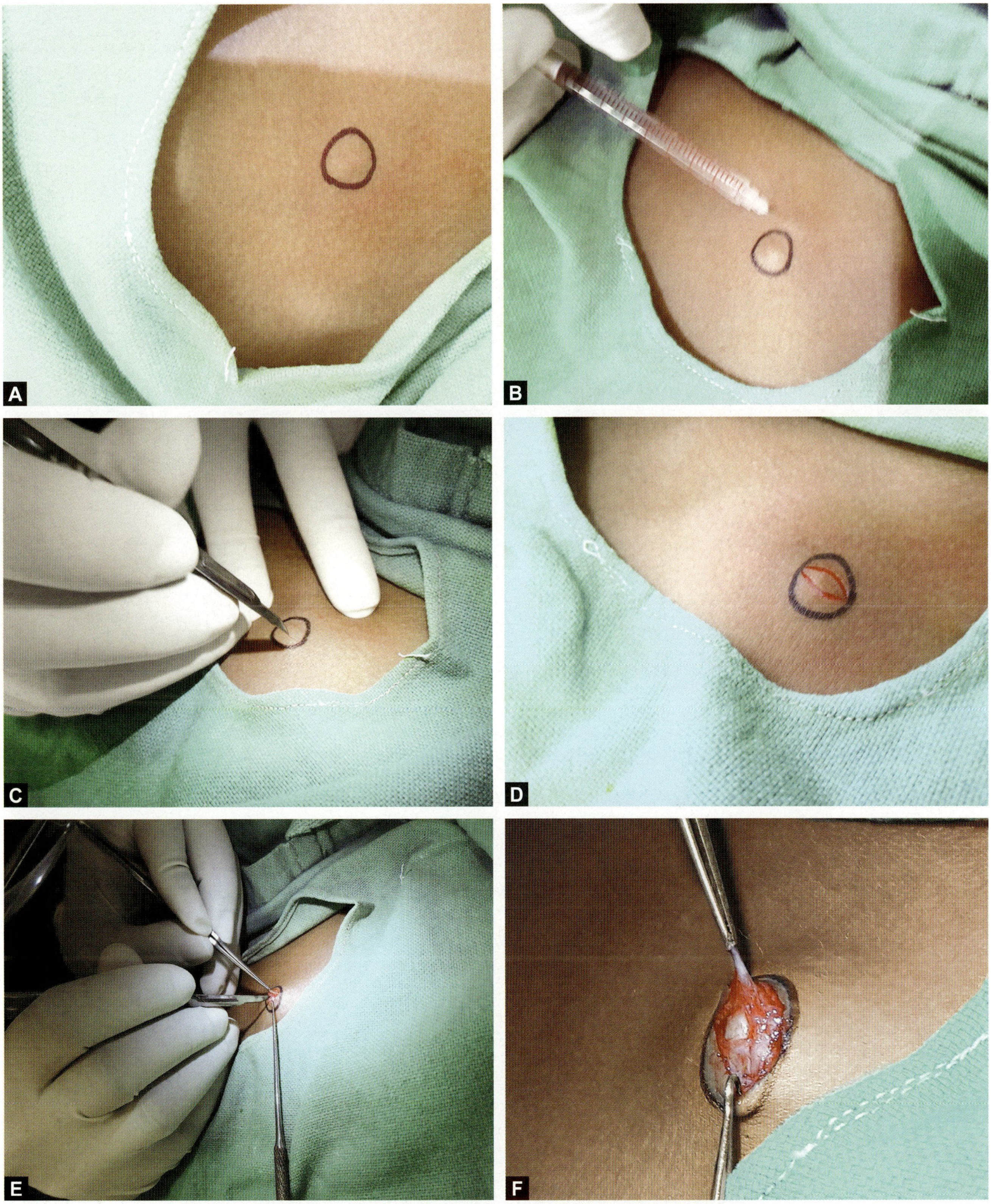

Figs. 6.22A to F: Sebaceous cyst removal by hydrodissection.

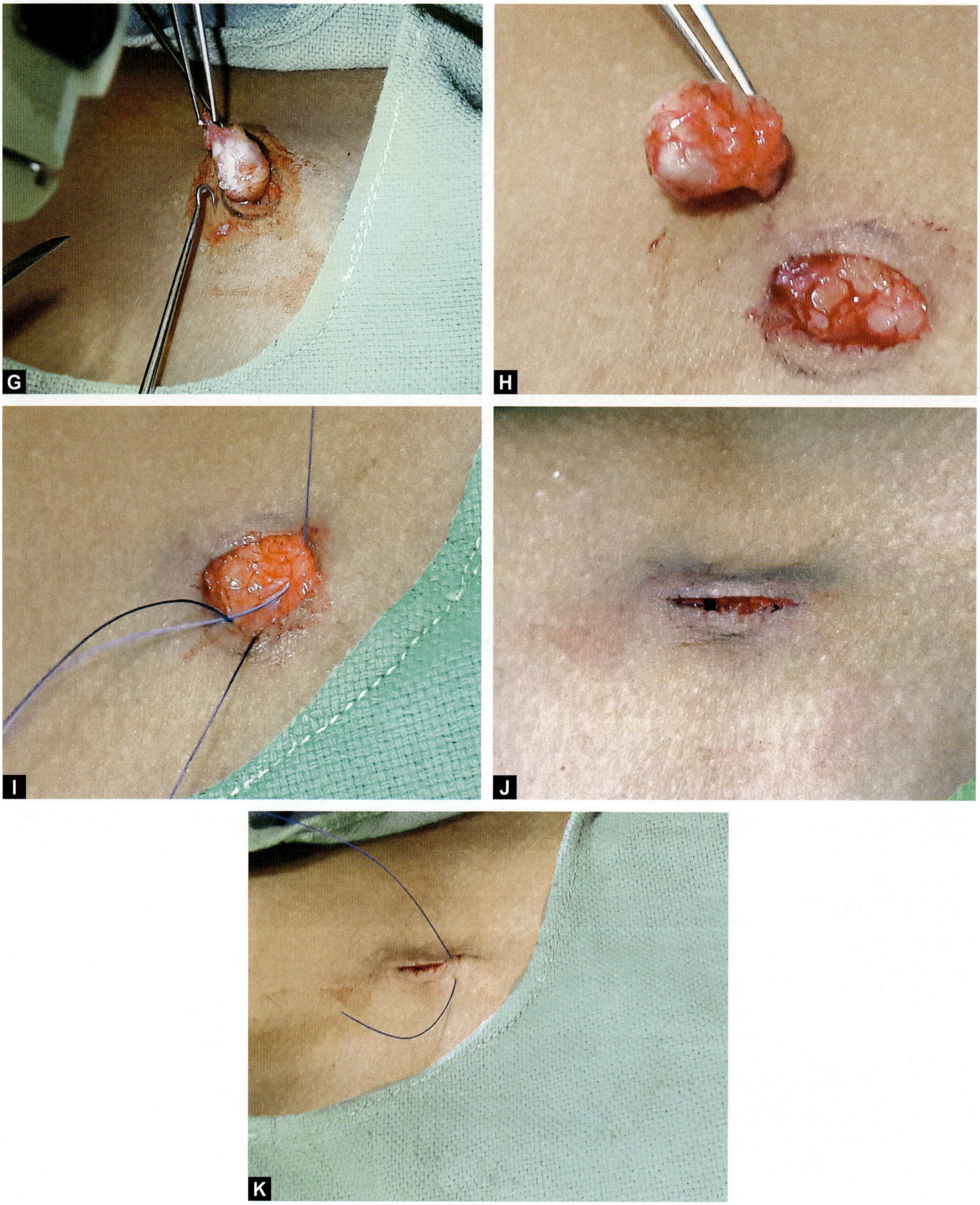

Figs. 6.22G to K: Hydrodissection of sebaceous cyst. Excision followed by suturing.

Steps

- Multiple punctures are made by using CO_2 laser to make hole 2 to 4 mm hole
- Gentle pressure is given to partially express out cyst contents
- Cavity is irrigated with 0.9% NaCl and inside wall is sterilized with povidone iodine
- Wound is sutured or glued
- After 1 month the mini hole technique is performed to remove the cyst wall

TIPS AND TRICKS

- Addition of a drop of phenol after the entire procedure to cause chemical destruction of any cyst wall remnant.
- Perilesional steroids one week before will help to localize the lesion.
- Placing of 2 iodine crystals in the center of the cyst. In next few weeks, the cyst becomes dark brown and hard and can be expressed easily from the skin.
- Taking of single suture to facilitate healing by primary intention and give a cosmetically better scar.

LIPOMA

Introduction

Lipomas are common benign soft-tissue neoplasms composed of fat cells. These tumors are often found where adipose tissue is present. They are the most common tumor of mesenchymal tissue and present as soft, immobile subcutaneous tumors that cause no symptoms, and as such, receive little attention from patients or physicians.

Solitary lipomas are classified into two types, superficial and deep seated/subfascial lipomas. Lipomas are rarely located within the muscles and between the muscles. The former is termed as "intramuscular lipoma" and later as "intermuscular lipoma." Incidence of intramuscular and intermuscular lipomas is 1.8% and 0.3% of fatty tumors, respectively.[1]

Radiolucency and poor vascularization are characteristics of lipomas on plain radiographic examination. However, lipomas with deep, large or unusual in locations and with neurovascular compression symptoms need radiographic evaluation such as MRI to identify and localize these tumors.[2]

Procedure

Preoperative Preparation

- Consent
- Photography
- Test dose.

Things to Avoid Prior to Surgery

- Alcohol, smoking
- Medication: anxiolytics, vitamin K.

Steps (Figs. 6.23A to H)[31-38]

- Part preparation
- Cleaned and draped
- Lesion outline marked with surgical pen
- RSTL is identified and marked for planned incision
- Field block anesthesia given along all margins
- BP handle no. 4 with no. 15 blade is used
- *Incision*: One half to one third the diameter of underlying lipoma—Smaller the incision, better is the cosmetic compatibility. Narrow hole extraction technique (NHET) is commonly *used the*se days, where a biopsy punch or just a stab incision with no. 11 blade can be done
- *Dissection*: Using a curved forceps, hemostasis in all directions is accomplished. Hydrodissection using normal saline or anaesthetic can be carried out.
- *Excision*: Once dissected free, a hemostat can be used to grasp the base and can be squeezed so that it can be removed in toto or in bits and pieces. If lipoma is too large incision can be extended
- *Closure*: Look out for any left out parts. Careful examination of base for any bleeders which can be cauterized accordingly. Two layered suturing to avoid dead space, inside with an absorbable suture (vicryl) and skin with a nonabsorbable sutures (prolene) perpendicular to RSTL
- *Drain*: It can be used, if dead space is more to prevent accumulation of serous fluid or hematoma formation
- *Dressing*: Topical antibiotic can be applied, followed by dry gauze application which in turn is covered by surgical pad and dynaplast with stretch perpendicular to incision.

Postoperative Care and Advice

- *Similar to* other procedures
- Frequent check for any discharge from drains, if used

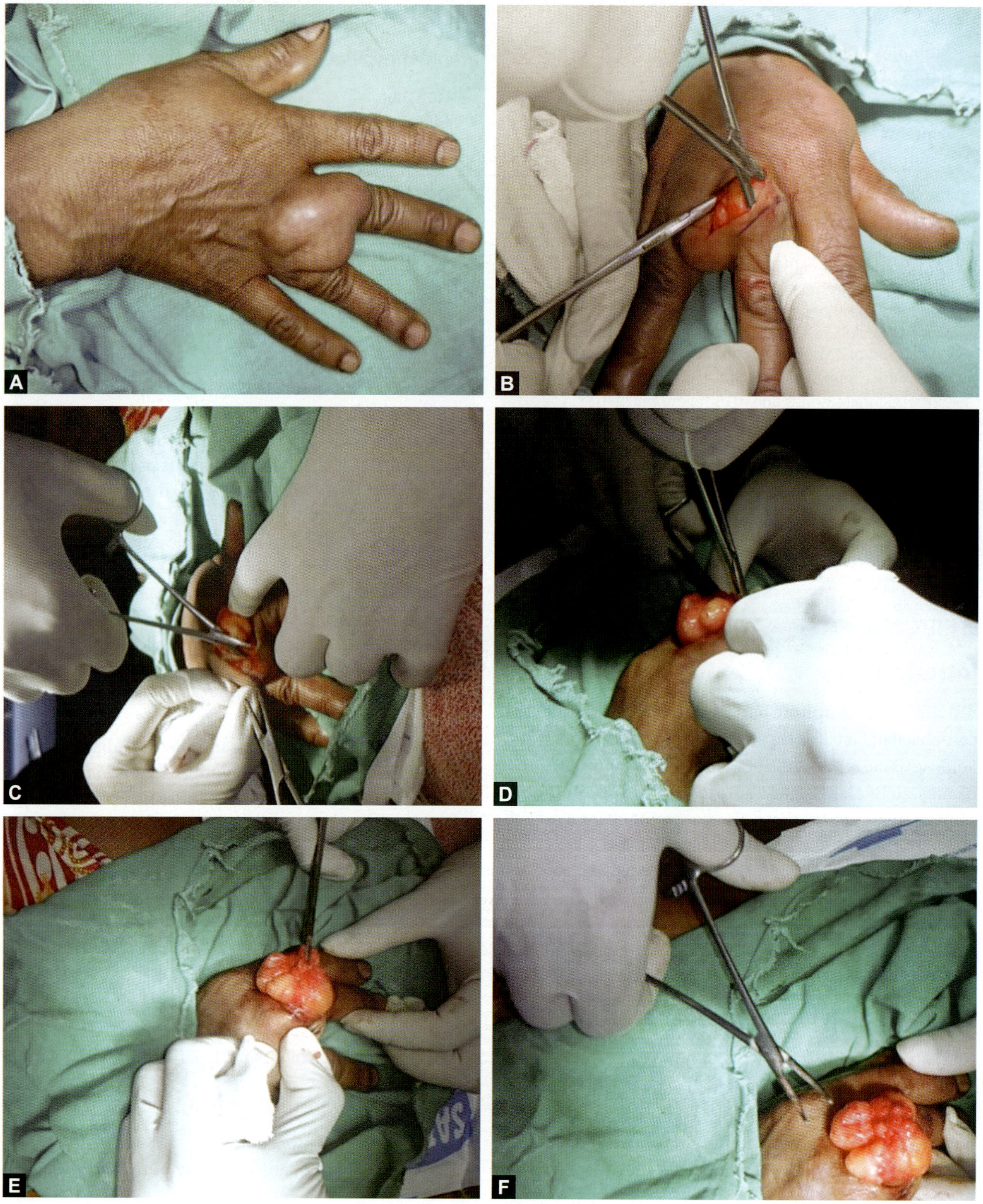

Figs. 6.23A to F

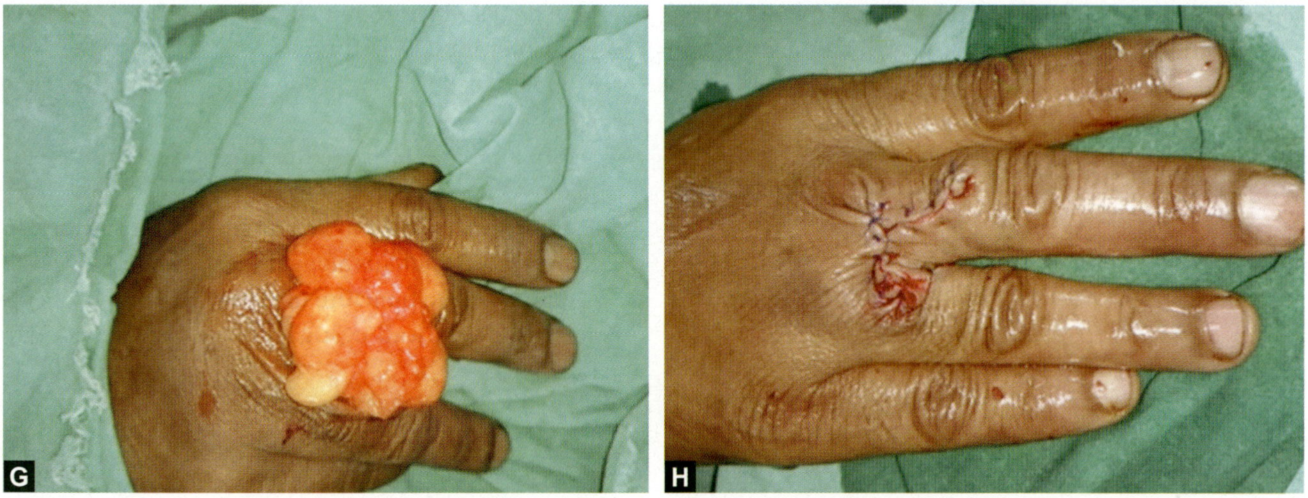

Figs. 6.23A to H: (A) A large lipoma on the dorsum of the hand. (B) A linear incision exposing the tumor. (C to G) Intraoperative images showing expressing out of tomor in totto. (H) Final closure.

- Drains can be removed after day 2 or 3
- Follow suture removal guidelines as described.

Special Situations and Modifications

Forehead Lipomas/Frontalis-associated Lipoma

Frontalis-associated lipoma arises in deeper tissue, as compared to traditional lipoma arising in subcutaneous tissue. They may arise in one of four locations: (1) within the frontalis muscle itself, (2) between the frontalis muscle and the deep investing fascia, (3) in the loose areolar tissue between the deep investing fascia of the frontalis muscle and the periosteum also called as "subgaleal lipomas," and (4) beneath the periosteum. Lipoma of forehead also can occur in temporalis muscle as infiltrating lipoma.

Removal of such intramuscular or deeper lipoma requires deeper incision onto fascia or muscle for complete excision than subcutaneous tumors. One must be careful regarding the anatomy of supratrochlear and supraorbital neurovascular bundles, frontalis muscle and aponeurosis.[3]

TIPS AND TRICKS

- When benign subcutaneous lesions in highly visible areas are excised directly, the resulting scar may be more disfiguring than the original lesion. Subcutaneous lesions can be excised through incisions located in areas that usually heal with minimal disfigurement. Incisions commonly employed in aesthetic surgery can be utilized to remove lesions of the face and breast with minimal complications and superior cosmetic results.[4]
- Marking of borders prior to infiltration of anesthesia is very important.
- Hydrodissection can fasten the excision speed.
- Finer dissection is utmost important as some times neurovascular bundles might have encapsulated lipomas; especially one has to be careful while handling lipomas on neck.
- Although clinically diagnosing lipomas are simple, FNAC should be done to confirm and document the diagnosis. In infiltrating or intramuscular types of lipoma, X-ray, CT, MRI should also be considered.
- Dead space closure is important either with double layered suturing or trimming of the lax skin in case of larger lipomas.
- Intralesional lipolytic agents have been used as mesotherapy. Following injections, 1 to 2 days erythema and edema and sometimes pain is seen. Then the lesions shrink over a period of time, however recurrence rates are very high.

Note: The injection of phosphatidylcholine (PDC) coupled with deoxycholate (DC) is a commonly studied pharmaceutical approach that has proven to be successful in reducing the size of lipomas.

STEATOCYSTOMA MULTIPLEX

Introduction

Steatocystoma multiplex is an uncommon benign cutaneous disorder. It was first described by Jamieson in 1873 and the name was given by Pringle in 1899. "Steato" and (Cyst) are Greek words which mean "fatty" and "bag". "Multi" and "Plex" are Latin words which mean "many networks".[39] This condition may be hereditary (as an autosomal dominant trait) or more commonly sporadic.[40] It usually begins in adolescence or early adult life.

Clinical Presentation

Steatocystomas can be solitary, usually multiple, recurrent, yellowish to skin-colored, dome-shaped, soft, mobile, dermal cystic papules and nodules, usually few millimeter diameter to some times bigger size, commonly asymptomatic, but might be pruritic or painful if infected.

The overlying epidermis is usually normal with no central punctum.[41] The trunk and proximal extremities are commonly involved sites, but lesions may appear anywhere, including the scrotum.[3] It can present with unusual variants: suppurative, papular, as steatocystoma multiplex conglobata or as a foreign body granuloma, and rarely, it may have a linear distribution.[42] If pricked, yellowish fluid can be expressed.

Steatocystoma is the only true 'sebaceous' cyst. It contains sebaceous lobules within the thin wall of the cyst, or it may have sebaceous ducts draining into the cyst cavity.

Differential Diagnosis

Eruptive vellus hair, multiple epidermoid cysts, lipomas, xanthomatosis, neurofibromatosis and syringomas are possible differentials.

Management

Medical line of treatment with isotretinoin has been tried with recurrences. Surgical modality with various techniques have been tried and CO_2 laser has been used to exteriorize and destroy the cysts with some success. Combination therapies have given significant results compared to individual treatments.

Surgical Techniques[43-46]

- Trepan with artery forceps
- Use no. 11 blade to incise lesions and artery forceps to remove the cystic wall
- Vein hooks with mosquito forceps
- Excision with skin grafting
- Tumor resection from inside with the frontal hairline approach
- Using a needle to puncture the cyst from one side followed by expression of its contents
- Radiofrequency used to make mini incisions to the cyst to express its contents along with its wall
- Cautery used to puncture the cyst with contents being squeezed and wall cyst gasped and extracted with forceps.

Scrotal Steatocystomas

- Puncturing and expression of contents using 18 gauge needle
- Incision with no. 11 blade followed by cyst wall removal with artery forceps
- Incision with RF followed by cyst removal with artery forceps
- Small lesions can be removed by shave excision followed by suturing
- Excisions using biopsy punches and suturing (Figs. 6.24A and B)
- Smaller elliptical incision, finer dissection and complete excision (Figs. 6. 25A and B)
- Excision followed by skin grafting
- Incision of one half, followed by dissection of cyst from below, complete excision and closure.

Tips

- Pudendal nerve block can be used, if multiple lesions have to be excised on scrotum
- Marking the borders prior to photography, if not visible
- Surgical marking prior to infiltrative anesthesia, as small lesions get masked
- FNAC confirmation and documentation.

EXCISION OF CORN

A corn or clavus is an area of well-circumscribed hyperkeratosis of the skin with a central, and often painful, keratin core which pains on vertical pressure. It is formed due to intermittent direct pressure over a limited area.

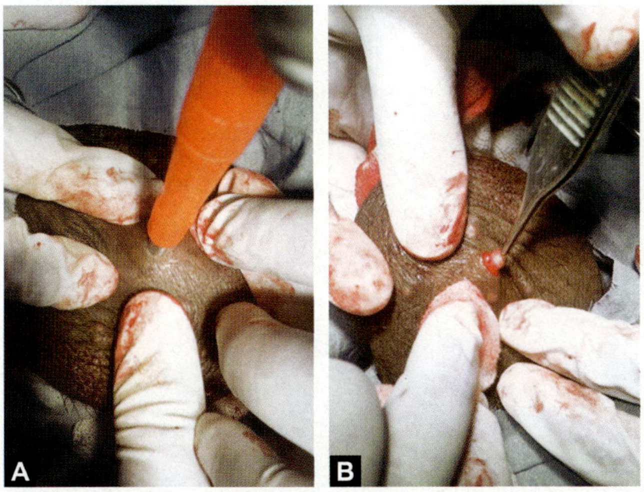

Figs. 6.24A and B: (A) Skin biopsy punch held perpendicular to skin and with gentle rotatory movement advanced downwards. (B) Lesion being excised after scoring the skin with punch.

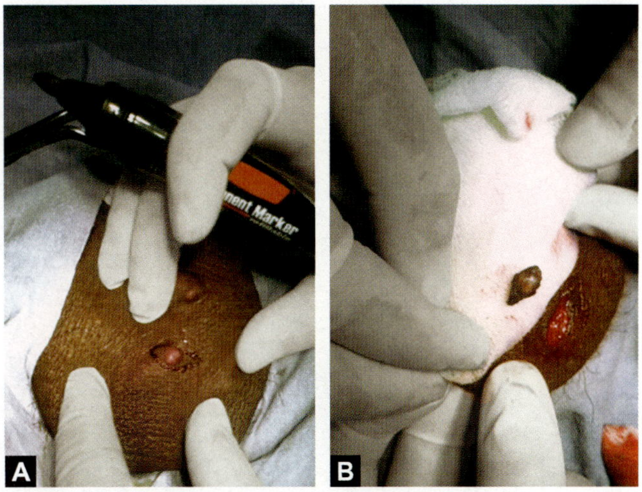

Figs. 6.25A and B: Elliptical excision and closure of steatocytoma multiplex of scrotum.

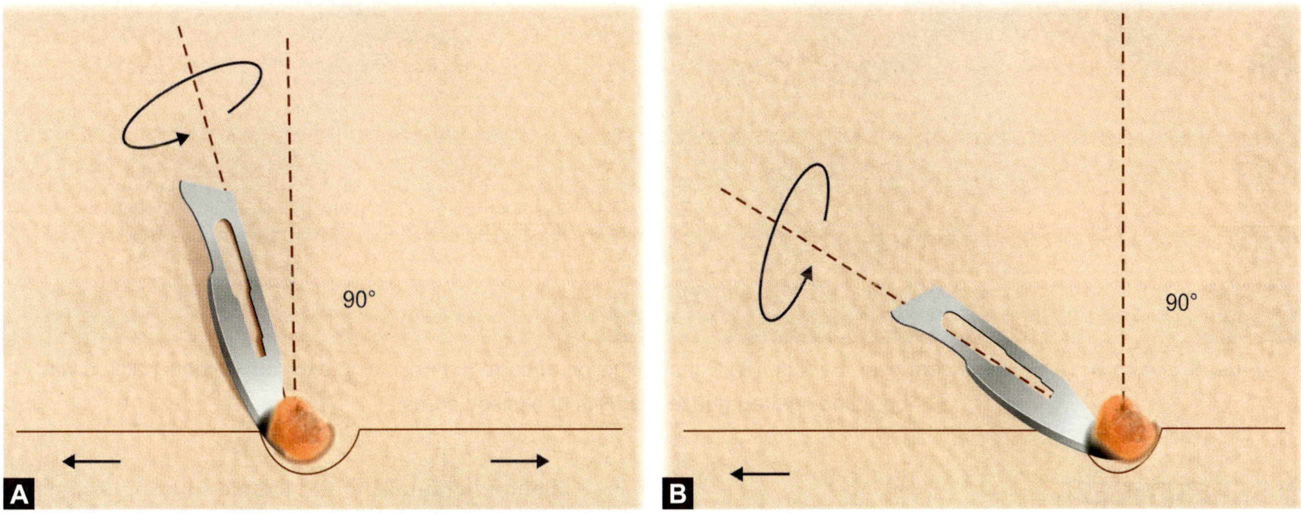

Figs. 6.26A and B: Corn excision with surgical blade.

Preoperative Evaluation

- Orthopedic problem to be corrected
- Footwear correction
- Peripheral vascular disease to be ruled out
- Blood sugar levels—to prevent nonhealing.

Step-by-Step Procedure

- 1% lignocaine is injected into the lesion and wait for 15 min.
- Corns can be excised using 11 no. blade or punch.
- With 11 no. blade incision is put along the corn margin. The blade is introduced at an angle deep to the level of corn base and rotated circumferentially to excise the cone of the corn (Figs. 6.26A and B).
- Similarly a skin biopsy punch kept perpendicular to skin surface and rotated downwards till entire cone is removed (Figs. 6.27A to D).
- The defect formed is packed with betadine soaked guaze.
- Compression dressing is provided.

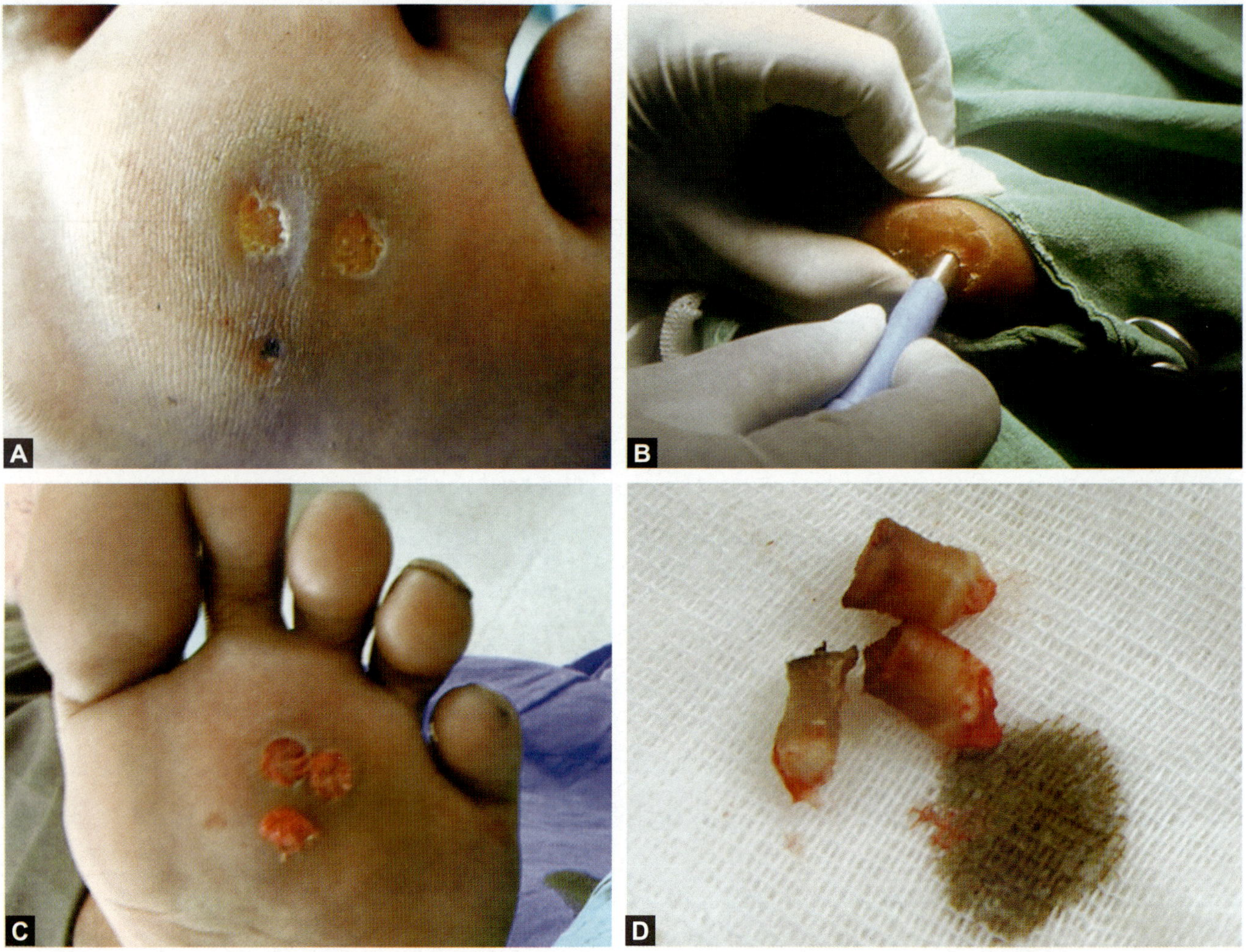

Figs. 6.27A to D: (A) Multiple corn over the foot. (B) Punch excision of corn. (C) Following excision defects packed with betadine soaked guaze. (D) Bits of excised corns.

REFERENCES

1. David W. Tumors of epidermis. In: Weedon's Skin Pathology, 3rd ed. 667-708.
2. Leboil PE, Berg G, Weedon D.WHO Classification of Tumors. Pathology and Genetics—Skin Tumors, 2003.
3. Bhide D. Simple dermatosurgical procedures biopsy, curettage and chemical cautery. ACSI Textbook on Cutaneous and Aesthetic Surgery, 1st ed. 2012; 228-44.
4. Menon RP, Crofts TJ. Teaching corner lumps and bumps: A practical guide to minor surgery for the surgical trainee. Malawi Medical J. 2014;23(2):54-7.
5. Saraf V, Raghunath S. Simple excision. ACSI Textbook on Cutaneous and Aesthetic Surgery, 1st ed. 2012; 214-26.
6. Webster RC, Smith RC. Cosmetic principles in surgery on face. J Dermatol Surg Oncol. 1978;4:397-402.
7. Goldberg LH. Cold steel surgery. The ellipse, principles and techniques of cutaneous surgery. 1996;165-70.
8. Odland PB, Murakami CS. Simple suturing techniques and knot tying. In; Wheeland RG (Ed). Cutaneous Surgery. 1994;178-88.
9. Hakverdi S, Balci DD, Dogramaci CA, et al. Retrospective analysis of basal cell carcinoma. Indian Dermatol Venereol Leprol. 2011;77(2):251.
10. Luz FB, Ferron C, Cardoso GP. Surgical treatment of BCC; an algorithm based on the literature. An Bras Dermatol. 2015;90(3):377-83.
11. Kimyai-Asadi A, Alam M, Goldberg LH, et al. Efficacy of narrow-margin excision of well-demarcated primary facial basal cell carcinoma. J Am Acad Dermatol. 2005;53:464-8.
12. Wetzig T, Woitek M, Eichhorn K, et al. Surgical excision of basal cell carcinoma with complete margin control: outcome at 5-years follow-up. Dermatol. 2010;220:363-9.
13. Bisson MA, Dunkin CS, Suvarna SK, Griffiths RW. Do plastic surgeons resect basal cell carcinomas too widely? A prospective study comparing surgical and histological margins. Br J Plast Surg. 2002;55:293-7.

14. Kumar P, Watson S, Brain AN, et al. Incomplete excision of basal cell carcinoma: a prospective multicentre audit. Br J Plast Surg. 2002;55:616-22.
15. Telfer NR, Colver GB, Morton CA. Guidelines for the management of basal cell carcinoma. Br J Dermatol. 2008;158(7):35-48.
16. Breuninger H, Dietz K. Prediction of subclinical tumor infiltration in basal cell carcinoma. J Dermatol Surg Oncol. 1991;17:574-8.
17. Wolf DJ, Zitelli JA. Surgical margins for basal cell carcinoma. Arch Dermatol. 1987; 123:340-4.
18. Kimyai-Asadi A, Goldberg LH, Peterson SR, et al. Efficacy of narrow-margin excision of well-demarcated primary facial basal cell carcinomas. J Am Acad Dermatol. 2005; 53: 464-8.
19. Nakayama M, Tabuchi K, Nakayama Y, Hara A. Basal cell carcinoma of head and neck. J Skin Cancer. doi;10.1155/2011/49610.
20. Johnson TM, Tromovitch TA, Swanson NA. Combined curettage and excision: a treatment method for primary basal cell carcinoma. J Am Acad Dermatol. 1991;24:613-17.
21. Chiller K, Passaro D, McCalmont T, Vin-Christian K. Efficacy of curettage before excision in clearing surgical margins of nonmelanoma skin cancer. Arch Dermatol. 2000;136: 1327-32.
22. Wollina U, Bennewitz A, Langner D. Basal cell carcinoma of outer nose. Overview on surgical techniques and analysis of 312 patients. J Cut Aesthetic Surgery. 2014;7;143-50.
23. Dourmishev LA, Rusinova D,1 Botev I. Clinical variants, stages, and management of basal cell carcinoma. Indian Dermatol Online J. 2013; 4(1):12-17.
24. Smeets NW, Kuijpers DI, Nelemans P, et al. Mohs' micrographic surgery for treatment of basal cell carcinoma of the face-results of a retrospective study and review of the literature. Br J Dermatol. 2004;151:141-7.
25. Roscher I, Brevig T, Mørk G, et al. Mohs surgery in basal cell carcinoma on the face. Tidsskr Nor Laegeforen. 2011;131: 2475-9.
26. Alcalay J. The value of Mohs surgery for treatment of nonmelanoma skin cancers. J Cutaneous and Aesthetic Surgery. 2012;5(1):1-2.
27. Smith V, Walton S. Treatment of facial BCC:A review. J Skin Cancer. 2011 ID 380371.
28. Zuber TJ. Minimal excision technique for epidermoid (sebaceous) cysts. Am Fam Physician. 2002;65(7):1409-12.
29. Moore RB, Fagan EB, Hulkower S, et al. What's the best treatment for sebaceous cysts? J Fam Pract. 2007;56(4):315-6.
30. Wu HL, Wang ES, Wu LJ, et al. A new procedure for treating a sebaceous cyst: removal of the cyst content with a laser punch and the cyst wall with a minimal postponed excision. Aesth Plast Surg. 2009;33:597-9.
31. Fletcher CD, Martin-Bates E. Intramuscular and intermuscular lipoma: Neglected diagnoses. Histopathology. 1988;12:275-87.
32. EgeaMartínez JM, Mena JF. Lipoma of the supraspinatus muscle causing impingement syndrome: a case report. J Shoulder Elbow Surg. 2009;18(4):e3-5.
33. Barde NG, Sacchidanand S, Madura C. Frontalis-associated lipoma: a rare case report. Indian J Dermatol. 2014;59(1): 96-8.
34. Peinert RA, Courtiss EH. Excision from a distance: a technique for removal of benign subcutaneous lesions. Plast Reconstr Surg. 1983;72(1):94-6.
35. Shemer A, Brawer S, Amichi B, Azhari H. Noninvasive lipoma size reduction using high-intensity focused ultrasound. Dermatol Surg. 2013;39(10):1446-51.
36. Self TH, Atkins D. Dramatic reduction in lipoma associated with statin therapy. J Am Acad Dermatol. 2008;58(2 Suppl):S30-1.
37. Janke J, Engeli S, Gorzelniak K, et al. Compounds used for 'injection lipolysis' destroy adipocytes and other cells found in adipose tissue. Obes Facts 2009;2(1):36-9.
38. Amber KT, Ovadia S, Camacho I. Injection therapy for the management of superficial subcutaneous lipomas. J Clin Aesthet Dermatol. 2014;7(6):46-8.
39. Borro DJ. Dictionary of Word Roots and Combining Forms. Mayfield Publishing Company: California. 1960.
40. Kaur T, Kanwar AJ. Steatocystoma multiplex in four successive generations. J Dermatol. 2003;30(7):559-61.
41. Gordon Spratt EA, Kaplan J, Patel RR, et al. Steatocystoma. Dermatol Online J. 2013;19(12): 20721.
42. Park Y, Cho S, Kang H. Congenital linear steatocystoma multiplex of the nose. Pediatr Dermatol. 2000;17(2):136-8.
43. Kanekura T, Kawamura K, Nishi M, Kanzaki T. A case of steatocystoma multiplex with prominent cysts on the scalp treated successfully using a simple surgical technique. J Dermatol. 1995;22(6):438-40.
44. Feinstein A, Trau H, Movshovitz M, Schewach-Millet M. Steatocystoma multiplex. Cutis. 1983;31(4): 425-7.
45. Duzova A, Senturk G. Suggestion for the treatment of steatocystoma multiplex located exclusively on the face. Int J Dermatol. 2004;43:60-2.
46. Choudhary S, Koley S, Salodkar A. A modified surgical technique for steatocystoma multiplex. J Cutan Aesthet Surg. 2010;3(1):25-8.

CHAPTER 7

Mole Surgery

Madura C, Pushpa KR

INTRODUCTION

Mole removal is one amongst the commonly performed dermatosurgical procedures. Mole or a melanocytic nevus is a benign cluster of melanocytic nevus cells arising as a result of proliferation of melanocytes at the dermoepidermal junction. Based on morphological and histopathological features nevi can be junctional, compound, intradermal,[1] or dysplastic (Figs. 7.1A to C). They can present as brownish black macules or papulonodular lesions anywhere on the body. Lesions often produce esthetic implications and hence mandate removal. Any recent increase in size, change of color or development of a new symptom in the mole induces fear of malignancy in patients and hence the requests for its removal. Up to 40% melanomas are associated with a precursor melanocytic nevus.[2] The single greatest predictor of risk for developing melanoma is the total number of nevi.[3] Patients also seek removal for mechanical/functional reasons but unesthetic appearance of the moles is the commonest indication for mole surgery (Table 7.1).

This chapter describes various treatment modalities, stressing on surgical techniques in stepwise manner sharing all tips and tricks to make surgical technique simple with the best esthetic outcome.

PATIENT SELECTION

Various modalities of mole removal exist and are often simple with a short learning curve. These include radiofrequency, dermabrasion, cold steel surgery and lasers (Table 7.2). Patients need to be counseled regarding the available methods, their relevance to a particular type of mole, side effects, postoperative care, resultant scar and chances of recurrence. As in any surgical procedure, informed consent should be obtained. Optimal results depend on choosing the right treatment modality and technique, based on type and site of mole, that offers both the patient and the treating physician a high degree of result-oriented satisfaction.

Extensive preoperative workup is usually not required for mole surgery. Blood investigations are done to rule out diabetes mellitus and bleeding disorders. There are no absolute contraindications for any of the techniques. As most of the procedures are for esthetic indications, procedure is deferred in case of active infection at the site or if diabetes is uncontrolled (Table 7.3). Radiofrequency is contraindicated in patients suffering from cardiac disease, patients with pacemakers and metallic prosthesis. Shave excision and punch techniques are contraindicated in suspected malignancy.

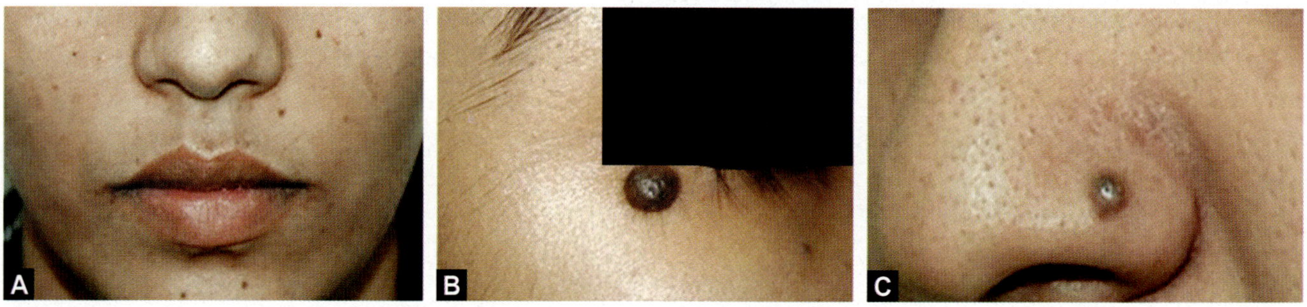

Figs. 7.1A to C: (A) Junctional nevi. (B) Compound nevus. (C) Intradermal nevus.
Courtesy: Cutis Academy, Bengaluru, Karnataka, India.

Table 7.1: Mole removal—indications.

• Aesthetic indication
• Mechanical irritation
• Suspicion of malignancy

Table 7.2: Treatment modalities for moles.

• Radiosurgery
• Cold steel surgery
• Dermabrasion
• Lasers
• Miscellaneous—curettage, cryotherapy

Table 7.3: Mole removal—contraindications.

• Active infection
• Keloidal tendency
• Bleeding diathesis
• Uncontrolled diabetes mellitus

Punch excision and grafting is contraindicated case of larger nevi, irregular nevi and lesions on mobile areas.

PRINCIPLES OF SURGERY FOR MOLES

- Method of mole removal depends on type, size, location and anticipated depth of the lesion.[4]
- An acquired melanocytic nevus should always be removed in toto to reduce the risk of recurrence and pseudomelanoma formation.
- Minimal or no damage should be done to the surrounding normal skin.
- Always try to achieve an esthetically acceptable scar.
- Any suspicion of dysplastic change in the nevus warrants excision biopsy followed by histopathological assessment (recent increase in size, ulceration, bleeding, change in color, appearance of new satellite lesions, palpable lymph nodes).

TYPES OF MOLE SURGERY

Radiofrequency Surgery

Radiofrequency is a type of electrosurgery and provides good control of tissue destruction and hence no or minimal lateral damage occurs to the skin when compared to electrocautery. It involves thermal ablation and destruction of tissue with a frequency of alternating current in the range of radio waves. It has four different modes—pure cutting, cutting-coagulation, coagulation and electrofulguration.[5] It is indicated in removal of junctional nevi, small elevated nevi, lesions around eyes, nose and mouth.

Instruments: Radiosurgical unit with tungsten electrodes (loop and pointed electrodes).

Procedure

- Topical EMLA cream is applied for 45 minutes-1 hour in case of multiple small superficial nevi and local anesthesia is achieved by infiltration of 1% lignocaine with adrenaline just below the lesion in case of deeper nevi.
- Surface of the lesion is cleaned with betadine solution and allowed to dry. Alcohol based cleansers are avoided.
- Appropriate sized probe (small tip electrode) is chosen with lower current settings.
- For small superficial lesions, the lesion is touched with pointed electrode in cutting mode and debris removed sequentially till all particles are completely removed (Figs. 7.2A and B). Cut-coagulation mode can also be used, however author prefers to use pure cutting mode as it is more precise and causes less damage to surrounding skin.
- Bigger lesions are removed using cutting or cutting-coagulation mode. The lesion is sequentially shaved from the superficial surface till its depth.
- Deep shave excision (pull through technique) can be used to remove dome shaped nevi and also dermal nevi. The lesion is ballooned with infiltration anesthesia. A wire loop electrode is anchored onto the lesion at desired depth.[4] With a single sweeping motion from one pole to another, the mole is removed in one mass. The lesion can be stabilized with forceps. No second pass is to be given. Wound heals by secondary intention, leaving behind a superficial scar.
- In case of persistence of mole, repeat radiosurgery can be done after 3 weeks.
- The advantages and disadvantages of radiosurgery are as given in Table 7.4.

Dermabrasion

Spot dermabrasion for mole removal is a less preferred and a less frequently done procedure. Mini sized, bullet or pear shaped diamond fraise dermabraders can be used

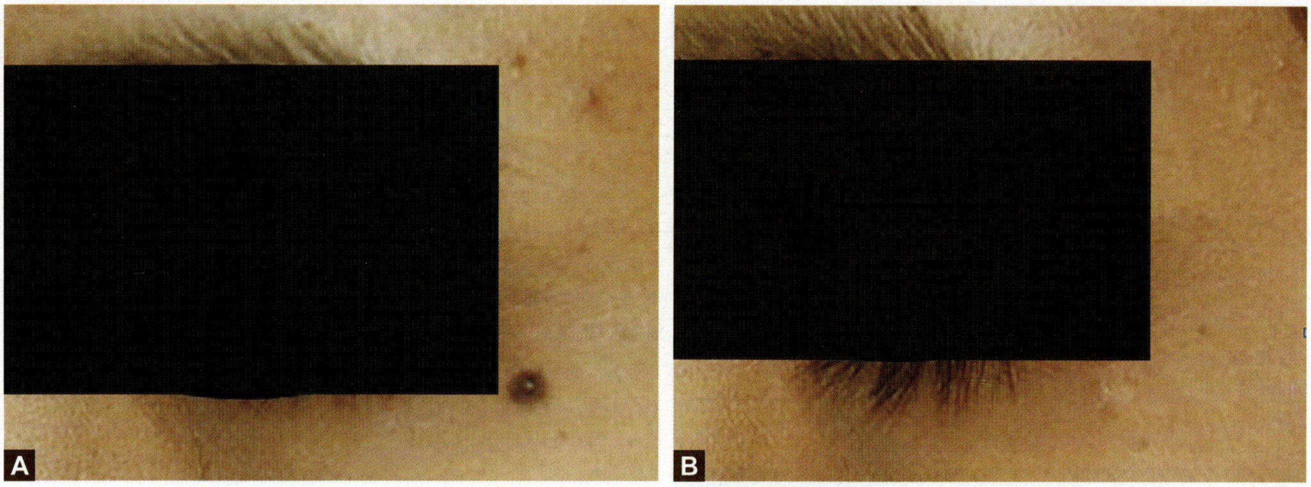

Figs. 7.2A and B: (A) Compound nevus. (B) Postradiofrequency at 3 weeks.
Courtesy: Cutis Academy, Bengaluru, Karnataka, India.

Table 7.4: Advantages and disadvantages of radiosurgery.

Advantages	*Disadvantages*
• Simple, short procedure • Ideal for small and superficial lesions (especially junctional nevi), lesions on eyelids, corners of mouth, nose and eyes • Easily available • Less tissue damage	• Pigmentary disturbances • Scarring (in case of larger lesions) • Recurrence • Cannot be used in cardiac patients with pace makers

for removal of small and superficial lesions under local anesthesia. Wound is allowed to heal by secondary intention and superficial scarring.[4]

Dermabrasion can also be used to reduce the bulk of the nevus in case of congenital melanocytic nevi awaiting surgery. It will decrease the rate of growth of nevus and thus reduce the final amount of tissue that needs to be removed. This will prevent the anatomical distortion and functional disability caused due to surgical treatment of congenital melanocytic nevi.

Cold Steel Surgery

Surgical technique is the most preferred technique of mole removal. It yields excellent cosmetic results and can be adapted for different sizes, shapes and depth of the nevi.[4]

Any nevi of more than 2.5 mm in size, dermal nevi and hairy nevi are the indications to resort to surgical techniques. The common steps are provided in Box 7.1 and various techniques are as given in Table 7.5. The size, site and type of mole, patient's preference and surgeon's skill determine the type of technique used.

Box 7.1: General steps of cold steel surgery.

- Patient needs to be counseled regarding the procedure and the resultant scar.
- Informed written consent taken for pre- and postoperative photography, local anesthesia and the surgical procedure.
- Lesion is marked with a skin marking pen before giving local anesthesia and technique of surgery decided accordingly.
- 1% lignocaine with adrenaline is injected just below the lesion and into the surrounding skin (approximately 1 cm into the surrounding normal skin).
- Operating site is painted with antiseptic and draped.

Table 7.5: Techniques of cold steel surgery.

- Shave excision
- Scissor excision
- Punch excision followed by secondary intention healing
- Punch excision and primary closure
- Punch excision and grafting
- Excision and primary closure
- Excision and full thickness skin grafting
- Excision and flap repair

Instruments: (Fig. 7.3)–No. 15 blade (excision), No. 22 blade (shave excision), No. 11 blade (circumferential excision), No. 3/No. 4 BP handle, razor blade (shave excision), Adson's toothed forceps, iris scissors, jeweller's forceps, manual metallic cylindrical punches/disposable punches of different sizes, skin hooks, blunt dissecting scissors, artery forceps, needle holders, 5-0 vicryl, 5-0/6-0 prolene (on face).

Shave Excision

Shave excision is always a deep shave excision (saucerisation) in case of mole removal. According to author, recurrence is more with superficial shave excision and hence not described here.

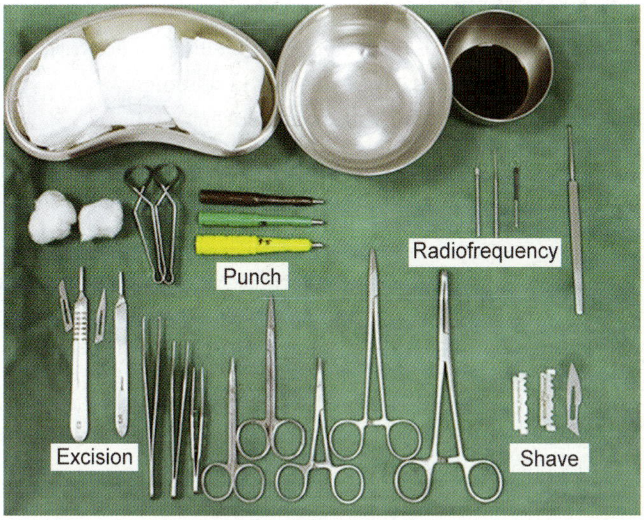

Fig. 7.3: Instruments used in radiosurgery and cold steel surgery.

Indications: Dome shaped nevi on flat surfaces like cheek, lesions on curved surfaces like nasolabial fold,[4] nose-cheek junction, mental crease (razor blade can be used) and lesions in esthetically important areas.

Procedure

- General steps of preparation 1–5 as mentioned earlier (*see* Box 7.1)
- Local anesthetic agent or normal saline is injected below the lesion to elevate it.
- The nevus is pinched up between the thumb and index fingers of the left hand.
- The perimeter of the mole is marked by scoring a very superficial incision with 11 or 15 number blade.
- Cutting edge of the scalpel blade (22/15 number blade based on size of nevi) is inserted horizontally through the incision.
- The blade is aligned to 30–45 degrees to the skin surface. With sweeping to and fro motion the lesion is cut from one pole to the other pole without slicing the normal skin (Figs. 7.4 and 7.5)
- Hemostasis is achieved by pressure and wound dressed with antibiotic ointment.[6]

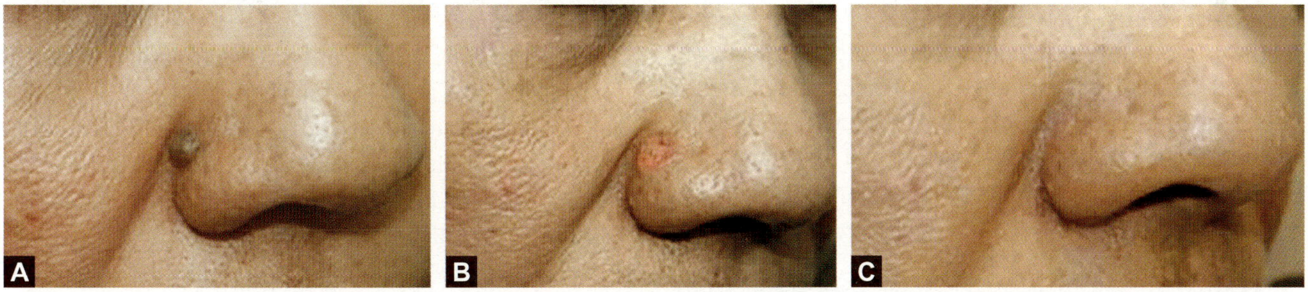

Figs. 7.4A to C: Shave excision. (A) Compound nevus. (B) After excision. (C) 8 weeks postexcision.
Courtesy: Cutis Academy, Bengaluru, Karnataka, India

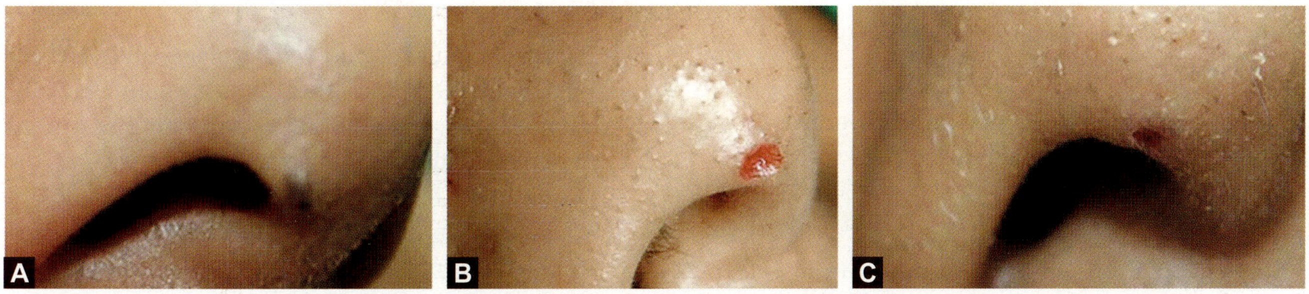

Figs. 7.5A to C: Punch excision of smaller nevus over nose. (A) Before. (B) After punch excision. (C) 5 days postexcision.
Courtesy: Cutis Academy, Bengaluru, Karnataka, India

Table 7.6: Advantages and disadvantages of shave excision.

Advantages	*Disadvantages*
Less skillful Lesser chance of scarring	Not useful in case of suspicion of malignancy, nonintact lesions Local indentation Depressed scar (in case of deep lesions)

Box 7.2: General steps of punch excision surgery.

Cylindrical punch of appropriate size which snuggly fits into the mole, encompasses it all around its circumference and accommodates the entire lesion is chosen before injecting local anesthesia

General steps of preparation 1–5 as mentioned earlier are carried out (*see* Box 7.1)

Advantages and disadvantages of Shave excision are provided in Table 7.6.

Scissor Excision

A pedunculated nevus can be snipped off at its stalk with iris scissors under local anesthesia. Hemostasis is achieved either by compression or with radiofrequency. Wound is left to heal by secondary intention and dressed with antibiotic ointment.

Punch Excision Surgery

Punch excision surgery is a simple and easy to master technique of mole removal. It is useful for removal of elevated nevi and nevi extending into subcutaneous tissue.[7] There are three techniques of punch excision surgery where a cylindrical metallic punch is used to make incision.

- Punch excision followed by secondary intention healing
- Punch excision and primary closure
- Punch excision and grafting

Manual metallic cylindrical punch with sharp edges used in skin punch biopsy is the key instrument in this technique (Box 7.2). Depending upon the size and depth of the lesion, punch of appropriate size is chosen.

Punch Excision Followed by Secondary Intention Healing

Indications: junctional nevi, nevi on concave areas like nose, ear, eye, temple, nevi ≤ 2 mm in size.

Procedure (Table 7.7, Figs. 7.4 and 7.5)

- Cylindrical punch is fitted onto the lesion, held perpendicular to the surface and the surrounding skin is stabilized by nondominant hand.
- Once stabilized, punch is driven through with rotatory movements in clockwise direction till the level of subcutaneous fat (a feel of giving away) to include the bulb of hair follicles, if any.
- If the mole is superficial, then scoring is done up to reticular dermis only.
- Nevus appears to float in the surrounding skin and is lifted up using iris toothed forceps and the base is cut using iris scissors. Wound is inspected for any leftover specks of mole which are cut using iris forceps and scissors.
- Hemostasis is achieved by pressure.
- Antibiotic ointment based pressure dressing is done. The lesion heals by secondary intention to leave slightly depressed scar.

Punch Excision and Closure

Melanocytic nevi less than 4.5 mm in size can be removed by punch excision and closure technique.

Indications: Lesions >2.0 mm and <4.5 mm in size on face, neck or elsewhere.

Procedure

- General steps of preparation as in Box 7.2.
- Cylindrical punch is fitted onto the lesion, held perpendicular to the surface and the nondominant hand stretches the surrounding skin perpendicular to the RSTL lines (Figs. 7.6A to C)
- Once stabilized, punch is driven through with rotatory movements in clockwise direction till the level of subcutaneous fat (a feel of giving away) to include the bulb of hair follicles, if any.
- Nevus appears to float in the surrounding skin and is lifted up using iris toothed forceps and the base cut using iris scissors (Fig. 7.6D). Wound is inspected for any leftover specks of mole/hair follicle, which are cut using iris forceps and scissors. Hemostasis is achieved by pressure.
- The circular punch defect will become slightly oval and align along RSTL lines after about 10 min (Fig. 7.6E). Using scalpel blade no.11/15 undermining is done circumferentially into the surrounding normal skin. This also facilitates its alignment along RSTL and lessens the wound tension. The wound is then easily closed in single layer with nonabsorbable suture material (prolene 6-0 for face/5-0 for lesions elsewhere), using simple interrupted sutures (Fig. 7.6F).

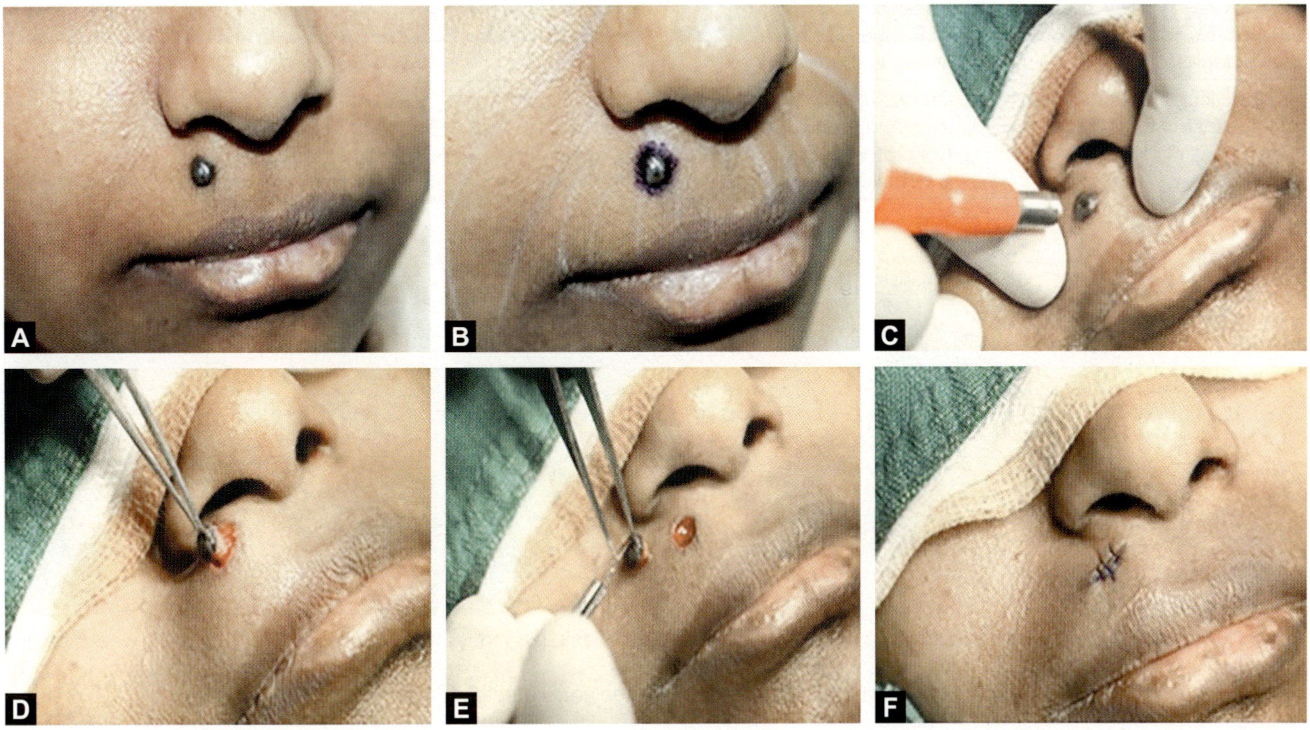

Figs. 7.6A to F: Steps of punch excision. (A) Compound nevus over upper lip. (B) Marking the RSTLs in the anatomic region. (C) Stabilising the surrounding skin by stretching the skin perpendicular to RSTL. (D) Excision of the nevus with the punch. (E) Wound bed after excision. (F) Suturing along RSTL.
Courtesy: Cutis Academy, Bengaluru, Karnataka, India

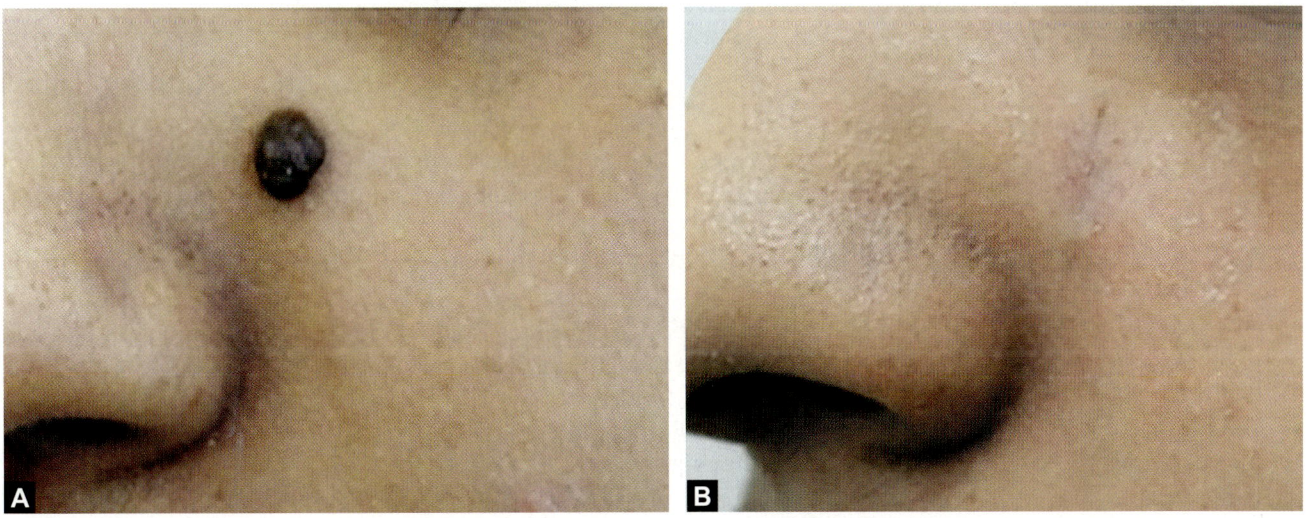

Figs. 7.7A and B: Punch excision and closure scar.

- If any dog ear formation occurs, it needs to be corrected. It is common while using punches of more than 4.5 mm.
- Antibiotic ointment is applied and dressing is done with steristrip. Dressing is removed on day 3. Suture removal can be done after 6 days on face. It heals with linear esthetically good scar (Figs. 7.7A and B).

Advantages and disadvantages of punch excision and closure are given in Table 7.8

Table 7.7: Punch excision followed by healing.

Advantages	*Disadvantages*
Less skillful, less time consuming Simple instruments required Scarring is minimal	Cannot be adopted to all sites and for bigger lesions Recurrence, if optimal care is not taken

Table 7.8: Punch excision and closure.

Advantages	*Disadvantages*
Simple, short procedure Minimal instruments required	Skill of suturing required Dog ear formation Recurrence Perilesional skin not available for analysis

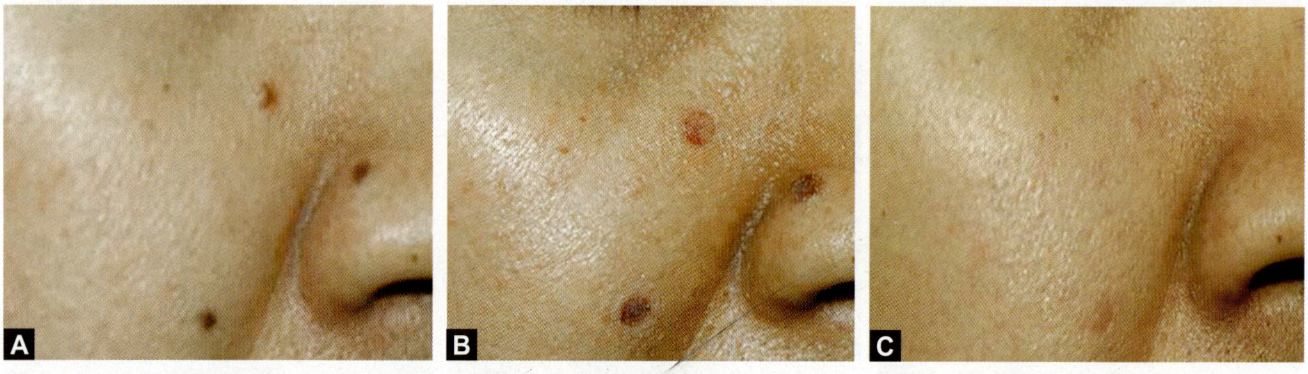

Figs. 7.8A to C: Punch excision and grafting. (A) Three nevi over right cheek. (B) 7 days after punch grafting (C) After 3 weeks healed excellently.
Courtesy: Cutis Academy, Bengaluru, Karnataka, India

Punch Excision and Grafting

Indications: Small superficial moles which extend up to papillary-reticular dermis junction, between 2 and 4 mm in size (sometimes up to 5 mm) on relatively less mobile areas like nose give good results, but it can be done elsewhere on face also.

Donor site: Postauricular area.

Procedure

- Nevus excised following the steps of punch excision (steps 1–4 as mentioned in the previous section)
- Same punch used to excise the nevus is used to harvest a circular graft from postauricular area. Scoring is done till the level of mid dermis.
- The harvested graft is then placed onto the recipient bed using small jewellers forceps after achieving hemostasis.
- Fat and any extradermis is trimmed from the base, so that the graft is exactly in level with the surrounding normal skin
- Graft is secured using cyanoacrylate glue. Glue is applied in 2 layers over the junction of graft and normal skin with a gap of 1–2 minutes in between.
- Smaller grafts can be secured by steri strip alone.

Table 7.9: Punch excision and grafting.

Advantages	*Disadvantages*
Simple procedure Less time consuming Better cosmetic results	Not useful in case of larger nevi, nevi over mobile areas

- Bigger grafts need to be secured with stay sutures (6-0/5-0 prolene)
- Antibiotic ointment based pressure dressing for larger lesions and steri strip dressing for smaller lesions are employed.
- Dressing is removed on day 5, it heals excellently (Figs. 7.8A to C).

Advantages and disadvantages of punch excision and grafting are given in Table 7.9.

Excision and Closure Surgery

Excision and closure, one of the basic dermatosurgical skills is the gold standard technique for mole removal.

Types

- Elliptical excision and closure
- Circumferential excision and closure

Indications: nevi > 4.5 mm in size, nevi over cosmetically important areas and lesions with suspected malignancy.

Box 7.3: Principles of elliptical excision.

- Long-axis of the ellipse should be placed parallel to RSTL.
- The length: width ratio of the ellipse should be 3:1 or 4:1 (Fig. 7.9A)
- Incisions should be placed taking into consideration the cosmetic units, parallel to/oblique to the free margins, in major skin folds like nasolabial fold, or in a permanent wrinkle (Fig. 7.9B)
- Repeated passes with scalpel blade should be avoided during incision to prevent 'staircasing' effect.
- Shape of the ellipse is altered according to the configuration of the lesion, it can be tangent to circle or fusiform.
- Free margin of 1–2 mm for benign lesions and 3–10 mm for malignant lesions is included along with the lesion.
- Defect should be of uniform depth both in the center and at the ends, scooping should be avoided.

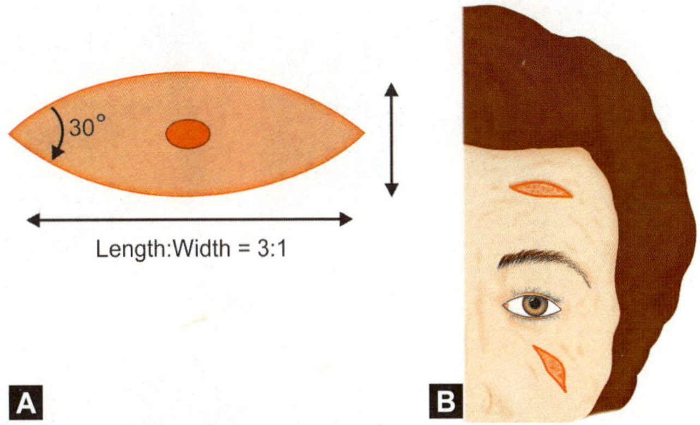

Figs. 7.9A and B: (A) Length:width ratio in elliptical excision. (B) Incision lines along RSTL.

Elliptical Excision and Closure[8] (Box 7.3)

Instruments: No. 3 BP handle, scalpel blade no.15, Adson's toothed forceps, skin hooks, iris scissors, blunt dissecting scissors, artery forceps, needle holder, 4-0 vicryl, 5-0/6-0 prolene, marking pen.

Preoperative workup to rule out diabetes mellitus, any bleeding disorders.

Procedure

- Written informed consent is taken after proper counseling regarding the procedure and the resultant scar (lengthier than the original lesion).
- Prior to giving local anesthesia an ellipse is marked, so as to enclose the nevus at the center of it.
- Lignocaine 1% with adrenaline is infiltrated subcutaneously as a field block and below the lesion.
- After stretching and stabilizing the skin with left hand, incision is made along the marked ellipse with 15 no blade perpendicular to the surface as a single pass from one apex to the other till the level of subcutaneous tissue.
- After incising, tissue at one end is grasped with forceps or skin hook and the base transected below the level of nevus by undercutting the tissue with scissors or scalpel.
- Undermining is done using blunt scissors or artery forceps for atleast 5–15 mm along the entire margin.
- Hemostasis is achieved with pressure.
- Wound is closed in two layers—deep buried interrupted intradermal sutures with absorbable 5-0 vicryl and percutaneous simple interrupted sutures with 5-0/6-0 nonabsorbable prolene sutures.
- If planning is proper dog ears never occur.
- Antibiotic based pressure dressing is applied which is removed on 2nd day. Suture removal is done on 7th day. It heals with esthetically superior scar (Figs. 7.10 and 7.11)

Modifications of elliptical excision like crescentic excision, S-plasty, M-plasty or diamond shaped incision is done depending on the size of the lesion and its location. Advantages and disadvantages of the procedure are provided in Table 7.10.

Circumferential Excision and Closure

Indications: larger moles in regions of skin where RSTL are not that apparent.

Procedure

- General steps of preparation as mentioned in Box 7.1.
- With scalpel blade no. 15/no. 11, perpendicular incision is made along the marked periphery of the lesion (Fig. 7.12A).
- Incision is extended till the base of the lesion all around (Fig. 7.12B).
- Lesion is lifted up with iris toothed forceps and cut at the base, using scalpel blade or iris scissors.
- Hemostasis achieved.
- Wound is undermined using scalpel blade all along the margins and wait for 5–10 minutes, so that it stretches along the RSTL
- Intradermal stitch is put with absorbable suture like vicryl 5-0 to decrease wound tension. If any dog ear occurs, correction is done and then sutured.

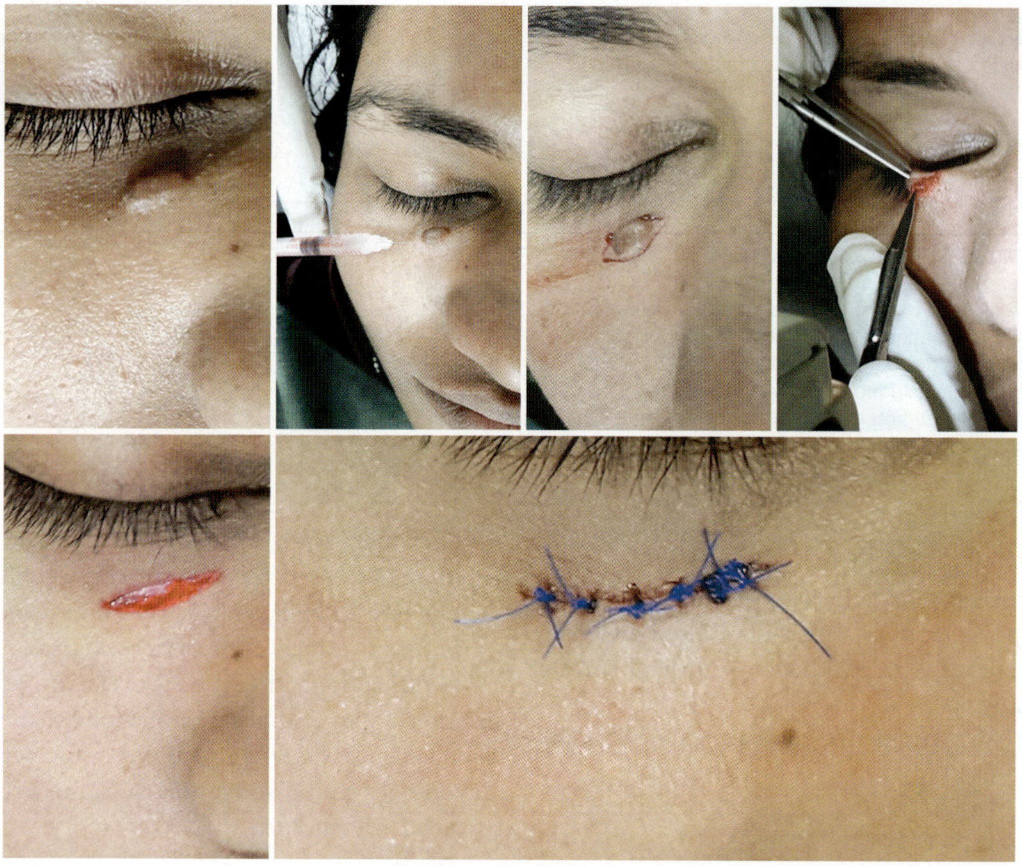

Fig. 7.10: Steps of excision and suture.

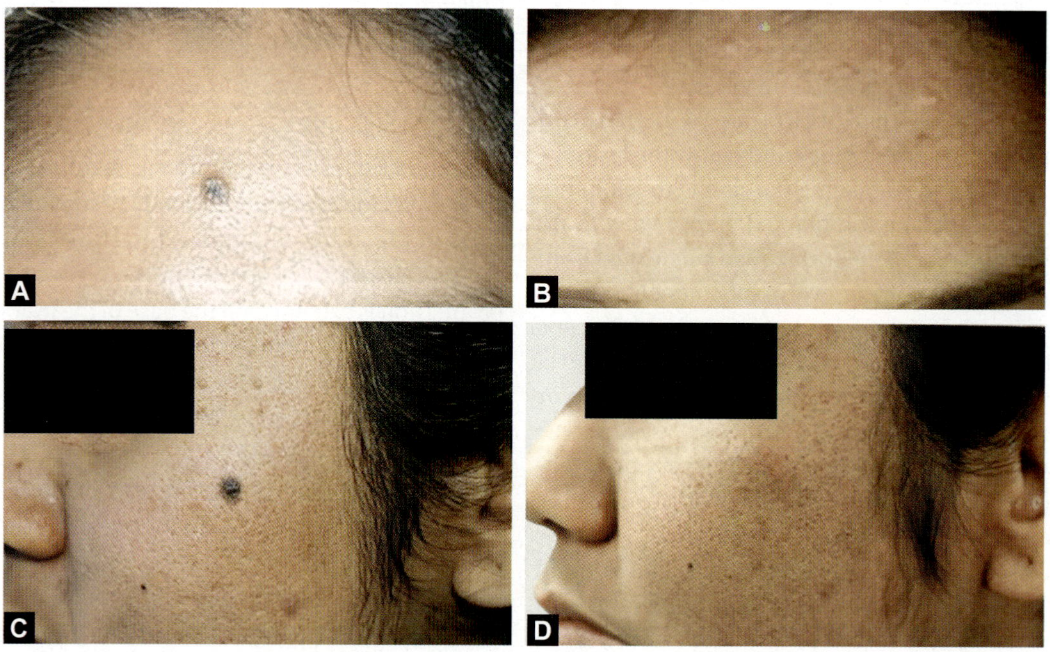

Figs. 7.11A to D: (A) Compound nevus. (B) After 3 weeks of excision. (C) Compound nevus over cheek. (D) Postexcision.
Courtesy: Cutis Academy, Bengaluru, Karnataka, India

Table 7.10: Advantages and disadvantages of elliptical excision.

Advantages	*Disadvantages*
• Depth of the excision is controllable • Dog ear formation is less • Both therapeutic and diagnostic • Malignant lesions/dysplastic nevi/lesions with suspicion of malignancy can be excised with free margins and subjected to analysis • Superior cosmetic results • Risk of recurrence is low	• Requires surgical skill • Recurrence, in case of incomplete removal[8] • Skin grafting/flap surgery is required for closure in case of larger lesion excision[8] (Figs. 7.13A to E)

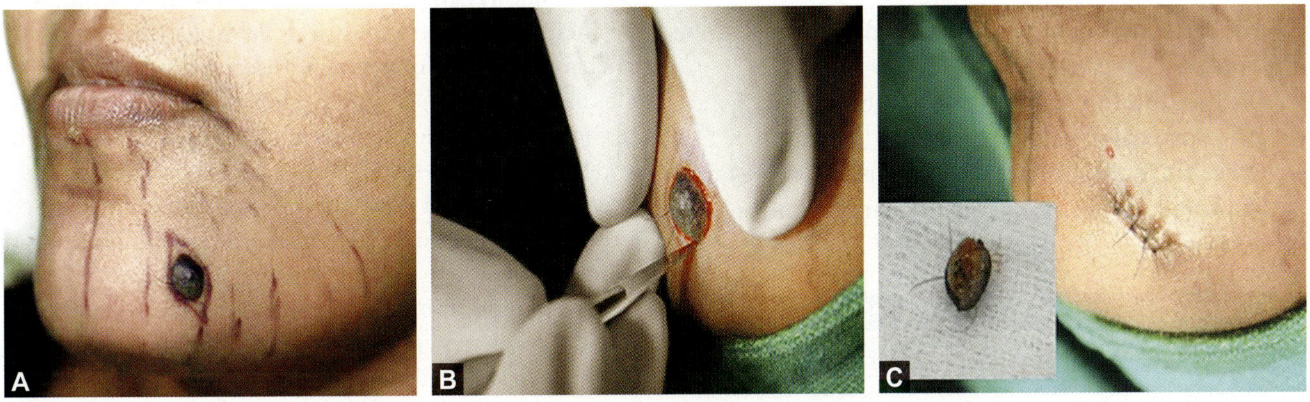

Figs. 7.12A to C: (A) Compound melanocytic nevus over chin, marking of RSTLs, plan can either be elliptical or circumferential excision. (B) Circumferential excision. (C) Wound closure along RSTL.
Courtesy: Cutis Academy, Bengaluru, Karnataka, India

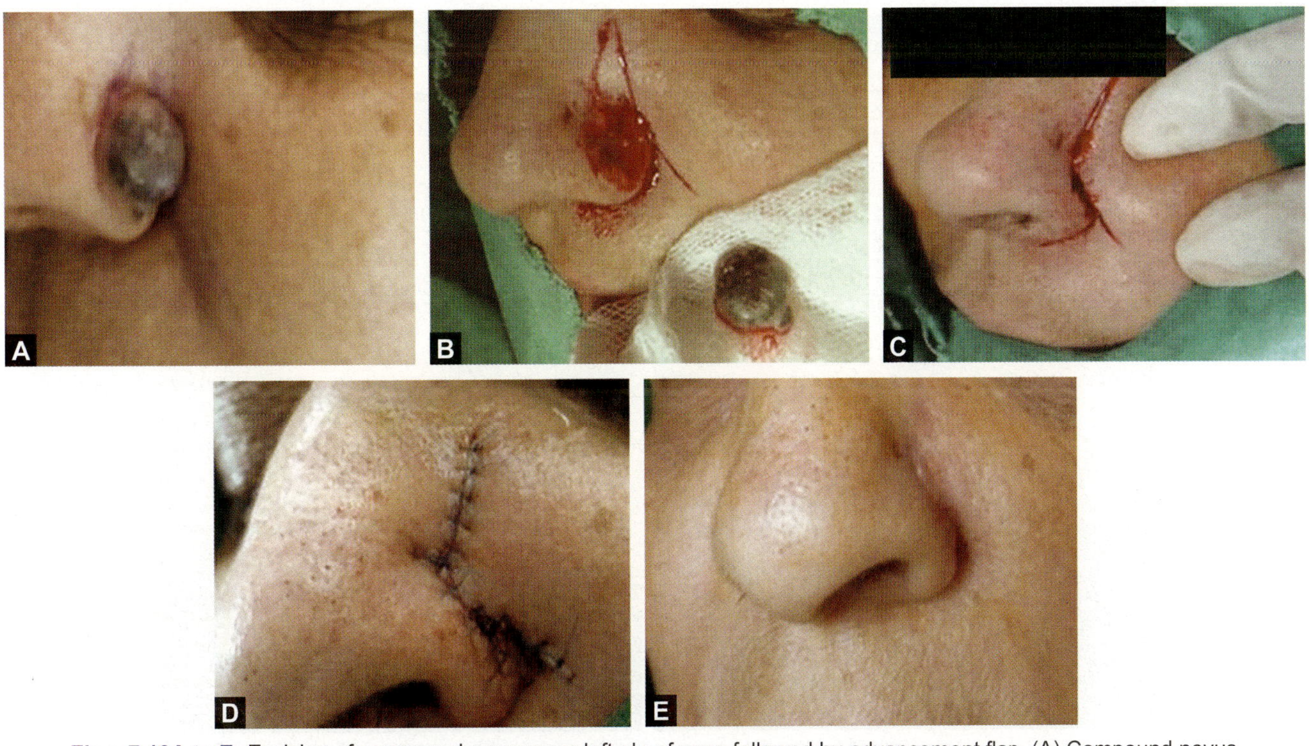

Figs. 7.13A to E: Excision of compound nevus over left ala of nose followed by advancement flap. (A) Compound nevus. (B) Circumferential excision. (C) Advancement flap. (D) Wound closure in two layers. (E) Three months postsurgery.

- Percutaneous suturing is done with simple interrupted sutures using prolene 5-0/6-0 (Fig. 7.12C).
- Antibiotic based pressure dressing done. It is removed after 48 hours and suture removal is done on 7th day. It heals with an esthetically better scar. Advantages and disadvantages of the procedure are provided in Table 7.11

POSTOPERATIVE CARE IN MOLE SURGERY

- Antibiotic ointment and pressure dressing are to be done postsurgery.
- Oral antibiotics and anti-inflammatory drugs are given for 5 days.
- Dressing is removed on 3rd postoperative day and inspected for any discharge, hematoma and wound dehiscence.

Table 7.11: Circumferential excision and closure.

Advantages	*Disadvantages*
• Skills of elliptical excision not required • Useful in regions where RSTL are not apparent • Length of the resultant scar is less	• Dog ear formation

- Open dressing with topical antibiotic creams or daily change of steri strip dressing is practiced by the patient
- Suture removal is done after 5–7 days.
- Steri strip dressing is continued for 3 weeks postsuture removal.

COMPLICATIONS OF MOLE SURGERY (TABLE 7.12)

Complications can be early or late. These are uncommon, if principles of surgery are strictly followed. Dog ears occur when more than 4.5 mm punch is used and in nonmalleable sites like forehead, nose and zygoma of cheek. They need to be corrected. Pseudo dog ears mostly resolve on their own. In case of wound dehiscence, it is left to heal by secondary intention. To avoid graft failure, grafts must be secured properly with adequate hemostasis, strict immobilization and dressings are to be removed after 7 days.

Late complications are often due to patient factors like keloidal tendency, excessive sun exposure, Fitzpatrick's type 4 and 5 skin and genetical background of poor wound healing. Therefore, proper selection of patient is a prime factor. Recurrences are known in case of shave excision and RF excisions (Figs. 7.15A and B). Cobble stoning

Table 7.12: Complications of mole surgery.

Early	*Late*
Pseudodog ears	Depression
Hematoma	Hyperpigmentation (Figs. 7.14A and B)
Wound margin necrosis	Dog ears
Wound dehiscence (Fig. 7.17C)	Atrophic scars
Secondary infection (Fig. 7.17B)	Hypertrophic scars, keloids, scar contractures
In case of punch grafting	Recurrence (Figs. 7.15 and 7.18)
Graft dislodgement	**In case of punch grafting**
Rejection of graft	Cobble stoning, depressed graft, color mismatch, donor site scarring

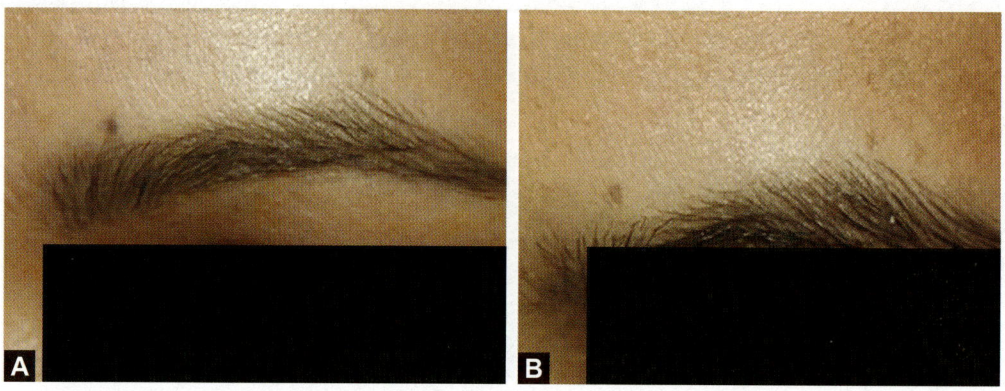

Figs. 7.14A and B: (A) Junctional nevus. (B) Postinflammatory hyperpigmentation post RF.
Source: Cutis Academy, Bengaluru, Karnataka, India

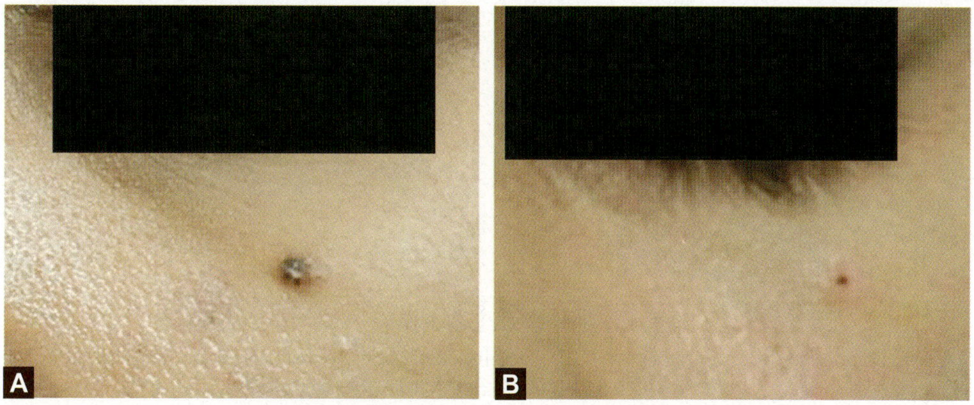

Figs. 7.15A and B: (A) Compound nevus. (B) Recurrence post RF.
Courtesy: Cutis Academy, Bengaluru, Karnataka, India

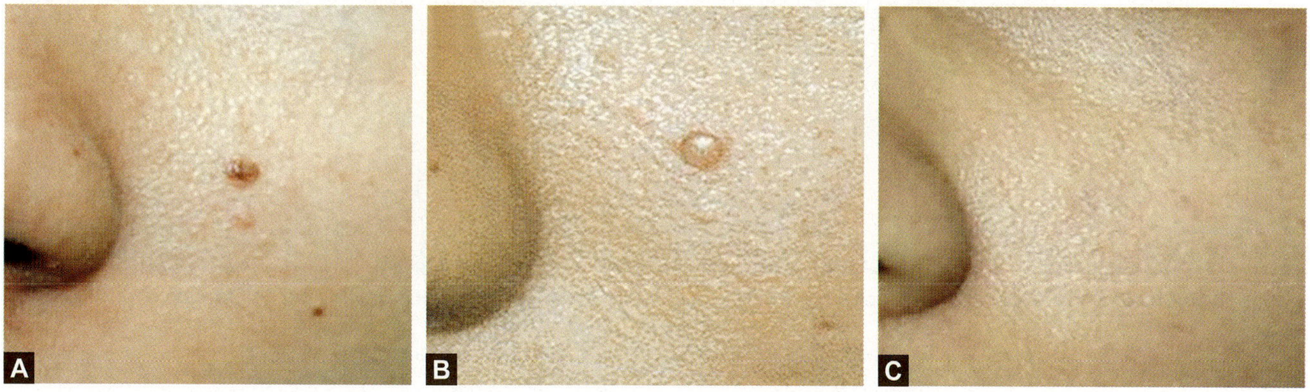

Figs. 7.16A to C: Punch excision and grafting. (A) Compound nevus over left cheek. (B) Seven days after punch grafting (C) After 3 months disappearance of cobblestoning with RF.
Courtesy: Cutis Academy, Bengaluru, Karnataka, India

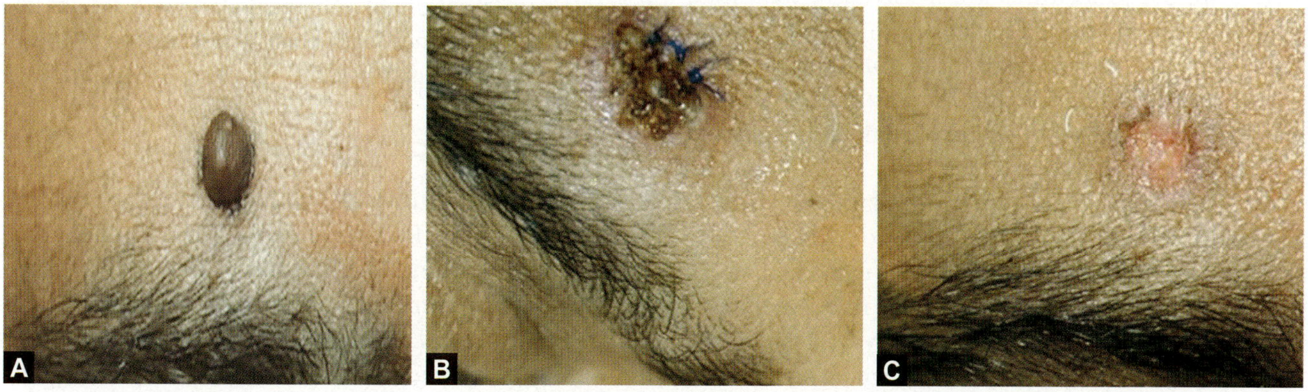

Figs. 7.17A to C: (A) Compound nevus over forehead. (B) Secondary infection postexcision. (C) Wound dehiscence.
Courtesy: Cutis Academy, Bengaluru, Karnataka, India

postgrafting is corrected by RF (Figs. 7.16A to C). Wound dehiscence can occur if especially infection occurs post surgery (Figs. 7.17A to C). Author has also experienced recurrences following excision of mole which was situated close (approximately 2–3 mm) to another mole which wasn't excised with it (Figs. 7.18A and B).

Miscellaneous treatment modalities: Cryotherapy and curettage.

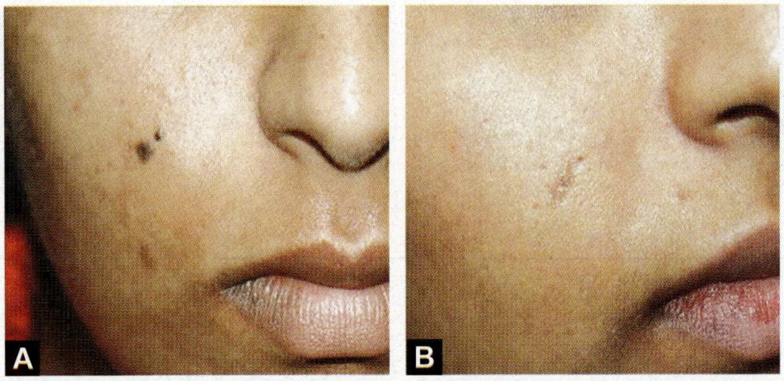

Figs. 7.18A and B: (A) Two compound nevi over right cheek. (B) Recurrence of larger nevi after excision (with smaller nevus left untouched).
Courtesy: Cutis Academy, Bengaluru, Karnataka, India

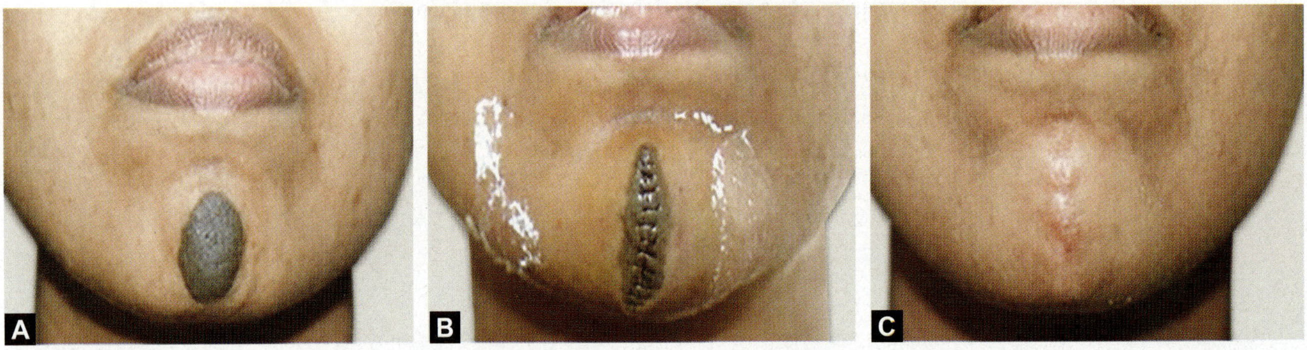

Figs. 7.19A to C: Serial excision of congenital melanocytic nevus over chin. (A) Before. (B) Nevus after 1st session of excision. (C) After 6 weeks of 2nd excision.
Courtesy: Cutis Academy, Bengaluru, Karnataka, India

CONGENITAL MELANOCYTIC NEVI

Nearly 2–3% of neonates suffer from congenital melanocytic nevi.[9] Multiple procedures are involved in treatment of larger nevi which includes excision, serial excision (Figs. 7.19A to C), tissue expansion, full-thickness skin grafting, expanded flaps and combination of lasers. Complications include contractures, functional impairment and pigmentary disturbances.

Congenital melanocytic nevi have a relatively high risk of becoming malignant. Prophylactic excision of all giant and large hairy nevi is indicated in infancy and early childhood.[11] An early aggressive approach lowers the risk of malignant melanoma.[12,13] Surgical excision results in the debulking of tissue at risk for the development of malignant melanoma.[9]

Therapeutic curettage can be done for giant melanocytic nevi. It is carried out from the center of the lesion to periphery as it is easier to find cleavage plane (below superficial dermis) at the center of the lesion than periphery. It is preferably carried out in neonates below or up to 2 months of age, as a one stage procedure under general anesthesia. This prevents malignancy arising at a later age.[10]

Serial excision can be done for larger nevi (size >1.5 cm), nevi located near anatomically important areas like eyes, nose and mouth. Conventional excision method is used to excise the nevus intramarginally. Adjacent skin is advanced by undermining sufficiently followed by wound closure. Repeat procedure is carried out serially once every 3–6 months.

Laser Surgery for Melanocytic Nevi

Reader is advised to refer to Chapter 42: "Lasers for Pigmented Lesions" for further details. The chromophore targeted by the laser in this context is melanin. The two basic class of lasers used are far infrared skin resurfacing lasers and pulsed lasers/IPLs.[14] Ideally a mixture of lasers should be used. Erbium Yag laser (2640 nm), 100 microsecond alexandrite laser (755 nm),[15] frequency doubled Nd:Yag laser, 1064 nm Qs Nd:YAG laser and carbon dioxide laser can be used.

Response to laser treatment is variable.[8] Common complications include hyperpigmentation, hypopigmentation, persistent erythema, atrophy, hypertrophic scarring and recurrence. Advantages of laser surgery are given in Table 7.13.

Table 7.13: Advantages of lasers surgery.

- Local anesthesia can be avoided
- Preferred in cardiac patients
- Less painful
- Provides bloodless field

Box 7.4: Tips and tricks for mole removal.

- During RF always select a proper electrode.
- Use pure cutting mode to avoid damage to surrounding skin.
- Do not coagulate base unnecessarily.
- Defer RF when mole is more than 3 mm or in mole having hair on it as it can cause depressed scar.
- For pedunculated nevi, punch smaller than the actual size of the lesion can be used to accommodate the entire nevus.
- The scoring with punch must always be complete, we must not lift up punch after scoring incompletely because when we do the second scoring we may create separate incision, it should be advanced through the original incision only, to avoid double scoring
- If the defect is small, bevel of 18 gauge needle can be used to do undermining with more precision and lesser chance of cutting through epidermis.
- Scoring with punch should be uniform throughout without ragged edges which can lead to irregular border and poor esthetic appearance after healing.

SUMMARY (BOX 7.4)

A good preoperative counseling, determining the type, size, depth and benign/malignant nature of the nevus, analyzing location of the nevus with respect to RSTL, cosmetic units, free margins of face, and its vicinity to facial orifices, choosing appropriate technique of surgery and meticulous execution of the surgical technique with proper handling of tissue will give optimal results.

REFERENCES

1. Valia RG, Jerajani HR, Amladi ST. Naevi and other developmental defects. IADVL Textbook and Atlas of Dermatology, Valia RG (Ed); 1st ed, Bombay: Bhalani Publishing House. 1994;1:114-50.
2. Becker D, Meier BC, Herlyn M. Proliferation of human melanomas is inhibited by antisense oligodeoxynucleotides targeted against basic fibroblast growth factor. The EMBO Journal. 1989:8;3685-91.
3. Navarani AA, Kolm I, Calvo X, et al. Trauma as triggering factor for development of melanocytic navi. Dermatology. 2010;220:291-6.
4. Savant SS. Mole surgery. Textbook of Dermatosurgery and Cosmetology, 2nd ed, Mumbai:ASCAD;2008: 644-9.
5. Savant SS. Radiosurgery. Textbook of Dermatosurgery and Cosmetology, 2nd ed, Mumbai: ASCAD;2008:305.
6. Savant SS. Skin biopsy techniques. Textbook of Dermatosurgery and Cosmetology, 2nd ed, Mumbai:ASCAD; 2008:75.
7. Sacchidanand S, Ramachander T. Melanocytic Nevi: Treatment Modalities. ACS(I) Textbook on Cutaneous and Aesthetic Surgery, 1st ed, New Delhi, Jaypee Brothers Medical Publishers. 2012;280-8.
8. Savant SS. Elliptical or fusiform excision and it's variations. Textbook of Dermatosurgery and Cosmetology, 2nd ed, Mumbai:ASCAD;2008:136-47.
9. Chauhan DS, Guruprasad Y. Congenital melanocytic nevus of upper eyelid. J Cutan Aesthet Surg. 2011;4:61-4.
10. DeRaeve LE, Roseuw DJ. Curettage of giant congenital melanocytic naevi in neonates: A decade later. Arch Dermatol. 2002;138:943-8.
11. Rhodes AR, Wood WC, Sober AJ, et al. Nonepidermal origin of malignant melanoma associated with giant congenital nevocellular nevus. Plast Reconstr Surg. 1981;67:782-90.
12. Huemer GM. The value of full-thickness skin grafts in reconstruction of the periorbital region. Plast Reconstr Surg. 2008;121:1857-8.
13. Bruce S, Bauer MD, Frank A, et al. An approach to excision of congenital giant pigmented nevi in infancy and early childhood. Plast Reconstr Surg. 1988;82:1012-21.
14. Sardana K. The science, reality, and ethics of treating common acquired melanocytic nevi (moles) with lasers. J Cutan Aesthet Surg. 2013;6:27-9.
15. Wang EC, Sen P, Goh CL, et al. Single treatment with 100-microsecond alexandrite laser clears selected acquired melanocytic nevi in type IV. Asian facial skin. J Cutan Aesthet Surg. 2013;6:21-6.

CHAPTER 8

Dermabrasion

Aarti Sarda, Abhishek De, Shilpa K

INTRODUCTION

Dermabrasion is defined as a dermatosurgical technique, typically performed in a professional medical setting by a dermatologist or plastic surgeon trained specifically in this procedure, where sequential planing of the raised, altered or otherwise normal skin with manual and/or electrical motorized abraders is carried out.[1]

Dermabrasion can be of 3 types—(a) microdermabrasion, (b) manual dermabrasion or (c) motor dermabrasion (Fig. 8.1).

a. Microdermabrasion is a nonsurgical cosmetic procedure that uses a mechanical medium for exfoliation to gently remove the outermost layer of dead skin cells from the epidermis.
b. In manual dermabrasion, Maneksha's hand-held manual dermabraders or sterilized sandpaper or salt crystals are used to abrade upper layers of skin. The advantage of manual dermabrasion is better depth control.
c. In motorized dermabraders stone or metallic dental burrs, wire brush or a diamond wheel with rough edges is attached to a micromotor machine which rotates at high speed. The advantage of motorized dermabrasion over manual dermabrasion is that this procedure is quicker and ideal for larger surface dermabrasion.

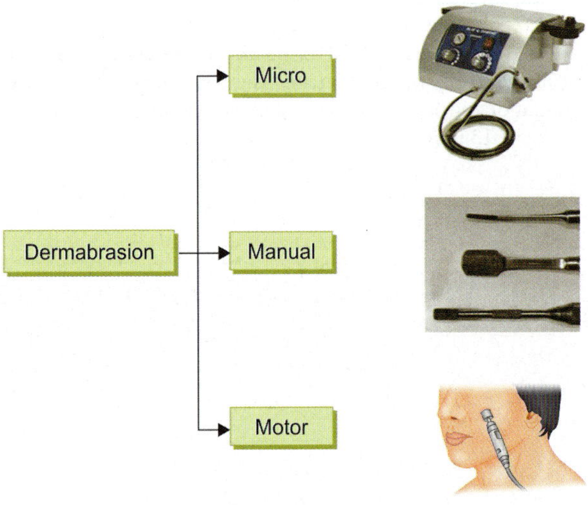

Fig. 8.1: Types of dermabrasion.

Dermabrasion involves controlled abrasion of the upper to mid layers of the skin and causes it to bleed. As the wound heals, new skin grows to replace the damaged skin that was removed during dermabrasion. Factors that affect the depth of the resurfacing include: how coarse the burr or brush is, how quickly it rotates, how much pressure is applied and for how long, and the condition and physical features of the skin.

HISTORY

Dermabrasion has been practiced for many years and till today, has not lost its place as a dermatosurgery office procedure, even with the advent of lasers.

Kromeyer[2] is credited with first using rasps or burrs with rotation in the early 1900s. He used carbon dioxide snow and ether spray as a refrigerant to freeze the skin prior to the procedures. Iverson,[3] in 1947, reported the successful treatment of tattoos with sandpaper. Kurten,[4] in 1953, treated a variety of conditions with a wire-brush dermabrasion machine. Kurten,[4] as well as other researchers, including Orentreich,[5] Burks,[6] Harmon and Yarborough,[7] Roenigk,[8] and Mandy et al.,[9] helped to refine the dermabrasion technique.[10,11]

PRINCIPLES (FIG. 8.2)

The skin is abraded from the epidermis through the papillary dermis up to the desired level (junction of upper and mid reticular dermis) creating a superficial wound which is allowed to heal by secondary intention, so as to achieve resurfacing effect, thus making the lesions/scar less conspicuous.[1] Re-epithelialization occurs via the underlying

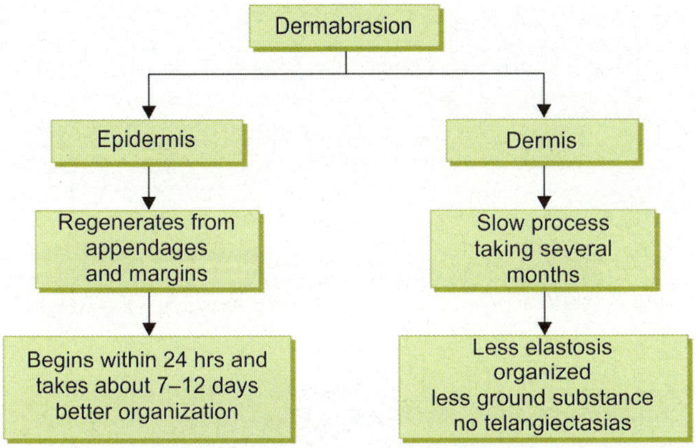

Fig. 8.2: Principles of dermabrasion.

adnexal structures. Dermabrasion is a "cold" form of ablation that minimizes vascular stimulation throughout the healing phase, allowing for a less intense postoperative erythema that regresses faster compared to other similar procedures. Re-epithelialization begins within 24 hours of dermabrasion and takes 8 to 12 days to complete. The new epidermis shows greater organization. There is collagen remodeling in the dermis with less elastosis. Clinically these changes result in an evenly contoured skin.

INDICATIONS[1,12-14]

Dermabrasion can be classified as spot or regional based on the area dermabraded.

- Scars—Acne, traumatic, surgical, varicella, smallpox
- Hyperkeratotic lesions—Lichen simplex chronicus, hypertrophic lichen planus, papular lichen amyloidosis, linear verrucous epidermal nevus, prurigo nodularis, Darier's disease.
- Tumors—Syringoma, trichoepithelioma, adenoma sebaceum, seborrheic keratosis, actinic keratosis, Bowen's disease, basal cell carcinoma, squamous cell carcinoma in situ.
- Pigmentary lesions—Epidermal nevi, melasma, freckles, lentigenes, tattoo, postinflammatory hyperpigmentation.
- Vitiligo surgeries—To denude the epithelium prior to suction blister grafts, ultrathin skin grafting, melanocyte and keratinocyte suspension.
- Miscellaneous—Fine wrinkling, rejuvenation, rhinophyma, resistant acne, porokeratosis, Hailey-Hailey disease, Fox-Fordyce disease, xanthelasma palpebrarum.

CONTRAINDICATIONS[14]

- Keloidal tendency
- Impaired wound healing
- Burn scars
- Active infection
- Bleeding disorder
- Recent treatment with isotretinoin in the last 6–12 months
- Prior radiation therapy
- Active herpes or bacterial infection
- Patients with unrealistic expectations.

EQUIPMENT

- Mechanical—Metallic dermabradors (Fig. 8.3), sandpaper (Fig. 8.4) (water paper no. 80,110)
- Electrical—Dermabrador or hand engine (Fig. 8.5)
- End pieces—Wire brushes, diamond fraises or serrated wheels, stone or metal burrs (Fig. 8.6)
- Barrier protection (mask, cap, gown, gloves, face shield).

PATIENT COUNSELING

- Explain the risk, complications, limitations and potential alternative procedures
- Sun protection is mandatory postprocedure for 3 to 6 months.

STEP-BY-STEP

- Priming (at least 2 to 6 weeks prior)
  - Sunscreens—to prevent postinflammatory hyperpigmentation
  - Topical retinoids—for faster postoperative healing and reduce chances of milia formation
  - Glycolic acid/hydroquinone—If patient has tendency to develop postinflammatory hyperpigmentation.
- Spot dermabrasion: 6 weeks prior to see healing pattern and possibility of complications
- Preoperative work up
  - History—Bleeding diasthesis, keloidal tendency, isotretinoin use, immunosuppressive agents, HIV, hepatitis B, herpes simplex infection, drug history (aspirin, etc.)
- Investigations—CBC, BT, CT, PT, blood sugar, hepatitis B and HIV serology, fitness for GA, if required
- Informed consent and photography

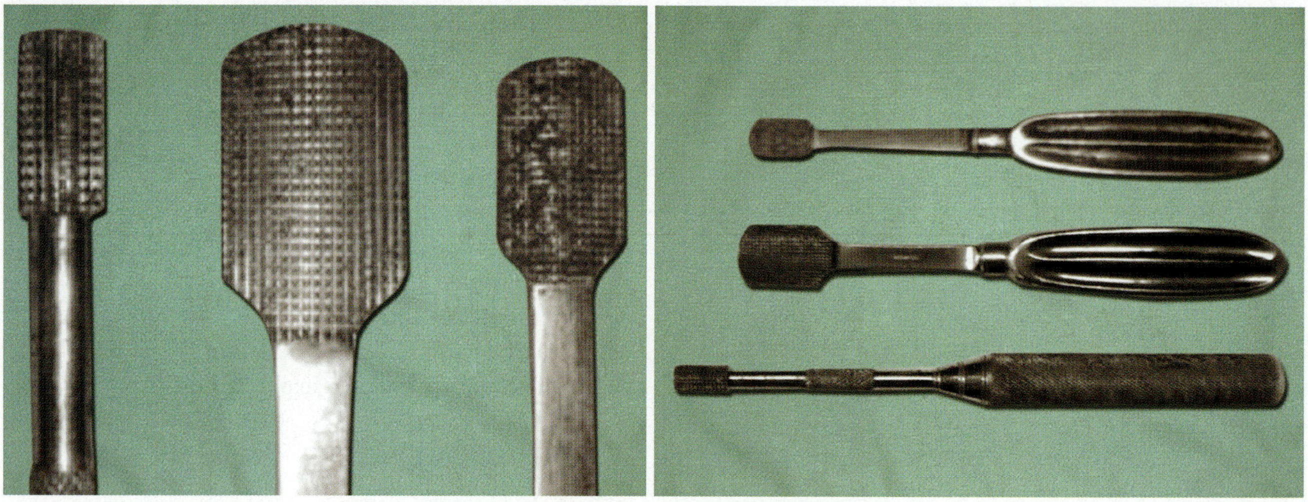

Fig. 8.3: Maneksha's manual dermabraders.

Fig. 8.4: Sandpapers used for manual dermabraders.

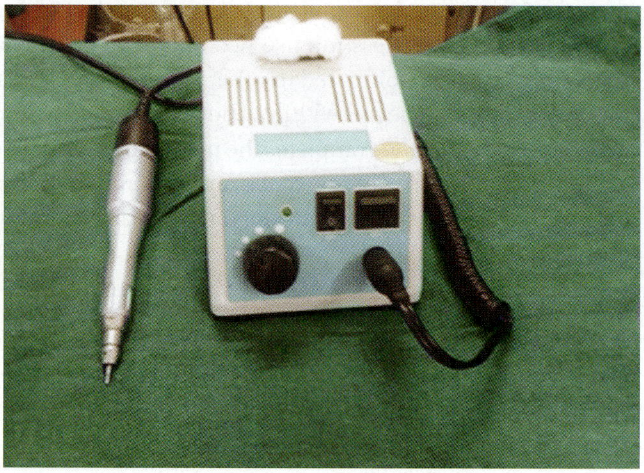

Fig. 8.5: Motor dermabraders.

- Room preparation—Appropriate lighting, proper ventilation, lighting, operating tables, and equipment for patient monitoring and/or anesthesia.
- Preoperative procedure:
  - Deep ice pick scars—subcision, punch excision, punch grafting
  - Depressed scars—soft tissue augmentation with fillers.
- Anesthesia: can be done under local anesthesia, regional block cryoanesthesia or general anesthesia. When the procedure is done under local anesthesia adrenaline should be avoided as the level of dermabrasion cannot be assessed because adrenaline-induced vasoconstriction
- Refrigerant topical anesthesia is used to help freeze the skin prior to the dermabrasion procedure.

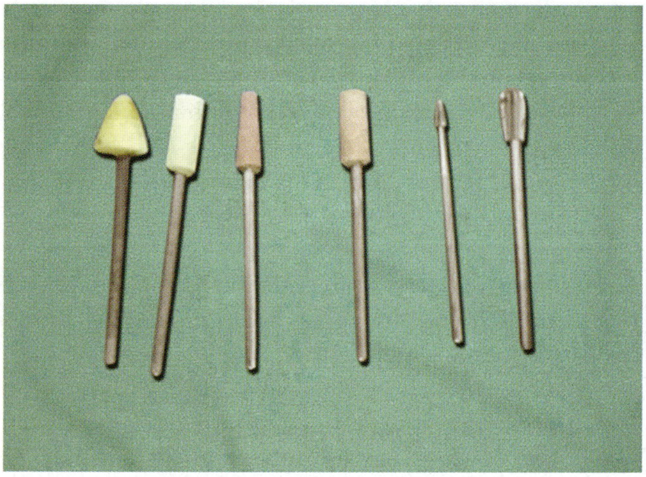

Fig. 8.6: Stone and metallic burrs.

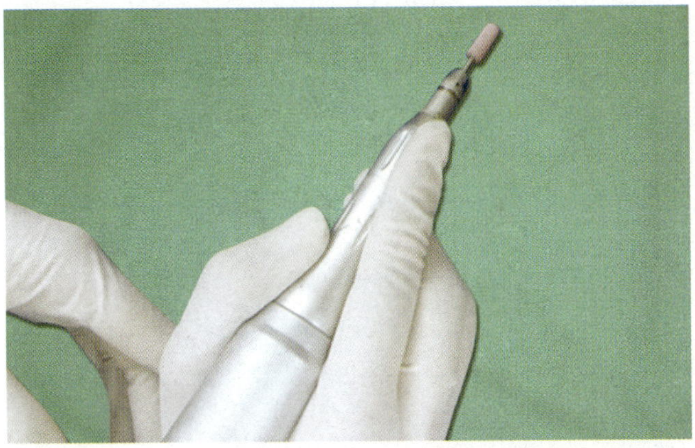

Fig. 8.7: Pen holding grip.

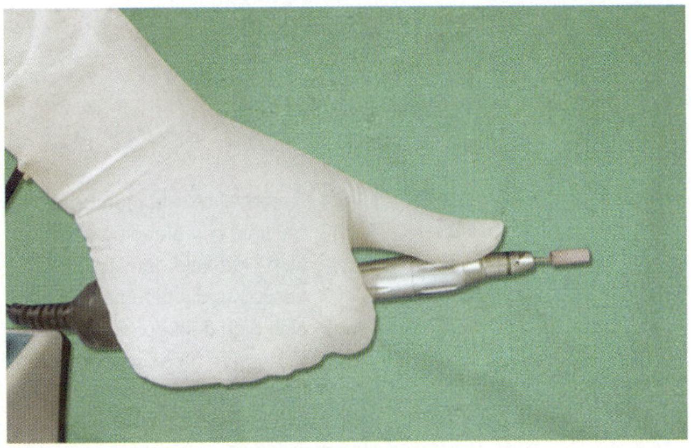

Fig. 8.8: Safety razor grip.

OPERATIVE PROCEDURE[1,14]

- Along with the universal precautions like wearing surgical masks to guard against sprayed blood and aerosolization of blood particles, wearing glasses is must. Even the patient's eyes must be covered with gauze after applying sterile ointment.
- While doing motor dermabrasion there are two methods of holding the handpiece: (a) pen holding grip (Fig. 8.7) and (b) safety razor grip (Fig. 8.8).
- Face is turned to one side and skin held taut by an assistant. Gentian violet is used to delineate the areas to be treated.
- Start dermabrading by marking submandibular border (either ears to the chin) with a wire-brush or diamond fraise.
- Establish the infraorbital margin by dermabrading downwards on the cheeks and sideburns.
- Dermabrade in the routine manner treating one anatomic unit at a time with feathering at potential lines of demarcation.
- The order (Fig. 8.9) can be right cheek, chin, left cheek, forehead, nose and upper lip. Abrade to adequate depth, i.e. junction of mid and deep papillary dermis. After this, mechanical dermabrasion can be done as it gives a better control, providing safety.
- Two quick passes with sandpaper can be done in same sequence to smoothen the surface.
- Hemostasis is achieved by ice cold sponges.
- Face is dressed with framycetin tulle or hydrocolloid dressing.
- Antibiotics and analgesics may be given after the procedure.

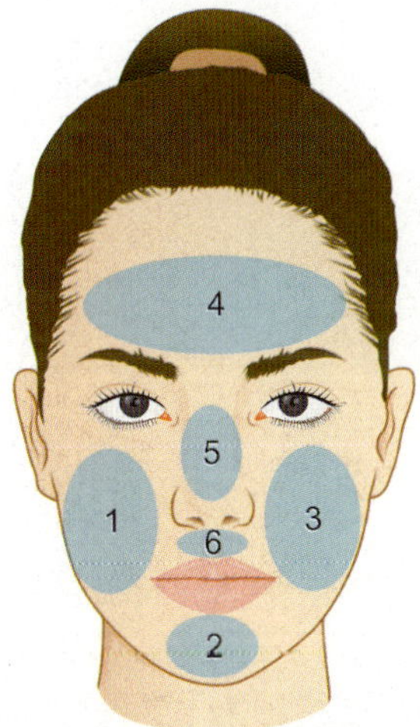

Fig. 8.9: Order of dermabrasion on face.

- Patient should avoid direct sunlight and apply sunscreen regularly
  - Dermabrasion level guide: Figure 8.10 shows schematic representation of level of dermabrasion
  - Large number of tiny pinpoint bleeding points: Superficial papillary dermis (Fig. 8.11).
  - Fewer number of larger bleeding points with gray-white ridging of collagen- junction of deep papillary and upper reticular dermis (Fig. 8.12).
  - Excessive bleeding with fraying or appearance of breaks in the parallel lines and ridges with a feeling of resistance—suggests the junction of upper and mid-reticular dermis (Fig. 8.13). Dermabrasion beyond this level can result in scarring.
  - Herniation of fat—Subcutis level (Fig. 8.14).

Dermabrasion done for verrucous epidermal nevus and tattoo are shown in Figures 8.15A to C.

1. Removal of skin pigment
2. Multiple tiny bleeding points with high field density
3. Large rapidly bleeding points with high field density
4. Excessive bleeding points feeling resistance breaks in parallel lines and ridges
5. Herniation of tiny fat

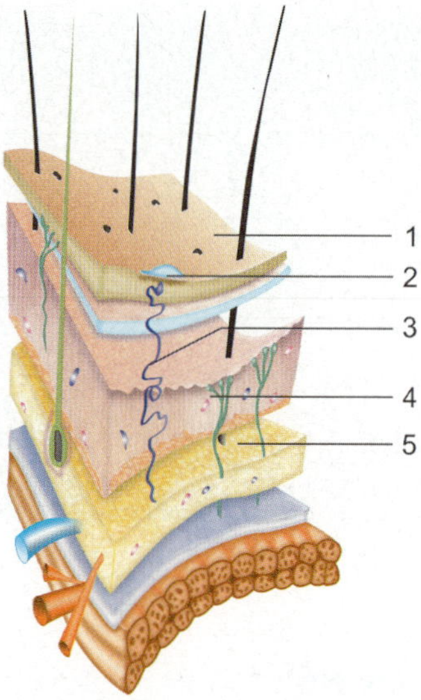

Fig. 8.10: Schematic representation of level of dermabrasion.

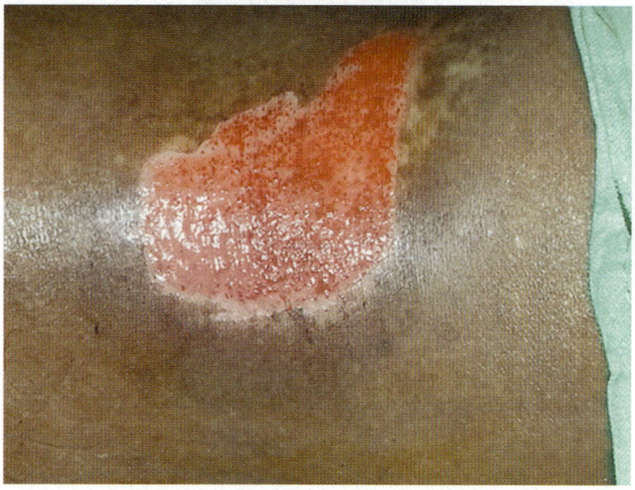

Fig. 8.11: Multiple tiny bleeding points with high field density.

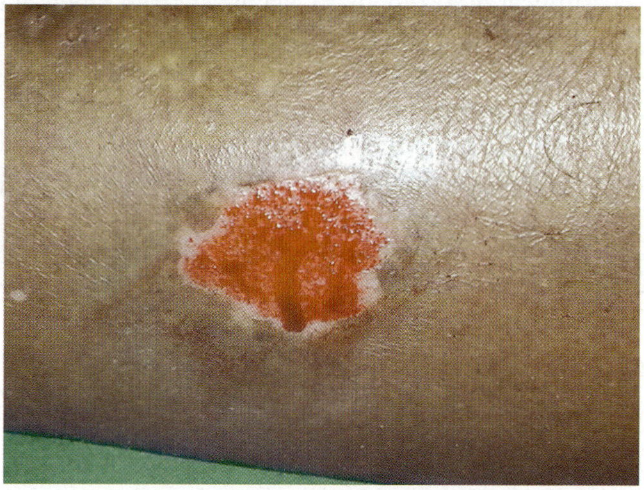

Fig. 8.12: Large rapidly bleeding points.

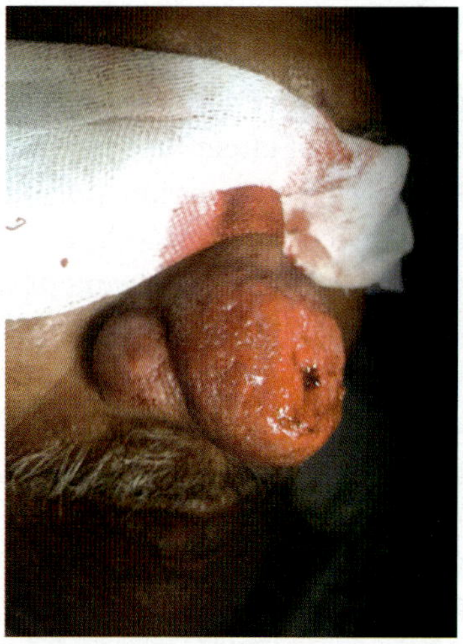

Fig. 8.13: Deeper level of dermabrasion in rhinophyma.

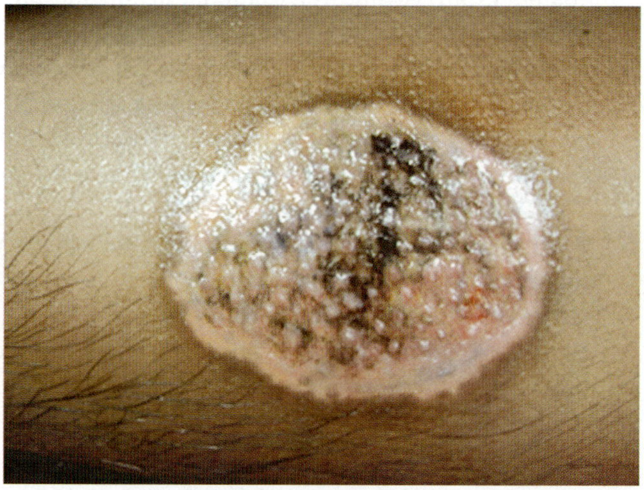

Fig. 8.14: Deeper dermabrasion with herniation of fat.

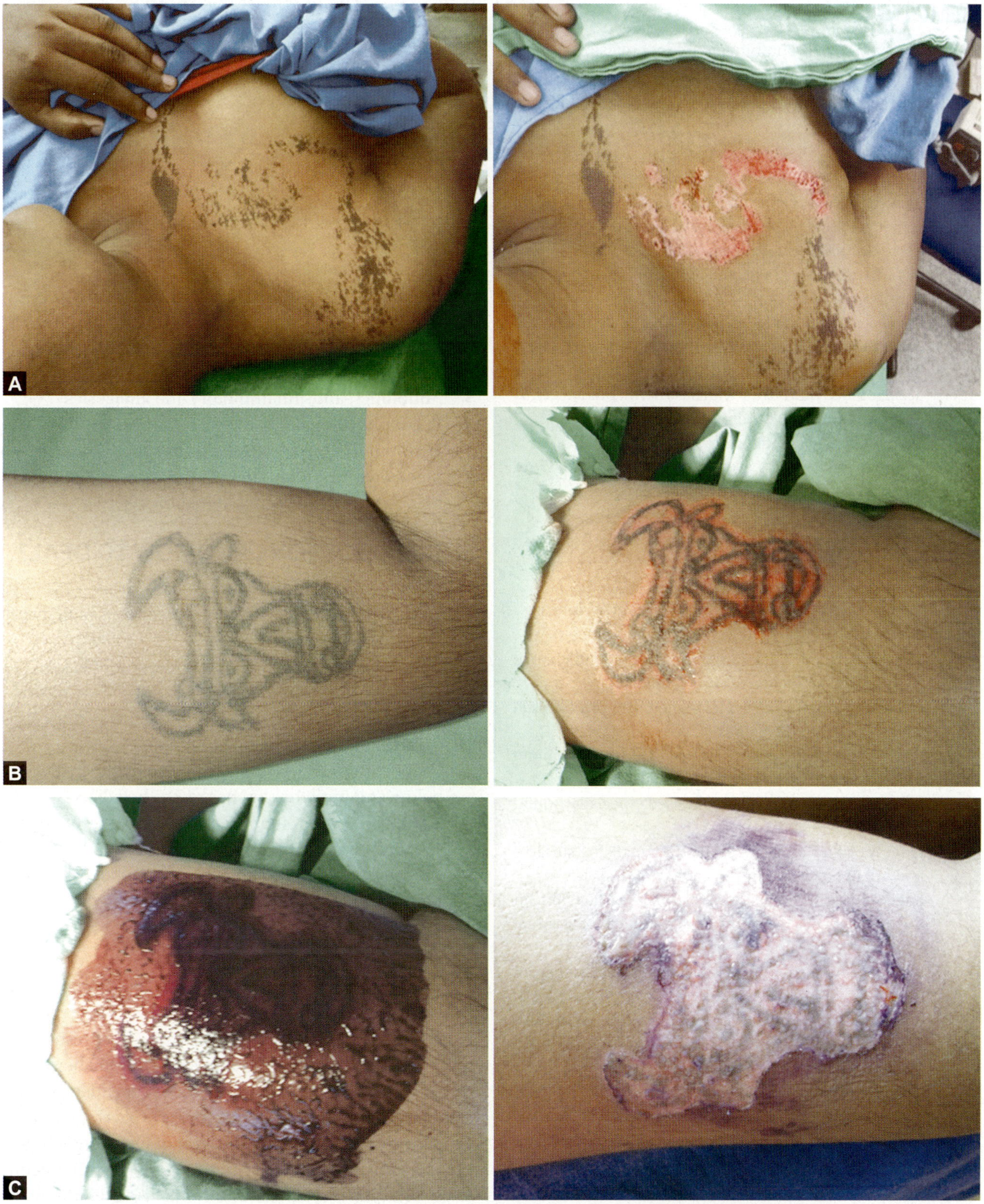

Figs. 8.15A to C: (A) Dermabrasion being done for linear verrucous epidermal nevus. (B and C) Dermabrasion done for tattoo with manual dermabraders and after gentian violet application.

MODIFICATIONS

Dermabrasion can be combined with scar revision surgeries and other resurfacing procedures like CO_2 laser. Scar revision procedure should be done 6 to 8 weeks prior to dermabrasion.

TIPS AND TRICKS

- Dermabrasion should not be done beyond the upper reticular dermis as injury beyond this plane can result in scarring. Excessive bleeding with fraying or appearance of breaks in the parallel lines and ridges with a feeling of resistance suggests the junction of upper and mid-reticular dermis.
- Pitted scars and raised lesions should be dermabraded in a circular fashion with pear-shaped diamond fraise.
- In depressed scars the shoulder of the scar should be dermabraded thoroughly with base dermabraded gently to decrease the shadowing effect (Fig. 8.16).
- Diamond fraises should be moved in steady, firm, back and forth strokes using even pressure throughout. Wire-brush end pieces are moved unidirectional.

Direction of rotation

Important in wire brush

Clockwise rotation	Deep resurfacing	Requires taut skin
Counter clockwise rotation	Superficial	Can be done on normal skin

- The movement of handpiece should be perpendicular to the direction of rotation of dermabraders.
- Conical or cylindrical dental stone burrs can be used when superficial dermabrasion is required.
- Wire brush should be used for deep scars and diamond fraise to feather the edges or plane more smoothly.
- Wire brushes should be carefully used especially around the eyes.
- Large metallic dermabradors are used for flatter surfaces and smaller ones for narrow surfaces and curves.
- Suggested rotational speeds of 15,000 to 20,000 rpm for the abrading heads result in a controlled gradual planing of the treated surface.
- The procedure of dermabrasion should be started from the outermost and dependent areas toward the central and upper most areas of the face to take the advantage of gravity and keep blood out of the next operative field.
- Dermabrasion should be planned in such a way that it should end at a natural fold, or at a relatively hidden site (e.g., at the nasolabial fold, at the hairline, or under the jaw line, respectively), so that the line of demarcation is not obvious.
- Feathering at the periphery of the area that is abraded by decreasing the number of strokes and the pressure on the handpiece gives the skin a more uniform appearance avoiding obvious demarcation line.

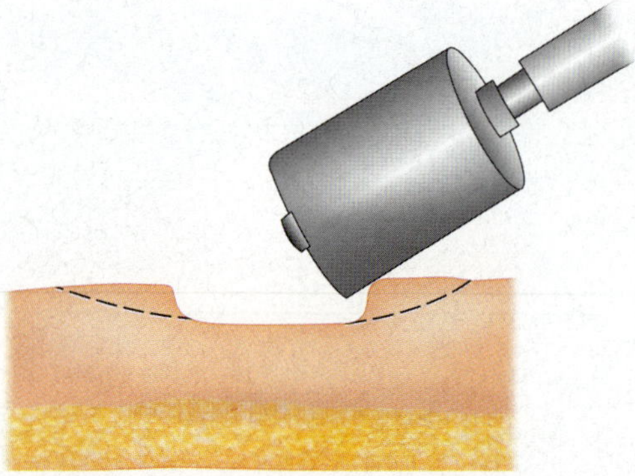

Fig. 8.16: Shouldering effect for atrophic scars.

POSTOPERATIVE CARE

- Antibiotics, anti-inflammatory and analgesics
- Regular dressings
- Hydroquinone-containing cream applied once daily at night after the 3rd month for 3 months postoperatively help to prevent hyperpigmentation disorders.

COMPLICATIONS AND HOW TO DEAL?

- Infections: folliculitis—Antibiotics
- Hypopigmentation—Wait for spontaneous repigmentation otherwise phototherapy
- Hyperpigmentation—Topical hydroquinone
- Hypertrophic scar (Figs. 8.17A to C)/Keloids—Intralesional steroid and silicone gel sheeting. Avoid dermabrading areas prone to develop keloids.
- Herpes simplex—Ask for history, oral antivirals 3 days before and until the skin has re-epithelialized
- Milia—Abrasive soaps, extraction, use of topical retinoids prior to and after dermabrasion
- Persistent erythema—It may be a precursor of hypertrophic scar. Treat with 1% hydrocortisone
- Telangiectasia.

CONCLUSION

With the advent of newer procedures including chemical exfoliation, laser resurfacing, nonablative laser resurfacing, and microdermabrasion, the popularity of dermabrasion has diminished. It is technique and operator dependent in which skill and expertise is essential in order to avoid complications. Proper patient selection, right level of abrasion and good postoperative are the requisites for a successful outcome (Figs. 8.18A and B). Dermabrasion remains a useful facial skin resurfacing and scar revision technique, particularly when performed by a trained and skilled surgeon.

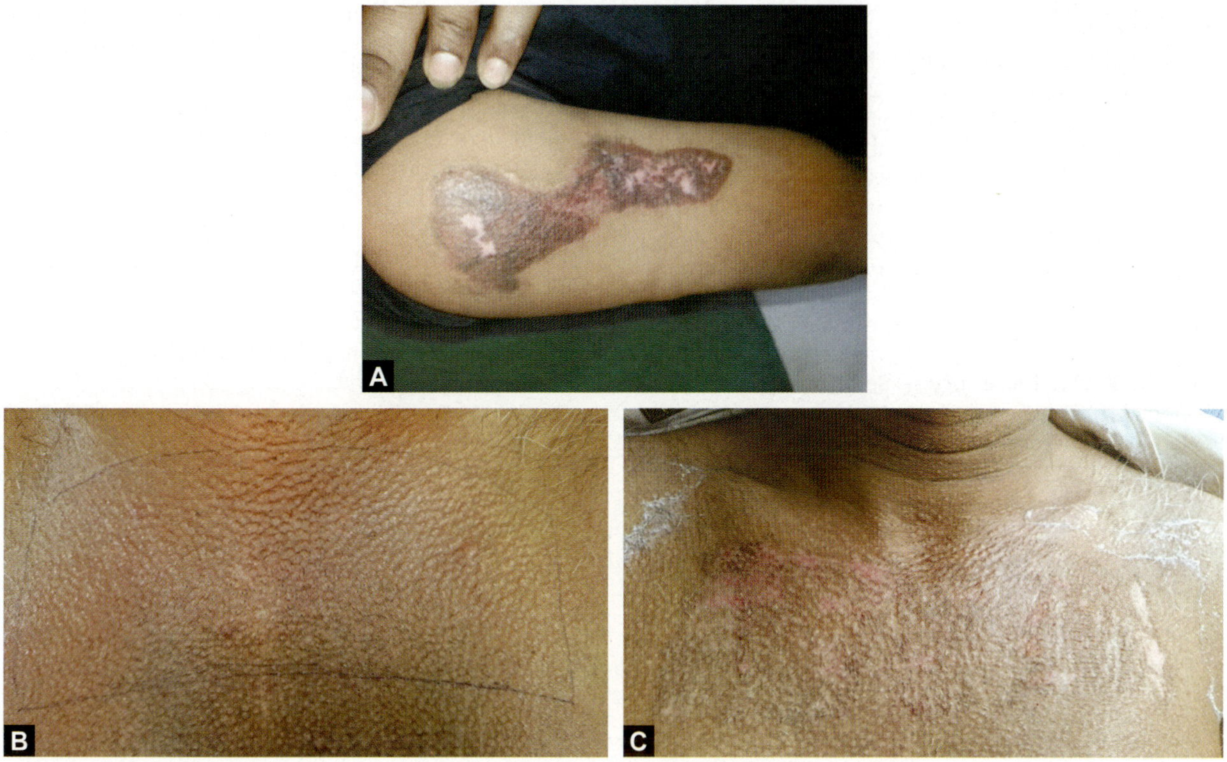

Figs. 8.17A to C: Hypertrophic scar due to deeper dermabrasion. (A) Hypertrophic scar on limbs. (B and C) Hypertrophic scar after dermabrasion on chest (pre and post).

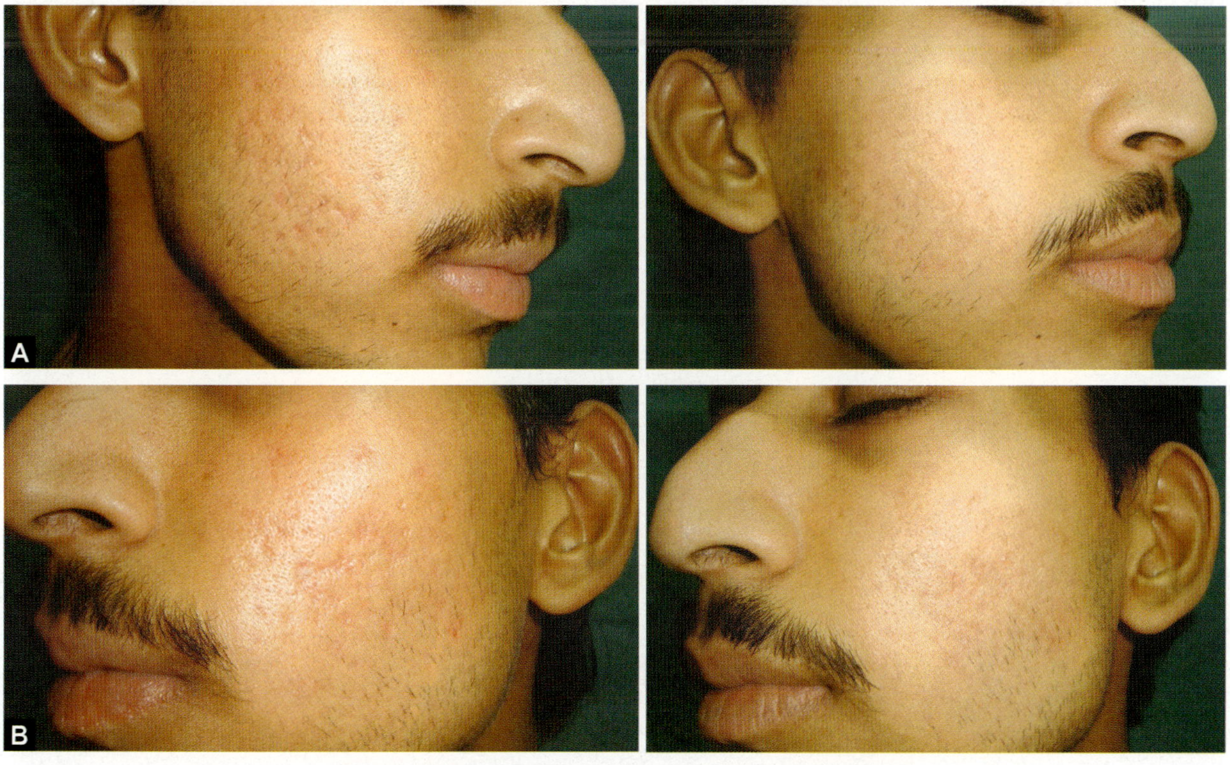

Figs. 8.18A and B: Succesful outcomes in dermabrasion.

REFERENCES

1. Savant S, Savant S, Deputy B. Dermabrasion. In: ACSI Textbook of Dermatosurgery, 2nd Ed. Jaypee Brothers Medical Publishers (P) Ltd. 2005;317-4.
2. Kromeyer E. Cosmetic treatment of skin complaints. New York: Oxford University Press. 1930.
3. Iverson PC. Surgical removal of traumatic tattoos of the face [abstract]. Plast Reconstr Surg. 1947;2:427.
4. Kurten A. Corrective surgical planing of the skin. Arch Dermatol Syphil. 1953;68:389-97.
5. Orentreich N. Dermabrasion. J Am Med Womens Assoc. 1969;24:331-6.
6. Burks JW. Wire brush surgery. Springfield (IL): Charles C. Thomas. 1956.
7. Harmon CB, Yarborough JM. Scar revision by dermabrasion. In: Roenigk NH, Roenigk RK (Eds). Dermatologic Surgery, 2nd ed. New York: Marcel Decker Inc. 1996;911-21.
8. Roenigk HH. Dermabrasion. In: Roenigk NH, Roenigk RK (Eds). Dermatologic Surgery, 2nd ed. New York: Marcel Decker Inc.1996;1089-2.
9. Mandy SH, Gross KKG, Yarborough JM. Guidelines of care for dermabrasion. J Am Acad Dermatol. 1994;31:654-7.
10. Mandy SH. Tretinoin in the preoperative and postoperative management of dermabrasion. J Am Acad Dermatol. 1996;15 (4 pt 2):878-9.
11. Lawrence N, Mandy S, Yarborough J. History of dermabrasion. Dermatol Surg. 2000;26:95-101.
12. Hanke CW, O'Brien JJ, Solow EB. Laboratory evaluation of skin refrigerants used in dermabrasion. J Dermatol Surg Oncol. 1985;11:45-9.
13. Gold M. Dermabrasion in dermatology. Am J Clin Dermatol. 2003;(7):467-71.
14. Khunger N. Dermabrasion. In: Sehgal V (Ed). Dermatologic Surgery Made Easy. 2006;142-53.

CHAPTER 9

Microneedling

Pradyumna Vaidya, Shilpa K

DEFINITION

Microneedling, also referred to as skin needling, collagen induction therapy or percutaneous collagen induction, suggests micro or "tiny" needling or "puncturing of the skin". It is a simple, minimally invasive technique used commonly in the treatment of acne scars, and functions by creating numerous punctures in the skin with the help of tiny needles. The hand-held dermaroller also serves as a cheap, safe and efficacious tool in the transdermal delivery of drugs.

The devices used for microneedling range from home-use rollers, stamps, micropen (Figs. 9.1A and B) and collagen pin to dermarollers. Both manual and electronic hand-held devices are now available. Multiple controlled skin injuries result in breakdown of old collagen strands and induces neocollagenesis with dermal revascularization.

THE EVOLUTION

The technique was first put forth by Montreal plastic surgeon Andre Camirand in 1990, who used tattoo gun without ink to needle abrade the postsurgical scars. The procedure evolved over the years and the instrument was modified to dermaroller by Des Fernandes. He introduced skin needling using roller for treating vertical perioral wrinkles at the Plastic Surgery Congress in Taipei in 2006 and coined the term "percutaneous collagen induction".

INDICATIONS OF MICRONEEDLING

- Scars:
  - Atrophic scars
  - Grade 2 and 3 boxcar and rolling scars post acne
  - Postsurgical scars/traumatic scars
  - Varicella scars
  - Hypertrophic scars—postburns.
- Skin rejuvenation:
  - Skin tightening
  - Fine lines/wrinkles/photoageing.
- Striae

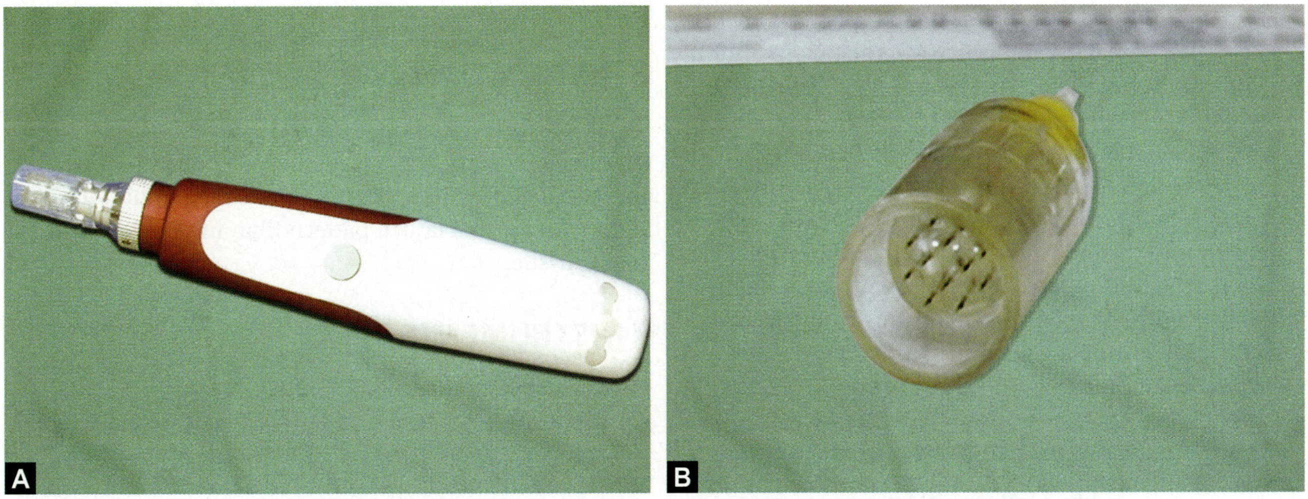

Figs. 9.1A and B: Dermapen and cartridge—a modified dermaroller for small or localized scars.

- Mesotherapy: Skin lightening, melasma, androgenetic alopecia, alopecia areata
- As combination therapy: with chemical peels, lasers, subcision, Botox and fillers.

CONTRAINDICATIONS

- Active acne vulgaris
- Infections—molluscum contagiosum, verrucae vulgaris and herpes simplex
- Solar keratosis
- Chronic skin diseases, such as eczema, psoriasis
- Patient on anticoagulants, steroids, isotretinoin, chemo/radiotherapy
- Pregnancy
- Tendency of keloids
- Collagen vascular diseases/autoimmune disorders
- History of previous treatments, such as blepharoplasty—may cause ectropion formation
- Cutaneous malignancy—to avoid spread.

PRINCIPLES OF MICRONEEDLING

The basic principle of microneedling is to trigger the process of neocollagenesis and neovascularization by creating multiple microwounds in the upper dermis using microneedles of different sizes and lengths.

The process of microneedling creates holes in the upper dermis, maintaining an intact epidermis. 15 passes with a standard dermaroller (192 needles, 200 μm length and 70 μm diameter) will result in approximately 250 holes/cm^2. These microwounds in the upper dermis stimulate the inflammatory process and trigger the normal healing cascade. The wound healing classically occurs in three phases. These include:

1. *Inflammatory phase*: Following trauma, platelets are first to respond releasing multiple chemokines including epidermal growth factors, fibronectin, fibrinogen, histamine, PDGF and serotonin. There is ingress of neutrophils which act as scavengers and decontaminate the wound. The macrophages secrete numerous enzymes and cytokines including collagenases which debride the wound, interleukins and tumor necrotic factors which stimulate fibroblasts to produce collagen and promote angiogenesis and transforming growth factor which stimulate keratinocytes.
2. *Proliferative phase*: During this phase, neutrophils are replaced by monocytes. Epithelialization takes place by migration of keratinocytes from surrounding intact skin and appendages. Angiogenesis occurs with endothelial cell migration to the site of wound. The granulation tissue appears on the second day which consists of fibroblasts. Fibroblasts differentiate to produce collagen 3, elastin, proteoglycans and glycosaminoglycans. Monocytes secrete fibroblast growth factor, TGF-alpha, TGF-beta, and platelet derived growth factor.
3. *Maturation phase*: This is phase of collagen remodelling. After almost 5 days postinjury, the fibronectin matrix is laid along the axis in which fibroblasts are aligned. There occurs reorientation of collagen in a parallel fashion and collagen deposition in upper dermis just below the basal layer of epidermis. In early phase, collagen 3 is predominantly deposited. As the wounds undergo maturation, collagen 3 is replaced by collagen 1 due to upregulation of TGFB3.

Another hypothesis proposed is based on 'Demarcation current' theory which triggers growth factors that stimulate healing phase. The potential difference at the site of injury causes migration of fibroblasts, their proliferation and collagen synthesis.

Microneedling widens the follicular infundibula to a significant extent, which enhances the transdermal penetration of drugs. In addition, in androgenetic alopecia, microneedling activates stem cells in the hair bulge area under wound healing conditions along with overexpression of hair growth-related genes, vascular endothelial growth factor, B catenin, etc.

In hypertrophic scars, matrix metalloproteinases play a vital role in cell proliferation following scar needling. TGF-β3 controls collagen fiber integration into skin's matrix while inhibitors of MMPs degrade excessive fibrotic tissue until degradation of surplus tissue is complete. Further, the capillaries and fibroblasts migrate into 'former' scar tissue and synthesize collagen 3 fibers which integrate into the skin matrix.

HISTOPATHOLOGY

Histological examination reveals around 40% thickening of stratum spinosum. There is increased collagen deposition and significantly more elastin. The collagen bundles are laid in the normal lattice pattern than in parallel bundles in scar tissue.

INSTRUMENTS

- **Dermaroller (Figs. 9.2A and B)**
  - Dermaroller is a simple hand-held drum-shaped roller.
  - It consists of a handle attached to a cylinder studded with 192 fine microneedles in 8 rows.

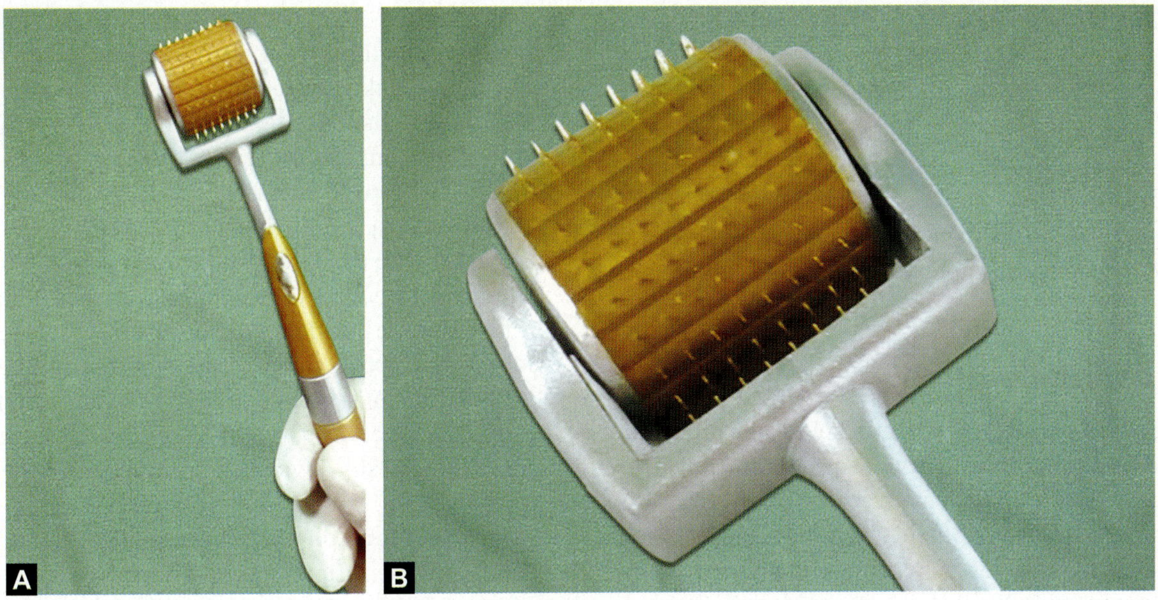

Figs. 9.2A and B: (A) Hand-held drum-shaped roller. (B) close up view showing 192 fine microneedles in 8 rows.

- The needles range from 0.5 to 3 mm in length with a diameter of 0.1 mm.
- The microneedles are synthesized by reactive ion etching techniques on silicon or medical grade stainless steel.
- High ratio of tip length versus diameter of 13:1 is an important property of good needles.
- Dermatologically preferred size is 1.5 mm (periorbital region 0.5 mm, deep scars: 2–3 mm).
- The needles are arranged radially at 15° in relation to roller center, so as to ensure uniform depth of penetration.
- Every needle penetrates at an angle and then goes deeper as the roller turns. Needle comes at a converse angle so that the paths are redirected and go into dermis for 1.5 to 2 mm. Depth also depends on the length of needles and pressure applied.
- Dermaroller is ideally presterilized by gamma irradiation. Resterilization in an autoclave or ultrasound is avoided as the needles lose their sharpness. The roller is kept in isopropyl alcohol for resterilization. Titanium needles are used instead of stainless steel especially for scalp.

- **Device modifications**
  - Home care dermarollers: These have a needle size less than 0.15 mm. and are used for transdermal delivery of substances like lipopeptides and antiaging agents. These can be used twice a week. These can be cleaned in hot tap water or using peptide-based roller cleansers.
  - Dermastamp: This miniature version of dermaroller (2 mm long and 0.12 mm diameter) is used in the treatment of localized scars like varicella scars. They may be either motorized or manual.
  - Automated dermarollers: These are battery operated with detachable heads. They can be used in multiple patients by changing the disposable heads.
  - Scalp rollers: Titanium needles are used instead of stainless steel needles.
  - LED dermarollers: Rollers with various lights 405 nm blue/590 nm yellow/560 nm green are available. They claim to give better results but no supporting data is available.
  - RF-based dermarollers: Radiofrequency-based rollers are the latest type of rollers available. These are used in indications like skin tightening, acne scars and skin rejuvenation.
  - Dermafrac: It is a newer modification combining microneedling with microdermabrasion, simultaneous deep tissue serum infusion, and light emitting diode (LED) therapy.

PROCEDURE OF MICRONEEDLING

Patient Selection

Proper patient selection is the key to success of microneedling. The patients who seek immediate dramatic results are likely to be disappointed and hence adequate counseling regarding the need for multiple sessions and expected percentage of improvement should be thoroughly emphasized.

Preoperative Care

Priming of the skin at least a month before any procedure is highly essential to prevent postinflammatory hyperpigmentation and other adverse effects.

- Priming involves use of topical glycolic acid, tretinoin or salicylic acid in low concentrations, which thins out the stratum corneum. Vitamin A and Vitamin C creams 1 month prior to the procedure helps in accelerating dermal collagen formation. Vitamin A controls release of TGFB3 in preference to TGFB1 and TGFB2 which is required for normal collagen synthesis. Scar collagen is regenerated secondary to TGFB1 and TGFB2 associated with thermal injury. Vitamin C helps in the production of normal dermal collagen.
- Patient should stop anticoagulant drugs at least 3 days before the procedure.
- Active acne should be treated prior to the procedure. Topical retinoids and clindamycin can be used to control acne. However, topical retinoids, should be stopped, at least a week before the procedure.
- Oral isotretinoin is to be ideally stopped 6 months before, to prevent scarring. However, this is a controversial issue.
- Any active infection like herpes simplex should be treated, as there are chances of flare ups of herpes labialis. So, patient with strong history of herpes labialis should receive prophylactic oral antivirals before the procedure.
- In the type 4 Indian skin, considering the chances of postinflammatory hyperpigmentation, chemical peels are sometimes recommended 21 days before the procedure. This will also enhance the efficacy of microneedling.

Preprocedure Preparation

- A written informed consent must be obtained prior to the procedure and before photographs.
- *Photographs*: Digital photographs to be taken in standard positions from front and sides prior to the procedure. Take photographs before every session, with same patient position. This makes pre- and post-procedure comparison easy.
- *Anesthesia*: Topical anesthesia, EMLA is to be applied 45 minutes to 1 hour before the procedure under occlusion with cellophane tape. After an hour, topical anesthetic is removed. The area to be treated is painted with antiseptic povidone- iodine and isopropyl alcohol solutions. Normal saline is used to cleanse the area treated with antiseptic, so as to prevent any irritation.
- *Patient positioning*: The procedure is done in a semisupine position with head elevated to 45° and eyes closed.
- *Technique (Figs. 9.3A to D)*: Dermaroller is held in the hand with a pen grip. The skin to be treated is stretched with one hand and the other hand is used to slide the roller. The roller is moved in a direction perpendicular to the stretching force. The depth of penetration increases with the stretching force. The roller is rolled in horizontal, vertical and oblique directions 6 to10 times, to cover an area of nearly 2 × 2 inches. This creates 250 to 300 holes/cm^2. Uniform controllable pin point bleeding spots are taken as the end point. Saline pads are further placed over the treated areas. The whole procedure takes around 15 to 20 minutes.

Points to Remember

- The entire procedure is operator dependent. Hence, choosing the proper needle size ensures proper depth of penetration. Usually, 1.5 to 2 mm long needles are used for the treatment of acne scars.
- The needles are sharp and penetrate the skin easily. The pressure applied plays a major role as more aggression can cause scarring and breakage of needles within the skin.
- Roll small areas at a time. This ensures proper movement of the roller and uniform depth of penetration.
- Bony areas like forehead and nose require lesser pressure.
- Periorbital areas being delicate have to be treated with special care. The roller length ideally should be 0.5 mm and fewer passes are given in this area. Aggressive movements can cause pain and sometimes edema and hematoma.
- Perioral areas have to be treated, after asking the patient to hold lips together. This will give a good stretch to the skin and make movements easy.

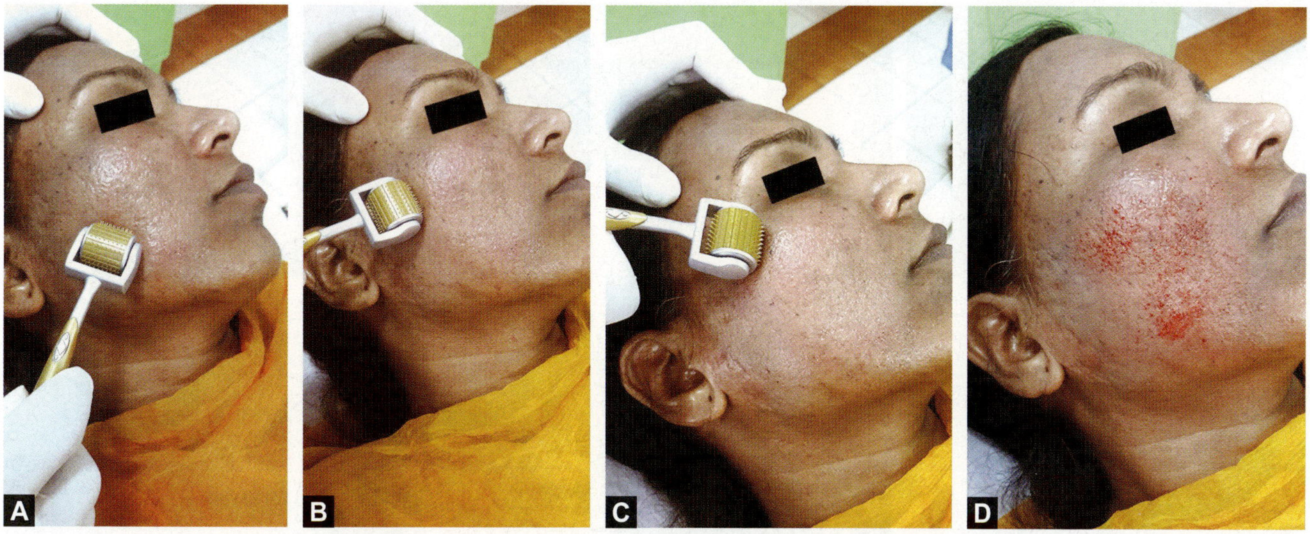

Figs. 9.3A to D: (A to C) Three directional movement and (D) Pinpoint bleeding.

- The pinpoint bleeding stops in minutes. The oozing can be wiped and minimized by keeping cold saline gauze over treated areas. This will also reduce the erythema and edema postprocedure.
- Microneedling creates multiple microwounds in epidermis and upper dermis keeping islands of normal stratum corneum in the intervening area intact. These epidermal microchannels close in minutes without any noticeable change in superficial layers.
- The treatment is to be repeated after 4 to 6 weeks. The gap between the sessions should be increased as the needle length increases. The patient should be thoroughly counseled regarding the outcome of procedure and need for multiple sessions.
- One roller is used per patient. The roller has to be properly cleaned after every use. Avoid repeated use (more than 4–5 times) as it can make needles blunt which in turn can cause more tissue damage, excessive bleeding, linear hypertrophic scars and hyperpigmentation. The needles tend to get blunt more easily in old fibrosed scars.
- Fresh scars (less than 1 year) respond better to the treatment.

POSTPROCEDURE CARE

- Saline gauzes are kept for 15 to 20 minutes.
- Topical antibiotic cream like mupirocin is applied immediately postprocedure.
- Local dressing is not required.
- Short course of systemic antibiotic is advisable to avoid secondary infection.
- Patient needs to be explained about changes likely to occur postprocedure. Facial erythema and oedema appears initially which lasts for 24 to 48 hours. Crusting and scab formation is noted by the 2nd or 3rd day which falls off by itself after 4 to 5 days without any mark or pigmentation. The downtime is relatively short with a dermaroller, as compared to other procedures.
- Strict sun protection is advised to avoid postinflammatory hyperpigmentation. Topical retinoids may be restarted after a gap of 10 days.
- Avoid use of cosmetics till a week or till the scabs fall off.
- Avoid use of scrubs, cleansers, soaps to the face. These can cause excessive dryness, irritation and further hyperpigmentation.

COMPLICATIONS (FIGS. 9.4A to D)

- Pain
- Reactivation of herpes simplex infection
- Superficial bacterial infections like impetigo
- Allergic contact dermatitis to needles
- Allergic granulomatous reactions
- Postinflammatory hyperpigmentation
- Bleeding and crusting
- Mild pain and discomfort
- Persistent erythema
- Tram-track effect—linear papular scars over bony prominences due to aggressive rolling.

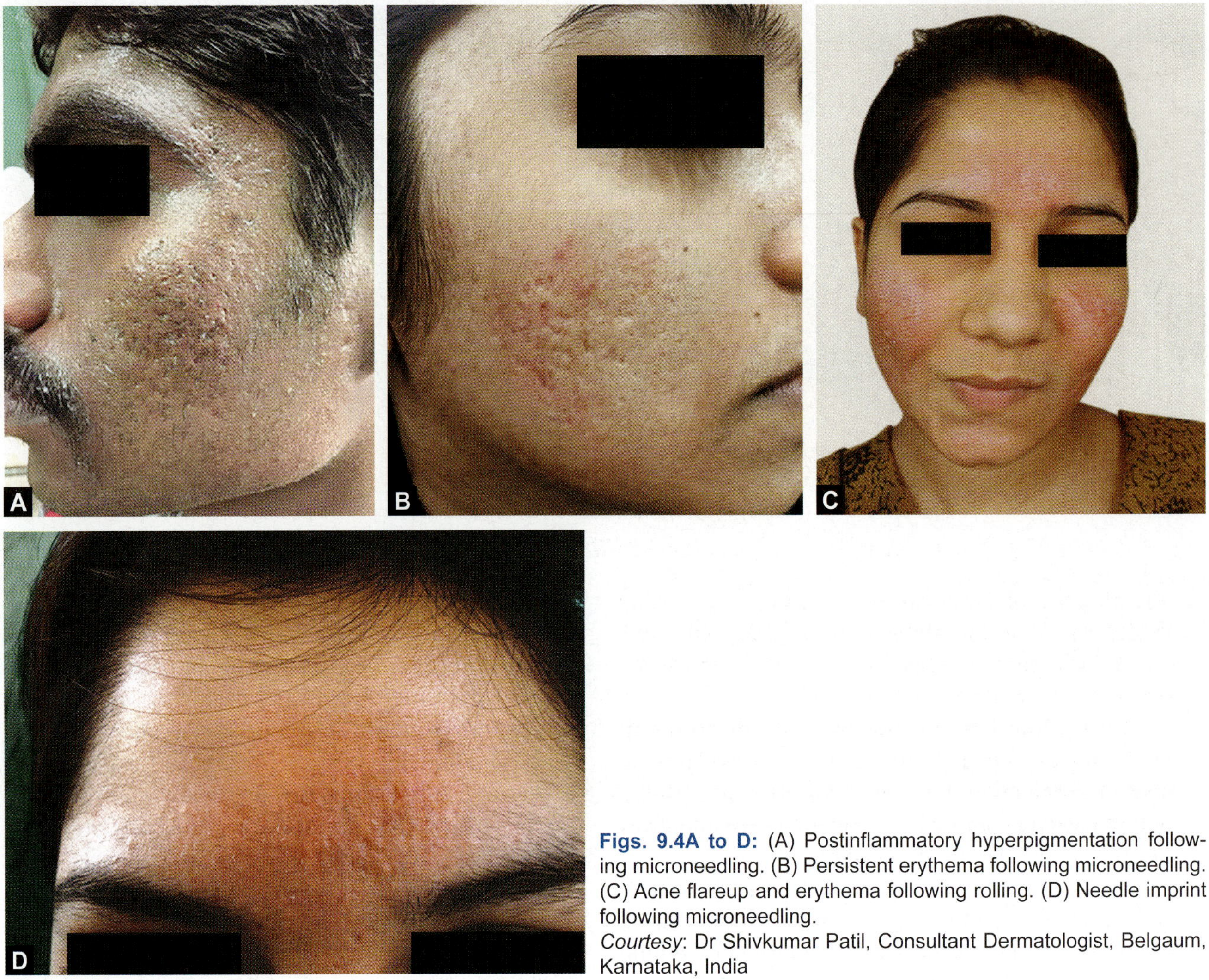

Figs. 9.4A to D: (A) Postinflammatory hyperpigmentation following microneedling. (B) Persistent erythema following microneedling. (C) Acne flareup and erythema following rolling. (D) Needle imprint following microneedling.
Courtesy: Dr Shivkumar Patil, Consultant Dermatologist, Belgaum, Karnataka, India

ADVANTAGES

- Downtime is less when compared to deep peels and other laser procedures.
- Microneedling is much more cost-effective than laser resurfacing techniques.
- Does not cause any skin damage.
- It can be done in any type of skin color.
- Office procedure which requires no hospitalization.
- Technique is easy to master.
- Low risk of PIH.
- Can be used in people with thin skin.
- Can be combined with other treatment modalities like peels, Botox, laser, etc.

DISADVANTAGES

- It is a minimally invasive procedure where multiple sessions are required.
- Expected outcome may not be as satisfactory as laser procedures, which are more invasive.
- The procedure is painful and requires topical anesthesia.
- Aggressive treatments can worsen scarring or produce needle imprints.
- Proper aseptic precautions are mandatory to prevent secondary infections.
- Not all types of scars respond well.
- Old fibrotic scars show a poor response.

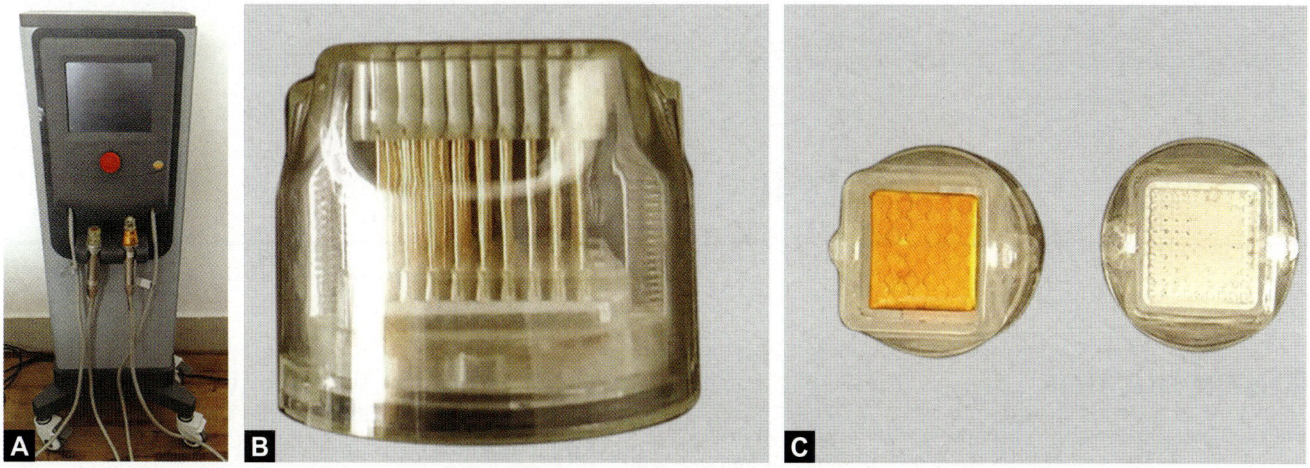

Figs. 9.5A to C: (A) Microneedling radiofrequency machine.(B and C) Microneedling radiofrequency cartridges.
Courtesy: Dr Akhilesh, Assistant Professor, Sapthagiri Medical College, Bengaluru, Karnataka, India.

INNOVATIONS

- Microneedling can be combined with other treatment modalities like peels, lasers/botox/dermal fillers and platelet rich plasma therapy.
- Radiofrequency based microneedling techniques are used for skin rejuvenation, tightening and acne scars (Figs. 9.5A to C).
- It is used to increase transdermal penetration of drugs. No efficacy studies are available.
- Dermarollers are used in mesotherapy for acne scars, both androgenetic alopecia and alopecia areata, to deliver drugs like Vitamin C, PRP, minoxidil and triamcinolone acetonide.
- Dermal fillers—Delivery becomes easy after microneedling to difficult areas like upper lip, vertical lines and small crow's feet.

CONCLUSION

The various modifications of dermaroller are now being widely used, besides its role in transdermal delivery of drugs. Though the dermaroller has its own set of limitations, microneedling enhances dermal neocollagenesis without compromising the epidermis. This makes it a safe, minimally invasive as well as a cost-effective solution in patients with superficial scarring.

CHAPTER 10

Platelet Rich Plasma

Swapnil Shah, Sukesh Mathapathi, Gautam Kumar Singh

INTRODUCTION

Platelet-rich plasma (PRP) is plasma which is rich in growth factors. It can also be referred to as autologous platelet gel. Another confusing term is platelet concentrate which denotes increased concentration of autologous platelets due to their suspension in smaller quantities of plasma achieved after centrifugation.[1] There is no consensus definition of PRP; it is arbitrarily defined as a volume of the plasma fraction of autologous blood where platelet concentration is usually more than 10,00,000 platelets/μL from the baseline.[2] Initial interest of PRP had started in oral surgery,[3] followed by sports medicine,[4] thereafter it become emerging therapeutic tools in many indications in dentistry, maxillofacial surgery, dermatology and esthetics. An article in New York Times gave this novel therapy a media hype describing, how 2 Pittsburg Steelers "used their own blood in an innovative injury treatment before winning the Super Bowl". The article cites several sports personalities who have been successfully treated similarly. It refers to PRP therapy as a means of delivering a "growth-factor cocktail" to injuries such as "tennis elbow" or "knee tendinitis".[5]

Although simultaneous researches have been started in many field of medicine, still scientifically proven evidences based on outcome in its efficacy is debatable. Cochrane review on use of PRP in musculoskeletal and soft tissue injuries is inconclusive. It concludes by saying "Overall, and for the individual clinical conditions, there is currently insufficient evidence to support the use of PRP for treating musculoskeletal or soft tissue injuries. There is need for standardization of PRP preparation methods".[6] Now, the PRP has become very essential for practising clinical dermatologists as well as for dermatosurgeons. This chapter aims to give comprehensive perspective of usage of PRP, methodology of preparation and their limitations.

PATHOPHYSIOLOGY OF PRP THERAPY

Platelets are natural sources of growth factors (GFs) and play a fundamental role in hemostasis. GFs, stored in platelet α-granules, are platelet- derived GF (PDGF), insulin- like GFf (IGF), vascular endothelial GF (VEGF), transforming growth factor β (TGF-β) and platelet- derived angiogenic factor (PDAF). The release of growth factors is usually triggered by activation of the platelets which can be most commonly initiated by variety of substances and stimuli like thrombin, collagen or calcium chloride. GFs are also involved in wound healing/regenerative processes like chemotaxis, proliferation, angiogenesis and differentiation.[7] It also contains plasma proteins, namely fibrin, fibronectin and vitronectin which act as scaffold for bone, connective tissue, epithelial migration.[8] The secreted growth factors which are released then bind to the respective transmembrane receptors expressed on the mesenchymal stem cells, fibroblasts, endothelial cells and epidermal cells.[3] This binding then induces various signal transduction pathways inside the cells leading to the expression of various gene sequencing function of cells-like proliferation of cells, bone formation and collagen synthesis. This enriches the wound healing process.[9] PRP also stimulates proliferation, differentiation of the stem cells in hair follicle bulge areas through multiple molecular mechanisms:[10]

- Upregulation of transcriptional activity of β-catenin which helps in differentiation of the stem cells into the hair follicle cells.
- Increase in bcl-2 levels, being antiapoptotic it prolongs survival of dermal papilla cells.
- Activation of Akt and ERK signalling pathways which prolongs survival of dermal papilla cells.
- Expression of FGF-7 in the dermal papilla cells which prolongs anagen phase of hair cycle.
- Increase in VEGF and PDGF level increases perifollicular vascular plexus.

Another field of interest is aesthetic dermatology. PRP can augment collagen remodelling through stimulation of removal of the photodamaged extracellular matrix components and inducing synthesis of the new collagen by the dermal fibroblasts through various molecular mechanisms:[11,12]

- Increased proliferation of human dermal fibroblasts.
- Increased expression of matrix metalloproteinase (MMP-1 and MMP-3) and removal of photodamaged ECM.
- Increased production of procollagen type I peptide and expression of collagen type I, alpha-I which help in synthesis of new collagen.
- Increases expression of G1 cell cycle regulators which accelerates wound healing.

PREPARATION OF PLATELET RICH PLASMA

It is a day care process performed under strict aseptic conditions as well as under optimum temperature regulations, i.e. 20 to 22°C after taking patient consent. In order to inhibit platelet aggregation, it is prepared with an anticoagulant, commonly using anticoagulant citrate dextrose solution formula A (ACD-A) or sodium citrate.[13]

BASIC PRINCIPLE OF PRP PROCEDURE

Centrifugation separates blood components due to their varying specific gravities, RBCs—heaviest, followed by WBCs, platelets—lightest. The first centrifugation which is usually a soft spin is done, so as to avoid spinning down of the platelets and also to isolate plasma. By this process platelets concentrate on the top of the buffy coat layer. The second spin which is the hard spin is a faster process and herein, the platelets are spinning down and they separate out as a pellet at the bottom of the tube from platelet poor plasma (PPP) above.[13]

STEP-WISE TECHNIQUE OF PLATELET RICH PLASMA PROCEDURE[14]

PRP Method

Flowchart 10.1 describes double centrifugation process in PRP. Whole blood (WB) is collected first in tubes which contain anticoagulants.

First spin step is then performed at a constant acceleration to mainly separate the RBCs from remaining WB volume. After first spin step, WB separates out into 3 layers: upper layer that mainly contains platelets and the WBC, intermediate thin layer known as buffy coat which is richer in WBCs and bottom layer which consists mostly RBCs. Second spin step is then done. 'G' for the second spin is to be just enough to help formation of the soft pellets (erythrocyte-platelet) at bottom of tube. Upper portion of volume composed mostly of the PPP (platelet-poor plasma) is removed. Pellets are therefore homogenized in lower third (5 mL of plasma) to create platelet-rich plasma (PRP). Items required in a resource poor set up and method of infiltration are hereby illustrated in the Figures 10.1 to 10.3 respectively.

Buffy Coat Method

Whole blood (WB) centrifuged at 'high speed' with a subsequent collection of buffy coat. Buffy coat contains a high concentration of the leukocytes. From small volume WB (10 mL), a thin layer of buffy coat can be produced. Difficulty lies in the separation of the thin buffy coat that contains mainly the white blood cells (WBCs) and the platelets, from underlying RBC layer.

TECHNIQUES OF PREPARATION

- Vaccutainer technique
- PRP method/buffy coat method
- Using commercially available PRP kits
- Modified syringe technique[15]

Vaccutainer Technique[14]

PRP Method

- Obtain WB by a venipuncture in the acid citrate dextrose (ACD) tubes.
- Do not chill out the blood during any time either before or during the platelet separation.
- Centrifuge blood using 'soft' spin.
- Transfer supernatant plasma containing the platelets into another of the sterile tubes (without anticoagulant).
- Centrifuge tube to higher speed (hard spin) to obtain the platelet concentrate.
- Lower 1/3rd is the PRP and upper 2/3rd is the plateletpoor plasma (PPP). At bottom of tube, platelet pellets are then formed.
- Remove the PPP and then suspend platelet pellets in minimum quantity of the plasma (2–4 mL) by mildly shaking the tube.

The authors use 1500 rpm × 5 min and 3000 rpm × 10 min as parameters for first and second spin respectively.

Buffy Coat Method

- WB to be stored at 20 to 24°C before centrifugation.
- Centrifuge the WB at 'high' speed.
- Three layers are then formed because of density: Bottom layer consists of RBCs, middle layer of platelets and the WBCs and top PPP layer.

Flowchart. 10.1: Explained in the pictorial itself.

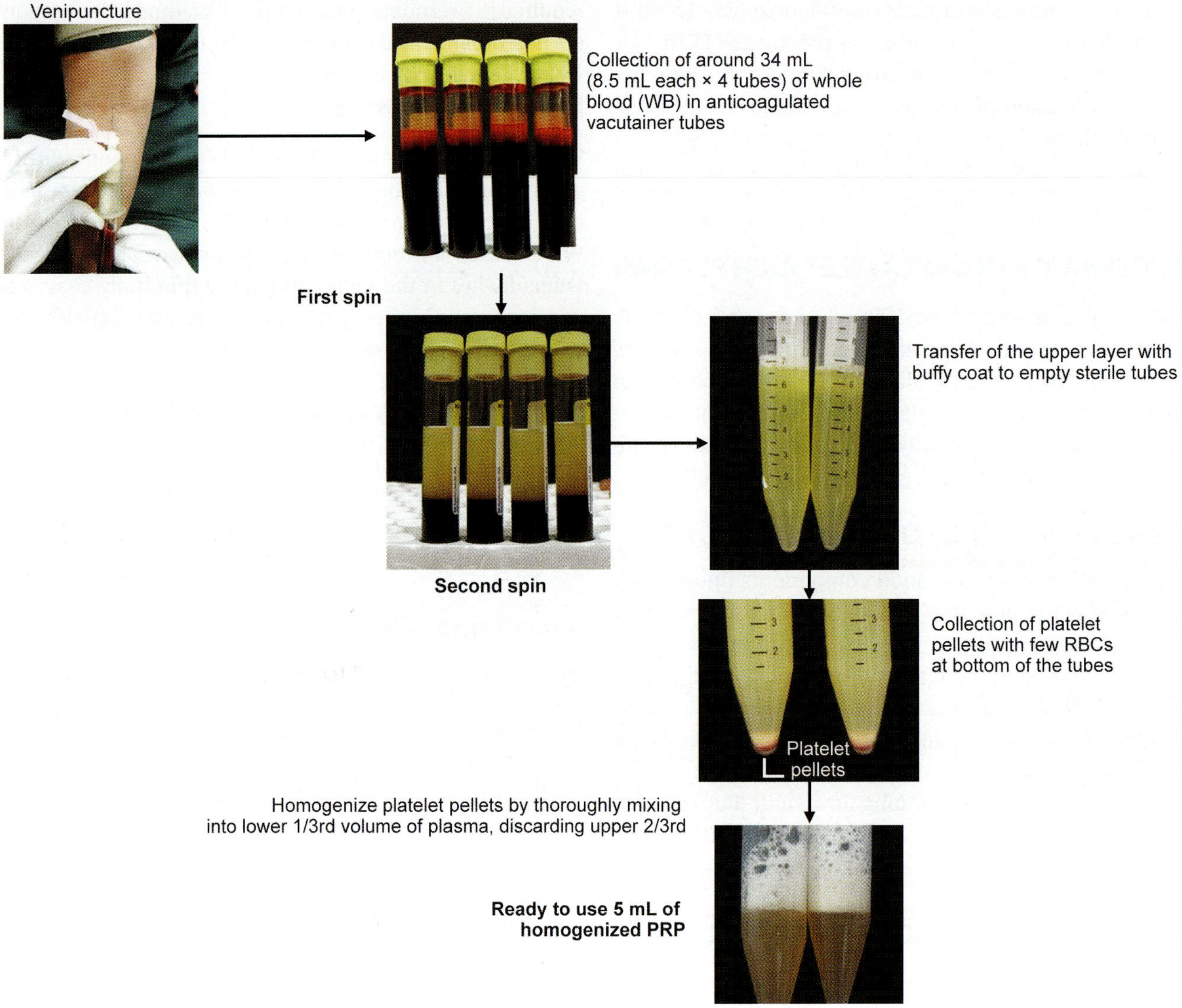

Courtesy: Dhurat R, Sukesh M.

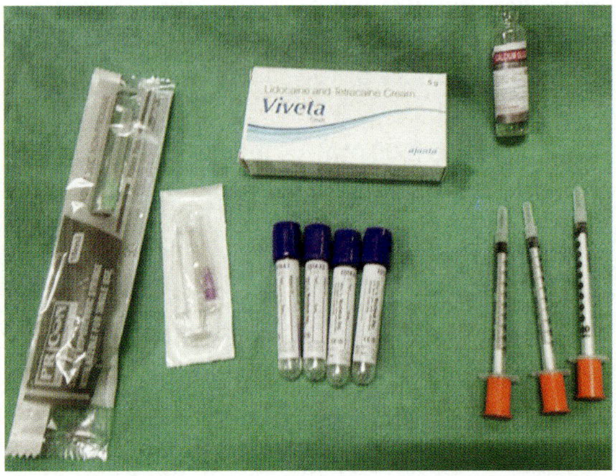

Fig. 10.1: Items used in making PRP in resource poor setting.

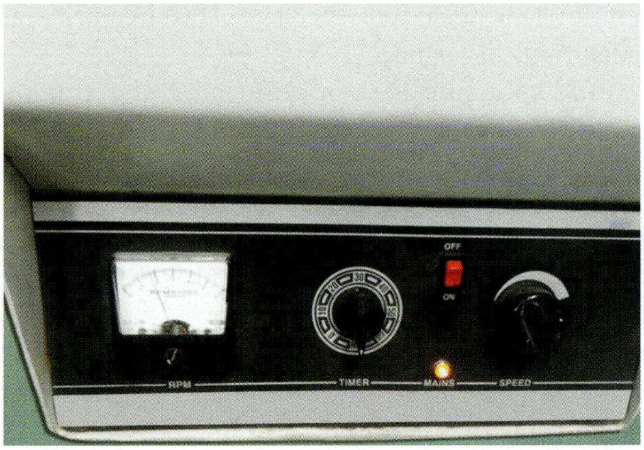

Fig. 10.2: Heavy duty centrifuge machine old pattern.

- Remove the supernatant plasma from top of container.
- Transfer buffy-coat layer to another of the sterile tubes.
- Centrifuge at a low speed to separate out WBCs or use the leukocyte filtration filter.

Using Commercially Available PRP Kits

There are lot of FDA approved commercial kits in market for the preparation of PRP. They used sterile endotoxin-free tubes of different kind. Most of these methods use single spin method.

The advantages of these kits are:

- Consistency in obtaining PRP.
- Closed systems, no risk of environmental contamination.

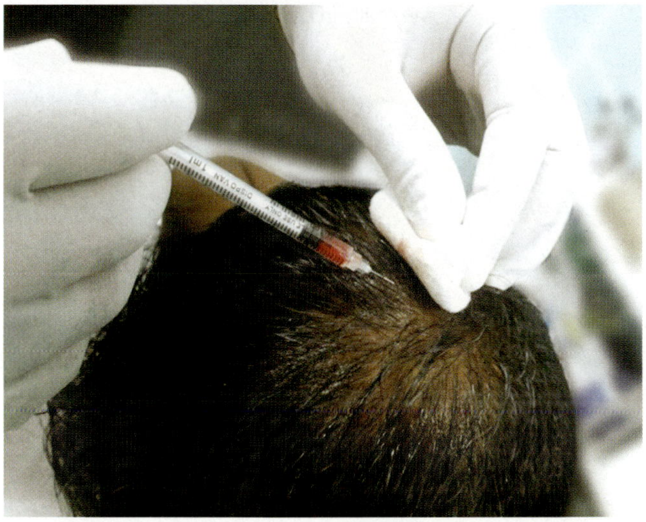

Fig. 10.3: Method of infiltration of platelet rich plasma.

- Fast, rapid harvesting.
- Chances of mixing with RBCs are minimal.

The disadvantages are:

- Expensive
- The final platelet concentrate obtained is only 1.5 to 2 times in most of the commercially available kits.

Modified Syringe Technique

The commercial kits for PRP are too expensive. The BD vacutainer are sterile but not endotoxin tested. BD do not recommend them for human injection use. Hypodermis syringes are sterile and endotoxin tested and can be used for human use. Mototsugu Fukaya et al describe this technique which is mentioned below to obtain easy PRP.[15]

The material required for the procedure:

- 5cc Luer lock hypodermis syringes.
- Syringe tip caps.
- 3-way connector.
- Scalp vein set.
- Sterile ACD-A solution.

Procedure (Figs. 10.4 to 10.9)

- Cut the finger guard of the syringes with sterile scissor so as to convert syringe into a tube.
- 0.5cc of ACD-A is taken in 2 tubes.
- 5cc of blood is withdrawn into syringes using a 19 no. scalp vein set.
- The tips of syringes are closed with sterile tip caps.
- The syringes are directly kept into the centrifuge with tips facing upward.

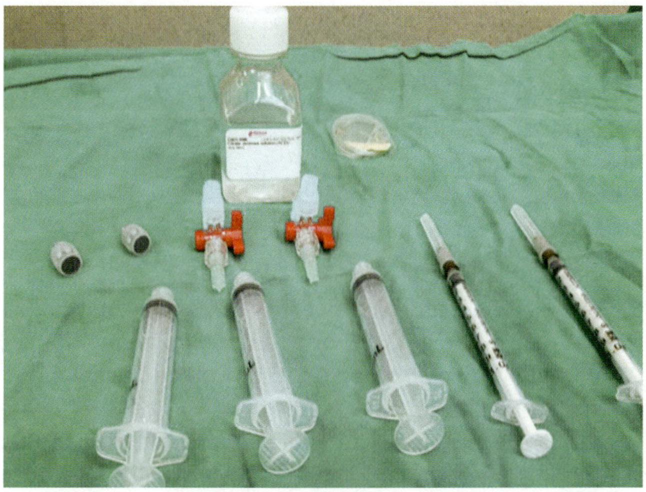

Fig. 10.4: Materials required.

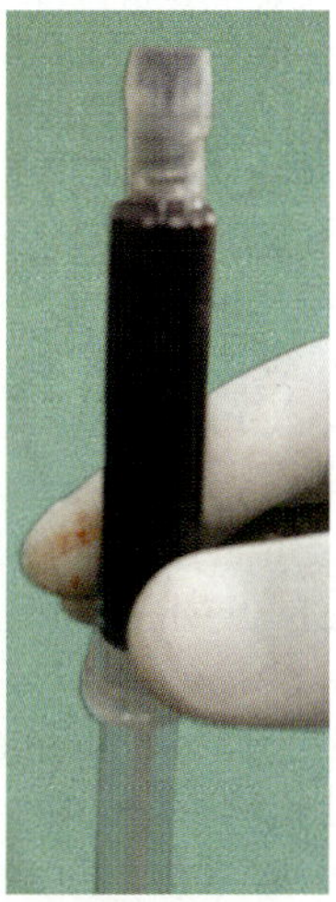

Fig. 10.5: Cut the finger guard.

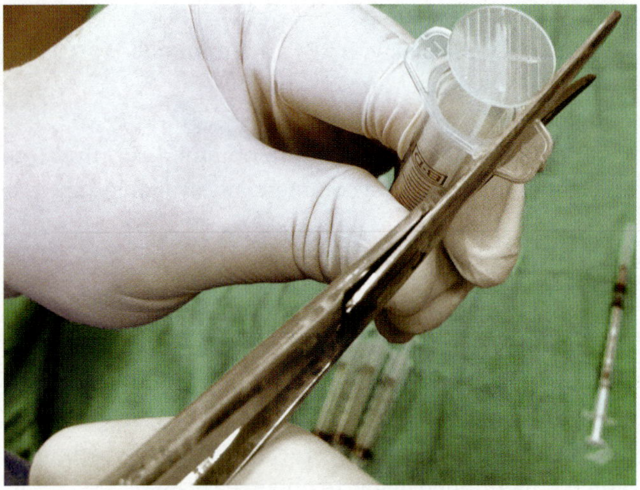

Fig. 10.6: Syringes are converted to tubes.

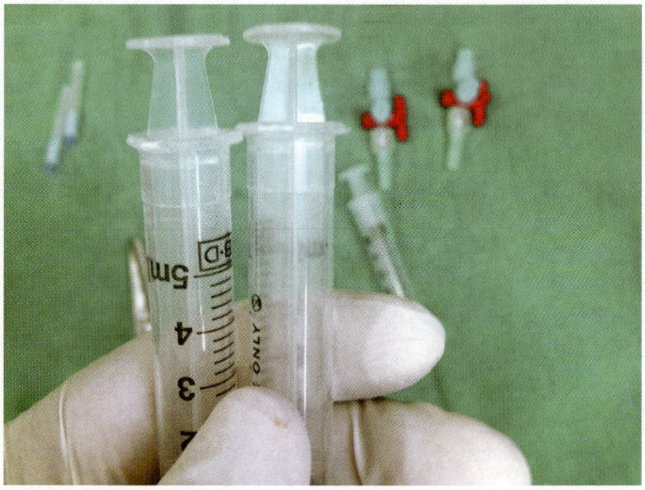

Fig. 10.7: Blood is collected, syringe cap applied and tube kept vertically in centrifuge.

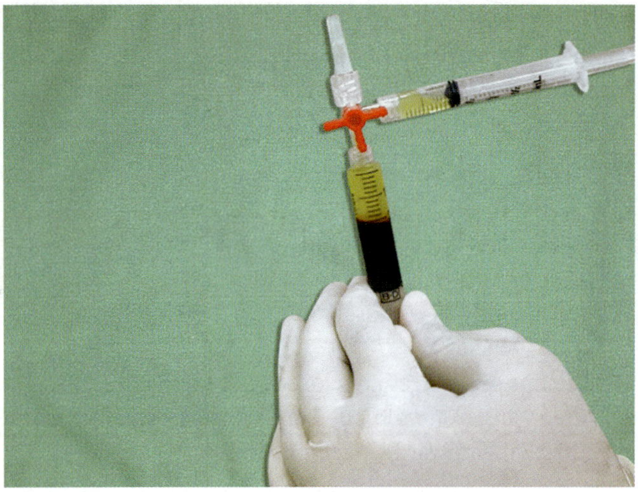

Fig. 10.8: After centrifugation—RBC layer below, thin buffy coat in middle and plasma with platelet layer above.

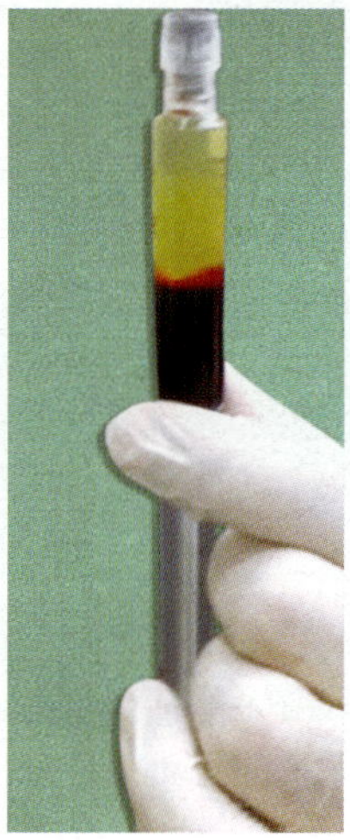

Fig. 10.9: 3-way connector applied and PRP is separated.

- Centrifuged with desired RPM. One can use single spin or double spin method.
- After centrifugation the blood is separated into lower RBC, buffy coat layer and PPP.
- 3-way connector is attached to the syringe tip. Upper end is closed. Another syringe is attached to the open end, and PPP is aspirated. Once a buffy coat is reached, tuberculin syringe is attached and the buffy coat is slowly aspirated, so as to obtain PRP.
- For better control of aspiration, one can attach an IV line extension set to the 3-way connector.
- Using another 3-way connector one can mix PPP and PRP in a tuberculin syringe.

Advantages

- Simple
- Cost effective
- Closed system, no risk of contamination
- Highly programmable.

Disadvantages

- Since syringes and commercial PRP tubes are not coated with silicone on their inner surface, platelet can get partially activated when they come in contact with the surface, and form a reversible clot.
- If we try to measure the platelet concentration at this time by an automated analyzer, we usually get a very low count. The only way to measure a true count is

by making a smear and counting platelets manually. However since the clot is reversible it does not alter the effectiveness of PRP.

ACTIVATION OF PLATELETS

Once obtained, platelets in PRP can be activated by using 10% calcium solution in the ratio of 1:9 (0.1 mL of 10% calcium chloride to 0.9 mL of PRP) or by using thrombin. The active secretion of prepackaged GFs begins within 10 minutes of clot initiation and 95% of the secretion is completed within 1 hour. Hence, PRP must be used on the treated site within 10 minutes of activation or else a gel would be formed making injection difficult. The concentrated platelets usually remain viable for upto 8 hours and is sterile, if placed on sterile surgical table.

TIPS AND TRICKS[14]

Following points are usually helpful in obtaining the optimum PRP concentrate:

- Temperature gradient of 12 to 20°C during centrifugation is required of optimum platelet recovery. Hence a refrigerated centrifuge is recommended.
- ACD>CPDA vacutainers are recommended for the procedure. EDTA tubes must be avoided as it causes platelet membrane damage. In addition PRP infiltration made in EDTA tubes are more painful.
- Blood is drawn in anticoagulant vacutainer tubes using the BD Eclipse™ blood collection needle (Ref: 368607; BD Biosciences, India) (Fig. 10.10). Set apart at least 1–2 mL for the baseline cell counting like RBCs, platelets, the WBCs and hematocrit. Donor percentage hematocrit (ratio of volume of RBCs to total volume of blood) is relevant to the plasma yield optimization. Blood with low percent hematocrit has generally more plasma available, so it dilutes the concentration of the platelets in plasma.
- Blood samples which are collected in ACD tubes are inverted 5 to 10 times for the proper mixing of anticoagulant and blood, otherwise small fibrin clots may then form, causing falsely decreased platelet counts.
- After the 1st spin, measure platelet count in the RBCs and supernatant to ensure the optimal separation of platelets from WB. If it does not happen, change parameters like rpm and time.
- After the first spin, if a large volume of plasma presents itself, then it would need a higher 'g' to concentrate the platelets at bottom of tube (law of the velocity).
- After the second spin, measure platelet count in the PPP and PRP after adequate racking of the tubes.
- If higher concentration of the platelets in the platelet poor plasma (upper layer) or a lower concentration in the PRP (bottom layer) is then observed, the parameters are then not optimal.
- PRP must be then separated from PPP soon after the centrifugation because concentrated platelets will then slowly diffuse into PPP over time and this would reduce platelet count of PRP preparation.
- For counting platelets in final PRP concentrate, it must then be resuspended for least of 5 to 10 min to allow for the equal distribution of platelets before the counting.

To obtain yield of platelet in the PRP more than 10 lakhs/mL, all variables like rpm, time and the temperature should be standardized with consistency of platelet concentrate maintained over the period. Various permutations and combinations with respect to the above factors have to be standardized with the available centrifuge machine to obtain the optimum yield of PRP.

TECHNIQUES OF PRP DELIVERY[13]

- Topical application of PRP.
- Intradermal injections by insulin syringes. The area to be injected is divided into grids and 0.1 mL is injected in each area, preferably 0.1 mL/cm^2 as used in intralesional triamcinolone injection.
- Combination treatments with fractional lasers, fillers and autologous fat.
- Along with microneedling/dermaroller.
- Topical application of PRP gel on ulcers.

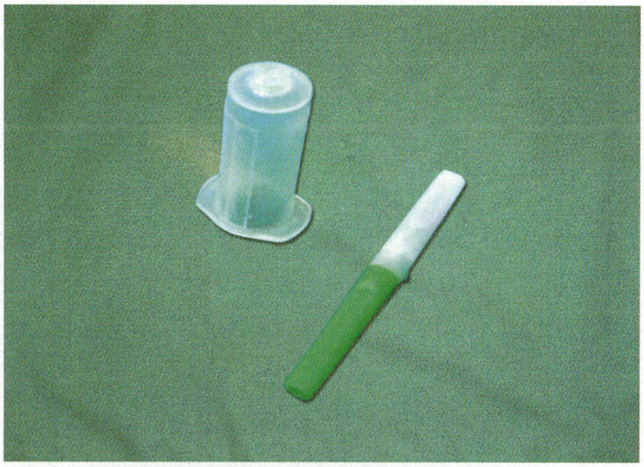

Fig. 10.10: Eclipse™ blood collection needle.

CLASSIFICATION OF PLATELET RICH PLASMA

According to classification proposed by author Ehrenfest et al., four main families of preparations can usually be defined, depending on cell content and fibrin architecture:[16]

- Pure PRP or leukocyte poor PRP products are the preparations without leukocytes and with low-density fibrin network after the activation. After the first spin, only the upper part of buffy coat is aspirated and the final concentrate has a large number of platelets with very few leukocytes.
- Leukocyte and PRP (L-PRP) products are preparations with leukocytes and with a low density fibrin network after activation. The entire buffy coat and the superficial layer of RBCs are aspirated out and this gives a final solution which is rich in leukocytes and platelets.
- Pure platelet-rich fibrin (P-PRF) or leukocyte poor platelet-rich fibrin preparations are without leukocytes and with a high-density fibrin network. As these products only exist in a strongly activated gelform, they cannot be injected or used like the traditional fibrin glues. This is derived from P-PRP. The P-PRP is mixed with activator and allowed to incubate for a small defined period of time. A stable P-PRF clot is obtained by this method.
- Leukocyte and the platelet-rich fibrin (L-PRF) or the second-generation PRP products are mainly preparations with the leukocytes and with high-density fibrin network. This is prepared from whole blood, by centrifuging without adding anticoagulant. The three layers that are collected in this manner include a top layer of cellular plasma, a base layer of RBC and a L-PRF clot in the middle.

INDICATIONS OF PRP IN DERMATOLOGY AND ESTHETICS

Rationale behind usage of PRP in field of dermatology and aesthetics is the knowledge that important roles are played by GFs which are involved in key stages of wound healing and regenerative processes including chemotaxis, proliferation, differentiation and angiogenesis. The diseases where pathogenesis is not clear or there are no effective therapies available at present, PRP gives ray of hope. PRP are being tried in many indications but credible evidences are still lacking. There are limited conditions where double-blind, controlled trials are available. Most of the literatures are uncontrolled studies, case series, or isolated cases. It has been combined with different types of ablative lasers for facial rejuvenation and management of acne scars. There are numerous drawback of PRP before it is considered an effective tool for dermatological and aesthetic usage. These are small sample sizes, wide variations in methods of preparation of PRP, inconsistent assessment tools for particular indications, lack of studies with negative outcome and bleak follow-up data. Photographs depicting the pre- and post- PRP therapy outcome from our clinical practises are illustrated in Figures 10.11 to 10.14. The indications for which PRP has been tried with promising results are enumerated below.

- Androgenetic alopecia[17-31]
- Alopecia areata[32-34]

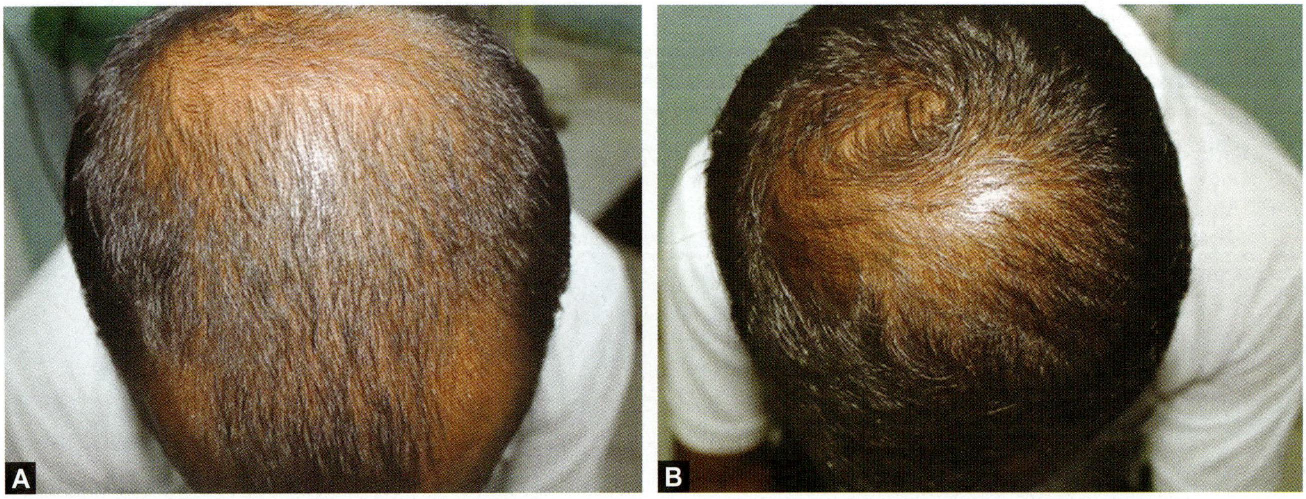

Figs. 10.11A and B: (A) A case of androgenetic alopecia before treatment; (B) Post four sitting of PRP along with minoxidil 5% lotion.

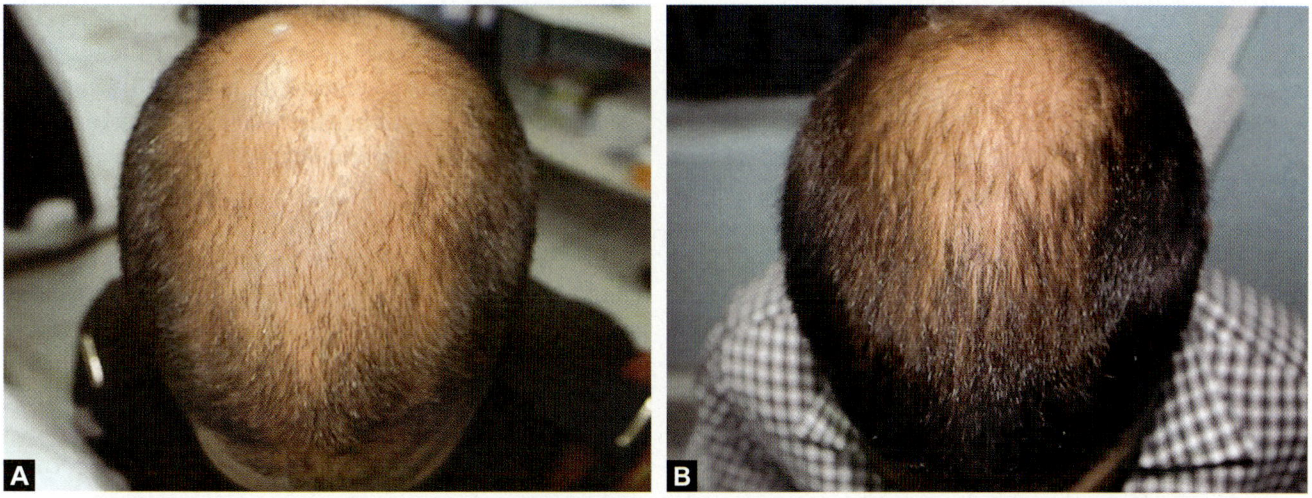

Figs. 10.12A and B: (A) A case of androgenetic alopecia before PRP. (B) Post PRP four sitting along with minoxidil 5% lotion.

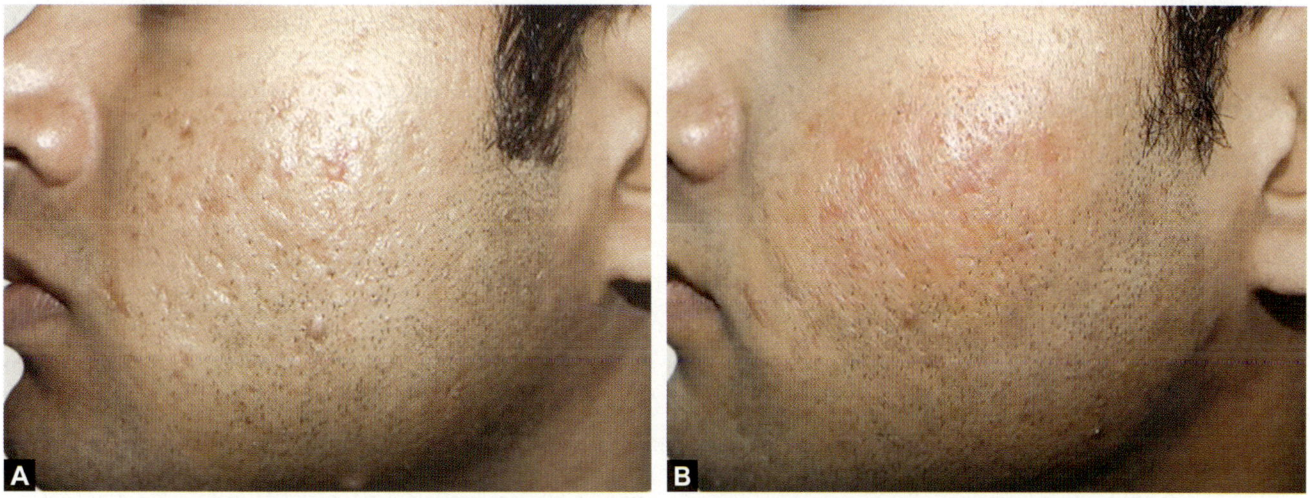

Figs. 10.13A and B: (A) Acne scars preoperation. (B) Acne scars post three sittings of PRP with dermaroller.

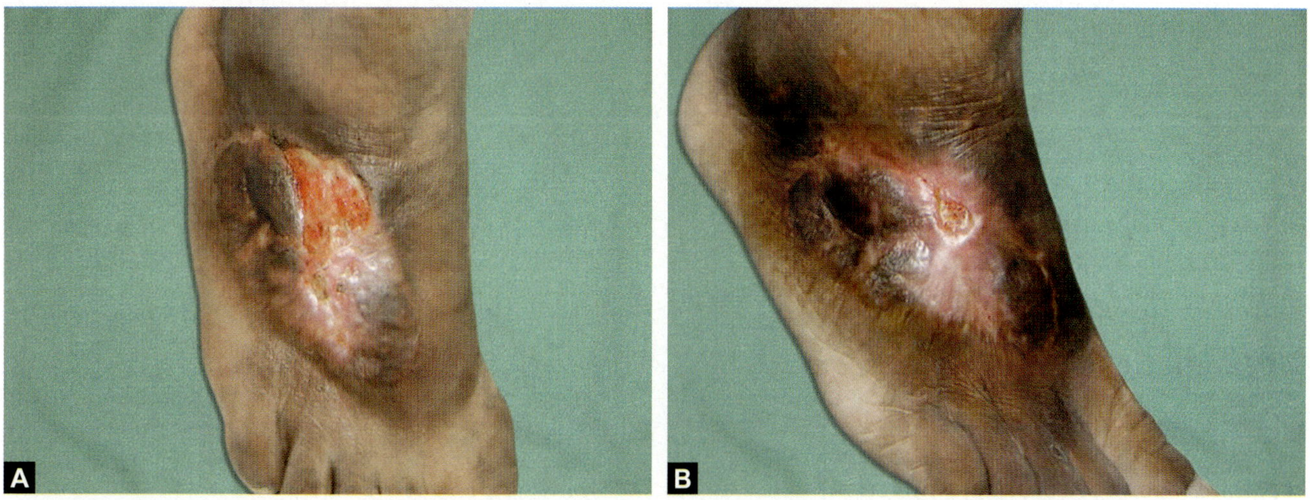

Figs. 10.14A and B: (A) Chronic nonhealing traumatic ulcer. (B) Chronic nonhealing ulcer post three sittings of intralesional PRP.

- Chronic ulcers of various aetiologies[35-41]
- Acne scars or traumatic scars and contour defects of face[42-46]
- Skin rejuvenation of face.[46-53]

  Statistically significant improvement in management of the acne and trauma scars as well as of contour defects of the face have been seen. However study conducted by Lee demonstrated that adding the platelet-rich plasma to fractional CO_2 laser treatment did not produce statistically significant synergistic effect and resulted in more severe side effects and a longer downtime.[47]
- Miscellaneous indications
  - Striae distensae[54-56]
  - Lichen sclerosus[57]
  - Lipodermatosclerosis[58]
  - Sensory improvement in peripheral neuropathy of leprosy[59]
  - Pyoderma gangrenosum.[60]

CONTRAINDICATIONS[13,14]

Absolute

- Platelet dysfunction syndrome, e.g. Bernard-Soulier syndrome, Wiskott-Aldrich syndrome
- Viral infections causing thrombocytopenia—herpes simplex, CMV, varicella-zoster, EBV, rubella, enterovirus, mumps, HIV, hepatitis
- Hemodynamically unstable as in cardiac complaints
- Local infection at site of procedure
- Systemic infections/sepsis.

Relative

- Corticosteroid injection at the treatment site within a month
- Consumption of NSAIDs, antiplatelet drugs within 5 days of procedure
- Systemic use of corticosteroids within last 2 weeks
- Alcohol and tobacco use
- Fever or illness recently
- Hematopoietic or bone cancer
- Hemoglobin <10 g/dL and platelet count < 1,05,000 per μL

COMPLICATIONS[13,14]

PRP is devoid of serious adverse effects being an autologous preparation, apart from few local injection site reactions—pain or secondary infection, and can be avoided with proper precautions. Scar-tissue formation and calcification are rare possibilities. Since PRP contains some RBCs, their deposition theoretically could lead to pigmentary changes due to deposition of hemosiderin. However, safety concerns with bovine thrombin have been raised about the potential transmission of Creutzfeldt-Jakob disease (mad-cow disease). Newer alternatives like human recombinant thrombin, thrombin receptor agonist peptide (TRAP), autologous thrombin (prepared simultaneously with some of the available kits) or type-I collagen have been explored. On the other hand, use of $CaCl_2$ as an activator, automatically eliminates the above risks.

CONCLUSION

The PRP has emerged as a newer therapeutic tool in the field of dermatology and aesthetics. Conditions like lichen sclerosus, striae distensae, lipodermatosclerosis, etc. where no contemporary therapies are effective; PRP has given ray of hope. Future of PRP is still full of challenges as there are very limited studies with credible evidences on different indications of dermatology as well as esthetics. There are wide variations in the methods of preparation of PRP, in different studies and commercially available kits. In addition, there is lack of standardization in commercially available centrifuge machines which are being used for preparation of PRP in routine clinical setting. Utmost care shall be taken to avoid contamination, proper biomedical waste disposal of tubes and handling of left over blood products during and postprocedures.

REFERENCES

1. Wang H-L, Avila G. Platelet rich plasma: myth or reality? European Journal of Dentistry. 2007;1(4):192-4.
2. Marx RE. Platelet rich plasma (PRP): What is PRP and what is not PRP? Implant Dent. 2001;10:225-8.
3. Marx RE, Carlson ER, Eichstaedt RM, Schimmele SR, Strauss JE, Georgeff KR. Platelet-rich plasma: Growth factor enhancement for bone grafts. Oral Surg Oral Med Oral Pathol Oral Radiol Endod. 1998;85:638-46.
4. Mishra A, Pavelko T. Treatment of chronic elbow tendinosis with buffered platelet-rich plasma. The American Journal of Sports Medicine. 2006;34(11):1774-8.
5. Schwarz A. A promising treatment for athletes, in blood. The New York Times, Sports Section.p A1, 2009.
6. Cochrane Database of Systematic Reviews 2014, Issue 4. Art. No.CD010071. DOI: 10.1002/14651858.CD010071.pub3.
7. Bennett NT, Schultz GS. Growth factors and wound healing: biochemical properties of growth factors and their receptors. Am J Surg. 1993;165:728-37.

8. Steed DL. The role of growth factors in wound healing. Surg Clin North Am. 1997;77:575-86.
9. Marx RE. Platelet-rich plasma: Evidence to support its use. J Oral Maxillofac Surg. 2004;62:489-96.
10. Li ZJ, Choi HI, Choi DK, Sohn KC, Im M, Seo YJ, et al. Autologous platelet-rich plasma: a potential therapeutic tool for Promoting Hair Growth. Dermatol Surg. 2012;38: 1040-6.
11. Kim DH, Je YJ, Kim CD, Lee YH, Seo YJ, Lee JH, et al. Can platelet-rich plasma be used for skin rejuvenation? Evaluation of effects of platelet-rich plasma on human dermal fibroblast. Ann Dermatol. 2011;23:424-31.
12. Cho JW, Kim SA, Lee KS. Platelet-rich plasma induces increased expression of G1 cell cycle regulators, type I collagen, and matrix metalloproteinase-1 in human skin fibroblasts. Int J Mol Med. 2012;29:32-6.
13. Arshdeep, Kumaran MS. Platelet-rich plasma in dermatology: boon or a bane? Indian J Dermatol Venereol Leprol. 2014;80: 5-14.
14. Dhurat R, Sukesh M. Principles and methods of preparation of platelet-rich plasma: a review and author's perspective. J Cut Aesth Surg. 2014;7(4):189-97.
15. Fukaya M, Ito A. A New economic method for preparing platelet-rich plasma; Plast Reconstr Surg Glob Open. 2014; 2(6):e162.
16. Dohan Ehrenfest DM, Rasmusson L, Albrektsson T. Classification of platelet concentrates: from pure platelet-rich plasma (P-PRP) to leucocyte- and platelet-rich fibrin (L-PRF). Trends Biotechnol. 2009;27:158-67.
17. Uebel CO, da Silva JB, Cantarelli D, Martins P. The role of platelet plasma growth factors in male pattern baldness surgery. Plast Reconstr Surg. 2006;118:1458-66.
18. Kang JS, Zheng Z, Choi MJ. The effect of CD34+ cell-containing autologous platelet-rich plasma injection on pattern hair loss: a preliminary study. J Eur Acad Dermatol Venereol. 2014;28:72-9.
19. Schiavone G, Raskovic D, Greco J. Platelet-rich plasma for androgenetic alopecia: A pilot study. Dermatol Surg. 2014;40:1010-19.
20. Khatu SS, More YE, Gokhale NR, Chavhan DC, Bendsure N. Platelet-rich plasma in androgenic alopecia: Myth or an effective tool. J Cutan Aesthet Surg. 2014;7:107-10.
21. Besti EE, Germain E, Kalbermatten DF, Tremp M, Emmenegger V. Platelet-rich plasma injection is effective and safe for the treatment of alopecia. Eur J Plast Surg. 2013;36:407-12.
22. Godse, Kiran. "Platelet rich plasma in androgenic alopecia: where do we stand?" J Cutan Aesthet Surg. 2014;7(2):110.
23. Gupta AK, Carviel JL. "Meta-analysis of efficacy of platelet-rich plasma therapy for androgenetic alopecia." J Dermatolog Treat. 2016:1-4.
24. Singhal P, Agarwal S, Dhot PS, Sayal SK. Efficacy of platelet-rich plasma in treatment of androgenic alopecia. Asian J Transfus Sci. 2015; 9(2):159-62.
25. Alexandros-Efstratios K, Dimitris R, Konstantinos K. Platelet-rich plasma as a potential treatment for noncicatricial alopecias. Int J Trichol. 2015;7:54-63.
26. Greco J, Brandt R. The effects of autologous platelet rich plasma and various growth factors on non-transplanted miniaturized hair. Hair Transplant Forum Int. 2009;19: 49-50.
27. Takikawa M, Nakamura S, Nakamura S, et al. Enhanced effect of platelet-rich plasma containing a new carrier on hair growth. Dermatol Surg. 2011;37:1721-9.
28. Park KY, Kim HK, Kim BJ, Kim MN. Letter: Platelet-rich plasma for treating male pattern baldness. Dermatol Surg. 2012;38:2042-4.
29. Gkini MA, Kouskoukis AE, Tripsianis G, Rigopoulos D, Kouskoukis K. Study of platelet-rich plasma injections in the treatment of androgenetic alopecia through an one-year period. J Cutan Aesthet Surg. 2014;7:213.
30. Greco J, Brandt R. Our experience with platelet rich plasma and hair restoration. Hum Trichology. 2010;1:49-53.
31. Gentile, Pietro, et al. "The Effect of Platelet Rich Plasma in Hair Regrowth: A Randomized PlaceboControlled Trial." Stem cells translational medicine. 2015;4(11):1317-23.
32. Trink A, Sorbellini E, Bezzola P, et al. A randomized, double-blind, placebo and active controlled, half- head study to evaluate the effects of plateletrich plasma on alopecia areata. Br J Dermatol. 2013;169:690-4.
33. Singh S. Role of platelet-rich plasma in chronic alopecia areata: Our centre experience. Indian J Plast Surg 2015; 48(1):57–9.
34. Kumar A, Sharma RP, Bali S, et al. Role of platelet rich plasma therapy in alopecia areataa prospective study. IJCMR. 2016;3(8):2499-2502.
35. Kathleen ML, Dardik A. Platelet-rich plasma: support for its use in wound healing. Yale J Biol Med. 2010;83(1): 1-9.
36. Setta S, Hany, et al. Platelet rich plasma versus plateletpoor plasma in the management of chronic diabetic foot ulcers: a comparative study. Int Wound J. 2011;8: 307-312.
37. Yotsu RR, Hagiwara S, Okochi H, et al. Case series of patients with chronic foot ulcers treated with autologous platelet-rich plasma. J Dermatol. 2015;42:288–295
38. Smiell JM, Wieman TJ, Steed DL, Perry BH, Sampson AR,Schwab BH. Efficacy and safety of becaplermin (recombinant human platelet-derived growth factor-BB) in patients with nonhealing, lower extremity diabetic ulcers: a combined analysis of four randomized studies. Wound Repair Regen. 1999;7:335-46.
39. Kim SA, Ryu HW, Lee KS, Cho JW. Application of platelet-rich plasma accelerates the wound healing process in acute and chronic ulcers through rapid migration and upregulation of cyclin A and CDK4 in HaCaT cells. Mol Med Rep. 2013;7: 476-80.
40. Martinez-Zapata MJ, Martí-Carvajal AJ, Solà I, Expósito JA, Bolíbar I, Rodríguez L, et al. Autologous platelet-rich plasma for treating chronic wounds. Cochrane Database Syst Rev Online. 2012;10:CD006899.
41. Conde-Montero E, Horcajada-Reales C, Clavo P, et al. Neuropathic ulcers in leprosy treated with intralesional platelet rich plasma. Int Wound J. 2014;1.
42. Cervelli V, Nicoli F, Spallone D, et al. Treatment of traumatic scars using fat grafts mixed with platelet-rich plasma, and

resurfacing of skin with the 1540 nm nonablative laser. Clin Exp Dermatol. 2012;37:55-61.
43. Oh IY, Kim BJ, Kim MN. Depressed facial scars successfully treated with autologous platelet-rich plasma and light-emitting diode phototherapy at 830 nm. Annals of Dermatology. 2014;26(3):417-8.
44. Sclafani AP. Platelet-rich fibrin matrix for improvement of deep nasolabial folds. J Cosmet Dermatol. 2010;9: 66-71.
45. Park KY, Kim IS, Kim BJ, Kim MN. Letter: Autologous fat grafting and platelet-rich plasma for treatment of facial contour defects. Dermatol Surg. 2012;38:1572-4.
46. Faghihi G, Keyvan S, Asilian A, Nouraei S, Behfar S, Nilforoushzadeh MA. Efficacy of autologous platelet-rich plasma combined with fractional ablative carbon dioxide resurfacing laser in treatment of facial atrophic acne scars: a split-face randomized clinical trial. Indian J Dermatol Venereol Leprol. 2016;82:162-8.
47. Lee JW, Kim BJ, Kim MN, Mun SK. The efficacy of autologous platelet rich plasma combined with ablative carbon dioxide fractional resurfacing for acne scars: a simultaneous split-face trial. Dermatol Surg. 2011;37:931-8.
48. Kim DH, Je YJ, Kim CD, et al. Can platelet-rich plasma be used for skin rejuvenation? Evaluation of effects of platelet-rich plasma on human dermal fibroblast. Annals of Dermatology. 2011;23(4):424-31.
49. Redaelli A, Romano D, Marcianó A. Face and neck revitalization with platelet-rich plasma (PRP): Clinical outcome in a series of 23 consecutively treated patients. J Drugs Dermatol. 2010;9:466-72.
50. Shin MK, Lee JH, Lee SJ, Kim NI. Platelet-rich plasma combined with fractional laser therapy for skin rejuvenation. Dermatol Surg. 2012;38:623-30.
51. Na JI, Choi JW, Choi HR, Jeong JB, Park KC, Youn SW, et al. Rapid healing and reduced erythema after ablative fractional carbon dioxide laser resurfacing combined with the application of autologous platelet-rich plasma. Dermatol Surg. 2011;37:463-8.
52. Kang BK, Lee JH, Shin MK, Kim NI. Infraorbital rejuvenation using PRP (platelet-rich plasma): A prospective, randomized, split-face trial. J Am Acad Dermatol. 2013;68:SAB24.
53. Mikhael NW, El-Esawy FM. Skin rejuvenation with autologous concentrated platelet-rich plasma. Egypt J Dermatol Venerol. 2014;34:5-9.
54. Kim IS, Park KY, Kim BJ, et al. Efficacy of intradermal radiofrequency combined with autologous platelet-rich plasma in striae distensae: A pilot study. Int J Dermatol. 2012;51:1253-8.
55. Suh DH, Lee SJ, Lee JH, et al. Treatment of striae distensae combined enhanced penetration platelet-rich plasma and ultrasound after plasma fractional radiofrequency. J Cosmet Laser Ther. 2012;14:272-6.
56. Ibrahim ZA, El-Tatawy RA, El-Samongy MA, Ali DA. Comparison between the efficacy and safety of plateletrich plasma vs. microdermabrasion in the treatment of striae distensae: clinical and histopathological study. Journal of Cosmetic Dermatology. 2015;14(4):336-46.
57. Casabona F, Priano V, Vallerino V, et al. New surgical approach to lichen sclerosus of the vulva: the role of adipose-derived mesenchymal cells and platelet-rich plasma in tissue regeneration. Plast Reconstr Surg. 2010;126:e210-1.
58. Jeong KH, Shin MK, Kim NI. Refractory lipodermatosclerosis treated with intralesional platelet-rich plasma. J Am Acad Dermatol. 2011;65:e157-8.
59. Anjayani S, Wirohadidjojo YW, Adam AM, et al. Sensory improvement of leprosy peripheral neuropathy in patients treated with perineural injection of platelet-rich plasma. Int J Dermatol. 2014;53:109–13.
60. Budamakuntla L, Suryanarayan S, Sarvajnamurthy SS, et al. Autologous platelet rich plasma in pyodermagangrenosum-Two case reports. Indian J Dermatol. 2015;60:204-5.

CHAPTER 11

Surgical Treatment of Acne Scars

Imran Majid, Syed Mubashir

INTRODUCTION

Acne vulgaris is one of the most common skin disorders seen in 85% of teenagers and 3% of people aged 35–44 years.[1] Studies have reported highly variable figures of frequency of scarring secondary to acne. This is because of differences in the evaluation method, recruitment and definition itself of the scars and, in particular, whether or not pigmentation and erythema are included in scarring assessment.[2,3] Post acne scarring is a common and a distressing condition with a significant negative impact on the quality of life.

Treatment of acne scars is a real therapeutic challenge. Most of the topical medications are mildly effective at the most and they are associated with troublesome side effects.

Many procedural treatments are employed to treat acne scars and the choice of procedure depends upon the availability of the treatment option, training and surgical expertise of the treating physician and the morphology and severity of scarring present. Procedures used to treat acne scars range from simple office procedures like peels and microdermabrasion to aggressive procedures like laser resurfacing and surgical treatment options. In many cases a combination of multiple treatment modalities are required to get a satisfactory therapeutic response.

Table 11.1: Classification of acne scars.

Atrophic acne scars	It is more common as compared to hypertrophic scars and can be broadly classified into three types
Ice pick scars	*Deep pitted scars exhibiting narrow opening with 0.5 mm or greater extension into the dermis, resembling a small hole*
Boxcar scars	*Most common, depressed, crateriform scars measures 3 to 4 mm or less in diameter*
Rolling scars	*Soft, distensible, depressed scars with wrinkled superficial base, can be small < 1 cm or large > 1 cm. Shallow scars may be subtle which become evident with lighting and when patient moves head.*[4]
Hypertrophic Scars	These are raised pink lesions with thick firm hyalinized tissue within the borders of tissue injury

TYPES OF ACNE SCARS

Acne scars are classified into the following morphological types (Table 11.1 and Fig. 11.1).

SCAR EVALUATION

Regarding the scar evaluation, two scales are most often used: Goodman and Baron scale (Table 11.2) and the ECCA (échelle d'évaluation clinique des cicatrices d'acné) scale (Table 11.3).

PRINCIPLES OF ACNE SCAR TREATMENT

- Acne scar treatment is complex and difficult. This is primarily due to two facts about acne scars: their depth (because of the localization in the deep dermis) and presence of underlying fibrosis.
- Fibrosis is really difficult to treat at any site and as the fibrotic process is present deep in the dermis it becomes even more difficult to manage it in acne scars.
- The underlying principle in acne scar management is to reduce the depth of the scars in order to minimize the shadow effect. In addition any dyspigmentation or irregularity of scar surface has to be managed to create a significant impact on the overall appearance of the scars.

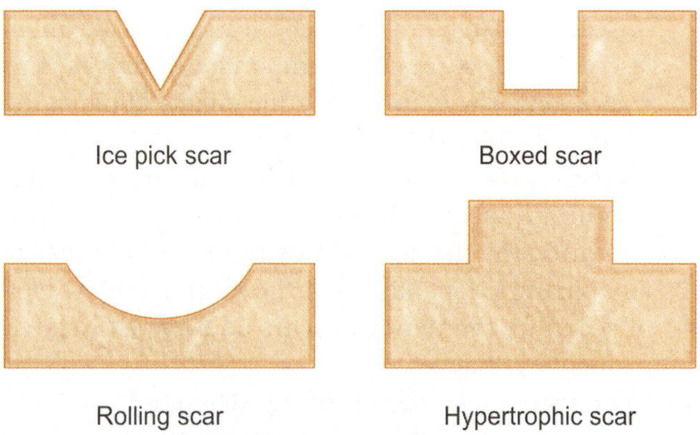

Fig. 11.1: Types of acne scars.

Table 11.2: Qualitative scarring grading system (Goodman and Baron).

Grades of post acne scarring	*Level of disease*	*Clinical features*
1	Macular	Those scars can be erythematous, hyper or hypopigmented flat marks.
2	Mild	Mild atrophic or hypertrophic scars that may not be obvious at social distance of 50 cm or greater and may be covered adequately by make up or the normal shadow of shaved beard hair in men or normal body hair, if extrafacial.
3	Moderate	Moderate atrophic or hypertrophic scarring that is obvious at social distances of 50 cm or greater and is not covered easily by make up or the normal shadow of shaved beard hair in men or body hair, if extrafacial, but is still able to be flattened by manual stretching of the skin (if atrophic).
4	Severe	Severe atrophic and hypertrophic scarring that is evident at social distance greater than 50 cm and is not covered easily by make up or the normal shadow of shaved beard hair in men or body hair, if extrafacial and is not able to be flattened by manual stretching of skin.

Table 11.3: Acne scars assessed by the ECCA (échelle d' évaluation clinique des cicatrices d'acné) scale.[5]

- V-shaped
- U-shaped
- M-shaped
- Superficial elastolysis
- Hypertrophic inflammatory scar
- Keloids

- It is very important to realize that scars are never eradicated and can never be changed into normal skin. Instead the aim of treating acne scars is to make them less visible at cosmetically important distances. This goes a long way in improving the quality of life of the affected individual.
- Majority of the patients with acne scars need a combination of different procedures to achieve a significant therapeutic response. The specific combination depends upon the morphological type of scarring, the depth of scars and any associated pigmentary changes.
- The different scars can be managed best by:
  - *Rolling scars*: Fractional laser resurfacing, microneedling
  - *Deep rolling or boxcar scars*: Need additional surgical procedures like subcision, punch elevation or excision. Dermal grafts or even fillers can be used in combination with fractional laser resurfacing to achieve good results in boxcar scars.
  - *Ice-pick scars*: Respond best to trichloroacetic acid—chemical reconstruction of skin scars (TCA CROSS) technique. This technique can also be combined with fractional laser resurfacing to improve the therapeutic response further.

PROCEDURES USED FOR TREATMENT OF ACNE SCARS

The main procedures employed for managing acne scars are as under:

- Microneedling
- Laser resurfacing
- Scar revision procedures
- Subcision
- Punch techniques
- TCA CROSS
- Dermal grafting
- Soft tissue augmentation with fat and fillers.

MICRONEEDLING

Microneedling is performed by using a dermaroller which is a hand held device consisting of 192 needles of 0.1 mm diameter in eight rows with length of the needle varying from 0.5 mm to 2 mm. Smaller versions of dermarollers are available for under-eye procedures.

Motorized dermastamps or dermapens can also be used which consist of needle cartridges attached to motor device and depth of the needles can be adjusted according to the depth of the scar to be treated.

Principle

Microneedling,[6-9] causes multiple tiny holes or micro-channels in the epidermis and dermis over the treated skin and this leads to a stimulation of healing process with resultant collagen production and remodeling of skin surface. The procedure is thus also called as percutaneous collagen induction therapy.

Indications

- Acne scars of Grade 2 to 3
- Rejuvenation using 0.5 mm dermaroller
- Recommended for rolling and boxcar scars.

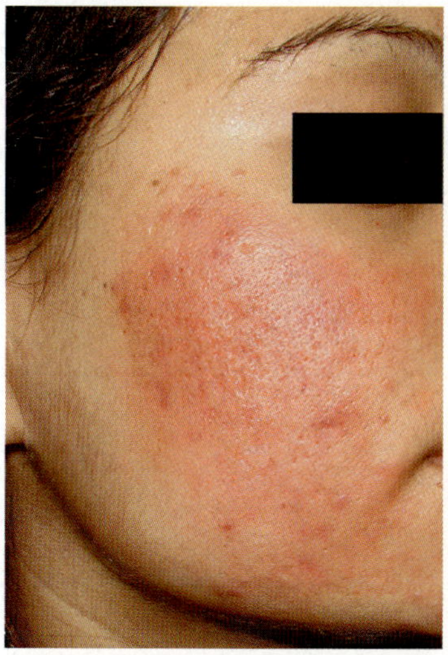

Fig. 11.2: Bleeding end point after dermaroller.

Contraindications

- Active herpes labialis
- Keloidal tendency
- Secondary infection or folliculitis
- Bleeding disorder.

Details of the Procedure

- Apply topical anesthesia under occlusion (eutectic mixture of prilocaine/tetracaine and lignocaine) and keep it for 45 minutes to 1 hour. Clean the affected area of the face or neck with betadine and then 70% ethanol.
- Roll the instrument (dermaroller) over the areas affected by the acne scars with your right hand while stretching the skin over the scar with the index finger and thumb of the left hand. The dermaroller should be held with a proper grip by the right hand and should be rolled over the area in different directions horizontally, vertically and diagonally right to left 4 to 5 times till pin point bleeding is visualized. Appearance of bleeding points is taken as the end-point of the procedure in acne scars (Fig. 11.2).
- Usually, the bleeding that occurs is self-limited and it is not essential to use anything to control the bleeding. After a few minutes the treated area is cleaned with water and dabbed dry.
- A simple noncomedogenic cream is applied on the treated area after the procedure. The patient is encouraged to use a broad-spectrum noncomedogenic sunscreen in the postoperative period.
- The procedure is repeated at intervals of 4–8 weeks and in usual cases a total of 3–4 sessions are performed. The idea of doing multiple sessions is to add to the healing response with each session (Figs. 11.3A to D).

Advantages of Microneedling

The main advantage of microneedling procedure is that it can be done as an office-based procedure and there is absolutely no down time associated with it. The patient can return to his or her duties within an hour after the procedure. Another important advantage is the safety profile of the procedure. No significant adverse effects are seen with the procedure and the only adverse effect noted in some cases is postinflammatory hyperpigmentation. Other adverse effects reported are activation of herpes simplex, infections and significant pain associated with the procedure.

Microneedling can be combined with platelet-rich plasma (PRP) or topical vitamin C serum to improve the therapeutic benefit.

Postprocedure Care

Patients may develop erythema and edema if more than 1.5 mm size of needle is used. There may be serous discharge in some cases. Patient need to be counseled about the post-procedure care and should apply antibiotic cream along with sun protection.

Therapeutic effect achieved with microneedling may not be evident immediately. It requires three to four sessions depending upon the type of scar and the depth of the scars to see any visible difference. It needs to be remembered that improvement of acne scars continues for at least 6 months after the end of treatment schedule. Thus the final assessment of results has to be done after 6 months of last session (Figs. 11.4A to D).

LASER RESURFACING FOR ACNE SCARS

Resurfacing lasers are one of the most popular devices used for treatment of acne scars at present. Fractional laser resurfacing with ablative or nonablative lasers has almost totally replaced traditional laser resurfacing for acne scars. This is because fractional lasers are not associated with any long-term troublesome adverse effects in usual cases while the therapeutic benefit is almost similar as with traditional resurfacing. Moreover, downtime is less with fractional lasers compared to nonfractional lasers.

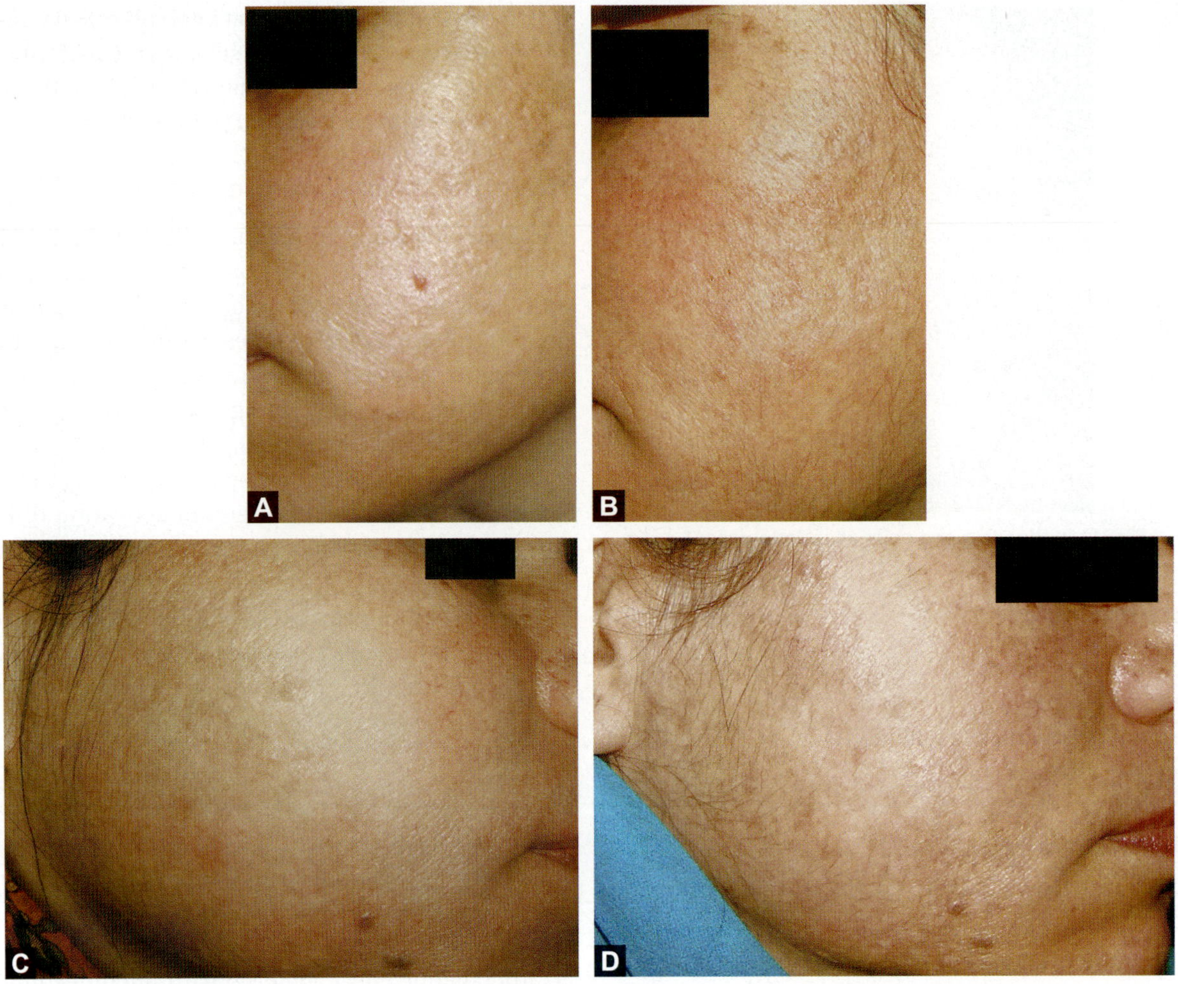

Figs. 11.3A to D: Pre- and post-treatment pictures after 4 sessions of dermaroller in acne scars.

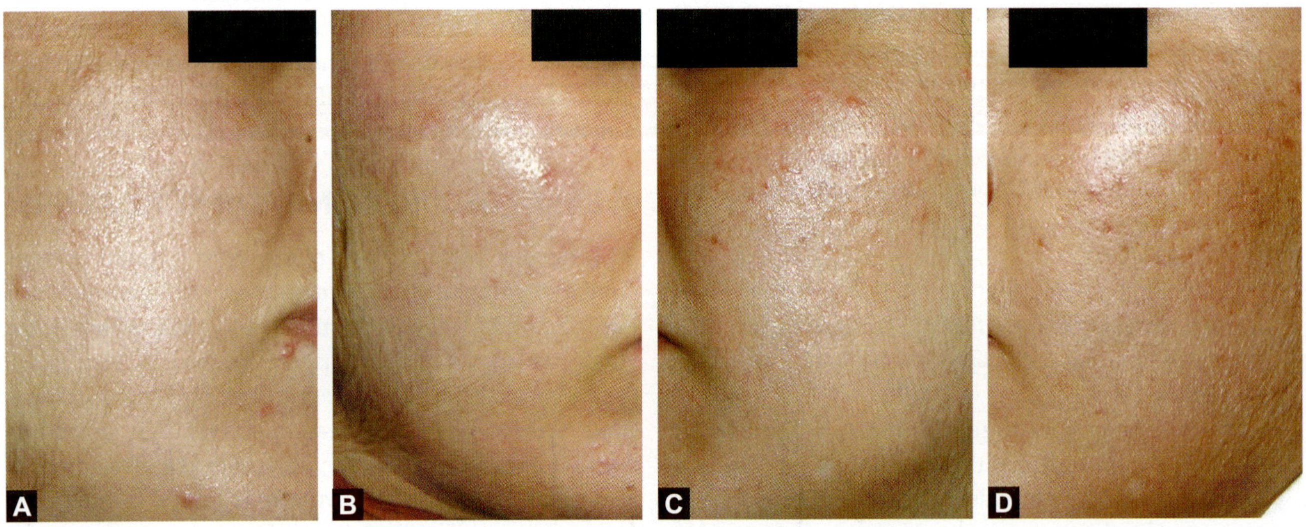

Figs. 11.4A to D: Dermaroller treatment—improvement continues for many months after treatment. (A and C) Preprocedure images (B and D) Post-treatment images after 6 months.

Fractional laser resurfacing for acne scars can be done by using either ablative lasers like Er:YAG or CO_2 lasers (Figs. 11.5A and B) or nonablative lasers like Erbium glass and Nd:YAG lasers.

Principles of Fractional Laser Resurfacing in Acne Scars

Fractional laser emits light in pixilated fashion to the skin producing small microscopic columns of thermal zones called microscopic treatment zones (MTZs).[10-11] Transepidermal elimination of the dermal-epidermal debris happens through these columns and this debris is known as microscopic epidermal necrotic debris (MENDs). Subsequently there is stimulation of re-epithelialization and stimulation of adjacent column of intact tissue to regenerate the treated area (Figs. 11.6A to D).

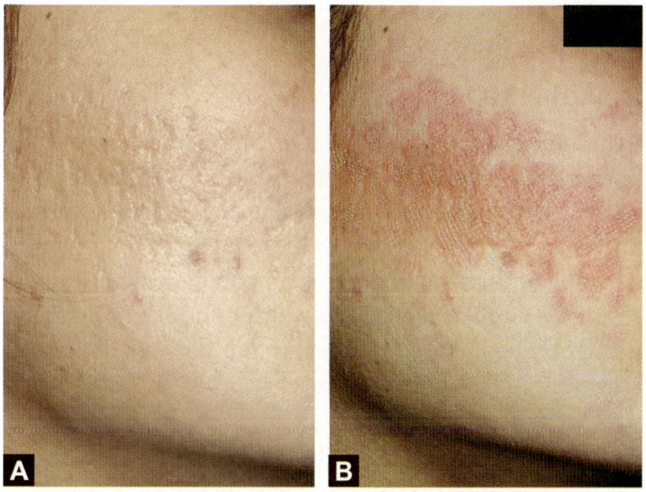

Figs. 11.5A and B: Postacne scars with immediate post-procedure look after CO_2 fractional laser treatment.

Preoperative Care

- Previous history of herpes labialis should receive prophylactic oral antivirals starting one day before fractional resurfacing and for 5 days postoperatively.
- History of bacterial infection should be treated with proper antibiotics.
- Patients having tendency for post inflammatory hyperpigmentation, test patch is advised, and priming should be done with topical retinoids along with depigmenting agents and strict sun protection.
- Patients having keloidal tendency or hypertrophic scars should be counseled regarding the risk involved. A test patch should be done and low fluence should be used during the procedure.

Steps of the Procedure

- Apply topical anesthesia under occlusion (eutectic mixture of prilocaine/tetracaine and lignocaine) and keep it for 45 minutes to 1 hour. Clean the affected area of the face or neck with betadine and then with normal saline.
- Wavelength related spectacles for surgeon, assistants and eye shield for patient have to be worn before the procedure is started.

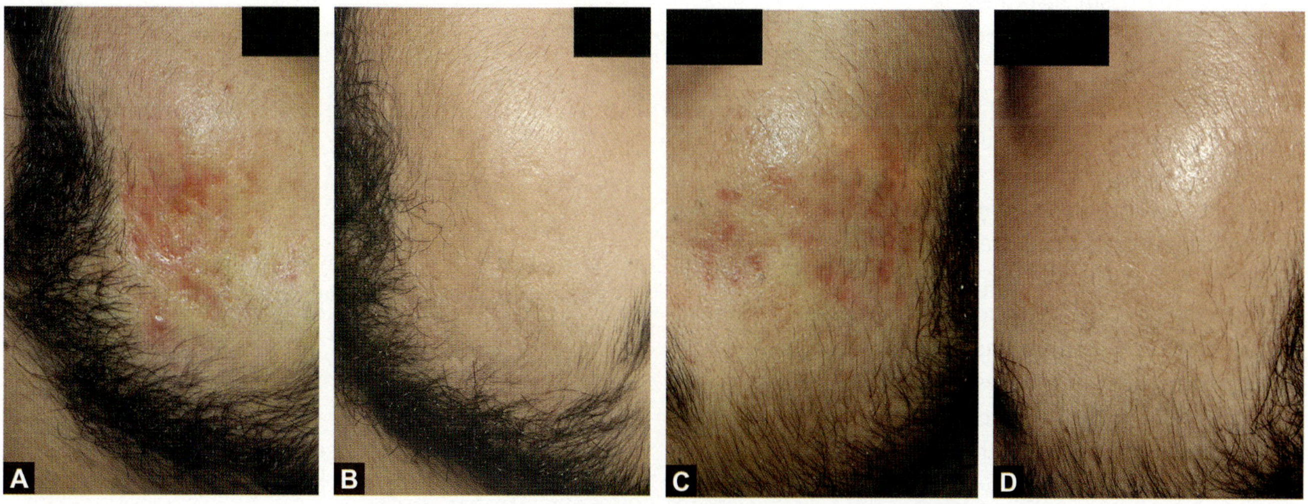

Figs. 11.6A to D: Vastly improved scars after fractional CO_2 treatment.

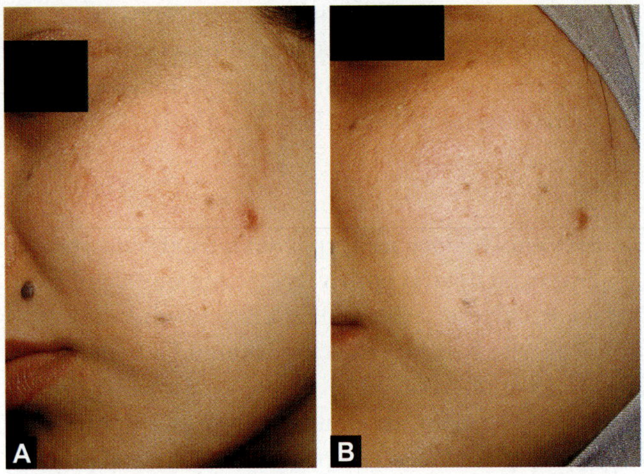

Figs. 11.7A and B: Improvement of scars after subcision.

- A smoke evacuator should be available in the procedure room and has to be used during the procedure as it removes the viral particles along with the smoke.
- Depending upon the type, size of the scar and skin type: fluence, mode, pulse width, frequency and shape of beam is selected.
- Shouldering of the scars needs to be done to get better results. However in case multiple passes are to be used, cleanse the treated area with a gauze to clear out the ablated tissue before giving the next pass.
- Usually a single pass of laser treatment is used.

Contraindications

- History of immunosuppression or active disease which will interfere in wound healing
- Active local or systemic infection
- Connective tissue disorders
- Lactation
- Photosensitive disorders
- Active psoriasis or vitiligo
- Body dysmorphic syndrome
- Unrealistic expectation
- *Patients on oral isotretinoin*: Fractional laser resurfacing is routinely contraindicated in patients on isotretinoin and a 6 months waiting period is usually advised especially in case of aggressive resurfacing. However, this recommendation has been challenged in many recent studies and studies have shown no significant increase in adverse effects in patients on low-dose isotretinoin therapy. Furthermore, in case of macular and superficial scars in a patient on isotretinoin, fractional laser resurfacing can be done safely.[12]

TIPS AND TRICKS

- Higher energies can be used at less treatment densities to reach deeper into the dermis without causing significant adverse effects.
- Using ice packs just before, during and after the procedure greatly minimizes the erythema and edema from fractional laser resurfacing.
- Always advise the patient to avoid picking at the crusts that form after the procedure as it can lead to postinflammatory pigmentation and scarring.
- Deep scars and ice pick scar's needs a combination approach with other procedures, such as chemical peels, subcision and trichloroacetic acid Chemical Reconstruction of Skin Scars (CROSS) technique.
- Double passes and shouldering of the scars is advised in case of deep scars.

SUBCISION

Subcision is a simple surgical technique used to cut the fibrous bands beneath the depressed scars. The aim is to minimize the adherence of the scar to the underlying tissue. The term was first used by Orentreich and Orentreich to describe a novel procedure of subcutaneous incisionless surgery.[7,13] Similar procedures were performed by Spangler using iris needle to cut fibrous strands beneath depressed scars (Figs. 11.7A and B).

Principle

The mechanism of action is believed to be:

- The surgical release of fibrotic band results in scar elevation

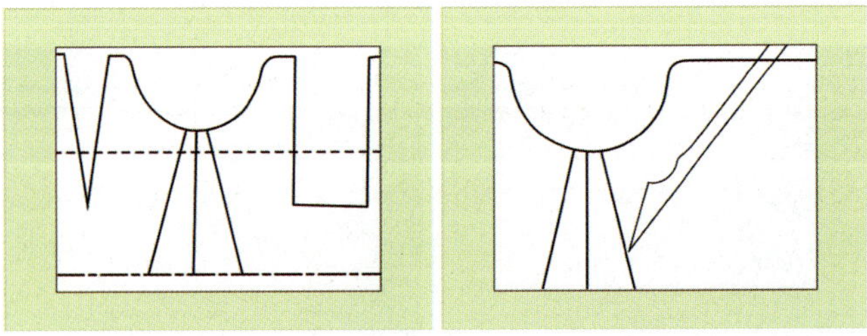

- The controlled trauma promotes new connective tissue formation under the defect, further elevating the scar.

Indications

- It is indicated for depressed rolling scars
- Scars most responsive to this technique are those scars that improve once skin is stretched.

Contraindications

- Keloidal tendency (relative)
- Secondary infection or folliculitis
- Bleeding disorder.

Steps of the Procedure

The steps of the procedure are as follows:

- Apply a topical anesthetic cream under occlusion as described in the microneedling section. Topical anesthesia under occlusion for two hours ensures proper anesthesia for deeper scars.
- Clean the affected area after sufficient anesthetic effect has been achieved.
- Mark the boundary of each scar that needs to be subcised.
- Needles ranging from 16 gauge to 23 gauge can be used, the best needle to perform subcision is 18 gauge. Apart from simple needles, Nokor needles and Iris knife have also been used for this procedure. The entry of the needle is through the edge of the scar and the bevel of the needle should face upwards and in a horizontal direction just below the dermal-subcutaneous junction plane.
- The needle should be moved gently to and fro in a sweeping manner and a snapping sound is heard as the fibrous bands are broken. Needle should be held firmly between index finger and thumb of right hand and skin should be stretched using left hand.
- Firm pressure using sterile gauge is used postoperatively for 5 to 6 minutes to achieve hemostasis.
- Another session can be repeated after 2 to 3 weeks depending upon the improvement.

Modifications

- Body of the needles can be bent at right angles as less force is required for to and fro motion of the needle.
- Iris knife has shown promising results in subcision.

TIPS AND TRICKS

- To prevent hematoma formation excess blood should be squeezed out which causes less swelling and a small hematoma.
- Always start the procedure from dependent position and move upwards.
- Scars which are close to each other can be subcized through single entry point by changing the direction of needle instead of making separate entry points.
- Avoid subcision of many scars in a single sitting to avoid gross edema.
- If punch excision and subcision are combined in the same session punch excision wound can be used as entry point for subcision of adjacent scars.
- If scar is heavily fibrosed, subcision at three points (triangulated approach) may be required.
- Subcision can be combined with other procedures like dermarollers, dermal grafts, subcutaneous fat grafts, along with ablative (fractional CO_2 and Erbium YAG lasers and nonablative lasers (Erbium Glass lasers).
- Care should be taken while doing subcision under the eyes and on the pinna. It may lead to large hematomas as skin under the eyes is too thin and fragile and hematomas on pinna can damage cartilage.

PUNCH TECHNIQUES

Punch techniques are used for acne scar revision surgeries depending upon the type of acne scars, size, color and textural irregularities. There are various types of acne scar revision surgeries using punches which include punch excision, punch floatation and punch replacement grafting.

Punch Excision

Indications

Ice pick and boxcar scars, of more than 3.5 mm in diameter.

Procedure

Depending upon the size of the scar various types of punches varying from 1.5 mm to 3 mm can be used. A proper outwards traction is needed for the punch during excision, so that an ellipse is formed and it runs parallel to the RSTL lines. The scar tissue is removed and the edges are sutured using prolene or nylon 6-0 and, if more than 2.5 mm vicryl 6-0 can be used for subcutaneous suture (Figs. 11.8A and B).

Punch Floatation

Indications

For boxcar scars less than 3 mm with no textural or color mismatch.

Procedure

Punch should be selected in such a way that inner diameter of the scar should lie along the punch. The punch should be rotated either clockwise or anticlockwise in a single direction which releases the bound down scar tissue and should not cross dermis. The plug formed should be elevated using fine nontraumatic forceps and can be positioned at a slight

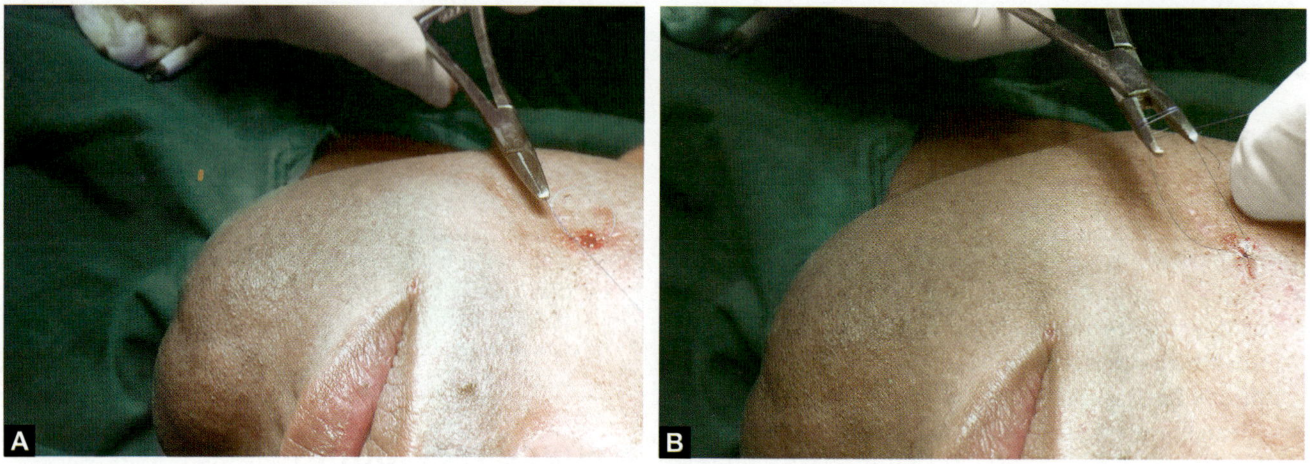

Figs. 11.8A and B: Suturing after scar excision.

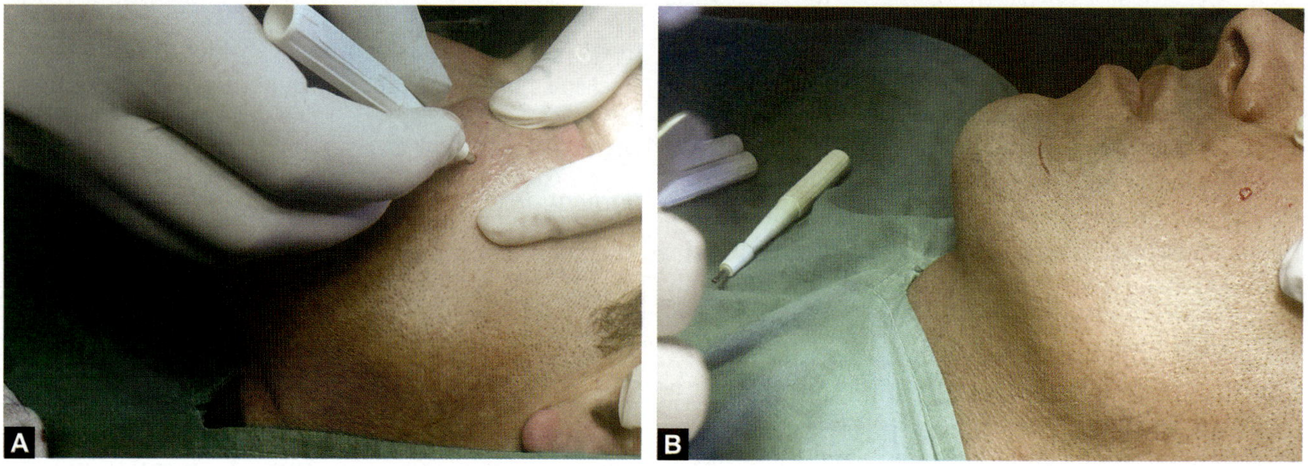

Figs. 11.9A and B: Scar punch excision and grafting (use of cyanoacrylate).

higher position than normal skin. The elevated punch can be secured in position by using cyanoacrylate tissue adhesive and can be further closed by Steri Strips.

Punch Replacement Grafting

Indication

It is used for deep, irregular scars and tethered boxcar scars with altered skin texture.

Procedure

In this technique scar plug is removed using a punch depending upon the size of the scar and replaced by a graft plug taken from the post auricular region or from inner side of the arm. If the scar is more than 1.5 mm in size then donor should be 0.5 mm larger than recipient plug, and if scar is less than 1.5 mm size, graft from the recipient area can be equal to the donor scar. Cyanoacrylate glue can be used as an adhesive for securing grafts (Figs. 11.9A and B).

Contraindications

- Keloidal tendency
- Color mismatch between donor and recipient area
- Bleeding disorders
- Active infection of the skin.

Postprocedure Care

Patient should be advised to make limited movement as aggressive chewing or movement may lead to poor graft intake and graft extrusion. Along with punch replacement or floatation, it can be combined with fractional lasers, chemical peels or PRP for a better outcome.

Tips or Precautions

- Scars more than 4 mm should not be posted for punch excision and closure as dog ear formation can occur.
- Scars which are very close to each other (< 5 mm distance) should not be excised and closed in a single sitting to avoid pull or traction over the suture line.
- Treat them at an interval of 4 weeks.
- Sutures should be removed within 5–7 days to avoid track marks.
- Ensure color match before grafting techniques.

TCA CROSS

Lee and colleagues reported use of high concentration (65% &100%) TCA in atrophic scars and termed it CROSS (Chemical Reconstruction of Skin Scars).[13,14] It is a self-neutralizing peeling agent and depending upon the concentration, can be used as a medium to deep peel.[14]

Indication

It is indicated for ice pick scars.

Principle

TCA causes coagulative necrosis of the cells in the epidermis and necrosis of collagen in papillary and reticular dermis which in turn leads to increase in collagen production causing its remodeling along with glycosaminoglycans and elastin deposition. Remodeling can continue for 4 to 6 months and leads to better outcome as far as results are concerned.

Procedure[15]

- It is advised to do a test patch in the post auricular area before doing TCA CROSS.
- The face is cleaned with spirit and degreased with acetone.
- Scars should be marked with surgical marker.
- Proper eye shield should be used and patient should lie down with face slightly projecting upwards.
- The skin is stretched
- 100% TCA is applied to the base of the scar using wooden toothpick whose tip can be tailored depending upon the size of scar till frosting appears which generally takes 10 to 15 seconds. The scar can be cleaned using dry spirit-postprocedure and face is to be washed with normal water.
- Patient should be counseled about the outcome of the procedure and strict photoprotection is recommended. The procedure can be repeated after 4 to 5 weeks.

Complications

Post inflammatory hyperpigmentation and hypopigmentation.

Tips

- Start from lower concentration of TCA and then escalate gradually.
- Use of epidermal growth factor topically helps faster healing.
- Pre procedure priming is must.
- While dipping tooth pick, care should be taken so that only the tip is in contact with TCA.
- Excess TCA to be removed to prevent spillage or dribbling.
- Scar should be stretched before applying to prevent contact of TCA to surrounding skin, so that TCA is in contact only with scar base.
- Avoid touching the shoulders of the scar with TCA as it may lead to increase in the scar diameter.

DERMAL GRAFTING

Dermal grafts have been used in the treatment of depressed scars as an autologous graft. Prior to dermal grafting scar should be subcised and depending upon the size of scar, grafts can be taken accordingly. These grafts should be devoid of epidermis and subcutaneous fat. The advantages of this procedure are as follows:

- Dermal grafts survival is better as compared to fat and nonpermanent filler.
- Less chances of allergic contact dermatitis
- Less susceptible to infection
- Cheaper alternative
- Can be tailored as per need of patient.

Procedure

Two types of techniques are used:

- Conventional technique
- Enzymatic separation.

Conventional Technique

Donor tissue is harvested either using biopsy punches or using dermatomes from post auricular area or inner side of arm. The graft should be devoid of epidermis and in case the defect is larger, fat can be taken along with dermis. The scar is subcised using 18 gauge needle and a pocket is created below the scar (Pocket technique). Through the entry a small nick is made through which the graft is placed placed inside the pocket below the scar with help of fine atraumatic forceps. Once complete correction is done entry wound can be sutured using prolene 6-0. (Dermal grafting for an atrophic scar is shown as a protocol and the procedure remains the same for acne scars—Figs. 11.10A to K).

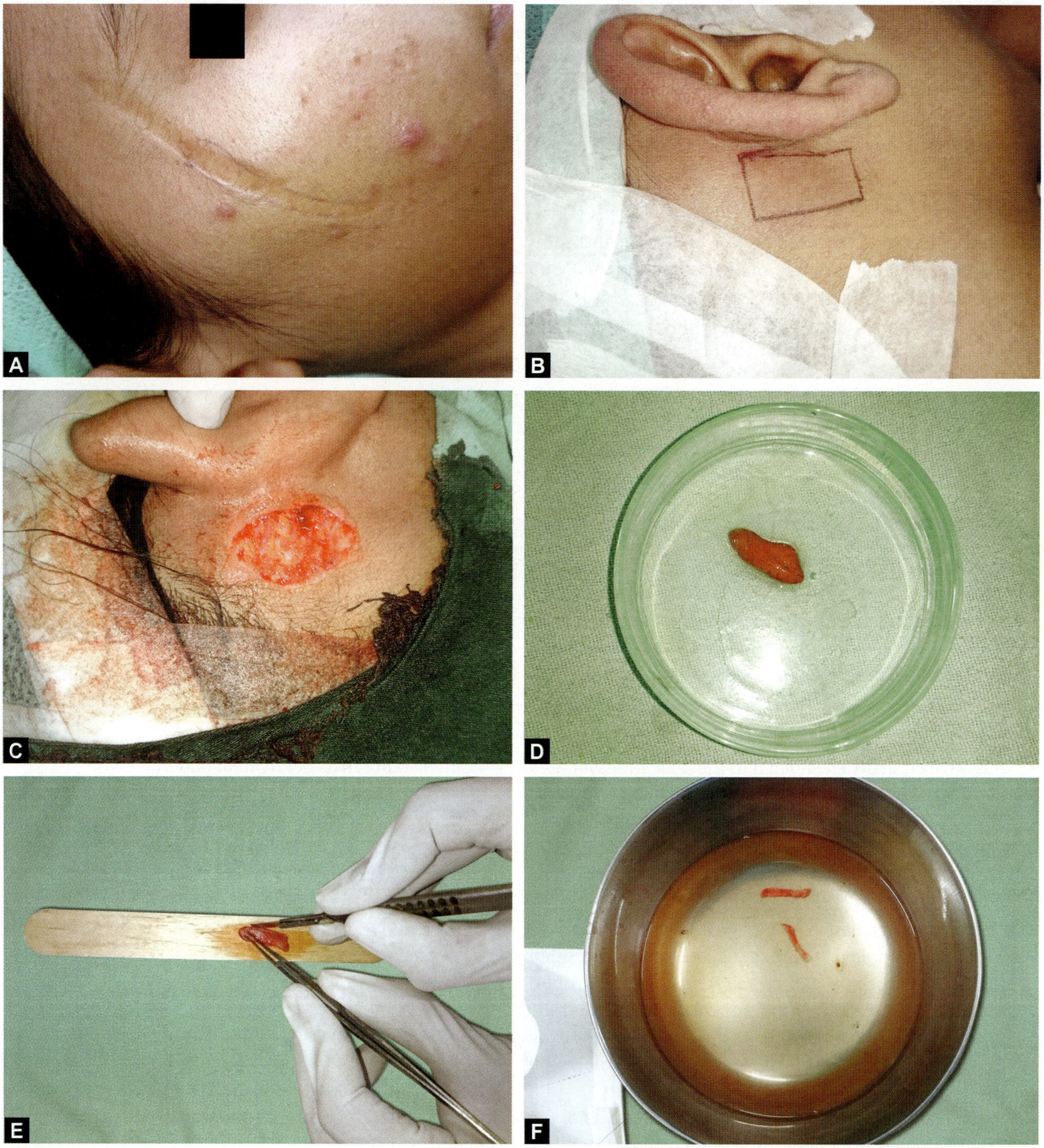

Figs. 11.10A to E: Dermal grafting. (A) Atrophic scar taken as a model to show dermal graft. (B) Donor area-postauricular region. (C) Donor graft taken. (D) Trypsinization. (E) Dermal portion alone separated. (F) Dermal portion.
Courtesy: Dr Shilpa K, Bangalore Medical College, Bengaluru, Karnataka, India

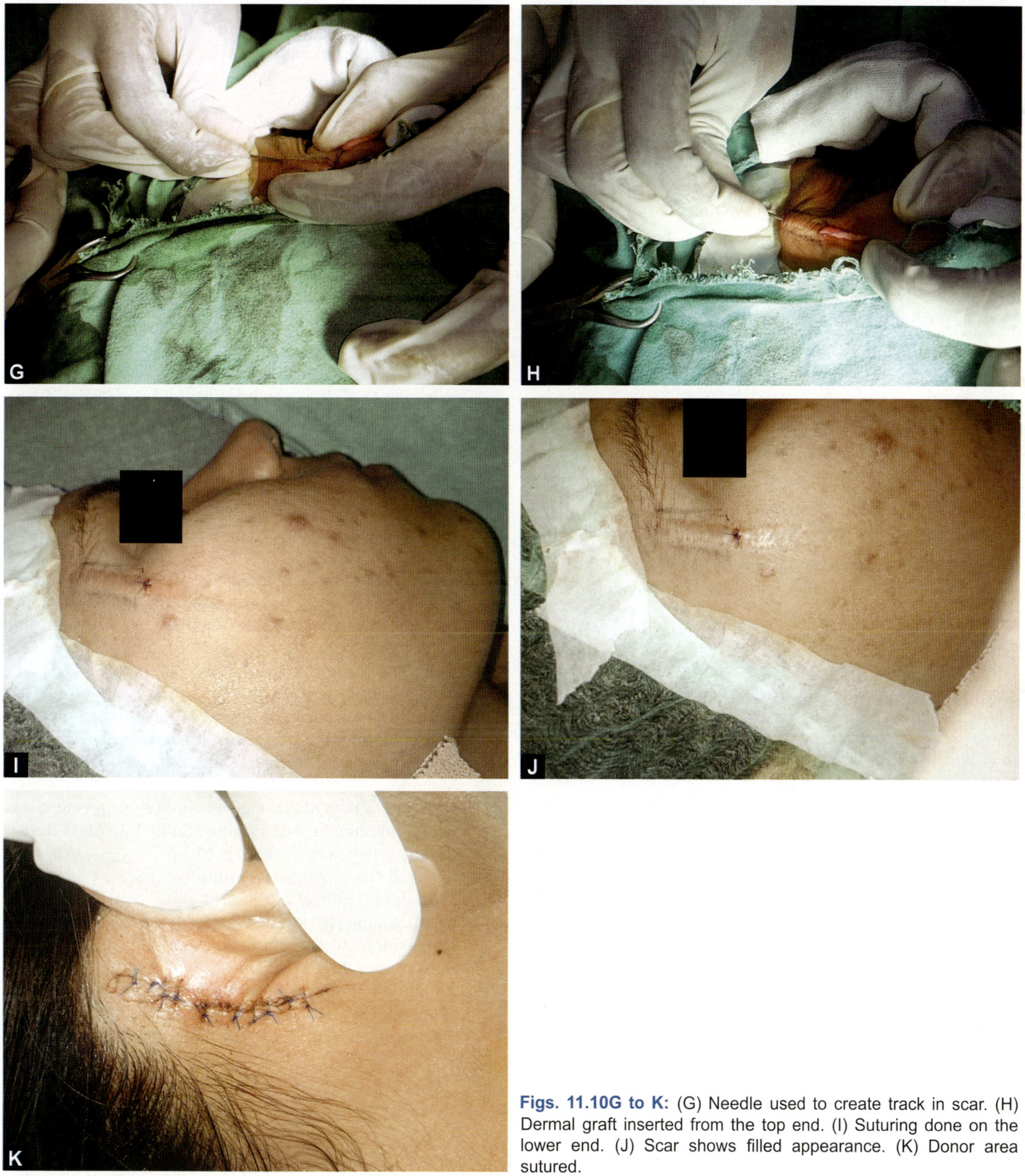

Figs. 11.10G to K: (G) Needle used to create track in scar. (H) Dermal graft inserted from the top end. (I) Suturing done on the lower end. (J) Scar shows filled appearance. (K) Donor area sutured.

Enzymatic Technique

Technique is same as conventional technique except for one step. This involves incubating the dermal graft with 0.25% trypsin for 45 minutes after harvesting to make the graft soft and supple so that it easily slides through the pocket. The dermal tissue which is whitish and soft can be used for filling the defect.

Table 11.4: Types of acne scars and treatment options.

Type of scar	*Treatment options*
Ice pick scars	TCA CROSS (<1.5 mm) Punch excision and suturing (> 1.5 mm)
Boxcar	Round scars-punch techniques Irregular scars- fractional laser, scar revisions
Rolling scars	Subcision with dermaroller, fractional laser
Other depressed scars	Fillers, dermal graft, fat injections, dermaroller
Hypertrophic scars	Intralesional steroids, cryorollers
Papular acne scars	Radiofrequency ablation

Tips

- Subcision two weeks prior to procedure helps in better take up and survival of graft.
- Bigger scar > 4 mm with normal epidermis can be considered for dermal grafting.
- Atrophic scars with altered skin texture, requires adjuvant resurfacing techniques for better outcome.
- Care should be taken to completely remove epidermis to prevent formation of cyst.
- Overcorrection should be avoided.

Other modalities of treatment of acne scars which can be combined with surgical procedures are:

- Chemical peels
- Microdermabrasion
- Soft tissue augmentation
- RF microneedling
- Botox for scars aggravated by muscle action

Summary of acne scar management is given in Table 11.4.

CONCLUSION

Treating acne scars is a challenge to the dermatologist and needs proper clinical judgment and requires multiple sittings and multimodality approach. Patient should be counseled about outcome of the surgery.

REFERENCES

1. White GM. Recent findings in the epidemiologic evidence, classification, and subtypes of acne vulgaris. J Am Acad Dermatol. 1998;39:s34-7.
2. Chivot M, Pawinh, Beylot C, et al. Acne scars: epidemiology, physiopathology, clinical features and treatment. Ann Dermatol Venereol. 2006;133:813-24.
3. Goodman GJ. Management of post acne scarring. What are the options for treatment? Am J Clin Dermatol. 2000;1:3-17.
4. Jacob CL, Dover JS, Kaminer MS. Acne scarring: a classification system and review of treatment options. J Am Acad Dermatol. 2001;45:109-17.
5. Dreno B, Khammari A, Orain N, et al. ECCA grading scale: an original validated acne scar grading scale for clinical practice in dermatology. Dermatology 2007;214:46-51.
6. Fernandes D. Minimally invasive percutaneous collagen induction. Oral Maxillofac Surg Clin North Am. 2005:17:51-63.
7. Orentreich DS, Orentreich N. Subcutaneous incisionless (subcision) surgery for the correction of depressed scars and wrinkles. Dermatol Surg. 1995:21:543-9.
8. Aust MC, Fernandes D, Kolokythas P, et al. Percutaneous collagen induction therapy. An alternative treatment for scars, wrinkles and skin laxity. Plast Reconstr Surg. 2008:26:192-9.
9. Majid I. Microneedling therapy in atrophic facial scars: an objective assessment. J Cutan Aesthet Surg. 2009;2:26-30.
10. Mainstein D, Herron GS, Sink RK, et al. Fractional photothermolysis: a new concept for cutaneous remodeling using microscopic patterns of thermal injury. Lasers Surg Med. 2004;34:426-38.
11. Hantash BM, Bedi VP, Sudireddy V, et al. Laser-induced transepidermal elimination of dermal content by fractional photothermolysis. J Biomed Opt. 2006;11:041115.
12. Mahadevappa OH, Mysore V, Viswanath V, et al. Surgical outcome in patients taking concomitant or recent intake of oral isotretinoin: a multicentric Study-ISO-AIMS study. J Cutan Aesthet Surg. 2016;9(2):106-12.
13. Good GJ. Therapeutic undermining of scars (Subcision). Australas J Dermatol 2001;42:114-7.
14. Lee JB, Chung WG, Kwahch H, et al. Focal treatment of acne scars with trichloroacetic acid: chemical reconstruction of skin scars method. Dermatol Surg. 2002;28:1017-21.
15. Khunger N, Bhardwaj D, Khunger M. Evaluation of CROSS technique with 100% TCA in the management of icepick acne scars in darker skin types. J Cosm Dermatol. 2011;10:51-7.

CHAPTER 12

Skin Grafting

Savitha AS, Sujala S Aradhya

INTRODUCTION

Skin grafting is a procedure that involves transfer of skin and its underlying tissue to another part of the body. It is usually indicated when wound closure by primary intention or by secondary healing would give suboptimal results.

INDICATIONS

- To close skin defects regardless of the cause
- Management of vitiligo—suction blister grafts, split thickness grafts
- Surgical removal of tattoo
- Ulcer management
- Cicatricial alopecia.

Classification of Skin Grafts (Figs. 12.1 and 12.2)

Composite grafts contain epidermis, dermis and part of the subcutaneous tissue, e.g. graft used in hair transplantation.[1]

The differences between split thickness skin graft (STSG) and full thickness skin graft (FTSG) are enlisted in Table 12.1.

STEPS OF GRAFT UPTAKE

The process by which the graft is incorporated in the recipient bed is called "Graft take". Graft take depends primarily on the speed and extent of vascular perfusion restoration in the graft.

1. **Imbibition:** The graft when harvested is completely separated from the donor area. Through plasmatic imbibition the graft is able to survive the immediate postgraft ischemic period until graft vasculature is re-established.[2] During initial 24 to 48 hours after skin grafting, graft receives nutrition through absorption of plasma from recipient wound bed via capillary action. Thinner grafts survive better at this stage as nutrition is absorbed over shorter distances. A fibrin network forms between graft and recipient bed. Clinically this stage is characterized by edema (Fig. 12.3A).

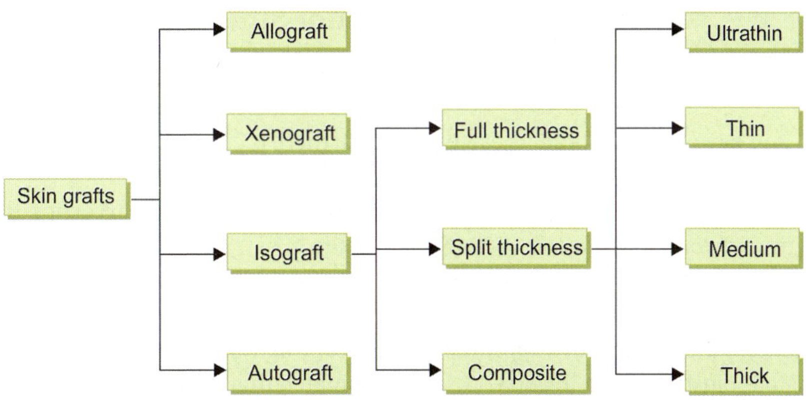

Fig. 12.1: Classification of skin grafts according to source and thickness.

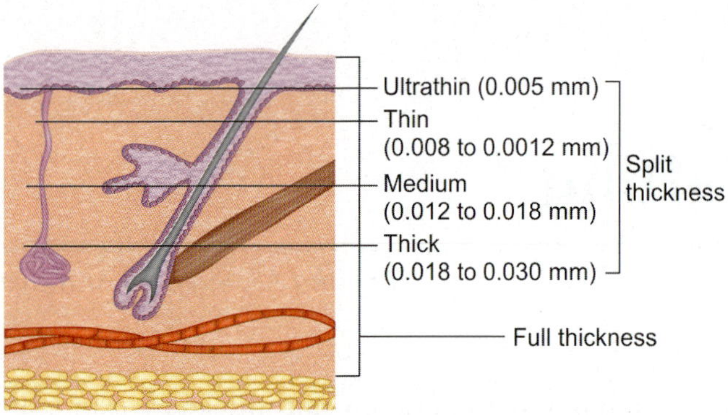

Fig. 12.2: Types of split thickness grafts.

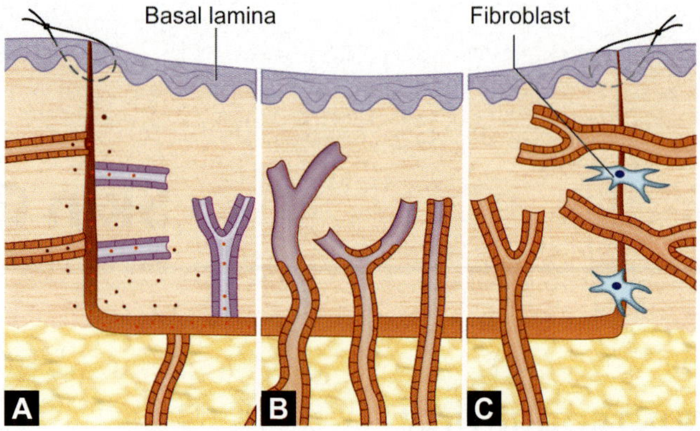

Figs. 12.3A to C: Steps of graft uptake.

Table 12.1: Differences between full thickness and split thickness grafts.

Full thickness skin graft	*Split thickness skin graft*
Contains entire epidermis and dermis	Contains entire epidermis and variable dermis
Common donor areas are above clavicle viz. preauricular, post-auricular, supraclavicular, upper eyelid, nasolabial fold; flexural skin namely inguinal folds, antecubital, axillary. Excess of skin obtained during surgical procedure like dog ear skin, standing cone skin can also be used. Donor area has to be sutured	Common donor areas are anterior, lateral, or medial part of the thigh, the buttock, or the medial aspect of the arm. The donor area heals by secondary intention
No need for special instruments	Dermatomes, Humby's knife, Silver's knife
Recipient areas are cosmetically important areas like head and neck, with small defects as there is good color and texture match with minimal secondary contraction.	Can be performed on any area where cosmesis is not a concern with almost no limitation of defect size. There is rapid uptake of graft with low nutritional requirement

2. and 3. **Inosculation and revascularization:** These two stages occur almost simultaneously. This phase starts at 48 to 72 hours. Vascular buds generate from recipient bed and through the fibrin network anastomoses with the undersurface of the graft. These anastomoses are called inosculation. Graft revascularization occurs faster in STSG, and is late in FTSG. Clinically there is a mottled appearance followed by erythematous blush (Figs. 12.3B and C)

4. **Keratinocyte activation phase:** There is activation and proliferation of keratinocytes during this phase that starts early and lasts up to four weeks. Epidermal keratinocytes undergo mitosis and the epidermis increases by seven-to eight-folds, seen clinically as scaling.[3]

Lymphatics develop in graft tissue at approx after 1 week. Reinnervation of graft may begin as early as first few weeks. Skin grafts show sensory recovery at 4 to 5 weeks postgrafting, but occasionally the sensation is delayed up to 5 months. Skin grafts may initially also be hyperalgesic.[4]

PROCEDURE

Preprocedure Work up

- Take an informed consent.
- If the patient is on NSAIDs or anticoagulants they should be stopped one week before the procedure.

Donor Site Selection

The selection of graft donor site is based on:

- Is it a full thickness or split thickness skin graft
- If there is color match between donor site and recipient site
- Adverse effects of harvesting the graft from particular site.[5]

An appropriate color match is important in head and neck reconstruction. Any skin graft taken below clavicles and applied above clavicle will result in a lifelong color mismatch that is extremely difficult to correct.[6]

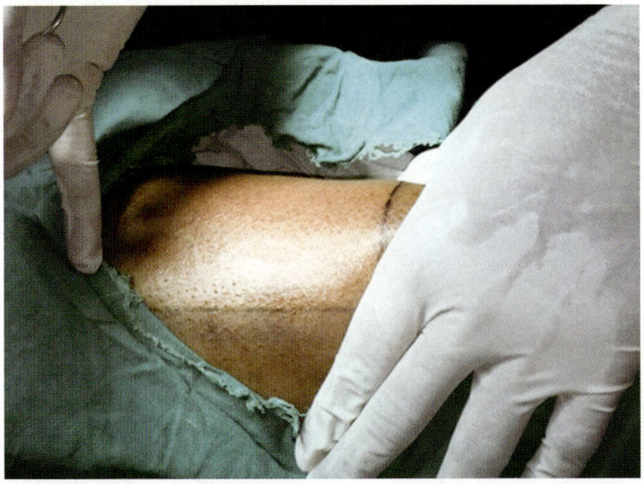

Fig. 12.4: The donor area preparation. Hair is trimmed, surgical preparation done and field block anesthesia is given.

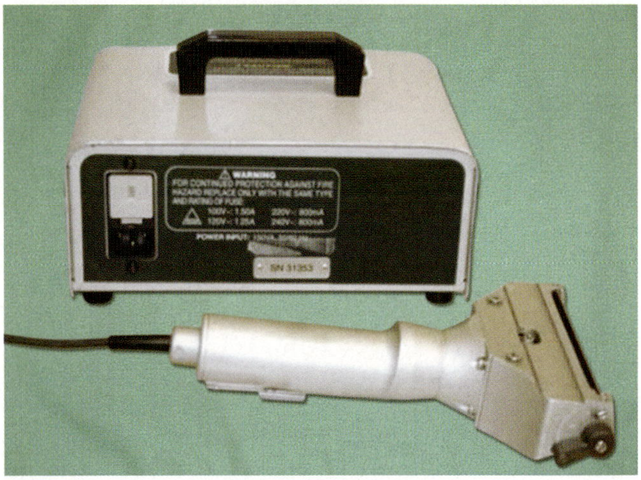

Fig. 12.5: Power dermatome.

Preparation of Recipient Site

- For wounds and nonhealing ulcers the recipient bed is debrided to remove slough, eschar, necrotic tissue or excessive granulation tissue.
- No preparation is needed for surgical wounds, e.g. following malignancy excision.
- For vitiligo surgeries the recipient bed has to be dermabraded either manually or with motor dermabrader till there are pinpoint bleeding points. The borders have to be dermabraded beyond the vitiligo lesions onto the normal skin. The terminal hair should be shaved or, waxed as they might lift up the graft (Fig. 12.4).[7]

SPLIT THICKNESS GRAFT

Harvesting Graft

- The donor site is surgically prepared and field block infiltration of local anesthesia (1–2% lignocaine) given.

  Few surgeons prefer to raise a wheal with local anesthesia to facilitate harvesting the graft. Topical anesthesia under occlusion can also be used. General anesthesia is preferred for extensive graft harvest. The size of the graft should be 10 to 25% larger than the defect to accommodate contraction.
- The graft may be harvested using a freehand technique or using power dermatomes (Fig. 12.5).

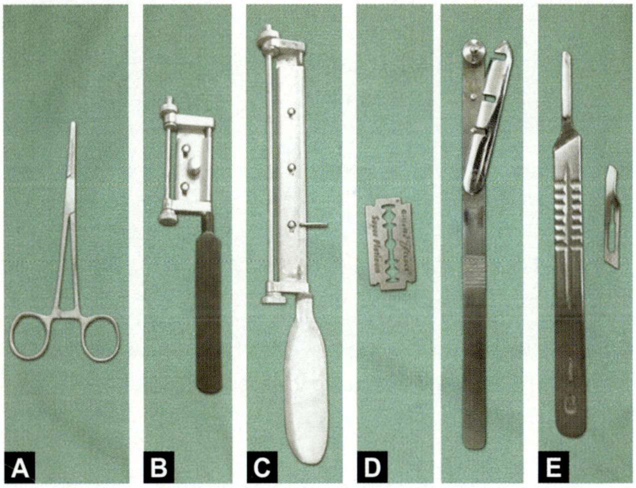

Figs. 12.6A to E: Instruments required for skin grafting: (A) Artery forceps. (B) Silver knife. (C) Humby's knife. (D and E) Blade handles.

- Instruments used with the freehand technique are Humby's knife, Silver knife, artery forceps with razor blade, scalpel blades (Figs. 12.6A to E).
- Betadine or other antibacterial solution used to prepare the donor site should be washed off with saline.
- The area is lubricated with mineral oil or normal saline, and the surgical assistant applies traction with folded gauze across the donor site and then placing it immediately in front of the graft site maintaining the traction on the entire area (Fig. 12.7).

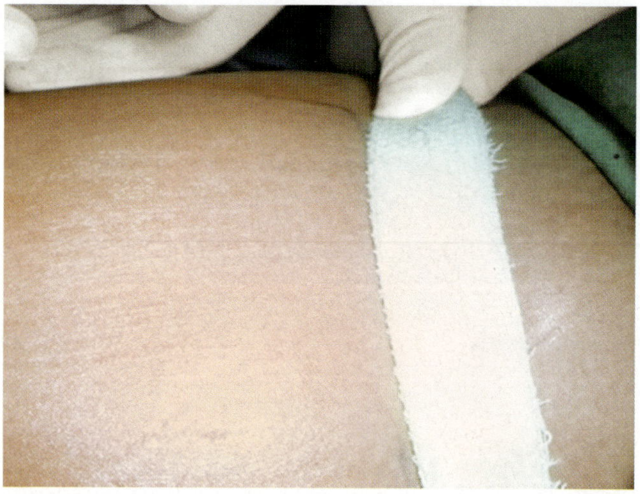

Fig. 12.7: Donor area is lubricated with traction on skin by gauze.

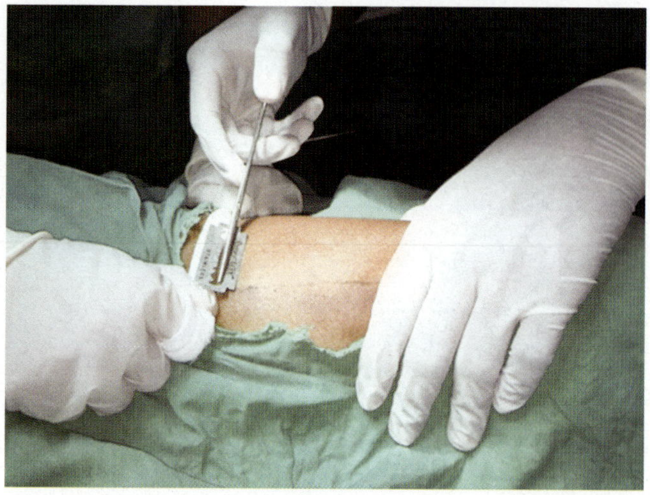

Fig. 12.8: The knife is applied to the skin at 30 to 45°.

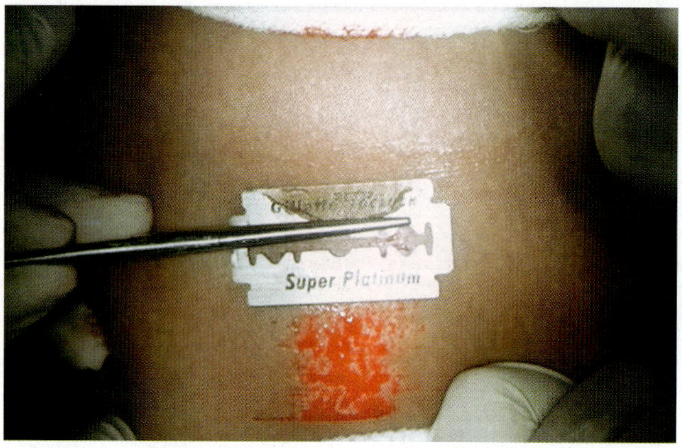

Fig. 12.9: Adequate thickness of STG.

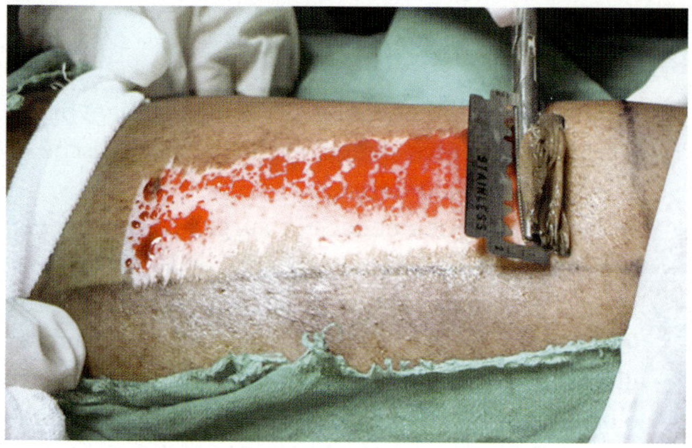

Fig. 12.10: With gentle to and fro motion advance the blade to take required amount of graft.

- The knife or dermatome is applied to the skin at 30 to 45° and try to keep it at 15 to 20° for thinner grafts (Fig. 12.8).

This angle determines the thickness of the graft. A thin layer of skin (epidermis with some of the underlying dermis) is taken. Both Humby's knife and dermatome can be adjusted to set thickness of graft. Usually the settings are set at 0.25 to 0.4 mm. By snuggly fitting the beveled edge of 10 no. blade into the opening, proper thickness of graft can be obtained.

Modifications

1. ***If you are using razor blade:***
   The print on the razor blade should be clearly visible from the top, if your graft is taken at right depth (Fig. 12. 9). Remember you are not taking full-thickness skin; some dermis must be left at the donor site for healing of donor area.
   With gentle to and fro motion advance the blade to take required amount of graft (Figs. 12.10 and 12.11).
2. ***If you are using a dermatome:***
   - Dermatome is to be held at an angle of 45° to the skin and is to held firmly against the skin after turning on the power.
   - The dermatome is slowly moved along the donor site in a smooth fashion till an adequate size graft is obtained.
   - Do not switch off the power of the dermatome till the graft is completely free from the donor site.
3. ***If you are using Humby's knife:***
   - Hold it with the sharp edge of the knife at an angle of 45° with the skin (Fig. 12.12).

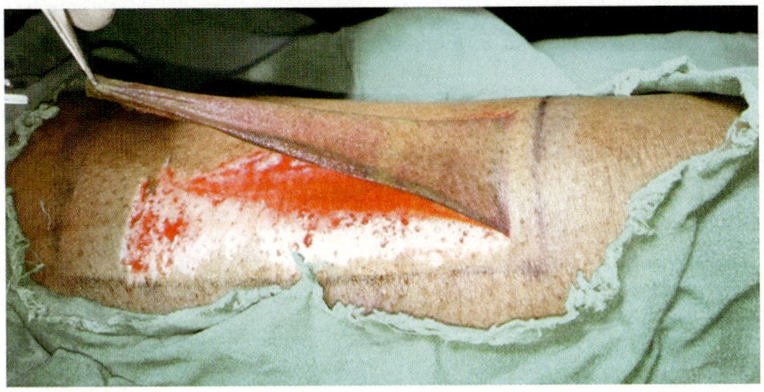

Fig. 12.11: STG.

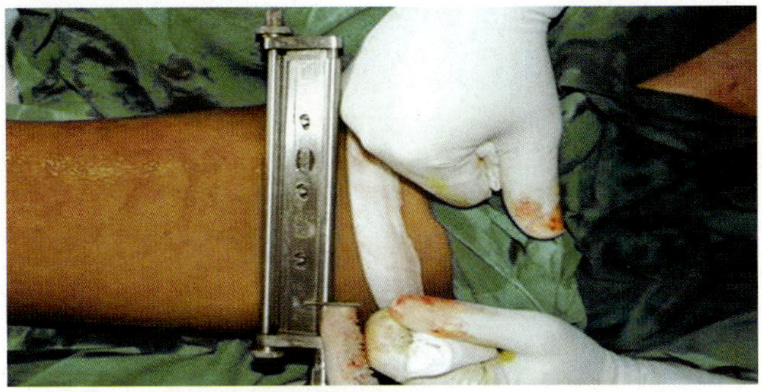

Fig. 12.12: Hold the knife at 45°.

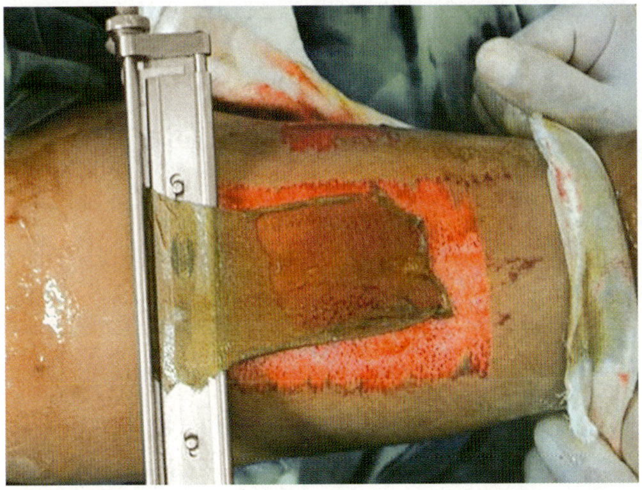

Fig. 12.13: Graft harvested by Humby's knife.

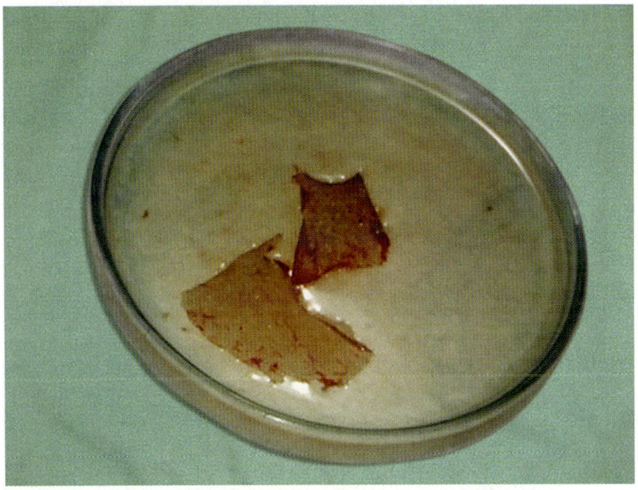

Fig. 12.14: Graft placed in a sterile Petri dish with saline.

- Run the knife over the tight skin with a back-and-forth motion (Fig. 12.13).
- After an adequate size graft is taken, the wrist is twisted into a supination position to remove the knife from the skin.
- The other option is to totally stop the knife movement and later cut out the graft from donor site from the edge of the blade using a scalpel.
- The knife has to be opened fully to get the skin graft totally off the knife.
- The graft is placed in a sterile Petri dish with normal saline (Fig. 12.14)

Advantages of Power Driven Dermatome

- Requires less expertise than freehand harvest
- Reduces harvest time
- Large graft can be taken
- Ultrathin grafts can be harvested

Expansion of STSG

- **Pinch graft:** A pinch graft is where whole graft of skin is broken up into many tiny pieces to increase edge area.[8]
- **Relay transplantation:** Here the graft is cut out into multiple strips which range from 3 to 6 mm in width and placed about 5 to 10 mm from each other. When the skin epithelium grows and becomes evident in about 5 to 7 days, the original strips obtained are removed and later transplanted, leaving the epithelial explants in place. The process may usually be repeated upto about 4 times.[9]
- **Meshing:** Slits or fenestrations are created on graft using scalpel blade to allow for the drainage of sero-sanguineous fluid and to accommodate minor expansion of graft. Contour of the meshed graft can be then adapted to fit recipient bed. A graft-meshing machine can also be used, which allows for expansion ratio of 3:1 to 9:1 (Fig. 12.15) Advantages of meshing are provided in Table 12.2.

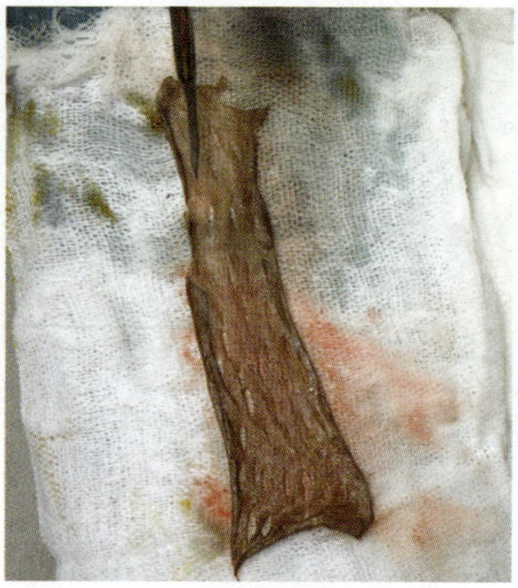

Fig. 12.15: Meshing the graft.

Table 12.2: Advantages and disadvantages of meshing graft.

Advantages	*Disadvantages*
Beneficial for highly mobile anatomic areas such as the knee, scrotum, or axillae because it easily fits irregular body folds.	Considerable area must heal by secondary intention
Considerable graft expansion	Cosmetic results are not ideal
Drainage of serosanguineous fluid	
If there is localized bacterial contamination, only a small area of the graft will be jeopardized	
Offers multiple areas of re-epithelialization	

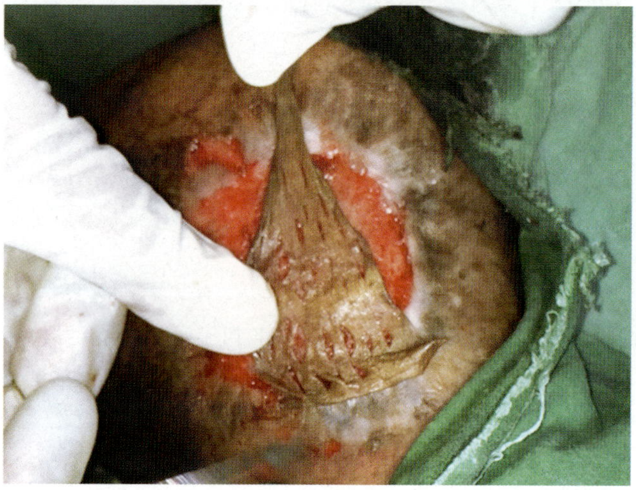

Fig. 12.16: Placement of meshed graft on clean ulcer bed.

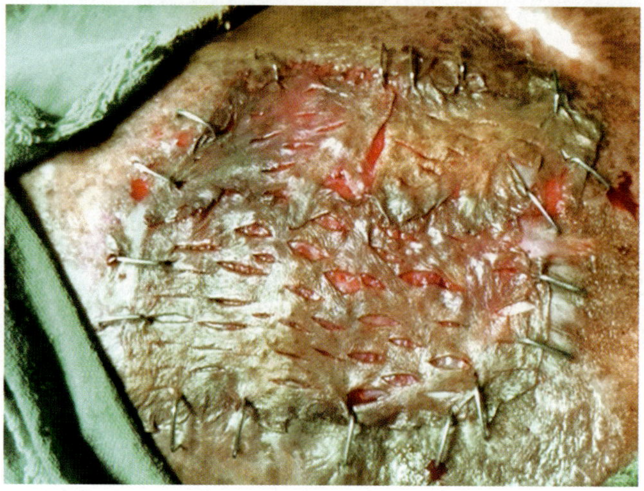

Fig. 12.17: The graft covers the entire wound bed.

Placement of Graft at Recipient Site

The harvested graft is trimmed to fit the donor site. The graft is placed with the dermal side down on the recipient bed. Clues to identify the dermal side are the brighter and whiter color and also curling in of the graft towards the dermal side. Some overlapping of the donor tissue with the recipient bed is acceptable. The graft is gently spread over the recipient side to cover it entirely without any wrinkling. The STSG is then secured in place by using interrupted sutures around the periphery or with surgical glue (Figs. 12.16 and 12.17).

A double layer vaseline gauze or framycetin dressing is placed on the graft. This is covered with either gauze pieces and an elastocrepe bandage or a tie over the bolster to aid in graft apposition to recipient bed.

Removal of Dressing

Dressing should ideally be kept on the wound for 3 to 5 days. It has to be checked daily. The dressing will have to be removed earlier in cases of more drainage or bad odor from the wound. When the dressing is being changed, extreme care has to be exercised not to pull off the graft from the wound. Using a saline soaked wet dressing helps to prevent sticking of the dressing. Hydrogen peroxide may be mixed with the saline too.

Aftercare

- Antibiotic ointment should be applied twice daily till the wound heals.
- Prevent sun exposure of the graft. Sunscreens are to be used over the graft one it is fully taken up.

- Patient has to be counselled to totally avoid smoking during the healing process. Smoking leads to death of skin grafts.

Management of Donor Site Wound

- Donor site should always be covered with a layer of antibiotic gauze. Thicker gauze layers are placed in a on top and dressing done.
- After 24 hours, outer gauze dressing and not antibiotic layer should be removed and area left open. Layer of antibiotic gauze will usually dry out over next 24 to 48 hours and gradually peel off as underlying wound heals.
- Emollients should be applied regularly and sunscreens to be used once wound heals completely.

FULL THICKNESS GRAFT (FIGS. 12.18 TO 12.27)

For FTSG, the defect size must be measured accurately. A template may be used to aid in measurement. Xylocaine is infiltrated into the donor area up to the level subcutaneous fat and the graft is excised using a scalpel.

A tie-over bolster dressing can be used to further stabilize the graft which is held in place using 5-0 silk sutures sewn into skin at opposing points around circumference of graft for 1 week. Free ends of silk suture are tied to one another over top of the bolster, and tight dressing is applied over entire bolster.

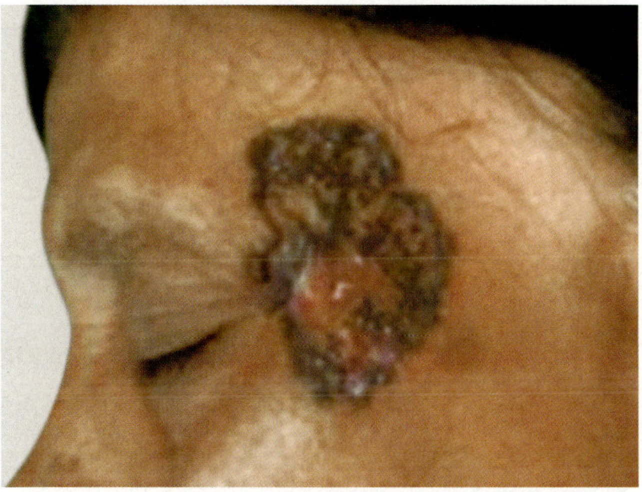

Fig. 12.18: Basal cell carcinoma on the temporal area.

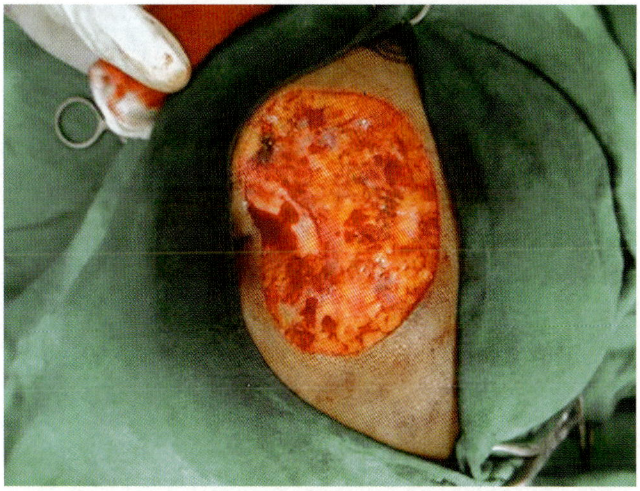

Fig. 12.19: The lesion is excised completely.

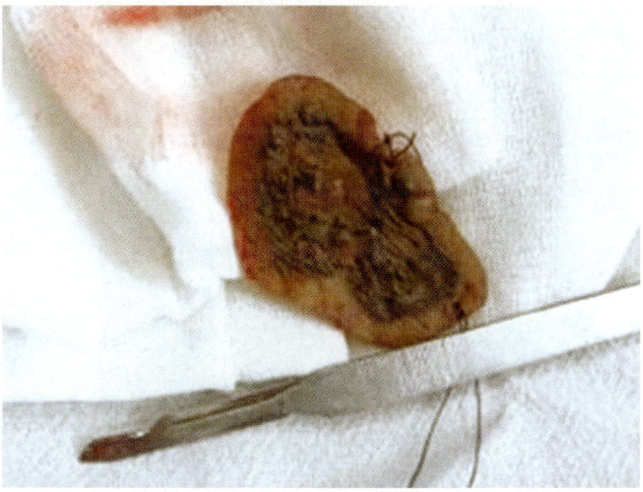

Fig. 12.20: Excised tissue.

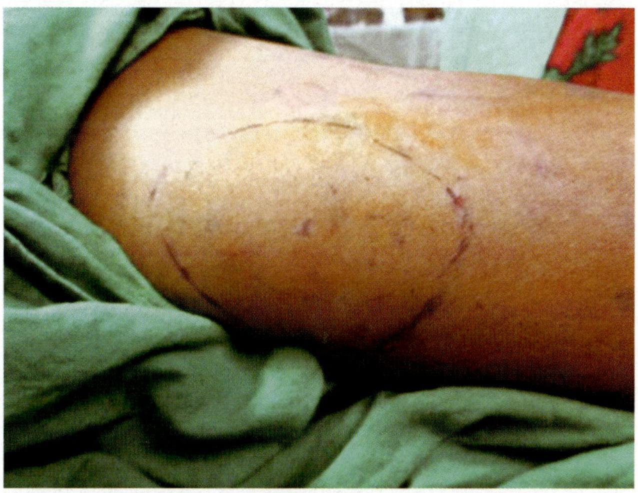

Fig. 12.21: Marking done on the donor area.

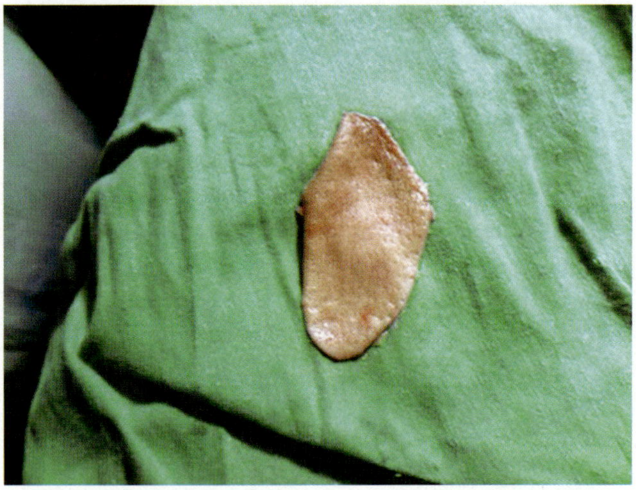

Fig. 12.22: Full thickness graft harvested.

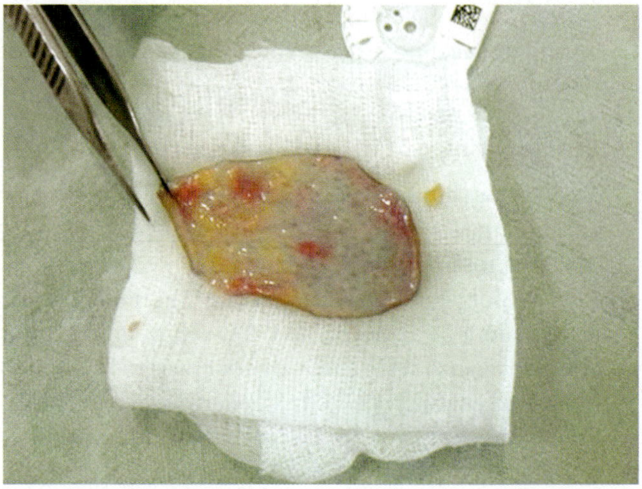

Fig. 12.23: Graft is defatted, which allows more efficient revascularization.

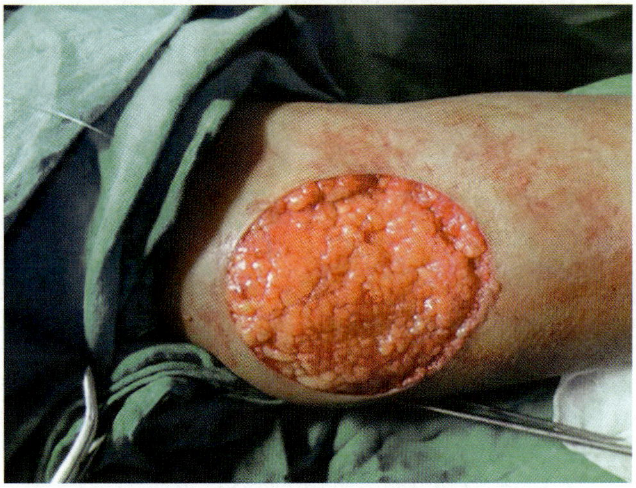

Fig. 12.24: Defect in donor area.

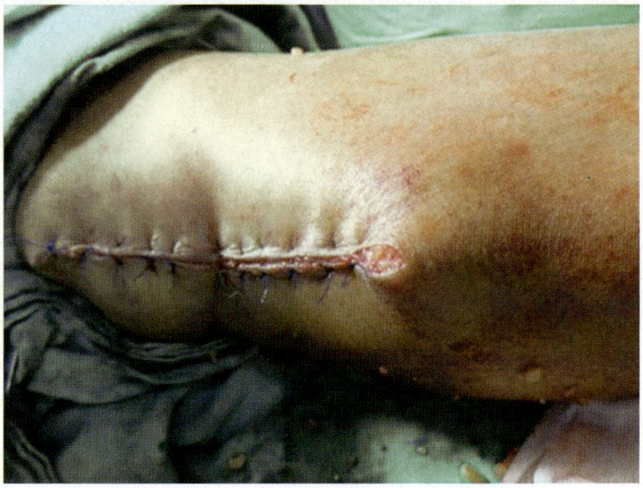

Fig. 12.25: Donor area sutured.

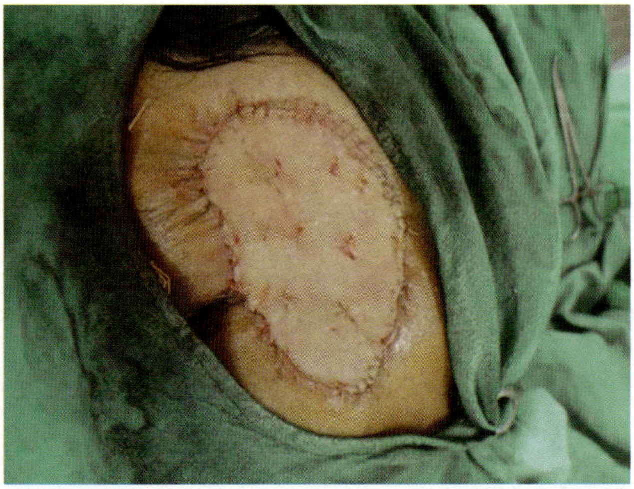

Fig. 12.26: Precise epidermal approximation is essential for optimal graft take and subsequent cosmetic results. The graft is trimmed and secured to the recipient site using interrupted sutures.

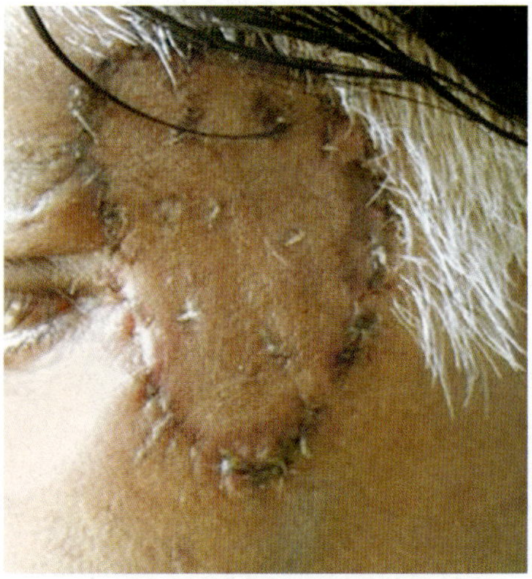

Fig. 12.27: On tenth postoperative day.

POSTOPERATIVE CARE

The patient is advised rest, preferably immobilization of the part for at least 3 days. Analgesics and antibiotics are given for 3 days. If a bolster dressing is not used, the graft can be inspected after 48 hours for hematoma or seroma. The dressing is removed in 7 to 10 days.

STSG will have light pink appearance and minimal crusting around edges of graft on removal of dressing on 7th day. Extensive black necrotic tissue or eschar involving part or all of the grafted skin signals partial or complete loss of graft. This eschar should not be then debrided because it functions as biologic dressing for underlying tissues.

Sun protection is advised to avoid hyperpigmentation after removal of the dressing for extended duration. Emollients may be prescribed for scaling.

GRAFT CONTRACTION

A skin graft begins to shrink immediately after the harvest.

- *Primary contraction*: This is passive and due to the recoil of the dermal elastic fibers. A *full thickness graft* loses about 40% of original area as a result of primary contraction and STSG about 20%.
- *Secondary contraction*: This occurs after transfer to recipient site during healing.

Full thickness grafts do not usually show secondary contraction. Split-thickness grafts inturn show considerable contraction. Greater the proportion of dermis, lesser the graft will contract.

CONTRAINDICATIONS

- Split thickness skin graft:
  - Areas of cosmetic importance like face and neck. FTSG is preferred
  - Over joints due to risk of contractures
  - Small defects which may heal better with primary closure, secondary intention or FTSG.
- Full thickness skin graft
  - Poor recipient area blood supply/avascular bed
  - Secondary infection
  - Large defect
  - Uncontrolled bleeding from the recipient area which may lead to graft failure.

COMPLICATIONS (TABLE 12.3)

The rate of complications varies between 8 to 30%[10]

- *Pain*: Analgesics have to be prescribed for at least 3 days after the procedure. Rule out infections at the donor and recipient site.
- *Hematoma or seroma*: Avoided by proper hemostasis and pressure dressings. Patients are advised to avoid vigorous activity for 7 to 10 days. If patients are on anticoagulants, it has to be stopped 1 to 2 weeks before the procedure. The wound can be inspected on 3rd day if a bolster dressing is not used. Hematoma if found has to be drained, else it will displace the graft and also act as a nidus for infection.
- Wound contracture may result in functional impairment when the graft is placed over a joint or an orifice, e.g. ectropion. Full thickness grafts have to be used in areas at risk of contractures.
- *Mismatch in texture, color, or topography*: These can be avoided with proper selection of the donor area. Graft hyperpigmentation occurs commonly. Photoprotection should be advised in the grafted area for extended periods. Spot dermabrasion or laser resurfacing can be used to flatten elevations.
- Perigraft halo in vitiligo and leukoderma.
- *Graft failure*: The graft appears necrotic with an eschar during dressing removal. Causes of graft failure are enumerated in Table 12.4.

Table 12.3: Complications.

Donor area	Early	Pain Bleeding Infection
	Late	Keloids Hypertrophic scars Pigment anomalies Paresthesias
Recipient area	Early	Pain Hematoma Seroma Graft displacement Infection
	Late	Graft failure Contractures Pigment mismatch Hyperpigmentation Loss of sensation, paresthesias Keloids, hypertrophic scars Stuck on tire appearance due to irregularity of graft spreading or rolling in of edges

Table 12.4: Causes of graft failure.

Technical errors	*Recipient bed factors*	*Patient factors*
Placement of dermal side up	Avascular bed /insufficient vascularity bone, cartilage	Systemic illness, immunosuppression
Very thick graft	Necrotic debris/slough	No rest/immobilization
Size mismatch	Hematoma/seroma	
Error in timing the graft	Infection	
Traumatic handling of graft	Graft displacement	

TIPS FOR GOOD GRAFT UPTAKE

- Full preoperative evaluation, stop anticoagulants.
- Choose a proper donor site with adequate color, texture and appendage match.
- Harvest adequate size graft, taking into consideration graft contraction.
- Atraumatic handling of the graft.
- Good vascularized recipient bed.
- Achieve close immobile contact between graft and bed. Adequate hemostasis to avoid hematoma/seroma.
- Pressure dressings.
- Reduced activity in postoperative period.

CONCLUSION

Skin grafting has to be well planned. In some areas healing by secondary intention would probably give a good outcome. Depending on the site, the size of the defect and the condition of the recipient bed, FTSG or STSG should be planned. Skin grafts also protect deeper vital structures such as bone or cartilage and keep them from becoming desiccated. Skin grafts speed healing time and may provide temporary coverage for a defect after surgery.

REFERENCES

1. Wheeland RG. Skin grafts. In:Roenigk RK, Ratz JL, Roenigk, Jr. HH (Eds). Current Techniques in Procedural Dermatology, 3rd ed. New York: Informa Healthcare. 2007;pp.527-36.
2. Rudolph R, Klein L. Healing processes in skin grafts. Surg Gynecol Obstet. 1973;136:641.
3. Savant SS. Skin grafting. In: Savant SS (Eds). Textbook of Dermatosurgery and Cosmetology, 2nd ed. Mumbai: ASCAD. 2005; pp.149-65.
4. Grabb WC. Basic techniques in plastic surgery (skin grafts). In: Grabb and Smith's Plastic Surgery, 3rd ed. Boston: Little Brown, 1979.
5. Thornton JF. Skin grafts and skin substitutes, Thorton JF, Goswan AA (Eds). Selected Readings in Plastic Surgery. 2004;10(1).
6. Kurul S. Is the groin region a good source for full-thickness skin graft? J Surg Oncol. 2001;77:281.
7. Khunger N, Khandari R. Thin split thickness skin grafting for vitiligo. In: Venkataram M (Eds). ACS(I) Textbook on Cutaneous and Aesthetic Surgery. New Delhi: Jaypee Brothers Medical Publishers (P) Ltd. 2012; pp.351-59
8. Christiansen J, Ek L, Tegner E. Pinch grafting of leg ulcers. A retrospective study of 412 treated ulcers in 146 patients. Acta Derm Venereol (Stockh). 1997;77:471.
9. Smahel J, Ganzoni N. Relay transplantation: a new method of expanding a free skin graft. Br J Plast Surg. 1975;28:49.
10. Henderson NJ, Fancourt M, Gilkison W, Kyle S, Mosquera D. Skin grafts: a rural general surgical perspective. ANZ J Surg. 2009;79(5):362-6.

CHAPTER 13

Scar Revision Techniques

Shilpa K, Biju Vasudevan

INTRODUCTION

The word scar is derived from the Greek word *eskhara,* which means scab. Scar is a lingering sign of damage or injury to skin. Scarring is an inevitable mark following healing of a wound or burn. Any wound that penetrates deeper than the epidermis, inflicted by biologic, chemical, or physical injury, results in healing by scar formation.

IDEAL SCAR

An ideal scar is the scar which is:[1]

- Level with the surrounding skin
- Soft
- Having good color match
- Narrow
- Lines of closure within or parallel to relaxed skin tension line (RSTL).

COUNSELING

- Foremost duty is to explain that no scar can be made to vanish completely
- Modified to make it more aesthetic and functionally viable
- Objective to be achieved should be explained
- Discuss all available invasive and noninvasive modalities.
- Patients with underlying psychiatric disease who blame their deformity for their psychological difficulties, who are soon to be married, who are involved in litigation related to their scar, are poor surgical candidates.

DEFINITION

Scar revision surgery refers to different types of procedures that are done to partially remove scar tissue, or to make the scar(s) less noticeable. The selection of procedure that is performed depends on the type of scar; its cause, location, and size; and the characteristics of the patient's skin.

SCAR REVISION TECHNIQUES

There are various techniques to improve the appearance of the scar, which include invasive and noninvasive techniques (Table 13.1). This chapter deals with only surgical/invasive scar revision techniques.

GENERAL PRINCIPLES OF SCAR REVISION

Timing of scar revision: Due to continuous collagen remodeling, it takes around 12–18 months for the scar to

Table 13.1: Scar revision techniques.

Noninvasive	*Invasive*
• Camouflage • Medications—(ILS, topical steroids, retinoic acid, placental extracts, allantoin, vitamin C, colchicine) • Massage • Silicone gel sheeting/silipos gel sheeting • Pressure garments/compressive dressings • Soft tissue augmentation • Cryotherapy • Electrical stimulation of skin • X-rays and Laser	• Fusiform/extramarginal scar excision • Intramarginal scar excision • Serial partial excision • Curvilinear S plasty • Z plasty • W plasty • Geometric broken line closure • V-Y plasty

mature and gain tensile strength of 70–80% of uninjured skin. Immature scars are prone to hypertrophy and give poor results after scar revision. However, if early intervention is needed, it is wiser to do it only after 8–12 weeks in adults and 6 months in children smaller than 7 years of age.[2]

Scar analysis: Scars that are usually taken up for revision are those which are:

- Wide (1–2 mm)
- Having length >2 cm
- Perpendicular to RSTL
- Crossing an esthetic unit of the face
- Webbed
- Hypertrophied
- Adjacent to, but not lying in, a favorable site
- Scars disturbing the functionality
- Pin cushioned scars
- Causing distortion of facial features
- Poor match to surrounding tissue (color, depth).

Scars should be analyzed in relation to the following aspects:

- Its anatomical location
- Its proximity to vital structures
- Direction with respect to local RSTL and cosmetic units
- Length, width and shape
- Contour (elevated, depressed, atrophic, hypertrophic or keloidal.
- Color (hypo/hyperpigmentation)
- Total number of scars.

Examination of the surrounding tissue should include:

- Local landmarks
- Tension in surrounding tissues
- Distortion of angle of eyes, mouth, vermilion border of lips
- Check for functional damage like ectropion, palmar contracture
- Skin texture, pigmentation, laxity, adnexal structures.

General Technical Considerations for Scar Revision

Anesthesia

Done under local anesthesia. Lignocaine with adrenaline is preferred for better hemostasis. Use of tumescent anesthesia reduces intraoperative bleeding.

Incision

Incisions can be made less visible by placing them at the junction of aesthetic subunits of the face. These junctions are the lines where there is a contour change on the face or at where the non-hair bearing skin meets the hair-bearing skin. The shadows that are cast from the changes in contour tend to hide the scars well. The hidden incisions that give better cosmetic camouflage are as follows:

Hidden incisions:

- *Hide incision in orifice*: Transconjunctival, sublabial, intranasal, etc.
- *Hide incision in hair*: Future balding tendency should be kept in mind when planning incision on the scalp.
- *Hide behind anatomic prominence*: For example retroauricular, submental.
- *Hide in junction of aesthetic subunits*: The shadow cast contour camouflages the scar
- Hide in relaxed skin tension lines (RSTLs).

Skin is stretched and stabilized by thumb and index finger of left hand. Incision is made perpendicular to the skin surface. In hair bearing areas, incision is put along the direction of hair follicle to prevent transection and permanent hair loss around the scar. A single pass or stroke of blade is desirable to prevent staircasing of the wound margin. The marked curve and angle should be strictly followed while incising to avoid nicking and cross hatching.

Tissue Handling

Tissues should be handled gently with minimal manipulation during surgery. Toothed and traumatic forceps should be avoided. Fine toothed forceps or skin hooks are preferred. Good hydration of wound margins using moist gauze should be maintained during surgery to promote wound healing and prevent excessive scarring.

Excision

Once complete incision is made, tissue or scar base is transected at the desired depth. Care should be taken that base is of uniform thickness. If there is excess tissue removal at the center, it results in scooping with pseudo-dog ear formation.

Undermining

It is a technique of detaching the epidermis and dermis from underlying subcutaneous fat and fascia. This helps to reduce tension on wound edges. About 1.5–2 cm width undermining will be sufficient.

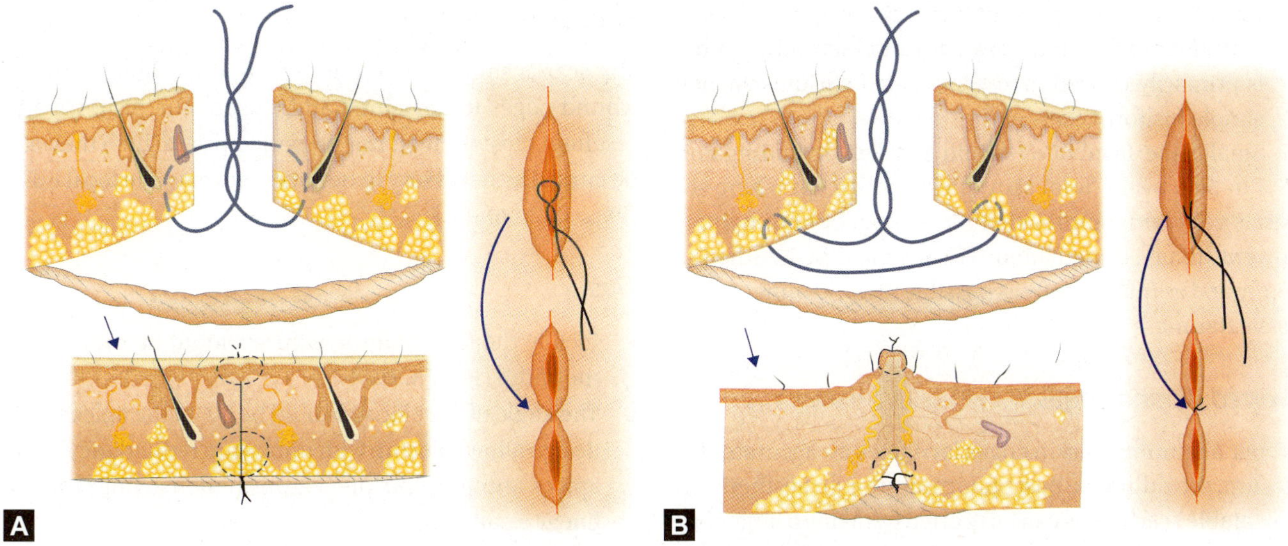

Figs. 13.1A and B: Layered wound repair.

Elimination of Dead Space

Dead space should be avoided to prevent hematoma formation. This can be achieved by layered closure.

Layered Wound Repair

Suturing the deep dermal layer with buried knots increases the strength of the wound repair. Traditionally, subcutaneous suture placement incorporates a small bite of dermis in a loop of fine absorbable suture, repeated many times along the wound edge. A modification of the technique is the placement of the subcutaneous suture 8 to 10 mm back on each side as shown in Figures 13.1A and B.

The advantage of this modified technique is:

- A greater degree of eversion is achieved
- No compromise on the wound edges as the suture is placed back from the edge
- Fewer stitches are required as each stitch exerts its influence over a greater distance
- More favorable wound healing.

This layered suture releases the tension from the interrupted superficial sutures and allows for early superficial suture removal to prevent cross hatching.

Elimination of Wound Edge Tension

Wounds heal with less scarring when tension is minimal. In addition, much finer suture material may be used, resulting in less wound edge trauma and scar formation. This is specially so when its only role is the precise alignment of the epidermal margins when the margins are already approximated. Proper undermining and subcuticular sutures reduce the wound edge tension.

Suture Material

Smaller the suture material better is the scar. It is better to use smallest possible suture based on the site, thickness and tension of the wound. Suture size 5/0 or 6/0 is appropriate for face and a size of 4/0 or 3/0 for trunk or limbs. For an atraumatic skin repair, a reverse cutting needle is more preferred (or cutting, if it is not available).

Suture Techniques

The different suture technique that are used in scar revision closure are simple interrupted, vertical mattress, or running locking configurations.

- Simple interrupted suturing technique has less chance to cause wound edema and impaired circulation[3] and helps in maintaining flap margin viability because of its spacing of normal tissue in between sutures along the wound margin. Wound margin eversion can also be achieved with this suture technique.
- The running locking suture technique helps in timesaving as it allows the surgeon to close a wound with multiple edges, such as with complex geometric broken line closure (GBLC) or running W-plasty. Running sutures are preferred over eyelids.[3,4]
- Do not pinch down the many running half-formed knots to maintain a viable blood supply.

- Superior eversion of wound margins can be achieved with the vertical mattress suturing technique and it is primarily is used in less angulated closures such as simple fusiform excision.

Small superficial bites should be taken, including only 25% to 50% of the total skin thickness, except where the skin is very thin. Sutures should be snug, but not tight, to prevent tissue strangulation. Tissues must be handled as gently and as infrequently as possible to avoid unnecessary tissue trauma.

Everted Wound Edges

Proper alignment of skin edges facilitates an accurate skin closure, providing the best opportunity for an aesthetically acceptable scar. Edges can be everted by taking a larger bite of the deeper dermis while inserting the needle vertically through the skin.

Good Hemostasis

Good hemostasis achieved by local anesthetic agent with adrenaline, gentle pressure, ligature or bipolar electrocautery.

Dressing

After closure is complete, a wound dressing should be applied. Semiocclusive dressings are preferred for several reasons.[5] First, they maintain warm environment and keep the wound surface hydrated, thus avoiding surface desiccation and eschar formation. They provide a physical barrier against microbial growth at the same time allowing gas exchange necessary for wound healing. Apart from these they also reduce the inflammatory infiltrate in healing wounds, apparently due to a reduction of necrotic elements which incite inflammation, thus keeping minimizing fibroblast proliferation and fibrogenesis.[6]

TYPES OF SCAR REVISION TECHNIQUES

Fusiform Elliptical Excision

Simple excision is the most basic scar-revision technique.

Indications

It is useful for small, round, elliptical, or stellate scars that lie:

- Within a hairline
- At the junction of two esthetic areas
- That parallel the RSTL and respects facial subunits.[7]

Principle/Technique

The scar is simply excised in a fusiform manner, and the wound edges undermined and closed. The fusiform and resultant closure need not be perfectly straight—they can be curved as necessary to better conform to the local RSTL (Figs. 13.2A and B).

Tips

- Ideally the length of the ellipse should be three times the width (Fig. 13.3).
- The angle of the ellipse should be 30° at the apices. This design allows closure with minimum redundancy at the apices and prevents dog ear formation giving rise to a linear clean scar.
- Extramarginal scar excision to be done to get normal tissue at the wound edges (unlike serial excision where its intramarginal.[2]
- M plasty can be done at the lateral edges to prevent lengthening of scar.

S-shaped modification of elliptical excision shown in Figures 13.4A to C.

Serial Excision

This technique is employed when the size, location, and elasticity of the scar and surrounding skin prevent complete excision and primary closure or when closure results in distortion of nearby structures.

Indication

Large scars in which the surrounding tissue laxity is insufficient for a single excision.[8]

Principle/Technique

Using above-mentioned simple conventional excision methods, the scar is partially excised (intramarginal) and the adjacent skin along with the remaining scar tissue is advanced by undermining sufficiently. Remaining scar excised in next sitting with complete removal of scar (extra marginal excision) (Figs. 13.5 and 13.6).

Tips

- Can move scar to better anatomic location
- Scar could be moved via serial excision to hairline

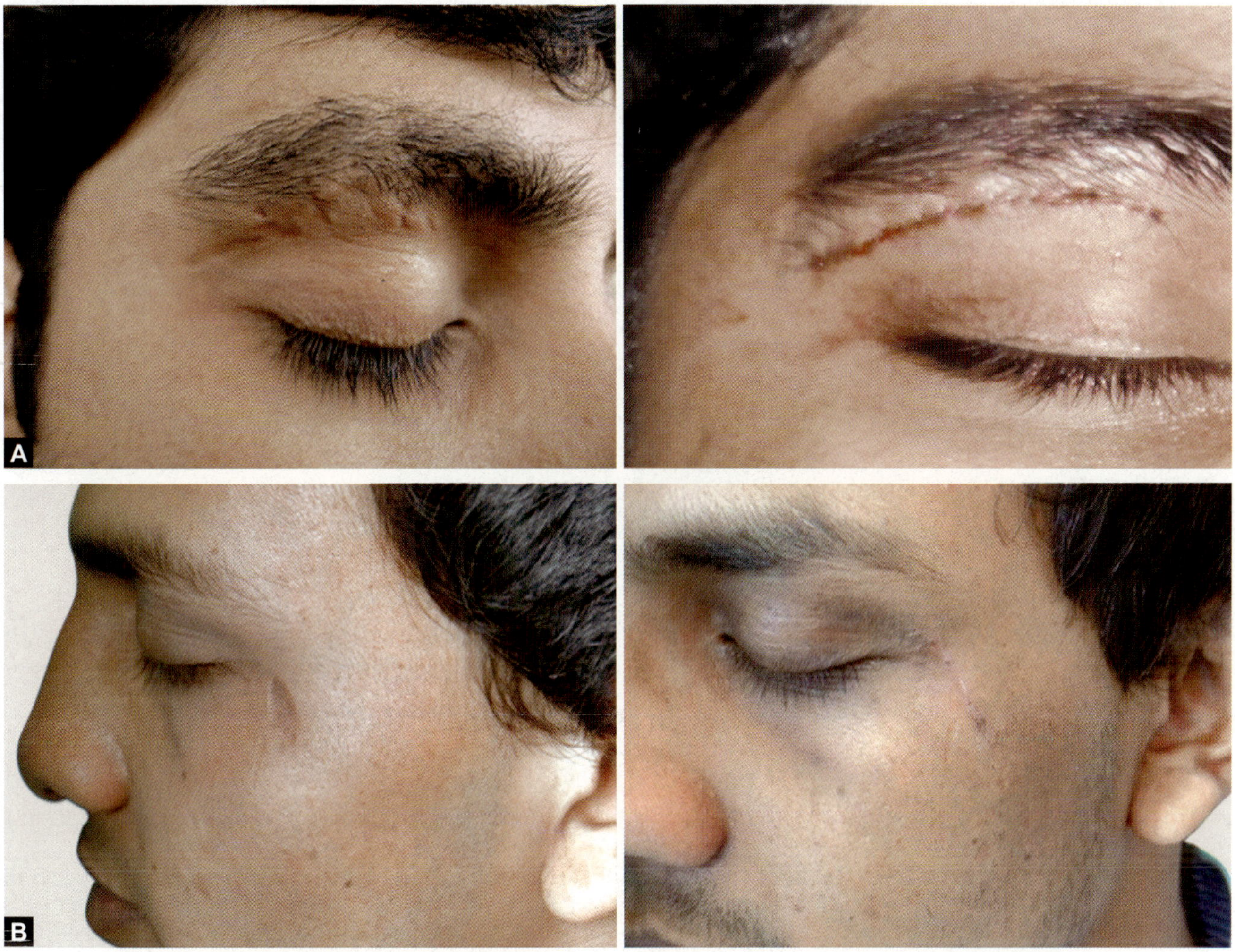

Figs. 13.2A and B: A linear scar along RSTL excised and closed primarily. (B) Another scar along RSTL closed with elliptical excision.

- Re-orient a scar along RSTL
- If the scar is very wide requiring more than two procedures better to consider tissue expansion technique as an alternate tool to reduce multiple excisions.[9]

Z-plasty

Z-plasty is an important scar revision technique used to improve the functional and cosmetic appearance of scars. Z-plasties can be functional when it is used to lengthen and relax scars as in severe contracted scars due to burns or cosmetic when it is used realign scars to make them less noticeable as in scars lying againt RSTL. They can be single or multiple depending on the length of the scar.

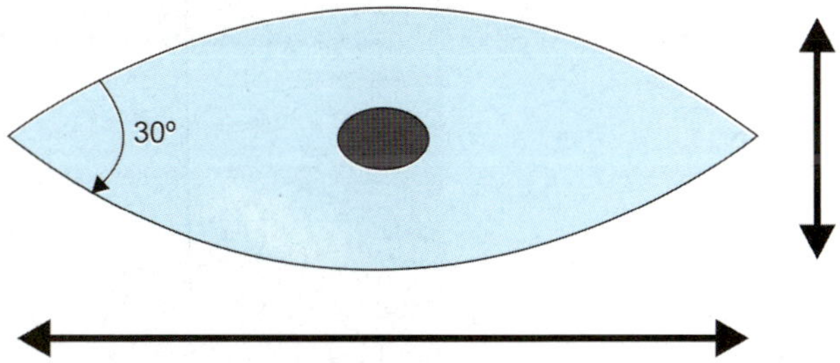

Fig. 13.3: Ratio of length and breadth in fusiform excision.

Indications

- Scar crossing relaxed skin tension lines
- Scar adjacent to esthetic units, such as the medial canthus or oral commissure
- Severe contracted scar, e.g. burns scar

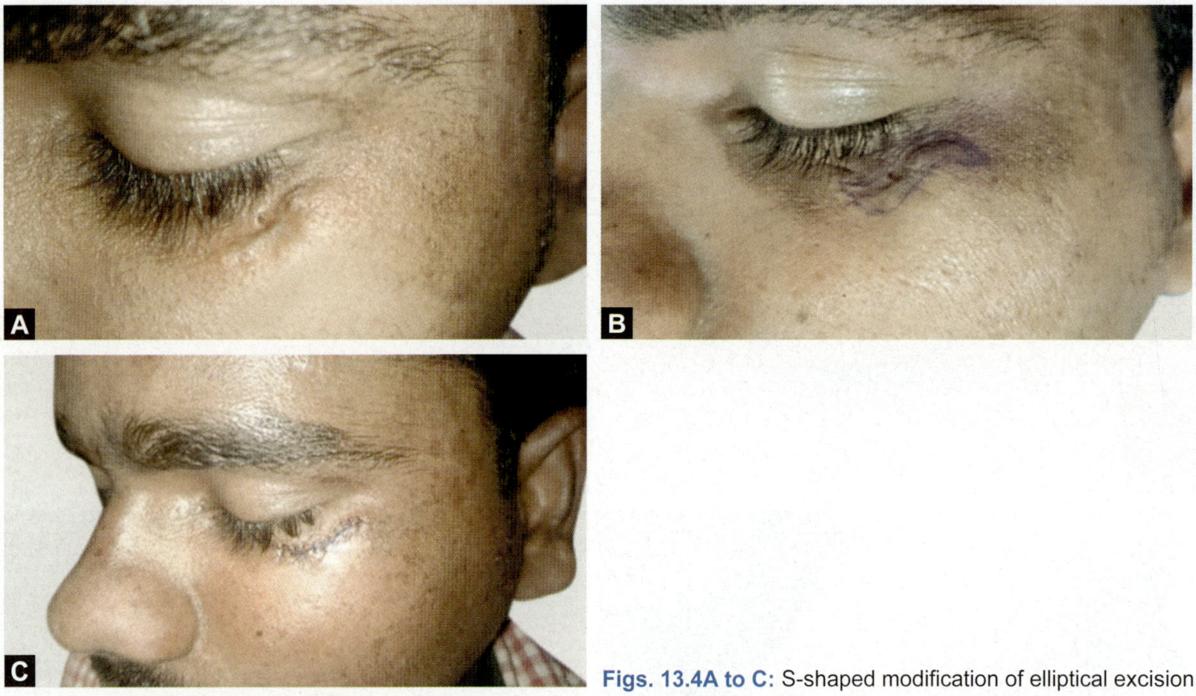

Figs. 13.4A to C: S-shaped modification of elliptical excision.

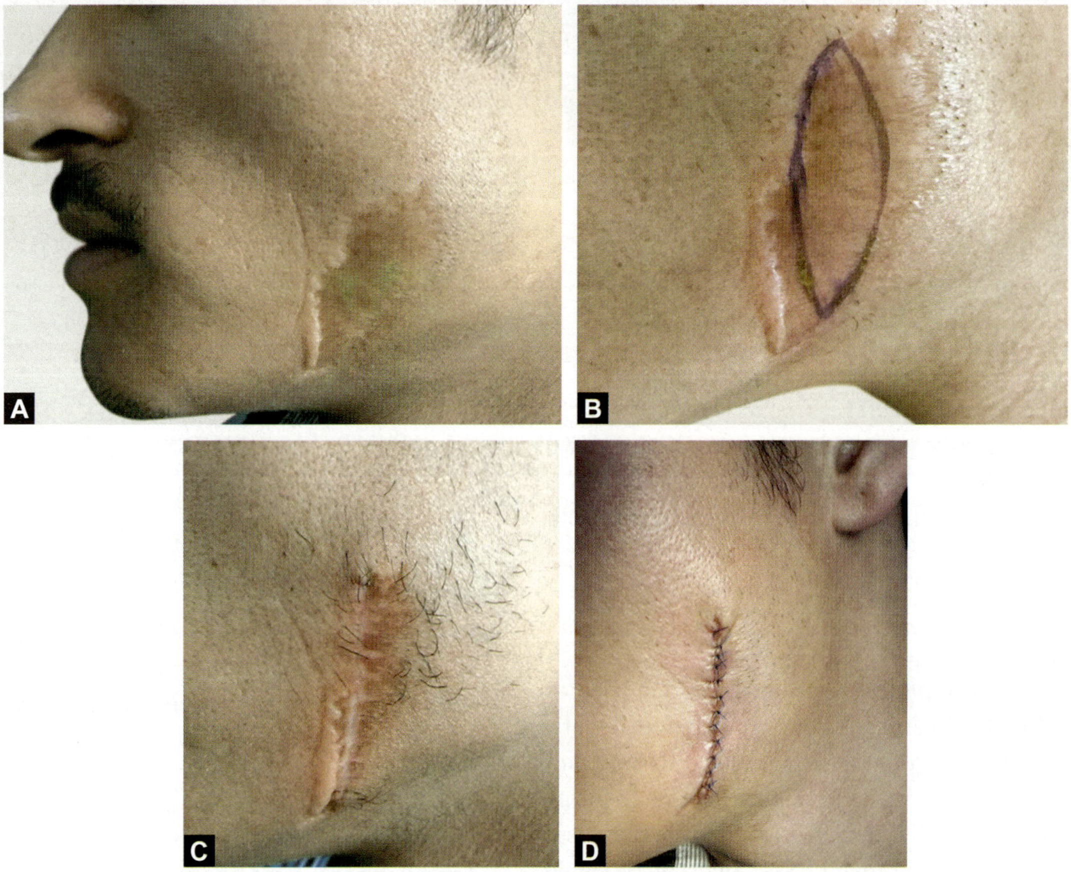

Figs. 13.5A to D: Serial excision of scar: (A) A large scar on the cheek. (B) Planned for partial excision. (C) After first serial excision the scar aligned along RSTL. (D) Scar completely excised in the second sitting with new scar along RSTL.

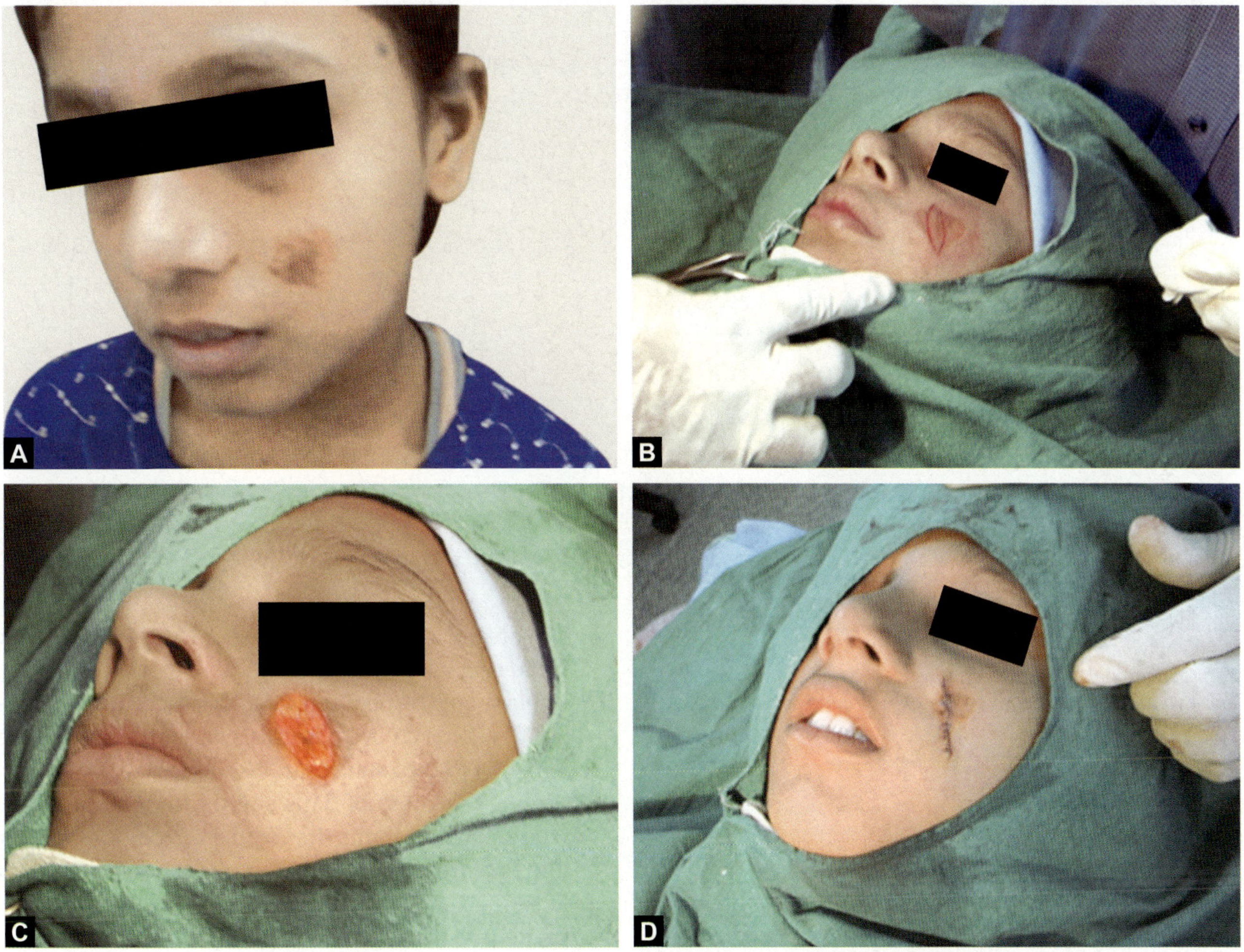

Figs. 13.6A to D: A large scar on the face being excised intramarginally in the first sitting.

- Linear scars, crossing the border of adjacent facial aesthetic unit (e.g. vermillion border)
- When scars crossing a concave surface (e.g. the medial canthus)
- Changing scar length (e.g. scar contracture of lip, eyelid, or neck)
- When scar vector needs to be changed (e.g. repositioning a scar across the nasolabial fold)
- Useful for correction of "trapdoor" or "pin-cushion" defects by repositioning malposed tissues
- Correction of webbed scars.

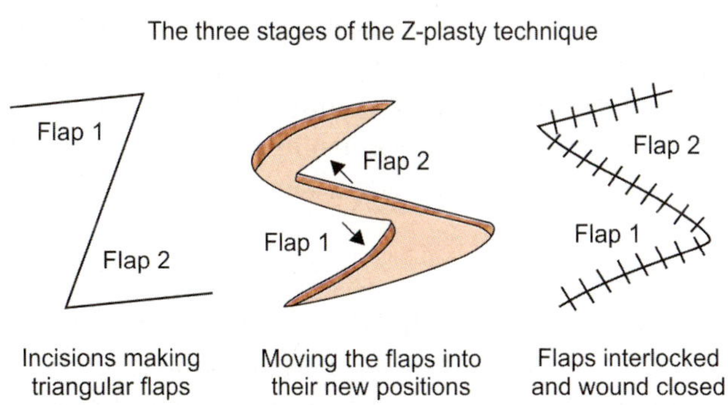

Fig. 13.7: Diagrammatic representation of Z plasty.

Principle

This technique diffuses tension by transposing triangular skin flaps, changing the direction of an abnormal scar to lie within RSTLs.[8] The central limb of the Z-shaped incision is put along the line of greatest tension or contraction, then two or more triangular flaps are raised on either sides of the two ends of the central limb and then transposed (Fig. 13.7). Two components which determine the outcome and tissue lengthening in Z-plasty are the length of

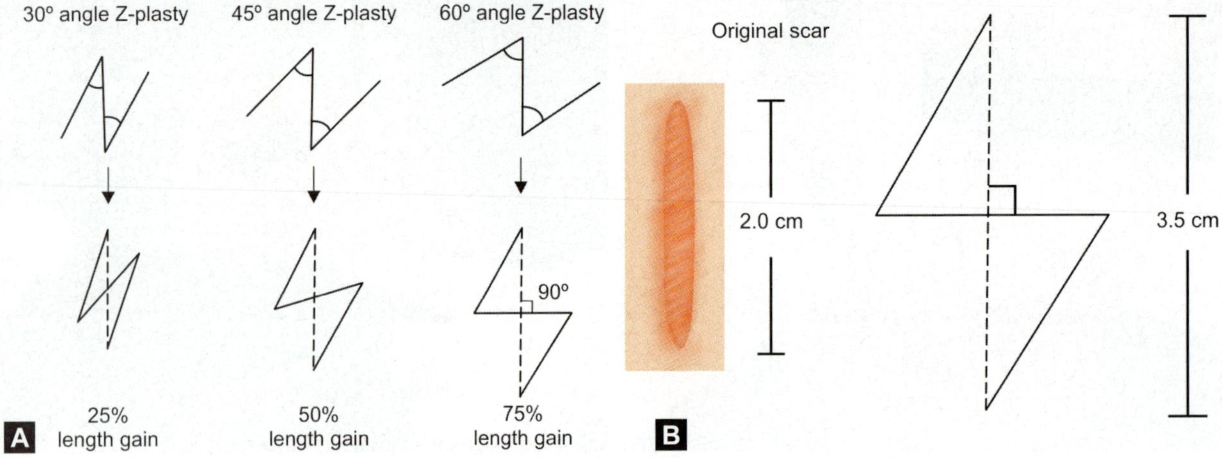

Figs. 13.8A and B: Diagrammatic representation of relation between angle and degree of lengthening.

Table 13.2: The relation between angle and degree of lengthening achieved in Z plasty.

Angle between central diagonal and two arms	*% increase in length*	*Change in orientation of the central limb*
30°	25%	45°
45°	50%	60°
60°	75%	90°
75°	100%	–
90°	125%	–

the center line of 'Z', called as the common diagonal and its angle with the two limbs at its edges (Figs. 13.8A and B). In scar revision, the original scar is used as the common diagonal and two arms of same length as the central line are extended in opposite directions. An angle of 60° is formed between the arms and the common diagonal. The angle determines the degree of lengthening of the tissue, the larger the angle, the greater the length gain (Table 13.2).

Technique

In performing Z-plasty, the original scar as the common limb of 'Z' is excised and an incision is made along the two outlined arms. The wound is widely undermined at the level of subcutaneous fat in order to loosen the scar. Then the direction of the common diagonal is changed into 'transverse diagonal' (the new scar is perpendicular to the original scar) by simultaneously lifting the full thickness triangular flaps of equal size and transposing them (Figs. 13.9A to D).

Tips

- Length and angle of two arms should be equal to avoid puckering.
- Angle should be between 45° and 60°. Too less an angle (>30°) can result in tip necrosis and greater the angle, lengthier the resultant scar.
- Proper thickness of flaps should be maintained. A very thick flap limits the degree of rotation and too thin flap may contracts and resultant outcome may be unsatisfactory. An ideal plane is between the subdermal plexus and the subcutaneous fatty tissue.
- Angles greater than 60° can be broken into multiple flaps
- Long scars can do with a series of Z-plasties (Figs. 13.10 and 13.11).

Modifications of Z plasty

- Double opposing Z-plasties
- Skew Z-plasty
- Half Z-plasty
- Four flap Z-plasty (Limberg flap)
- Planimetric Z-plasty
- S-plasty
- Jumping man procedure.

W plasty

Indications[10]

- For linear scar measuring greater than 2 cm which are at an angle > 35° to the RSTLs.

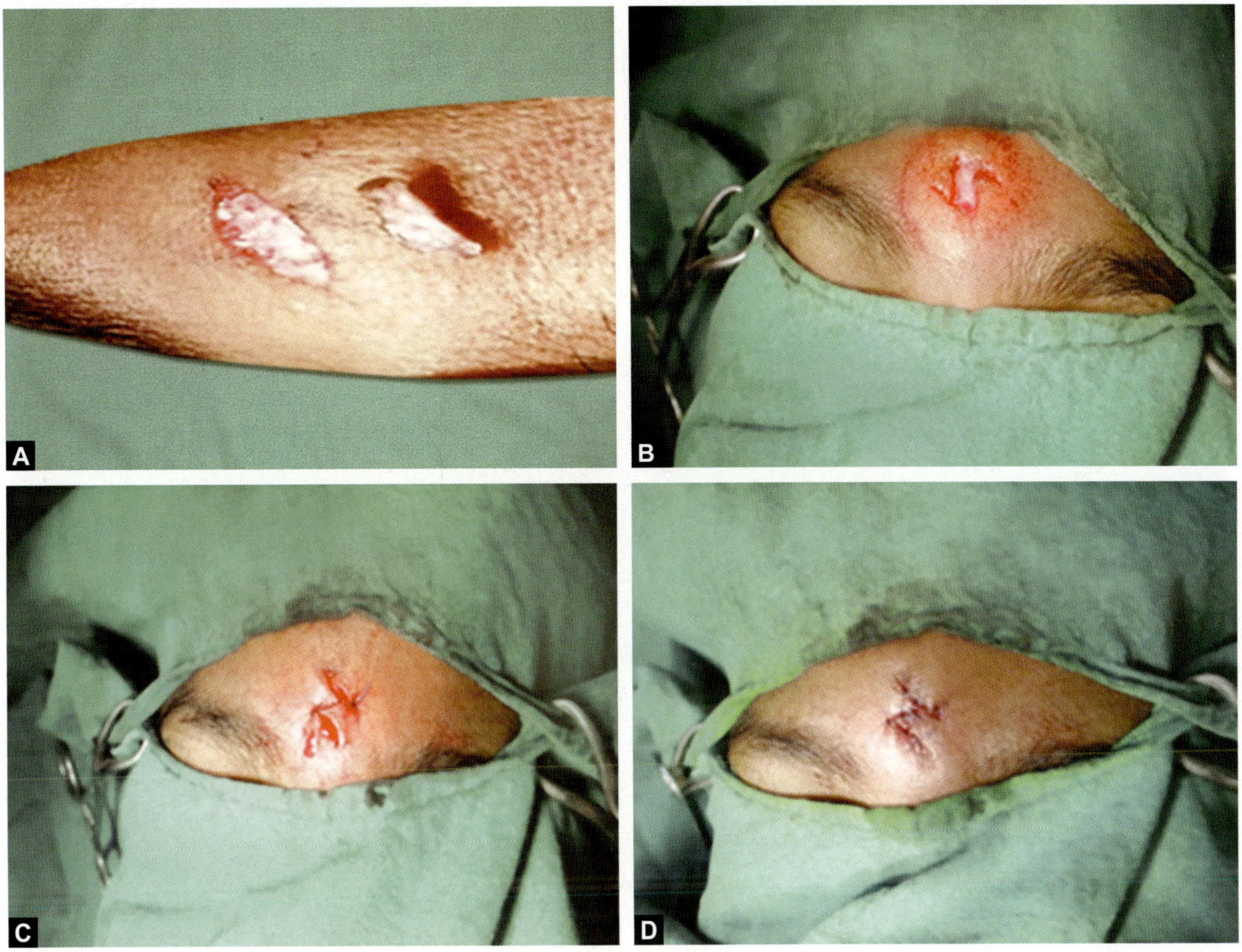

Figs. 13.9A to D: (A) A vertical scar (perpendicular to RSTL) on forehead after excision. (B) Two limbs of equal length on either side of central limb. (C) The flaps are transposed. (D) Final closure of Z-plasty.

- Short scars present on relatively unforgiving areas like the forehead and cheeks.
- Helpful in curved scars.
- Closures in pretrichial areas (following a browlift or forehead flap).
- Closure over curved surfaces like the inferior mandibular border.

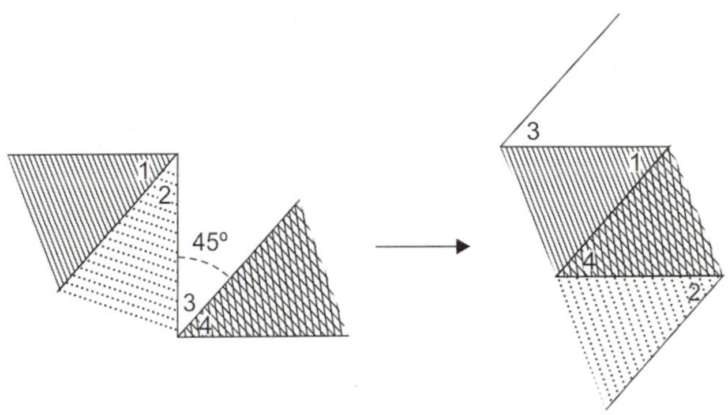

Fig. 13.10: Diagrammatic representation of series of Z-plasties.

Principle

The eye is always drawn towards straight lines. Straight scars are more likely to cause contracture. The principle behind W-plasty is that the visibility of an irregular, broken line is less due to insignificant light reflection and less easier for the eyes to follow as compared to a straight scar.[10]Another advantage of these W-plasties is that they break up a linear scar into an accordion pattern, which has much greater elasticity and allows the skin more movement during contraction, thus contributing to facial expression.[11]

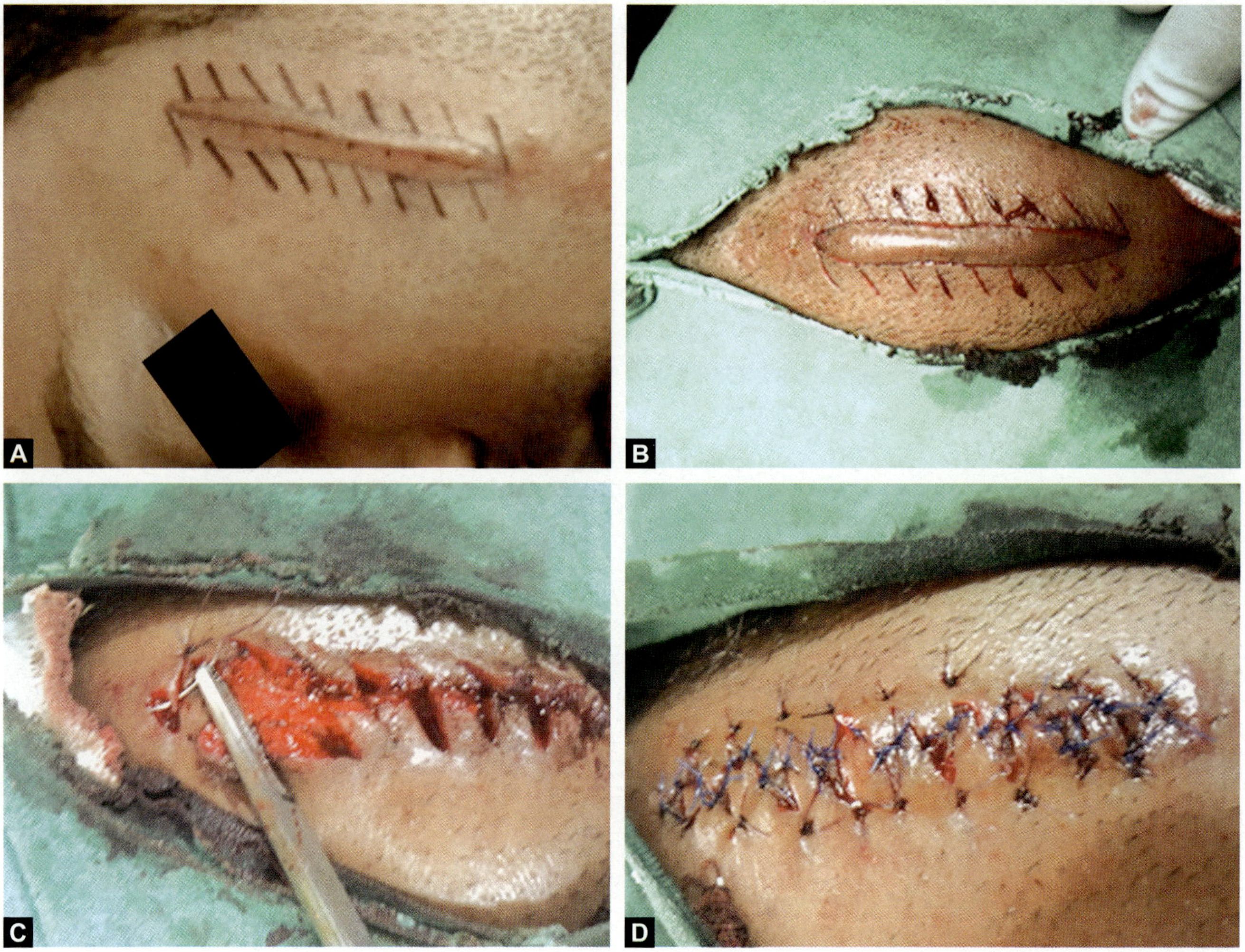

Figs. 13.11A to D: (A) A long linear scar against RSTL on left cheek with planning for serial Z-plasty. (B) Scar being excised along with raising of multiple limbs on either side of the scars. (C) Flaps being transposed. Image also shows tip suture. (D) Closure with multiple Z-plasty.

Technique

In W-plasty series of consecutive triangles are made on one side of the scar with its mirror image on the other side. After excising the scars along these lines and undermining it, re-approximation is done by interdigitating the triangles to form a single zigzag line (Figs. 13.12 to 13.14).

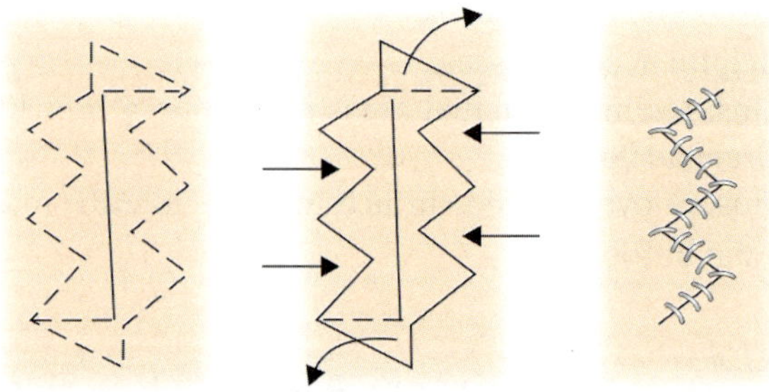

Fig. 13.12: Diagrammatic representation of W-plasty.

Tips

- No. 11 blade is most helpful
- Try to place segments in RSTLs
- The 'dots' of the apex of the triangles are placed 5–6 mm apart from each other and at a distance of 3–7 mm from the scar line. A distance of less than 3 mm is too small to avoid the scar appearing to be a straight line and one greater than 7 mm will create a separately visible scar.[10]
- Gillies corner stitch may be helpful; simple stitch is the other option.

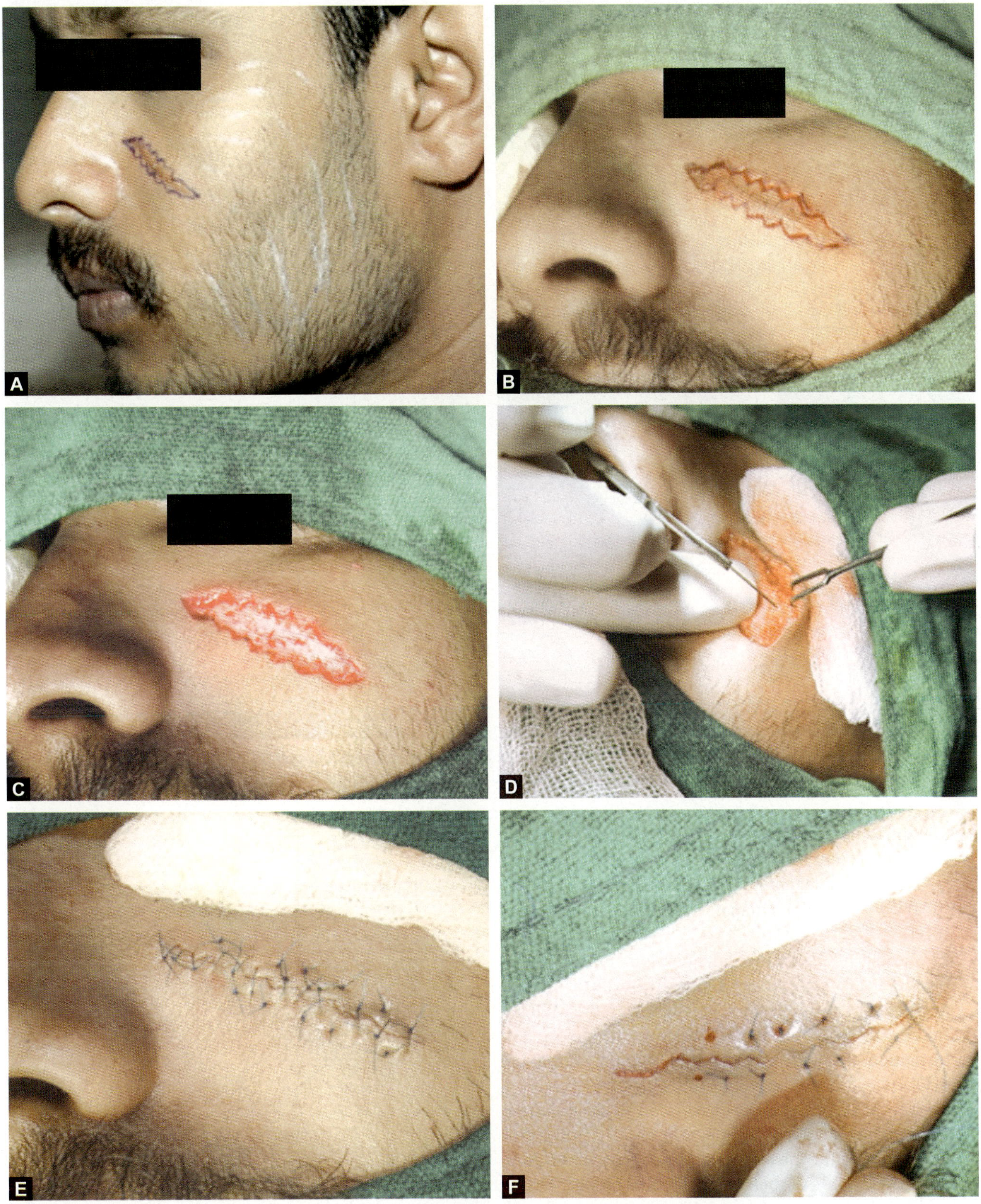

Figs. 13.13A to F: A linear scar against RSTL excised and closed with W-plasty.
Courtesy: Dr Madura C, Consultant, Cutis Academy, Bengaluru, Karnataka, India

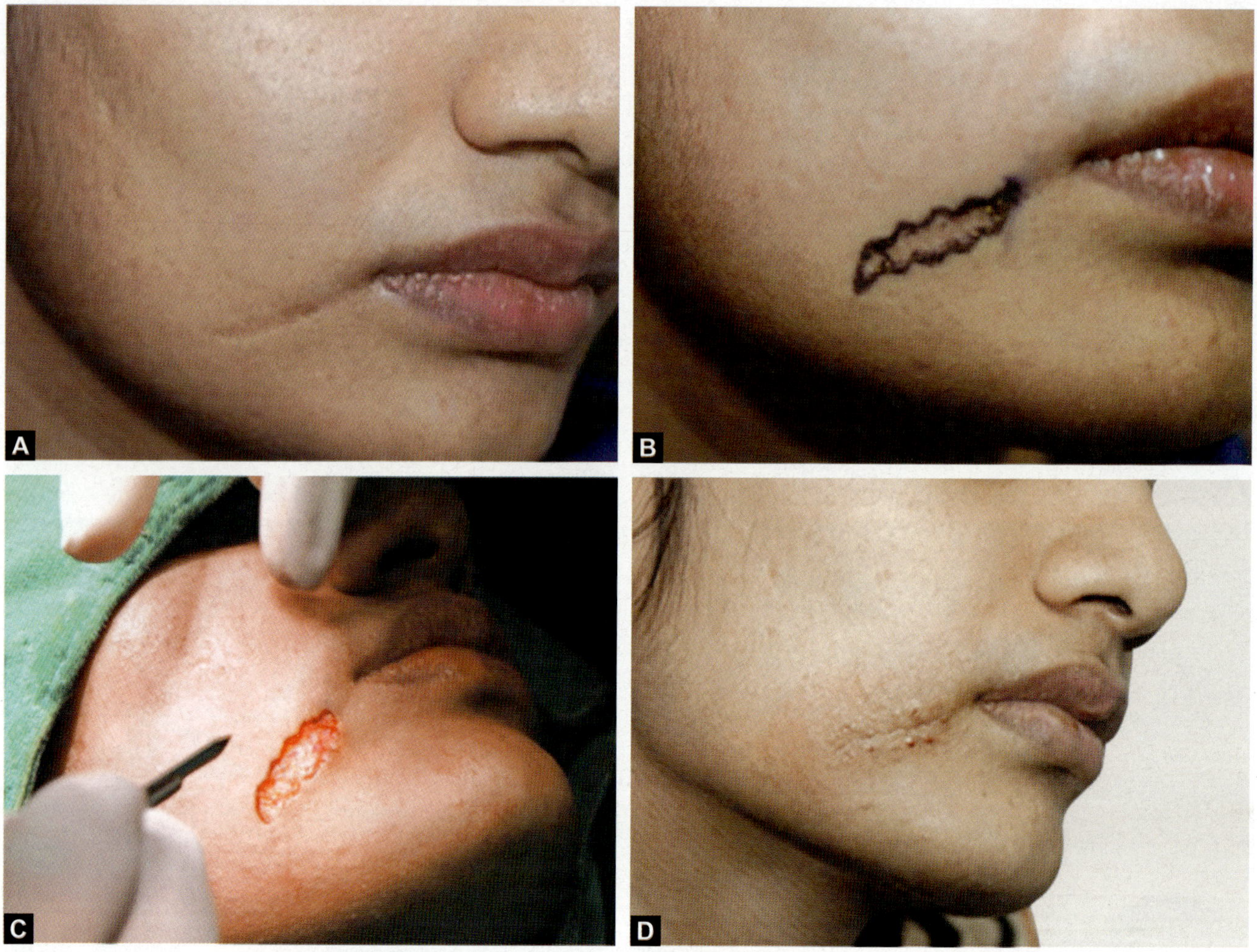

Figs. 13.14A to D: A linear scar against RSTL excised and closed with W-plasty.
Courtesy: Dr Madura C, Consultant, Cutis Academy, Bengaluru, Karnataka, India

- The limbs of each triangle should be 3–5 mm long as length of < 3 mm will not break the scar adequately and > 5 mm will make it more conspicuous.
- Ideally one arm of the triangle should be parallel to the RSTLs.
- The angle of the triangular apex is usually angled between 60° and 90° and should be determined according to the angle the scar makes with the RSTLs.
- In order to avoid 'dog ear' or 'standing cone deformity' formation, the angle at the ends of W-plasty should be < 30°.
- To prevent extension of the incision, an M-plasty can be done at the end of the incision.
- For curved scars, when cutting the flaps on a curved scar, make the flaps on the outside of the curve broader based and less acutely angled in order to keep the number of flaps on each side equal (Fig. 13.15).

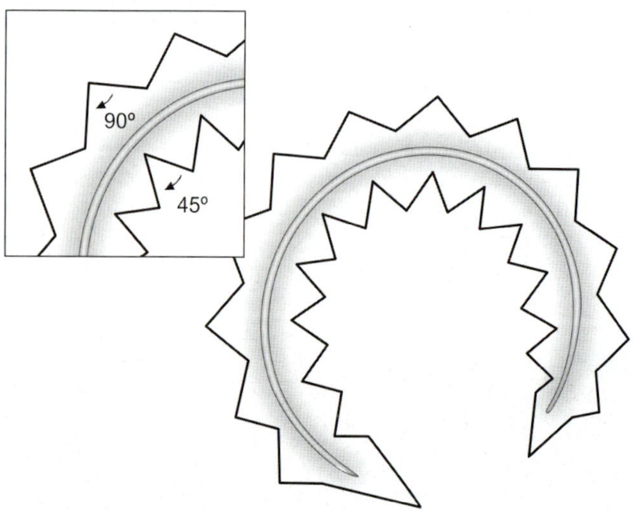

Fig. 13.15: Diagrammatic representation of W-plasty for curvilinear scar.

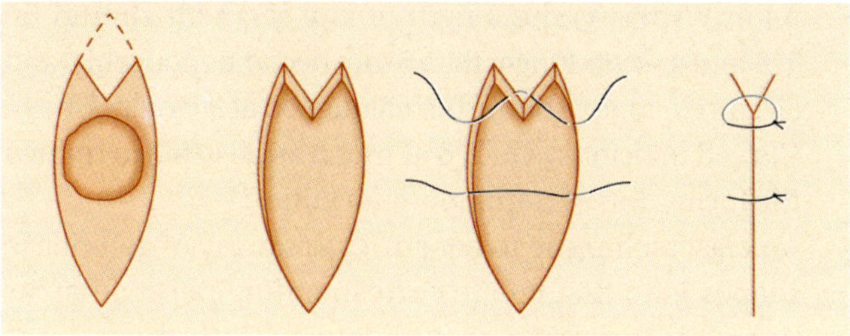

Fig. 13.16: Diagrammatic representation of M-plasty.

M-plasty

It is a useful technique to preserve healthy tissue, especially near the orifices thus reducing the risk of secondary tissue deformity.[12]

Principle

In M-plasty, there is a simple modification of simple fusiform excision in which instead of one, two separate 30° angles are created at the edges. This preserves the surrounding healthy tissue approximately by 50% at the same time reducing the length of suture line. It also prevents "dog ears" ear formation, which can be caused by an attempt to close of round defects; because this action compresses the tissue at angulated points and forces it upward and outward resulting in standing cones (Fig. 13.16).[13]

Technique

To construct the M-plasty, midpoint of the line joining the tip of central vertical line and lateral apex is marked. The proximal part forms the one side of triangle.The second side is drawn from this midpoint to the most lateral edge of the scar on both sides thus creating two triangles of 30° each (Figs. 13.17A and B). The lateral most point of tissue at the wound edges is centrally advanced into the wound as in a V-Y advancement maneuver, so that the overall length of the wound is shortened, (Figs. 13.18A and B).

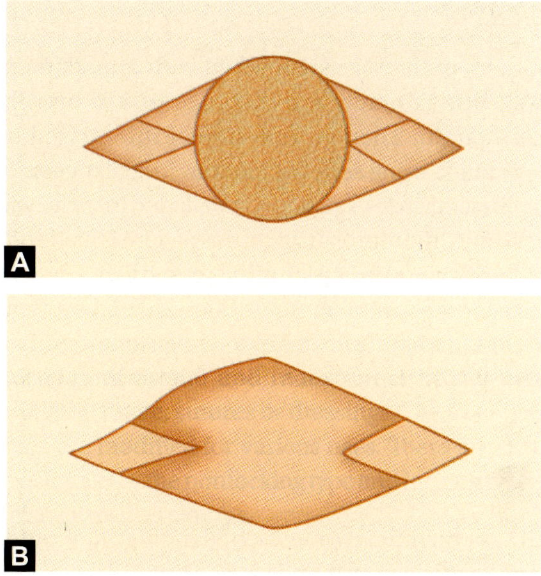

Figs. 13.17A and B: Designing for M-plasty.

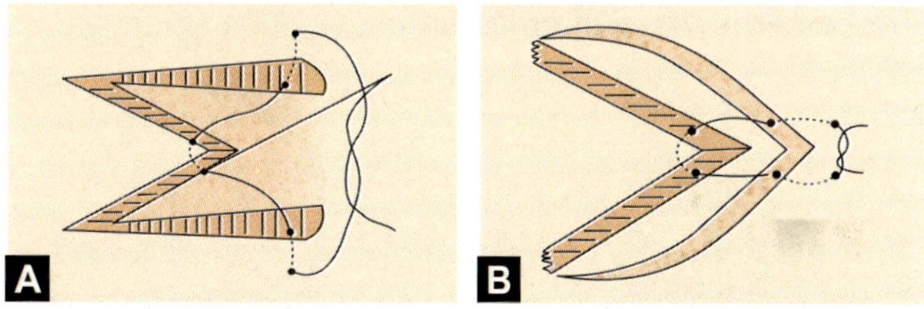

Figs. 13.18A and B: M-plasty closing as in V-Y advancement.

Indications

- When the angle created at the lateral wound, margin is greater than 30°.
- When preserving healthy surrounding tissue is essential.
- To decrease the formation of dog ear.
- Broad scar which result in longer scar.

Geometric Broken-Line Closure (GBLC)

While W-plasty is a regularly irregular scar revision technique, geometric broken-line closure (GBLC) is an irregularly irregular technique that provides maximum camouflage of longer scars, more than that due to W-plasty. In GBLC, triangular flaps of a W-plasty are substituted by a series of randomly ordered irregular geometric shapes.[10]An irregularly irregular configurations render the scar less visible as compared to regularly regular W-plasty. Like W-plasty, GBLC also does not lengthen the scar.

Indications

- Relatively longer scars of >4 cm[11] that are at an angle ≥ 45° to the RSTLs.
- Scars involving a convex or a concave surface.

Principle

The irregularly irregular pattern of the incision line of GBLC is less predictable than the regularly irregular line of W-plasty due to its random twists and turns which makes it difficult for the eyes to follow. However, it is more time consuming and technically more difficult than W-plasty.

Technique

The borders of the scar are marked with a marking pen. A dotted line is made at a distance of 3–6 mm from the scar margin. Then on one side of the excised scar, outline is made using series of random irregular geometric designs like semicircles, squares, rectangle and triangles within the dotted line. The mirror image of this pattern is made on the other side, creating a succession of interposed flaps (Fig. 13.19). After excising the scars along these lines and undermining it, wound edges are approximated by interdigitating the different geometric shaped flaps on each side to form an irregular line of closure.[2]

Tips

- GBLC is technically more challenging. It should be planned meticulously and carried out.
- Incisions are made perpendicular to the skin surface using a No-11 scalpel blade as it ensures precise geometric shape interdigitation.

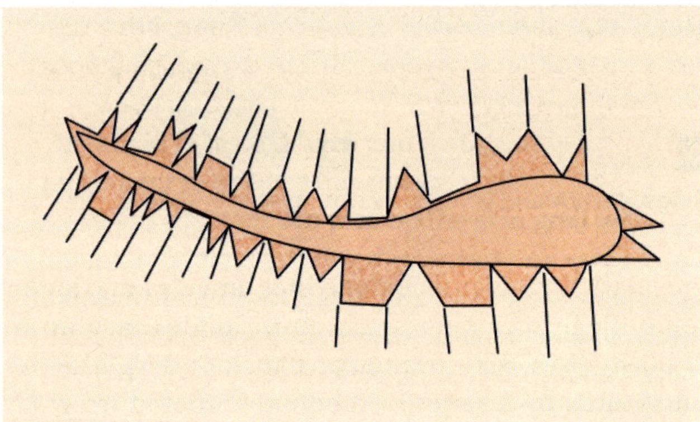

Fig. 13.19: Diagrammatic representation of series of GBLC.

- As in W-plasty, the length of any segment should be 3–6 mm as scars longer than 6 mm becomes noticable, and all corner angles should be maintained at 90° or less.
- Curved incisions avoided as much as possible to reduce the formation of trapdoor deformities.
- An easy technique to construct this array of geometric shapes is to first create corresponding perpendicular lines on each side of the wound. With these lines different geometric shapes are created in such a way that the corresponding shapes on either side interlock in the final closure.
- If the scar is curvilinear, the size of the geometric shapes is kept smaller on the concave side than on the convex counterpart. For example, outer triangles on convex side must be larger in both side length and angle than their inner curve on concave sides.

V-Y Plasty

This technique is used on periorificial areas or free margins such as the eyelid and to eliminate minor notches in the perioral or nose area. It provides additional tissue for an area with a deficiency. The lengthening effect on the scar is similar to that of a Z-plasty, except that the additional skin is advanced instead of transposed.[14] Thus, beneficial for the correction of wounds that have contracted around the eye or mouth (Fig. 13.20).

Technique

- A "V" shaped incision is made into the skin encompassing the scar.
- The skin on either side of the "V" is undermined, advanced, and closed as a "Y".

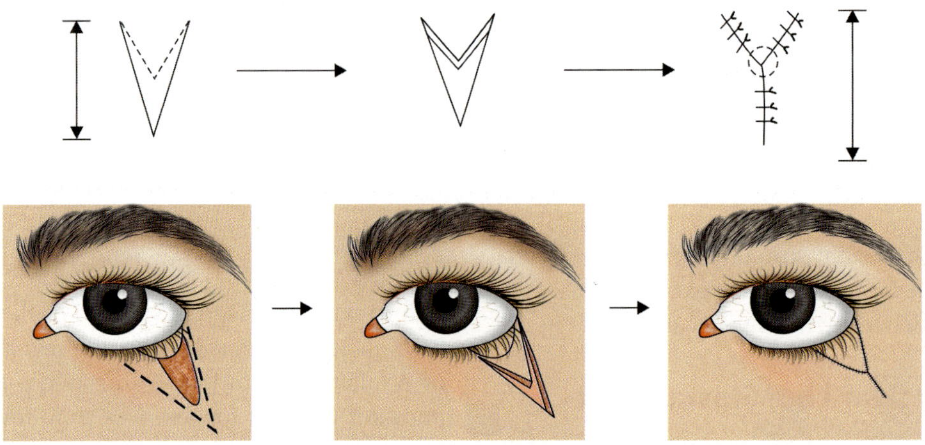

Fig. 13.20: Diagrammatic representation of V-Y plasty.

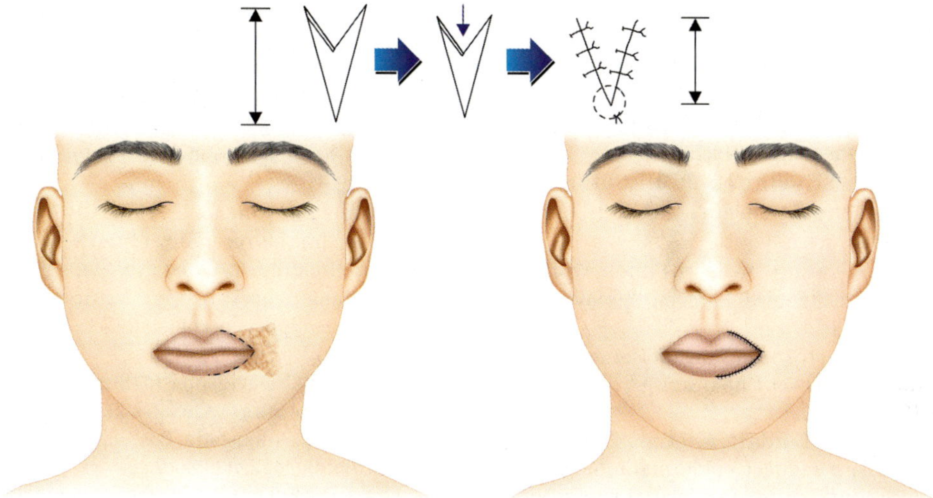

Fig. 13.21: Diagrammatic representation of Y-V plasty.

- The flap is closed with a three-point suture to avoid lip necrosis.

Tips

- The lengthening of the scar depends on the size of the V.

Y-V Plasty

The Y-V incision is made in a Y-shape, and the tip of the triangular flap is advanced. This variation of the V-Y flap is used to move the oral commissures laterally when some defect has pulled the commissure toward the midline (Fig. 13.21).

COMPLICATIONS OF SCAR REVISION AND TIPS TO PREVENT THEM

The complications of scar revision and the tips to prevent them are listed in Table 13.3.

Table 13.3: Scar revision: Complications and prevention.

Complications	*Tips to prevent them*
Immediate complications	
Hematoma formation	• Proper hemostasis during surgery. • Pressure dressing • Avoid dead space during closure • A small drain should be left in place, if risk is high
Secondary infection	• Aseptic precautions during surgery • Antibiotics to be started on the day of surgery
Wound dehiscence	• Avoid excessive tension of epidermal sutures • Place good dermal sutures to relieve the epidermal tension • Use of steristrips.
Delayed complications	
Hyperpigmentation	• Proper sun protection • Use of sunscreens • Depigmenting agents
Scar widening	• Proper placement of suture and delaying suture removal in areas prone to stretch and increased movement • Dermal/subcuticular sutures can be done with sutures like PDS which persists for longer time thus preventing widening • Postoperative use of botox temporarily paralysis the underlying muscle, so that pull on the scar is prevented • Postoperative use of steristrips for 6 weeks
Hypertrophic scar/keloid	• Intralesional steroid injection should be given prophylactically after scar revision for those who have the tendency

CONCLUSION

Scar revision techniques serve to improve a scar's functional capability, enhance cosmetic appearance, or both. No single method is ideal for every patient or every scar type. Careful selection of each is needed and they can be used in combination with each other or with adjunctive therapies for optimal results. A dermatologist should be well versed in the plethora of options available.

REFERENCES

1. Watson D, Reuther MS. Scar revision techniques-pearls and pitfalls. Facial Plast Surg. 2012;28:487-91.
2. Garg S, Dahiya N, Gupta S. Surgical scar revision: An overview. J Cutan Aesthet Surg. 2014;7:3-13.
3. Kudur MH, Pai SB, Sripathi H, et al. Sutures and suturing techniques in skin closure. Indian J Dermatol Venereol Leprol. 2009;75:425-34.
4. Popkin GL, Robins P. Closure of skin wounds. Workshop Manual for Basic Dermatological Surgery. Kenilworth: NJ. Schering, Inc. 1983:18-36
5. Zhai H, Maibach HI. Effect of occlusion and semi-occlusion on experimental skin wound healing: A reevaluation. Wounds. 2007;19(10):270-6.
6. Kloeters O, Schierle C, Tandara A, et al. The use of a semi-occlusive dressing reduces epidermal inflammatory cytokine expression and mitigates dermal proliferation and inflammation in a rat incisional model.Wound Repair Regen. 2008;16(4):568-75.
7. Moran ML. Scar revision. Otolaryngol Clin North Am. 2001;34:767-80.
8. Batra RS. Surgical techniques for scar revision: Advances in dermatologic surgery. Skin Therapy Letter. 2005;10(4):4-7.
9. Mostafapour SP, Murakami CS. Tissue expansion and serial excision in scar revision. Facial Plast Surg. 2001;17(4): 245-52.
10. Rodgers BJ, Williams EF, Hove CR. W-plasty and geometric broken line closure. Facial Plast Surg. 2001;17:239-44.
11. Pérez-Bustillo A, González-Sixto, Rodríguez-Prieto MA. Surgical principles for achieving a functional and cosmetically acceptable scar. Actas Dermosifiliogr. 2013;104: 17-28.
12. Webster RC, Davidson TM, Smith RC. M-plasty techniques. J. Dermatol Surg. 1976;2(5):393-6.
13. M-plastiapós-ajustada. Post-adjusted M-plasty. Surg Cosmet Dermatol. 2012;4(1):80-2.
14. Leake DS, Baker SR. Scar revision and local flap refinement. In: Baker SR (Ed). Local flaps in Facial Reconstruction, 2nd edition. Mosby/Elsevier, Inc. Philadelphia. pp. 723-60.

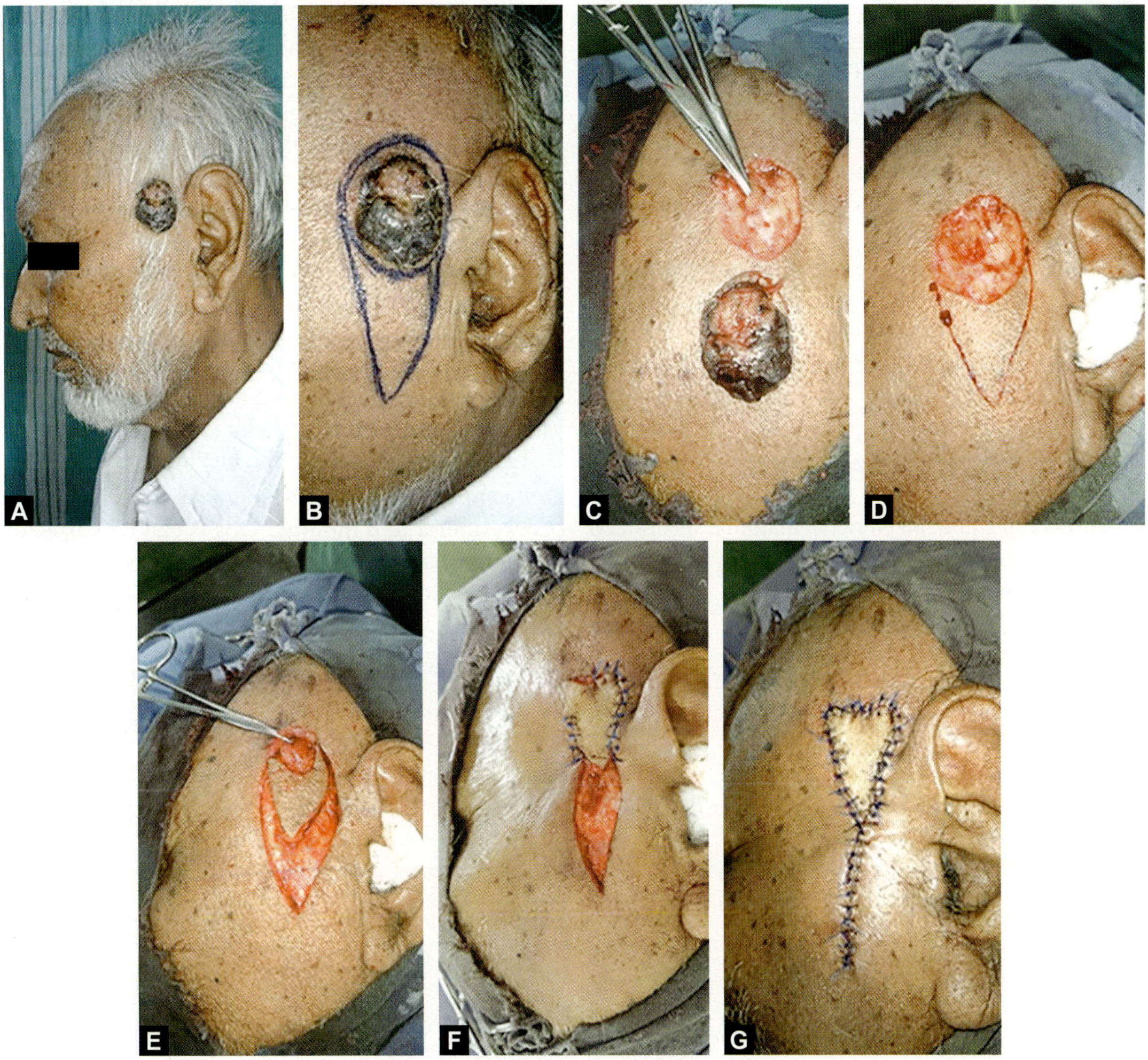

Figs. 14.16A to G: V-Y plasty.

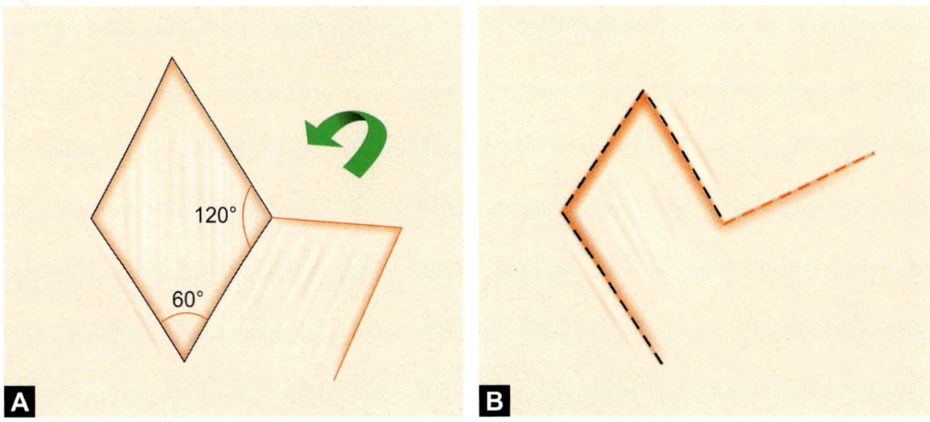

Figs. 14.17A and B: Rhomboid flap.

Tips

- Place the longitudinal axis of the rhomboid parallel to the line of maximal extensibility.
- All sides of the rhomboid should be equal.
- All sides of the flap should be equal.
- The angle of the rhomboid can be changed according to the shape of lesion.
- As many as four flaps can be raised for one rhomboid defect. But the side with minimum skin tension and better cosmetic outcome is selected.
- 2 cases of rhomboid flap are demonstrated in Figures 14.18 and 14.19.

COMPLICATIONS OF FLAP SURGERY

Immediate complication: Bleeding, hematoma, secondary infection, failure of flap and flap necrosis are the common side effects encountered.

- Bleeding is minimized by used of tumescent anesthesia, lignocaine 1% with adrenaline and postoperative pressure dressing.
- Hematoma can be prevented by placing a pen rose drain. Large hematoma has to be evacuated by removing few sutures.
- Strict aseptic precaution with postoperative antibiotics prevents infection.
- Appropriate thickness of flap with minimum wound tension decreases the risk of flap necrosis. Any pallor or bluish discoloration of wound 1 to 2 days after surgery indicates impending necrosis. Once necrosis of flap occurs, the sutures are removed and the wound is allowed to heal with secondary intention. PRP (platelet-rich plasma) aids in wound healing.

Late complications: Pin-cushioning or trap door deformity occurs after 2 to 3 months. This is can be corrected by injecting 10 mg/mL of triamcinolone into the base, every month for 3 to 4 months.

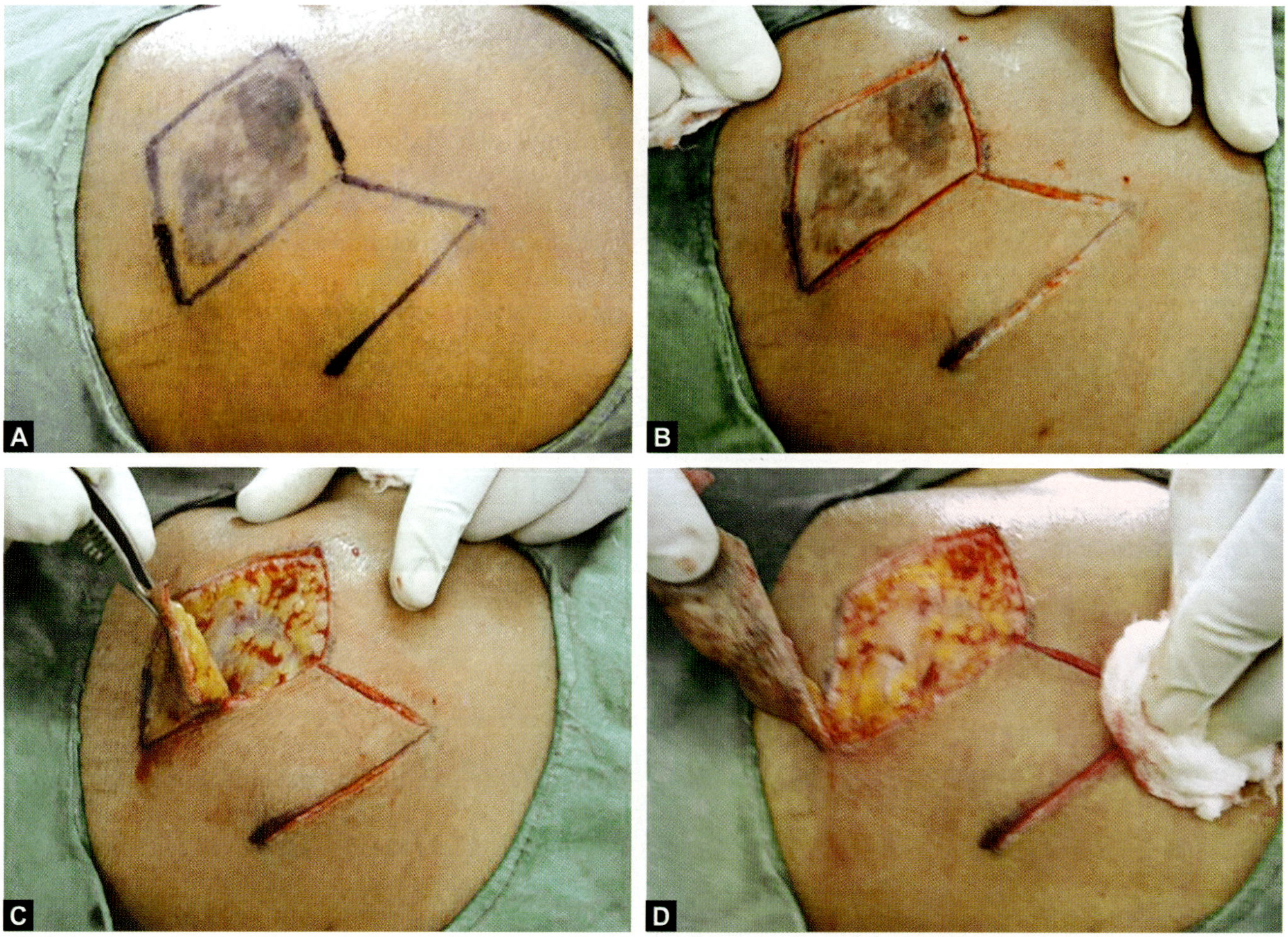

Figs. 14.18A to D

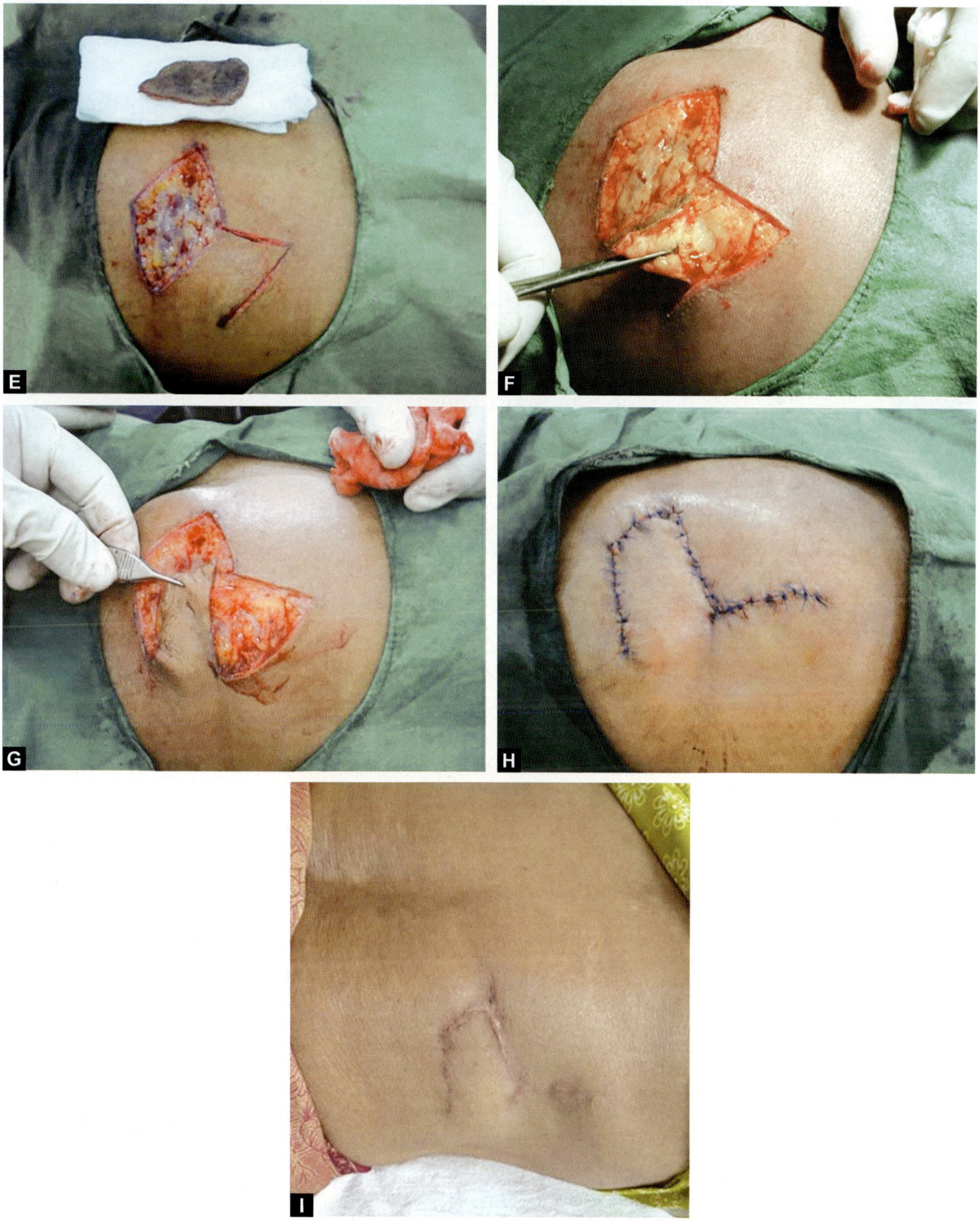

Figs. 14.18A to I: Steps of rhomboid flap.

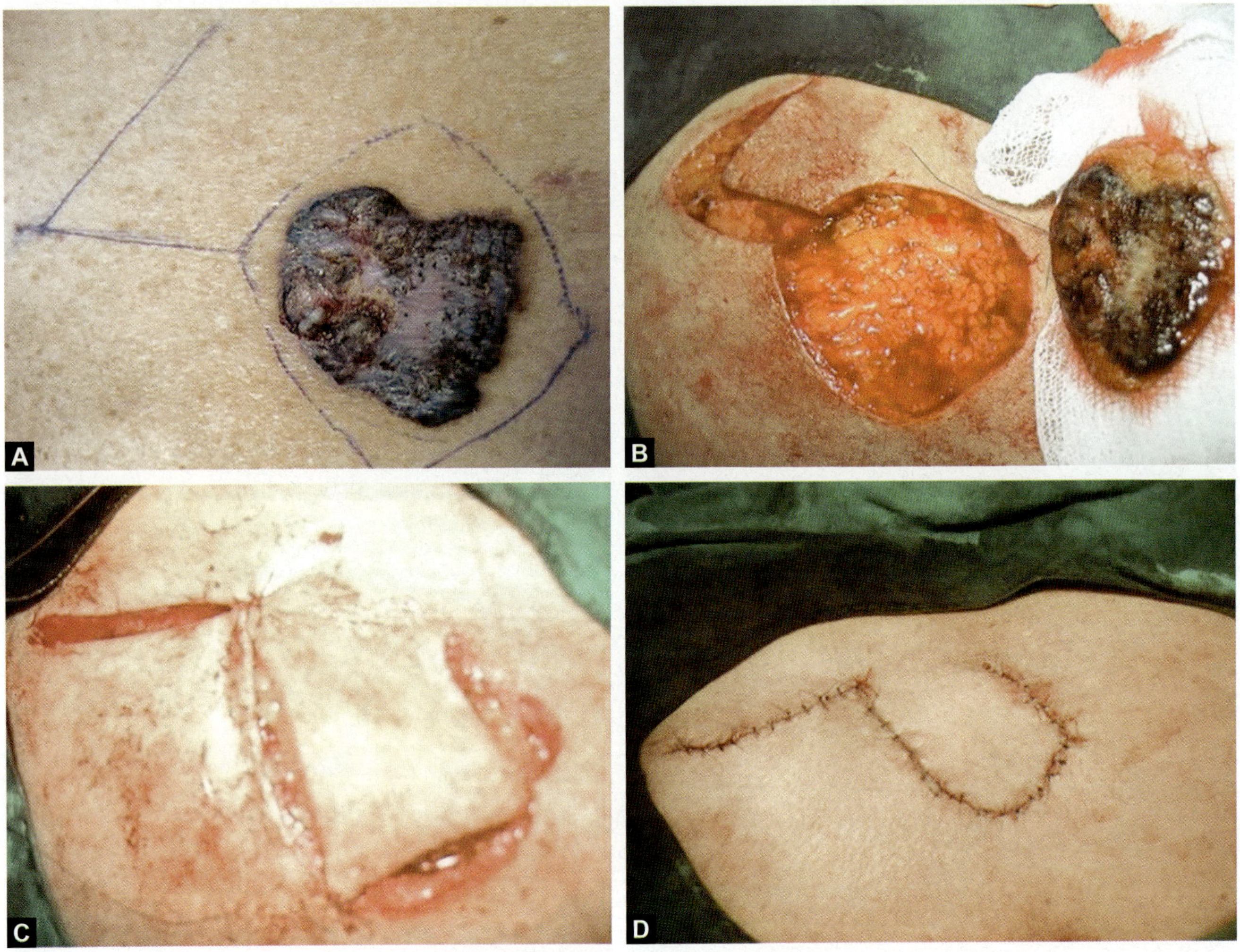

Figs. 14.19A to D: Results of rhomboid flap.

REFERENCES

1. Murakami CS, Nishioka GJ. Essential concepts in the design of local skin flaps. Facial Plast Surg. Clin North Am. 1996;4:455–68.
2. Baker SA. Rotation flap. In: Baker SA (Ed). Local Flaps and Reconstruction 2nd ed. Philadelphia: Elsevier;2007 107-11.
3. Baker SA. Advancement flap. In: Baker SA (Ed). Local Flaps and Reconstruction , 2nd ed. Philadelphia:Elsevier. 2007; 157-62.
4. Redondo P. Repair of large defects in the forehead using a median forehead rotation flap and advancement lateral U-shaped flap. Dermatol Surg. 2006;32(6):843-6.
5. Krishnan R, Garman M, Nunez-Gussman J, et al. Advancement flaps: a basic theme with many variations. Dermatol Surg. 2005;31(8 Pt 2):986-94.
6. Moody BR, Sengelmann RD. Standing cone avoidance via advancement flap modification. Dermatol Surg. 2002;28:632-5.
7. Stevens C, Tan L, Kassir R, Calhoun K. Biomechanics of A-TO-T flap design. Laryngoscope. 1999;109:113–7.
8. Jackson IT. Local flap reconstruction of defects after excision of nonmelanoma skin cancer. Clin Plast Surg. 1997;24:747-67.
9. O'Donnell M, Briggs C, Condon KC. The horn flap: a curved V-Y advancement flap with lateral pedicle. Br J Plast Surg. 1992;45:42-3.
10. Dini M, Innocenti A, Lo Russo G, et al. The use of the V-Y fasciocutaneous island advancement flap in reconstructing postsurgical defects of the leg. Dermatol Surg. 2001;27:44–6.
11. Robbins TH. The "deep pedicle" V-Y advancement flap. Plast Reconstr Surg. 2004;113:463-4.
12. Zook EG, Van Beek AL, Russell RC et al. V-Y advancement flap for facial defects. Plast Reconstr Surg. 1980;65:786–97.
13. Limberg A. Mathematical principles of local plastic procedures on the surface of the human body. Leningrad: Medgis. 1946.
14. Turan T, Kuran I, Ozcan H, et al. Geometric limit of multiple local Limberg flaps: a flap design. Plast Reconstr Surg. 1999;104(6):1675–8.
15. Chasmar LR. The versatile rhomboid (Limberg) flap. Can J Plast Surg. 2007 Summer; 15(2): 67-71.

CHAPTER 15

Surgical Management of Leg Ulcers

Umashankar Nagaraju, Priyanka Agarwal, Anagha Ramesh, Abhilasha MD

INTRODUCTION

An ulcer is a break in the continuity of the covering epithelium, either skin or mucous membrane due to molecular death.[1] They are also defined as wounds with a full thickness depth having slow healing tendency.[2] Complete loss of epidermis and often portions of the dermis and even subcutaneous fat result in ulcers of skin.[3]

1% in the adult population to 3 to 5% in the population over 65 years of age is the average prevalence of leg ulcers.[4,5] Peak prevalence is between 60 and 80 years of age.[6] Leg ulcers can be painful, debilitating and can be recurrent affecting the patient's quality of life. Leg ulcers pose an economic burden on both the patient and society. One important problem in management of leg ulcers is its multifactorial etiology and associated comorbidities. Causes for leg ulcer are listed in Table 15.1. Venous leg ulcers correspond to 60 to 80% of all leg ulcers.[7]

A correct diagnosis aids to avoid inappropriate treatment which in turn delays wound healing and also causing deterioration of wound.

Table 15.1: Causes for leg ulcer.[8]

Venous disease
Venous hypertension
Varicose veins, deep-vein thrombosis, venous obstruction, congenital vascular malformations, Klippel-Trenaunay syndrome
Arterial disease
Atherosclerosis, diabetes, hypertension, embolism, calcific uremic arteriopathy (calciphylaxis)
Skin cancer
Basal and squamous cell carcinoma, melanoma or any fungating tumor
Vasculitis
Connective tissue diseases, e.g. systemic lupus erythematosus, rheumatoid disease and, progressive systemic sclerosis. Necrotizing leukocytoclastic vasculitis, ANCA-associated disorders, polyarteritis nodosa
Livedoid vasculopathy, cryoglobulinemia
Hematological disorders
Coagulation states, e.g. factor V Leiden, protein C or S deficiency, hyperhomocysteinemia, antithrombin III deficiency, sickle cell disease, thalassemia, spherocytosis, antiphospholipid syndrome, myeloproliferative disorders, e.g. polycythemia rubra vera, thrombocythemia
Emboli
Cholesterol, platelets, tumor cells, infective
Loss of sensation
Leprosy, diabetes, spina bifida
Infections
Diabetes, osteomyelitis, Buruli ulcer, fungal infections, syphilis, mycobacteria, leishmaniasis, acute 'desert' sore, necrotizing fasciitis and cellulitis
Trauma
Physical, e.g. pressure sore, chemical or thermal (e.g. burns or cold injury), self-harm, intravenous drug use
Drugs/therapy
Radiation, hydroxycarbamide, ergotamine, iododerma
Skin disorders
Pyoderma gangrenosum, Necrobiosis lipoidica,scleroderma, Graft-versus-host disease, blistering disorders (e.g. pemphigoid)
Bites and stings
Insects, snake, scorpion
Genetic
Prolidase deficiency, Klinefelter's syndrome

DEFINITION OF CHRONIC LEG ULCER

A chronic leg ulcer is defined as any ulcer below the knee including the foot, that does not heal within a 6-week period.[9,10]

MANAGEMENT OF CHRONIC LEG ULCER

Various modalities of treatment including conservative, medical, and surgical have been described for management of leg ulcers. However the challenge is to deal with chronic leg ulcers which can be better dealt surgically after taking care of the primary etiology (e.g. diabetes, varicose veins, arteriosclerosis) and educating the patient about the risk factors (smoking, alcohol) which if not taken care off will push the patient into vicious cycle of recurrence.

INVESTIGATIONS[8,11,12]

It is the key to correct diagnosis and appropriate treatment when chosen correctly.

Routine Investigations

- Hemoglobin (Hb%), erythrocyte sedimentation rate (ESR), total count and differential count, hemogram, bleeding time and clotting time
- Fasting blood sugar, postprandial blood sugar
- Liver function test
- Serum creatinine, blood urea
- Bone marrow
- Lipid profile
- Lupus erythematosus cell test
- Blood VDRL test
- Serum electrolytes
- Serum albumin, transferrin
- Rheumatoid factor, autoantibodies, C-reactive protein
- Urine examination
- Examination of discharge from ulcers: Culture and sensitivity of bacteria/fungus. They have to be treated with proper antibiotics and antifungals.
- Biopsy and histopathological examination from ulcer site.

Radiological Examination

- X-ray should be taken to find out any bony abnormalities and/or osteomyelitis of the underlying bone
- Chest X-ray and ECG/ 2D ECHO.

Special Investigations

- Photoplethysmography
- Doppler ultrasound—arterial and venous
- Duplex imaging
- Venography
- Radioisotope tests
- Arteriography
- Digital subtraction angiography (DSA)
- Pulse oximetry
- Toe brachial pressure index (TBPI)
- Transcutaneous oxygen.

GENERAL MEASURES FOR MANAGEMENT OF COMMON LEG ULCERS[13,14]

Venous—Leg elevation
Compression therapy
Aspirin
Pentoxifylline.

Arterial—Revascularization
Antiplatelet medications
Management of risk factors.

Neuropathic—Off loading of pressure
Recommending MCR (microcellulose rubber) Footwear
Strict control of diabetes.

SURGICAL MANAGEMENT OF LEG ULCERS

Various techniques employed can be classified as:

- **Debridement**
  - Surgical
  - Laser assisted.
- **Skin grafting**
  - Split skin graft
  - Pinch graft
  - Postage stamp graft.
- **Platelet concentrates**
  - Platelet-rich plasma (PRP)
  - Platelet-rich fibrin matrix (PRFM).
- **Flaps:** Flaps suitable for chronic leg ulcers include local flaps like advancement, rotation, or transposition which can be V-Y, rhomboid, and bilobed flaps.

DEBRIDEMENT

Debridement is the most essential and first measure to be considered in any ulcer management. Necrotic tissue and foreign material may serve as a nidus for infection and thereby delay wound healing.[15-17] Hence, wound debridement by removing the necrotic tissue, foreign debris, and reducing the bacterial load on the wound surface, is important in chronic leg ulcer management.[18]

Various debridement techniques are available. Mechanical methods of debridement include surgical sharp debridement, pulse lavage, ultrasound disruption of debris, and high-pressure water jet dissection of the wound surface. More gradual and potentially less effective methods of debridement include the use of topical enzymatic ointments, maggots, or endogenous proteases under occlusion for autolytic cleaning of the wound bed.[19-23] Laser debridement using fractional CO_2 laser,[24] or Erbium-doped yttrium-aluminum-garnet (Er:YAG) laser[25] is one of the lesser known wound debridement techniques as of date, but holding great promise for future.

Principles/Techniques

- Debridement serves to clear biofilms, reduce bacterial burden, and stimulate the repair process.[18]
- Debridement also converts the physiology of the wound from that of a chronic lesion to an acute one.[26]

Methods

Conservative Sharp Wound Debridement (CSWD)

Surgical/sharp debridement using a scalpel or a curette is considered the optimal method for rapidly cleaning the ulcer, removing loose avascular tissue and converting a chronic wound to an acute wound.[18,27]

Sharp debridement can be performed at the bedside by trained health care professionals using surgical instruments including scalpel, blade no. 15, scissors and curette.[28]

Scalpel Technique

Steps

Instruments required: High quality scalpel (either disposable or reusable), blade size 10 or 15, scissors and forceps capable of grasping and holding necrotic tissue. A probe is also useful for assessing the track and depth (Fig. 15.1A).[27]

- It can be performed under topical or local anesthesia. Topical anesthesia includes application of cream comprised of lidocaine and prilocaine which has to be applied to the wound for 30 to 45 minutes prior to onset of procedure. Local anesthesia is performed by giving ring block using injection 1% Lignocaine. General anesthesia can be given when deep debridement is performed (Fig. 15.1B).[27]
- Scalpel should be held like a pen. Necrotic tissue is lifted with the forceps and the necrotic tissue should be cut with the scalpel holding it parallel to or angled away from the wound bed. Cut should be made tangentially removing the necrotic tissue in layers rather than by piecemeal excision (Figs. 15.1C and D).[27]
- Once debridement is complete, the wound bed is flushed with normal saline of lukewarm temperature (Fig. 15.1E).
- Primary dressing is done with nonabsorbable dressing material like paraffin tulle dressing (Fig. 15.1F), which is covered by secondary dressing with slightly saline-moistened gauze.
- Simple analgesics can be prescribed for pain relief.
- Dressing can be changed after a week.

Complications

There is an increased risk of postdebridement hemorrhage from damage to underlying blood vessels; hence must be performed by a clinician competent in dealing with it. The risk is increased in:[29]

- Patients taking anticoagulants: They are advised to discontinue four days prior to the procedure.
- Wounds that are located in the gaiter area of the leg due to close proximity to the long saphenous vein.

Curette Technique

Instruments required: sharp circular curette of size 4 or 7.

Steps

- Anesthesia is similar to the method described above under scalpel technique (Fig. 15.2A).
- Debridement should be performed using a sharp circular curette of size 4 or 7 with the patient in a reclining or supine position.
- Curette should be held like a pen at 10 to 200 angle towards the area to be debrided. The skin-wound base is stretched with the nondominant hand, and the curette is to be moved toward soneself, scraping away loose, nonviable tissue (Fig. 15.2B).
- Flushing the wound with normal saline and dressing is similar to scalpel technique (Fig. 15.2C).
- Primary dressing is done with nonabsorbable dressing material like paraffin tulle dressing (Fig. 15.2D) which is covered by secondary dressing with slightly saline-moistened gauze.

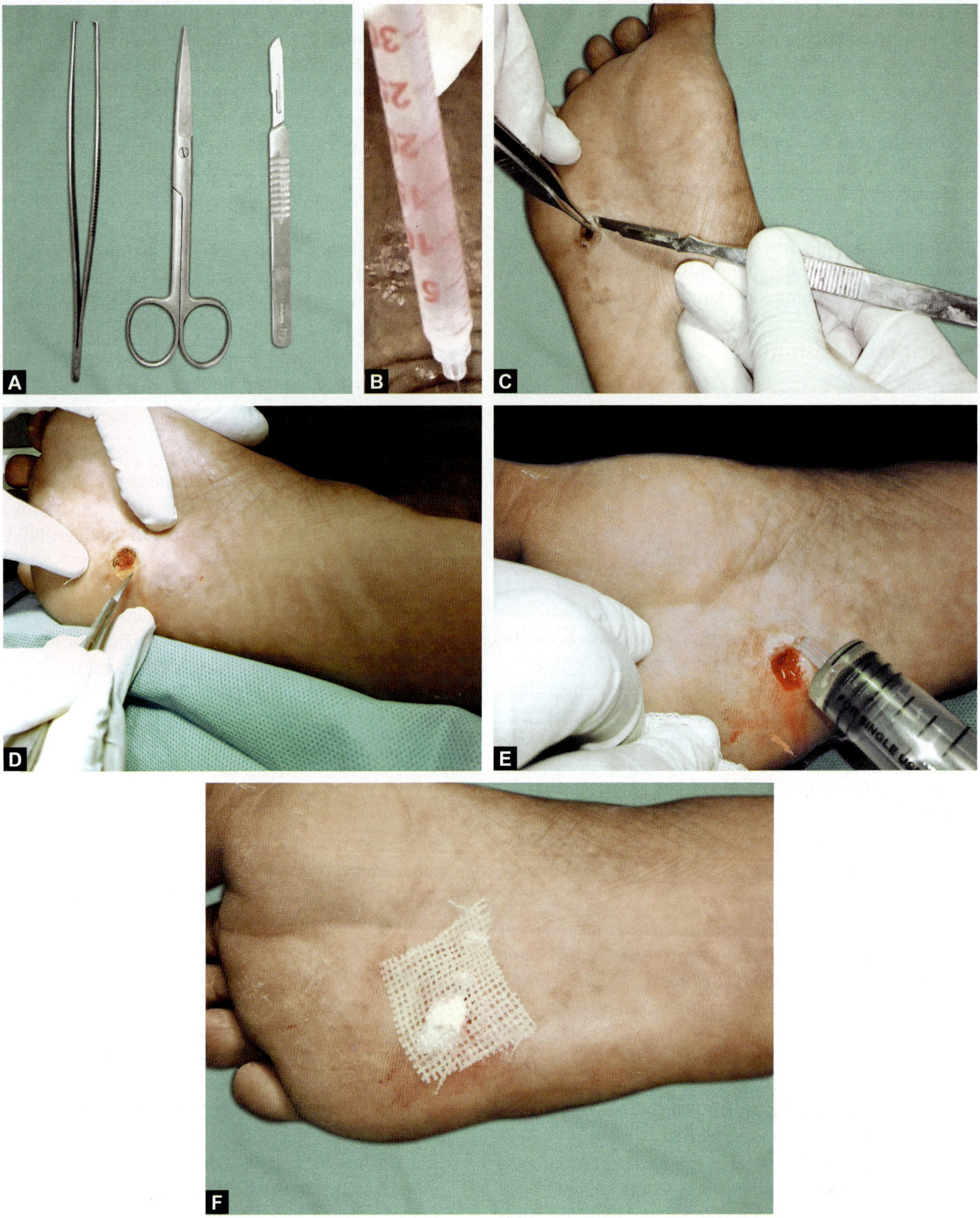

Figs. 15.1A to F: Steps of scalpel debridement of leg ulcer.

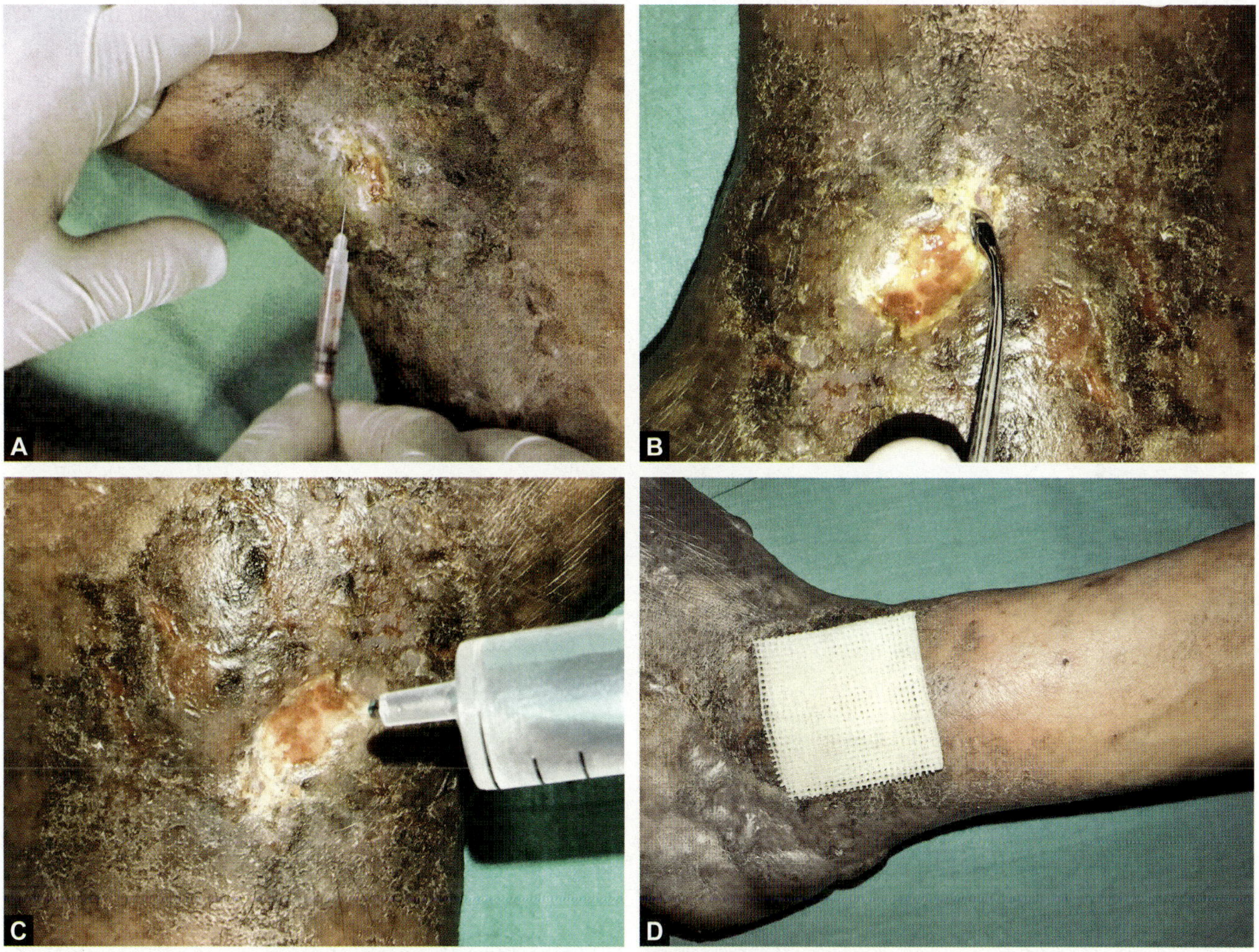

Figs. 15.2A to D: Steps of curette debridement of leg ulcer.

Tips[27,29]

- Care should be taken to avoid the sensitive ulcer edges. The aim is to remove the slough, nonviable tissue, any avascular fibrous tissue down to the vascular base.
- Particular care must be taken with anesthetic areas, such as neuropathic limb or diabetic foot, as the protective mechanism of pain is absent.
- An increased risk of bleeding is associated with surgical/sharp debridement. When pressure fails to control bleeding, other methods employed include pressure coupled with hemostatic dressing (e.g. Kaltostat) and suturing at the bleeding point.
- Sharp debridement may not be suitable for patients with underlying clotting abnormality, bleeding disorder or on anticoagulant medication, malignant wounds as there is risk of dissemination and uncontrolled hemorrhage.
- Special care should be taken in terminally ill patients.

Laser Debridement

Laser debridement is based on controlled vaporization of superficial layers of the wound bed containing unwanted microbial and necrotic particles. The depth of the tissue ablation depends on the type of laser as well as the number of passes one performs, and ranges from 2 to 150 μm per pass.[25]

Lasers used include fractional CO_2 laser,[24] or Erbium-doped yttrium-aluminum-garnet (Er:YAG) laser.[25]

Principles

Laser debridement acts by multiple postulated mechanisms:

- Improving the pliability of the tissue at the wound edge and adjacent skin, there is an increase in oxygen and circulation to the wound, encouraging more rapid healing.[30]

- Causes microdebridement of the wound bed, creating acute injury cytokines that may stimulate the healing process.[30]
- Disrupts the bacterial biofilm that is commonly present in wounds and that may impede wound healing.[31,32]
- Stimulate collagen remodeling.[33]
- The fractional laser may also remove necrotic and senescent cells that inhibit wound healing.[31,32]

Steps

The steps in brief for carrying out fractional CO_2 laser debridement include:[30]

- Anesthesia, if required is similar to the method described above under scalpel technique.
- The wound base should be treated at 30 mJ and 5% density (Fig. 15.3A). The entire wound edge and 1 to 2 cm of the normal surrounding skin should be treated at 50 mJ and 5% density (Fig. 15.3B).
- One pass should be completed at 150 Hz per treatment.
- Flushing the wound with normal saline and dressing is similar to scalpel technique (Figs. 15.3C and D).

Advantages of Laser Debridement Over Mechanical Debridement

- Precision and uniformity of tissue ablation by lasers reduces trauma to wound bed.
- Procedural pain is another limiting factor commonly associated with sharp debridement whereas laser debridement is well-tolerated with only mild discomfort noted.[30]

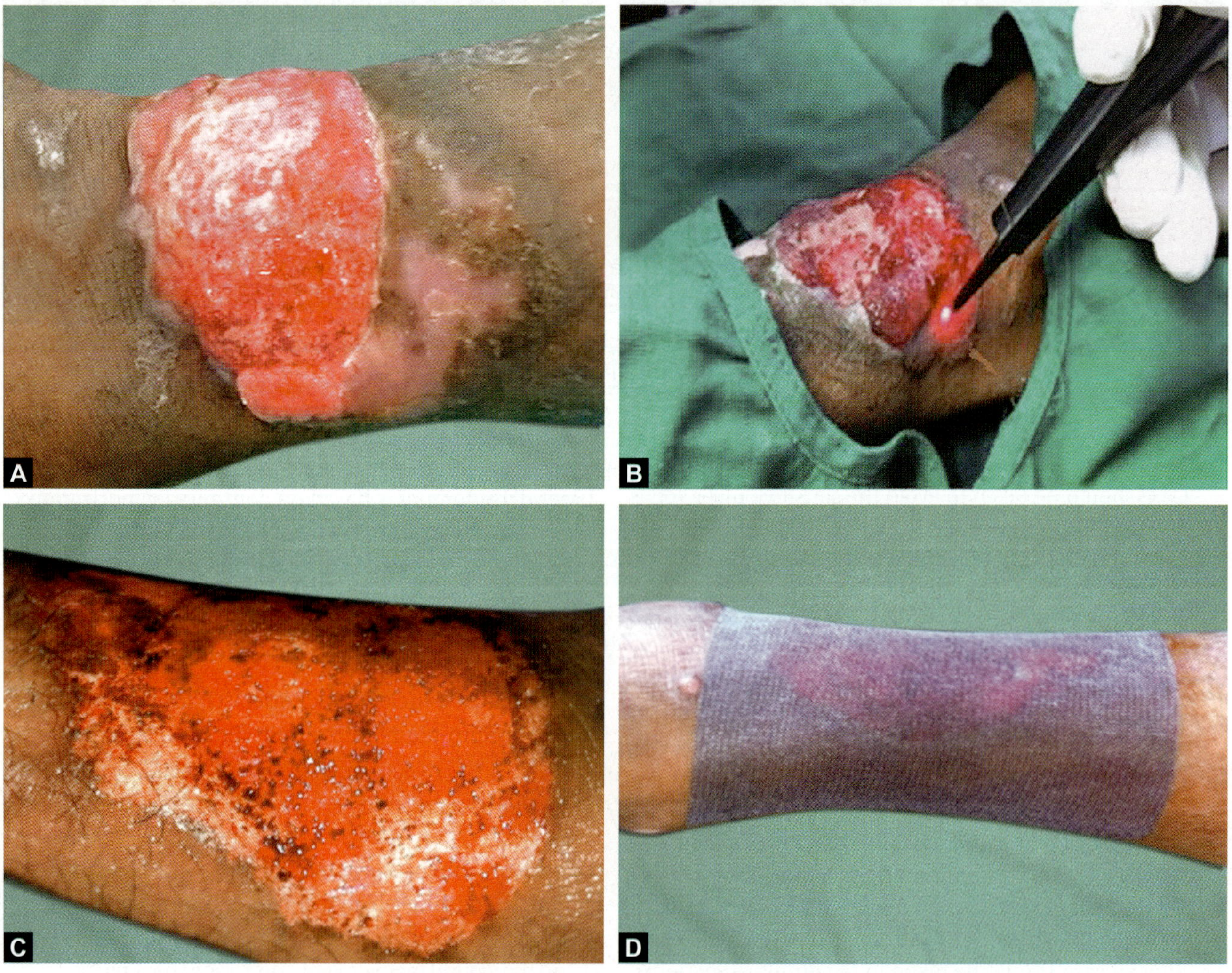

Figs. 15.3A to D: Laser debridement of leg ulcer.

Tips

Lasers, such as pulsed dye laser can be used for treating hypertrophic granulation tissue as well which is one of the cause for nonhealing ulcers.[34,35]

SKIN GRAFT

Skin grafts are indicated when nonsurgical measures fail to re-epithelialize the wound bed.

Principles

The mechanisms by which skin grafts helps wound healing are:

- Tissue replacement.[36]
- The epidermal cells produce cytokines, adhesion molecules, growth factors, and basement membrane components, which are essential to wound healing.[37,38]
- Antimicrobial effect.[39]

General Measures

- If the patient is on anticoagulants, discontinue 4 days prior to the grafting.
- Grafting is to be done only on healthy ulcers.
- Ulcer is debrided to remove any necrotic tissue, if present.

Graft Techniques

Split Thickness Skin Graft (STSG)[40,41]

Principle: An STSG consists of epidermis and a variable amount of superficial to deep dermis. As the dermis is responsible for the viscoelastic property of the skin, it is crucial for stability of the future skin.[40]

There are three biological changes which are observed following skin grafting:[41]

- *Graft take and adherence*: The first 72 hours after placement of the graft are the most crucial for graft uptake as fibrin bonding occurs during this time. The fibrin bonding is followed by onset of vascular anastomosis and fibrovascular growth. The graft imbibes wound exudate by capillary action through the sponge-like structure of the graft dermis and through the dermal blood vessels. This prevents graft desiccation, maintains graft vessel patency and provides nourishment for the graft.
- *Graft revascularization*—It begins 2 to 3 days postgrafting. This stage involves establishment of direct anastomoses between graft and recipient blood vessels, a process known as inosculation.
- *Contracture*—Graft contracture can occur immediately after harvesting the graft or after grafting at the recipient site. This occurs due to contraction of the elastic fibers. Myofibroblasts are said to be responsible for graft contraction.

Variants of split thickness skin grafts: This include thin, thick and full STSGs.[40]

Thin STSGs: It includes the epidermis and a thin layer of the dermis. They do not include the full length of appendages and are therefore unlikely to grow hair or to develop full sweat gland function.

Thick STSGs: It includes more dermis with a greater number of full hair follicles and glandular structures. These grafts will likely develop some hair growth and sweat gland function about 2 to 3 months after grafting. Thick STSGs are commonly selected to cover areas of high mechanical friction, such as joints, palms and soles.

Full thickness skin graft: Skin grafts thicker than 0.6 mm usually correspond to full-thickness skin grafts and are called Wolfe-Krause grafts.

Indications[40]

Thin STSG

- Debrided burn wounds
- Chronic wounds with less vascularized wound beds
- Acute well-vascularized wounds
- Exposed flap areas

Thick STSG: Same as thin STSG.

Full thickness skin graft: Noninfected, well-vascularized wound beds.

Instruments required: Humby's skin grafting knife, Padget's or Davol's dermatome, straight artery forceps with a razor blade or Silver's razor blade holding knife, Graft spreading rods or spatulas, nontraumatizing ring forceps, surgical glue: Cyanoacrylate adhesive (N-butyl 2-cyanoacrylate)/6-0 prolene, iris scissors, sterile Petri dishes (Fig. 15.4A).

Steps[40,41]

- Procedure is done under local, spinal or general anesthesia.
- Sites from where STSGs are harvested are shown in Figure 15.4B. Preferred sites include anterolateral aspect of thigh, the arms or the abdomen.

- The donor area is cleansed with povidone-iodine and surgical spirit.
- To reduce bleeding during skin harvest, infiltrate the donor site area primarily with epinephrine diluted in saline subcutaneously (tumescent technique).
- The size of the graft needed should be accurately measured prior to harvest.
- If small to medium-sized areas of skin are needed, skin grafts can be harvested using either a sterile razor blade mounted on a Kocher's forceps or a blade holding instrument. Alternatively a hand dermatome, Silver's knife, Humby's knife or a motor driven Zimmer dermatome can also be used (Figs. 15.4C and D).
- To avoid contamination of the donor site from the ulcer, the donor site should be covered first after harvesting the skin graft or consider a separate set of instruments for the donor site.
- The graft thickness can be adjusted by a lever near the end of the dermatome between 0.1 and 1.0 mm.
- The skin over the donor area is stretched and the cutting edge of the surgical knife is held at 15 to 300 angle to the skin surface and sunk to the desired depth and device should be moved from distal to proximal with uniform pressure and speed.
- The blade is moved back and forth gently by sawing movement to obtain a translucent graft.
- A second assistant can pick up the skin graft with two anatomical forceps during the harvest process to avoid damage of the graft (Fig. 15.4E).
- If the desired length is taken, the dermatome will cut the edge when elevating it while running the motor.
- It is vital to keep the graft moist with saline-impregnated gauze till it is grafted.
- Larger skin grafts should be incised with an 11 knife multiple times to allow wound fluid drainage and prevent collections between the skin graft and the wound bed (Fig. 15.4F).
- Graft is placed and spread uniformly on the ulcer bed with dermal side down (Figs. 15.4G and H). It is secured with simple stay sutures using 6-0 prolene or with surgical glue (Fig. 15.4I).
- Site is covered with a paraffin tulle dressing and slightly saline-moistened gauze (Fig. 15.4J).
- Postoperatively the patients should remain still, but immobilization not required.
- On the grafted ulcer, only the outer dressing should be changed daily whereas the donor site should be left untouched for a week.
- Dressing on both donor and recipient areas will be removed after a week (Fig. 15.4K). Sutures are removed if they are used.

Complications[40]

- The donor site usually heals with obvious scarring, discoloration and might undergo contraction.
- *Thin STSG*: Contraction of the skin graft may be a disadvantage. Quality of graft is limited because of minimal dermal thickness.
- *Thick STSG*: It slows the donor site re-epithelialization.
- *Full thickness skin graft*: Limited availability and graft rejection is higher in a less vascularized wound bed.

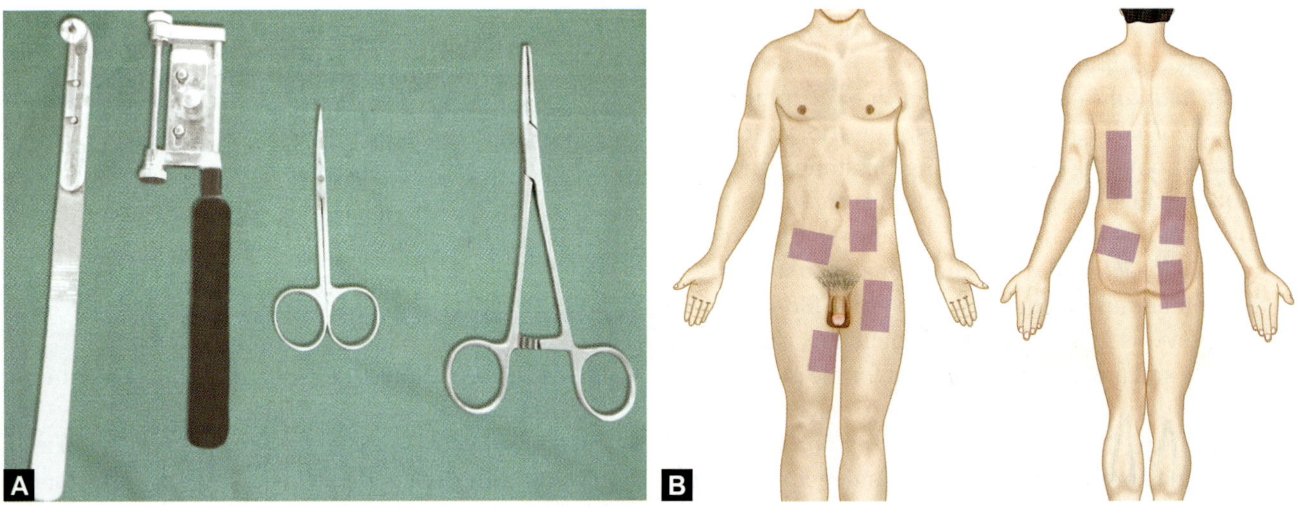

Figs. 15.4A and B: Instruments required for and donor areas for skin grafting respectively.

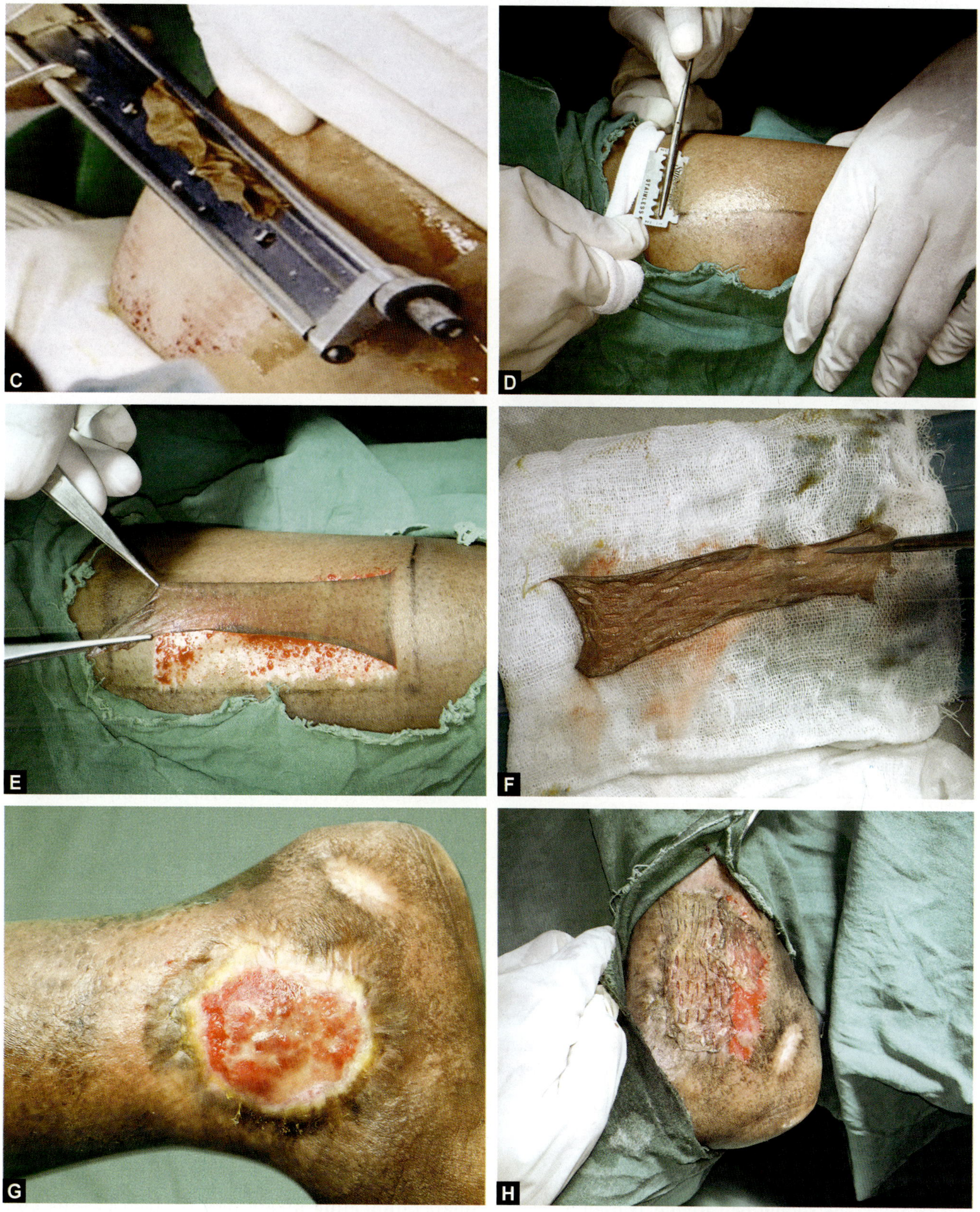

Figs. 15.4C to H: Steps of skin grafting from taking of graft to placing it at donor site.

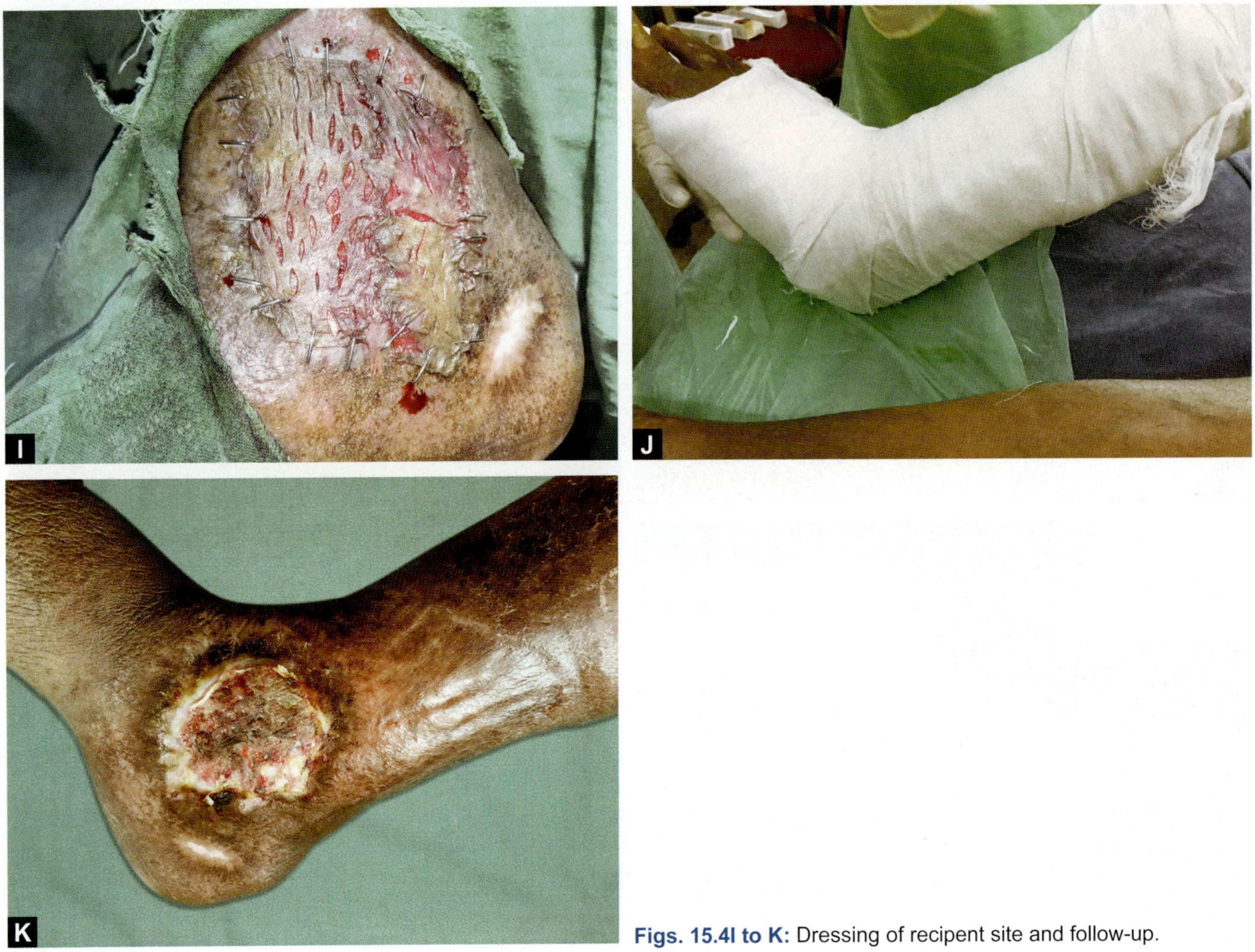

Figs. 15.4I to K: Dressing of recipent site and follow-up.

Advantages[41]

- *Thin STSG*: It allows faster donor site re-epithelialization, multiple possibilities to reharvest from the same area and good graft uptake.
- *Thick STSG*: Secondary graft contraction is less compared to thin STSG. Grafts are more stable because of thicker dermal layer and results in good graft uptake (Figs. 15.5A to C).
- *Full thickness skin graft*: Secondary graft contraction is almost minimal. It results in excellent skin quality, stability, hair regrowth and skin appendage function.

Tips[40]

- Hair regrowth is common in thick STSGs and hence, the donor site should be carefully chosen to avoid unpleasant hair growth.
- Thick grafts should be avoided in unhealthy wound beds such as in chronic ulcers because of decreased nutrient diffusion.

Pinch Graft

Reverdin first introduced the technique of lifting the epidermis with a needle and the lifted epidermis was cut and transplanted to the granulating wound bed. He called this technique as "epidermic grafting".[42] It is now widely known as the "pinch graft." John Staige Davis expanded on Reverdin's concept by adding dermis along with the epidermal graft which he claimed to give a better result as it is more like normal skin.[43-45]

Indications[46,47]

Small nonhealing ulcers particularly, venous and neuropathic.

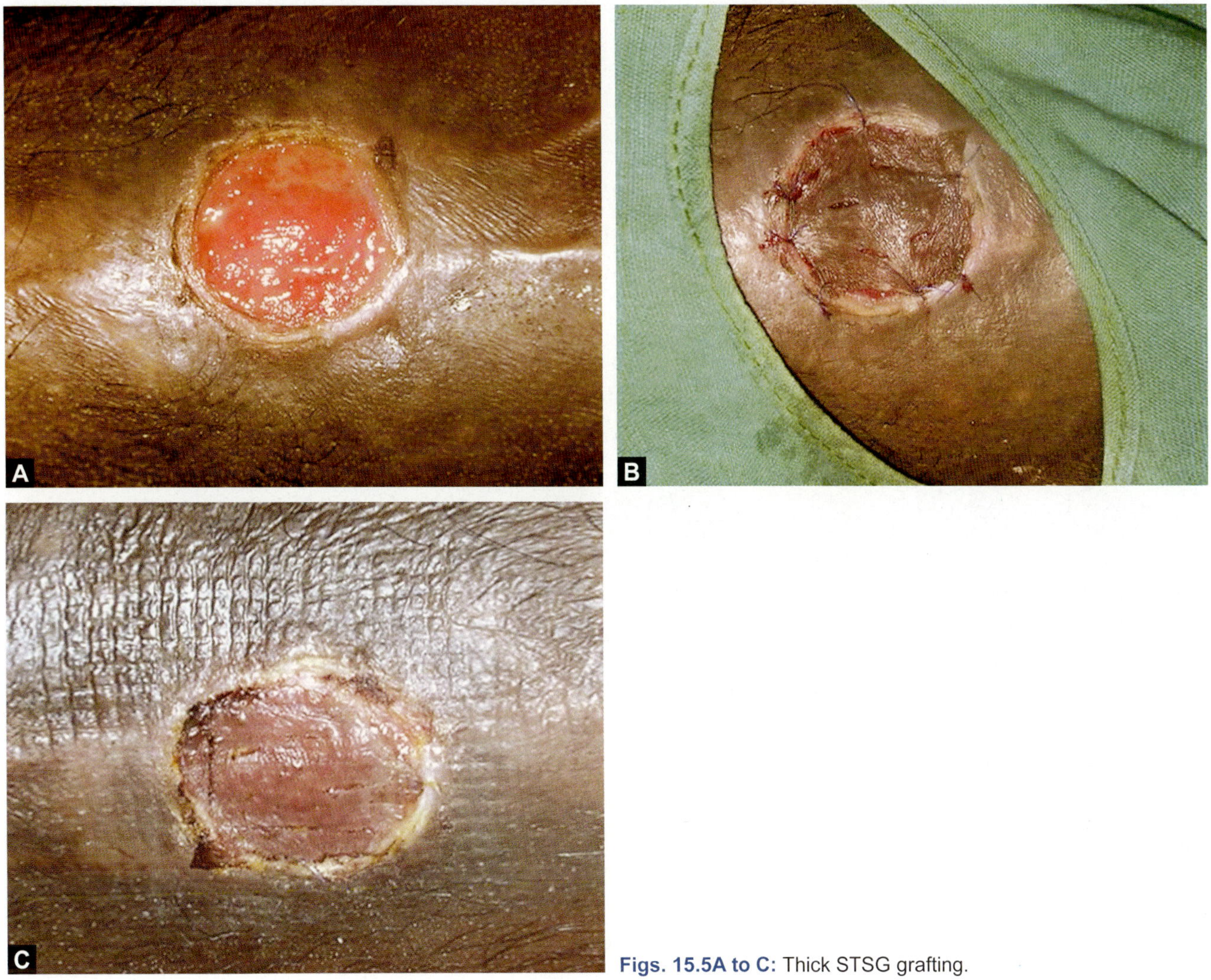

Figs. 15.5A to C: Thick STSG grafting.

Principle[46]

Pinch grafting involves harvesting small discs of skin and applying them evenly across an epithelial defect to enable epithelialization from the wound edge and the skin islands.

Instruments required: Hypodermic needle, no. 11 Parker blade.

Steps[47,48] *(Figs. 15.6A to D)*

- Appropriate donor area would be anterior aspect of the thigh.
- 1% injection lidocaine is injected to donor area so that number of wheals are raised.
- The point of a hypodermic needle should be inserted into the wheal at an angle and raised to form a conical fold of skin.
- The grafts are harvested by cutting the base of the cone using no. 11 Parker blade thus obtaining skin grafts 3 to 5 mm in diameter each.
- These pinched grafts are placed on the ulcer bed with dermal side down.
- Multiple grafts are placed on the ulcer bed, spacing them few millimeters apart from one other and covered with a silicone or paraffin tulle dressing and slightly saline-moistened gauze.
- Postoperatively the patients should remain still, but immobilization is not required.
- On the grafted ulcer, only the outer dressing should be changed daily whereas the donor site should be left untouched for a week.
- Dressing on both donor and recipient areas will be removed after a week.

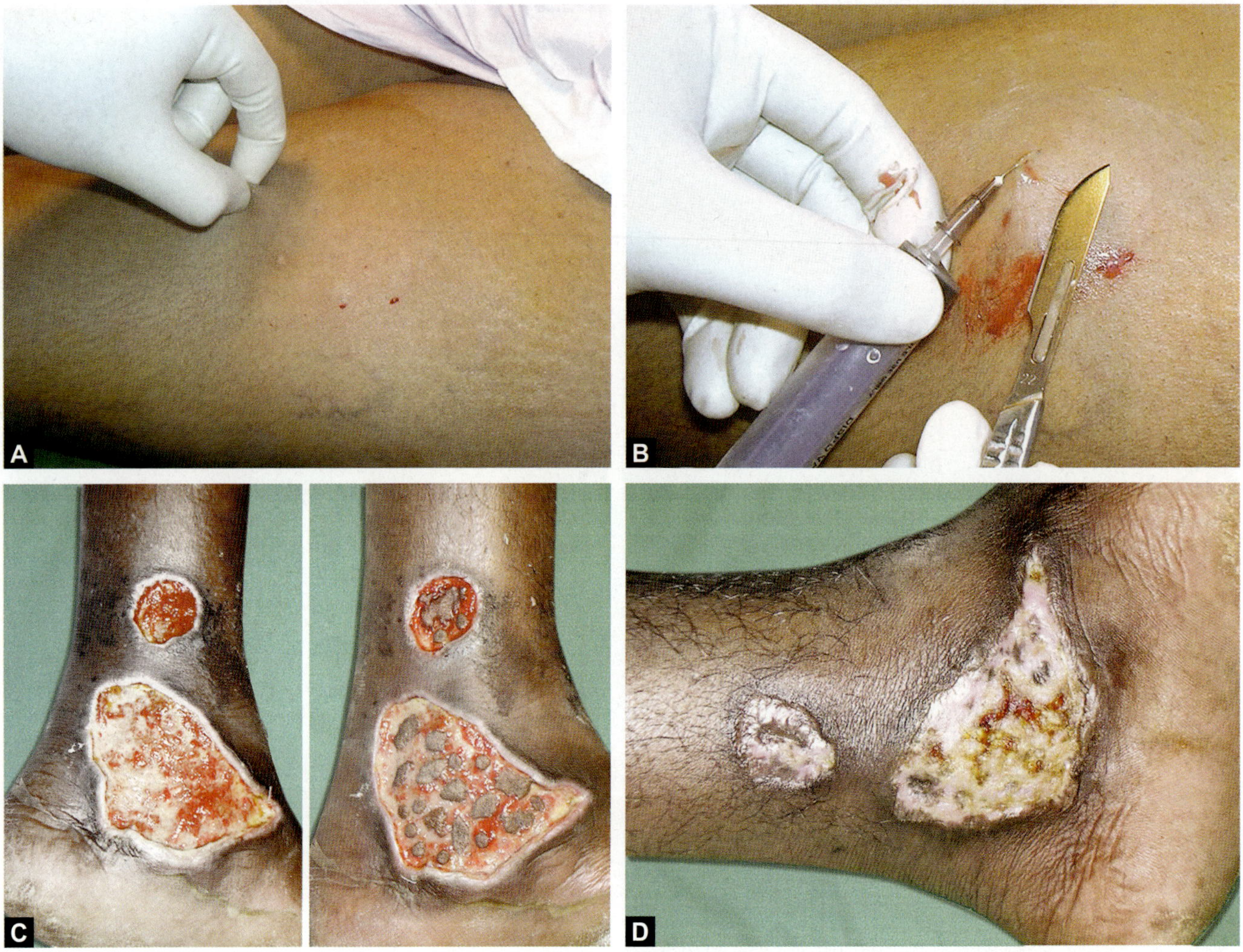

Figs. 15.6A to D: Steps of pinch grafting.

Disadvantages

- Donor area which is used to harvest full-thickness skin pieces, is virtually removed from future use for grafts.[46]
- If the grafts are to be placed close together, a large donor area may be needed.[49]
- Less reliable on wounds greater than 4.6 cm^2 in size.[50]
- Poor cosmetic results because of the nonuniform distribution of the grafts. May result in cobblestoning.

Advantages

- Simple and inexpensive.
- Full-thickness skin offers better resistance to pressure and infection.
- No complex machinery involved, a needle point and no. 11 Parker blade are the only necessary requirements to perform the procedure.

Tips

- If the patient has a venous ulcer, a compression bandage should be applied as well.[51]
- If the patient is a diabetic with injection sites on the thigh, the grafts should be taken more distally or laterally.

Patch/Postage Stamp Graft (Figs. 15.7 to 15.9)

Patch graft technique was first described by Gabarro in 1943. These are the grafts obtained by Split thickness technique which are cut into postage stamp size, i.e. 2 to 3 cm^2 and are placed over the prepared ulcer bed, spaced 1 to 2 mm apart followed by dressing with double layer of framycetin tulle.[52]

The patch/postage stamp methods have now become overshadowed with the advent of dermatomes to produce mesh skin grafts.

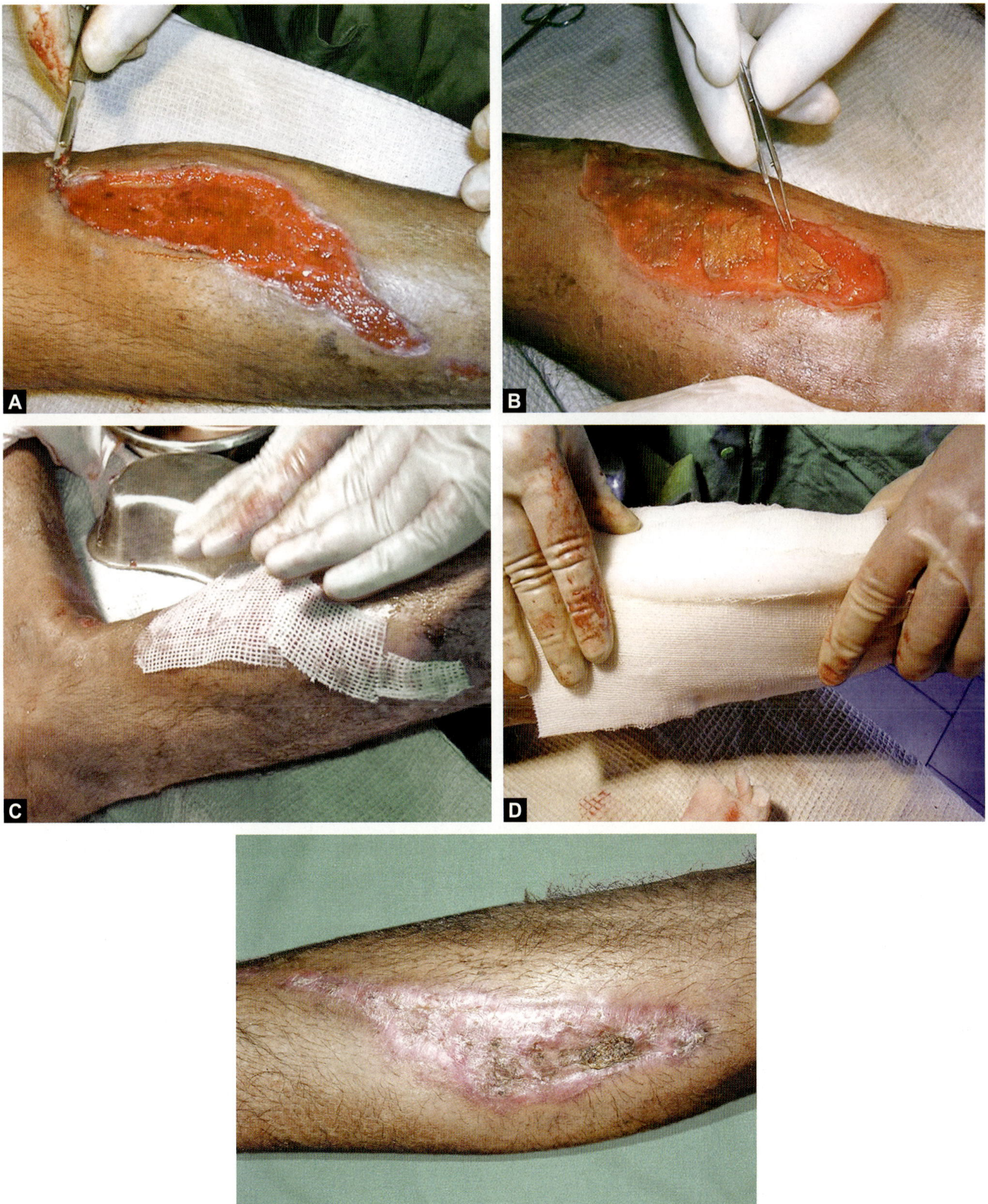

Figs. 15.7A to E: Steps of patch grafting.

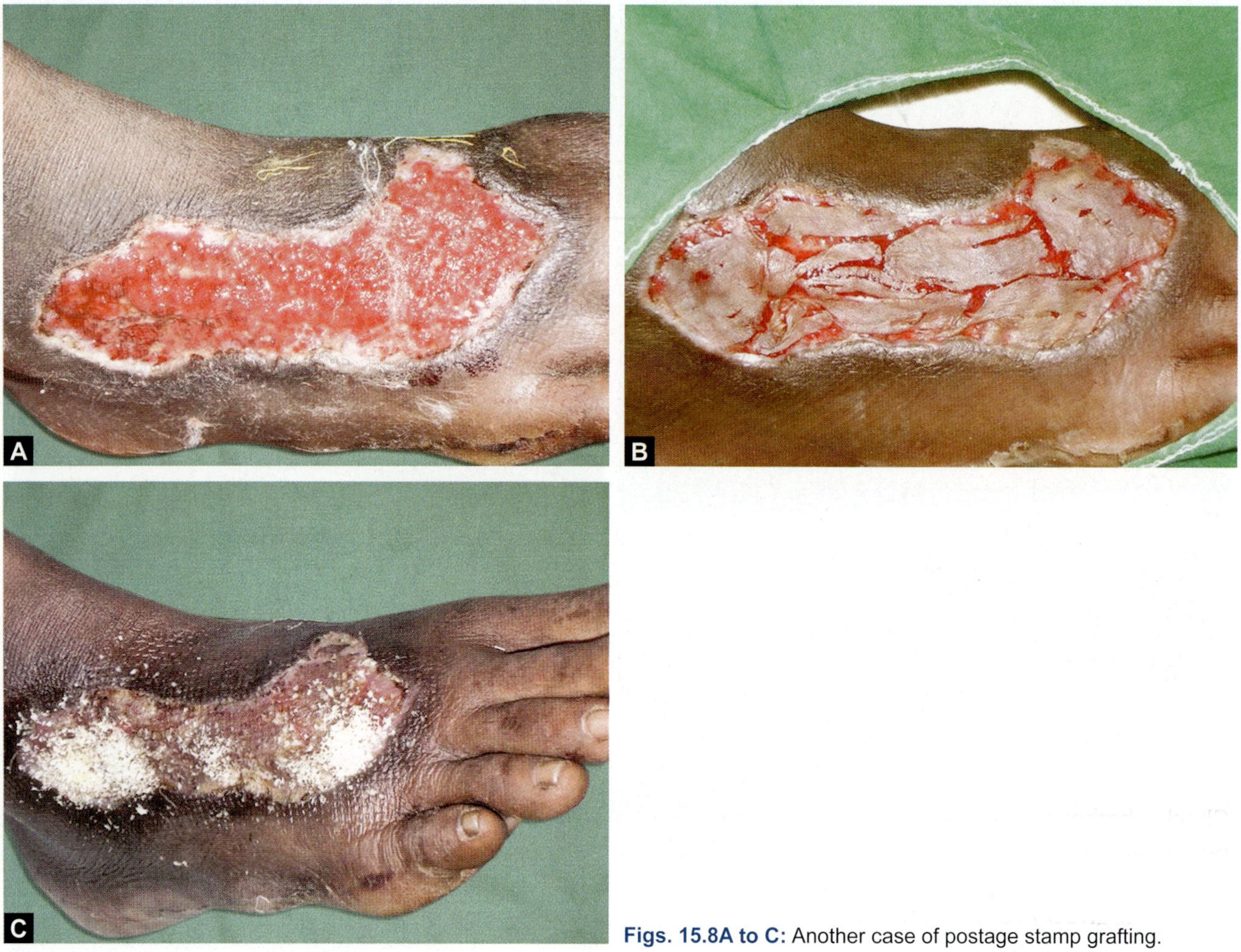

Figs. 15.8A to C: Another case of postage stamp grafting.

PLATELET CONCENTRATES

Platelet-rich Plasma

Platelet-rich plasma (PRP)[53-59]: In addition to use in the treatment of chronic skin and soft tissue ulcerations,[60-62] the usage of PRP in periodontal and oral surgery,[63-66] maxillofacial surgery, orthopedic and trauma surgery,[67-69] cosmetic and plastic surgery,[69,70] spinal surgery, heart bypass surgery, and burns[71] have been reported.

Mechanism of Action of Platelet-rich Plasma

PRP functions as tissue sealant, drug delivery system,[72] and along with platelets, they help wound healing by the release of growth factors which are active locally.[59,73-80] These growth factors help tissue healing and its regeneration.[70,81] Platelets in PRP also play roles in improving host defense mechanisms and have antimicrobial activity.[82,83]

Procedure[84,85]

Whole blood from patient is initially centrifuged at low speed to separate out plasma from packed RBC and then at higher speed to separate out PRP from the platelet-poor plasma. This platelet concentrate is then activated with thrombin or calcium, resulting in formation of platelet gel. PRP to be called so should contain at least 1 million platelets/μL.

Principles of PRP Preparation

PRP is prepared by differential centrifugation wherein acceleration forces are adjusted to concentrate specific cellular components based on different specific gravities.

In manual double spin method, platelet-rich plasma is separated from whole blood by 'light-spin' centrifugation and subsequently the platelets are concentrated by 'heavy-spin' centrifugation with removal of the supernatant plasma.[86]

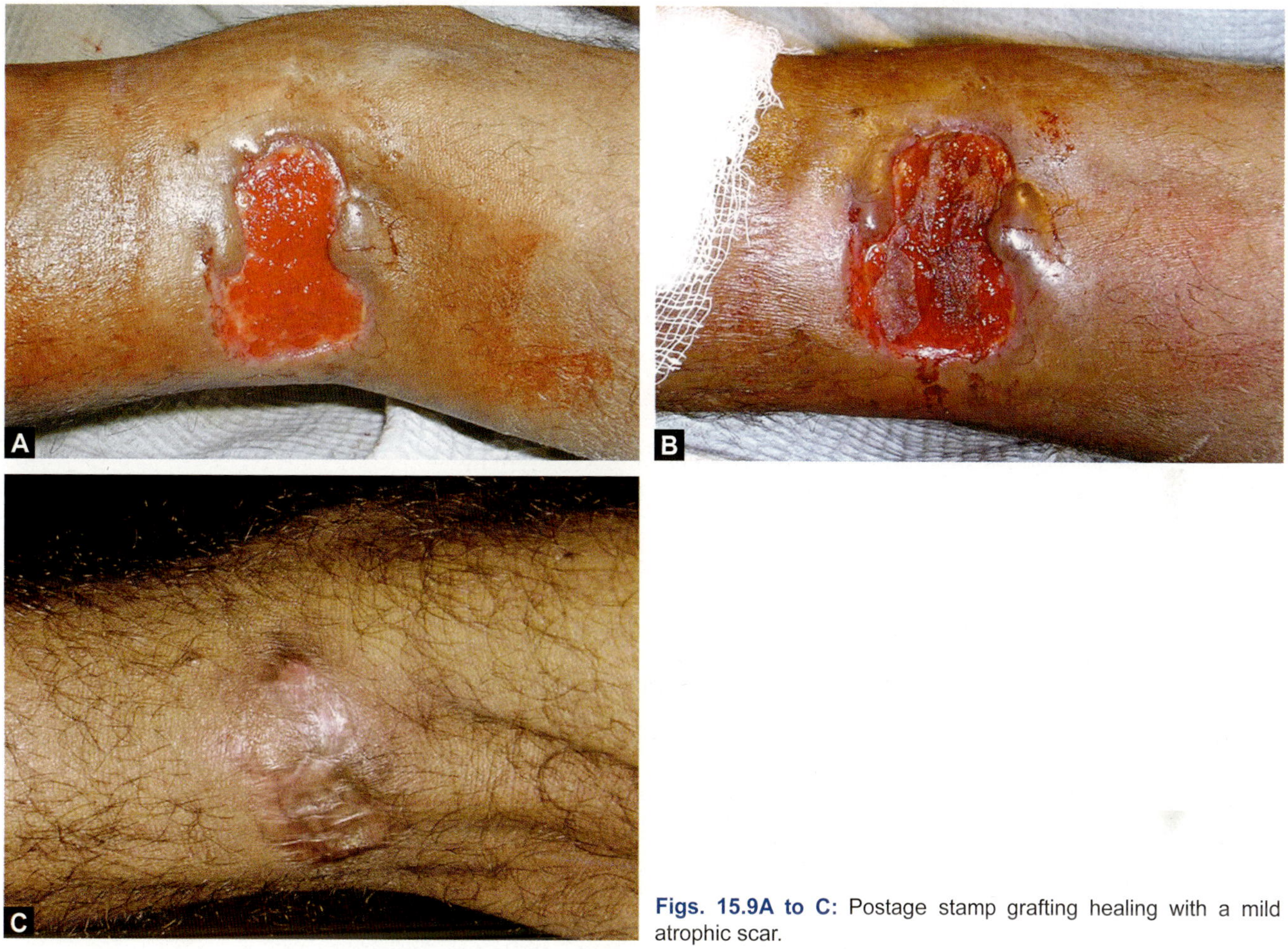

Figs. 15.9A to C: Postage stamp grafting healing with a mild atrophic scar.

Instruments required: Table top centrifuge, acid citrate dextrose (ACD) tubes, sterile tubes without anticoagulant (Figs. 15.10A and B).

PRP Method[87,88]

- Whole blood is obtained by venipuncture in acid citrate dextrose (ACD) tubes.
- Centrifuge the blood using a 'soft' spin. (2000 rpm at 8–10 mins).
- Transfer the supernatant plasma containing platelets into another sterile tube (without anticoagulant) (Fig. 15.10C).
- Centrifuge tube at a higher speed (a hard spin - 4000 rpm at 10–15 mins) to obtain a platelet concentrate.
- The lower 1/3rd is PRP and upper 2/3rd is platelet-poor plasma (PPP). At the bottom of the tube, platelet pellets are formed.
- Remove PPP and suspend the platelet pellets in a minimum quantity of plasma (2–4 mL) by gently shaking the tube.

Buffy Coat Method

- Whole blood should be stored at 20°C to 24°C before centrifugation. It is centrifuged at a 'high' speed.
- Three layers are formed because of its density: The bottom layer consisting of RBCs, the middle layer consisting of platelets and WBCs, and the top PPP layer (Fig. 15.10D).
- Supernatant plasma is removed from the top of the container.
- The buffy-coat layer is transferred to another sterile tube and centrifuged once again at low speed to separate WBCs or use leukocyte filtration filter.
- Calcium chloride ($CaCl_2$) or thrombin can be used in the proportion of 0.1 mL of $CaCl_2$ per 0.9 mL of PRP.[89] as an "activator" to trigger coagulation and hence degranulation of growth factors to yield "activated PRP".[90]

Applying PRP on Ulcer

The activated PRP should be applied onto the wound after proper surgical debridement and dressing is done with a nonabsorbent dressing (paraffin gauze) (Fig. 15.10E). Some amount can also be injected at the edges of the ulcer. This process is repeated once weekly for 6 weeks.

Factors Influencing PRP Yield

Various factors influence the yield of PRP such as amount of blood drawn; speed, time and temperature of centrifugation; and use of anticoagulants.

- 10–15 mL whole blood yields 1–1.5 mL PRP on an average.
- The process must be carried out under strict aseptic conditions as well as optimum temperature regulations, i.e. 20°C to 22°C.
- The clotting process is influenced from the time of the blood drawn. To avoid unintentional activation of platelets, most protocols use large bore needles (>22) to draw the blood.[91]
- The active secretion of prepackaged GFs begins within 10 minutes of clot initiation and 95% of the secretion is completed within 1 hour.[92] Hence, PRP must be used on the treated site within 10 minutes of activation.
- The concentrated platelets remain viable for up to 8 hours and sterile, if placed on a sterile surgical table.
- Do not use EDTA as anticoagulant because it could damage the platelet membrane. Anticoagulants with citrate and dextrose of sodium citrate are recommended.[93]
- Do not chill the blood at any time before or during platelet separation.[94]

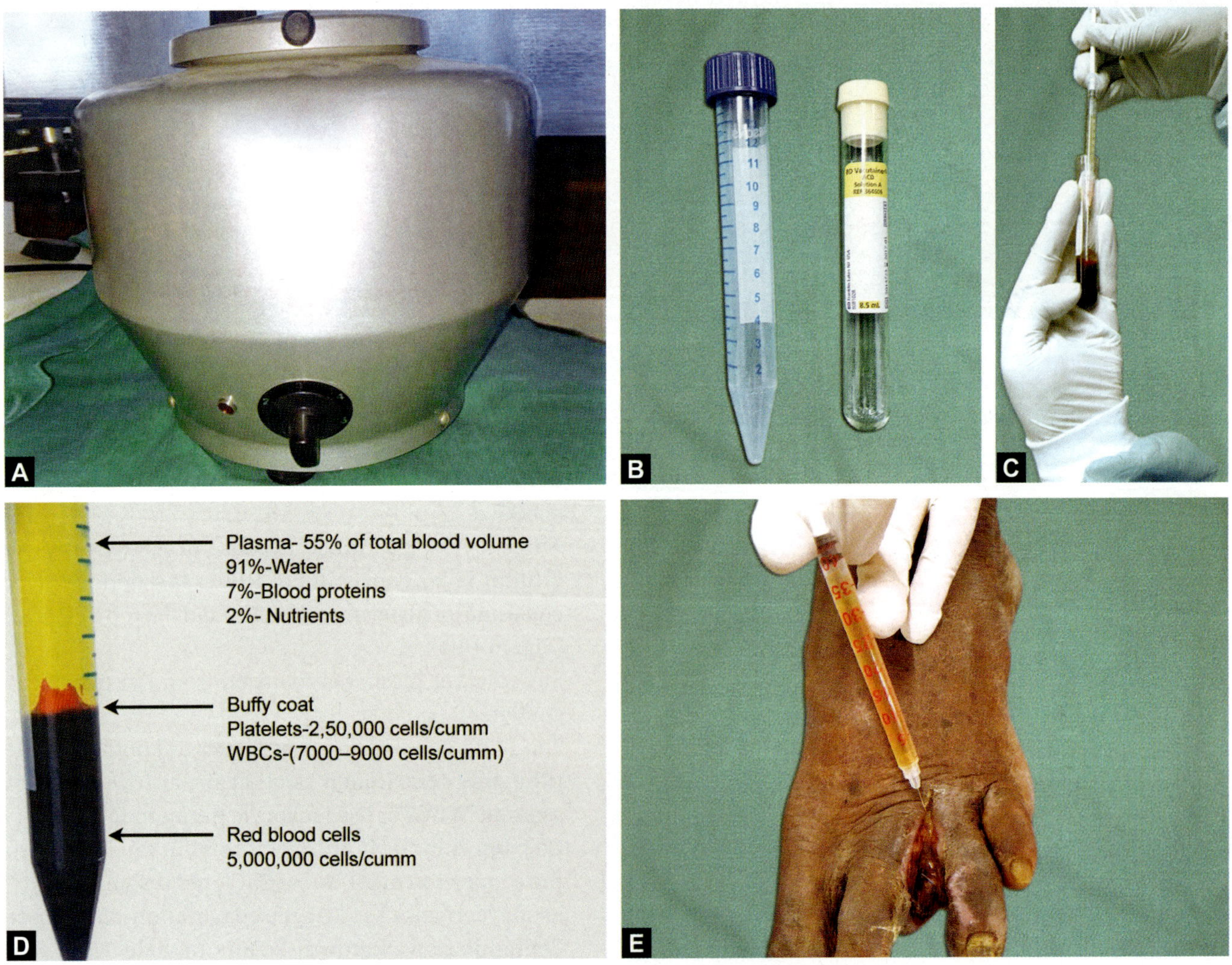

Figs. 15.10A to E: Steps of PRP in managing leg ulcer.

Platelet-rich Fibrin Matrix (PRFM)

PRFM belongs to second generation of platelet concentrates with simplified preparation and without any biochemical blood handling.[95] PRF is an autologous healing biomaterial, incorporating in a matrix of autologous fibrin mostly comprised of leukocytes, platelets and growth factors harvested from a simple blood sample.[96,97] Platelet-rich fibrin (PRF) was first developed by Choukroun et al. in 2001 at France for use in oral and maxillofacial surgery.[98]

Principle of PRF Formation

PRF is just centrifuged blood without any anticoagulant or bovine thrombin. The absence of anticoagulant leads to activation in a few minutes of most platelets of the blood sample in contact with the tube walls that leads to release of the coagulation cascades. Fibrinogen is initially concentrated in the upper part of the tube, before the circulating thrombin transforms it into fibrin. A fibrin clot is thus obtained in the middle of the tube, just between the red corpuscles at the bottom and acellular plasma at the top. Platelets are theoretically trapped massively in the fibrin meshes.

Mechanism of Action

- Slow release of growth factors from PRF matrix results in more stem cell migration and the healing program efficiently.[99]
- PRF matrix (PRFM) effectively induces endothelial cell proliferation and improves wound angiogenesis in chronic wounds, thus assists in healing of chronic ulcers.[100]

Uses

- PRFM can be used to promote wound healing, bone regeneration, graft stabilization, wound sealing and hemostasis.
- It also yields fruitful results in chronic trophic ulcers when coupled with adequate paring of lesions.

Contraindications

Patients having history of bleeding disorders, anemia, and other hematological disorders, platelet count less than 1.5 lakhs/mm^3, on anticoagulant medications (aspirin, warfarin, heparin), uncontrolled diabetes mellitus and malignant ulcers.

Instruments required: Table top centrifuge, sterile tubes without anticoagulant, sterile tweezers/scissors.

Steps

- Primary infection, if any should be taken care by antibiotic based on culture sensitivity and debridement of ulcer as required.

  Under strict aseptic precautions 10 mL of venous blood should be drawn by venipuncture and added to a sterile centrifugation tube devoid of anticoagulant. Quantity of blood required should be adjusted based on size of ulcer. In our experience, 10 mL of blood was sufficient to extract PRFM that could cover an area upto 9.42 cm^2.
- Centrifugation should be carried out at 3000 rpm (approx. 400 g) for 10 min.
- Following this, three layers will be obtained: upper straw-colored platelet poor plasma (PPP), red-colored lower fraction containing red blood cells (RBCs), and the middle fraction containing the fibrin matrix (Fig. 15.11A).
- PPP should be discarded.
- PRFM should be separated from red corpuscles at the base (Figs. 15.11B and C), preserving a small red blood cell layer, using a sterile tweezers/scissors then transferred onto a sterile saline soaked gauze (Fig. 15.11D).
- Middle membrane so obtained should be compressed between two gauze pieces gently, spread to make uniform thin layer and applied on a healthy wound followed by application of a secondary non-absorbable dressing (Figs. 15.11E and F).
- Adequate rest should be ensured during the treatment course.
- Procedure can be repeated every week as per requirement.

Tips

The success of PRF technique entirely depends on the speed of blood collection and transfer to the centrifuge. Quick handling is important. Sample collection and transfer to centrifuge should be quick and is the only way to obtain a clinically usable PRF matrix.

Delay in this steps results in polymerization of fibrin in a diffuse way in the tube and only a small blood clot without consistency will be obtained.

Advantages of PRFM over PRP[101]

- In PRFM there is no biochemical handling of blood.
- It is simplified and cost-effective process.
- Does not require the use of bovine thrombin and anticoagulants.
- Favorable healing due to slow polymerization.
- More efficient cell migration and proliferation.

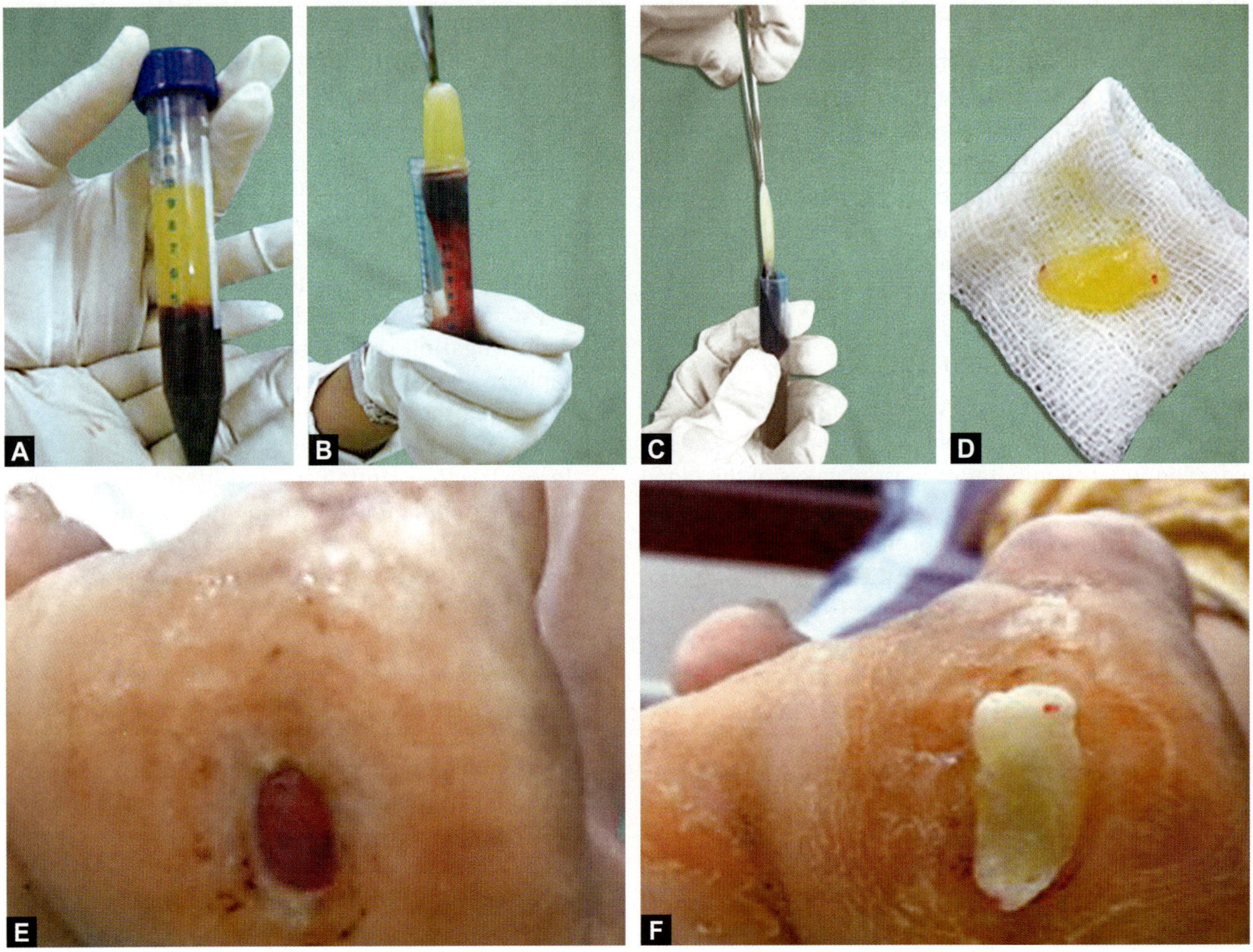

Figs. 15.11A to F: Steps of platelet rich fibrin matrix treatment in leg ulcer.

FLAPS

Classification[102-107]

Many types of flaps have been described based on:

- Composition like skin flap, muscle flap, bone flap, fascia flap.
- Location like local, distal and regional flaps.
- Vascular pattern like random, axial, pedicled and free flaps.

Among these, local flaps are more suitable for leg ulcers particularly trophic ulcers. Local flaps are raised from the tissue adjacent to the primary defect. It is moved to the defect by rotation, advancement or transposition. Specific examples of local skin flaps are the V-Y, rhomboid, and bilobed flaps.

Survival

The success of a flap depends on its survival and also on its ability to achieve the goals of reconstruction. The failure of a flap results ultimately from vascular compromise or the inability to achieve the goals of reconstruction. Factors influencing the survival of the flaps include: tension, kinking, compression, vascular, thrombosis and infection.[108]

Complications

Common complications include hematoma, necrosis of flap, contracture, and gaping of the defect which heals slowly by secondary intention.

Disadvantages

- Not advised in areas of compromised healing
- Patients on radiation therapy
- Size is limited by location of flap.

Advantages

- Simple and inexpensive
- Quick and easy to perform.

CONCLUSION

Proper diagnosis of chronic leg ulcers prior to considering surgical modalities of treatment is vital. Surgical options should be considered when medical mode of treatment has not been effective or when there is absolute indication for surgery. Combination of medical and surgical line of treatment should be considered in certain conditions particularly while treating ulcers of infective causes. Surgical treatment of venous ulcer should always be combined with compression therapy. It is important to debride and keep the ulcer healthy before considering any surgical options. Many instances may demand combination of various surgical methods described above in a given patient.

REFERENCES

1. Bhat SM. Ulcer. In: SRB's Manual of Surgery, 3rd ed. Panama: Jaypee Brothers Medical Publishers (P) Ltd. 2009;14-29.
2. Mekkes JR, Loots MA, Van Der Wal AC, et al. Causes, investigation and treatment of leg ulceration. Br J Dermatol. 2003;148(3):388-401.
3. Van Gent WB, Wilschut ED, Wittens C. Management of venous ulcer disease. BMJ. 2010;341:c6045.
4. Ryan TJ. The epidemiology of leg ulcers. In: Westerhof W (Ed). Leg Ulcers: Diagnosis and Treatment. Amsterdam: Elsevier Science Publishers BV. 1993:19-27.
5. Baker SR, Stacey MC, Jopp-McKay AG, et al. Epidemiology of chronic venous ulcers. Br J Surg. 1991;78:864-7.
6. Gonsalves CF. Venous leg ulcers. Tech VascInterv Radiol. 2003;6(3):132-6.
7. O'Meara S, Al-Kurdi D, Ologun Y, et al. Antibiotics and antiseptics for venous leg ulcers. Cochrane Database Syst Rev. 2013;(12):CD003557
8. Mortimer PS, Burnand KG, Neumann HAM. Disease of the veins and arteries: leg ulcers. In: Burns T, Breathnach S, Cox N, Griffiths C,(Eds). Rook's Textbook of Dermatology. 8th ed. Oxford: Wiley-Blackwell. 2010;47:p.1-58.
9. In: Burns T, Breathnach S, Cox N, Griffiths C, (Eds). Rook's Textbook of Dermatology, 8th ed. Oxford: Wiley-Blackwell. 2010;47:p.1-58.
10. Adeyi A, Muzerengi S, Gupta I. Leg ulcers in older people: a review of management. J Med Pract. 2009;2:21-8.
11. Bergqvist D, Lindholm C, Nelzén O. Chronic leg ulcers: the impact of venous disease. J Vasc Surg. 1999;29:752-5.
12. Das S. Examination of an ulcer. In: A manual on clinical surgery. 6th ed. Kolkata. 4:45-54.
13. Rao R, Shenoi SD. Diseases of arteries, veins and lymphatics. IADVL Textbook of Dermatology, Volume 1. 3rd ed. Bhalani Publishing House. 2008;24:716-35.
14. Aydin A, Shenbagamurthi S, Brem H. Lower extremity ulcers: venous, arterial, or diabetic? Emergency Medicine. 2009;41(8):18-24.
15. Collins L, Seraj S. Diagnosis and treatment of venous ulcers. Am Fam Physician. 2010;81(8):989-96.
16. Lipsky BA, Berendt AR, Deery HG, et al. Infectious Diseases Society of America Diagnosis and treatment of Diabetic Foot Infections. Clin Infect Dis. 2004;39:885-910.
17. Armstrong DG, Lipsky BA. Diabetic foot infections: stepwise medical and surgical management. Int Wound J. 2004;1: 123-32.
18. Armstrong DG, Lavery LA, Nixon BP, et al. It is not what you put on, but what you take off: techniques for debriding and offloading the diabetic foot wound. Clin Infect Dis. 2004;39:S92-9.
19. Cardinal M, Eisenbud DE, Armstrong DG, et al. Serial surgical debridement: a retrospective study on clinical outcomes in chronic lower extremity wounds. Wound Repair Regen. 2009;17(3):306-11.
20. Sherman RA. Maggot therapy for treating diabetic foot ulcers unresponsive to conventional therapy. Diabetes Care. 2003;26:446-51.
21. Annoni F, Rosina M, Chiurazzi D, et al. The effects of a hydrocolloid dressing on bacterial growth and the healing process of leg ulcers. IntAngiol. 1989;8:224-8.
22. Barr JE, Day AL, Weaver VA, et al. Assessing clinical efficacy of a hydrocolloid/alginate dressing on full-thickness pressure ulcers. Ostomy Wound Manage. 1995;41:28-30, 32,34-6 passim.
23. Friedman SJ, Su WP. Management of leg ulcers with hydrocolloid occlusive dressing. Arch Dermatol. 1984;120:1329-36.
24. Smith J. Debridement of diabetic foot ulcers. Cochrane Database Syst Rev. 2002. CD003556.
25. Stellar S, Meijer R, Waila S, et al. Carbon dioxide laser debridement of decubitus ulcers: followed by immediate rotation flap or skin graft closure. Ann Surg. 1974;179(2):230-7.
26. Alster TS, Lupton JR. Erbium:YAG cutaneous laser resurfacing. Dermatol Clin. 2001;19(3):453-66.
27. Attinger CE, Bulan E, Blume PA. Surgical debridement: the key to successful wound healing and reconstruction. ClinPodiatr Med Surg. 2000;17:599-630.
28. Vowden KR, Vowden P. Wound debridement, Part 2: Sharp techniques. J Wound Care. 1999;8(6):291-4.
29. NICE. Guidance on the use of debriding agents and specialist care clinics for difficult to heal surgical wounds, 2001.
30. Williams D, Enoch S, Miller D, et al. Effect of sharp debridement using curette on recalcitrant nonhealing venous leg ulcers: A concurrently controlled, prospective cohort study. Wound Repair Regen. 2005;13(2):131-7.
31. Phillips TJ, Morton LM, Uebelhoer NS, et al. Ablative Fractional carbon dioxide laser in the treatment of chronic, posttraumatic, lower-extremity ulcers in elderly patients. JAMA Dermatol. 2015;151(8):868-71.
32. Steed DL. Debridement. Am J Surg. 2004;187(5A):71S-74S.
33. Leaper DJ, Schultz G, Carville K, et al. Extending the TIME concept: what have we learned in the past 10 years? Int Wound J. 2012;9(suppl 2):1-19.
34. Ozog DM, Liu A, Chaffins ML, et al. Evaluation of clinical results, histological architecture, and collagen expression following treatment of mature burn scars with a fractional carbon dioxide laser. JAMA Dermatol. 2013;149(1):50-7.

35. Moody MN, Landau JM, Goldberg LH, et al. 595 nm long pulsed dye laser with a hydrocolloid dressing for the treatment of hypergranulation tissue on the scalp in postsurgical defects. Dermatol Online J. 2011;17(7):2.
36. Wang SQ, Goldberg LH. Pulsed dye laser for the treatment of hypergranulation tissue with chronic ulcer in postsurgical defects. J Drugs Dermatol. 2007;6(12):1191-4.
37. Turczynski R, Tarpila E. Treatment of leg ulcers with split skin grafts: early and late results. Scand J Plast Reconstr Surg Hand Surg. 1999;33(3):301-5.
38. Kirsner RS, Falanga V, Kerdel FA, et al. Skin grafts as pharmacological agents: pre-wounding of the donor site. Br J Dermatol. 1996;135:292-6.
39. Triquet B, Ruffieux P, Mainetti C, et al. Topical haemotherapy for leg ulcers. Dermatology. 1994;189:418-20.
40. Maier K, Ehrhardt G, Frevert J. Antibacterial activity of cultured human keratinocytes. Arch Dermatol Res. 1992;284(2):119-21.
41. Saja S, Pietramaggiori S, Pietramaggiori G, et al. Skin graft. In: Neligan PC, Gurtner GC (Eds). Plastic Surgery. Volume One: Principles. 3rd ed. Elsevier Inc. 2013;17:p318-38.
42. Khunger N, Kandhari R. Thin split thickness skin grafting for vitiligo. In: Venkataram M (Eds). Textbook on Cutaneous and aesthetic surgery.1st ed. Jaypee Brothers Medical Publishers (p) Ltd. 2012;24D: p 351-9.
43. Reverdin JL. Skin grafts-experience derived from the service of Dr Guyon at Hospital Necker. Bull Soc IMP of Chir of Paris. 1869;10:511-5.
44. Davis JS. Address of the president: the story of plastic surgery. Ann Surg. 1941;113(5):641-56.
45. Davis JS. The use of small deep skin grafts. JAMA. 1914;63: 985-9.
46. Davis JS. The small deep graft: relationship to the true reverdin graft. Ann Surg. 1929;89(6):902-16.
47. Biswas A, Bharara M, Hurst C, et al. The micrograft concept for wound healing: strategies and applications. J Diabetes Sci Technol. 2010;4(4):808-19.
48. Oien RF, Hansen BU, Håkansson A. Pinch grafting of leg ulcers in primary care. Acta DermVenereol. 1998;78(6):438-9.
49. Jayashree R, Rai R, Srinivas CR. Leg ulcers. In: Venkataram M (Eds). Textbook on Cutaneous and Aesthetic Surgery, 1st ed. Jaypee Brothers Medical Publishers (p) Ltd. 2012;28: p 472-83.
50. Gabarro P. A new method of grafting. Br Med J. 1943;1:723-4.
51. Oien RF, Håkansson A, Hansen BU, et al. Pinch grafting of chronic leg ulcers in primary care: fourteen years' experience. Acta Derm Venereol. 2002;82(4):275-8.
52. Hjerppe A, Sane M, Huhtala H, et al. Pinch grafting of chronic leg ulcers: a retrospective analysis of 104 patients with 169 ulcers. J Wound Care. 2010;19(1):37-40.
53. Malhotra S, Kaur A, Sargodhia P, et al. Evaluation of postage stamp skin grafting in the treatment of nonhealing leg ulcers. The Internet Journal of Dermatology. 2008;7(1):1-7.
54. Mehta S, Watson JT. Platelet rich concentrate: basic science and current clinical applications. J Orthop Trauma. 2008;22(6): 432-8.
55. Marx RE. Platelet-rich plasma (PRP): what is PRP and what is not PRP? Implant Dent. 2001;10(4):225-8.
56. Driver VR, Hanft J, Fylling CP, et al. Autologel Diabetic Foot Ulcer Study Group. A prospective, randomized, controlled trial of autologous platelet-rich plasma gel for the treatment of diabetic foot ulcers. Ostomy Wound Manage. 2006;52(6):68-70, 72, 74 passim.
57. Petrova N, Edmonds M. Emerging drugs for diabetic foot ulcers. Expert Opin Emerg Drugs. 2006;11(4):709-24.
58. Millington JT, Norris TW. Effective treatment strategies for diabetic foot wounds. J Fam Pract. 2000;49(11 Suppl):S40-S48.
59. Steed DL, Goslen JB, Holloway GA, et al. Randomized prospective double-blind trial in healing chronic diabetic foot ulcers. CT-102 activated platelet supernatant, topical versus placebo. Diabetes Care. 1992;15(11):1598-1604.
60. Everts PA, Brown Mahoney C, Hoffmann JJ, et al. Platelet-rich plasma preparation using three devices: implications for platelet activation and platelet growth factor release. Growth Factors. 2006;24(3):165-71.
61. Pietrzak WS, Eppley BL. Platelet rich plasma: biology and new technology. J Craniofac Surg. 2005;16(6):1043-54.
62. Eppley BL, Pietrzak WS, Blanton M. Platelet-rich plasma: a review of biology and applications in plastic surgery. Plast Reconstr Surg. 2006;118(6):147e-159e.
63. Salemi S, Rinaldi C, Manna F, et al. Reconstruction of lower leg skin ulcer with autologous adipose tissue and platelet-rich plasma. J Plast Reconstr Aesthet Surg. 2008;61(12):1565-7.
64. Lindeboom JA, Mathura KR, Aartman IH, et al. Influence of the application of platelet-enriched plasma in oral mucosal wound healing. Clin Oral Implants Res. 2007;18(1):133-9.
65. El-Sharkawy H, Kantarci A, Deady J, et al. Platelet-rich plasma: growth factors and pro- and anti-inflammatory properties. J Periodontol. 2007;78(4):661-9.
66. Nikolidakis D, Jansen JA. The biology of platelet-rich plasma and its application in oral surgery: literature review. Tissue Eng Part B Rev. 2008;14(3):249-58.
67. Shashikiran ND, Reddy VV, Yavagal CM, et al. Applications of platelet-rich plasma (PRP) in contemporary pediatric dentistry. J Clin Pediatr Dent. 2006;30(4):283-6.
68. Wrotniak M, Bielecki T, Gazdzik TS. Current opinion about using the platelet-rich gel in orthopaedics and trauma surgery. Ortop Traumatol Rehabil. 2007;9(3):227-38.
69. Mishra A, Woodall J Jr, Vieira A. Treatment of tendon and muscle using platelet-rich plasma. Clin Sports Med. 2009;28(1):113-25.
70. Frechette JP, Martineau I, Gagnon G. Platelet-rich plasmas: growth factor content and roles in wound healing. J Dent Res. 2005;84(5):434-9.
71. Bhanot S, Alex JC. Current applications of platelet gels in facial plastic surgery. Facial Plast Surg. 2002;18(1):27-33.
72. Henderson JL, Cupp CL, Ross EV, et al. The effects of autologous platelet gel on wound healing. Ear Nose Throat J. 2003;82(8):598- 602.
73. Eppley BL, Woodell JE, Higgins J. Platelet quantification and growth factor analysis from platelet-rich plasma: implications for wound healing. Plast Reconstr Surg. 2004;114(6):1502-8

74. Knighton DR, Ciresi KF, Fiegel VD, et al. Classification and treatment of chronic nonhealing wounds. Successful treatment with autologous platelet-derived wound healing factors (PDWHF). Ann Surg. 1986;204(3):322-30.
75. Knighton DR, Doucette M, Fiegel VD, et al. The use of platelet derived wound healing formula in human clinical trials. Prog Clin Biol Res. 1988;266:319-29.
76. Marx RE. Platelet-rich plasma: evidence to support its use. J Oral Maxillofac Surg. 2004;62(4):489-96.
77. Pietramaggiori G, Kaipainen A, Czeczuga JM, et al. Freeze-dried platelet-rich plasma shows beneficial healing properties in chronic wounds. Wound Repair Regen. 2006;14(5): 573-80.
78. Gonshor A. Technique for producing platelet-rich plasma and platelet concentrate: background and process. Int J Periodontics Restorative Dent. 2002;22(6):547-57.
79. Robson MC, Phillips LG, Thomason A. et al. Recombinant human platelet-derived growth factor-BB for the treatment of chronic pressure ulcers. Ann Plast Surg. 1992;29(3): 193-201.
80. Weibrich G, Kleis WK, Kunz-Kostomanolakis M, et al. Correlation of platelet concentration in platelet-rich plasma to the extraction method, age, sex, and platelet count of the donor. Int J Oral Maxillofac Implants. 2001;16(5):693-9.
81. Harrison P, Cramer EM. Platelet alpha-granules. Blood Rev. 1993;7(1):52-62.
82. McAleer JP, Sharma S, Kaplan EM, et al. Use of autologous platelet concentrate in a nonhealing lower extremity wound. Adv Skin Wound Care. 2006;19(7):354-63.
83. Bielecki TM, Gazdzik TS, Arendt J, et al. Antibacterial effect of autologous platelet gel enriched with growth factors and other active substances: an in vitro study. J Bone Joint Surg Br. 2007;89(3):417-20.
84. Tang YQ, Yeaman MR, Selsted ME. Antimicrobial peptides from human platelets. Infect Immun. 2002;70(12): 6524-33.
85. Gandhi A, Bibbo C, Pinzur M, et al. The role of platelet-rich plasma in foot and ankle surgery. Foot Ankle Clin. 2005;10(4):621-37.
86. Rozman P, Bolta Z. Use of platelet growth factors in treating wounds and soft-tissue injuries. Acta Dermatovenerol Alp Panonica Adriat. 2007;16(4):156-65.
87. American Association of Blood Banks technical manual committee. Method 6.11: Preparation of platelets from whole blood. In: Vengelen-Tyler V (Ed). AABB Technical Manual, 13th ed. Bethesda (MD): American Association of Blood Banks.1999; p.725.
88. Sweeny J, Grossman BJ. Blood collection, storage and component preparation methods. In: Brecher M, (Ed). Technical Manual. 14th ed. Bethesda MD: American Association of Blood Banks (AABB) 2002;955-8. 14.
89. Welsh WJ. Autologous platelet gel: Clinical function and usage in plastic surgery. Cosmetic Derm. 2000;11:13-9.
90. Mikhael NW, El-Esawy FM. Skin rejuvenation with autologous concentrated platelet-rich plasma. Egypt J DermatolVenerol. 2014;34:5-9
91. Arshdeep, Kumaran MS. Platelet-rich plasma in dermatology: Boon or a bane? Indian J. Dermatol Venereol Leprol. 2014;80:5-14.
92. Marlovits S, Mousavi M, Gabler C, et al. A new simplified technique for producing platelet-rich plasma: A short technical note. Eur Spine J. 13:102-06.
93. Kevy S, Jacobson M. Preparation of growth factors enriched autologous platelet gel. Proceedings of the 27th Annual Meeting of Service Biomaterials, April 2001.
94. Anitua E, Prado R, Sánchez M, et al. Platelet-rich-plasma: Preparation and formulation. Oper Tech Orthop. 2012;22:25-32.
95. Dhurat R, Sukesh MS. Principles and methods of preparation of platelet-rich plasma: A review and author's perspective. J Cutan Aesthet Surg. 2014;7:189.
96. Dohan DM, Choukroun J, Diss A, et al. Platelet-rich fibrin (PRF): a second-generation platelet concentrate. Part I: technological concepts and evolution. Oral Surg Oral Med Oral Pathol Oral Radiol Endod. 2006;101(3):e37-44.
97. Dohan DM, Choukroun J, Diss A, et al. Platelet-rich fibrin (PRF): a second-generation platelet concentrate. Part II: platelet-related biologic features. Oral Surg Oral Med Oral Pathol Oral Radiol Endod. 2006;101: e45-50.
98. Dohan DM, Choukroun J, Diss A, et al. Platelet-rich fibrin (PRF):a second-generation platelet concentrate. Part III: leucocyte activation: a new feature for platelet concentrates? Oral Surg Oral Med Oral Pathol Oral Radiol Endod. 2006;101:e51-55.
99. Choukroun J, Adda F, Schoeffler C, et al. An opportunity in perio-implantology (in French): the PRF. Implantodontie 2001;42:55-62.
100. Naik B, Karunakar P, Jayadev M, et al. Role of platelet rich fibrin in wound healing: a critical review. J Conserv Dent. 2013;16:284-93.
101. Roy S, Driggs J, Elgharably H, et al. Platelet-rich fibrin matrix improves wound angiogenesis via inducing endothelial cell proliferation. Wound Repair Regen. 2011;19:753-66.
102. Toffler M, Toscano N, Holtzclaw D, et al. Introducing Choukroun's platelet rich fibrin (PRF) to the reconstructive surgery milieu. J Implant Adv Clin Dent. 2009;1:21-30.
103. Cormack GC, Lamberty BGH: The Arterial Anatomy of Skin Flaps. London, Churchill Livingstone, 1986.
104. Menick FJ: Aesthetic refinements in use of forehead for nasal reconstruction: the paramedian forehead flap. Clin Plast Surg. 1990;17:4.
105. Mathes, SJ. Reconstructive Surgery: Principles, Anatomy and Techniques. New York, Elsevier Science, 1997.
106. McCarthy JG. (ed). Plastic Surgery, vol.1. New York: Elsevier Science, 1990.
107. Russell, RC, Zamboni WA. Manual of Free Flaps New York: Elsevier Science, 2001.
108. Serafin, D. Atlas of Microsurgical Composite Tissue Transplantation. New York: Elsevier Science, 1996.

CHAPTER 16

Tissue Grafting Techniques in Vitiligo

Koushik Lahiri, Anupam Das

INTRODUCTION

Vitiligo is a fairly common dermatosis encountered in our day-to-day practice. It is characterized by the development of white patches in any part of the body. There are multiple treatment options for vitiligo, but medical strategies are often unsatisfactory. Many cases require surgical management, commonest one being tissue grafting. In this chapter, we shall briefly review the techniques of tissue grafting, namely autologous minipunch grafting, suction blister graft and thin split thickness skin grafting.

PRINCIPLE

The etiopathogenesis of vitiligo involves the absence of melanocytes in the affected skin. Thus, the backbone of any surgical therapy is based on the introduction of melanocytes into the affected areas, with a hope that these newly introduced melanocytes will function as epidermal melanin units, subsequently leading to pigmentation of the skin.[1]

The choice of the method is based on a number of factors like site of the lesion, number, duration, availability of the equipments, and expertise of the dermatosurgeon and most importantly, the stability of the disease. Stability is defined as absence of new lesions, no increase in the size of pre-existing lesions, evidence suggestive of repigmentation and no signs of Koebner phenomenon. According to Indian Association of Dermatologists, Venereologists and Leprologists (IADVL) taskforce for standard guidelines of dermatosurgical procedures, surgery may be taken up for patient with disease which is at least stable for 1 year.[2]

INDICATIONS[2,3]

- Minipunch grafting is indicated for the treatment of small irregular vitiliginous patches over the acral areas, palms and soles, although this method works excellent in most of the parts of the body.
- Suction blister grafting works good in small areas like lips, eyelids, etc.
- The most commonly employed technique is thin split thickness skin grafting which is suitable for large areas, including some difficult areas like eyelids, nipple-areola complex, genitalia, etc.

AUTOLOGOUS MINIPUNCH GRAFTING

This technique is the easiest and the most user friendly surgical method of treatment of vitiligo. This method produces magical results, if the sites are properly chosen and post-procedure advice is followed religiously.

History

- 1804: Baronio described successful skin grafting in sheep
- 1941: Lewin and Peck published autograft transplantation in guinea pigs[4]
- 1972: Norman Orentriech reported autograft transplantation in human[5]
- 1976: Labuono and Shatin reported similar results in discoid lupus erythematosus[6]
- 1978: Falabella reported the successful results of superficial split thickness grafts[7]
- 1995: Behl claimed comparatively better results with thin Thiersch grafting[8]
- 1995: Falabella combined both epidermal graft and mini graft.[9]

Procedure[10-16]

- Patient is properly assessed regarding the feasibility of the procedure, with special attention to the stability of the disease. A written informed consent from the patient, followed by pre-treatment photographs is taken.
- The recipient area is prepared using strict aseptic precautions and the area is anesthetized using 2% lignocaine ± adrenaline, depending on the site.

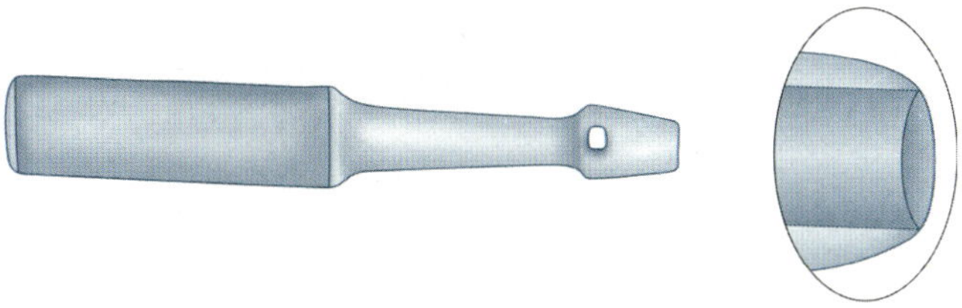

Fig. 16.1: Keye's punch.[36]

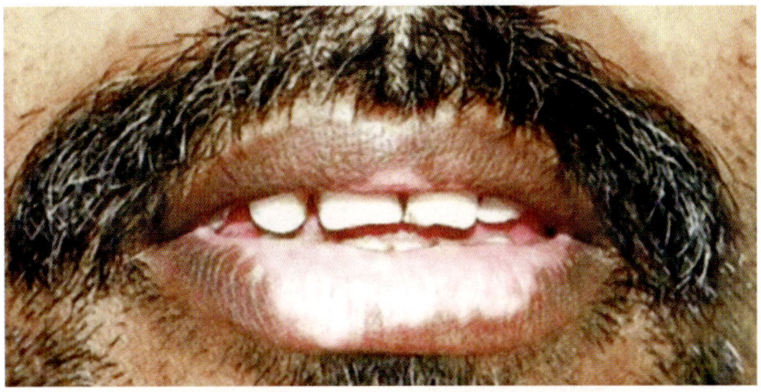

Fig. 16.2: Lip vitiligo.[36]

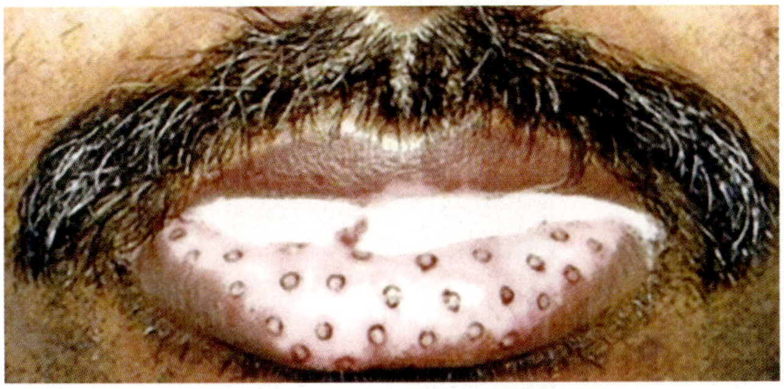

Fig. 16.3: Proper positioning of the graft.[36]

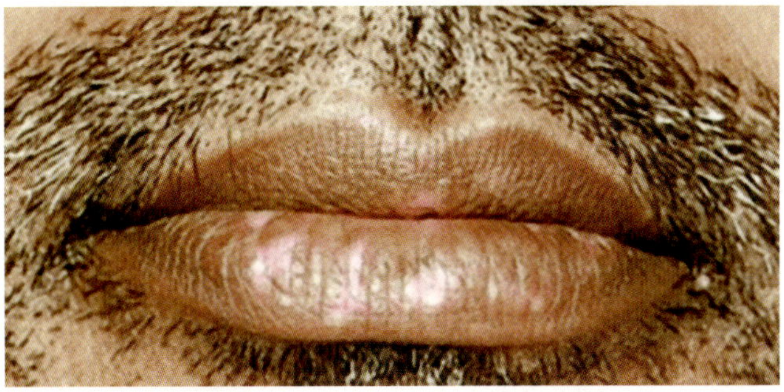

Fig. 16.4: Repigmentation of lip vitiligo achieved after 9 months.[36]

- The site of placement of the grafts must be chosen wisely to avoid any perigraft halo. Usually, border of lesion is preferred and grafts are placed at a distance of usually 5–10 mm from each other.
- The most commonly preferred donor area is upper lateral aspect thigh or gluteal region. The punches are placed close to one another, so that maximum grafts can be obtained from selected donor area. Punch of same size is preferred for both recipient and donor area. Keye's punch is shown as in Figure 16.1.
- Grafts are taken from donor area and placed carefully on recipient area, with special focus on placement of grafts, avoidance of folding of edges and most importantly, of not placing grafts upside down. Tip of scissors are preferred to place the graft precisely.
- Hemostasis is attained by pressing saline soaked gauze piece over recipient area, followed by three layered dressing from inside out using nonadherent paraffin-embedded sterile gauze, sterile Surgipad and a bio-occlusive Micropore. Donor area dressing is done using Surgipad and Micropore only.
- Dressings are opened on recipient area to check for dislodgement of the grafts after 24–72 hours and re-opened on the 7th day to check for uptake of grafts.
- Postsurgically,[2] weeks later patients are prescribed (PUVA or PUVASOL or NBUVB). The entire grafted area is then expected to develop pigmentation by 3–6 months. Pretreatment and the post-treatment photographs have been shown in Figures 16.2 to 16.10.

Complications[11-13,16,17]

- *Recipient site*: Cobblestoning, polka dot appearance, color mismatch, graft rejection (common in vitiligo diathesis due to herpes labialis), perigraft halo, depigmentation of grafted area, graft dislodgement, keloid and hypertrophic scar.
- *Donor site*: Keloid, scarring, contact dermatitis, etc.

Avoiding Complications

- *Cobble stoning*: It is the most frequently faced complication even in the most experienced hands. Same size of Punch needle may be taken to get snugly fitting grafts. A smaller donor punch size of 1 to 1.5 mm prevents cobblestoning. The donor graft may be slightly bigger and thinner, with least dermal tissue. For this the donor tissue should be cut closer to graft, away from the underlying skin (preferably with the distal end of a curved scissor, the

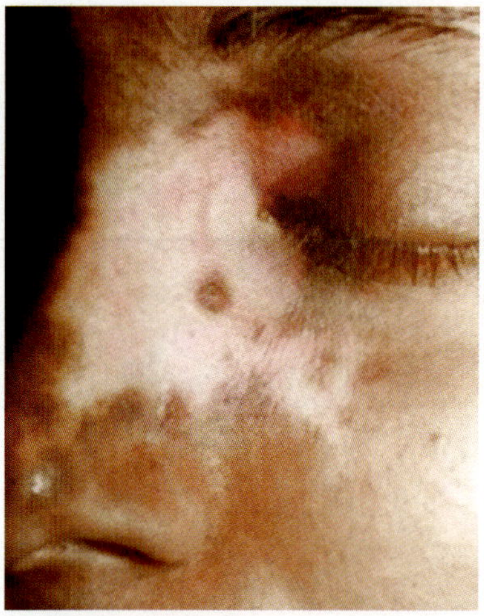

Fig. 16.5: Segmental vitiligo over the face.[36]

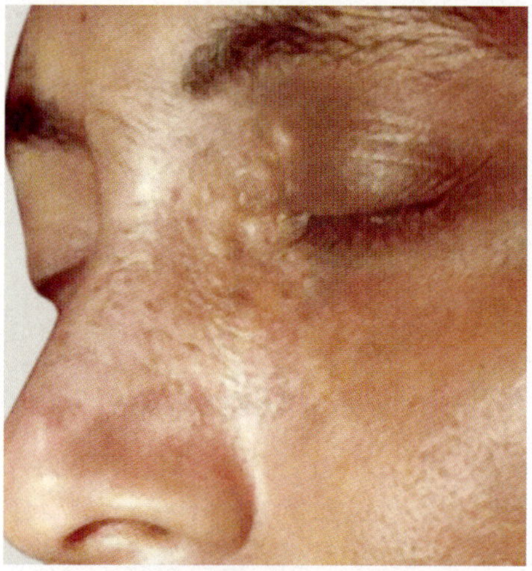

Fig. 16.6: Repigmentation of segmental vitiligo after 6 months.[36]

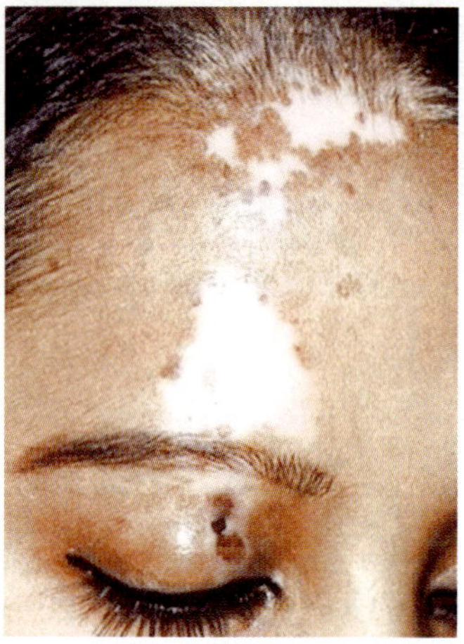

Fig. 16.7: Segmental vitiligo on the forehead.[36]

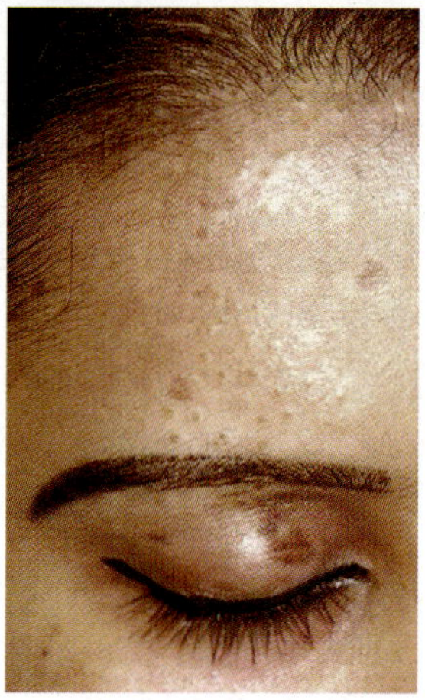

Fig. 16.8: Repigmentation of forehead vitiligo after 5 months.[36]

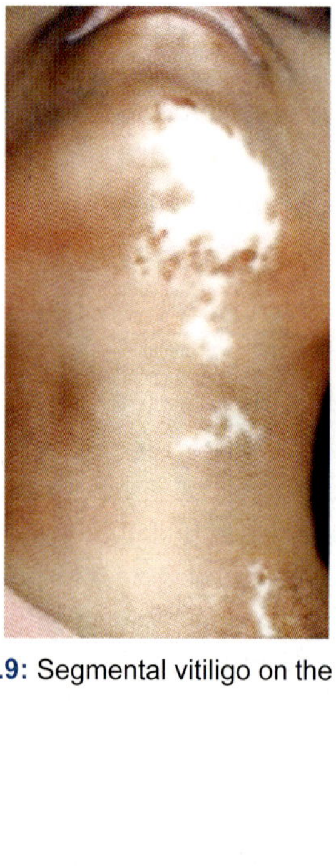

Fig. 16.9: Segmental vitiligo on the neck.[36]

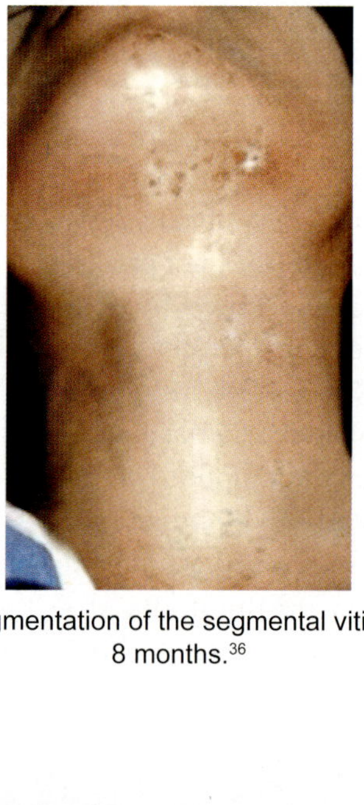

Fig. 16.10: Repigmentation of the segmental vitiligo of neck after 8 months.[36]

thinnest part or the blade). This approximately helps to calculate the depth of donor and recipient area.

- A variable rotation technique to achieve different depths in case of donor and recipient can be used. For the donor area use 10–20 rotations (moderate pressure as we do in case of punch biopsy), to reach only up to upper dermis. And for the recipient area, 15–25 rotations (clockwise and anticlockwise), depending on the site to reach till the mid dermis.
- *Prevention of polka dot appearance*: The grafts should be placed in a brick laying fashion at a distance of 1 punch diameter from each other, to allow a random spread of pigmentation v/s a predictable linear placement of graft (like creating anterior hairline in hair transplantation).
- Perigraft halo can be prevented by dermabrading 1–2 mm in the margin of normal skin, placing the grafts initially all along the periphery and also 1–2 mm inside the outer border of recipient area.

Comments[18,19]

This is undoubtedly one of the easiest and most commonly done surgery for vitiligo which can be performed on any part of the body but side effects are quite common and a perfect match may not occur even, if the procedure is performed by expert professionals. Besides, post procedure phototherapy is mandatory and scarring of donor site is frequent.

SUCTION BLISTER ROOF GRAFTING

In this procedure, a negative pressure is created at the donor site as a result of which a blister is created. Later on, the blister roof is grafted onto the recipient site. Thus method is suited for small and stable vitiliginous lesions, especially face.[2,20]

Procedure[21-24]

- Apart from the common equipments, the pre-requisite for the procedure is the availability of disposable syringes (10 cc/20 cc and 50 cc) and 3-way cannulas.
- Strict aseptic preparation of the donor site (medial forearm, medial upper arm, medial posterior thigh etc.) is done.
- The area is infiltrated with 1% xylocaine as a field block ± topical anesthesia (EMLA).
- Plunger of the 10 cc/20 cc syringe is removed and it is attached to one end of the 3-way cannula, following which the inferior part of the barrel of the syringe is positioned over the donor site.
- 50 cc syringe is taken and the needle end is attached to another adaptor of the 3-way cannula of the 20 cc syringe.
- The 3-way cannula is unlocked and the air within 20 cc syringe is sucked out with the help of 50 cc syringe and a negative pressure is created.
- The cannula is locked and the air is aspirated from 50 cc syringe, cannula is again unlocked and the air is re-sucked to further increase the negative pressure inside the 20 cc syringe.
- Cannula is locked once again and 50 cc syringe is disconnected, which ensures that a constant negative pressure is maintained inside the 20 cc syringe (Fig. 16.11).
- Within 1–3 hours, blisters are formed. Cannula is unlocked and syringes are disconnected (Fig. 16.12).
- Recipient site is prepared using dermabrasion, radiofrequency, laser, PUVA, cryotherapy etc.
- Blister is removed from the donor site, cleaned with normal saline and placed over the recipient area from the thumb and spread with the help of forceps. All the grafts are placed similarly.
- The graft is pressed using a sterile moist gauze. Pressure dressing is done with double layer antibiotic ointment soaked cotton, moist gauze and crepe bandage.
- Dressing is removed on Day 7. Care is taken to avoid tearing of the graft from the area. The elastocrepe plaster

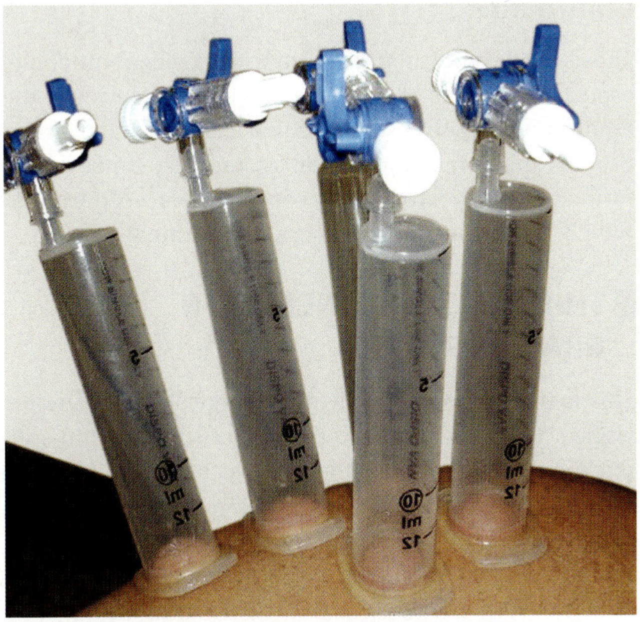

Fig. 16.11: Method of raising suction blisters.[23]

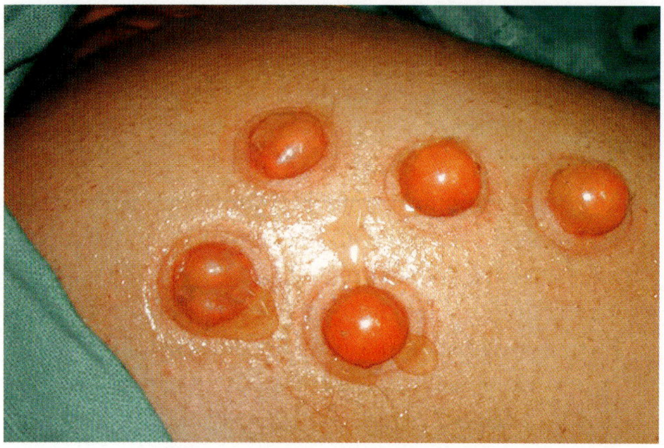

Fig. 16.12: Formation of blisters after 2 hours of suction.[23]

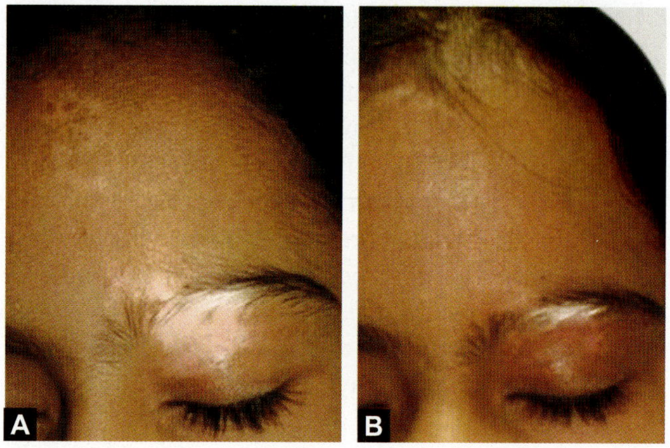

Figs. 16.13A and B: (A) Stable resistant zosteriform vitiligo; (B) Repigmentation achieved 3 months after suction blister grafting. Note the persistence of leukotrichia.[23]

is lifted up from corner and slowly detached from the underlying dressing. The gauze piece and cotton are soaked with normal saline and removed slowly one after the other. Redressing is carried out for Day 8–10 and the dressing is finally removed on Day 10.

- Complete repigmentation is usually achieved within 3 months (Figs. 16.13A and B).

Complications

Although rare, bruising, hematoma, infections and graft rejection may happen in unfortunate circumstances.

Comments[1]

This is a safe surgical procedure with excellent outcome, especially in cases of lip and eyelid vitiligo. However, the limiting factor for this surgery is that it is a time-consuming process and in rare circumstances, the blister may not be formed and we may have to convert the procedure into punch grafting or split thickness skin grafting.

THIN SPLIT THICKNESS SKIN GRAFTING (STSG)

This is the most commonly done surgical procedure for vitiligo.[25] When it comes to the rate of success, thin split thickness skin grafting is the most successful of all types of surgery. However, STSG requires special training and surgical skills. It involves the transfer of the graft (0.1–0.7 mm thickness) containing epidermis and superficial part of dermis from the donor area to the recipient vitiliginous patch. This is followed by graft uptake and adherence, revascularization and contracture. It is used for stable vitiligo, post burns leukoderma, post herpes leukoderma, contact leukoderma, post discoid lupus erythematosus, leucoderma, piebaldism, etc.

History

- 1964: Behl reported the use of thin Thiersch skin graft[26,27]
- 1995: Kahn et al. treated vitiligo using dermabrasion and epidermal sheet grafting[28,29]
- 1997: Olsson and Juhlin used epidermal sheet grafts for piebaldism and vitiligo.[30]

Prerequisites[2,15,31-34]

Selection of patients is a crucial step in this procedure. Since immobilization of the grafted site is mandatory as a part of the postoperative care, certain parts like fingers, elbows, knees, toes, etc. are not suitable recipient sites. However, this technique works excellent for large vitiliginous patches which are not possible to treat by autologous minipunch grafting or suction blister roof grafting. Equipments include dermabrader (manual or electrical), Humby's skin grafting knife, Padget's or Davol's dermatome, artery forceps, cyanoacrylate adhesive (surgical glue), etc.

Procedure[1]

- Shave the donor and recipient areas prior to the procedure. This is mandatory because areas with thick hair lead to lifting up of the graft and subsequent dislodgement.

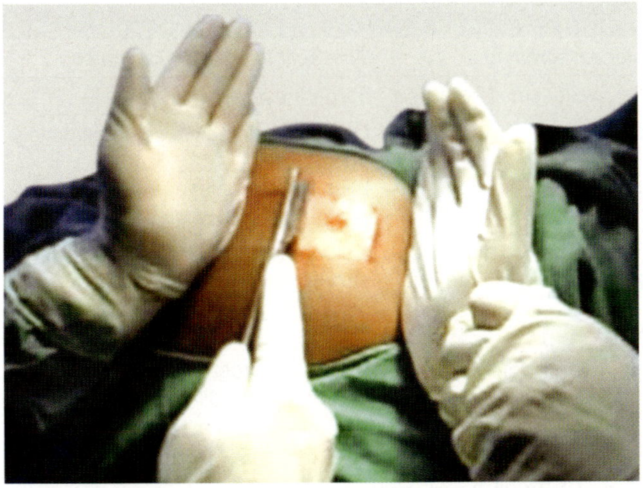

Fig. 16.14: Harvesting a thin split thickness graft.[23]

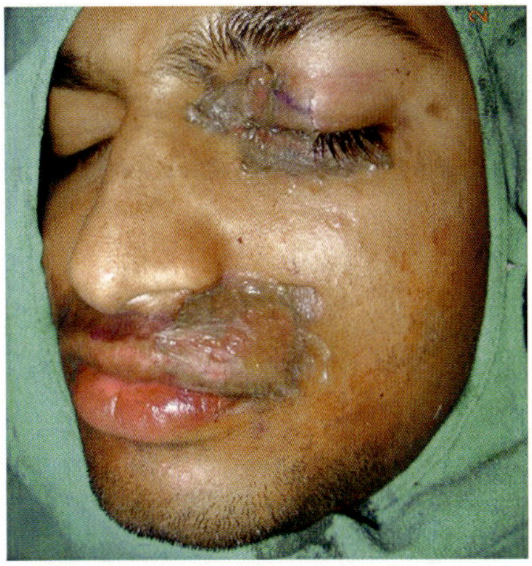

Fig. 16.15: Cyanoacrylate adhesive for immobilization of the graft.[23]

- Gluteal area is considered to be the best donor site because of cosmetic reasons. Other options include anterolateral thigh, arms, abdomen, etc.
- *Modification*: Anterolateral thigh is more practical, because of large straight area, less postoperative difficulty to the patient.
- Donor area is anesthetized using EMLA cream or 2% lignocaine or field block with 1% lignocaine. The anesthesia should not be given very superficially lest it may cause dimpling of skin and difficult manoeuvering ability of blade.
- The donor site is hydrated using normal saline and the area is stretched before commencement of harvesting of the graft.
- Split thickness skin graft of uniform thickness is procured from the area using a sterile blade or a hand dermatome (Fig. 16.14).
- A simple hand held Dermatome using an autoclaved shaving blade can be used, preferably the one with a longer handle.
- Enter the skin at nearly 10–20° angle (with the assistant giving countertraction). Gradually move the blade swiftly but steadily preferably by stopping breath for a moment. Maintain the correct depth, which can be judged by the clearly visible writings on the blade from above and pin point bleeding below.
- The harvested graft is transferred in to a sterile petridish containing normal saline and hemostasis is secured in the donor area.
- Donor area is dressed, preferably using semiocclusive dressing which ensures re-epithelialization within 10 days and least chances of infection and complications in comparison to other dressings.
- Recipient vitiliginous area is properly cleaned and anesthetized using infiltration of 1% lignocaine or topical anesthetic cream under occlusion or general anesthesia.
- The area is abraded using an electric or manual dermabrader or ultrapulse CO_2 laser or Er:YAG laser.
- The graft is then transferred to the dermabraded area, ensuring that there is no air, blood, water, serum or debris trapped beneath the graft.
- The grafted site is properly immobilized at least for the first 72 hours. Surgical glue (octyl-2-cyanoacrylate) usually serves the purpose of immobilization (Fig. 16.15). Alternatively, pressure dressings may be employed for the same.
- Anti-inflammatory drugs and antibiotics are prescribed for 7 days. However, the dressing is opened and checked after 24 hours to check for the presence of any hematoma, seroma, dislodgement of graft. Dressing is reopened on Day 7.
- STSG provides excellent cosmetic results and repigmentation is usually achieved with 3–6 months.

Complications[25]

- *Recipient site*: Graft rejection due to the accumulation of the air bubbles and serum,secondary infection, hyperpigmentation, perigraft halo, stuck on tyre patch appearance, hypertrophy, milia, vitiligo diathesis.
- *Donor site*: Postinflammatory hypo or hyperpigmentation, scarring.

Table 16.1: Comparison between the various tissue methods of grafting.

Salient point	*Autologous mini punch grafting*	*Suction blister roof grafting*	*Thin split thickness skin grafting*
Preferred site	Acral areas, palms, soles	Mucosae, lip, eyelid, small areas	Large areas, eyelids, genitalia
Advantages	Easy and fast method Suitable for any site Only method for palms	Excellent cosmesis Scarring is negligible Suitable for mucosal areas	Color match achieved immediately after surgery Less time consuming
Disadvantages	Cobblestoning is common Phototherapy is mandatory Color mismatch is frequent	Time consuming Blister may not be formed and procedure may be a complete failure	Surgical skills required Color mismatch, perigraft halo, milia, stuck-on appearance may occur

Comments

This is undoubtedly one of the most popular surgical methods for treating vitiligo. It gives excellent results in most of the cases. Even, repigmentation of leukotrichia can be achieved using this technique. Besides, it is a less time consuming procedure in comparison to punch grafting and suction blister grafting. However, if performed by persons lacking precise surgical skills, complications may happen.

The procedures have been compared in a tabular form (Table 16.1).[35,36]

ACKNOWLEDGMENTS

1. Lahiri K, Malakar S, Sarma N, et al. Repigmentation of vitiligo with punch grafting and narrow-band UV-B (311 nm—a prospective study. Int J Dermatol. 2006;45:649-55.
2. Malakar S. Lahiri K. Minigrafting for vitiligo. In: Gupta S, Olsson MJ, Kanwar AJ, Ortonne JP (Eds). Surgical Management of Vitiligo. 1st ed. Oxford: Blackwell Publishing; 2007. pp. 87-95.
3. Malakar S, Lahiri K. Spontaneous repigmentation in vitiligo: why it is important. Int J Dermatol. 2006;45:478-9.
4. Lahiri K. Evolution and evaluation of autologous mini punch grafting in vitiligo. Indian J Dermatol. 2009;54:159-67.
5. Khunger N, Kathuria SD, Ramesh V. Tissue grafts in vitiligo surgery—past, present, and future. Indian J Dermatol. 2009;54:150-8.

REFERENCES

1. Mysore V, Lahiri K. Overview of vitiligo surgery. In: Mysore V. (Ed). ACS(I) Textbook on Cutaneous and Aesthetic Surgery. 1st ed. New Delhi: Jaypee Medical Brothers (P) Ltd; 2012. pp. 327-33.
2. Parsad D, Gupta S. Standard guidelines of care for vitiligo surgery. Indian J Dermatol Venereol Leprol 2008;74(Suppl S1):37-45.
3. Falabella R. Surgical treatment of vitiligo: why, when and how. J Eur Acad Dermatol Venereol. 2003;17:518-20.
4. Lewin ML, Peck SM. Pigment studies in skin grafts on experimental animals. J Invest Dermatol. 1941;4:504.
5. Orentreich N, Selmanowitz VJ. Autograft repigmentation of leukoderma. Arch Dermatol. 1972;105:734-6.
6. Labuono P, Shatin H. Transplantation of hair bulbs and melanocytes into leucodermic scars. J Dermatol Surg Oncol. 1976;2:53-5.
7. Falabella R. Repigmentation of leucoderma by minigrafts of normally pigmented, autologous skin. J Dermatol Surg Oncol. 1978:4:916-9.
8. Behl PN. Repigmentation of segmental vitiligo by autologous mini grafting. J Am Acad Dermatol. 1985;12:118-9.
9. Falabella R, Barona M, Escobar C, et al. Surgical combination therapy for vitiligo and piebaldism. Dermatol Surg. 1995;21:852-7.
10. Falabella R. Repigmentation of segmental vitiligo by autologous minigrafting. J Am Acad Dermatol. 1983;9:514-21.
11. Lahiri K. Autologous mini punch grafting in vitiligo. In: Mysore V. (Ed). ACS(I) Textbook on Cutaneous and Aesthetic Surgery. 1st ed. New Delhi: Jaypee Medical Brothers (P) Ltd; 2012. pp. 334-43.
12. Lahiri K, Sengupta SR. Treatment of stable and recalcitrant depigmented skin conditions by autologous punch grafting. Indian J Dermatol Venereol Leprol 1997;63:11-4.
13. Malakar S, Dhar S. Treatment of stable and recalcitrant vitiligo by autologous miniature punch grafting: a prospective study of 1,000 patients. Dermatology. 1999;198:133-9.
14. Skouge JW, Morison WL, Diwan RV, et al. Autografting and PUVA. A combination therapy for vitiligo. Dermatol Surg Oncol. 1992;18:357-60.
15. Hann SK, Im S, Bong HW, et al. Treatment of stable vitiligo with autologous epidermal grafting and PUVA. J Am Acad Dermatol. 1995;32:943-8.
16. Lahiri K, Malakar S, Sarma N, et al. Repigmentation of vitiligo with punch grafting and narrow-band UV-B (311 nm—a prospective study. Int J Dermatol. 2006;45:649-55.
17. Malakar S, Lahiri K. Spontaneous repigmentation in vitiligo: why it is important. Int J Dermatol. 2006;45:478-9.
18. Lahiri K, Malakar S. The concept of stability of vitiligo. In: Gupta S, Olsson MJ, Kanwar AJ, Ortonne JP (Eds). Surgical Management of Vitiligo. 1st ed. Oxford: Blackwell Publishing; 2007. pp. 49-55.
19. Malakar S. Lahiri K. Minigrafting for vitiligo. In: Gupta S, Olsson MJ, Kanwar AJ, Ortonne JP (Eds). Surgical Management of Vitiligo. 1st ed. Oxford: Blackwell Publishing; 2007. pp. 87-95.

20. Lahiri K. Stability in vitiligo? what's that? J Cutan Aesthet Surg. 2009;2:38-40.
21. Gupta S, Jain VK, Saraswat PK. Suction blister epidermal grafting versus punch skin grafting in recalcitrant and stable vitiligo. Dermatol Surg. 1999;25:955-8.
22. Hanumanthaiah HC. Suction blister roof grafting. In: Mysore V. (Ed). ACS(I) Textbook on Cutaneous and Aesthetic Surgery. 1st ed. New Delhi: Jaypee Medical Brothers (P) Ltd; 2012. pp. 344-50.
23. Khunger N, Kathuria SD, Ramesh V. Tissue grafts in vitiligo surgery—past, present, and future. Indian J Dermatol. 2009;54:150-8.
24. Savant SS. Surgical therapy of vitiligo: current status. Indian J Dermatol Venereol Leprol 2005;71:307-10.
25. Khunger N. Recent advances in the surgical treatment of vitiligo. In: Ghosh S. (Ed). In Recent Advances in Dermatology. Vol 2. New Delhi: Jaypee Medical Brothers (P) Ltd; 2007. pp. 319-40.
26. Falabella R. History and chronology of development of surgical therapies for vitiligo. In: Gupta S, Olsson MS, Kanwar AJ, Ortonne JP (Eds). Surgical Management of Vitiligo. 1st ed. Massachusetts, USA: Blackwell Publishing; 2007. pp. 41-8.
27. Behl PN. Treatment of vitiligo with homologous thin Thiersch grafts. Curr Med Pract. 1964;8:218-21.
28. Kahn A, Cohen M. Vitiligo: Treatment by dermabrasion and epithelial sheet grafting. J Am Acad Dermatol. 1995;33:646-8.
29. Kahn AM, Cohen MJ. Repigmentation in vitiligo patients: melanocyte transfer via ultra-thin grafts. Dermatol Surg. 1998;24:365-8.
30. Olsson MJ, Juhlin L. Epidermal sheet grafts for repigmentation of vitiligo and piebaldism, with a review of surgical techniques. Acta Derm Venereol. 1997;77:463-6.
31. Mutalik S, Ginzburg A. Surgical management of stable vitiligo: a review with personal experience. Dermatol Surg. 2000;26:248-54.
32. Falabella R, Escobar C, Borrero I. Treatment of refractory and stable vitiligo by transplantation of in vitro cultured epidermal autografts bearing melanocytes. J Am Acad Dermatol. 1992;26(2 Pt 1):230-6.
33. Falabella R, Arrunategui A, Barona MI, et al. The minigrafting test for vitiligo: detection of stable lesions for melanocyte transplantation. J Am Acad Dermatol. 1995;32:228-32.
34. Khunger N, Kandhari K. Thin split thickness skin grafting for vitiligo. In: Mysore V. (Ed). ACS(I) Textbook on Cutaneous and Aesthetic Surgery. 1st ed. New Delhi: Jaypee Medical Brothers (P) Ltd; 2012. pp. 351-59.
35. T Salim. Surgical management of vitiligo. In: Lahiri K, Chatterjee M, Sarkar R. (Eds). Pigmentary Disorders: A Comprehensive Compendium. 1st ed. New Delhi: Jaypee Medical Brothers (P) Ltd; 2014. pp. 227-40.
36. Lahiri K. Evolution and evaluation of autologous mini punch grafting in vitiligo. Indian J Dermatol. 2009;54: 159-67.

CHAPTER 17

Modifications of Tissue Grafting Techniques for Vitiligo

Debjit Kar

SUCTION BLISTER GRAFTING[1]

Site selection: The donor site selected is either the medial upper arm, flexor aspect of the forearm,[2] or the thigh and gluteal area. Take donor blister from a more cosmetically acceptable area (the author's choice being anterolateral aspect of thigh, because of easier accessibility, large area available and postoperative convenience for the patient).

Choice of anesthesia: Again, the choice depends on the operating surgeon. We can use topical anesthesia, local anesthesia or no anesthesia at all. Topical anesthesia (Prilocaine plus lignocaine), is applied simultaneously on the donor and recipient area as a uniform thick paste (Fig. 17.1). This saves time and obviates the need for local anesthesia before dermabrasion of the recipient area. The author uses a combination of local and topical anesthesia when large number of lesions or a giga session is planned. A 23 G spinal needle can be used alternatively to give field block with a mixture of lignocaine and bupivacaine (1:1), to anesthetize large area in giga sessions.

Inducing Blisters: Prolonged suction causes a column of negative pressure, resulting in a split at the dermoepidermal junction, and blister formation. In the modified syringe-assisted technique, a 20 mL syringe, with its piston removed, is inverted and a 3-way connector is attached at the needle end. Negative pressure of about 300 to 400 mm Hg, monitored by a pressure gauge, is created by aspiration of air with a 50 mL syringe.[4] Alternatively this pressure is achieved approximately by giving a suction upto 30 mL to 40 mL in 50 mL syringes.[3] The required suction pressure to form a blister varies with the age of the patient, varying between 500 mm Hg in adolescents to 400 mm Hg in adults and 300 mm Hg in an elderly patient.[4] We have to keep checking the formation of vesicles (before formation of blisters) (Fig. 17.2).

Suction is maintained until a single blister of sufficient size is formed or few vesicles form (approx 50 to 70% of the area), which is the end point. Multiple syringes can be used, depending on the size of graft needed. The time taken for blister formation depends on the site of donor area, diameter of the suction syringe, temperature of the site, and the negative pressure obtained. In general, a 20 mL syringe, with a negative suction pressure of –400 mm Hg (equivalent to 38.4 ± 6.7 mL in a 50 mL syringe- withdraw the piston of 50 mL syringe up to 30 mL to 40 mL mark), results in blister formationin about 1 to 2 hours.

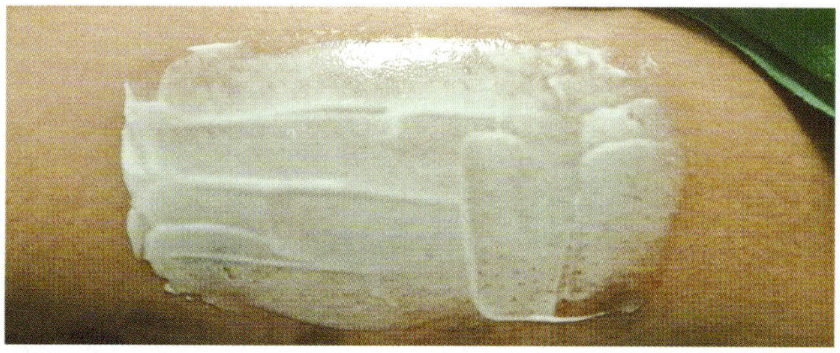

Fig. 17.1: Thick uniform layer of topical anesthesia on donor and recipient site before start of procedure.

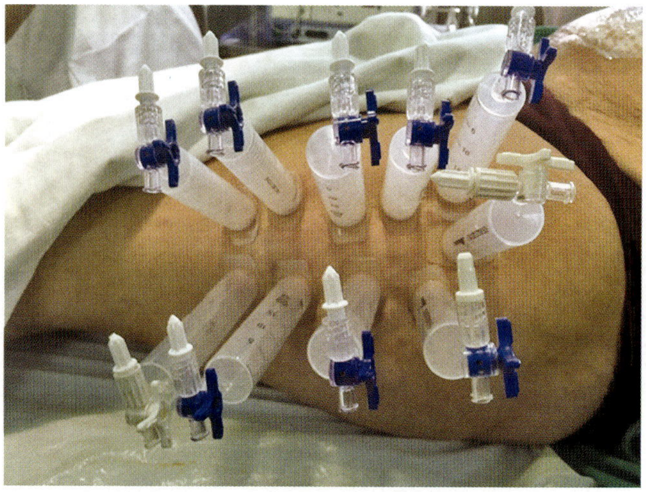

Fig. 17.2: 20 mL syringes with 3-way connector placed on donor site with negative pressure to induce blisters.

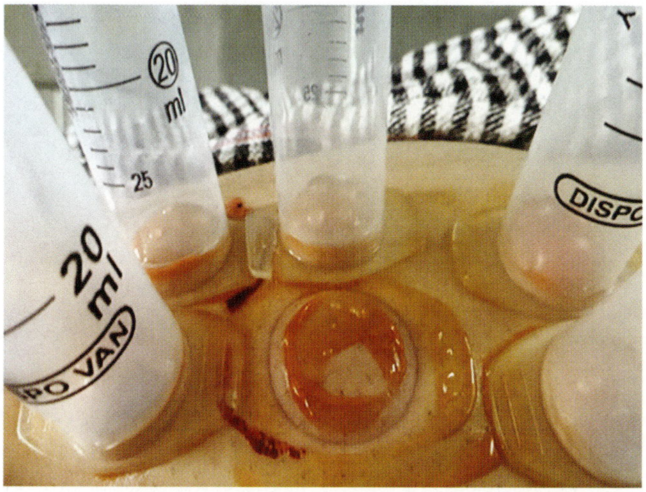

Fig. 17.3: The on-off technique: Removing the syringe without or less vesicle formation and replacing it at the same position with higher pressure.

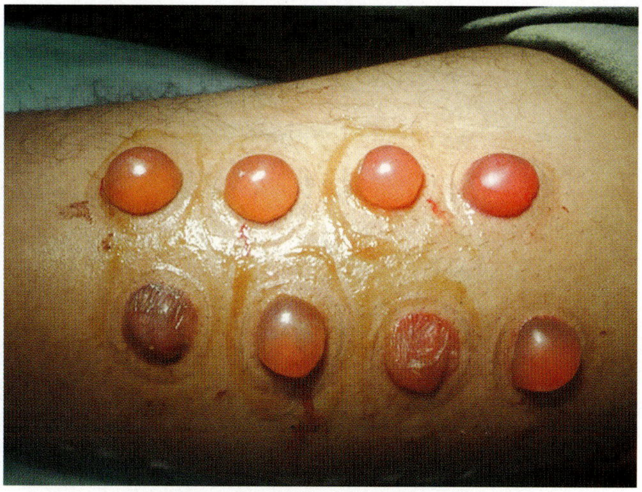

Fig. 17.4: Well-formed blisters.

Troubleshooting

Nonformation of Blisters and Vesicles

To avoid such a situation, use in and out technique, and frequent monitoring. Sometimes there is no formation of blister in one or more suction cups, even after few hours. Check whether you are getting enough pressure while pulling the piston. If not, there can be air leakage at the following points: (1) base of suction pressure: tell your assistant to give firm downward pressure and seal the base with petroleum jelly, (2) 3-way cannula: check for any cracks and never reuse a 3-way cannula, and (3) pressure release at the rubber seal of the piston of 50 mL syringe: in such a case discard the syringe and use a new one.

On-off technique (author's own): 1 or 2 suction cups may not form vesicles or blisters or may lag behind. In such cases, just release the pressure from the 3-way connector. Remove the syringe and replace it at the same place with 5 to 10 mL, higher pressure. This can also be done for suction cups with very small vesicles, just remove and replace with higher pressure (Fig. 17.3).

Reducing the time of blister formation: Various methods have been used to reduce the time of blister formation, as this is the main limiting factor in suction blister grafting. A hair dryer, room heater all have been used in the past by various workers to decrease the time of blister formation. The author prefers a simple inexpensive way of giving subcutaneous injection of 5 mL normal saline, every 10 minutes right underneath the suction cups (subcutaneous) which leads to blister formation within 1 to 1.5 hours (Fig. 17.4).

Occasional hemorrhagic blisters may be formed which does not affect the final results.

Handling of Grafts

The periphery of the blister is then cut with fine iris scissors, a sterile glass slide is placed coated with paraffin, on the blister, and the graft is then gently everted onto the glass slide (preferably near one edge for easy maneuverability in graft placement) with the help of a fine forceps, with the dermal side facing upwards. Other workers have suggested other means of graft cutting and placement on recipient area, i.e. cutting the graft and placement on gloved finger of the operating surgeon.[5] The graft can be rolled on to a 5 mL syringe with dermal side upwards and rolled back on to the recipient area, so that the dermal side faces down. Alternatively, the paper that sandwiches the sterile petrolatum-soaked gauze (which is used for dressing the donor site) can be used. Press the sticky surface of the paper on the donor graft site to transfer the blister roof to the paper. The blister roof along with the paper can be easily cut with surgical scissors to obtain linear or any other desirable shape of grafts, which is otherwise difficult on a glass slide (Fig. 17.5).[6]

Recipient Site

The recipient site is prepared by denuding the area by dermabrasion using a high-speed motor-driven dermabrader with a diamond fraise. A manual dermabrader

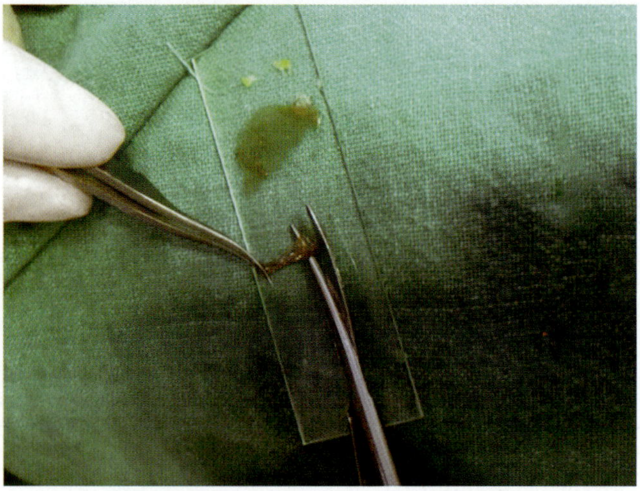

Fig. 17.5: Resizing graft on glass slide.

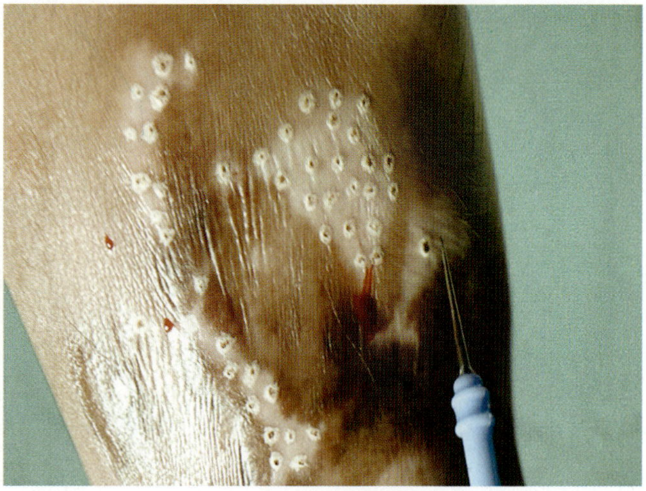

Fig. 17.6: Fulguration of recipient site before dermabrasion.

may also be used, though it is time-consuming, especially in dorsum of hands and feet. A radiofrequency cauterization machine can be used in such difficult areas. Multiple fulguration points (Fig. 17.6) at a very low power setting (to avoid damaging the dermis) can be done before starting motorized or manual dermabrasion, which hastens the process and makes the process much easier especially with manual dermabraders (so that beginners need not invest in a costly laser machine before starting suction blister grafting!!!).

The end-point of dermabrasion is the appearance of pinpoint bleeding. Other modalities such as erbium:yttrium-aluminium-garnet (Er:YAG) laser or CO_2 laser have also been used to denude the recipient area (makes thing really simple but for the inhibitory costs!!!). Whatever the method the recipient area should be dermabraded 0.5 cm beyond the depigmented area to take care of postoperative perigraft halo. The author prefers giving radial tangential slits, at the periphery of grafts to prevent graft folding, increasing surface area and preventing perigraft halo (Fig. 17.7).

Transfer of Grafts to Recipient Site

The grafts are transferred onto the recipient site by everting the slide and maneuvering the graft with the dermal side down. The author prefers leaving the grafts for 5 to 10 minutes (along with maintaining hydration), allowing the graft to adhere to the recipient bed with the serous oozing from the recipient site, avoiding the use of tissue glue. Tissue glue at the edges may be used in mobile area (e.g. breast, penis, mouth) and dressed with a nonadherent dressing.

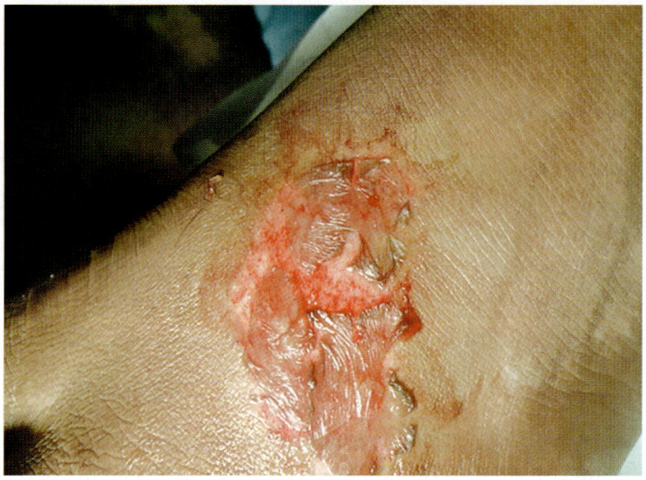

Fig. 17.7: Radial tangential slits to prevent graft folding at margin and postoperative perigraft halo.

Maintaining intraoperative hydration of placed grafts to prevent desiccation cannot be overemphasized (especially in giga sessions), by simply sprinkling few drops of normal saline intermittently on all grafted areas.

Dressing

The author prefers a *3 layer* dressing. The first layer: a gauze impregnated with Soframycin or paraffin, the second layer of moist gauze, third layer of dry gauze. This helps in maintaining postoperative hydration and better graft survival. Bandaging is done with a Dynaplast. The bandage is removed on day 5 (as melanocyte migration takes 48–72 hours).

Repigmentation takes about 2 to 3 months with or without medical line of treatment.

CONCLUSION

Excellent repigmentation, lesser learning curve, minimum chances of complication and being one of the most economical options, suction blister grafting still continues to be a excellent surgical modality for vitiligo surgeons, in the era of cellular grafting.

REFERENCES

1. Li J, Fu WW, Zheng ZZ, et al. Suction blister epidermal grafting using a modified suction method in the treatment of stable vitiligo: a retrospective study. Dermatol Surg. 2011;37: 999-1006.
2. Laxmisha C, Thappa DM. Reliable site for suction induction and harvesting. Indian J Dermatol Venerol Leprol. 2005; 71:321-4.
3. Gupta S, Shroff S, Gupta S. Modified technique of suction blistering for epidermal grafting. Int J Dermatol. 1999;38: 306-9.
4. Khunger N, Lahiri K, Mysore V. Vitiligo surgery: Surgery of the skin. Robinson JK, Hanke CW, Siegel DM, Fratila, editors. 3rd Edn. Elsivier Saunders. 2015;688-701.
5. Laxmisha C, Thappa DM. Surgical Pearl Gloved finger as a transport platform for epidermal graft of suction blister. J Am Acad Dermatol. 2007;57:S118-9.
6. Ashique KT, Srinivas CR. Resizing blister roof grafts for vitiligo surgeries. J Am Acad Dermatol. 2014;71:e39-40.

CHAPTER 18

Cellular Grafting Techniques

Somesh Gupta, Suman Patra, Debdeep Mitra, Akshi Bansal

INTRODUCTION

Vitiligo is a common acquired depigmenting disorder characterized by, the presence of depigmented or white patches, and histologically by complete or near complete absence of functional melanocytes in affected areas. Notably, it is a disease of cosmetic concern with much social stigma.

Both surgical and nonsurgical therapies have been employed in the management of vitiligo. Surgical methods are useful when the disease is recalcitrant to medical therapies and stable for at least 1 to 2 years.

Vitiligo surgery has reached an interesting stage in its development where apart from patients with vitiligo being treated surgically, a wise decision should be taken as to which patients, at what stage of their disease, and by which techniques have to be operated. The progressive development from one technique to another is always in search for the best outcome.

PRINCIPLES OF CELLULAR GRAFTING FOR VITILIGO IN BRIEF

Principle of surgical technique is to introduce melanocytes into the lesional skin, which will then establish and function as an epidermal melanin unit, so as to produce repigmentation of vitiligo lesion. Although tissue grafts are the mainstay of treatment for vitiligo at present, they have a number of disadvantages. Therefore, various cellular grafting techniques have been introduced to overcome this. In cellular grafting techniques, either noncultured or cultured cell suspensions of melanocytes or both melanocytes and keratinocytes are transferred to the lesional skin in place of whole tissue. It helps to cover larger recipient areas due to spreadability of the suspension.The donor: recipient ratio is much larger than tissue grafts.Therefore in cultured suspensions, the donor melanocyte number can be exponentially expanded to cover areas several times the donor area. Application of the cell suspension is much easier when compared to application of grafts, especially in difficult to treat areas such as ear, umbilicus, genitals, etc. It has been suggested that necessity for immobilization is less in the case of cellular grafts. Postoperative color match is excellent, blending of treated area with surrounding normal skin is better than other procedures. The small area of the donor harvesting reduces much of the postoperative pain and morbidity.

PRINCIPLE FOR USING HAIR FOLLICLE AS SOURCE OF MELANOCYTES

Follicular melanocytes are functionally and morphologically of 2 different types: pigmented melanocytes present in infundibulum and the bulb, and amelanotic melanocytes present in the outer root sheath (ORS) of middle and lower hair follicles.

The outer root sheath and bulge areas of the hair follicle contain amelanotic, DOPA-negative "inactive" melanocytes (proposed to be melanocyte stem cells), these ORS melanocytes are mainly responsible for pigmentation of hair. They also serve as the reservoir of epidermal melanocytes during re-epithelialization following the loss of epidermis and for re-pigmentation in vitiligo. These cells divide and migrate upward along surface of hair follicle, to nearby epidermis where they move radially and lead to repigmentation of the surrounding skin. The finding that not only did melanocytes reside in hair follicles but could also, in addition, migrate to surrounding skin was another landmark observation. These findings suggested that inactive melanocytes in the ORS of the hair follicle could be potentially harvested and cultivated for therapeutic purposes in vitiligo.

Follicular melanocytes are more active, but only during anagen phase (cyclical activity).They are larger, having more dendrites and more number of melanosomes, more extensive Golgi and endoplasmic reticulum. It also has greater melanocyte to keratinocyte ratio 1:1 to 1:6 compared to 1: 36 in epidermis.

TYPES OF CELLULAR GRAFTING TECHNIQUES

Cellular grafting techniques described till now are:

- Noncultured cell suspensions:
  - Epidermal/basal cell rich suspensions
  - Follicular (EHF-ORS-CS = extracted hair follicle outer root sheath cell suspension) suspensions.
- Cultured melanocyte/keratinocyte grafts:
  - Epidermal (melanocyte/keratinocyte) grafts
  - Follicular-based grafts.

Procedure of cellular grafting technique composed of:

- Harvesting of graft
- Preparation of suspension
- Preparation of recipient area
- Transfer of suspension to recipient area.

We will be discussing all the procedures in these headings.

Basic Requirements

- Laminar flow hood (if the procedure is done in aseptic operating room, this may not be needed) (Fig. 18.1).
- Incubator to maintain temperature and 5% CO_2 (ordinary incubator is a good economic replacement of this) (Fig. 18.2).
- DMEM medium (Dulbecco's modified eagle medium) (Fig. 18.3).
- Trypsin-ethylenediaminetetraacetic acid (EDTA) solution [0.25% trypsin and 0.02% EDTA] solution (Fig. 18.4)
- Phosphate buffered saline (Fig. 18.5)
- Centrifugation machine (Fig. 18.6)
- Petri-dishes (Fig. 18.7).

Noncultured Epidermal Suspension

1. About one-tenth the size of the recipient area is selected as the donor site. Hairy skin over the lateral side of the thigh is preferred. The donor area is cleansed, shaved and anesthetized with 2% lignocaine (Figs. 18.8 and 18.9). A split-thickness skin graft is taken with the help of a shaving blade and straight artery forceps (Figs. 18.10A to C). Other instruments like Humby's knife can also be used.

   The skin specimen is transferred under aseptic conditions to a container with normal saline or DMEM

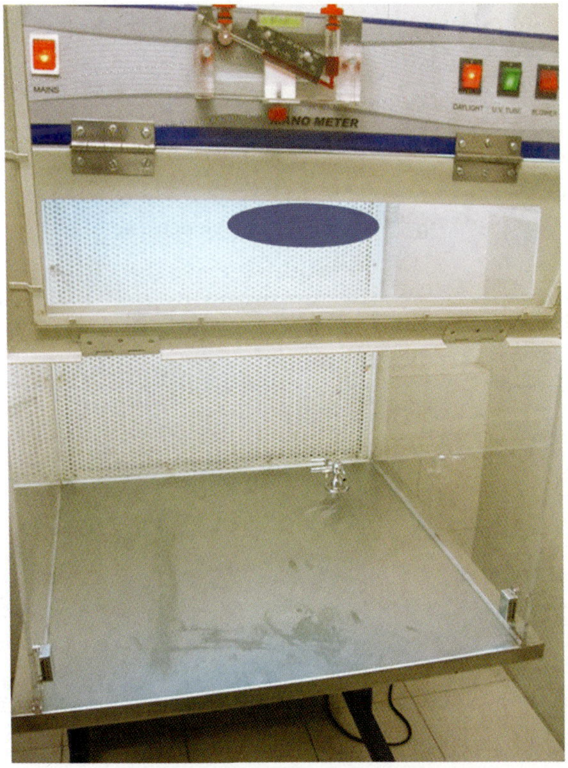

Fig.18.1: Laminar flow hood.

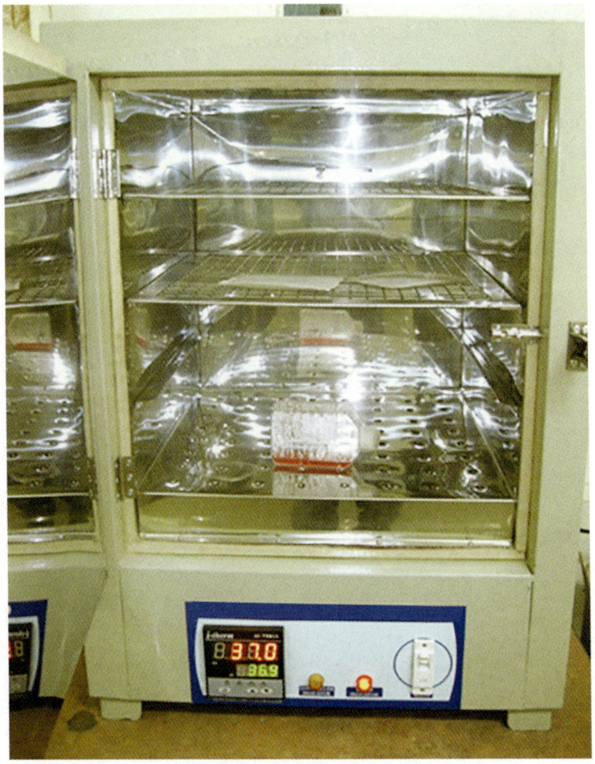

Fig.18.2: Incubator.

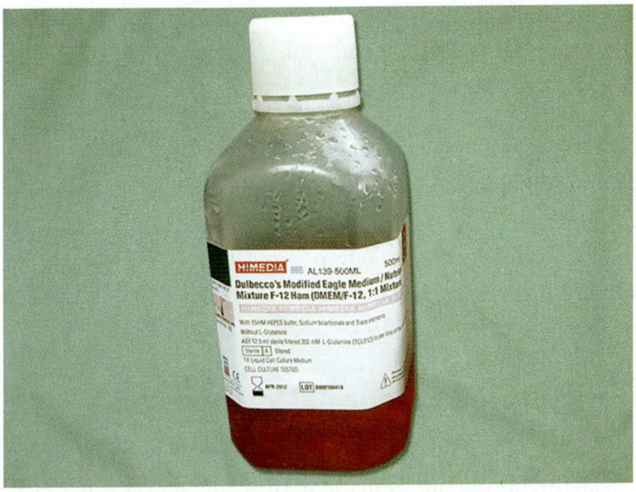

Fig.18.3: DMEM medium (Dulbecco's modified eagle medium).

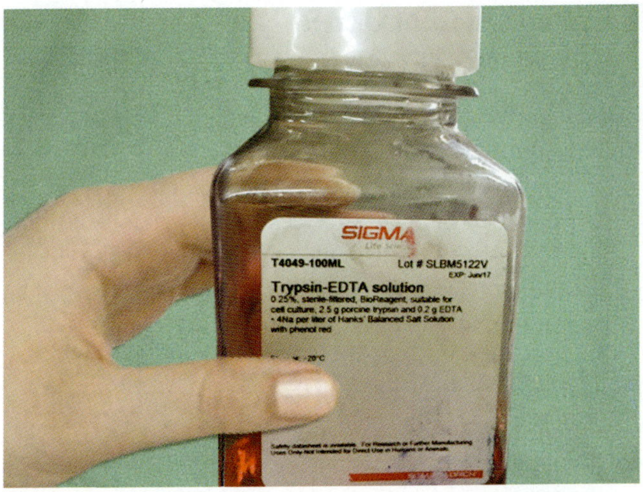

Fig.18.4: Trypsin–ethylenediaminetetraacetic acid (EDTA) solution (0.25% trypsin and 0.02% EDTA) solution.

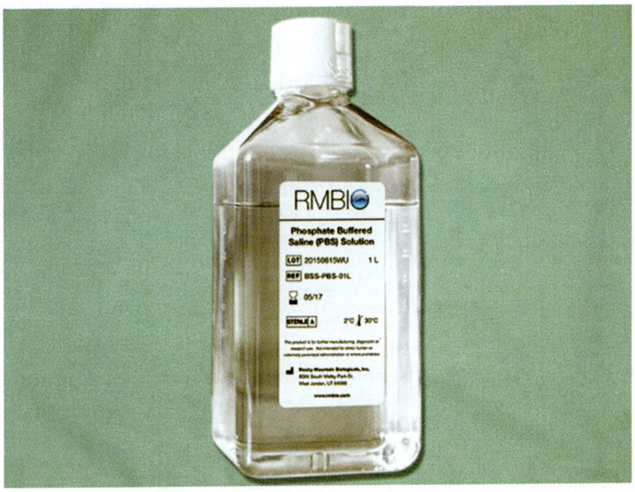

Fig.18.5: Phosphate buffered saline.

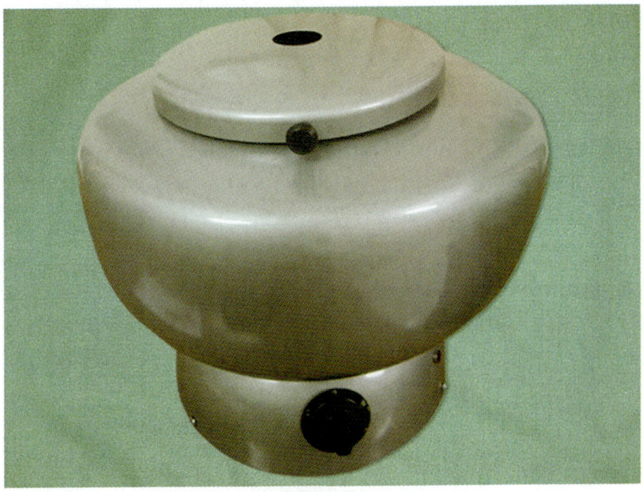

Fig.18.6: Centrifugation machine.

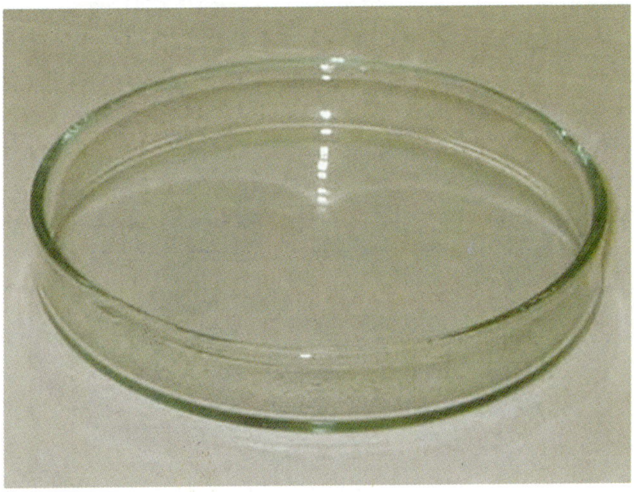

Fig.18.7: Petri dish.

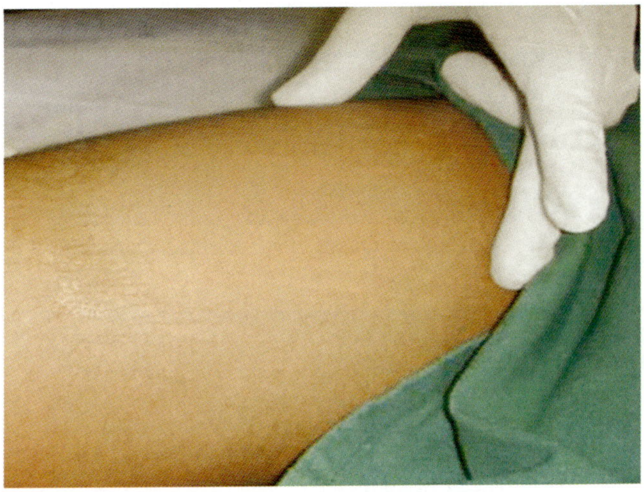

Fig.18.8: Donor area is cleansed and shaved.

medium and transferred to the laboratory (Figs. 18.11A and B).

2. The graft is transferred to a Petri dish where trypsin-ethylenediaminetetraacetic acid (EDTA) solution (0.25% trypsin and 0.02% EDTA) is added and incubated at 37° with 5% CO_2 for 45 minutes. The time of incubation varies in each individual case, depending on the thickness of the graft and the activity of the enzyme (Fig. 18.12).

   After incubation, the trypsin/EDTA solution is removed and 3 mL (15°C) of 0.5 mg/mL trypsin inhibitor in PBS or PBS alone is added to the Petri dish to terminate the trypsin reaction.

   The epidermis is removed from the dermis with the help of one curved fine pointed forceps and one straight fine-pointed forceps (Figs. 18.13A to C), and the epidermal parts are transferred to a test tube containing

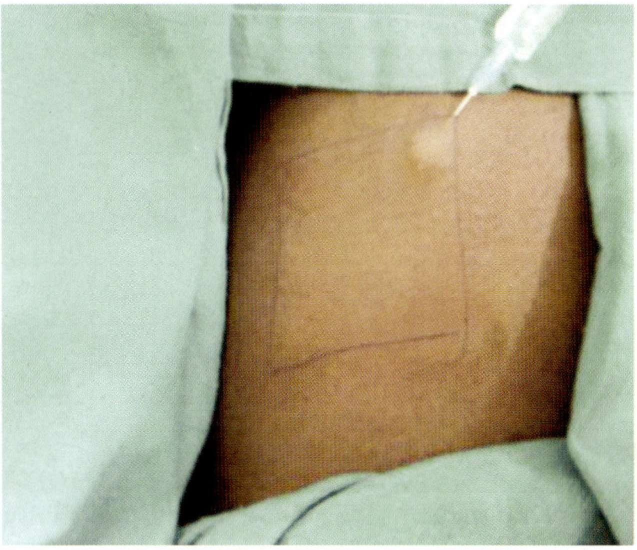

Fig.18.9: Donor area infiltrated with 2% lignocaine.

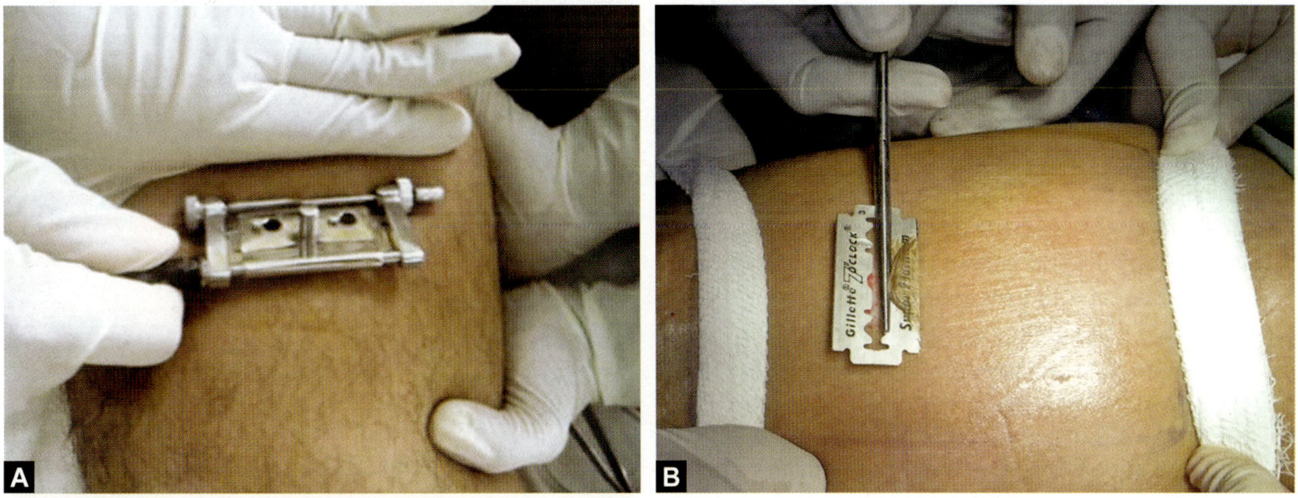

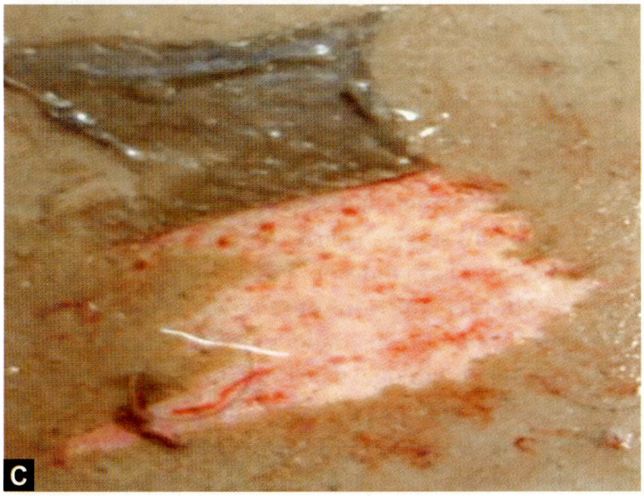

Figs.18.10A to C: Obtaining a split thickness graft.

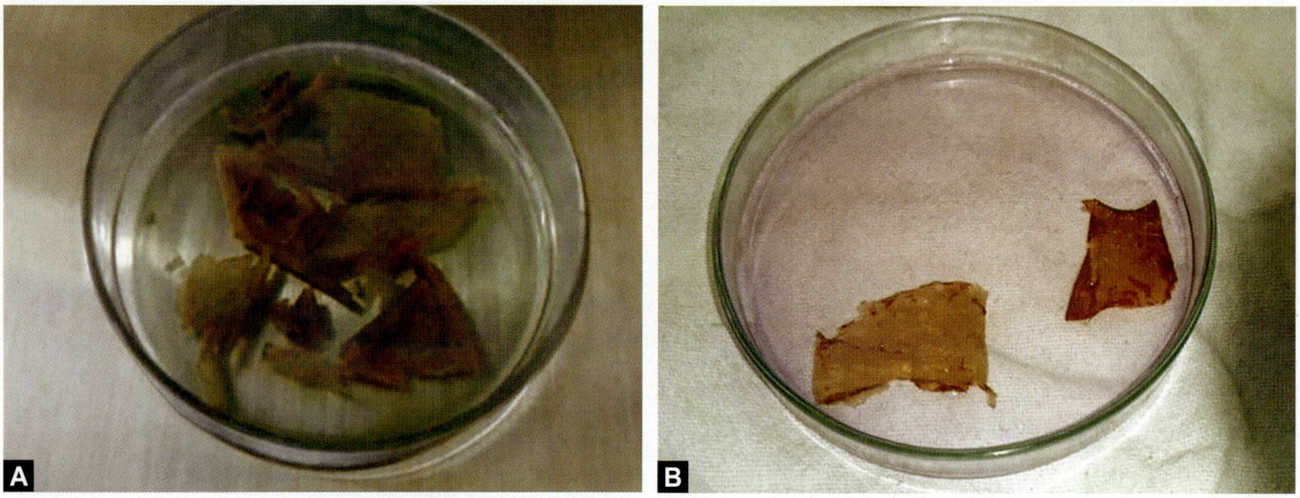

Figs.18.11A and B: (A) Skin grafts transferred to DMEM media with epidermal surface floating upwards. (B) NCES graft in trypsin EDTA.

5 mL of Dulbecco's modified eagle medium and vortex mixed (a form of rigorous mechanical separation) for 15 seconds.The dermal pieces are then removed with the tip of a Pasteur pipette or with the help of a hooked forceps and discarded (Fig. 18.14).

The basal cell layer side of the epidermal pieces is scraped with a curved jeweller's forceps to free the cells and the pieces are then minced to smaller fragments. The remaining epidermal fragments, now mainly consisting of stratum corneum and stratum granulosum, are removed from the test tube and discarded.

The rich cell containing solution in the Petri dish is transferred to the test-tube, the Petri dish is then rinsed twice with a small volume of DMEM or PBS, which is also transferred to the test tube, gently mixed with a pipette. Sometimes it may be difficult to pellet the cells due to free DNA and collagen, which form mucous-like structures. In such cases, the contents of the test tube should be run up and down a few times in a Pasteur pipette with sharp glass-edge. This will cut the mucous into shorter fragments which will facilitate the formation of a pellet when centrifuged.

The suspension is then centrifuged at 78 g for 5 minutes. The supernatant is then discarded and the pellet, containing cells from the stratum basale and the lower half of the stratum spinosum, which are rich in melanocytes, is taken (Fig. 18.15).

Around 0.5 to 2 mL of PBS or DMEM according to recipient area is added to the pellet of melanocytes to make a suspension of noncultured epidermal cells.

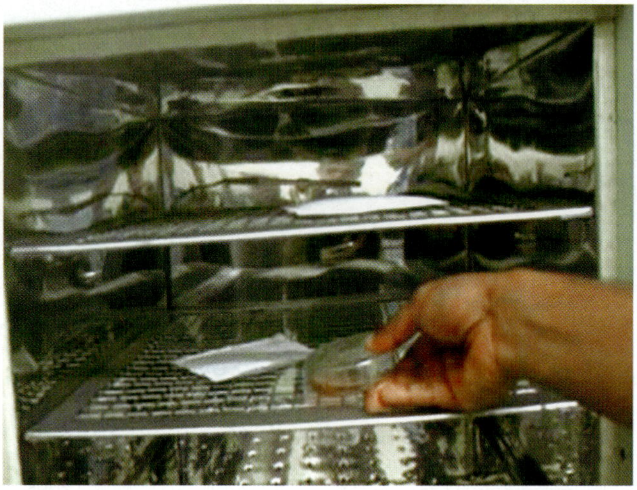

Fig.18.12: Sample incubated at 37°C for 1 hour in trypsin EDTA solution.

Avoid larger volumes because of the risk that the cells will float out onto the sides of the lesion. If found necessary, it is much easier in a later stage to add some more medium to the tube/syringe to produce right viscosity, or be able to cover an extensive area.

3. Shave the recipient site, clean with povidone-iodine solution and surgical spirit and anaesthetize with 2% lignocaine. Dermabrasion is done using a motorized dermabrader until the punctate bleeding is seen. Dermabrasion is extended 5 mm beyond the margins to prevent perilesional halo (Figs. 18.16A and B).
4. The NCES is carefully transferred to recipient site with a tuberculin syringe and 18-gauge needle (Figs. 18.17A and B).

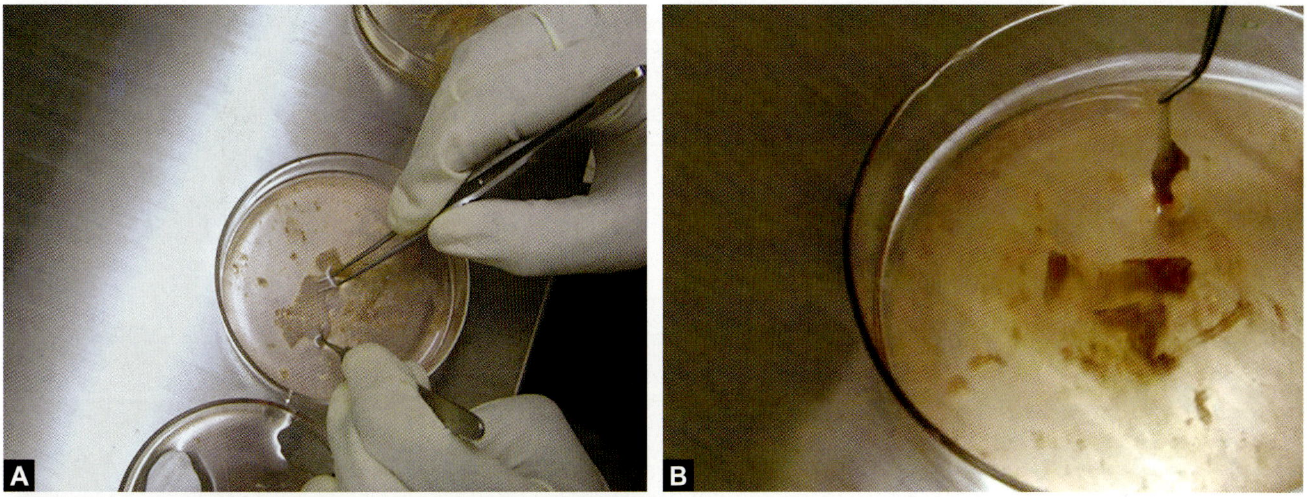

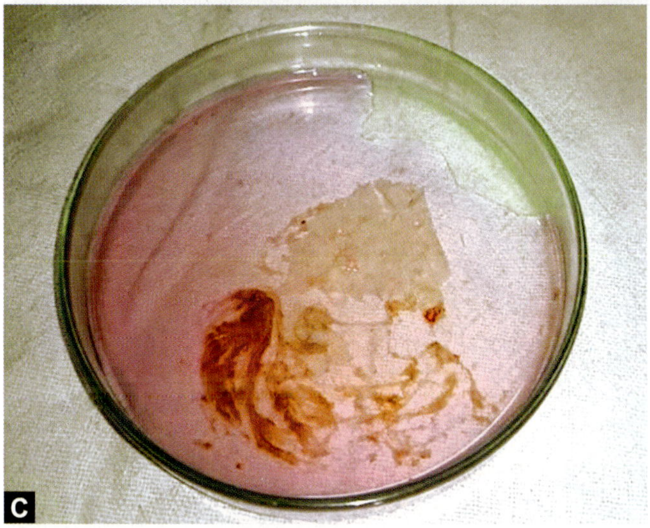

Figs.18.13A to C: (A and B) Epidermis is removed from the dermis. (C) NCES graft post teasing.

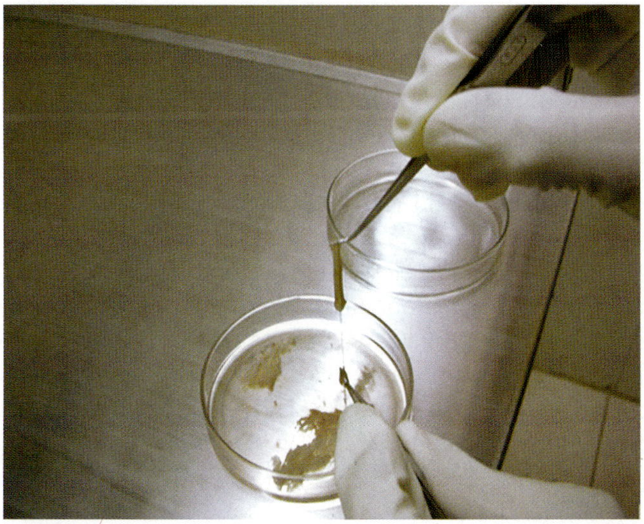

Fig.18.14: Discarding the unwanted epidermal and dermal parts.

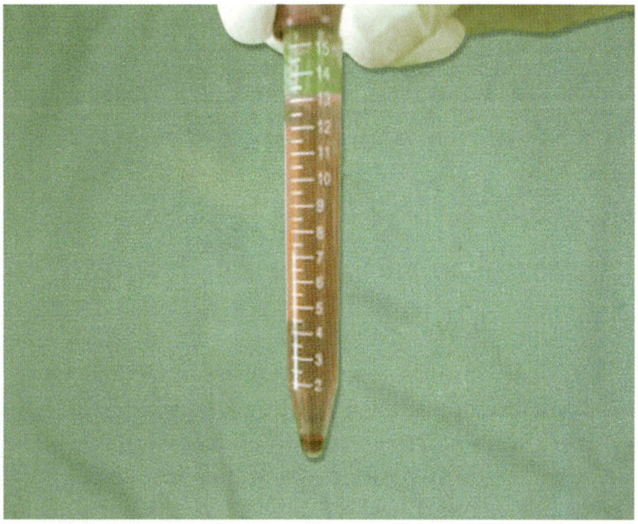

Fig.18.15: Obtaining a cell pellet after centrifugation.

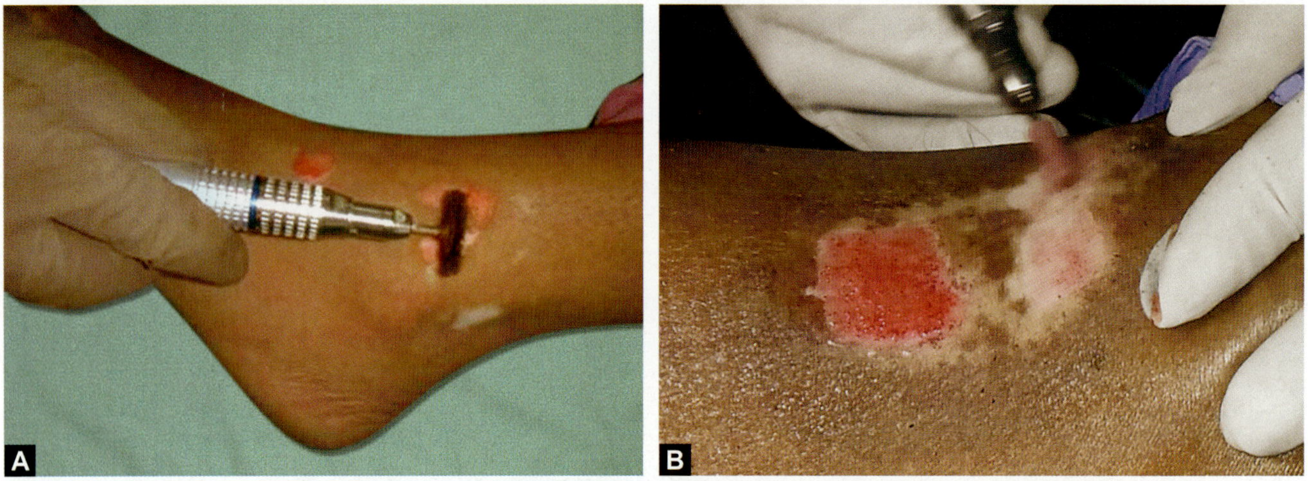

Figs.18.16A and B: (A) Dermabrasion of the recipient area. (B) Dermabrasion— preparation of the recipient site using cylindrical burr.

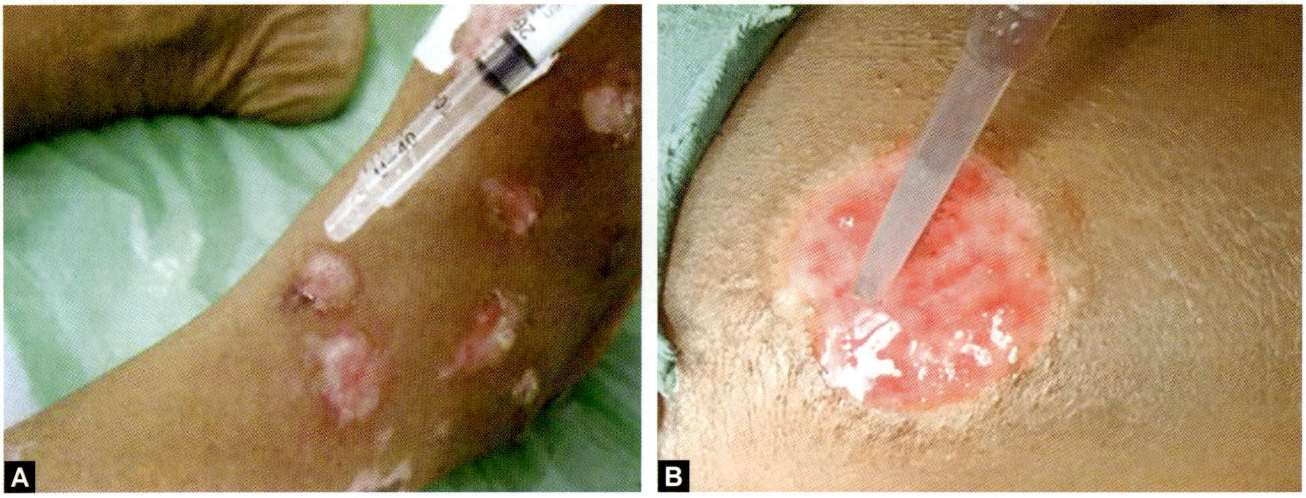

Figs.18.17A and B: (A) NCES is transferred to the recipient site. (B) Spreading suspension in NCES.

A three layered dressing consisting of dry collagen sheet (Neuskin-F), Vaseline-chlorhexidine gauze, and sterile surgical pad is placed over recipient site (Figs. 18.18 and 18.19).

Modifications of NCES Technique

- *Cold trypsinization*: Treatment at high trypsin concentrations at 37°C followed by vigorous agitationleads to complete separation of epidermis. However, this leads to lower number of intact cells which exhibit numerous vacuoles throughout the cytoplasm. Whereas mild trypsinization of the epidermis with or without EDTA at low enzyme concentration and 4°C produces an incomplete dissociation, thereby giving higher yield of single viable cells. The beneficial effect of this can be explained by the fact that endocytotic uptake of the trypsin is negligible at 4°C, whereas at 37°C trypsin taken up persists in cells for up to 48 hours.
- Hyaluronic acid (HA) can be used to increase the viscosity of the suspension, it acts as biodegradable cell carrier. HA increases adherence of the cells to grafted surface. This method has been introduced by Van Geel in 2001 (Figs. 18.20A to C).
- Various other modalities have been used for preparation of the recipient site with good result but there is no comparative study.
  - Er : YAG laser
  - Short pulse CO_2 laser

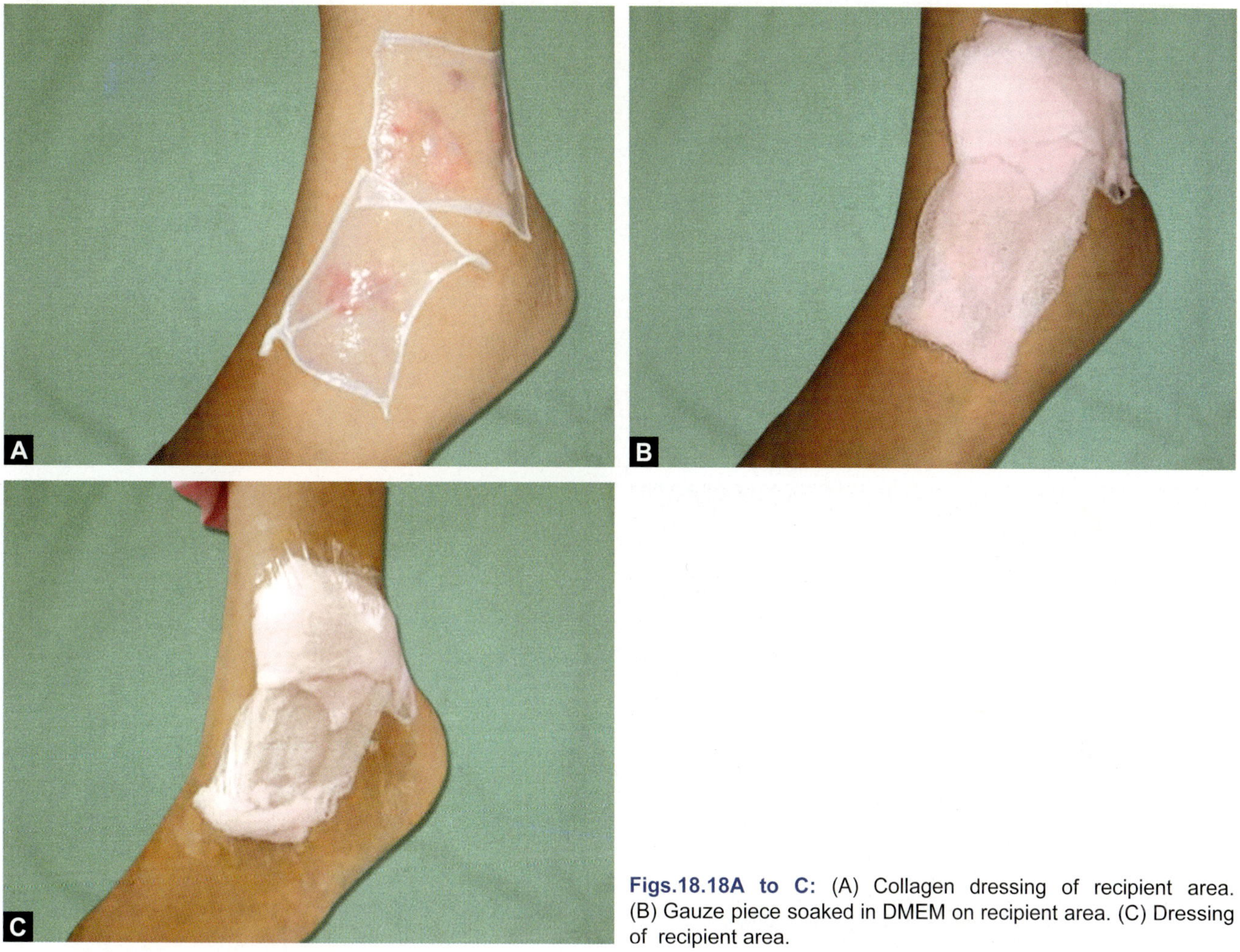

Figs.18.18A to C: (A) Collagen dressing of recipient area. (B) Gauze piece soaked in DMEM on recipient area. (C) Dressing of recipient area.

 - Diathermy
 - Ultrasonic abrasion.

- Enzymes other than trypsin like 0.1 to 0.25% dispase II solution can be used for separation of dermis and epidermis and sample is incubated for 16 to 24 hours at 4°C. Dispase splits epidermis from dermis along basement membrane, thus epidermal stem cells located in the basal layer can be isolated with less loss.
- Various antibiotics and antifungals can be incorporated in DMEM medium to prevent infections.
- Intraepidermal injection of dissociated epidermal cell suspension by Khodadadi et al. Autologous dissociated epidermal cell suspension (110–2,000 cells/mm^2 with approximately 1.5% melanocytes) is prepared. To avoid any side effects of transplantation technique, such as scar formation and Koëbner phenomenon, cells are injected intraepidermally.

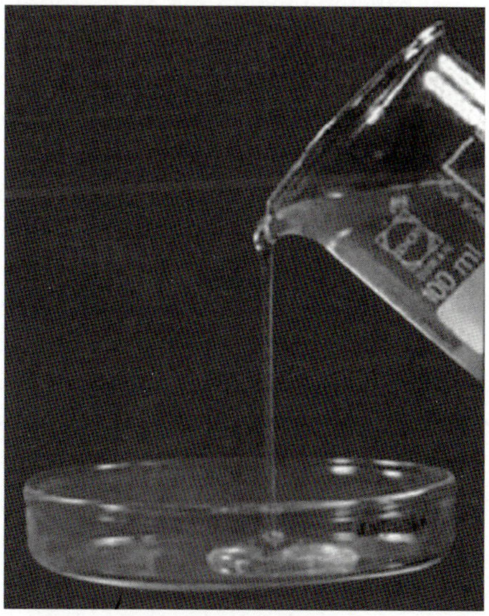

Fig.18.19: Hydroxy methylcellulose gel for viscosity.

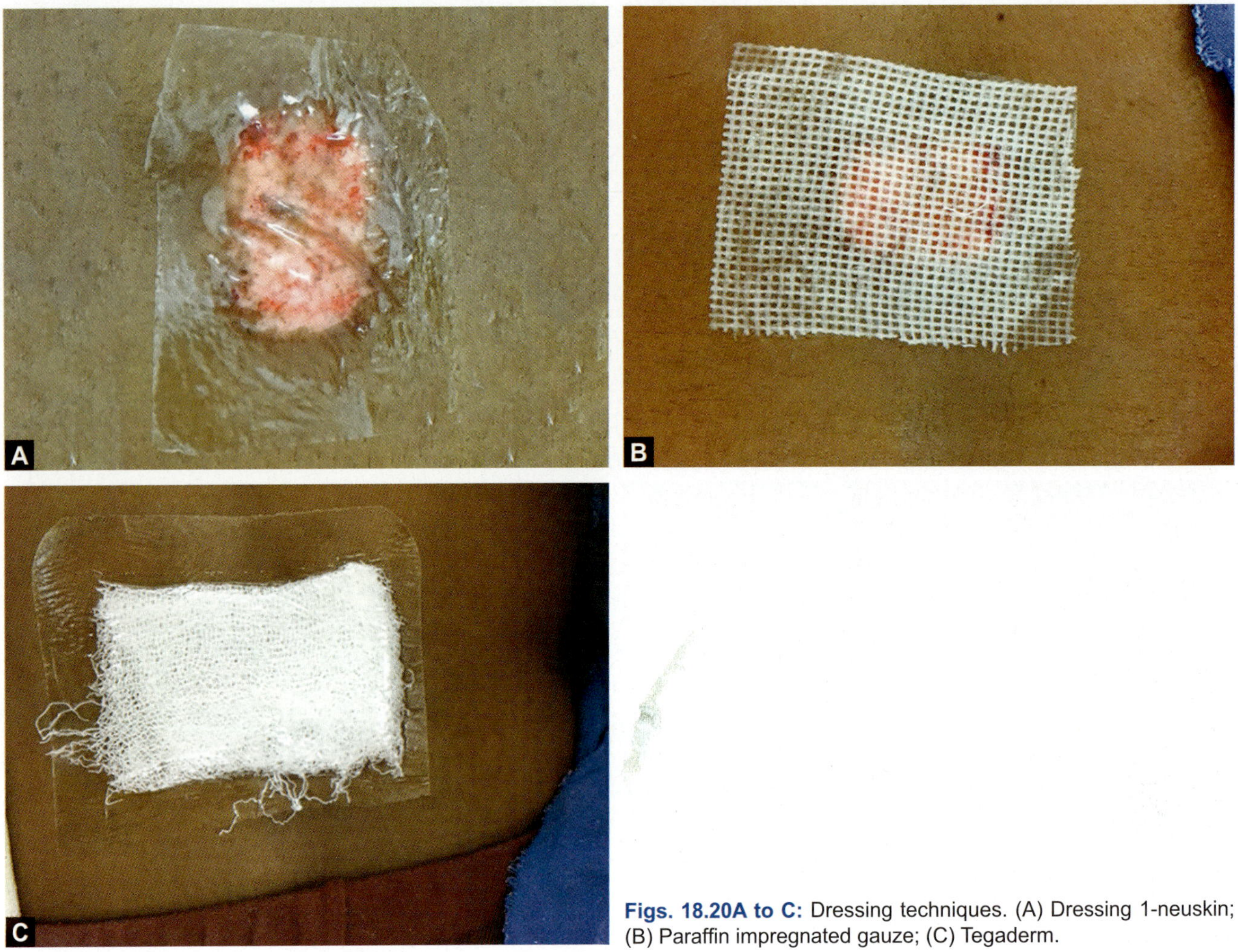

Figs. 18.20A to C: Dressing techniques. (A) Dressing 1-neuskin; (B) Paraffin impregnated gauze; (C) Tegaderm.

- Epidermal brushing technique NCES modification—This is a novel, minimally invasive, scarless technique of harvesting tissue for the noncultured epidermal cell suspension. The donor skin is superficially dermabraded with a manual dermabrader until pinpoint bleeding appears. Discard initial brushings of the superficial horny layers. The remaining epidermal brushings on dermabrader and donor skin are then transferred to sterile test tube, furthur processing in lab is same as that of the NCES. The donor site heals well without scarring or pigmentary changes and can be reused for future harvesting. Epidermal brushings without trypsinization have been used as tissue graft previously in vitiligo, however, pigmentation is cosmetically less satis factory.

Tips to achieve better results in nonculture melanocyte transplant are:

- Ensure that the trypsinization is complete. For this purpose, both the time of incubation and maintenance of a proper temperature in the incubator is important. If trypsinization is not complete, it is better to reincubate the donor graft for some more time. Two types of trypsinization have been described in the literature—cold and hot trypsinization. Though the former is claimed to give a better yield of cellular constituents, the latter is more commonly followed in India as it is less time consuming.
- Ensure that the graft suspension is not too 'fluidy'. Use of hyaluronic acid gels has been recommended in such situations to increase the viscosity or thickness of the graft suspension.
- Spread the solution evenly and uniformly over the dermabraded area to minimize the chances of a non-uniform repigmentation.
- The cellular component in the suspension needs to be maintained at an ideal level to prevent hyper- or hypopigmentation at the recipient area. A donor to

recipient ratio of 1:10 has been considered ideal to prevent this complication but the same is yet to be scientifically validated.

- Use of collagen dressings is also encouraged to improve the pigmentation achieved with the procedure.
- Another way to know the size of the graft needed is to measure the number of melanocytes in the cellular suspension; a count of 210 to 250 cells per mm^2 has been seen to be ideal for the procedure. In study by Sobhy et al transplanted melanocytic cell count/ mm^2 ranged between 210 to 300 cells per mm^2 donor skin graft which was enough to induce repigmentation. Similar results were seen in study conducted by Tegta et al who found that the optimal melanocytes count for repigmentation was 210 to 250 cells/mm^2 donor skin graft.
- The lack of pigmentation at periphery of transplanted skin observed in few patients is due to residual activity of some melanocyte-destroying factors and not due to the technical procedure,.Another hypothesis is that inflow of keratinocytes from the pigmented border does not allow the transplanted pigment cells to remain where they were seeded. This influx of keratinocytes at the margins appear as a white rim which can be treated by extending the dermabrasion beyond lesion boundary or performing another session of transplantation of frozen autologous melanocytes which was not used in first session. Similar observation was noted by Olsson et al who found that the white rim decreased in patients treated with the epithelial sheets compared with those patients treated with the cell free in suspension.

Some more points that can be considered as pearls in this procedure are:

- Use of trypsin inhibitor can be avoided by washing the grafts after trypsinization in DMEM or any other suitable medium twice or thrice. This cuts down the cost of the procedure to a great extent as the most expensive reagent in the whole procedure is the trypsin inhibitor only.
- Even patient's own serum can be used as an alternate to DMEM medium with equally good results. This modification has even been claimed to improve the viscosity of the cellular suspension.

Follicular (EHF-ORS-CS = Extracted Hair Follicle Outer Root Sheath Cell Suspension)

- "Follicular unit extraction" (FUE) is used for obtaining follicular tissue. Trim the hairs to a length of approximately 2 mm (Fig. 18.21A). Field block anesthesia with 2% lignocaine is infiltrated in the skin encircling the area chosen for FUE. To obtain follicular units, a 0.8 to 1 mm punch is rotated in the direction of the hair follicle until it reaches the mid-dermis (Fig. 18.21B). To avoid transection, care is taken not to go into the subcutaneous space of the hair follicle. The follicular unit is then gently pulled out using hair follicle holding forceps by holding the skin surrounding the hair shaft(s). Transected hair follicles are discarded. Depending on there cepient area, approximately 15 to 25 pigmented follicles are extracted per subject

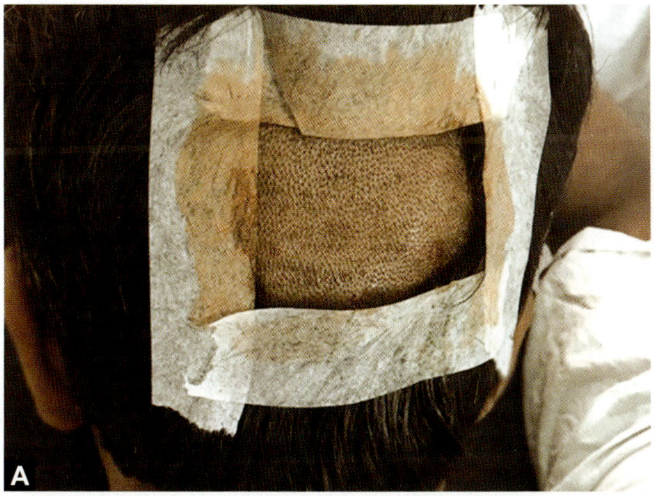

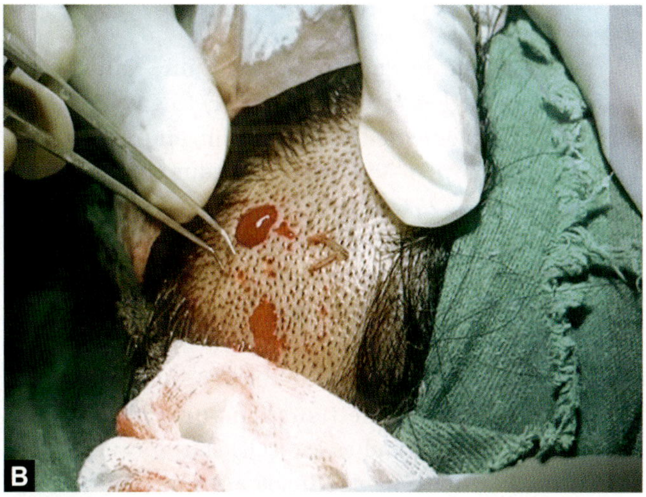

Figs. 18.21A and B: (A) NCFCS donor site. (B) NCFCS—Harvesting the graft (FUE).

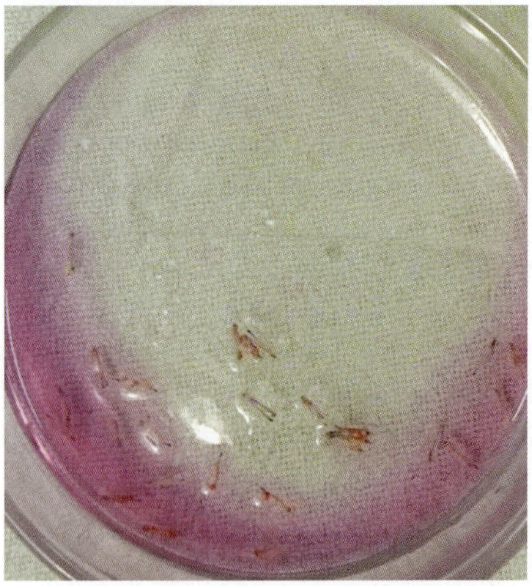

Fig. 18.22: NCFCS graft after 1st incubation in trypsin EDTA.

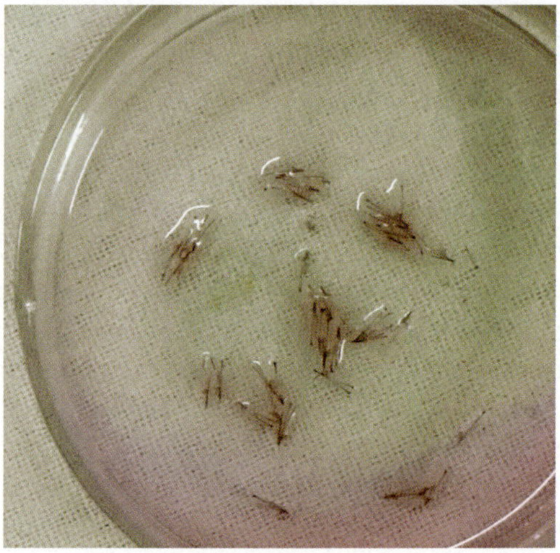

Fig. 18.23: NCFCS graft after 3rd incubation.

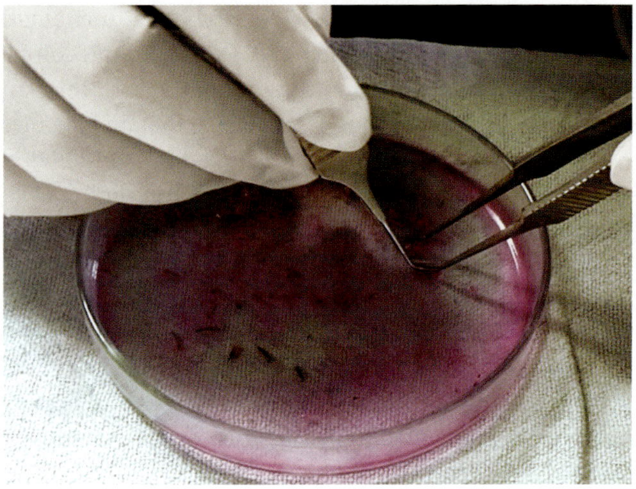

Fig. 18.24: Teasing the hair follicles.

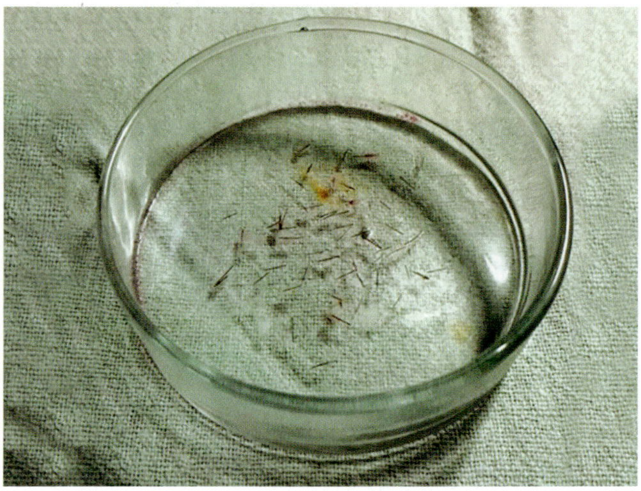

Fig. 18.25: Naked hair shafts after separation.

and collected in Petri dish containing Dulbecco's modified Eagle's medium (DMEM) (Sigma-Aldrich) pH 7.2, supplemented with penicillin, amphotericin-B and streptomycin. The entire procedure of FUE takes approximately 25 to 30 minutes.

- The extracted hair follicles are transported to laboratory under sterile conditions and washed thrice with phosphate-buffered saline containing antimycotics and antibiotics. The follicles are incubated with 0.025% trypsin–0.025% EDTA at 37°C for 90 minutes to prepare single cell suspension (Fig. 18.22). Within 15 to 20 minutes the cells start loosening up. Every 30 minute hair follicles are placed in a new tube containing trypsin–EDTA and trypsin inhibitor (Sigma-Aldrich) is added in the previous tube to terminate the reaction (Fig. 18.23). This is done to prevent digestion of the separated cells by trypsin. After cell separation only thin keratinous shafts of hair are left which are discarded (Figs. 18.24 and 18.25). The cell suspensions of all three tubes are combined in a single tube and it is filtered through a 70 μ cell strainer to obtain a single cell suspension. This final cell suspension is then centrifuged for 5 minutes at 1000 rpm to obtain the cell pellet, which is resuspended in small amount of DMEM and transported to operation theater for transplantation. The procedure of cell suspension preparation takes approximately 2 to 3 hours.

A smear of a representative sample can be subjected to cytological examination so as to ensure that cells

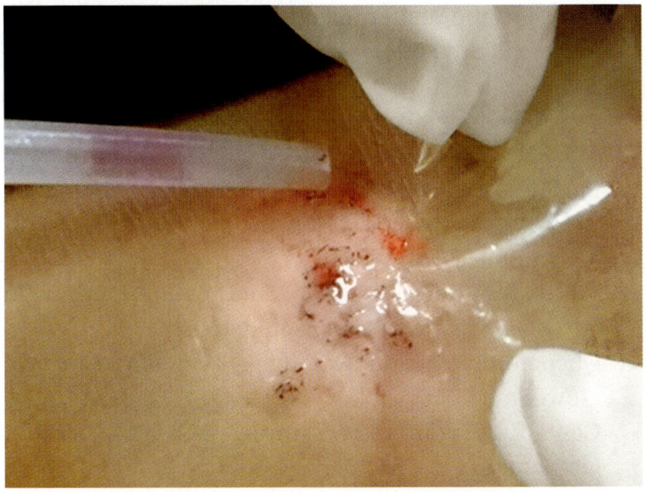

Fig. 18.26: Spreading suspension in NCFCS.

used for transplantation have a normal morphology and special staining with HMB45 antibody can be done to visualize the percentage of melanized cells.

- Recipient vitiligo patch is anesthetized first by using the topical anesthetic cream (EMLA) followed by infiltrating a small amount of local anaesthetic (2% lignocaine). The recipient site is dermabraded superficially by motorized dermabrader fitted with a stone burr or diamond fraise. The depth of dermabrasion is determined by the bleeding pattern and dermabrasion is stopped once pinpoint bleeding appears. The prepared hair follicle suspension is spread uniformly over the de-epidermized area with the use of a pipette (Fig. 18.26). The suspension is then covered with a collagen dressing of fish origin. The dressing is removed on the 8th day. Complete re-epithelialization takes around 2 to 3 weeks.

Modifications

Cell suspension of the 'plucked' hair follicles was done in one study and found to be effective although the cell count was less.

In Vivo Noncultured Epidermal Suspension

In this case, using standard procedure for suction blisters, blisters are raised on lateral aspect of patient's upper thigh. The blister fluid is aspirated using a 24G hypodermic needle attached to a 2 mL syringe and is introduced into the adjacent skin subcutaneously into blister cavity through its floor. With needle still in place, syringe is detached and replaced with another syringe having 1 mL 0.25% trypsinand EDTA solution. Within 45 minutes, keratinocytes and basal melanocytes get detached to form a cellular suspension inside blister cavity, this fluid is aspirated and transferred to a Petri dish, along with excised roofs of blister cavities after gently scraping the dermal side to release the remaining basal cells into suspension. The blister roofs are replaced back on donor sites as biological dressings, while cell suspension is transferred onto the dermabraded patches of vitiligo lesions.

The advantages of this procedure are:

- The viability of cells are >99%; much more than other cell suspension techniques.
- There is no lag period between harvesting and transplantation.
- Minimal handling of tissue outside body: so risk of contamination is negligible.
- No specialized training or lab equipment required; useful in smaller centers that lack infrastructure.
- Trypsin has no effect on dermal tissue on floor of blister, thus donor site heals well.

Four Compartment Method of NCES

This is a modification of standard NCES technique. The cell suspension is prepared from a split-thickness graft, which is transferred to a four compartment (FC) Petri dish. In the first compartment, trypsinization is performed. Compartments 2 and 3 are for the first and second washings with phosphate buffered saline (PBS) respectively. In compartment 4, the dermis is gently separated from the epidermis using sterile forceps. In order to form a homogeneous single-cell suspension, it is aspirated several times with the help of a sterile syringe. The suspension is then used for transplantation in vitiligo.

Procedure of Melanocyte Culture

Preparing Reagents

- *Preparation of transportation media for collecting skin biopsies*: The medium for collecting skin tissue is composed of sterile solution of Hanks balanced salt solution (HBSS) without calcium and magnesium containing 10% antibiotic antimycotic (100X) solution. Transportation media is kept in an aliquotin a laminar hood and storedat 4°C till further use.
- *Preparation of 0.25% dispase II solution*: Dissolve 0.125 g of dispase II in 50 mL of melanocyte growth

media. Sterilize the enzyme solution through a 0.22 micrometer filter and store at 4°C for up to 1 month.

- *Preparation of 0.1% trypsin solution*: Prepare 0.1% solution by dissolving 2 mL of 2.5% trypsin stock solution with 48 mL of versene solution. Filter and sterilize through a 0.22 micrometer filter, make 10 mL aliquot and store at 4°C.
- *Preparing melanocyte and keratinocyte growth media*: Reconstitute the melanocyte medium by adding the supplements provided with the media bottle. First thaw the supplements at 37°C, add the thawed supplements into the main media bottle, mix the contents gently and aliquot into smaller volumes (e.g. 50 mL) for later use. Store at 4°C until further use.

Method (Figs. 18.27A to D)

Sterilizing the Skin Biopsies (Day 1 Processing)

Note: All steps are performed in a laminar flow hood:

Starting material skin biopsies

- All skin biopsies (sample) are collected in sterile 15 mL centrifuge tube containing 5 mL transportation media.
- The samples are washed once with transportation solution. Cut the skin into smaller pieces (approx. 5 × 5 mm) using the surgical scalpel blade (this step is optional according to expertise).
- Skin pieces are transferred into the tube containing 5 mL of 70% ethanol solution. Shake it for 1 minute. The solution is discarded. This step is repeated thrice. Then the samples are washed with 5 mL HBSS solution. This step is also repeated thrice.
- 5 mL of 0.1% dispase solution (for enzymatic separation of epidermis) is added and incubated in the refrigerator at 4°C for 16 to 24 hours.

Making Epidermal Cell Suspension (Day 2 Processing)

- Tube containing the sample is washed with HBSS solution after removing from the refrigerator.
- The tissue is poured into a sterile Petri dish containing HBSS solution. The epidermis (thin, brownish, translucent layer) is separated from dermis (thick, white, opaque layer) using a pair of forceps.

Note: do not attempt to pull parts of the epidermis that stay firmly attached to the dermis, as this will increase the risk of fibroblast contamination. This can be achieved instead by incubating the sample a little longer in dispase solution.

- Collect epidermis layer in tissue culture Petri dish containing 5 mL of the 0.1% trypsin solution. If large sheets of the epidermis come off, then gently cut it into smaller pieces (approx 2 × 2 mm). Mince the skin pieces with a surgical scalpel. The remaining dermis is discarded immediately.
- Transfer the collected minced epidermal pieces from the Petri dish in to a 15 mL centrifuge tube containing 5 mL of 0.1% trypsin solution. Incubate the tube at 37°C for 5 minutes.
- Vortex the tube or use repeated pipette motions to release the single cells from epidermis.
- Quench the reaction by adding 10 mL of melanocyte growth medium.
- Centrifuge again for 5 minutes at 1000 g at room temperature.
- Aspirate the supernatant carefully as this, may contain pieces of stratum corneum. Resuspend the pellet in 2 mL melanocyte growth media.
- Transfer the epidermal cell suspension in a T25 cell culture flask. Add 3 mL melanocyte growth medium to make the total media volume 5 mL. Incubate at 37°C for 48 to 72 hours in 5% carbon dioxide without disturbance.

Note: The epidermal cell suspension contains both melanocytes and keratinocytes.

Subsequent Maintenance of Melanocyte Cultures

Wash cultures with melanocyte growth media on the 3rd day to remove nonadherent cells and fragments of stratum corneum. Medium change should be performed twice a week there after. Primary cultures established from skin biopsies (1.5 × 1.5 cm) usually reach 70% confluence within 8 to 10 days after 2nd processing. At this point, small clusters of keratinocytes are seen as well.

Note: Avoid cell cultures from becoming fully confluent. Always subculture at 70 to 80% confluency. Keratinocytes are alive but grow slowly in melanocyte growth medium.

Differential Trypsinization of Melanocytes (To Remove Contaminating Keratinocytes)

Semiconfluent melanocytes and keratinocytes appear 7 to 8 days after initial plating of epidermal cell suspension. To obtain pure melanocyte cultures, differential trypsinization method is used as explained below:

- Remove medium and wash cells in 1 to 2 mL HBSS solution.
- Swirl the flask gently around to rinse away the media.
- Add 0.5 mL of 0.1% trypsin- versene solution at room temperature for 1 to 2 minutes.

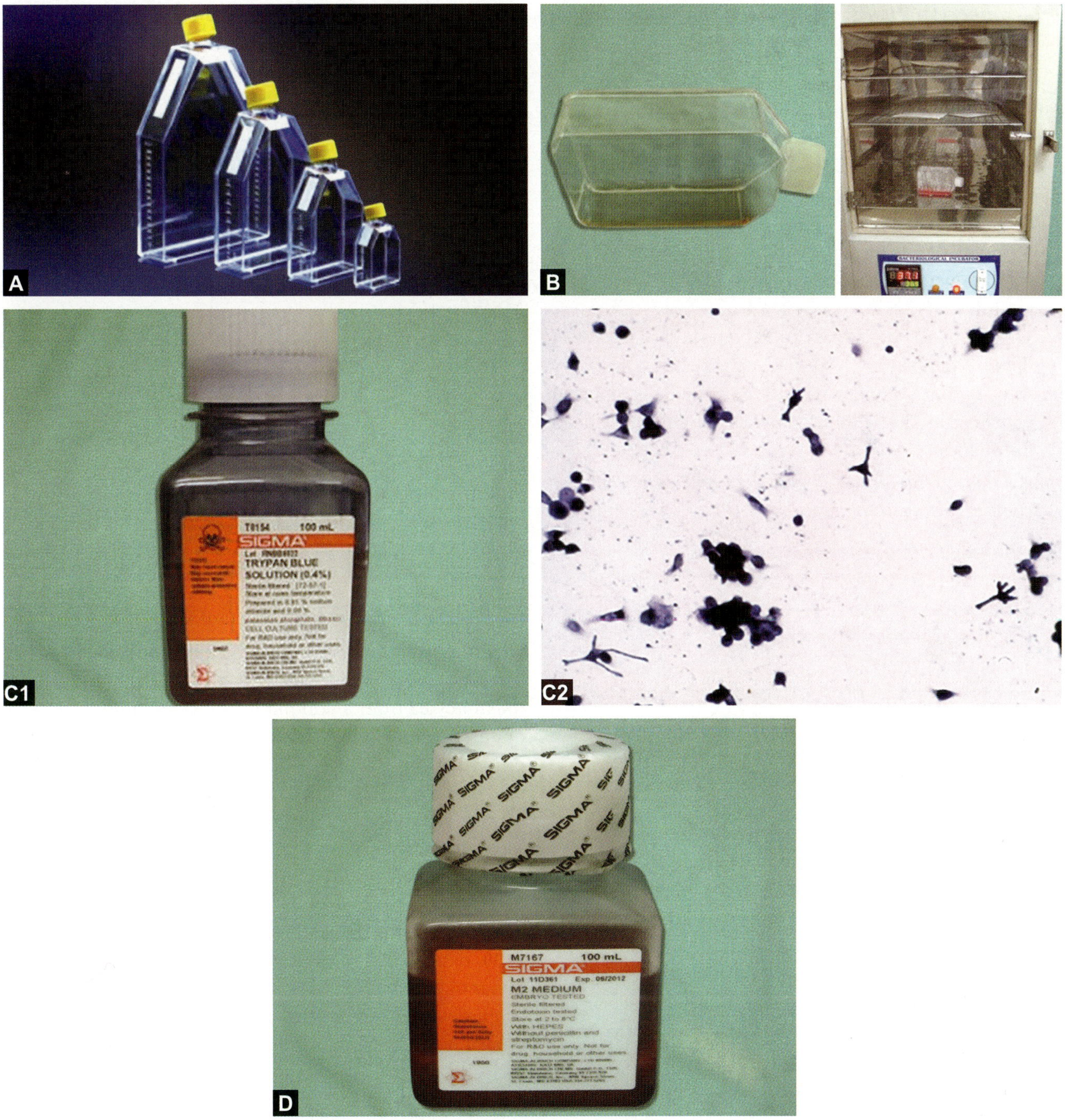

Figs. 18.27A to D: (A) T25 tissue culture flask. (B) Melanocyte culture. (C) Checking viability of melanocytes (1) Trypan blue, (2) Viable melanocytes. (D) M2 medium: Melanocyte culture.

- When cells detach, quench the trypsin with 5 mL of melanocyte growth media.
- Centrifuge the cells in a 15 mL falcon at 1000 g for 5 minutes.
- Resuspend the cell pellet thus obtained in 2 mL melanocyte growth medium. Plate the cells in a sterile 25 cm^2 tissue culture flask containing 4 mL melanocyte growth media.
- Place in 37°C with 5% carbon dioxide incubator.

Note: Melanocytes are weakly adherent cells and quickly retract their dendrites upon short trypsinization, leaving relatively strongly adherent keratinocytes behind.

Keratinocytes leftover in the flank can be subcultured in keratinocyte media.

Antibiotic Selection for Getting Pure Melanocyte Cultures: Differential trypsinization removes any contaminating keratinocytes. It is important to remove contaminating fibroblasts as well from the flask by giving a 24-hour geneticin treatment (given after 1st passage).

- Geneticin (G418) is added to the culture for removing fibroblasts growing along with the melanocytes.
- G418 is used at a concentration of 400 microgram per mL.
- Treatment of G418 is given for 24 hours at 37°C in carbon dioxide incubator.
- After 24 hours, geneticin containing media is replaced with fresh media (without geneticin) to remove the dead fibroblasts.

Note: Single treatment with geneticin efficiently removes contaminating fibroblasts.

Subculturing Primary Melanocyte Cultures

Starting material: 70 to 80% confluent melanocyte culture (T25 flask):

- Discard the media of the culture.
- Wash once with HBSS.
- Add 500 microliter of 0.1% trypsin.
- Incubate for 1 minute at room temperature.
- Quench with 500 microliter trypsin inhibitor or with 5 mL melanocyte growth media.
- Transfer in a 15 mL falcon.
- Centrifuge at 1000 g, 5 minute at room temperature.
- Discard supernatant very carefully.
- Resuspend pellet in 1 mL melanocyte growth media.
- Transfer the resuspended cells in a single T75 cell culture flask containing 9 mL melanocyte growth media (or in 3 T25 flasks containing 4 mL melanocyte growth media in each flask.
- Incubate at 37°C in 5% carbon dioxide incubator until confluent.

Counting of Cells

- For setting an experiment, trypsinize cells as mentioned above.
- Resuspend the cell pellet thus obtained in 1 mL melanocyte growth media.
- Count cells in a hemocytometer after appropriate dilution with trypan blue dye. Typically, 10 microliter cell suspension is directly placed on a coverslip (dilution factor 1) placed on hemocytometer and cell counting is done in 16 squares of the chamber.
- Multiply the cell number obtained with the dilution factor and by a factor of 10,000 to get no of cells per mL. For instance, if the average cell count is 120 (in 16 squares) and dilution factor is 1, then the number of cells/mL would be $120 \times 1 \times 10^4$ cells/mL or 12×10^5 cells/mL. Finally, seed the cells into flasks or tissue culture plate accordingly for further studies.

Transfer of Melanocytes to Recipient Area: This step is same as other previous procedures as in NCES.

Modifications

It has been seen that keratinocytes present along with melanocytes provide favorable milieu for proliferation of melanocytes. But presence of greater number of melanocyte can be inhibitory to melanocytes. So, it can be proposed in future to coculture keratinocytes and melanocytes differently and mix in an optimum proportion and transfer to the recipient area.

Innovation

Hair Follicle can be Used as a Source of Melanocyte for Culture

Dieckmann et al reported a technically simple method (the "explant" method) for isolation and culture of follicular melanocytes from a comparatively small amount of raw material. Here, 30 to 60 anagen hair follicles have to be plucked from patient's scalp and cultivated under low oxygen pressure (5%). After a short period of time, cells of various types grow out from the ORS of hair follicles. Most of the cells other than melanocytes are eliminated under selected culture conditions and almost 100% pure population of melanocytes has been achieved, which is confirmed by the IHC for melanocyte specific markers, e.g. S100, tyrosinase 1, and premelanosomal antigens. These melanocytes derived from the ORS have the capacity to proliferate up to 2 months. This method does not require enzymatic treatment, which is potentially unfavorable for the cells.

Savkovic et al used modifications, i.e. DLM melanocyte medium, microdissection (excision of the proximal part of hair follicle), with subsequent use of collagenase and geneticin treatments, and maintenance of purity of the melanocyte culture by differential trypsinization. The basis for each of these modifications is as follows:

- DLM melanocyte medium—with low serum content is an excellent base for explants method.
- Microdissection—fibroblasts divide quickly, competitively out-selecting the slower dividing

melanocytes, excision of the proximal fibroblast-rich part of hair follicle; lowers the nutritional and spatial competition of fibroblasts in the culture.

- Collagenase—partial digestion of the follicular collagen by collagenase loosens the extracellular matrix, leading to accelerated cell migration from the ORS pool.
- Geneticin—inhibits protein synthesis, thus efficiently removes keratinocytes and fibroblasts from the culture, leaving behind melanocytes at their lower protein synthesis pace unharmed.
- Differential trypsinization maintains the purity of the melanocyte culture. This is because melanocytes are weakly adherent and quickly retract dendrocytes upon a short period of trypsinization, and get released into the suspension quickly, as compared to the more adherent melanocytes and keratinocytes. This was found to increase the melanocyte yield by 20%, and lowered non- melanocytes by 14.15%, which was statistically significant ($p < 0.05$) to very highly statistically significant ($p < 0.005$). This lead to a higher yield, faster growth and differentiation, higher yield of desired cells and out-selection of competing cells, which further resulted in the time necessary to cultivate 10^6 melanocytes by 50%, compared to the explants method of Dieckmann.

Complications and Disadvantages Encountered

- Disadvantages of cell-based therapy include cost, feasibility, training requirements and paucity of data.
- There are some safety concerns of cultured autografts. Mutagenicity and possible risk of cancer have been cited as potential risks. 12-tetradecanoylphorbol 13-acetate (TPA) had been previously used in the culture medium, and since this is a tumor-promotor, concerns about its long-term safety have been expressed. Nevertheless, the recent availability of TPA-free and serum-free media is a possible solution to this problem. β FGF has been used as a substitute and is believed to provide satisfactory results. The presence of cyclic adenosine monophosphate elevating agents (such as isobutylmethylxanthine and cholera toxin) is also essential for the growth of melanocytes in the absence of TPA.
- Chance of possible infections are more due to more tissue handling, so performing the steps in an aseptic environment inside laminar hood is essential.

CONCLUSION

With the advancement in various techniques, and horizontal spread of training, vitiligo surgeries are more frequently practiced, especially in Asian countries. Compared to tissue graft technique, the use of cultured or noncultured cellular suspension is a step ahead in providing improved cosmetic results. It also eliminates many limitations of tissue-grafting methods. Although the cultured methods appeared more promising and appealing, they have their own limitations beingrestricted to research centers and universities due to the requirement for a specialized laboratory, highly-trained personnel, inventory of culture media and additives and associated cost escalations. The surgical therapies are being increasingly accepted in the management of vitiligo both by physicians and patients. Despite the advances in the technique, there are experiences of partial or complete failures even in patients with stable vitiligo. This may be due to the absence of any parameter to determine the degree of immunological activity. Further research in the understanding of the pathogenesis of vitiligo will help us to determine stability and prognosis of surgical treatment. Histological and immunological evidence suggest that melanocytes from clinically normal skin may also be defective, which may be one of the reasons for the failure to repigment following the surgery. To conclude the main future directions in surgical management should be: increasing effectiveness, minimizing adverse effects, improvement of outcomes and maintenance of pigmentation.

CHAPTER 19

Modifications of Cellular Techniques for Difficult Vitiligo

Munish Paul

INTRODUCTION

What is Difficult Vitiligo?

Everything about vitiligo is difficult.

Vitiligo is an autoimmune disease which can start at any age and has an unpredictable nature. A person might develop a single vitiligo patch which may stay stable for years and then start spreading or it might have a progressive spread right from the word go, the pace of which can vary from a slow burn to explosive spread which is unfortunate for the patient and for the treating physician who at times faces the brunt of the patient's emotions and frustrations.

The only thing that is predictable in vitiligo is its absolute unpredictable nature. In most patients, the disease can be best controlled/slowed down with the use of various immunosuppressive drugs, phototherapy and topicals. Majority of the patients would require some form of treatment all throughout their lives.

Medical treatment is successful usually in vitiligo patches that have pigmented hair. Such hair contain the reservoir of melanocytes and on stimulation with UV rays in the form of UVB therapy/PUVA/PUVAsol, the patch would recover pigmentation in a perifollicular distribution. Melanin production occurs also from the viable active melanocytes present in the margin of the vitiligo patch leading to repigmentation from the margins.

Hence areas that fall in below mentioned list will be labeled to treat as difficult to treat vitiligo.

Acral Vitiligo

- Fingers, toes
- Lips, nipples, periareolar, genitalia, perianal
- Dorsum of the hand and feet
- Lateral and medial malleolus, knees, elbows
- Vitiligo patch with leukotrichia
- Segmental vitiligo especially, if overlying hair are non-pigmented
- Patient who has achieved partial repigmentation with medical treatment and now is left with a mottled appearance.

Why are These Areas Difficult?

- Absence of viable melanocytes in the skin and the absence of hair follicles.
- Presence of disease activity. Even though most of the patches seem to be stable, the acral areas will show a slow spread hence resulting in surgical failure in these cases.
- Acral areas are more difficult to operate, i.e. it is difficult to dermabrade the acral areas for example, the finger tips, lips, penis and it is also difficult to retain the transplanted grafts whether tissue or cellular.
- If adequate depths are not achieved while deepithelializing the recipient area, and area is not adequately immobilized, the cell/graft uptakes will be poor and thus result in partial or poor repigmentation.

Wisdom: When to Say no?

When treating the difficult vitiligo, it is important for the treating dermatologist to understand that beyond a certain limit, medical treatment will not repigment patches and the injudicious and long-term use of systemic steroids, immunosuppressive, UV radiations is not only futile but is exposing the patient to innumerable risks and side effects The only option is surgical replacement of melanocytes and the wise dermatologist is the one who knows when to withhold medical therapy and go ahead with the surgical management.

Only patches that have been stable for at least one year should be taken up for surgery.

Patients having extensive vitiligo, i.e. more than 30% body surface area, acral actively spreading vitiligo, universal vitiligo, patients with comorbidities, i.e. diabetes, hypertension, elderly age should be taken up judiciously for treatment and at times the only viable option may be use of concealer creams or depigmentation in very extensive cases.

What are the Choices, if We Finally Decide to Operate?

Surgical Procedures

- Melanocyte replacement procedures:
  - *Tissue grafting*: Minipunch grafting,[7,8] ultrathin split thickness grafting,[9] blister grafting,[10] hair follicle grafts, smash grafts
  - *Cellular grafting*: Cultured[11] and noncultured autologous cell suspensions[12]
- Procedures in which melanocytes are not being replaced, i.e. tattooing, excision and closure, dermabrasion or chemabrasion.

The Golden Question

How to choose a surgical modality, i.e. which type of procedure is best suited for which area?

When a surgical procedure is being planned, it is borne in the mind that the end result should match as close to the surrounding skin in terms of texture and color matching, with no alteration in the functionality of the recipient area with minimum scarring over the donor area.

All the above mentioned procedures can produce varying amount of repigmentation but have their own advantages and disadvantages.

Autologous noncultured melanocyte keratinocyte cell suspension scores over most techniques in almost all the difficult sites mentioned and gives consistently good repigmentation with excellent color and texture matching. The exceptions are the lips (blister grafting), angles of the lip (tattooing), labia majora (excision and closure), where the first choices are different.

However centers not performing this surgery can use other techniques as per their training and experience.

Site of vitiligo	Suitable surgical modality
Eyebrows, beard area	FUE
Upper eyelids, lips	Suction blister graft
Angle of mouth	Tattooing, MPG
Areola	MPG
Palms and soles	MPG
Labia majora	FUE, excision and closure, tattooing
Scrotum	SBG, ECS, excision and closure

How do We Plan the Surgery?

Preoperative Counseling and Informed Consent[13]

The entire process involves a detailed history and physical examination of the patient followed by counseling about the procedure and the pre and postoperative care.

A detailed consent form elaborating the procedure and possible complications should be signed by the patient and an attendant. The consent form should specifically state the limitations of the procedure, and the possibility that the disease can become unstable again in the future and there can be a loss of pigment on other sites as well as operated sites. The patient is also counseled that he/she may require additional medical treatments and or phototherapy postprocedure to stimulate pigmentation on the operated patches and that it can take a few months to a year for significant repigmentation and color match to occur.

Preoperative laboratory studies include complete hemogram, bleeding and clotting time (or prothrombin and activated partial thromboplastin time), thyroid profile, LFT, KFT, serum electrolytes, chest X-ray PA view and ECG in adults. Screening for antibodies for hepatitis B, C and HIV is recommended.

Anesthesia

Small areas are managed under topical and or local anesthesia in an OT as a day care procedure.

If a case is being done under local, lignocaine (2%) with or without adrenaline is generally used. Maximum dosage that can be used is 4.5 mg/kg (up to 300 mg) and with epinephrine 7 mg/kg (up to 500 mg). Larger areas may need regional blocks or IV sedation.

Tips

- Topical EMLA cream can be applied to donor and recipient area.
- If local injectable anesthesia is used, then plain lignocaine is used for recipient area.

Procedure: Autologous Melanocyte Cell Suspension[14]

The basic equipments, dressings and other requirements for this technique are as given in Figures 19.1 to 19.4.

The steps involved in this process are:

- Harvesting a skin graft from the thigh
- Trypsinization and cell separation
- Dermabrasion of the recipient (vitiligo) site
- Transfer and fixing of melanocyte rich cell suspension

Harvesting of Skin Graft

The lateral aspect of the gluteal region is selected as the donor area. The size of the split-thickness donor skin

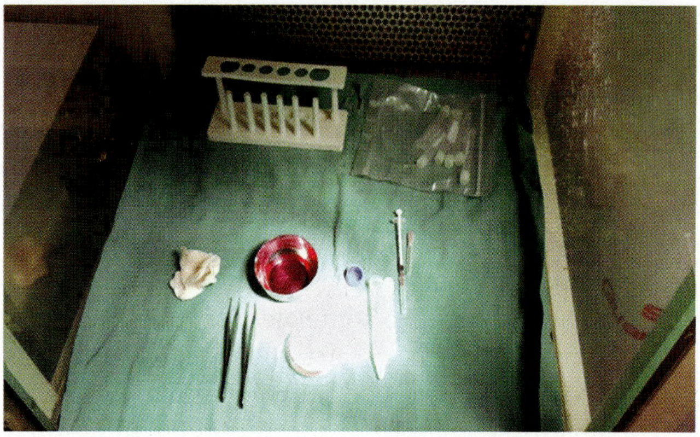

Fig. 19.1: Laminar air flow for cell separation.

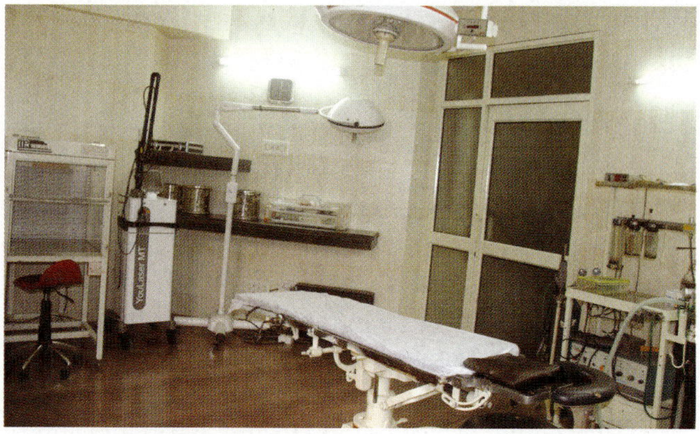

Fig. 19.2: OT setting with laminar airflow, CO_2 laser.

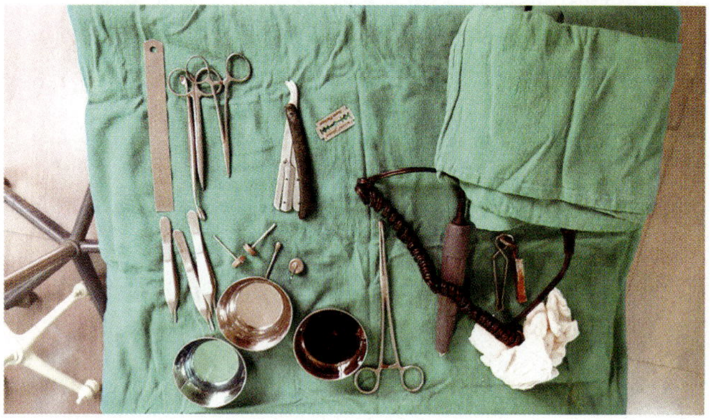

Fig. 19.3: Basic equipments for cell transfer.

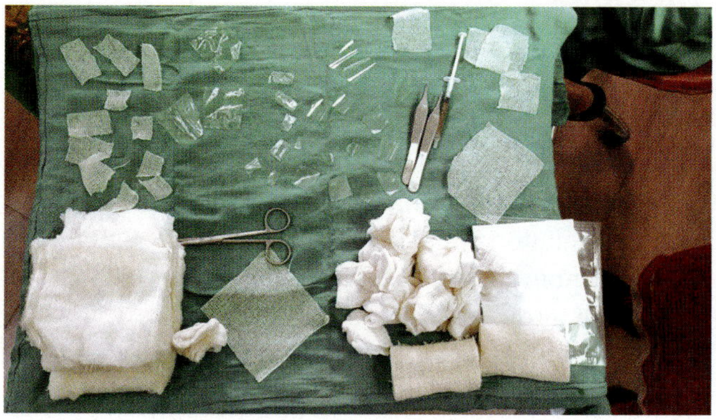

Fig. 19.4: Dressing materials collagen, paraffin, gauze and pad.

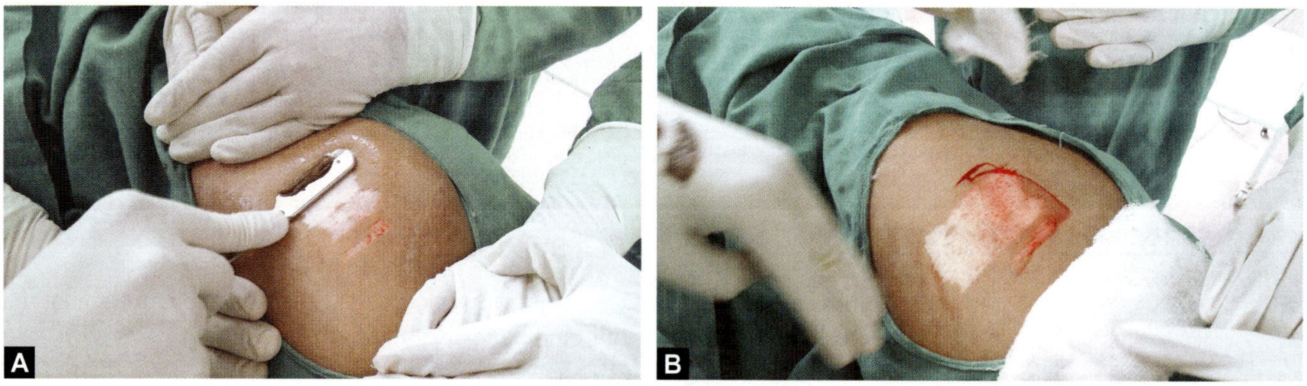

Figs. 19.5A and B: (A) Harvesting the graft (B) Donor area bleeding level.

taken is one-tenth of the recipient area. Under aseptic precautions, a very superficial sample is harvested using a shaving blade held in straight Kocher's forceps (Figs. 19.5A and B). The donor area is dressed with liquid paraffin dressing tulle (Fairlee™) and sterile gauze pad.

Trypsinization and Cell Separation Technique

The cell separation is done under aseptic precautions in a laminar flow bench kept in the operation theatre. The skin sample harvested is transferred to a Petri dish containing 5 mL of the 0.2% w/v trypsin solution, epidermal side facing upwards, and incubated for 45 min at 37°C (Fig. 19.6). After 45 min, the epidermis is separated from the dermis (Figs. 19.7A and B) and transferred (epidermis) to a test tube containing 2 ml of Dulbecco's modified Eagle medium: Nutrient Mixture F-12 (DMEMF/12) medium (Life Technologies) and vortex mixed for 15 seconds.

The epidermis is further broken into smaller pieces in a Petri dish and washed with the DMEM F/12 medium and finally transferred to a test tube containing the DMEM F/12 medium (Figs. 19.8A and B) and centrifuged for 6 min. The supernatant is discarded and the pellet is suspended in a 1 mL insulin syringe (Fig. 19.9). The final volume prepared varies from 0.2 to 0.5 mL depending on the size of the area to be treated.

Dermabrasion of the Recipient Site

The recipient site is abraded with a dermabrader fitted with a diamond fraise wheel (Delasco™) (Fig. 19.10). While operating close to the eye, inside the ear, penile shaft and other sensitive sites, erbium YAG laser or CO_2 laser is used

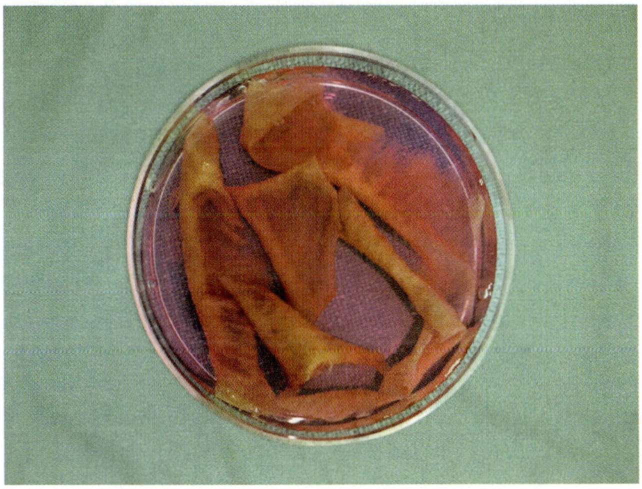

Fig. 19.6: Skin graft trypsinized dermal side down.

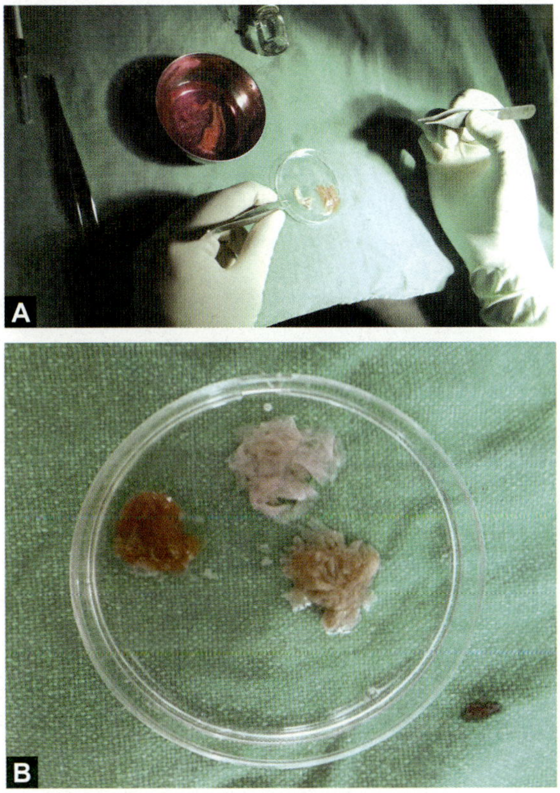

Figs. 19.7A and B: (A) Teasing the dermis from the epidermis (B) Complete separation dermis, epidermal fractions.

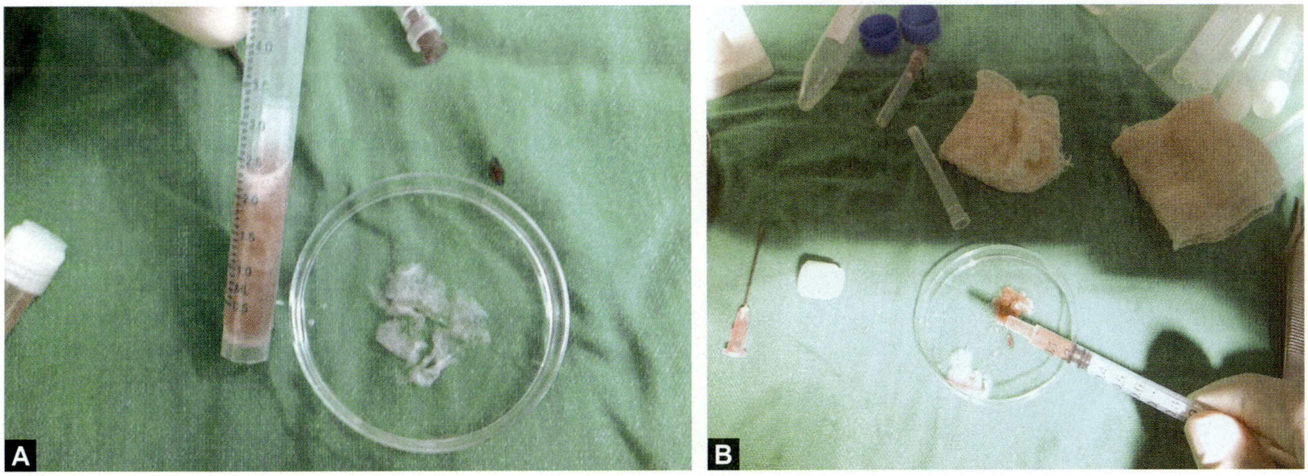

Figs. 19.8A and B: (A) Epidermis suspended in DMEM for centrifugation (B) Final separations.

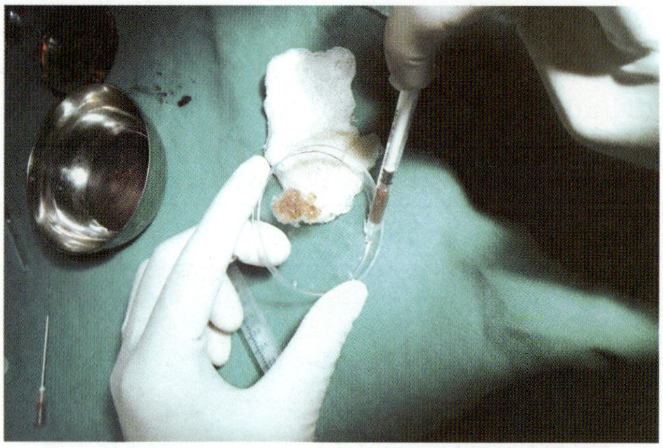

Fig. 19.9: Stratum basale and granulosum aspirated.

in an ablative mode. The endpoint of ablation is pinpoint bleeding. Hemostasis is achieved and the ablated area is covered with saline-soaked gauze pieces (Fig. 19.11).

Transplantation Technique

The cell suspension is spread evenly on the dermabraded area and covered with collagen dressing to hold the cells applied. This is covered with liquid paraffin and gauze pieces and finally bandaged (Figs. 19.12A and B). Patients are instructed to lie still in the same position for at least 1 hour to ensure cell fixation and then shifted to a room and further instructed to avoid excessive movements of the treated area for at least 6 hours.

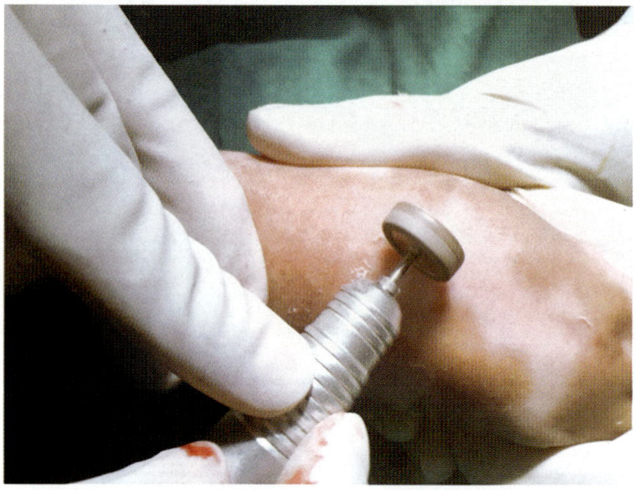

Fig. 19.10: Hand dermabrasion.

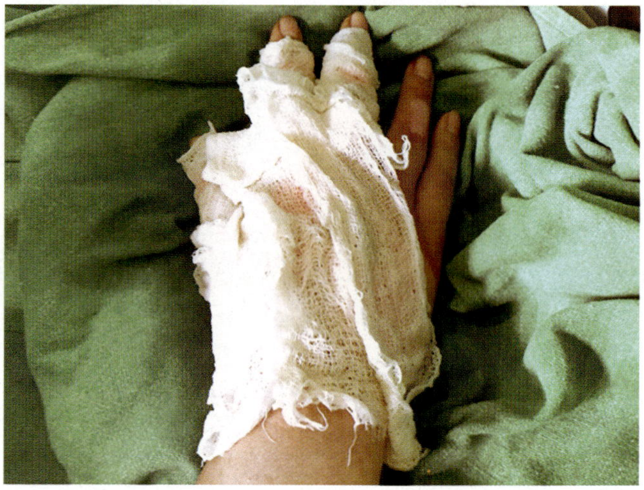

Fig. 19.11: Dermabraded area covered with wet gauze.

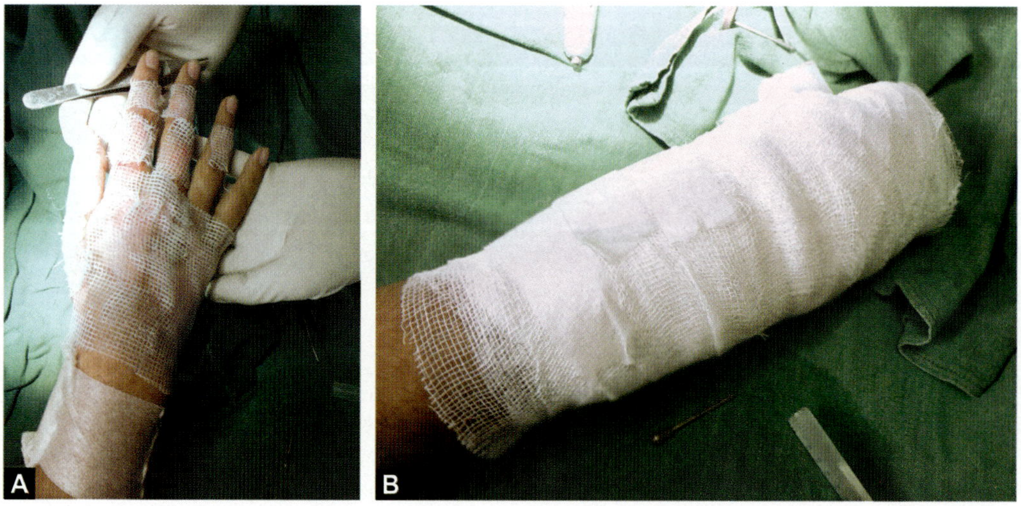

Figs. 19.12A and B: (A) Cell suspension applied area dressed with collagen and paraffin. (B) Bandaging done.

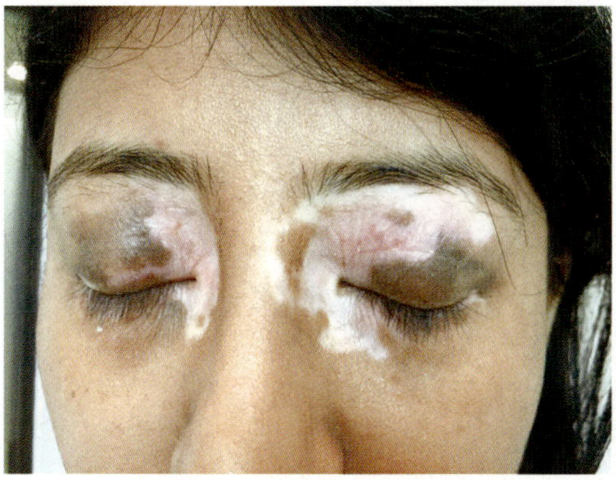

Fig. 19.13: Vitiligo eyelids.

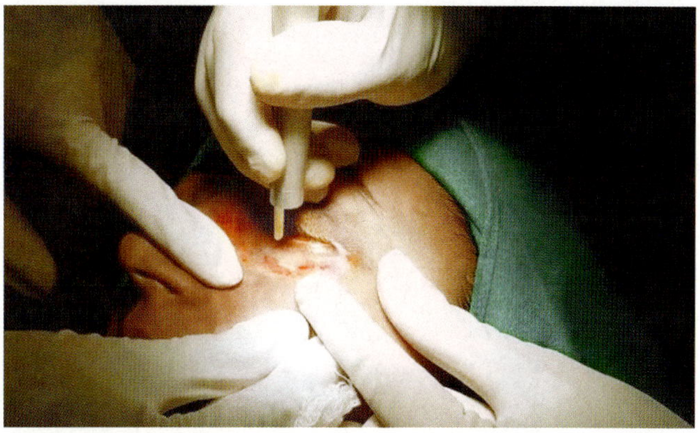

Fig. 19.14: Eyelid being resurfaced with CO_2 laser.

Postprocedure Instructions

All patients are instructed to take complete rest and avoid all vigorous physical activities. Patients are prescribed oral antibacterial agents for 5 days and nonsteroidal anti-inflammatory drugs (NSAIDs) for 3 days. The dressings are removed after 1 week in most cases. Patients are asked to follow-up at weeks 1 and 3, and then at 3-month intervals.

How to Modify the Procedure for Specific Areas?

Certain modifications and fine tuning have to be done on some specific sites to help in dermabrasion and retaining the cells transferred. These techniques can be used to improve the results over these areas.

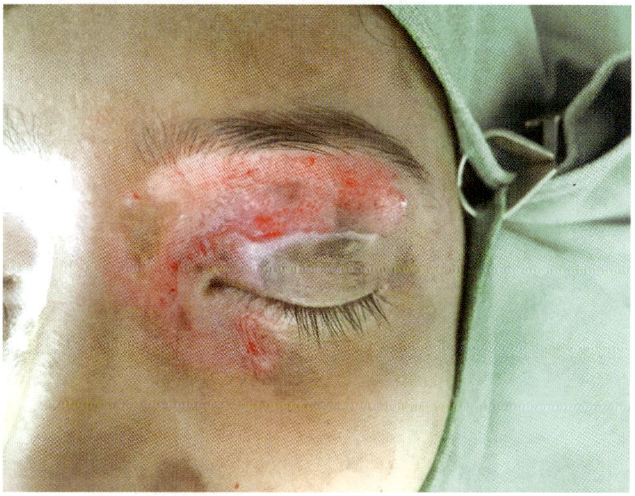

Fig. 19.15: Resurfacing of the eyelid.

Modifications of the Procedure: Periorbital Region (Fig. 19.13)

Dermabrasion over the eyes is started with larger wheel burrs, and when we move close to the eyelid margin, shift to smaller cylindrical burrs and finally when doing next to the eyelashes a CO_2 or Erbium YAG Laser should be used (Figs. 19.14 and 19.15). The eyelid should be stretched well and the dermabrasion should be very superficial as the skin is very thin. A corneal shield can be placed while deploying lasers in these areas.

Following dermabrasion hemostasis is achieved and area is covered with saline soaked gauze which should be wetted frequently. The dermabraded bed should never be left to become dry.

Immobilization for small areas: Only a dry collagen sheet should be applied and it can be left open. While doing larger area, e.g. a full eyelid, apply small bits of collagen, followed by paraffin, gauze, pad and then close with hypo allergic micropore tape. The eye is closed for 7 days. Patient should be counseled that, if there is any pain or irritation they should report earlier.

Removal of dressing: It is very vital that on day 7 postoperative, the dressings are removed carefully after soaking in normal saline. In most cases the collagen would be digested at day 7. If it is still persisting it should not be peeled off and the patient should be instructed that they can take bath, wet the area and let the collagen shed on its own, which will occur spontaneously after few days. If the recipient area has not healed, a redressing only with paraffin dressing may be done for another 3 days. By then it would heal in almost all the cases.

A case which showed good repigmentation is shown in Figures 19.16A and B.

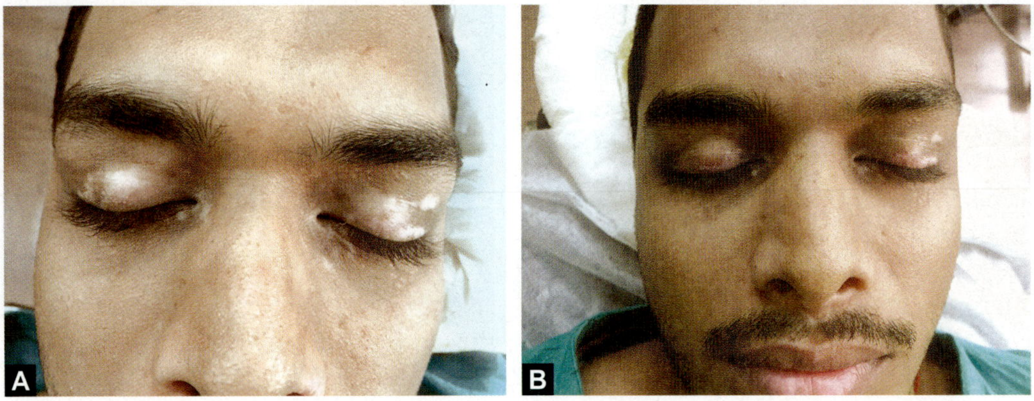

Figs. 19.16A and B: Vitiligo eyelids: (A) Preoperative. (B) Partial repigmentation post-MCT.

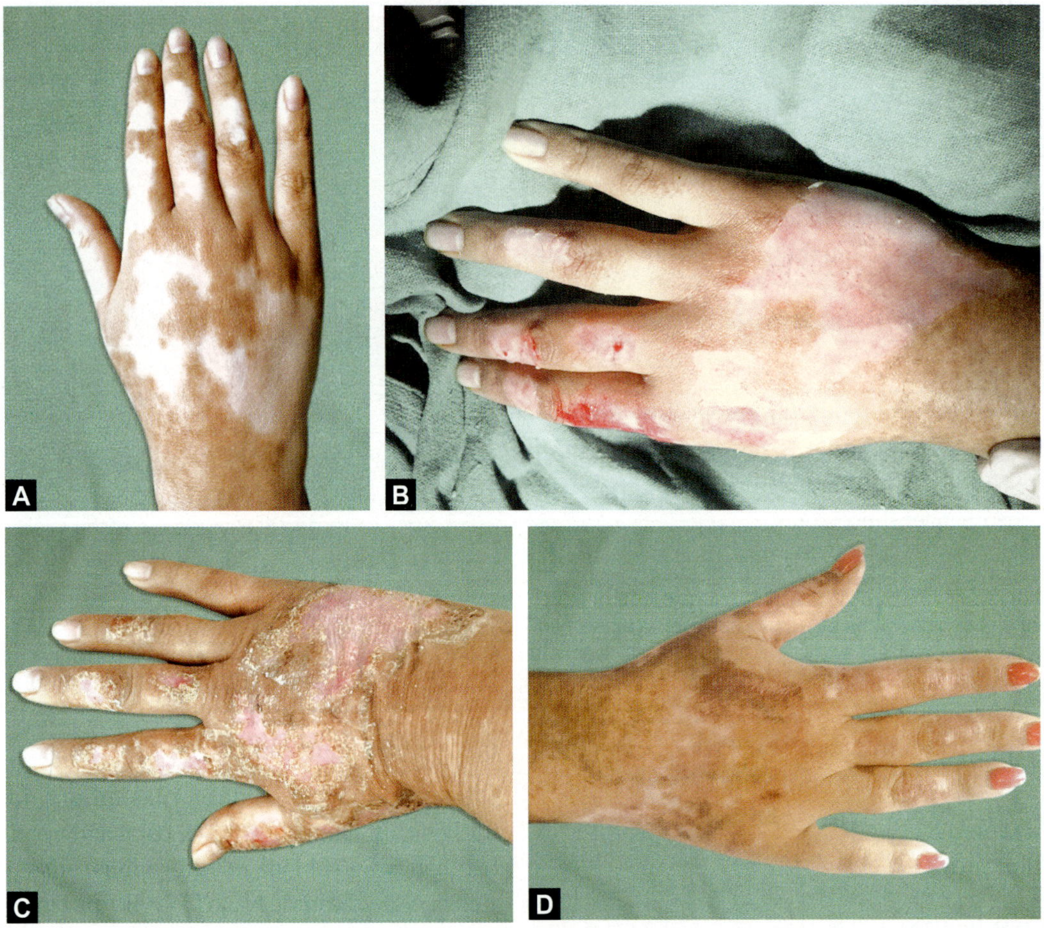

Figs. 19.17A to D: (A) Hand preoperative. (B) Hand dermabraded. (C) Day 7 wound healed. (D) Repigmentation.

Modifications of the Procedure: Finger Tips (Figs. 19.17A to D)

Dermabrasion over the fingers is started with larger wheel burrs, and when we move close to the periungual areas smaller cylindrical burrs should be used. The dermabrasion depth has to be controlled carefully to deepithelialized only the epidermis. A very deep dermabrasion will definitely result in hypertrophic scars and rarely contractures. Following dermabrasion, hemostasis has to be achieved.

Each finger is bandaged separately and area is covered with saline soaked gauze which should be wetted frequently. The dermabraded bed should never be left to become dry.

Immobilization: Dry collagen sheet should be applied to hold the cell suspension followed by paraffin dressings, wet gauze, dry gauze, surgical pads and then all fingers are bandaged together. This provides the best splinting. The hand is bandaged for 7 days. Patient should be counseled that if there is any pain or irritation, they should report earlier than 7 days.

Removal of dressing: It is very vital that on day 7 postoperative the dressings are removed carefully after soaking in normal saline. In most cases the collagen would be digested at day 7. If it is still persisting, it should not be peeled off and the patient should be instructed that they can take bath, wet the area and let the collagen shed on its own: which will occur spontaneously after few days. If the recipient area has not healed, a redressing only with paraffin dressing may be done for another 3 days: by then it would heal in almost all the cases.

Few procedures done on fingertips and hands are highlighted in Figures 19.18 and 19.19.

Modifications of the Procedure: Lips

If we have a patient who presents with only vitiligo over the lip, a suction blister grafting would be the first treatment of choice (Representative images of procedure on lips are shown in Figs. 19.20A to G), since the cell suspension technique has an issue of the cell suspension running away; however, if we have a patient who has other body parts as well-being operated, then the NCES can be performed (Fig. 19.21).

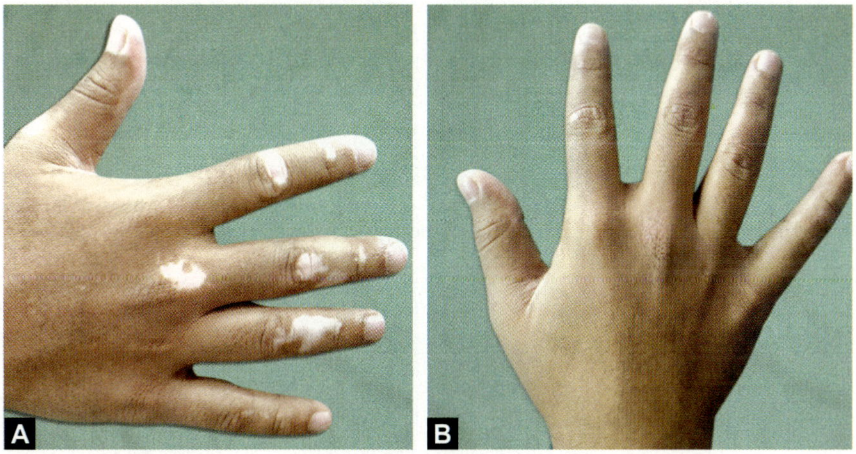

Figs. 19.18A and B: A case with good repigmentation on the dorsum of fingers by NCES.

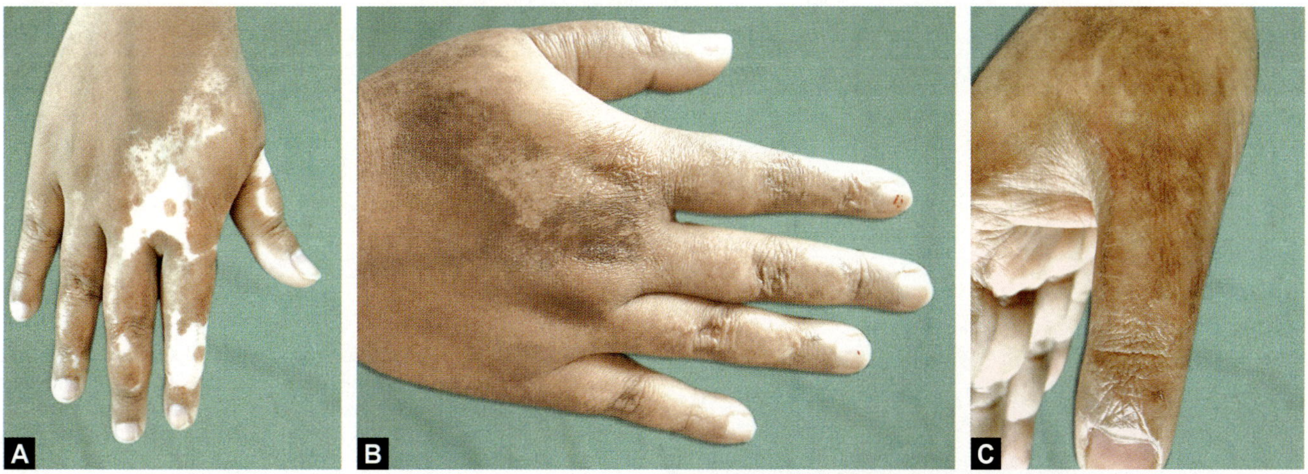

Figs. 19.19A to C: Good repigmentation following NCES technique on the dorsum of hand.

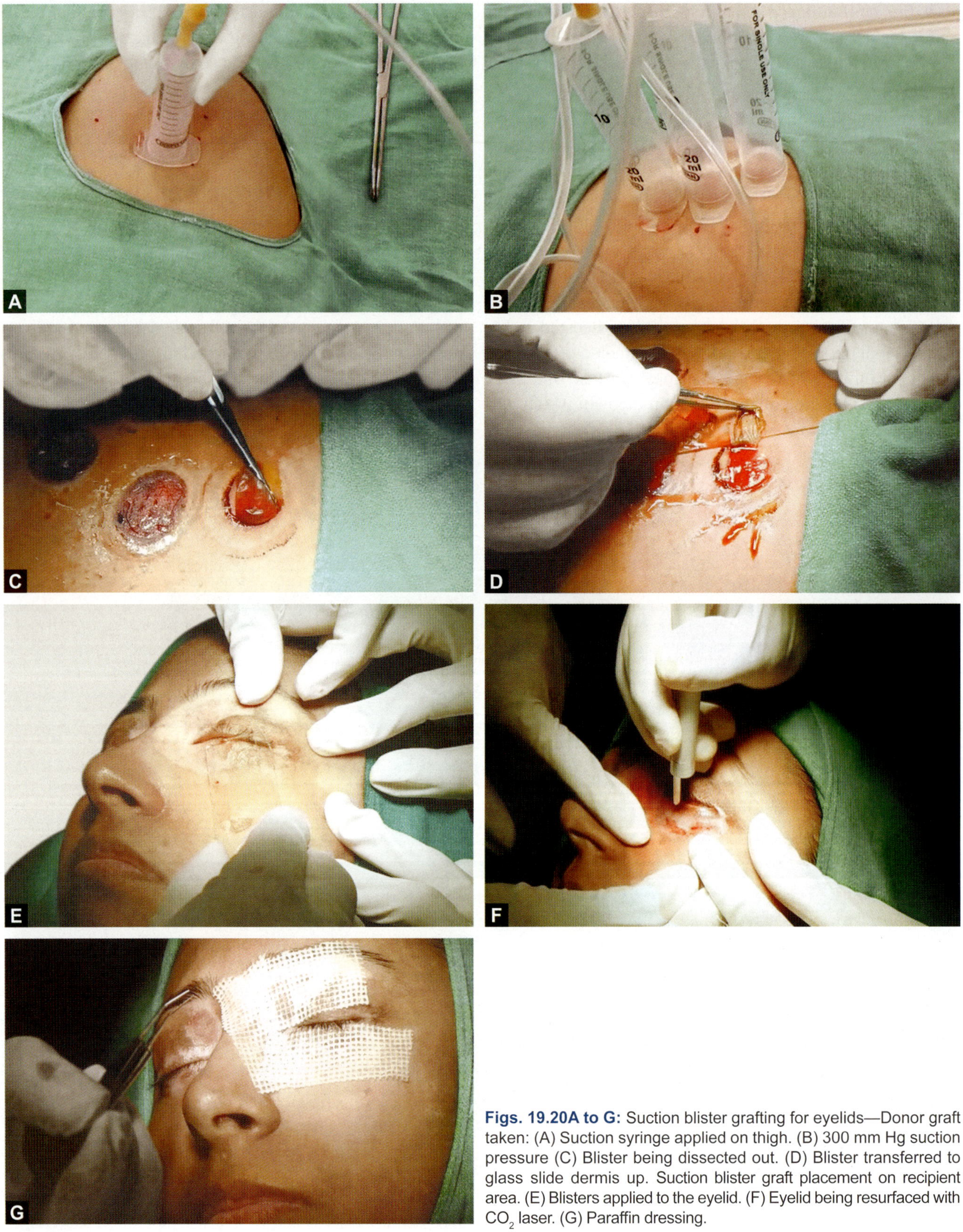

Figs. 19.20A to G: Suction blister grafting for eyelids—Donor graft taken: (A) Suction syringe applied on thigh. (B) 300 mm Hg suction pressure (C) Blister being dissected out. (D) Blister transferred to glass slide dermis up. Suction blister graft placement on recipient area. (E) Blisters applied to the eyelid. (F) Eyelid being resurfaced with CO_2 laser. (G) Paraffin dressing.

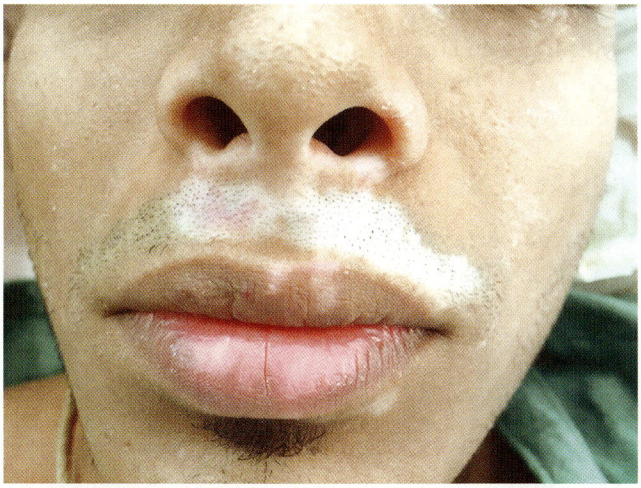

Fig. 19.21: NCES preferred, if multiple areas like in this patient are involved.

Anesthesia: An infraorbital block is used to anesthetize upper lip (three and half method) and mental nerve block is used to anesthetize lower lip (four and a half method).

Dermabrasion: Over the lips is started with larger wheel burrs. Putting wet gauze inside the mouth makes the lip taught and easier to dermabrade. The dermabrasion depth has to be controlled carefully to deepithelialize only the upper mucosa. Very deep dermabrasion will definitely result in scars. CO_2 or erbium YAG laser can also be used to remove the top mucosal layer.

Following dermabrasion, hemostasis is achieved and then tie over sutures are placed with 4–0 prolene. Lip is then covered with saline soaked gauze which should be wetted frequently. The dermabraded bed should never be left to become dry.

Immobilization: Blister grafts cut out according to the size and shape of the dermabraded areas of the lip are then placed over the recipient area, followed by paraffin dressings over which the prolene 4–0 is tied to secure the grafts. This is followed by gauze, pad, and micropore dressing respectively.

If a cell suspension is applied then it is made thick by adding methylcellulose and then dry collagen sheets are applied to hold the cell suspension followed by paraffin dressings. Prolene is tied over the dressing followed by gauze, surgical pads and micropore dressing successively upwards.

The lip is bandaged for 7 days. Patient should be counseled that if there is any pain or irritation they should report earlier. Patients are advised to take liquid or semisolid diet and avoid contamination of the dressing as far as possible.

Removal of dressing: It is very vital that on day 7 post-procedure, the dressings are removed carefully after soaking in normal saline. The sutures are cut and gently removed to avoid dislodgement of the grafts. In most cases the collagen would be digested by day 7. If it is still persisting, it should not be peeled off and the patient should be instructed that they can take bath, wet the area and let the collagen shed on its own, which will occur spontaneously after few days.

Modifications of the Procedure: Penis and Scrotum

Operating the vitiligo area over the penis/scrotum requires couple of modifications and expertise, since there are certain specific issues:

- The length and girth of the penis will keep varying
- Temperature, anxiety, sleep: all can alter the tumescence of penis
- Scrotum skin can considerably contract and expand
- The skin over the penis is very thin and a very superficial dermabrasion needs to be performed.

Dermabrasion over the penis and scrotum is done with pear shaped burr while the assistant is holding the skin taught. CO_2 or erbium YAG laser use will have a better controlled depth of dermabrasion, on this site. The dermabrasion depth has to be controlled carefully.

Immobilization: Following dermabrasion, hemostasis is achieved. After the cell suspension is applied, it is covered with dry collagen sheets which are cut into small pieces for which we have coined the term pixel collagen. This is especially helpful in this site because the collagen can then move with the increase or decrease in the length or girth of the penis or the scrotum. This is followed by gauze, pad and micropore dressing successively. It is advisable to admit the patient for a day or two, so that the area is adequately immobilized.

Drugs like diazepam can be given to reduce the erections.

The area is bandaged for 7 days. Patient should be counseled that, if there is any pain or irritation they should report earlier. Patients are advised to void urine carefully and avoid contamination of the dressing as far as possible. Some patients may be catheterized for initial 2–3 days.

Removal of dressing: It is very vital that on day 7 post-operative the dressings are removed carefully after soaking in normal saline. In most cases, the collagen would be digested at day 7. If it is still persisting it should not be peeled off and the patient should be instructed that they can take bath, wet the area and let the collagen shed on its own which will occur spontaneously after few days. If the patient has vitiligo patches only on the scrotum then a simple excision and closure can give good results considering this area has considerable laxity.

Modifications of the Procedure: Labia Majora/Minora

In spite of the concealed areas of the female genitalia, some patients insist on getting this area treated. It is difficult to hold any kind of grafts, i.e. punches, split thickness, NCES in this area and the preferred choice of treatment is to tattoo the area.

Tattooing or micropigmentation is a process in which artificial pigments are introduced into the mid-dermis level of the vitiligo lesion.

The other option is to *excise and close* the vitiligo patch. It will always end up with just a linear suture scar line and given the laxity present in this area, it heals very well.

Since labia majora is hairy region, FUE is another option.

CHALLENGING CASES

A very difficult case of segmental vitiligo after NCES is depicted in Figures 19.22A to J.

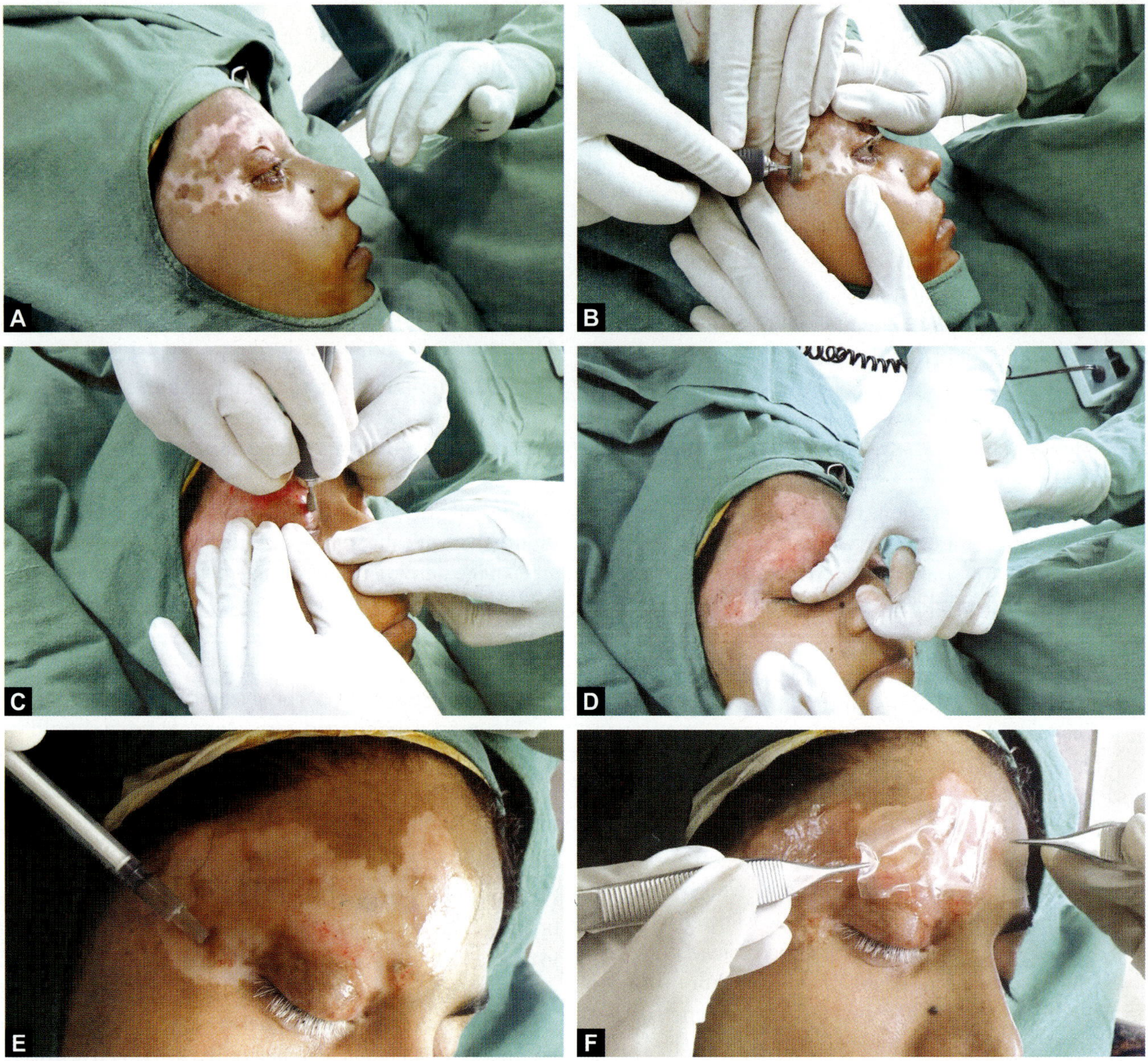

Figs. 19.22A to F: Difficult case of segmental vitiligo: (A) Vitiligo preoperative. (B) Recipient area being dermabraded with diamond burs. NCES being done: (C) Pear bur to dermabrade the upper eyelid. (D) Even dermabrasion up to papillary dermis. (E) Cell suspension being applied. (F) Dry collagen sheet applied to hold the suspension.

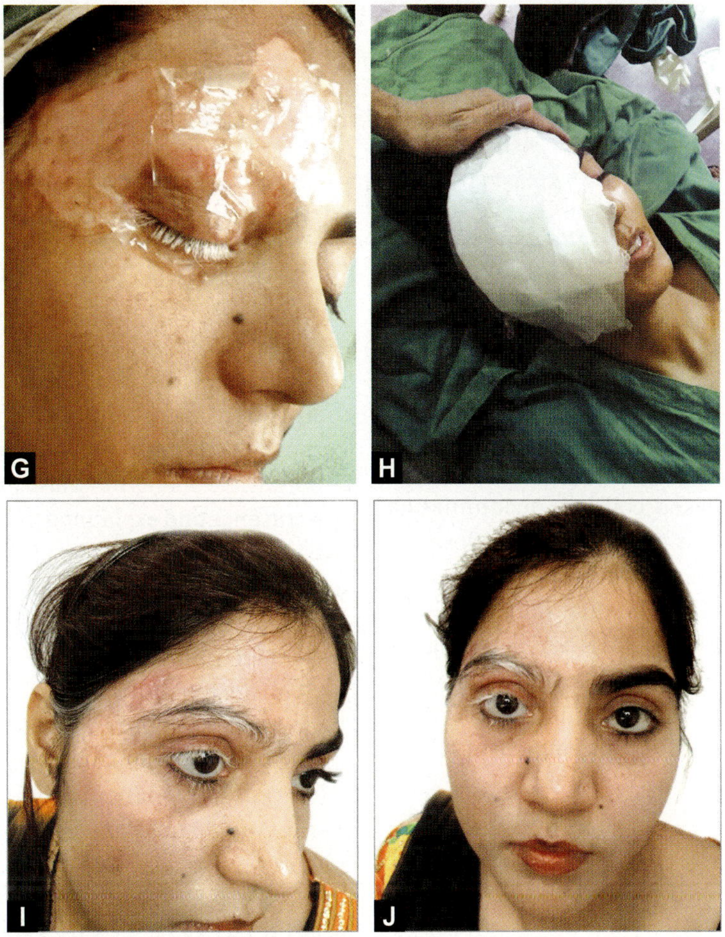

Figs. 19.22G to J: (G) Entire area covered with the collagen sheet. (H) Gauze, pad, micropore, close the eye for immobilization. (I) Postoperative 2. (J) Postoperative.

CONCLUSION

Every patient of vitiligo is a different challenge and the treatment whether surgical or medical should be customized according to the type, extent and stability of the disease. Consideration also needs to be given to the medical history, i.e. age, family history, comorbidities, e.g. diabetes, hypertension, etc. With the advent of vitiligo surgery, the difficult to treat vitiligo have become easier to deal. Careful case selection, detailed history taking, examination, patient counseling and choosing the right procedure for the specific site is imperative for a favorable outcome.

CHAPTER 20

Practical Tips for Management of Keloids and Hypertrophic Scars

Sharad Mutalik, Meenaz Khoja

INTRODUCTION

Keloids are fibroproliferative scars that occur due to imbalance between matrix degradation and collagen synthesis resulting in increased collagen accumulation along the wound tissue or scar tissue. Keloids differ from hypertrophic scars for the fact that hypertrophic scars do not cross the margins of the original injury and can possibly regress spontaneously.[1] Keloids have an unsightly appearance and cause functional deformities leading to psychological distress in patients, apart from other symptoms of pruritus and pain. Hence, treatment of keloids becomes essential.

Keloids and hypertrophic scars respond to same modalities of treatment discussed below, however, hypertrophic scars are relatively less disfiguring and more amenable to treatment.

Common sites of occurrence of keloids include the chest or presternal area, shoulders, back, breasts and the pinna, amongst others.

PRINCIPLES OF DERMATOSURGICAL MANAGEMENT OF KELOIDS (TABLE 20.1)

While the management of keloids involves several modalities, it may be important to combine more than one form of treatment as no single form of treatment may be exclusively effective. Keloids commonly have high recurrence rates and are difficult to treat or eliminate completely. Pretreatment counseling of the patient that it may not be possible to deliver 'completely scarless normal looking skin' is of paramount importance. Patients must also understand about possibility of recurrence and explaining this would reduce medicolegal hassles. However, in most patients, especially those with ear keloids, cosmetically acceptable results can be obtained with combined surgical treatment and postsurgical measures to prevent recurrence.

With treatment, it is indeed possible to significantly flatten the keloids, normalize the thickness of skin, improve the texture as well as eliminate symptoms of pain and pruritus.

Importantly, patients with keloidal tendency should be cautioned about any elective procedures in the future and preventive measures should be instituted.

MODALITIES FOR TREATMENT OF KELOIDS

Various modalities have been described which include invasive and noninvasive methods and these have been listed in Table 20.2.

DETAILED PROCEDURE FOR DERMATOSURGICAL MANAGEMENT OF KELOIDS

Intralesional injections: This has been the first line of management of keloids. Intralesional injections of

Table 20.1: Principles of dermatosurgical management of keloids.

- Adequate pretreatment counseling of the patient and use of combined modalities of treatment wherever applicable to hasten response/prevent recurrence
- In case of planned excision of keloid (e.g. ear keloids), the resection of keloidal tissue must be as complete as possible
- Skin closure—with decreased wound tension
- Maintain asepsis and prevention of infection
- Proactive postoperative measures to prevent recurrence
- Preventive measures to be instituted in patients with keloidal tendency while opting for elective procedures.

Table 20.2: Modalities for treatment of keloids.

Noninvasive/Semi-invasive	*Invasive*
• Topical treatments: Topical Mitomycin C, Imiquimod (postexcision), Silicone gel cream • Silicone gel sheets • Surface cryotherapy • Intralesional injection: triamcinolone, 5-fluorouracil, verapamil • Radiation therapy • Pulse Dye Laser	• Surgical excision of the Keloid • Intralesional cryotherapy

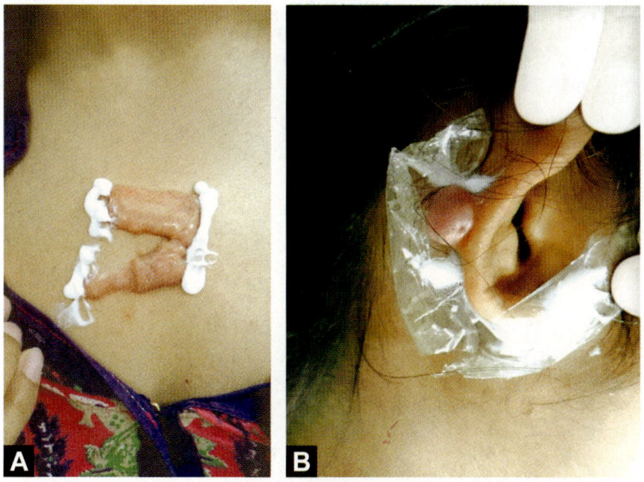

Figs. 20.1A and B: Applying topical anesthesia cream at the borders of the keloid.

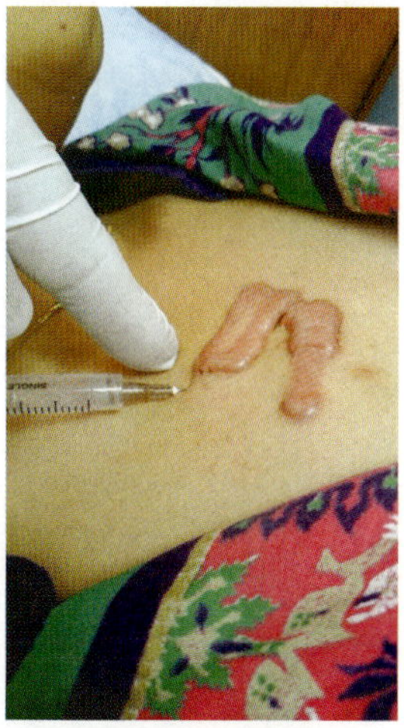

Fig. 20.2: Injecting local anesthesia.

triamcinolone acetonide, 5-fluorouracil (5FU)/bleomycin may appear to be an easy office-based procedure, but certainly helps in achieving significant aesthetic improvement if carried out in a systematic manner at regular and adequate intervals.

Steps of Intralesional Injection

Step 1: Administering Local Anesthesia

Allocate more time in administration of local anesthesia so that the pain factor is significantly reduced and actual injection time is also reduced, which in turn increases the comfort level of the patient and the clinician. This helps to increase the patient compliance in completing the prolonged treatment.

It is advisable to call the patient 90 minutes before the scheduled procedure time. Apply EMLA (eutectic mixture of local anesthesia) cream under occlusion at the borders of the lesion (Figs. 20.1A and B). Wait for 90 minutes. Use ice packs, hand held vibrator/massager which further reduce the pain.

Step 2: Infiltrate Local Anesthesia

Load a disposable luer-lock syringe with Inj. Lignocaine 2% + Inj. Ropivacaine 0.2% + normal saline in a ratio of 2:1:1 with a small bore 26 gauge 0.5 inch needle (Fig. 20.2). With Ropivacaine the anesthesia lasts for at least 6 to 8 hours, so there is no post-injection pain.

Pierce the skin and raise a wheal. Change the needle and infiltrate using a long needle (25 G × 1½") through the wheal slowly (after aspirating, to ensure avoidance of intravenous injection). Cover the entire area to achieve field block (Figs. 20.3A to C). Regional/nerve blocks should be used while treating sensitive areas like forehead and ear (Figs. 20.4A and B).

Step3: For Inflamed, Hard Keloid

Inj. Triamcinolone acetonide 40 mg/mL or 10 mg/mL (depending on the size and thickness of the keloid) + Inj. 5 Fluorouracil 50 mg/mL (Maximum 2 vials of 40 mg or 4 vials of 10 mg with 1 mL of 5 FU). For smaller keloids, use insulin syringe and 10 mg/mL triamcinolone acetonide. Use a luer-lock syringe with a wide bore long needle (23 G × 1½ inches). Luer-lock syringe prevents spillage/splash while injecting against resistance of thick keloidal tissue.

Pierce the normal skin, then enter the bulk of keloid. Squeeze the keloid with thumb and index finger of the non-dependent hand in order to restrict the injected medication to the keloid. Otherwise injected medication spreads to the surrounding normal skin, may enter the lymphatics as well. It can cause atrophy, hypopigmentation or depigmentation, telangiectasia and sepsis.

Always make it a practice to aspirate before injecting. Injection should neither be too superficial nor too deep.

Step 4: Apply Gentle Pressure with Sterile Gauze

Repeat the procedure every 4–6 weeks till the keloid flattens completely and merges with the surrounding normal skin.

***Adverse effects*:** If 5-FU (FFU) is injected too superficially, it can lead to ulceration and necrosis of the skin. Injection spilling in the surrounding skin can produce atrophy and depigmentation along the lymphatics.

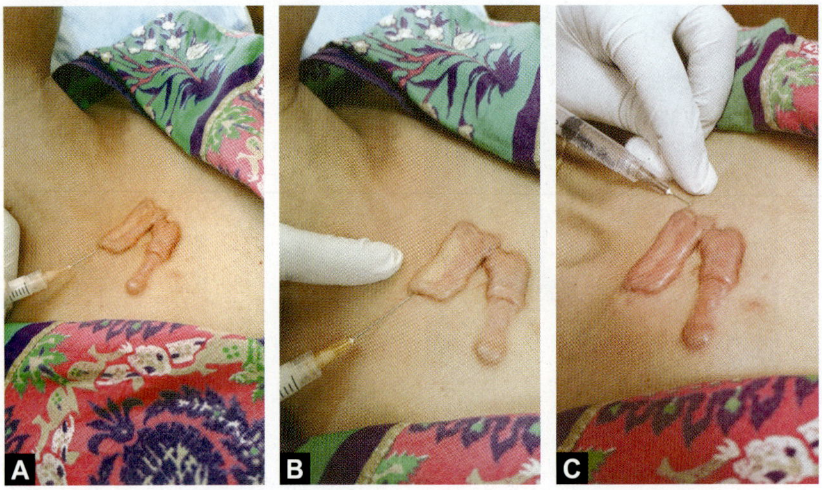

Figs. 20.3A to C: Steps of injecting local anesthesia.

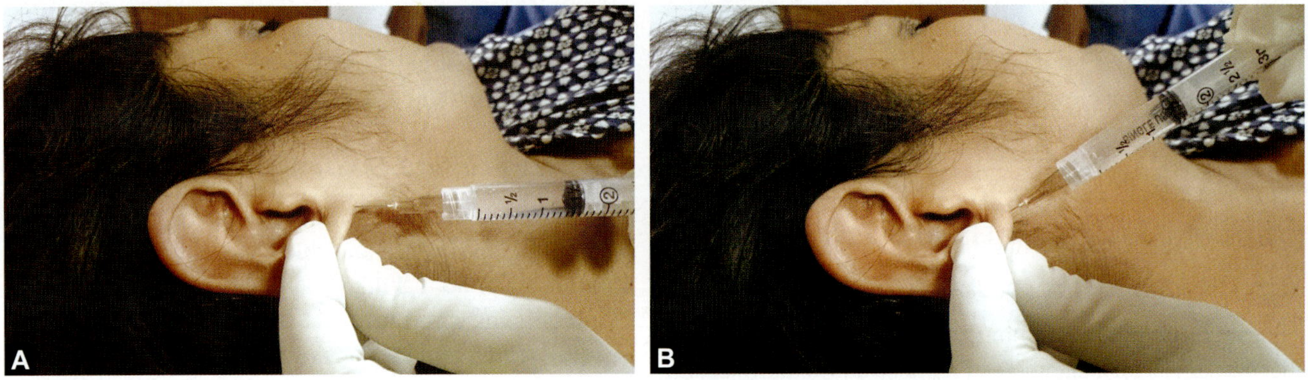

Figs. 20.4A and B: Regional block for the ear.

After complete flattening of keloid occurs, silicone gel dressing under compression is advised for 3 to 6 months in order to prevent recurrence. Clamps are also desirable for the keloids (Fig. 20.5).

***Silicone gel topical/sheet*:** According to the Cochrane review 2006, the evidence to support silicone gel sheeting in treatment of keloids and hypertrophic scars was found to be limited. However, many randomised controlled trials (RCTs) have shown a positive influence of silicone gel sheeting in the treatment of hypertrophic scars and keloids. They not only prevent recurrences, but promote faster involution. Silicone gel sheets must be worn for at least 2 to 12 months after surgical/definitive treatment for about 12 to 24 hours daily.[2]

***Radiation therapy*:** Superficial X-ray, electron beam therapy and brachytherapy are different radiation modalities known to be used in treatment of keloids, with brachytherapy being the most effective.[3,4] Radiation therapy is best performed after surgical excision of the keloid to prevent recurrence and elaborated in the section under ear keloids.

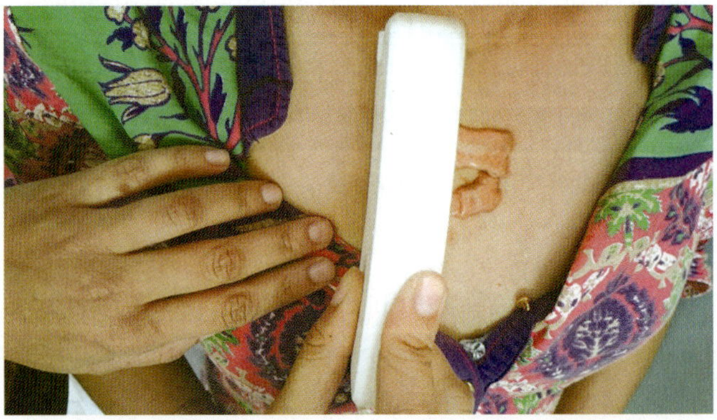

Fig. 20.5: Regular assessment of treatment efficacy.

***Pulse dye laser*:** With hemoglobin as the target chromophore, treatment with pulse dye laser helps in the destruction

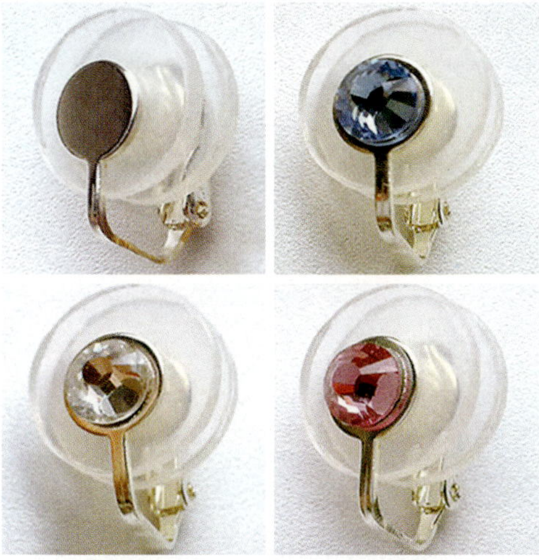

Fig. 20.6: Pressure earrings.

of the vessels within the keloid and those supplying it. As a result there is tissue hypoxia followed by cytokine stimulation and collagenolysis. This ultimately results in volume reduction of the keloids.[3] With or without intralesional steroids combined, pulse dye laser treatment is a useful modality for moderate improvement of keloids with a very good side effect profile and patient compliance.[5] Pulsed dye laser or QsNdYAG laser can also be used to reduce the hard consistency and bulkiness of the keloid.

***Pressure therapy*:** This is best suited for auricular keloids where pressure can be applied from the front and countered from behind to build an abutment. This can be done in the form of silicone gel custom made pressure clips,[6] or simple pressing type pressure earrings (Fig. 20.6). The pressure applied should be 20 to 30 mm Hg and should be applied to comfort levels to avoid skin necrosis.[7] It is a form of adjuvant treatment with minimal risk, best initiated about 2 weeks postsurgery after suture removal to prevent recurrence and maintain contour of ear lobe. For larger keloids on the limbs or trunk, compression garments may be used.[3]

Surgical Excision of Keloids

Excision of keloids is associated with high recurrence rates and is not done routinely in dermatosurgical practice. Froelich et al. report that recurrence rates of keloids range between 45% and 100% when treated with surgical excision without adjuvant measures.[8]

Auricular keloids are best treated with surgical excision combined with adjuvant therapies to prevent recurrence. The details of the same are discussed in the section on ear keloids. However, keloids associated with extensive burn injuries, chemical injuries, or injuries and keloids resulting in contractures and restriction of joint movement are usually operated upon by the plastic surgeon along with skin grafting and adjuvant measures to prevent recurrence. The details of this are beyond the scope of this chapter.

Cryosurgery

This includes spray cryotherapy and intralesional cryosurgery using needle cryoprobe. Nascent keloids are supposedly more responsive to treatment with cryotherapy.[8] Cryotherapy helps to soften the keloid thereby making intralesional injection easier. At the same time, it can leave behind hypo or depigmentation at the treated site. Intralesional cryotherapy is another option to overcome this untoward effect.

Spray cryotherapy: This is often combined with intralesional steroid injections.

- Spray cryotherapy must be performed first as it induces mild inflammation and edema in the keloid.
- It is advisable to wait for 15 to 30 minutes after spray cryotherapy prior to intralesional injection.
- This facilitates the subsequent insertion of the needle and injection of the steroid into the edematous keloid, while it also reduces the pain for the patient.

Intralesional cryosugery using needle cryoprobe: This was described by Har-Shai and colleagues.[9]

- An 18 G hypodermic needle is inserted into the keloid through its substance, parallel to the surface of the skin. A wide bored spinal needle may be used alternatively. The entry and the exit points may be marked before inserting the needles as shown in the Figure 20.7A. More than one needle may be inserted simultaneously in larger keloids and the distance between these should be 1 cm.
- The sharp end of the needle may be secured with small plastic tubes, which prevents injury to the dermatosurgeon as well as the patient (Fig. 20.7B).
- The needle hub is then attached to the nozzle of the cryogun and fed with the cryogen (Fig. 20.7C). The cryogen flows through the needle which immediately cools the surrounding keloidal tissue. The flow of the cryogen is stopped when the keloid freezes and appears white and there is formation of white cryoball at the points where needle enters and exits the keloid (Fig. 20.7 D).
- Allow the tissue to thaw for 2 to 3 minutes and then withdraw the needles carefully (Fig. 20.7E).
- This may be followed by intralesional steroid injection (Fig. 20.7F).

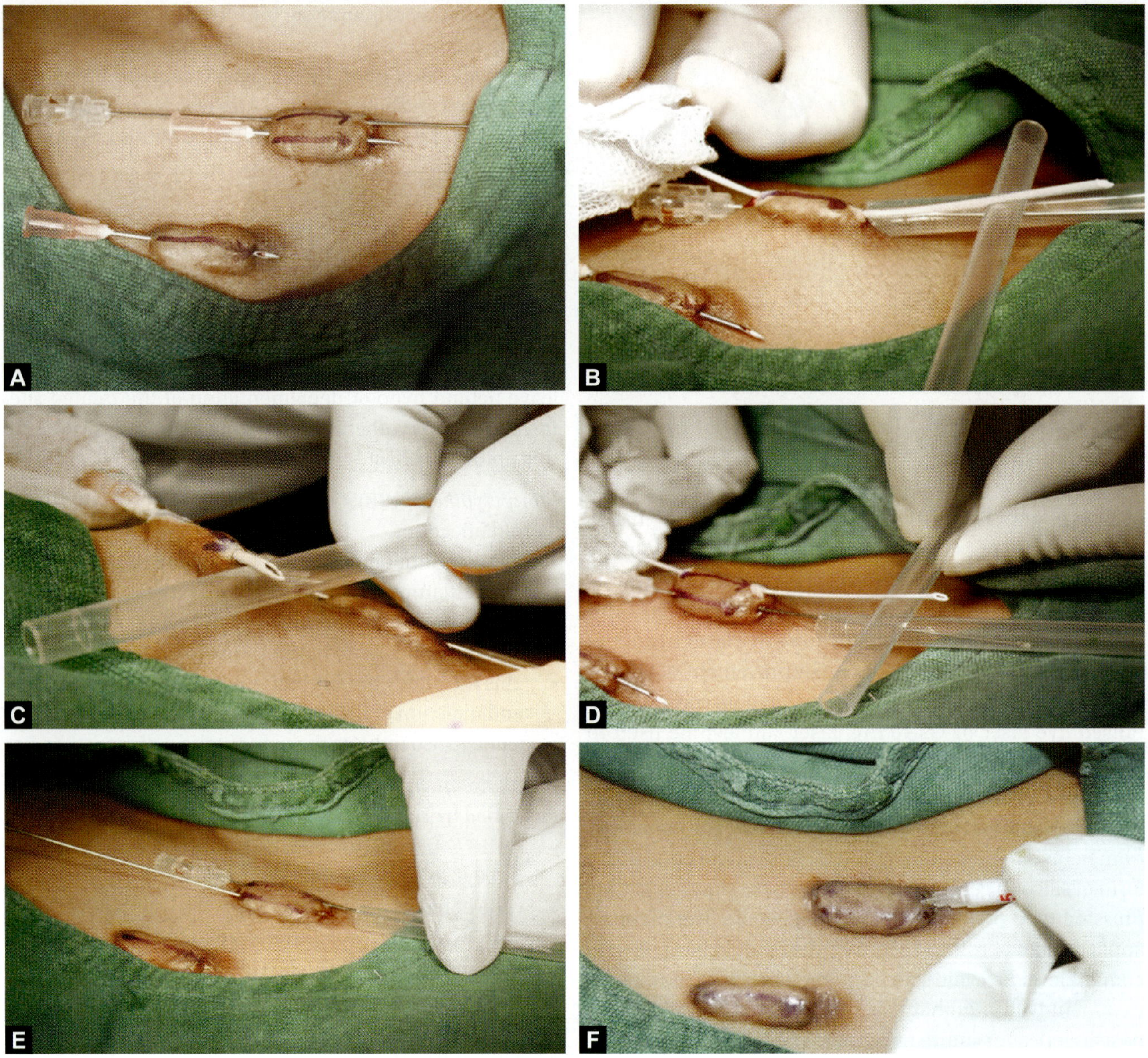

Figs. 20.7A to F: Steps of intralesional cryotherapy.

Advantages

- Relatively simple treatment and less painful
- Economical
- Spray cryotherapy alone may be practised in children who often have needle phobia
- Intralesional cryotherapy does not cause surface epithelial damage, thus lesser chances of depigmentation.

Har-shai et al. reported marked efficacy with lasting keloid volume reduction with single treatment and no evidence of permanent hypopigmentation, recurrence, active bleeding or infection in patients who had received intralesional cryotherapy using cryoprobe.[9]

Disadvantages and Side Effects

- Spray cryotherapy may cause hypopigmentation or depigmentation of the skin of the keloid. Hence, it may not be preferable for keloids on the head and neck and other exposed areas. The hypopigmentation or depigmentation may be permanent or transient with repigmentation occurring within a few months.

- Epidermolysis with blister formation with excessive burning sensation and pain felt by the patient
- Practical issues associated with procuring and storing the cryogen has limited the availability of cryotherapy to fewer centers or institutions.

Innovative Treatments

- Fractional CO_2 laser may be safely used in keloid treatment and it mainly improves the pliability and softness of keloids and hypertrophic scars.[10] Use of fractional CO_2 laser followed by application of topical corticosteroid creams is a useful alternative, especially in patients not willing to take intralesional steroids. Fractional CO_2 treatment forms channels and alternative route for the corticosteroid enabling better penetration and efficacy at the deeper dermal level and lesser epidermal side effects. The proposed mechanism by which fractional CO_2 works is possibly with the involvement of matrix metalloprotease 9 (MMP9) and by stimulating collagen remodeling with the formation of thinner and well-organized collagen bundles which is apparent at least 3 months post-treatment.[10] Fractional CO_2 or Erbium YAG laser can also be used for transdermal drug delivery.
- *Postburns keloids*: In the experience of the author and his colleagues, microneedling with dermaroller over the areas of postburns keloids which may or may not be followed by application of platelet rich plasma topically is a promising therapy for treatment of postburns keloids to achieve some degree of flattening and softening of the keloid. However, currently, there are no published studies regarding the same. Microneedling may possibly work in the same manner as fractional CO_2 laser does in improving the pliability of the keloids and enabling enhanced delivery of topically applied corticosteroid cream.
- *Long pulse Nd: YAG laser*: Mysore et al. reported improvement in hypertrophic scars and keloids by about 30% in Vancouver scar score (VSS) with 3 sessions of long pulse Nd: Yag laser done three weeks apart[11].

CONCLUSION

Treating keloids is a Herculean task! It is frustrating and challenging for the patient as well as the treating clinician. Various treatment modalities give temporary results and recurrence is known.

Response to treatment varies according to the consistency of keloid, anatomical distribution and the treatment method used. Counseling plays an important role in the treatment of keloids. At the outset, it must be explained that multiple sessions are required for complete flattening of the keloids, which may take as long as 2 to 3 years. It should also be emphasized that the keloids may flatten completely, but some visible difference between the normal skin and the keloidal skin will remain despite the treatment. Cryotherapy, intralesional injections and silicone gel dressings play a major role in treating keloids and hypertrophic scars. Each method has its set of pros and cons.

Recurrence rate is 100% after excision of keloids over most of the anatomical sites. Debulking with electrocautery/radiofrequency/ablative laser, results in the recurrence of keloid with substantial increase in the pretreatment size. Use of these modalities should be strictly avoided while treating keloids.

REFERENCES

1. Bayat A, McGrouther DA, Ferguson MWJ. Skin scarring. BMJ. 2003;11;326(7380):88-92.
2. Mustoe TA. Evolution of silicone therapy and mechanism of action in scar management. Aesthetic Plast Surg. 2008;32(1):82-92.
3. Mutalik S. Treatment of keloids and hypertrophic scars. Indian J Dermatol Venereol Leprol. 2005;71(1):3-8.
4. Mankowski P, Kanevsky J, Tomlinson J, et al. Optimizing radiotherapy for keloids: A meta-analysis systematic review comparing recurrence rates between different radiation modalities. Ann Plast Surg. 2017;78(4):403-11.
5. Stephanides S, Rai S, August P, et al. Treatment of refractory keloids with pulsed dye laser alone and with rotational pulsed dye laser and intralesional corticosteroids: A retrospective case series. Laser Ther. 2011;20(4):279-86.
6. Tanaydin V, Beugels J, Piatkowski A, et al. Efficacy of custom-made pressure clips for ear keloid treatment after surgical excision. J Plast Reconstr Aesthetic Surg JPRAS. 2016;69(1):115–21.
7. Walliczek U, Engel S, Weiss C, et al. Clinical outcome and quality of life after a multimodal therapy approach to ear keloids. JAMA Facial Plast Surg. 2015;17(5):333–9.
8. Froelich K, Staudenmaier R, Kleinsasser N, et al. Therapy of auricular keloids: review of different treatment modalities and proposal for a therapeutic algorithm. Eur Arch Oto-Rhino-Laryngol Off J Eur Fed Oto-Rhino-Laryngol Soc EUFOS Affil Ger Soc Oto-Rhino-Laryngol - Head Neck Surg. 2007;264(12):1497–508.
9. Har-Shai Y, Sabo E, Rohde E, et al. Intralesional cryosurgery enhances the involution of recalcitrant auricular keloids: a new clinical approach supported by experimental studies. Wound Repair Regen Off Publ Wound Heal Soc Eur Tissue Repair Soc. 2006;14(1):18–27.
10. Azzam OA, Bassiouny DA, El-Hawary MS, et al. Treatment of hypertrophic scars and keloids by fractional carbon dioxide laser: a clinical, histological, and immunohistochemical study. Lasers Med Sci. 2016;31(1):9–18.
11. LA & HA Journal | Laser and Health Academy [Internet]. [cited 2017 Mar 22]. Available from: http://www.laserandhealthacademy.com/en/journal/?id=1980&type2.

CHAPTER 21

Surgical Management of Earlobe Keloids

Govind Mittal, Biju Vasudevan

INTRODUCTION

The pinna or the external ear can be divided into a cartilaginous upper portion and noncartilaginous pendulous end called the earlobe which is formed by a wedge of adipose tissue.

The incidence of keloids after ear-piercing is around 2.5%.[1] Ear-piercing brings about a contact between deeper dermis layers with more superficial skin layers which could be the reason behind keloid formation (Table 21.1).[2] Incidence is 15 times greater in darker skin types than in white skinned races.

Slobodkin reported that keloids that develop after ear-piercing are more common over the posterior aspect of the pinna than the anterior aspect.[2]

The pinna may be affected with cutaneous tumors and other conditions like cauliflower ear, cystic lesions, etc. thus suspected keloids should be evaluated with an eye on differential diagnoses.

Various forms of treatments have been used for ear keloids including nonsurgical measures and surgical excision. Nonsurgical treatment includes intralesional injection of steroids/5-FU, silicone gel sheeting, post- operative radiotherapy and pressure therapy. Although nonsurgical forms of treatment may be effective in reducing the size of the keloid, they me be cosmetically ineffective, thus making surgical treatment as the preferred line of treatment in patients with ear keloid. Patients must be counseled about possibility of recurrence, persistent palpable nodules postoperatively and the need for regular follow-ups and monitoring.

Classification of Ear Keloids

- Keloids involving the earlobe (noncartilaginous portion of the pinna)—These are further classified according to the Chang-Park classification below.
- Keloids involving the pinna in areas other than the ear-lobe/keloids involving the helical rim (cartilaginous portion of the pinna).

According to the Chang-Park classification,[3] the ear- lobe keloids could be classified into five types as listed in Table 21.2.

A keloid may be referred to as pedunculated or sessile depending on the amount of surface contact of the keloid with the normal skin of pinna. The keloid is called sessile if the diameter of the mass of contact of the keloid with the skin of the pinna exceeds 2/3rd of the largest diameter of the keloids.[3]

The classification of ear keloids according to morphology assists surgeons in choosing the appropriate surgical method and further management.[4]

Principles of Ear Keloid Surgery

Kim et al.[5] have mentioned five As and one B in closure technique for surgical treatment of ear keloids.

- Asepsis
- Atraumatic technique
- Absence of raw surface
- Accurate approximation of wound margin
- Avoidance of tension
- Bleeding control.

Table 21.1: Etiology of ear keloid.

Anything involving **deep dermal injury**
- Ear-piercings (most common)
- Postelective surgery
- Trauma
- Burns

Miscellaneous–acne, mosquito bite, etc.

Table 21.2: Chang-Park classification of earlobe keloids.

- Type I—Pedunculated with 3 subtypes—Type IA, IB, IC
  - IA—Pedunculated anterior surface
  - IB—Pedunculated posterior surface
  - IC—Both surfaces
- Type II—Sessile, single nodular pattern
- Type III—Sessile, multinodular pattern
- Type IV—Buried
- Type V—Mixeds

The principles of surgical management of ear keloids are listed in Table 21.3.

Local Anesthesia for the Pinna

The pinna can be anesthetized by giving the diamond block (Fig. 21.1).

- 1% lignocaine with adrenaline is infiltrated by using 1.5 inch 26-g needle by introducing it at the inferior end of the pinna where it is attached to the cheek, and directed anteriorly and injected as the needle is withdrawn.
- The needle need not be removed completely and with the same skin puncture, the needle is directed posteriorly along the retroauricular groove.
- The same procedure can be done for the superior end of the pinna attachment, if keloids involving the helical rim are being operated upon.

Table 21.3: Principles of ear keloid surgery.

- Meticulous surgical planning to preserve cosmetic auricular structure in view of scanty subcutaneous tissue.[6]
- Preservation of volume and contour of the pinna/earlobe.
- Resection of keloidal tissue—as completely as possible.
- Skin closure with or without flap should be done with minimal tension. Redistribution of tension along the wound edges or along margins of the flap contributes to reduced rate of recurrence.
- Strict asepsis and postoperative antibiotics to prevent secondary infection.
- Postoperative measures to/institution of nonsurgical measures prevent recurrence.

Efforts must be taken to treat ear keloids in a single surgical procedure. This is important as a second or revision surgery may be hindered by the small volume of earlobe being available.[7]

- Inflitration of the periphery of the keloid with 0.5% lignocaine with 1:200,000 adrenaline helps in providing a less bloody field. This facilitates dissection and creation of a flap.
- Alternatively the pinna can also be anesthetized by giving a combination of the following:
  - Auriculotemporal nerve block (Fig. 21.2) where the area between the root of the helix and the tragus is infiltrated in order to anesthetize the helix and tragus.
  - Infiltration along the retroauricular area (Fig. 21.3) from just behind the earlobe (as in diamond block) to anesthetize the earlobe and lateral helix supplied by the greater auricular and less occipital nerves.

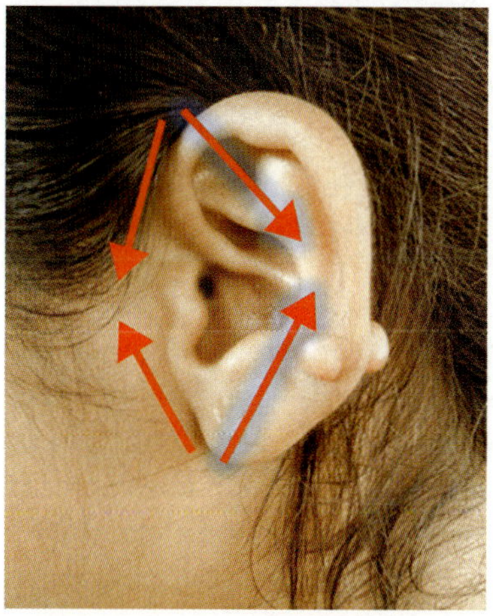

Fig. 21.1: Diamond block technique of anesthetizing the pinna. The blue are around the red arrow indicates that the earlobe is folded forwards and anesthetic is injected into the retroauricular groove.

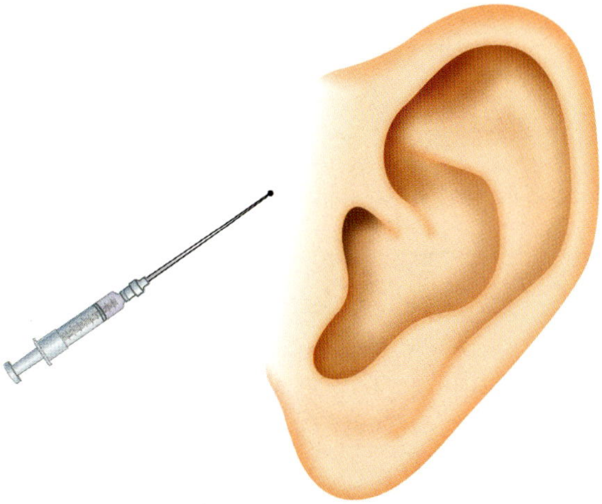

Fig. 21.2: Auriculotemporal nerve block.

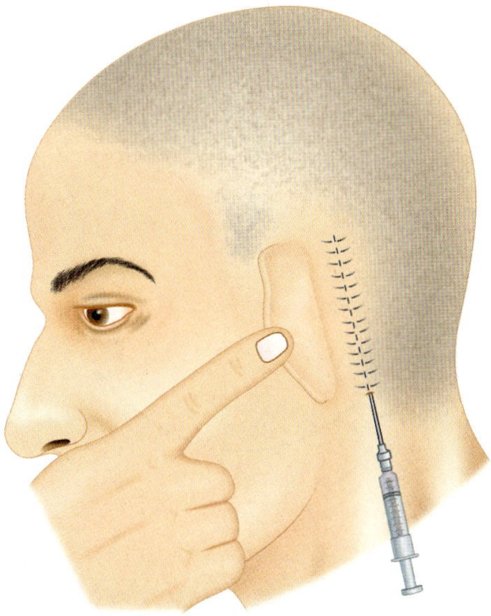

Fig. 21.3: Infiltration along the retroauricular area.

Steps to be Followed as Routine for All Ear Keloid Surgeries

- The scalp hair must be secured with a surgical cap and the preauricular hair lock be safely tucked in the same and secured with micropore tape.
- The external auditory canal (EAC) can be stuffed gently with a cotton ball smeared with petroleum jelly. This will prevent betadine/saline/blood from entering the EAC.
- A bipolar cautery can be used for hemostasis if necessary.
- Tissue handling—In surgeries where flaps are raised, the flap created should be handled with minimal manipulation, preferably with fine toothed forceps or skin hooks. Traumatic forceps should be avoided.
- Intraoperatively, triamcinolone acetonide to be injected along the edges of resection and line of wound closure to prevent chances of recurrence of keloid.
- After the procedure a pressure dressing to be applied.

Surgical Techniques for Management of Ear Keloids

The techniques for ear keloid surgery could be broadly classified as extramarginal excision and intramarginal excision.

Simple total excision of keloids or **extramarginal excision** is associated with high rates of recurrence due to reproliferation of keloidal tissue along the line of incision closed under tension. However, standard keloidectomy and radical keloidectomy which are types of **extramarginal excision**, may be the procedure of choice in specific types of ear keloids where closure can be achieved without tension.

In ear keloids where surgical excision may result in large defects and simple excision and closure without tension is not possible, **intramarginal excision**,[8] is the preferred technique in such cases. This surgical technique involves creation of a fillet flap by sharp dissection of the keloid from the native overlying expanded skin. This skin can be trimmed and is available for tension-free closure of the defect. Thus elimination of "closure under tension" in intramarginal excision ensures reduced chances of recurrence and better cosmesis.

It is important to note that every keloid of the ear is different and depending on the size and extent of the keloid, the surgical plan should be tailored.

Standard Keloidectomy

- Pedunculated keloids have a narrow base and can be excised rather with ease by standard keloidectomy (Fig. 21.4).
- Using the 135° angle between the skin and the scalpel blade, a sequential bevel elliptical incision is made at the base of the keloid right at the peduncle.
- The keloid is excised in toto followed by primary closure of the surgical wound.

Radical Keloidectomy

- This is preferred for sessile keloids (Types II and III).
- It involves a full thickness wedge excision (Figs. 21.5 and 21.6), if the keloidal mass has extended over the entire lobule surface.

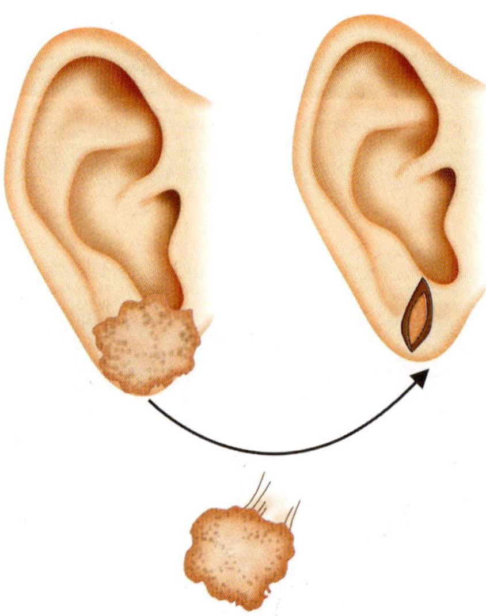

Fig. 21.4: Standard keloidectomy.

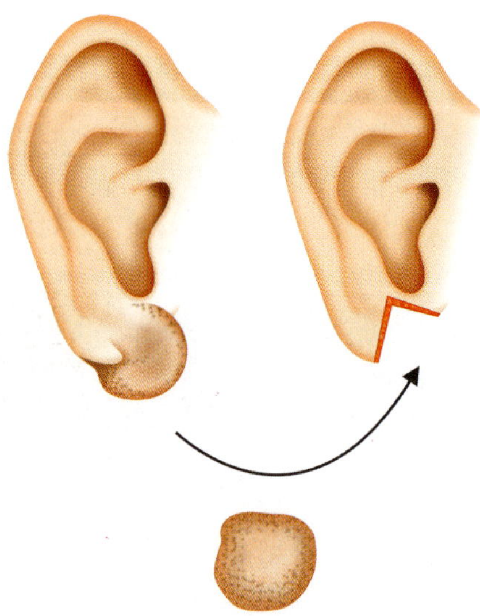

Fig. 21.5: Radical keloidectomy.

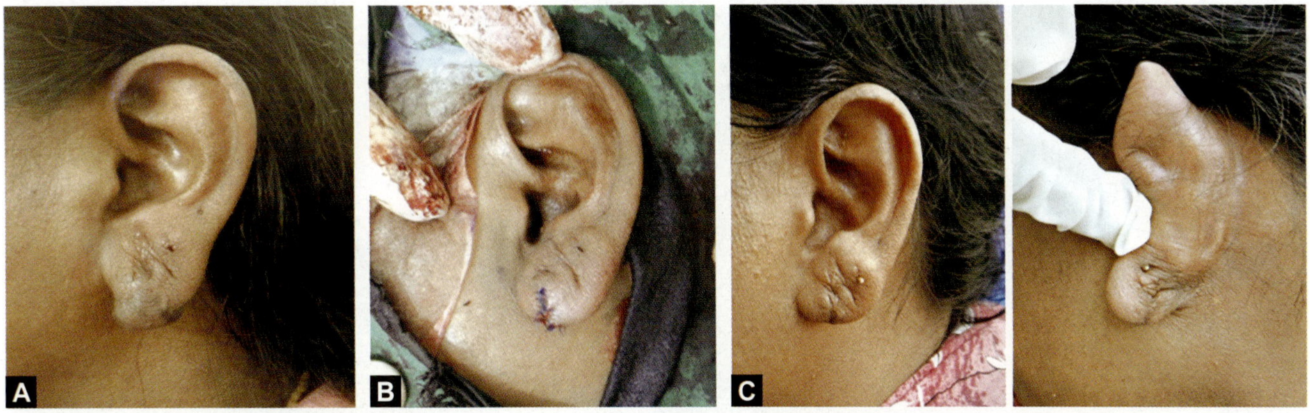

Figs. 21.6A to C: (A) Recurrent sessile keloid involving the entire thickness of the earlobe, preoperative. (B) Immediate postoperative photograph postradical keloidectomy by wedge excision of the keloid. (C) Three months after radical keloidectomy.

- Complete removal of the fibrotic tissue is important to prevent recurrence.
- Some cases of wedge excision of large earlobe keloids may involve earlobe reconstruction with V-Y advancement flap from the cheek.[9]

Excision of Park Type IV or Buried Earlobe Keloid

Pure buried types of keloids are best diagnosed on palpation since they are usually not raised more than 3 mm from the surface and show minimal color or contour change externally on the skin surface. These are more often present along the anterior aspect of the earlobe or along the noncartilaginous outer and upper extension of earlobe adjoining the antihelix. These are usually less that 5 mm in size and can be easily excised by punch excision and primary closure.

- ***Through and through (punch) excision and keloid core extirpation (Figs. 21.7A to D)***: This may be preferred if the keloid is thicker and extending through the entire tract of the original ear-piercing from the anterior to the posterior cutaneous wall of the earlobe. A scalpel with no. 15 BP blade can be used to dissect the keloidal mass from the rest of the earlobe tissue if needed after the punch has been used to incise into the earlobe.

  It is better to choose the smallest punch size suitable to excise the keloid. This will ensure that circular defect created in the anterior and posterior cutaneous wall can be closed primarily with a smaller aesthetic scar, without dog ear formation. Instead of a punch excision, the excision may be performed by a standard elliptical excision on the anterior and posterior earlobe walls.

  One must minimize the amount of normal earlobe tissue excised along with the (buried) keloid so as to prevent volume loss of the earlobe.

  Steps
  - The small buried keloid is located; a sponge holding forceps is used to provide a blood less field (Fig. 21.7A).
  - The keloid if small can be localized in the loop or eye of the forceps and the punch is passed through it, from the anterior wall and exiting from the posterior wall and thus keloid is excised in toto including the tract (Figs. 21.7B to D).
  - The defect is then sutured using 6-0 prolene interrupted simple sutures anteriorly and posteriorly.
- ***Single-sided punch excision (Figs. 21.8A and B)***: In patients where the buried keloid is small or the sessile keloid is small and predominantly situated closer to either the anterior or posterior cutaneous wall of the earlobe; punch excision can also be done respectively from the anterior or posterior aspect of the earlobe without a complete through and through incision. This is followed by primary closure on the respective aspect of the earlobe. This technique may involve higher chances of recurrence since the entire tract of pierced earlobe is not excised.

Keloid Core Extirpation

(Figures involving this technique will be found in surgical case discussions below)

This was described by Lee et al.[10] as an intramarginal surgical treatment for both keloids involving the auricle or

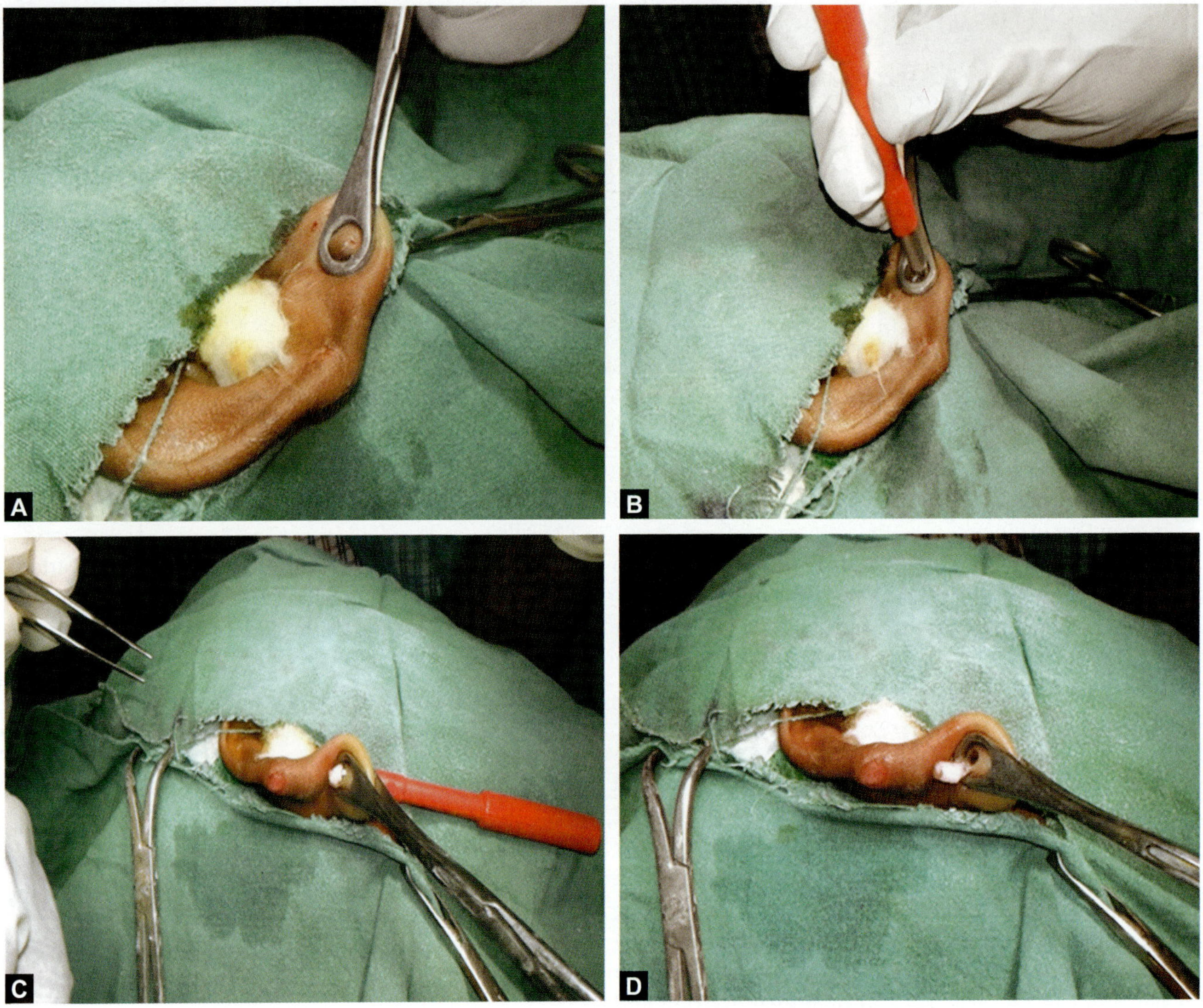

Figs. 21.7A to D: Steps of punch excision of a keloid.

elsewhere in the body. The principle of the surgery involves excision of core keloidal tissue and use the keloid rind flap to close the defect.

- An incision is made along the circumference of the keloid, about 1 mm internal to the outer edge of the keloid (intramarginal).
- A flap of skin referred to as the keloid rind flap is thus raised and separated from the fibrous keloid core.
- The keloid rind flap includes epidermis, dermis and the rich subcapsular vascular plexus which is located just deep to the fibrous capsule of the keloid.
- This is followed by extirpation of the keloid core and only a thin margin of scar tissue is left behind.
- The defect is then closed by resurfacing the surrounding skin with the flap raised.

Lee et al.[10] reported high levels of patient satisfaction in those treated with core extirpation for ear keloids, without any flap related complication (congestion, necrosis and flap loss) and a nonrecurrence in 87.5% of the patients. Keloid core extirpation technique has been reported to be excellent in preventing recurrence of keloid with no adjuvant therapy after surgery.[6,10]

Keloids of the Helical Rim

(Figures involving this technique will be found in step surgical case discussions below)

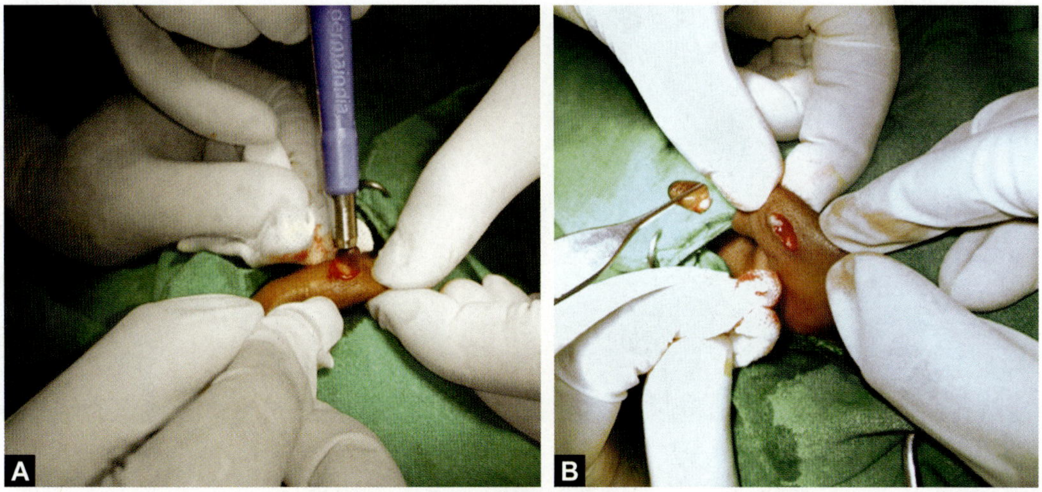

Figs. 21.8A and B: (A) The punch introduced from the posterior aspect around a small buried keloid protruding posteriorly. (B) The keloid is excised by punch excision.

Keloids of the rim are tough to manage since the helix has a thin, curved cartilage and has a unique three dimensional structure, which is important to maintain in order to give esthetically acceptable results postsurgery. Due to the above reasons, it is important to preserve the skin over the keloid especially in the helix area and hence intramarginal excision or intralesional excision of the rim keloids is commonly preferred. This involves full thickness excision or shaving off the bulk of the keloid while maintaining a thin rim of keloid and skin overlying it in order to close the defect (rind fillet flap). While shaving off the keloidal core, it is important to remove the scar tissue till deeper healthy tissue is visualized, however, care must be taken so as to not damage the perichondrium.

Modifications

Various techniques have been performed for surgical management of keloids across the globe and some modifications have been mentioned below.

X-shaped excision: Qi et al.[11] described the novel method with the following steps.

- X-shaped incision drawn on the keloid
- Elevation of four isocentric triangular flaps of epidermis and dermis with the subdermal plexus
- The exposed underlying keloid is dissected and carefully separated from the cartilaginous framework
- The flaps are transposed, followed by approximation with 6-0 prolene sutures.

Use of autograft postkeloid excision: Ziccardi and Lamphier,[12] reported the use of full thickness autograft skin separated from excised dumbell-shaped ear keloid in order to close a large defect involving the posterior lobe of the earlobe. No recurrence was reported during 6 months of follow-up postsurgery.

Subcutaneous island pedicle flap: Hatoko et al. reported the use of subcutaneous island pedicle flap created at the posterior aspect of the pinna.[13]

BRIEF DISCUSSION OF THE DERMATO-SURGICAL PROCEDURE PERFORMED FOR SOME EAR KELOIDS

Case 1 (Figs. 21.9A to F)

- This patient presented with a mixed type of keloid with both protuberant anterior and posterior extent (Figs. 21.9A and B). Since an area of normal skin along the lower end of the helix was noted between the anterior and the posterior keloidal growth, it was planned to be retained and used for resurfacing the flaps after excision of the keloid.
- A C-shaped incision was made intramarginally along the outer aspect of the anterolaterally extending keloid and a flap of skin was raised (Fig. 21.9C). The keloidal scar tissue was excised. The excess skin from the flap (Fig. 21.9D) was trimmed with a small curved scissors to ensure adequate approximation of the edges. The keloid in the posterior aspect was excised in similar fashion.
- The two flaps thus created were sutured with 6-0 interrupted prolene sutures to the normal intervening skin of the helix and upper part of the earlobe (Figs. 21.9E and F).

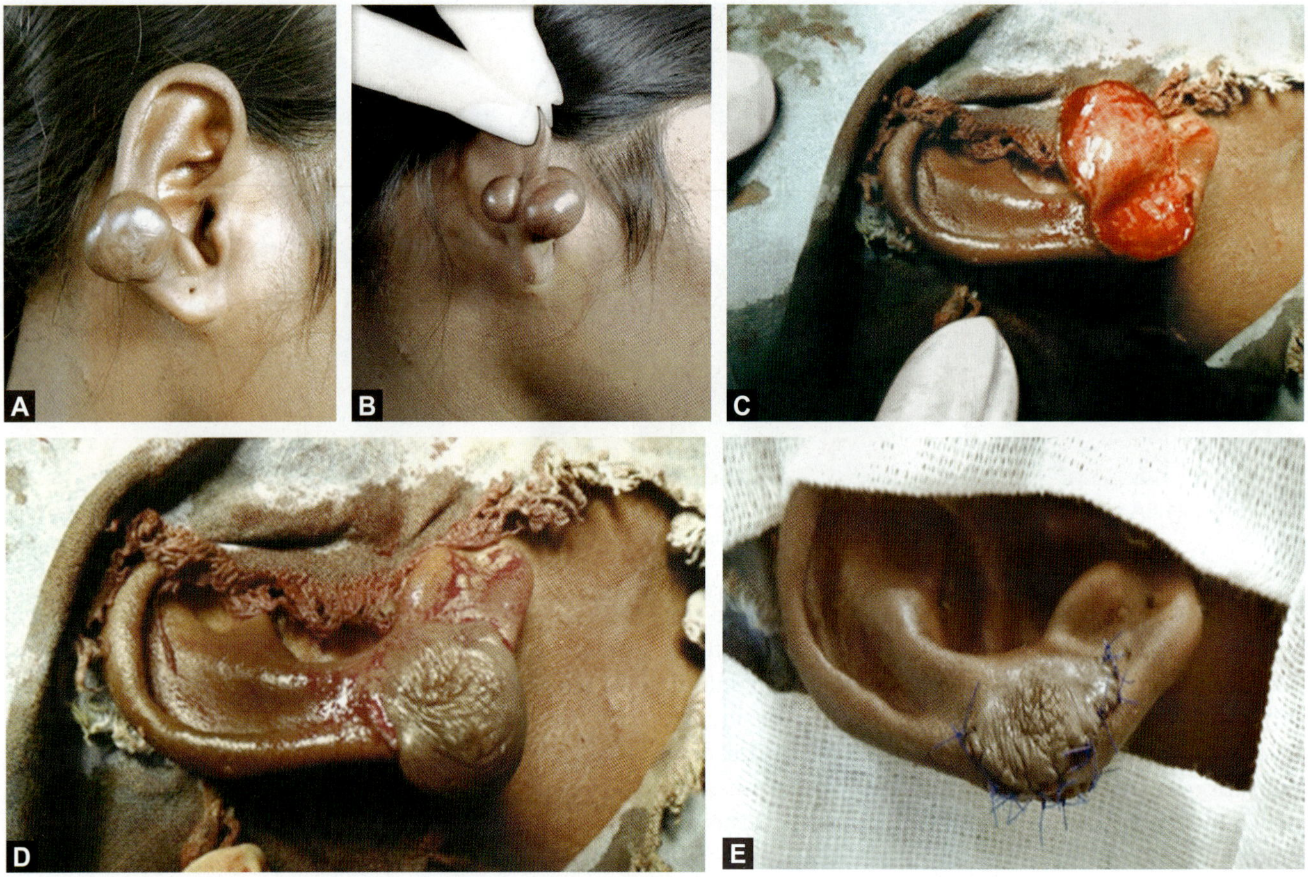

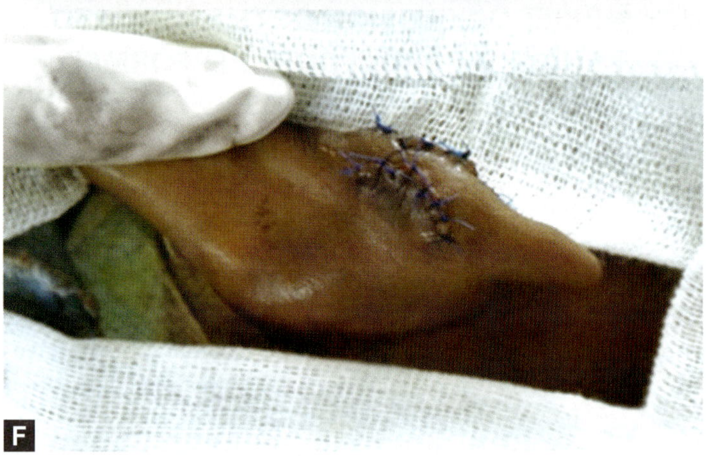

Figs. 21.9A to F: (A to D) Dumbell ear keloid: Flaps raised and preparation for suturing. (E and F) Flaps sutured.

Case 2 (Figs. 21.10A to I)

- The patient in Figure 21.10A presented with keloid on the margin of the helix which developed after a mosquito bite.
- For intramarginal excision, the incision was planned on the lateral aspect of the keloid in such a way, that the rind fillet flap was raised on the anterior aspect (Fig. 21.10B). The keloid core was incised through a wedged elliptical incision from the posterior part of the keloid and the core was removed (Fig. 21.10C).
- The rind fillet flap rised anteriorly was folded along the margin of the helix and after necessary trimming of the margins to suit the contour, the flap was resurfaced with the posterior margin using 6-0 prolene interrupted sutures (Figs. 21.10D to F).

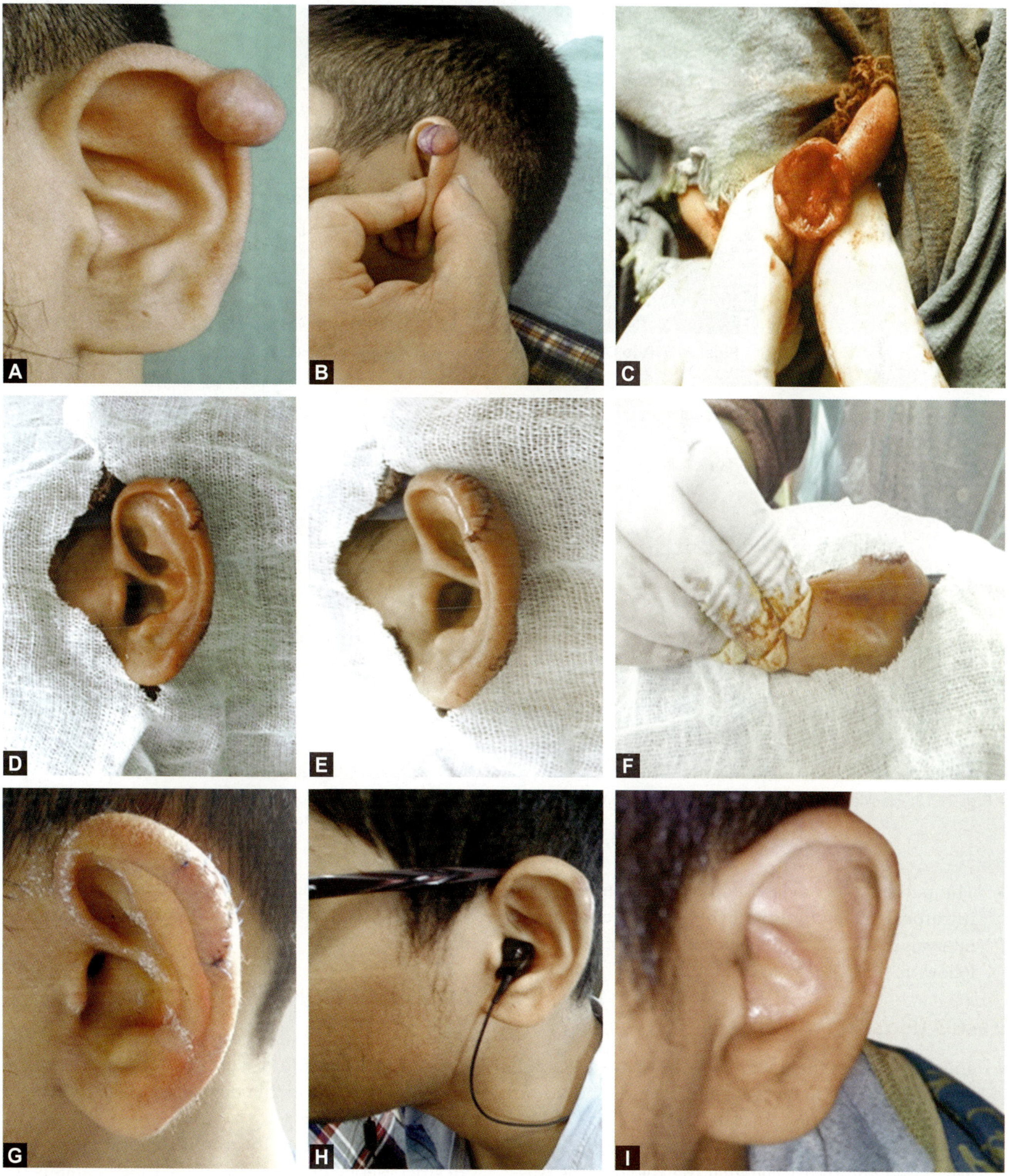

Figs. 21.10A to I: (A to F) Steps of flap raising and suturing. (G) 2 days postsurgery. (H) 3 weeks postsurgery. (I) 2 months postsurgery.

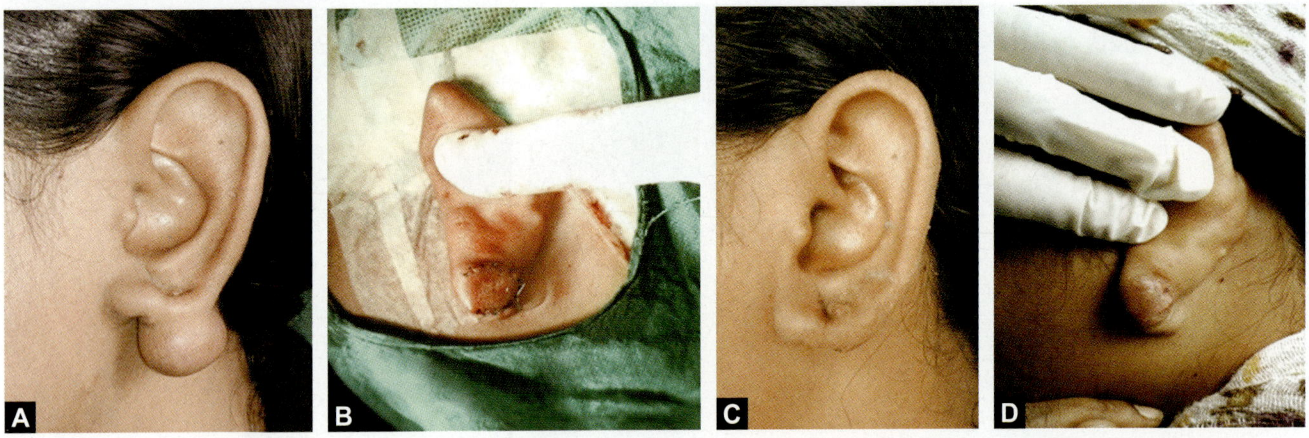

Figs. 21.11A to D: Steps of excision of a berry-shaped keloid.

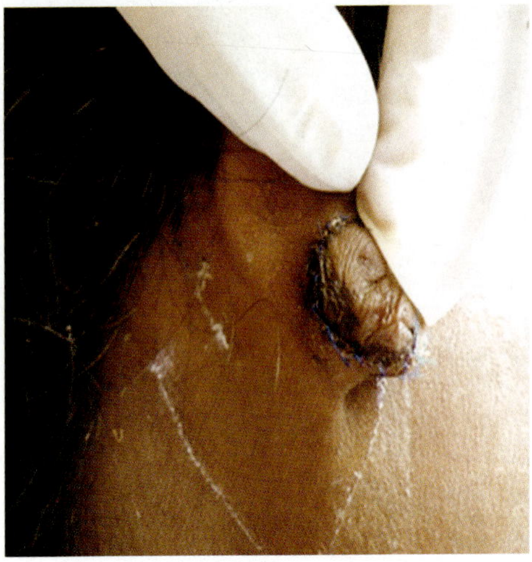

Fig. 21.12: Blackish discoloration noticed along the C-shaped suture line.

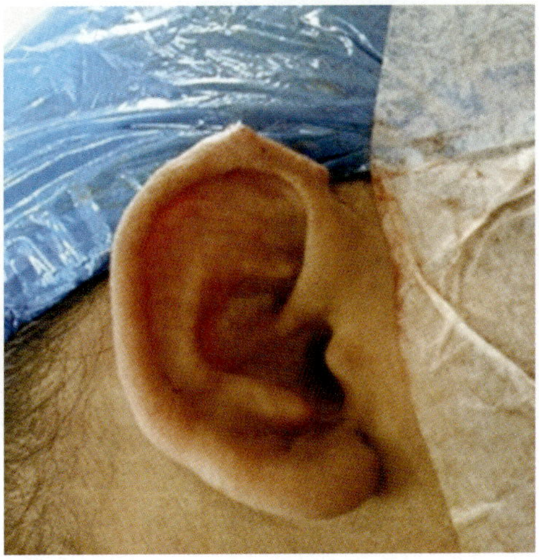

Fig. 21.13: Dog ear formation leading to a sharp edge on superior surface.

- The patient was advised adjuvant treatment with intrafocal triamcinolone acetonide injections at intervals of 3 weeks and the patient was doing fine on follow-up (Figs. 21.10G to I).

Case 3 (Figs. 21.11A to D)

- This patient presented with a "berry-shaped" keloid which was found to be "hanging" from the posterior wall of the earlobe (Fig. 21.11A).
- This was excised by making a C-shaped incision; a flap was raised and resurfaced after the keloid tissue was excised. It was closed using 6-0 interrupted prolene sutures (Fig. 21.11B).
- At follow-up on 14th day postsurgery, the sutures were removed and the patient was doing fine. The "berry" had gone! (Figs. 21.11C and D). The residual keloidal nodularity was managed with intralesional steroid injections.

COMPLICATIONS

- Epidermal necrosis, flap necrosis—This can occur due to increased tension or very closely placed sutures (Fig. 21.12) or due to thin flap raised lacking sufficient arterial supply.
- Secondary infection—This can be minimized by used of strict aseptic precautions during surgery and use of intraoperative and postoperative course of antibiotics.
- Dog ear formation (Fig. 21.13)—This can be prevented by planning the incision well, adequate resection of keloidal tissue from the base and edges of the flap

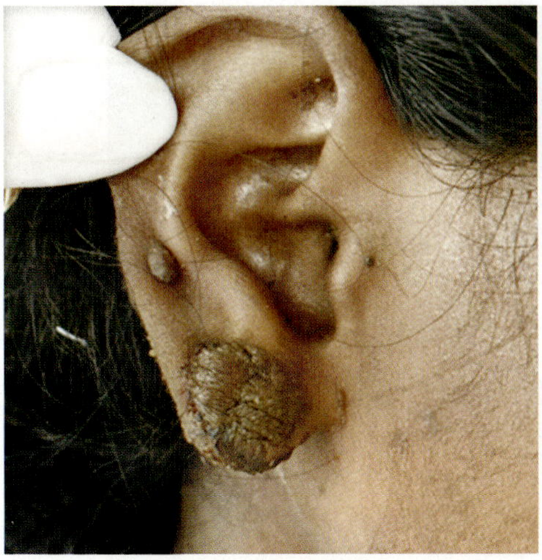

Fig. 21.14: Color mismatch of flap.

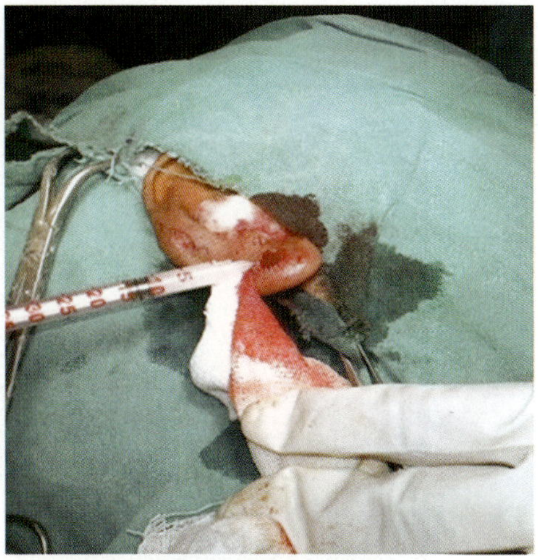

Fig. 21.15: Intraoperative dose of triamcinolone acetonide after excision of the keloid.

and adjusting the flap length and pedicle width before suturing. Dog ear once noticed, should be corrected. Dog ear correction can be challenging in a three dimensional structure such as the pinna.

- Color mismatch of the flap—The skin overlying the keloid is atrophic and discolored due to prolonged stretching caused by growth of fibrous tissue. In most instances of intramarginal excision, the same skin is used to raise the flap which thus appears different in color and texture from surrounding skin (Fig. 21.14). This however, improves with time and topical depigmenting agents can be used.
- Recurrence of keloid—Recurrence has been defined as any elevation of the scar or extension of the keloid beyond the original surgical field.[12] Recurrence of keloids postsurgery is a rule rather than exception.[10] This necessitates long-term follow-up of patients after surgery for duration of 1 to 2 years.[22] Recurrence rates are different for keloids involving the earlobe and the auricle. Ogawa et al. reported recurrence rate of 5.7% in earlobe keloid as against 38.5% in patients with keloid in the auricle excluding the earlobe, when the two were treated with surgical excision followed by electron beam radiation.[14]

PREVENTION OF RECURRENCE OF EAR KELOIDS POSTSURGERY

- Intraoperative triamcinolone acetonide injection (Fig. 21.15) followed by monthly local injections for up to six months largely reduces the incidence of postexcision recurrence of keloids. However, there are incidences of delayed recurrence and the patient is advised to be on regular follow-up for 6 to 12 months.
- Intralesional steroid may also be combined with 5-Fluorouracil (5-FU). However, 5-FU combination is preferably avoided during the intraoperative dose of steroid since it may further prolong wound healing.
- Intralesional verapamil injection may be administered at concentration of 2.5 mg/mL (depending on the size of the keloid—0.5 mL to 2 mL per session) initiated 2 weeks postsurgery and then repeated after a month post-resection.[15] Verapamil being a calcium channel blocker is helpful as an adjunctive measure in preventing relapse as the molecular mechanics of formation of extracellular matrix involves calcium antagonism.
- Radiation therapy—This is most often delivered post-operatively. However, combining preoperative radiotherapy, one day prior to extralesional keloid excision and followed by postoperative radiotherapy (sandwich technique) has been reported to be effective with low recurrence rates.[8] According to a randomized, prospective trial, postoperative radiotherapy was found to have a lower recurrence rate of 12.5% as against 33% in patients who were treated with postoperative intralesional steroid injections.[16] The recommended dosage is 10–15 Gy over 2 to 3 fractions and the overall reported recurrence is about 4%.[18] Therapy was found to be maximally beneficial when administered within 48 hours of surgery.[7]
- Cotton pledgets soaked in mitomycin-C (0.4 mg/5 mL) can be placed in the defect for 4 minutes immediately after surgical excision of the keloid core, prior to primary

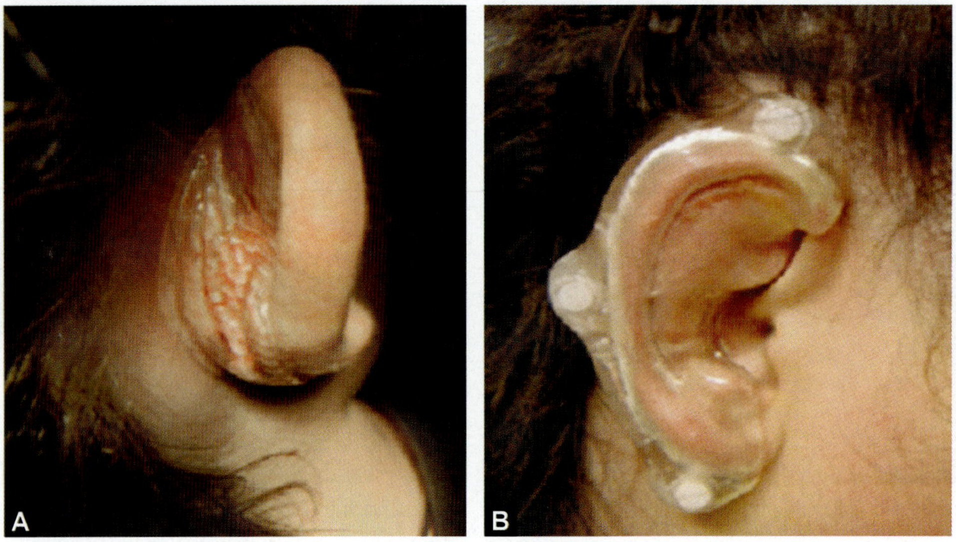

Figs. 21.16A and B: Application of the compressive device. (A) Application of the silicone gel sheet. (B) Fixing of the oyster shells (with kind permission from Quintessenz Zahntechnik).

closure. This technique was reported to have a 90% success rate in prevention of recurrence in a 10 patient cohort study followed for a mean of 8 months.[17]

- Mitomycin-C applied topically postexcision has been reported to reduce the rate of recurrence.
- Imiquimod application—5% imiquimod cream, applied daily over night for 8 hours for a period of 8 weeks, after healing of the surgical wound, has been reported to reduce postoperative recurrence of keloids. Patients should be cautioned about possible local irritation and redness.

 When radiation treatment or intralesional steroids are not available or suitable in particular patients, it has been has shown that topical application of mitomycin-C and imiquimod postsurgical excision has a recurrence rate of 16.5% and 24.7% respectively.

- Pressure therapy and silicone gel sheets—This can be done in the form of custom made silicone gel pressure clips[5] (Figs. 21.16A and B), magnetic disks or simple pressing type pressure earrings. The pressure applied should be 20 to 30 mm Hg and should be applied to comfort levels to avoid skin necrosis.[18-22] It is a form of adjuvant treatment with minimal risk, best initiated about 2 weeks postsurgery after suture removal to prevent recurrence and maintain contour of earlobe. Tanaydin et al. reported a recurrence rate of 29.5% when pressure-adjustable silicone ear clips were worn for 12 hours/day postsurgical excision for a duration on 6 to 18 months.[23]

TIPS AND TRICKS

- In very large irregular earlobe keloids, it may be advisable to treat with few sessions of intralesional triamcinolone acetonide injection in order to reduce the size of the keloid before it is taken up for surgery.
- A chalazion clamp or sponge holding forceps may be gently held proximal to the keloid, so as to reduce the bleeding and provide a clear field (Fig. 21.17).
- The intraoperative dose of triamcinolone injection may often trickle away with the oozing margins of the operative wound after excision of the keloid. In order to ensure sufficient delivery of the drug, the injection may be given (using an insulin syringe) after the surgical defect is closed and margins resurfaced. The injection is given along the walls and margins of the closed defect and also through the freshly sutured surgical incision between two sutures.
- During suture removal, it is always advisable to remove the alternate sutures first and look for any gaping. If the surgical wound has healed well and complete adhesion of the adjoining skin edges has taken place, all sutures can be removed at once.

Further, even after suture removal if there are small areas of gaping, or even otherwise, dressing with "Steristrips" may be advised.

Other Modalities of Treatments for Ear Keloid

- Collagenase injections may be given along with compression or pressure therapy as described by Bae-Harboe and colleagues.

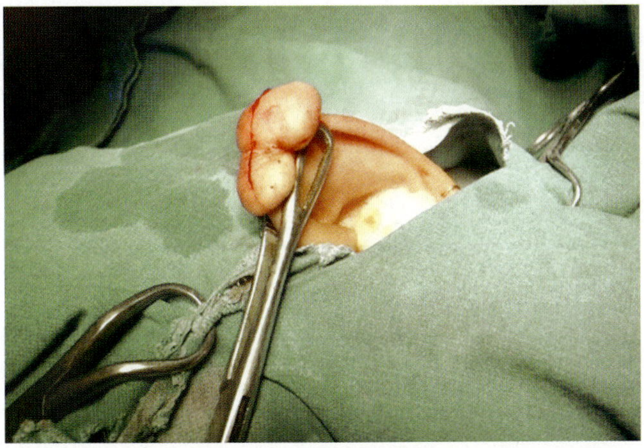

Fig. 21.17: Sponge holding forceps being used to grip the pinna, proximal to the keloid— *without traumatizing the ear cartilage* in order to reduce intraoperative bleeding).

- Radiofrequency tissue volume reduction (RFTVR)— This is a novel, minimally invasive treatment option for treatment of keloids of the auricle. It is a technology that induces extensive fibrosis at the target tissues and hence causes volume reduction over one to several sessions. It may be combined with intralesional steroid injections.[24-26]

REFERENCES

1. Zuber TJ, DeWitt DE. Earlobe keloids. Am Fam Physician. 1994;49(8):1835-41.
2. Slobodkin D. Why more keloids on back than on front of earlobe. Lancet Lond Engl. 1990;335(8694):923-4.
3. Park TH, Seo SW, Kim JK, et al. Earlobe keloids: classification according to gross morphology determines proper surgical approach. Dermatol Surg Off Publ Am Soc Dermatol Surg Al. 2012;38(3):406-12.
4. Park SY, Lee GH, Park JM, et al. Clinical characteristics of auricular keloids treated with surgical excision. Korean J Audiol. 2012;16(3):134-7.
5. Kim DY, Kim ES, Eo SR, et al. A surgical approach for earlobe keloid: keloid fillet flap. Plast Reconstr Surg. 2004;113(6):1668-74.
6. Watson D, Panuganti B. Treating scars in the auricle region. Facial Plast Surg Clin N Am. 2017;25(1):73-81.
7. Akaishi S, Ogawa R, Hyakusoku H. Management of ear keloids. Plast Reconstr Surg. 2008;122(2):670-1.
8. Walliczek U, Engel S, Weiss C, et al. Clinical outcome and quality of life after a multimodal therapy approach to ear keloids. JAMA Facial Plast Surg. 2015;17(5):333-9.
9. Ogawa R, Huang C, Akaishi S, et al. Analysis of surgical treatments for earlobe keloids: analysis of 174 lesions in 145 patients. Plast Reconstr Surg. 2013;132(5):818e-825e.
10. Lee Y, Minn KW, Baek RM, et al. A new surgical treatment of keloid: keloid core excision. Ann Plast Surg. 2001;46(2):135-40.
11. Qi Z, Liang W, Wang Y, et al. 'X'-shaped incision and keloid skin-flap resurfacing: a new surgical method for auricle keloid excision and reconstruction. Dermatol Surg Off Publ Am Soc Dermatol Surg Al. 2012;38(8):1378-82.
12. Ziccardi VB, Lamphier J. Use of keloid skin as an autograft for earlobe reconstruction after excision. Oral Surg Oral Med Oral Pathol Oral Radiol Endod. 2000;89(6):674-5.
13. Hatoko M, Kuwahara M, Shiba A, et al. Earlobe reconstruction using a subcutaneous island pedicle flap after resection of 'earlobe keloid'. Dermatol Surg Off Publ Am Soc Dermatol Surg Al. 1998;24(2):257-61.
14. Ogawa R, Miyashita T, Hyakusoku H, et al. Postoperative radiation protocol for keloids and hypertrophic scars: statistical analysis of 370 sites followed for over 18 months. Ann Plast Surg. 2007;59(6):688-91.
15. Lawrence WT. Treatment of earlobe keloids with surgery plus adjuvant intralesional verapamil and pressure earrings. Ann Plast Surg. 1996;37(2):167-9.
16. Stahl S, Barnea Y, Weiss J, et al. Treatment of earlobe keloids by extralesional excision combined with preoperative and postoperative 'sandwich' radiotherapy. Plast Reconstr Surg. 2010;125(1):135-41.
17. Sclafani AP, Gordon L, Chadha M, et al. Prevention of earlobe keloid recurrence with postoperative corticosteroid injections versus radiation therapy: a randomized, prospective study and review of the literature. Dermatol Surg Off Publ Am Soc Dermatol Surg Al. 1996;22(6):569-74.
18. Froelich K, Staudenmaier R, Kleinsasser N, et al. Therapy of auricular keloids: review of different treatment modalities and proposal for a therapeutic algorithm. Eur Arch Oto-Rhino-Laryngol Off J Eur Fed Oto-Rhino-Laryngol Soc EUFOS Affil Ger Soc Oto-Rhino-Laryngol-Head Neck Surg. 2007;264(12):1497-508.
19. Stewart CE, Kim JY. Application of mitomycin-C for head and neck keloids. Otolaryngol—Head Neck Surg Off J Am Acad Otolaryngol-Head Neck Surg. 2006;135(6):946-50.
20. Chi SG, Kim JY, Lee WJ, et al. Ear keloids as a primary candidate for the application of mitomycin C after shave excision: in vivo and in vitro study. Dermatol Surg Off Publ Am Soc Dermatol Surg Al. 2011;37(2):168-75.
21. Martin-García RF, Busquets AC. Postsurgical use of imiquimod 5% cream in the prevention of earlobe keloid recurrences: results of an open-label, pilot study. Dermatol Surg Off Publ Am Soc Dermatol Surg Al. 2005;31(11 Pt 1):1394-8.
22. Shin JY, Yun SK, Roh SG, et al. Efficacy of 2 representative topical agents to prevent keloid recurrence after surgical excision. J Oral Maxillofac Surg Off J Am Assoc Oral Maxillofac Surg. 2016;6:7.
23. Tanaydin V, Beugels J, Piatkowski A, et al. Efficacy of custom-made pressure clips for ear keloid treatment after surgical excision. J Plast Reconstr Aesthetic Surg JPRAS. 2016;69(1):115-21.
24. Chang CH, Song JY, Park JH, et al. The efficacy of magnetic disks for the treatment of earlobe hypertrophic scar. Ann Plast Surg. 2005;54(5):566-9.
25. Bae-Harboe Y-SC, Harboe-Schmidt JE, Graber E, et al. Collagenase followed by compression for the treatment of earlobe keloids. Dermatol Surg Off Publ Am Soc Dermatol Surg Al. 2014;40(5):519-24.
26. Fruth K, Gouveris H, Kuelkens C, et al. Radiofrequency tissue volume reduction for treatment of auricle keloids. The Laryngoscope. 2011;121(6):1233-6.

CHAPTER 22

Earlobe Repair

Nitin Barde

INTRODUCTION

Earlobe piercing has been performed among both sexes since ancient times for religious, social, and cosmetic purposes[1] Earlobe tear/cleft is a relatively common problem which results from different forms of trauma: abuse, entanglement in telephone cord, babies pulling earrings, trauma while using hair brushes, and clothing, wearing of heavy jewellery, huge decorative objects or even heavy earrings.

Torn earlobes, referred to as cleft or split earlobes can be classified into mostly 2 types: congenital and traumatic.[2] Congenital clefts may be anterior, posterior or sagittal.[3,4] Traumatic clefts may be complete or incomplete. All these variants may be for one ear or both.

Earlobe clefts may also be classified based on length of the tear into 3 types:[5] Type 1—Here the cleft does not extend to more than half the distance between the actual ear piercing and the lower margin of earlobe; Type 2—Here the cleft extends more than half this distance; Type 3—Here the cleft extends till the lower margin totally splitting earlobe. Repair of a torn earlobe is a common procedure encountered in dermatosurgery.

PRINCIPLES OF THE SURGICAL PROCEDURE

Although earlobe repair looks like a simple procedure, accuracy is important in carrying it out. While suturing, even, if one edge is off by a mm, it becomes cosmetically unacceptable leading to patient's dissatisfaction. The patient may have a requirement that she may want to wear earrings as soon as possible which will lead to pressure on the repaired lobe predisposing it to partially healed wound and repeat tears.[6]

Principles

- Freshen the margins of tear by removing the entire epithelial lining of piercing tract along with the earlobe tear. The original hole is closed by suturing to minimize chance of recurrence.
- Convert the partial tear into a complete tear, especially if >75% of the distance between piercing and lower margin is already torn. This will lead to better strength of the wound with better cosmetic results.
- Using single or multiple Z-plasties along vertical axis of complete tear for repair has 2 advantages: first, they will give strength to the repair by adding layers of zigzagging to the scar tissue; second, Z-plasty will ensure vertical elongation, which will prevent the indentation of the earlobe margin because of scar contracture later.
- While repairing complete tear, one should always mark a line along center of the earlobe margin before infiltrating the anesthetic solution and close the inferior margin first. This gives a proper three-dimensional alignment and makes it easier to close remainder of tear.
- The closing of earlobe margins must be done with overcorrected everted sutures. This will allow the margin to end up flat after healing thus avoiding indentation due to scar contracture
- Do not pierce the earlobe again for at least 3 months.[6]

SURGICAL PROCEDURE

Multiple techniques have been proposed for repair of the torn earlobe. We will describe procedure in 2 steps: Surgical repair for:

- Complete earlobe tear
- Partial earlobe tear.

Preoperative workup including relevant blood investigations, consent and photographs are taken.

Complete Earlobe Tear

Steps

- Cleanse the entire earlobe area with Betadine solution and place sterile drapes around the field (Fig. 22.1).

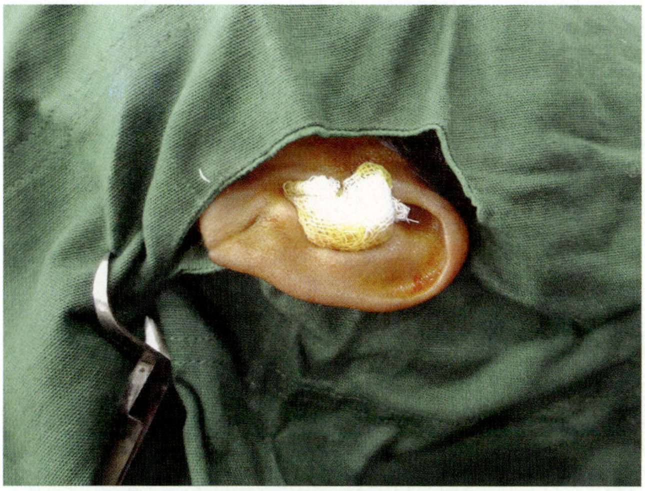

Fig. 22.1: Cleansing and draping of earlobe.

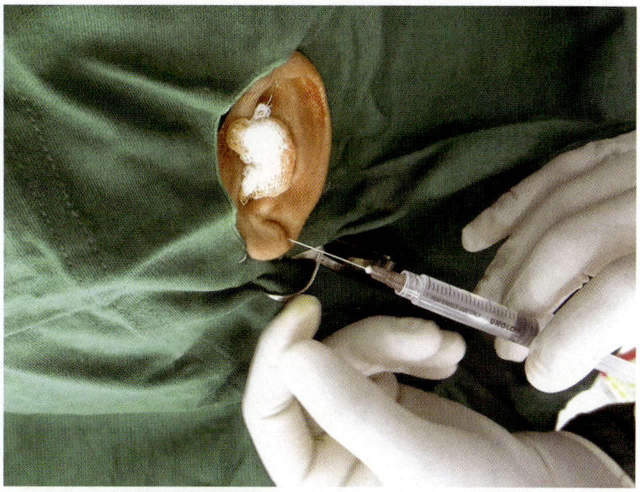

Fig. 22.2: Administration of local anesthesia.

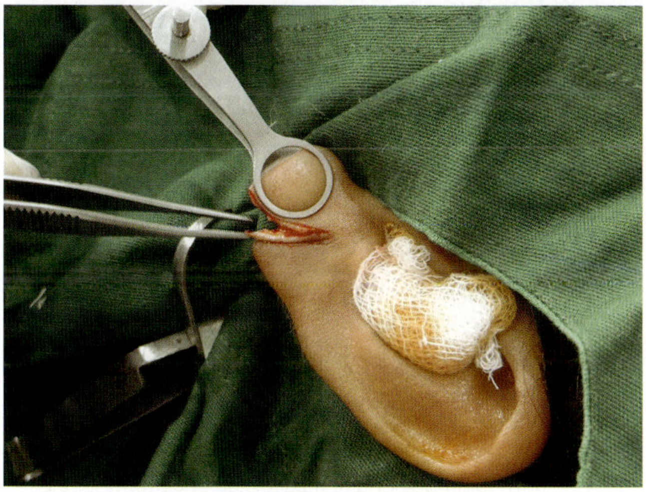

Fig. 22.3: Incision of epithelial tract.

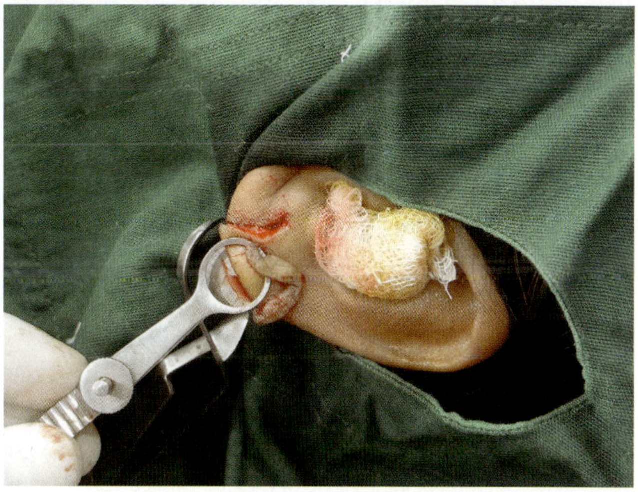

Fig. 22.4: Excision of epithelial tract.

- Mark the surgical area—The marking of surgical area should be done with surgical marker before infiltration of anesthesia, since after infiltration, area becomes distorted. The marking of inferior margin of earlobe is important since wrong suturing can change the shape of earlobe.
- Infiltration of local anesthesia—The anesthetic solution used for infiltration is lignocaine 2% with adrenaline in 1:100000 dilutions. The addition of hyaluronidase is helpful for enhancing spread of anesthesia (Fig. 22.2).
- With scalpel blade No. 15, an incision is given on the marked margin (inverted V shape) and the complete epithelial tract is removed (Figs. 22.3 and 22.4).
- The wound margins are undermined for 1-2 mm to achieve good eversion of margins.
- The suturing of inferior margin of lobule is critical in aligning the inferior border and ensuring symmetrical closure (Figs. 22.5A and B).
- The suturing of lateral surface is done first, because closing medial surface first may result in any soft tissue abnormality on the lateral surface. This will also hide any minor irregularity behind the earlobe (Fig. 22.6).
- The suturing of medial surface is done next. For suturing purpose 6-0/5-0 polypropylene or nylon suture is used (Fig. 22.7).
- The area is cleaned and dressed with antibiotic ointment.

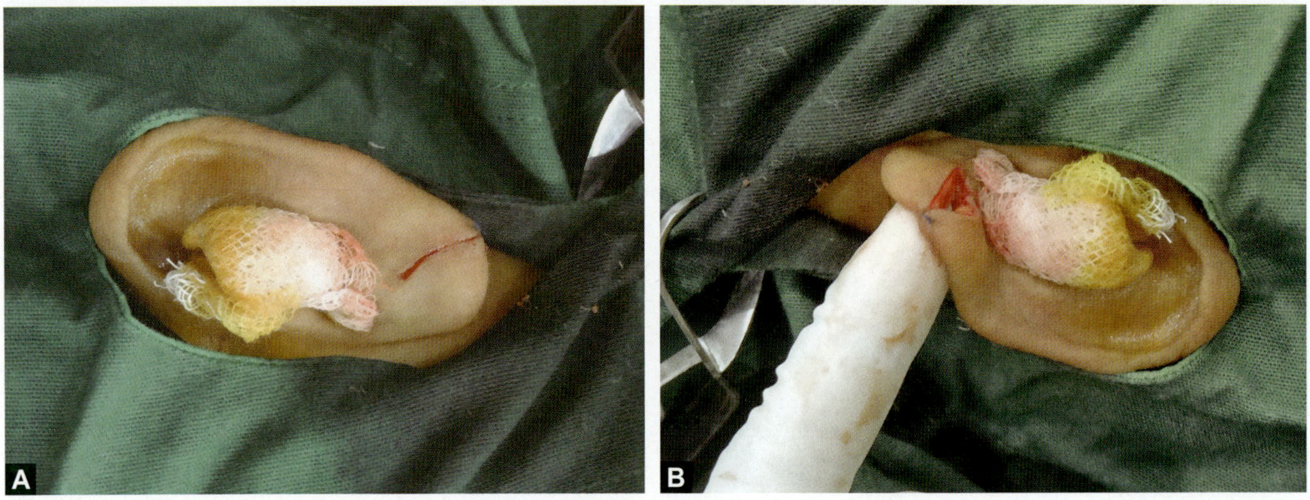

Figs. 22.5A and B: Stitch at inferior margin of earlobe.

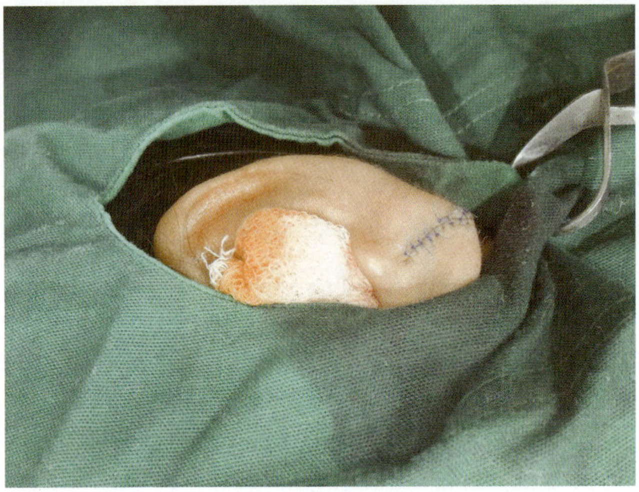

Fig. 22.6: Suturing of lateral side of earlobe with polypropylene 6–0 simple interrupted sutures.

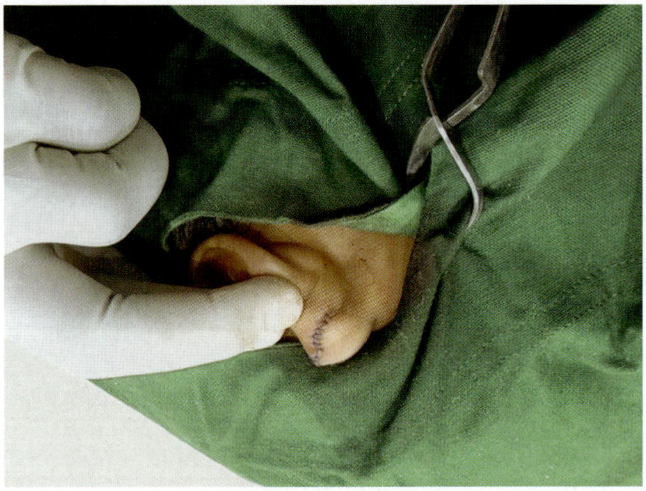

Fig. 22.7: Suturing of medial side of earlobe.

Postoperative Care and Instructions

- The postoperative care includes cleaning of the area and antibiotic application for 5–7 days.
- The suture removal is done on day 5–7.
- Ear piercing is done after 12 weeks.

Incomplete Earlobe Tear

Steps

- Steps 1 to 3 are same as mentioned above (Figs. 22.8 and 22.9).
- Assessment of an incomplete tear:
  - For tears >75% of distance between piercing and earlobe margin: convert to a complete tear.
  - For partial tears <60–75% of distance between piercing and earlobe margin:
    - If the tear is small, the epithelial tract can be removed with surgical blade no 15 and closed in a straight line with polypropylene or nylon 6–0 sutures in two or three layers (Figs. 22.10 to 22.13).
    - If the tear is large, it can be closed with broken line closure or W-plasty.

Modifications

- For stabilizing the earlobe while cutting the epithelial tract:

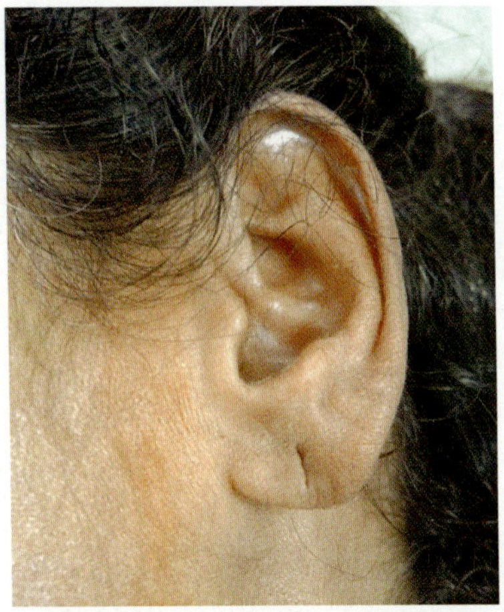

Fig. 22.8: Incomplete earlobe tear.

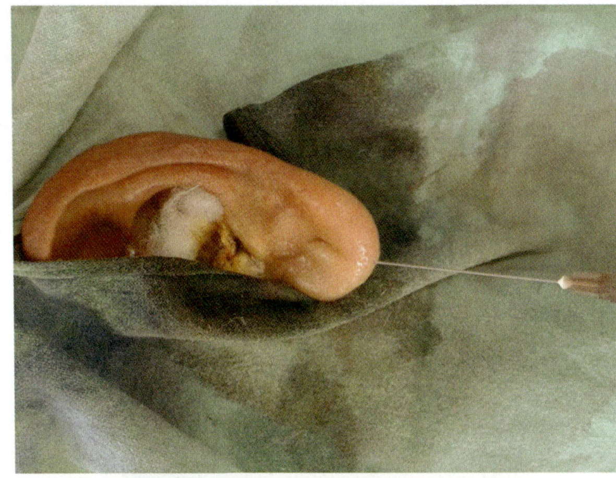

Fig. 22.9: Infiltration of local anesthesia.

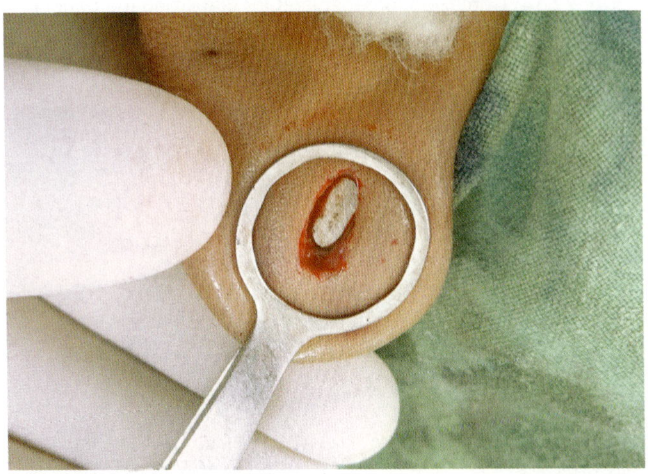

Fig. 22.10: Excision of complete epithelial tract stabilized with chalazion forceps.

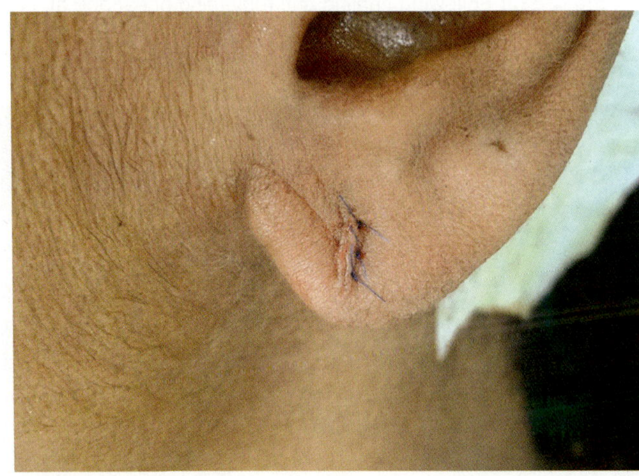

Fig. 22.11: Closure in two layers with polypropylene 6–0 simple interrupted sutures.

- *Chalazion clamp*: It is used for partial tears. In the punch technique, the wound edges are freshened with a punch. Using a chalazion clamp, the earlobe can be held in a stable manner before using the punch (Fig. 22.14).[7]
- *Tongue depressor*: While repairing the cleft, the tongue depressor can be used as a base (firm surface) posteriorly on which the earlobe can be placed to freshen up the wound edges (Figs. 22.15A and B).[8]
- *6–0 prolene stay suture*: 6–0 prolene suture is affixed to each inferior free margin of the earlobe for stabilization. As a surgical assistant applies gentle tension, the margins are scored using a No. #15 blade, followed by excision using iris scissors.[9]

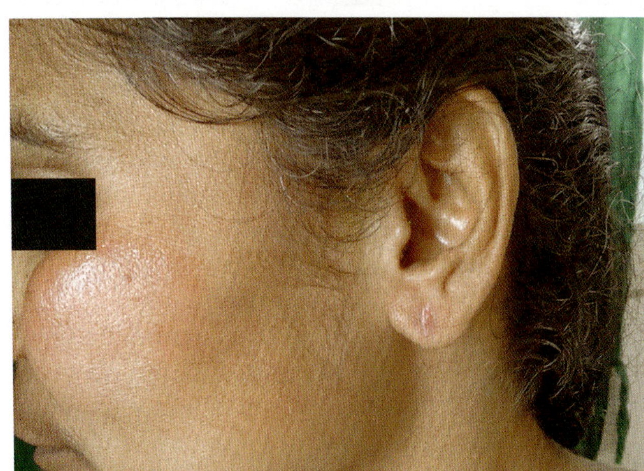

Fig. 22.12: Immediately after suture removal.

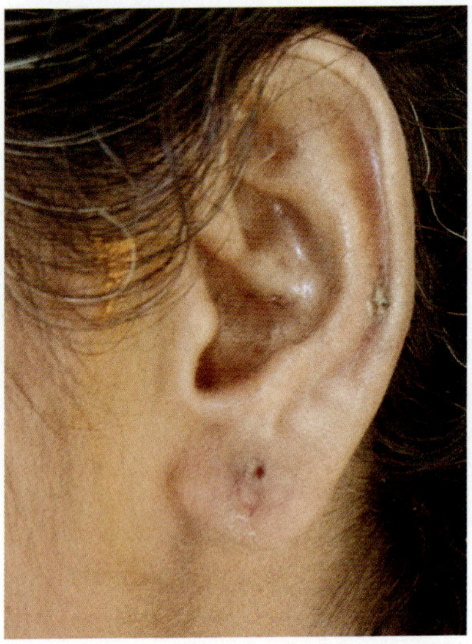

Fig. 22.13: Following healing and repiercing of earlobe at different site.

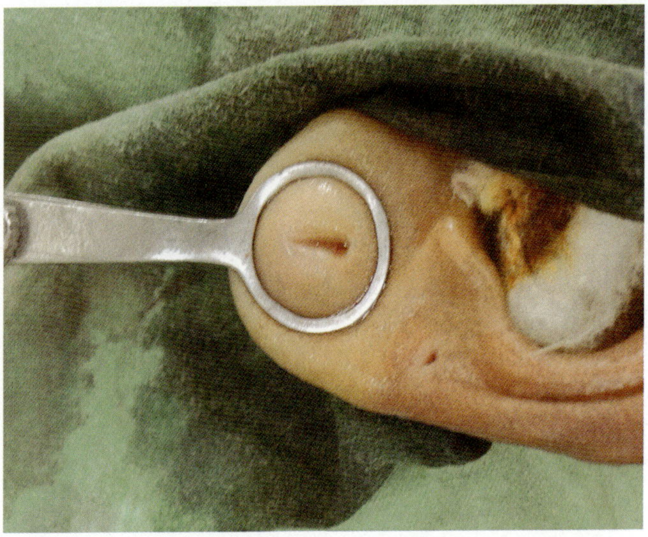

Fig. 22.14: Chalazion forceps used for stabilizing the earlobe.

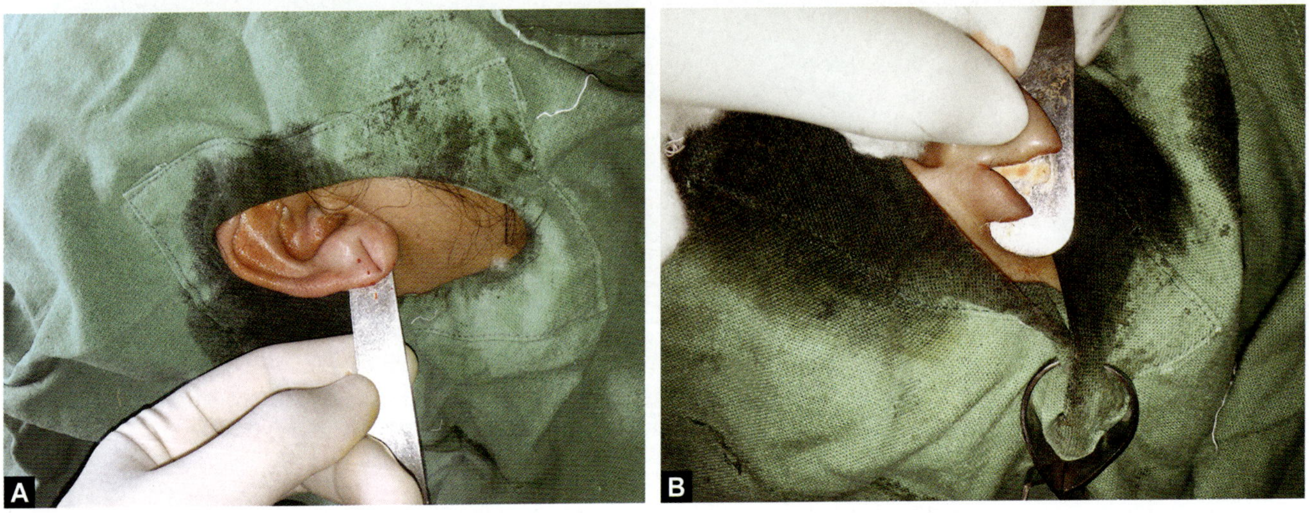

Figs. 22.15A and B: Tongue depressor used for stabilizing earlobe.

- *Skin hook*: This simple instrument which also can be used to stabilize earlobe. The skin hook can be used to hold the inferior margin of lobe. Once stabilized the margins can be freshened with surgical blade.
- To prevent notching of inferior margin:
  - *Z-plasty*: Employing this technique permits a single layer, side to side closure at inferior margin of the earlobe and allows redirection of vector of wound contraction, there by decreasing the risk of notching. Additionally, as the flaps are very small, tip stitches are not required (Fig. 22.16).[10]
  - *L specular plasty*: The lines are marked both side of cleft, to produce two mirrored "L" designs. The lines end up usually in an "L" design on inferoanterior side of cleft. On the opposite/other side, a reversed defect is drawn. The excision is made according to the surgical markings drawn. Nonabsorbable interrupted sutures (4/0, 5/0) are used to close the wound both medially and laterally along the length of the wound itself.[11]
  - *V-plasty*: In this, two V-flap variants are used. In one, 3 mm V-shaped socket is cut from the fat on one side of the split earlobe. On the other side of split earlobe,

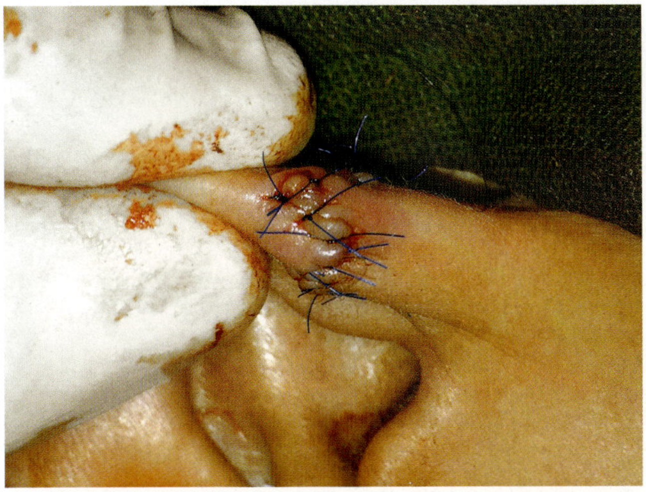

Fig. 22.16: Z-plasty at inferior margin of earlobe.

an inverted V-shaped joint is cut into the fat to receive the opposite side. The flaps are sutured with simple interrupted suture.[12]

- For strengthening the tract of earlobe repair:
  - *Deep polypropylene*: After the optimum site for ear repiercing is identified, a sterile 6-0 or 5-0 polypropylene suture is placed as a buried, nonabsorbable dermal suture a few millimeters inferior to this point. Any suture elevation resultant to wound contraction is offset by the deep suture placement. The suture should be oriented horizontally with respect to the long axis of the ear, penetrating a few millimeters into the dermis on each side. The usage of small caliber suture (5-0, 6-0) will minimize the likelihood of extrusion and palpability of sutures, and also avoid its placement in close approximation to the epidermis.
- For cutting the epithelial tract:
  - *Punch technique*: this is useful in cases of partial earlobe repair. This technique simultaneously removes the preexisting hole and creates a non-epithelialized tract is subsequently sutured.[7]
  - *Modified punch technique*: Here, the 18 gauge needle is used as a guide for trimming the edges with a Mayo's scissors. After aligning the punch properly, the needle plastic base is positioned just posterior to the lobe, and then the cut needle is put into the cleft. The punch is positioned just anterior to lobe and using the cut needle as a guide, it is firmly pushed against the plastic needle base. A small cylinder of skin and deeper tissue including the epithelial tract connecting the anterior and posterior holes is removed with much ease.[13]
  - *Guidewire punch technique*: In this modification, a guidewire is used to precisely cut the epithelial tract with punch. A guidewire is inserted into the earring hole which guides the proper placement of a punch.[14]
  - *Radiocautery technique*: A radiocautery probe with a precision tip or an epilator probe can be used to make the incision to create a nonepithelialized tract. This modality allows for a pressure-less incision as the probe does not cut by pressure.
  - *Laser technique*: A diode laser (frequency of 2.5 W and wavelength of 850 nm) maybe used for skin incision instead of surgical blade. Rest of the procedure is completed in a usual manner. With the use of a laser for the initial incision, the bleeding is very minimal, fine suture line can be obtained, time taken to complete the procedure is significantly less, use of epinephrine can be avoided and dose of local anesthetic used will be lesser.
- Keeping the earlobe tract intact: In this modification we can use a sterile IV cannula for keeping the tract intact. While doing partial earlobe repair once the epithelial tract is excised, the tract is closed with 6-0 polypropylene suture leaving the uppermost part of defect open. A cannula with trocar is put through the ear hole, then one end of a sterile spare suture is put in the beveled edge of trocar. The trocar is pulled out of the cannula. As the trocar is extracted, suture will follow through to the other end of cannula. The hub of cannula is now cut and both ends of suture are tied to each other. The rest of epithelial tract is now closed leaving one intact hole in earlobe (Figs. 22.17A and B).

Complications

The potential complications of earlobe repair include:

- *Bleeding*: Managed with external pressure.
- *Infection*: Managed with antibiotics and proper wound care.
- *Notching of earlobe*: Corrected with scar revision.
- *Hypertrophic scar*: Managed with intralesional corticosteroids, silicone gel sheets, cryotherapy or laser therapy.
- *Keloid*: Requires combination approach. It may be dealt with by surgical excision, intralesional corticosteroids, intralesional interferon, silicone gel sheeting, cryotherapy or laser therapy.

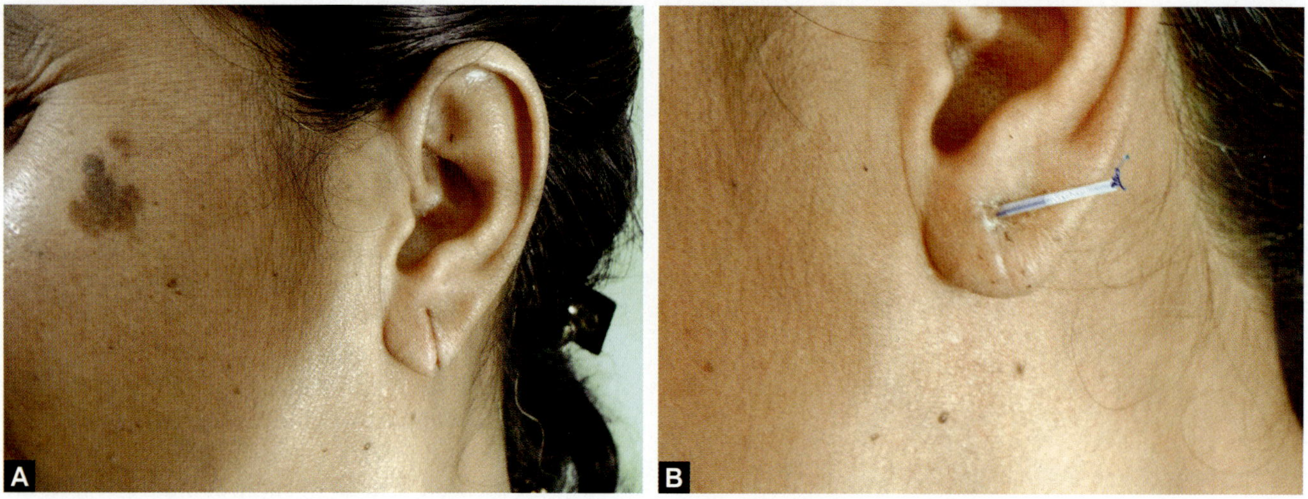

Figs. 22.17A and B: (A) Complete earlobe tear. (B) Preserving the tract for use.

Prevention of Earlobe Tears

- Avoid wearing heavy earrings for longer time periods
- Remove heavy earrings when using the telephone
- Remove earrings at the hair salon
- Be aware that small children and babies are attracted to earrings
- Do not allow children to wear small loop or dangling earrings
- Remove your earrings before removing upper clothing, like sweaters.

REFERENCES

1. Raveendran SS, Amarasinghe L. The mystery of the split earlobe. Plast Reconstr Surg. 2004;114:1903-9
2. Maral T, Tuncali D, Ozgur F, et al. A technique for the repair of simple congenital earlobe clefts. Ann Plast Surg. 1996;37:326-31.
3. Vujevich J, Goldberg LH, Obagi S. Repair of partial andcomplete earlobe clefts: a review of 21 methods. J Drugs Dermatol. 2007;6(7):695-9.
4. Zoltie N. Split earlobes: a method of repair preserving the hole. Plast Reconstr Surg. 1987;80:619-21.
5. Munro-Ashman D, MacDonald A, Feiwel M. Split earlobe syndrome. Contact Dermat. 1975;1:393-4.
6. Enzer YR. Repair of the torn earlobe. In: Hartstein ME, Massry GG, Holds JB (Eds), Pearls and Pitfalls in Cosmetic Oculoplastic Surgery. Newyork: Springer; 2015. pp. 595-598.
7. Tan EC. Punch technique: an alternative approach to the repair of pierced earlobe deformities. J Dermatol Surg Oncol 1989;15:270-2.
8. Smith C, Glaser DA. Surgical Pearl: Repair of split or deformed ear lobe with a tongue depressor blade for stabilization during surgery. J Am Acad Dermatol. 1998;38:990-1.
9. Beschloss JK, Toren KL, Bingham JL. Earlobe stabilization with 6-0 suture for repair of a complete split. Dermatol Surg. 2011;37:848-9.
10. Casson P. How do you repair split earlobe? J Dermatol Surg. 1976;2:21.
11. Chiummariello S, Iera M, Arleo S, et al. L-specular plasty versus double-round plasty: two new techniques for earlobe split repair. Aesth Plast Surg. 2011;35:398-401.
12. Kalimuthu R, Larson BJ, Lewis N. Earlobe repair: a new technique. Plast Reconstr Surg. 1984;74:299-300.
13. Dessy L, Buccheri E, Anniboletti T. Modified punch technique for incomplete earlobe cleft repair. Aesth Plast Surg. 2006;30:731-2.
14. Taher M, Metelitsa A, Salopek TG. Earlobe repair assisted by guidewire punch technique: a useful method to remove unwanted epithelial tracts caused by body piercing. J Am Acad Dermatol. 2004;51:93-4.

CHAPTER 23

Nerve Biopsy

BM Shashikumar, Divya Gorur, Syed Mubashir, Amrita Hongal

INTRODUCTION

Nerve biopsy is an invasive procedure in which a nerve is sectioned either partially or fully to diagnose potentially treatable causes of neuropathy. The histopathological evaluation of a nerve biopsy specimen is often the final and important step in the diagnostic work-up while evaluating a case of neuropathy of unknown origin.[1] Etiology of a peripheral neuropathy is difficult to ascertain in many cases and nerve biopsy may be essential to confirm diagnosis when all other available diagnostic methods fail to establish the diagnosis.

INDICATIONS

Though it is an invasive procedure, a nerve biopsy is advocated when:

- There is progressive neuropathy
- Threatens to become debilitating
- Other noninvasive tests fail to identify a cause.

Common indications for nerve biopsy are enumerated in Table 23.1.[1-3]

Table 23.1: Indications for nerve biopsy.

Genetic	Charcot-Marie-Tooth (CMT) disease Hereditary motor and sensory neuropathies Familial amyloid neuropathy Giant axonal neuropathy Infantile and juvenile neuroaxonal dystrophy (Seitelberger disease)
Vasculitides	Polyarteritis nodosa Microscopic polyangiitis Churg-Strauss syndrome Rheumatoid arthritis
Infectious neuropathies	Leprosy Herpes zoster and simplex Human immunodeficiency virus (HIV) Lyme disease or borrelia neuropathy
Inflammatory and immune alterations	Sarcoidosis Ganglionitis Chronic inflammatory demyelinating polyradiculoneuropathy (CIDP) Monoclonal gammopathy
Storage disorders	Amyloidosis Glycogen storage disorders
Metabolic disorders	Diabetic uremic, nutritional neuropathies
Toxic neuropathies	Amiodarone Chloroquine Antiretroviral drugs Industrial agents like n-hexane, methyl n-butyl ketone, acrylamide
Tumors	Primary and secondary nerve tumors—schwannomas, neurofibromas Malignant peripheral nerve sheath tumors Paraneoplastic neuropathy
Ischemic injury of nerve	Chronic nerve compression
Others	

PREPARATION

- Before considering nerve biopsy other less invasive investigations should be considered to know the cause of pathology.
- In a situation of thickened nerve with infective etiology like Hansen's disease, even fine needle aspiration cytology (FNAC) of the affected nerve can offer some diagnostic help; but negative aspiration findings cannot rule out the diagnosis.
- Nerve conduction studies and electromyography must be carried out along with other investigations to rule out or diagnose various other differential diagnoses. Other tests like ESR, liver function tests, renal function tests and genetic screening should also be done.[4]
- Complete blood count, clotting parameters depending on history should also be done. Written informed consent for the procedure should be obtained, clearly indicating the possible clinical diagnoses, the need for the biopsy, the procedure involved and the possible consequences and risks associated with the procedure.
- All preoperative evaluations, pre- and postoperative instructions and medications are similar to other minor surgical procedures.

Table 23.2: Site of nerve biopsy.[2-4]

Nerve	*Site of incision*	*Indication*	*Remarks*
Distal sural nerve	Behind the lateral malleolus	Vasculitis, Hansen's disease	With minimal postoperative problems or complications
Superficial peroneal (fibular) nerve	Junction of the middle and distal thirds of leg on lateral aspects	Vasculitis	Through the same incision, the peroneus brevis muscle can be accessed
Medial sural nerve	Junction of the gastrocnemius muscle bellies	Vasculitis	Concomitant gastrocnemius muscle biopsy can be done. Very minimal sensory loss
Distal superficial radial nerve (radial cutaneous nerve)	Anatomical snuff box	Upper limb neuropathy, including Hansen's disease	Visible scar, neuroma common, no major postprocedure complications
Dorsal cutaneous branch of the ulnar nerve	Wrist	Upper limb neuropathy, including Hansen's disease	
Obturator nerve biopsy	4 inches distal to the pubis bone over medial aspect of thigh	Useful to differentiate motor neuropathies and lower motor neuron diseases like Guillain-Barré syndrome, motor neuron disease, and mixed neuropathy with prominent motor symptoms	Very rarely done. Concomitant gracilis muscle biopsy is taken
Greater auricular nerve	Sternocleidomastoid muscle at the upper and lateral aspect of the neck	Hansen's disease	Considered rarely for biopsy

SELECTION OF BIOPSY SITE

- Nerve biopsy is performed most often on a sensory nerve. Rarely the biopsy of combined nerve and muscle or nerve supplying to muscle which is either suspected to be affected or located nearer to the site of affection on the body is carried out.
- Partial fascicular biopsy of a mixed cutaneous and motor nerve trunk is practiced very rarely in special and unavoidable situations.
- Nerve biopsy should be done from the cutaneous nerve which has a known replicable anatomical location and course and also should be readily accessible.
- In comparison with full thickness nerve biopsy, fascicular biopsy causes fewer complications or less sensory deficit, but provides less tissue for analysis. This is especially important, if focally accentuated lesions including inflammatory processes are looked for. Such foci are less likely to be detected if just a portion of the nerve is examined. Therefore, biopsy of the complete cross-section of the nerve is recommended wherever possible.[5]
- The minimum recommended length of the biopsied nerve segment should be 5 cm.[2] Less than minimum length may give unsatisfactory results.

Table 23.2 summarizes the common nerve biopsied along with site and indication.

Combined nerve and muscle biopsies can be obtained by the same skin incision, but in separate pieces. The possibility of detecting inflammatory changes, in particular vasculitis, is significantly higher in a combined biopsy compared to either nerve or muscle biopsy alone. In addition, other disorders that can affect both nerve and muscle such as amyloidosis and certain hereditary diseases including neuropathy and myopathies can benefit by combined biopsy. While evaluating a patient with pure motor neuropathy, nerve biopsy should preferably be done from a nerve supplying a muscle which has little functional importance (e.g. the nerve to gracilis).

BIOPSY SAMPLE HANDLING[2]

The nerve biopsy samples are prepared in three different ways to fully assess the tissue for diagnostic purposes (Table 23.3).

COMPLICATIONS

The rate of complications varies in different from centers and with expertise of surgeon. Surgery-related complications are persistent pain, dysesthesia, paresthesia, allodynia, sensory impairment and neuroma (Table 23.4). In case of pure cutaneous nerves biopsy like biopsy of sural or radial cutaneous nerves, except for paresthesia/ anesthesia over the small area supplied by the respective

Table 23.3: Biopsy sample handling.

Segment	*Length*	*Method of fixation/processing*	*Uses*
1st piece	0.5 cm	Formalin-fixed, paraffin-embedded	H and E and special stain is useful in diagnosing vasculitis, amyloidosis, sarcoidosis, leprosy, lymphoma
2nd piece	0.5 cm	Transported in Michel's medium and frozen	Staining of light chains is useful in diagnosis of amyloidosis
3rd piece	2–2.5 cm	Glutaraldehyde fixed for transverse semithin plastic sections	Useful for analysis of myelinated fibers

Table 23.4: Complications of nerve biopsy and its prevention.[2-4,6-8]

Complication	*Prevention*
Hematoma	Stopping anticoagulants at least 1 week prior to surgery, good hemostasis, postoperative pressure dressing and limb elevation
Muscle herniation (only if motor nerves deep to muscles are biopsied)	Proper closer of fascia
Wound dehiscence	Adequate rest and support
Wound infection	Adequate antibiotics
Neuroma	Ends of transected nerve to be sutured into surrounding muscle
Pain, dysesthesia, paresthesia	Leg to be immobilized in plaster cast for 7–10 days

nerve biopsied, no major side/adverse effects are reported. Many a times, it has been reported that the nerve trunks get reunited and may re-establish the sensations.

SURAL NERVE BIOPSY

Nerve biopsy has been a time tested well-established diagnostic procedure for the evaluation of peripheral neuropathies. Leprosy is one of the most common treatable causes of peripheral neuropathy but diagnosing leprosy in the absence of typical dermatological features is challenging. Despite the availability of many diagnostic tools like, nerve conduction studies, electromyelogram, ultrasound examination, imaging techniques, etc. the best diagnosis of Hansen's disease is mainly by clinical examination. In a situation where both clinical examination and other diagnostic tests cannot either confirm or rule out Hansen's disease, nerve biopsy becomes crucial as it is the most conclusive diagnostic test. Thus, the nerve biopsy may give useful information in diagnosing pure neuritic form of Hansen's diseases.

The sural nerve is the most preferred site of biopsy because:[6]

- It is a purely sensory nerve and there is no risk of motor loss following biopsy.
- Resulting sensory loss is small and confined to an area on the dorsolateral aspect of the foot.
- It is readily accessible and easy to identify at the level of the lateral malleolus.
- Its structure has been studied extensively in both health and disease conditions.

Anatomy of Sural Nerve[4] (Fig. 23.1)

Sural nerve is a pure sensory nerve which supplies sensation to dorsolateral aspect of foot and the ankle region. Marriage of the medial sural nerve, which is a branch of tibial nerve (6 cm proximal to fibular head), with the lateral cutaneous sural nerve (common peroneal nerve branch), forms the distal sural nerve. The two branches join in distal 1/3rd of leg proximal to lateral malleolus. Distally, the nerve passes in subcutaneous fat along a fascial sling between deep crural fascia and superficial fascia adjacent to the short saphenous vein and lateral to Achilles tendon.

Anatomical Variation

Sometimes medial and lateral branches may join to for sural nerve in the popliteal fossa in 12% cases rather distally.[8] Other anatomical variations like early union of the two branches or nonunion of the two branches may also be seen. Very rarely the sural nerve may be fully absent.[9]

Procedure

- After obtaining informed written consent, the part is prepared, draped and surface anatomy of the nerve to be biopsied should be marked (Figs. 23.2 to 23.4). The planned incision site is anesthetized with infiltration of local anesthetic agent. Patient is asked to flex the leg at around 30° at the knee and ankle must be slightly everted (at 90°) to keep sural nerve under a slight tension. This help in better localization of nerve.
- A superficial, vertical incision is made halfway between the Achilles tendon and the lateral border of fibula, starting at lateral malleolus and then extending it 5 cm upwards along course of Langer Line following nerve (Fig. 23.5).

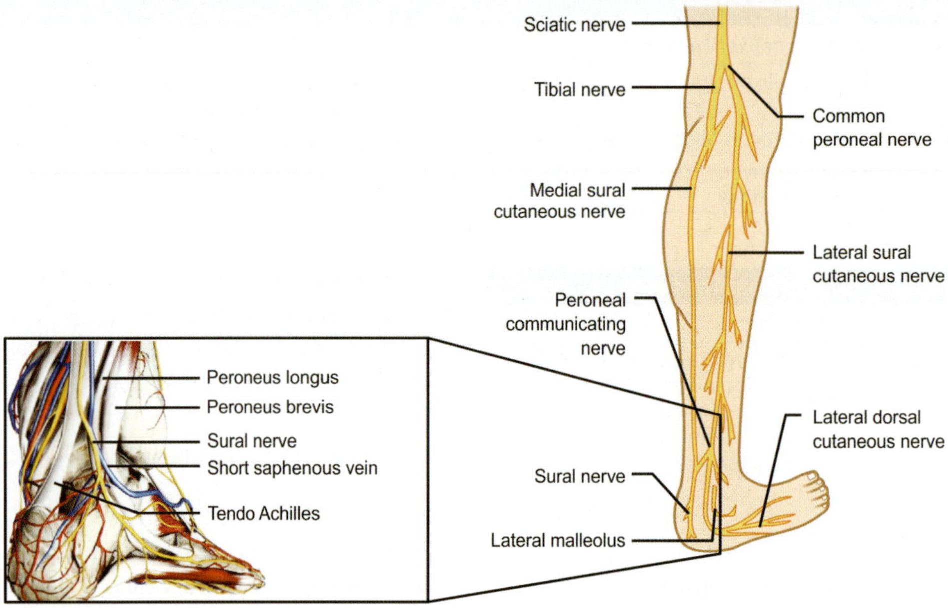

Fig. 23.1: Anatomy of sural nerve.

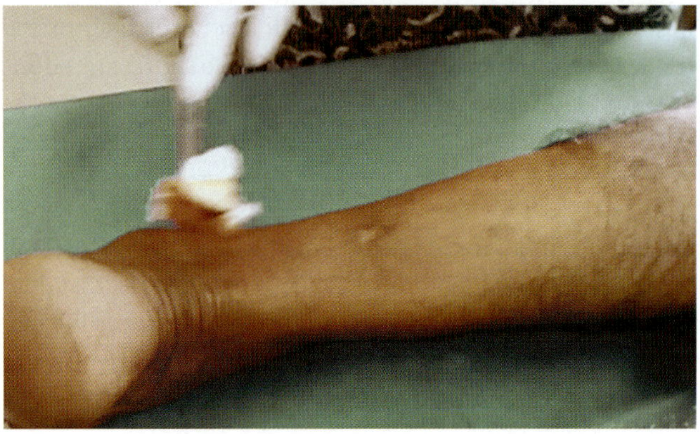

Fig. 23.2: Surgical preparation of the area.

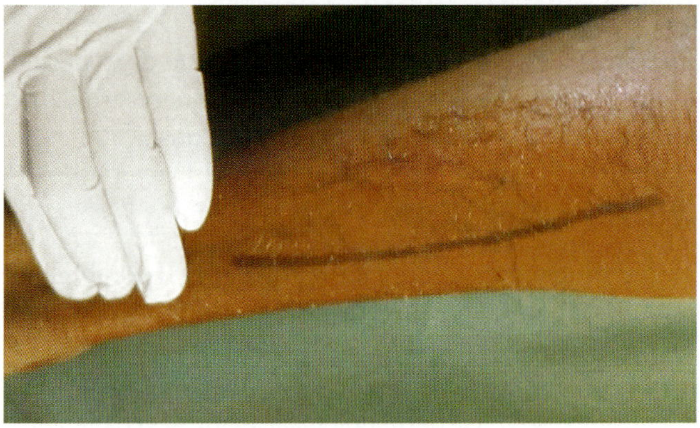

Fig. 23.3: Surface marking of sural nerve.

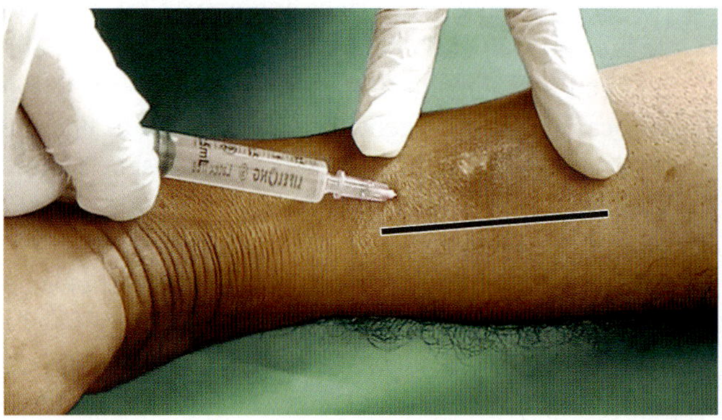

Fig. 23.4: Infiltration of anesthesia along the course of the nerve.

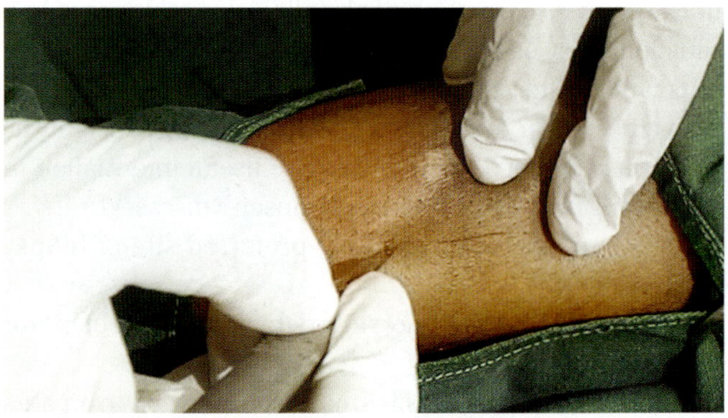

Fig. 23.5: Incision placed along the marking.

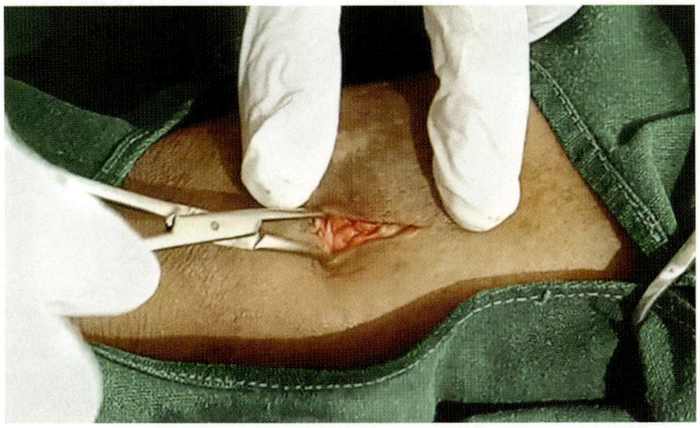

Fig. 23.6: Blunt dissection of fascia.

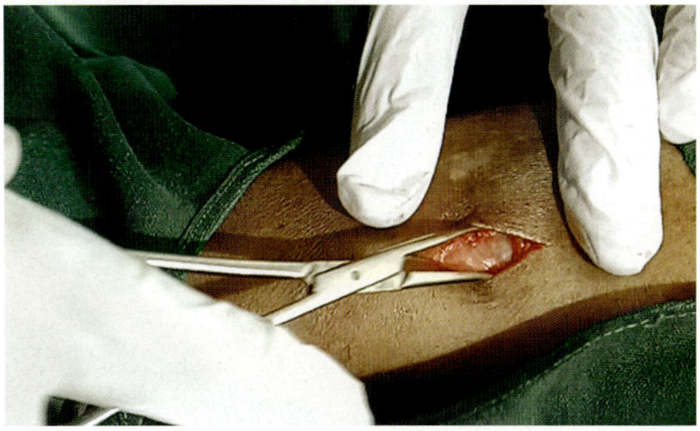

Fig. 23.7: Blunt dissection of fascia.

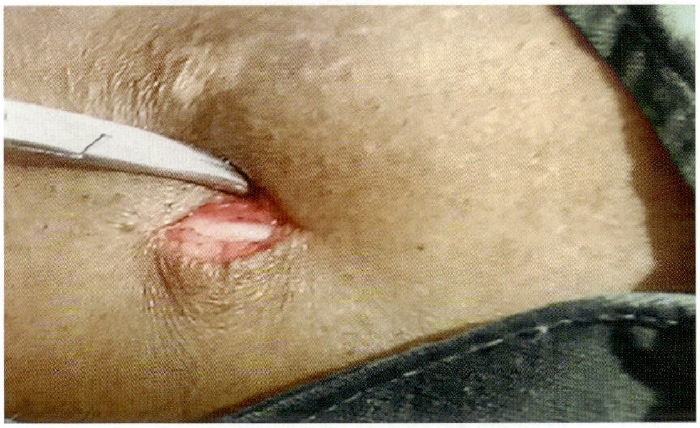

Fig. 23.8: Dissect till the vein is visible.

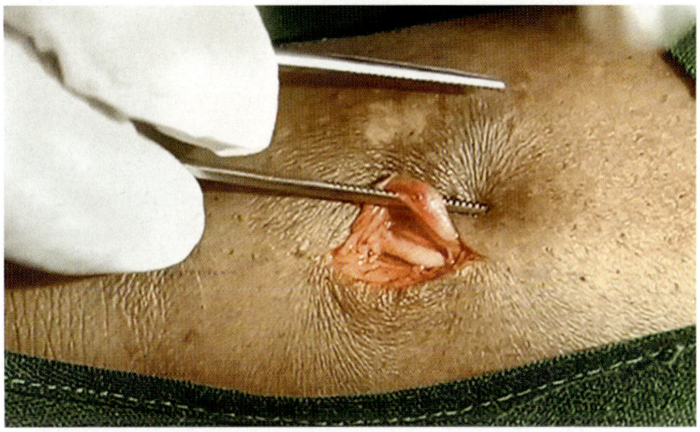

Fig. 23.9: Sural nerve lies medial to the vein, and is visible beneath the retracted saphenous vein.

- Using sharper dissection and with careful undermining of the tissues, dissection is carried out in the superficial fascia until lesser saphenous vein is properly identified. This is retracted posteriorly and the sural nerve reveals itself just medial to this.[10] Care should be taken to preserve saphenous vein (Figs. 23.6 to 23.10).
- Before sectioning the nerve, local anesthetic can be injected into proximal part of nerve to recude the pain that may occur with sectioning.
- A 3.0 nylon suture is then placed through the nerve proximally: Utmost care must be taken to see that nerve is very minimally handled/manipulated by using the proximal suture (Fig. 23.11).
- The nerve is sharply cut proximally first to prevent pain, and distal end is subsequently sectioned with a scalpel (scissors are not preferred as it can produce compression trauma artifact). The nerve is left alone or buried into the adjacent muscle. In case of fascicular biopsy, a few fascicles are separated and sectioned (Figs. 23.12 to 23.14).
- The wound is sutured in layers (Fig. 23.15).

The specimen is processed as mentioned in Table 23.3.

Differentiating nerve from vessel[6]
- Nerve is glistening white and solid in appearance, if examined carefully, fascicles can be visualized (Fig. 23.16).
- Vessels will have true lumen and tributaries.
- Nerve has pattern of alternating longitudinal lighter and darker bands.

Postoperative Care

Immediate postoperatively, look for appropriate hemostasis and possibility of hematoma if any. They are advised to keep the wound dry for 48 hours and avoid strenuous activity for 2 weeks. Optionally, leg can be immobilized in a plaster cast for 7 to 10 days. Skin sutures may be removed after 10 days. Appropriate antibiotics and anti-inflammatory drugs are to be given for a short duration (5–7 days).

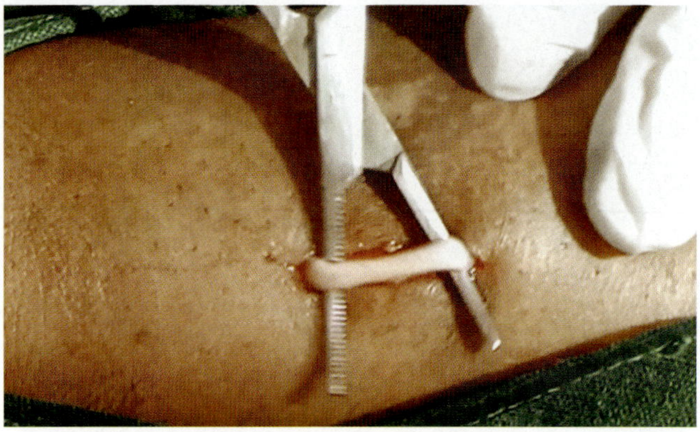

Fig. 23.10: Dissected sural nerve.

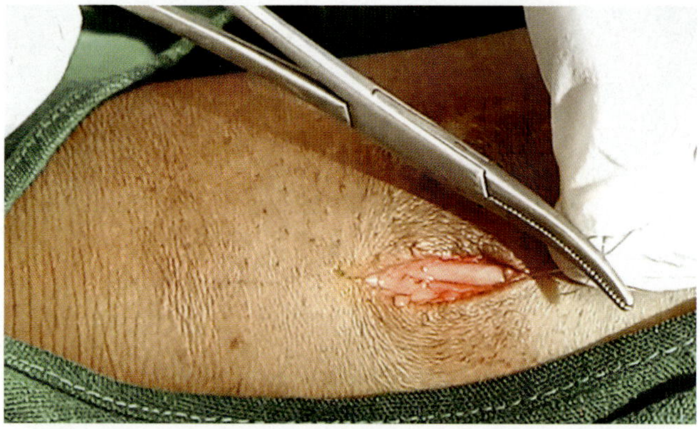

Fig. 23.11: Suture is tied proximally for easy manipulation.

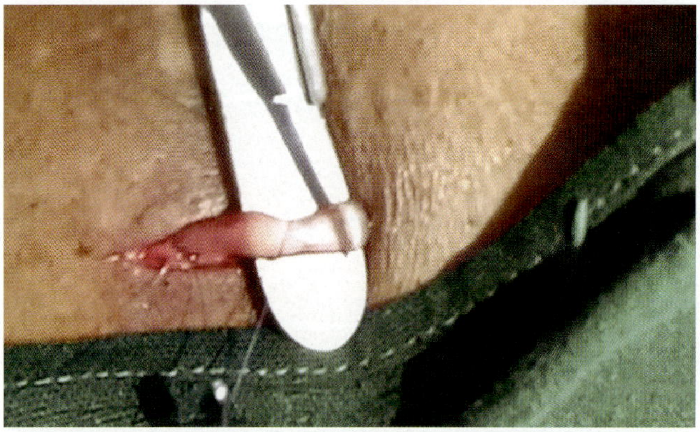

Fig. 23.12: Proximal portion cut with scalpel.

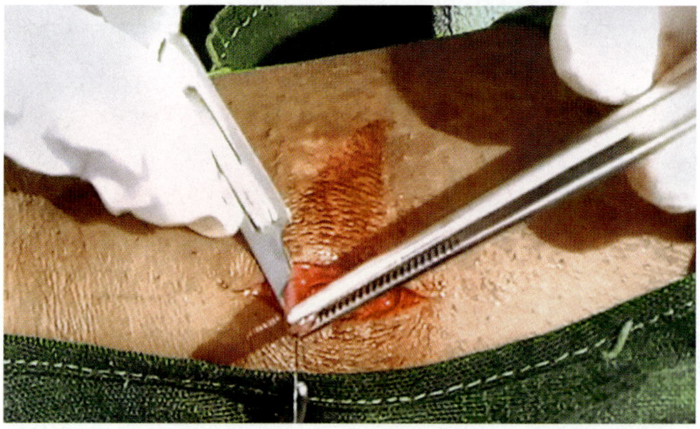

Fig. 23.13: Distal end cut with scalpel.

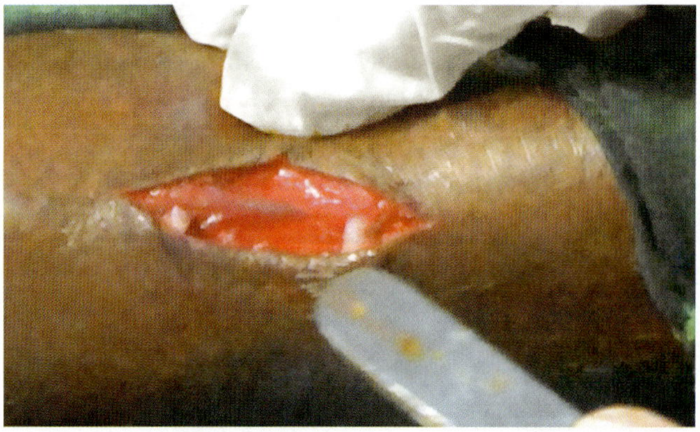

Fig. 23.14: Vein is visible with transected ends of nerve.

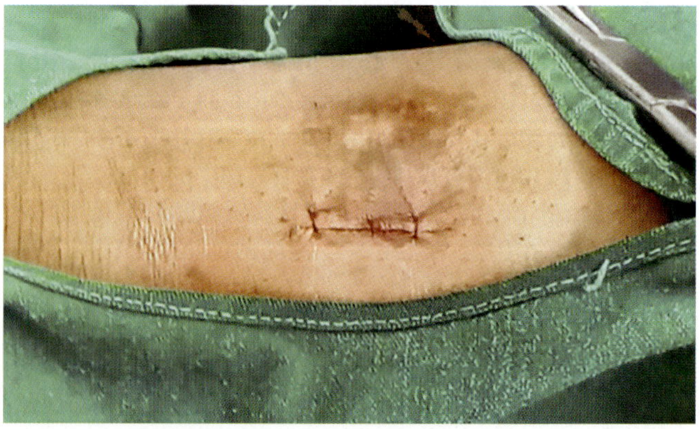

Fig. 23.15: Wound closed in layers.

DISTAL SUPERFICIAL RADIAL NERVE BIOPSY[4]

Anatomy

The distal superficial radial nerve is direct continuation of the radial nerve. It goes below the brachioradialis muscle in the anterolateral aspect of the forearm. Here it pierces the deep fascia along the distal part of the forearm where it lies in the subcutaneous plane. Nerve can then be normally palpated directly over the distal radius, or in the anatomical snuff box which lies laterally over the extensor carpi radialis longus. Above anatomical landmarks aid in the

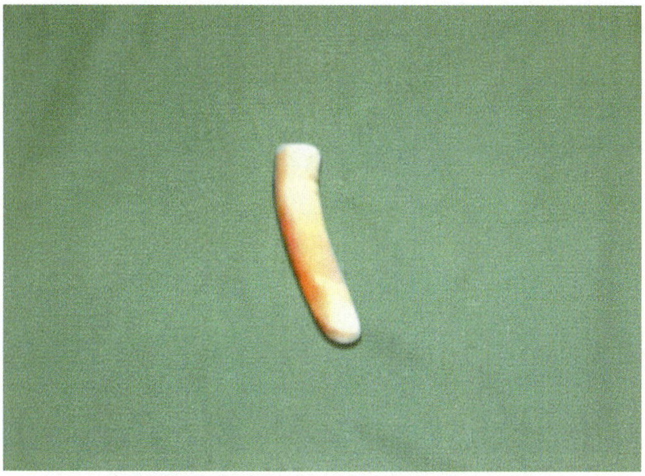

Fig. 23.16: Nerve bit to be sent to laboratory.

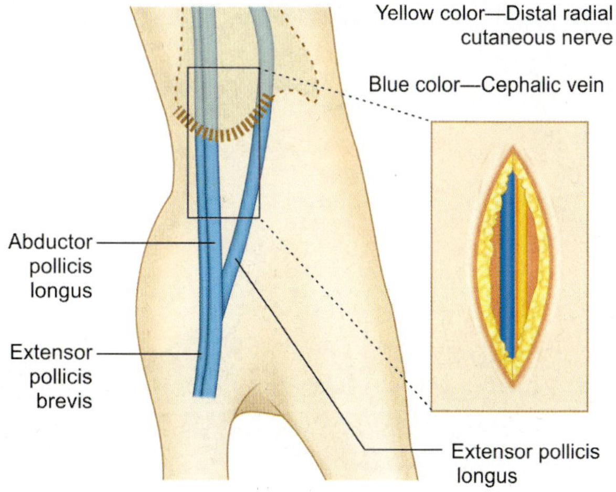

Fig. 23.17: Anatomy of radial cutaneous nerve.

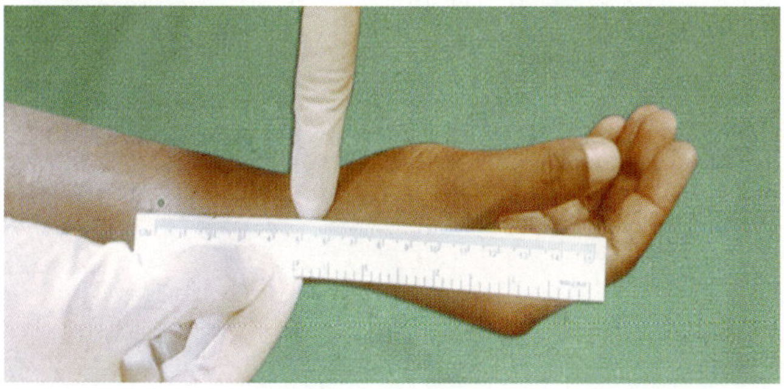

Fig. 23.18: Marking of incision for radial cutaneous nerve, 5 cm proximal to radial styloid process.

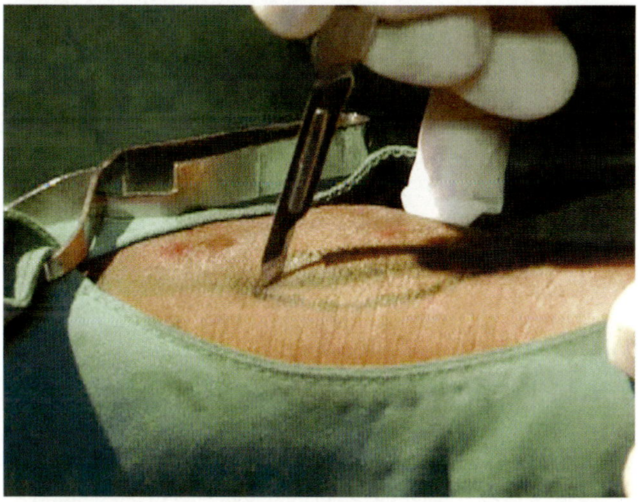

Fig. 23.19: Marking the site of radial cutaneous nerve biopsy and incising the site.

planning of the biopsy. The anatomical snuff box is bounded posteriorly by the extensor pollicis longus tendon, anteriorly by tendons of extensor pollicis brevis and abductor pollicis longus and proximally by the syloid process of radius, while floor is formed by both trapezium and scaphoid (Fig. 23.17).

Procedure (Figs. 23.18 to 23.26)

Preoperative preparations are same as described above. Area around anatomical snuff box is cleaned and draped. The operating field is then infiltrated with 1% lignocaine. Identify and mark the course of radial artery to avoid injury or accidental cutting. Anterolaterally, a longitudinal or a transverse incision is placed over the distal radius/ anatomical snuff box. The cephalic veins lying medially are retracted to visualize the nerve lying superficial to the extensor retinaculum. The nerve is ligated proximally (3–5 cm of nerve is resected mostly in total thickness or partial thickness, if it is grossly thickened). After achieving hemostasis, wound is closed in layers. Postoperative care is done as described above.

TIPS TO THE SURGERY

- Sural nerve is the commonest nerve biopsied by a dermatologist, mainly to rule out Hansen's disease.
- Knowing proper anatomy and variation is crucial before planning surgery.
- Gentle handling of nerve with blunt dissection is crucial.
- Sharp section of nerve is important.

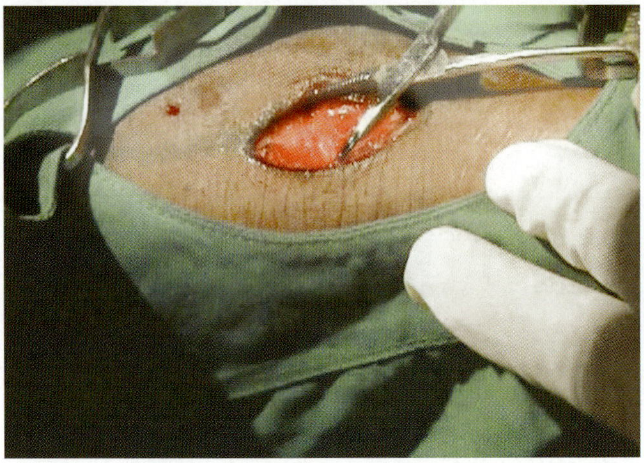

Fig. 23.20: Widening the incision site.

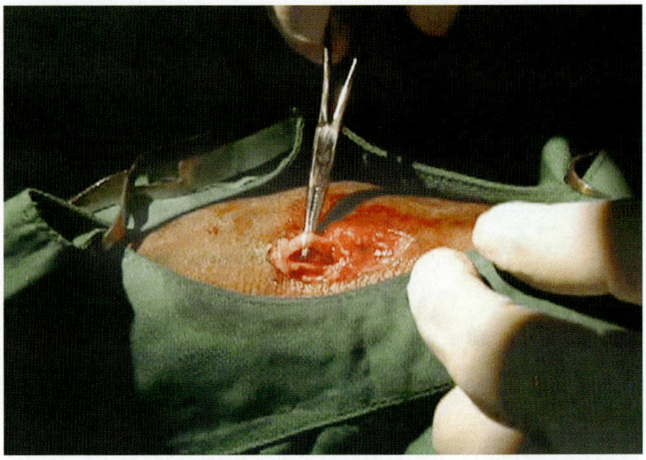

Fig. 23.21: Radial cutaneous nerve exposed.

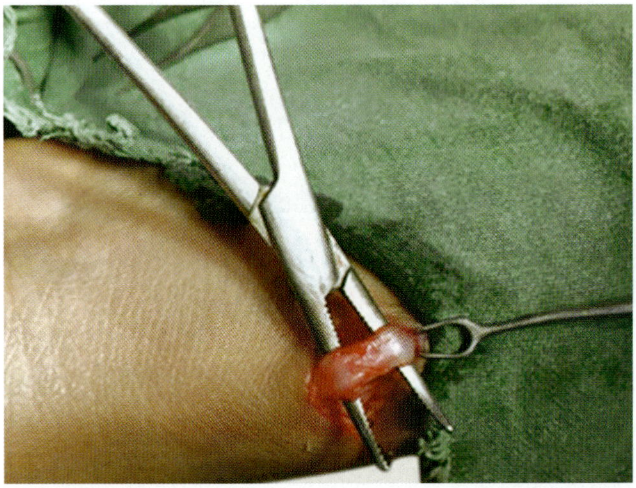

Fig. 23.22: Thickened radial cutaneous nerve exposed.

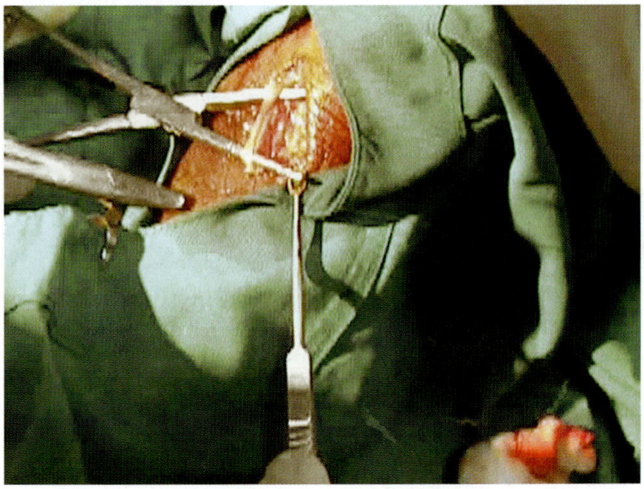

Fig. 23.23: Ligated proximally.

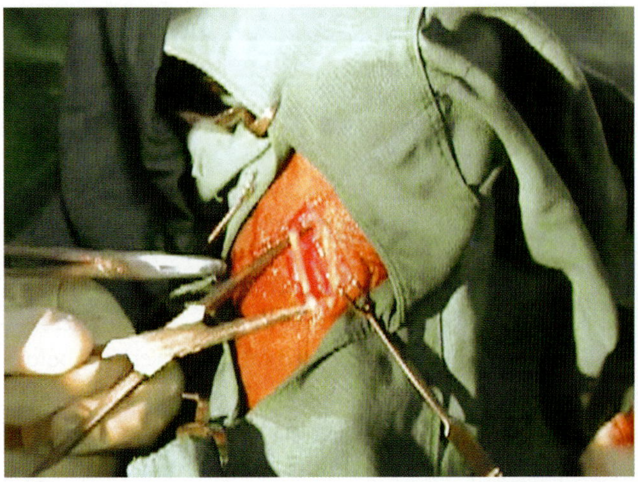

Fig. 23.24: The full segment of nerve exposed.

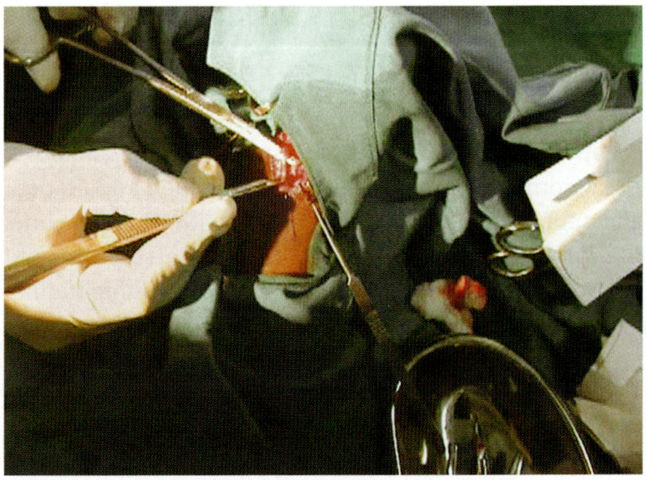

Fig. 23.25: Portion of nerve excised.

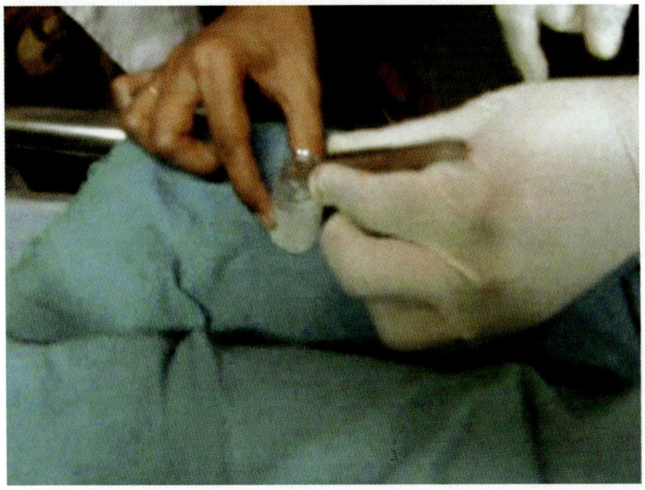

Fig. 23.26: Nerve part being sent in formalin bottle.

Key Messages

- Nerve biopsy is a key diagnostic procedure to definitely diagnose pure neuritic leprosy in a situation of diagnostic dilemma (either to confirm or to rule out neuritic leprosy).
- Commonly performed on a pure cutaneous nerve like sural nerve or radial cutaneous nerve. Biopsy of mixed or motors nerve is done very rarely in special circumstances.
- Complete circumference of the nerve taken for biopsy is better than taking a few fascicles. However partial thickness nerve biopsy may be done, if the cutaneous nerve trunk is grossly thickened.
- Nerve biopsy can also be done for the diagnosis of vasculitis, inflammatory, congenital or metabolic disorder.

REFERENCES

1. Sommer C, Brandner S, Dyck PJ, et al. 147th ENMC international workshop: guideline on processing and evaluation of sural nerve biopsies, 15-17 December 2006, Naarden, The Netherlands. Neuromuscul Disord. 2008;18:90-6.
2. Weis J1, Brandner S, Lammens M, et al. Processing of nerve biopsies: a practical guide for neuropathologists. Clin Neuropathol. 2012;31:7-23.
3. Vallat JM, Funalot B, Magy L. Nerve biopsy: requirements for diagnosis and clinical value. Acta Neuropathol. 2011;121: 313-26.
4. Hart MG1, Santarius T, Trivedi RA. Muscle and nerve biopsy for the neurosurgical trainee. Br J Neurosurg. 2013;27: 727-34.
5. Pollock M, Nukada H, Taylor P, et al. Comparison between fascicular and whole sural nerve biopsy. Ann Neurol. 1983;13:65-8.
6. Ginsberg L, King R, Orrell R. How to do it? Nerve Biopsy Pract Neurol. 2003;3:306-12.
7. Mellgren SI, Lindal S. Nerve biopsy—some comments on procedures and indications. Acta Neurol Scand Suppl. 2011; 124: 64-70.
8. Ducic I, West J. A modifed approach to sural nerve biopsy: minimizing complications. Ann Plast Surg. 2009;62: 220-2.
9. Devi SK, Sharmila BP, Susan PJ, Gajendra K. Variant formation of sural nerve and its distribution at the dorsum of the foot. Int J AnatomVar. 2009;1:33-4.
10. Bevilacqua NJ, Rogers LC, Malik RA, et al. Technique of the sural nerve biopsy. J Foot Ankle Surg. 2007;46:139-42.

CHAPTER 24

Nail Surgery

Chander Grover, Nirmal B Krishna

INTRODUCTION

Nail surgery has generated great interest among dermatologists in the last decade. It is needed as an aid in diagnosis, to treat infections, to alleviate pain in the nail unit, to correct deformities, to excise tumors and to achieve cosmesis.

A proper understanding of nail anatomy is the first step towards performing successful nail surgery. Along with this, selection of appropriate instruments; establishing good hemostasis; ensuring proper anesthesia; proper surgical technique; and postoperative care ensures good results.

This chapter aims to summarize the practice essentials before undertaking any nail surgery procedures. Each surgery is summarized step wise and supported by intra-operative photographs essential nuances. Each section also includes practical tips from authors who have engaged in years of successful nail surgery.

ESSENTIAL PREREQUISITES FOR NAIL SURGERY

There are a certain basic essentials needed to ensure appropriate surgical outcome. These are over and above those required for any other dermatosurgical technique. These include:

Surgical Anatomy of Nail

A practical understanding of the nail unit anatomy is essential to prevent long-term scarring after any surgical procedure. Dermatologists are at a vantage position in this respect. The surgical anatomy of the nail is highlighted in Figures 24.1A and B. The important surgical units are explained here.

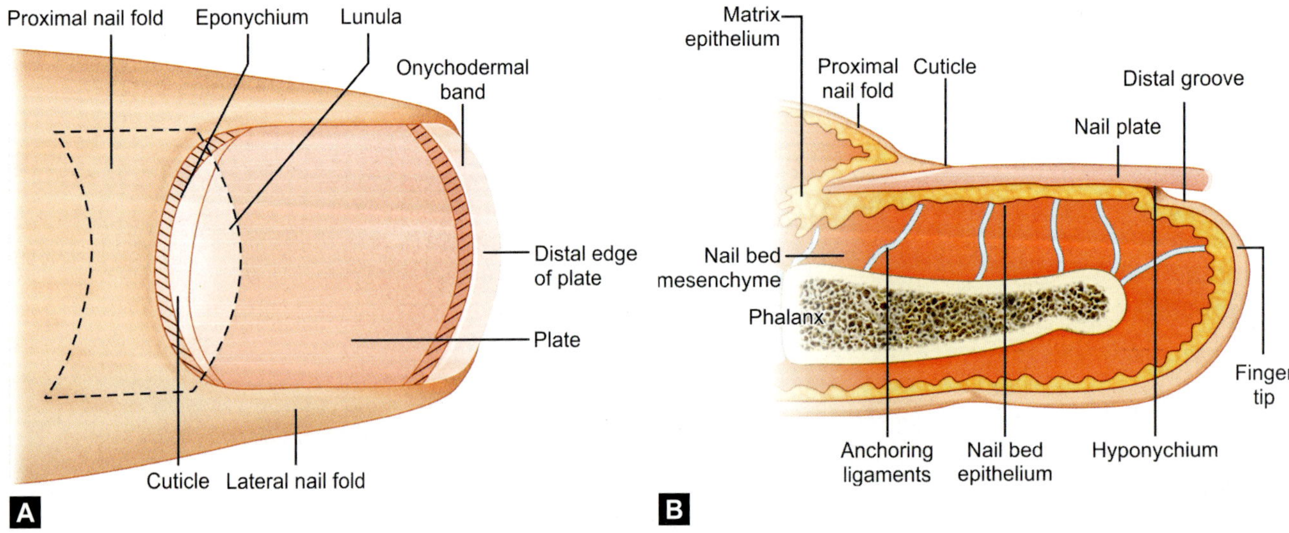

Figs. 24.1A and B: Surgical anatomy of nail. (A) Dorsal view of the nail plate structure. While operating, respect the boundaries of lunula. (B) Sagittal section of the nail unit. The nail fold structure with the nail plate is seen. The underlying nail matrix and nail bed epithelium is visualized.

Nail Plate

It is a flat, translucent, convex, hard structure derived almost exclusively from nail matrix. Proximal matrix produces the dorsal part of nail plate and distal matrix produces the ventral part of nail plate. Nail bed probably also contributes to a small part of nail plate undersurface. Nail plate overlying the lunula is loosely attached while that over the nail bed is firmly attached.

Nail Matrix

It is the germinative portion of the nail unit which has two parts namely dorsal and ventral matrix. The dorsal matrix continues proximally and laterally to form the lateral matrix horns. Lunula is the distal most part of ventral matrix that is visible through the nail plate in larger nails like the thumb and middle finger. Boundary of lunula should be left intact in nail surgery as shape of distal border of lunula determines the shape of nail.

Nail Bed

It extends from the distal lunula to the hyponychium. Lateral nail folds form the lateral borders of nail bed. It has parallel longitudinal ridges that interlock with the grooves over the ventral surface of the nail plate. The dermis has a rich vascular network, hence bleeds a lot on manipulation. This rich network along with the presence of glomus cells is responsible for temperature regulation. Nail bed lacks adipose tissue and sits directly over the periosteum of the underlying phalanx.

Proximal Nail Fold

It is a continuation of dorsal skin of digit and has two surfaces dorsal and ventral. Cuticle is present at the junction of the two surfaces.

Blood Supply

Both the radial and the ulnar arteries supply deep and superficial palmar arcades, which in turn give rise to digital vessels. Each digit is supplied by the palmar and the dorsal digital arteries, lying on the sides of the digits. The palmar digital arteries are the predominant source of blood supply of the digits. Dorsal digital arteries, which are branches of radial artery, also contribute to the digital blood supply. These lateral digital arteries ultimately supply the nail unit formation by forming superficial (dorsal nail fold arcade), proximal and distal subungual arcades.

Nerve Supply

Nail unit is innervated by branches of median, ulnar and radial nerves. This is derived from the two laterally positioned sensory nerves—dorsal and palmar. Palmar digital nerves innervates index, middle and ring finger tips. Thumb, little finger and toe tips are innervated by dorsal digital nerve.[1]

TIPS AND TRICKS

- Anesthesia for nail surgery can be achieved by blocking the laterally placed digital nerves. This can be achieved by proximal digital block technique which works on the laterally placed neurovascular bundle.
- Similarly, any excessive bleeding from the nail bed can be controlled by applying sustained pressure laterally at the base of the digit. The same effect is achieved by a tourniquet.
- While operating on the nail unit, the boundaries of the nail matrix (as explained above) should be respected as far as possible. This helps in preventing postoperative scarring.

Patient Considerations

Patients undergoing nail surgery should be assessed for factors predisposing to poor peripheral circulation or those which can impair healing. These include but are not restricted to diabetes mellitus, peripheral vascular disease, collagen vascular disease, bleeding diathesis, prosthetic heart valves and immunosuppression. Simultaneous drug intake that prolong bleeding (NSAIDs, anticoagulants), affect healing (steroids), affect anesthesia (β-blockers, phenothiazine, monoamine oxidase inhibitors) and allergy to lignocaine should also be noted.

Affected finger is examined for color change and compared with the other side. General physical examination to assess for signs of infection and systemic examination to assess for any associated diseases should also be performed. Dermatoscopy is an important tool to exclude associated collagen vascular diseases through nail fold capillaroscopy, infections and nail tumors. Ultrasound and magnetic resonance imaging (MRI) are also helpful in the evaluation of soft tissue and phalanx of the nail unit.[2]

TIPS AND TRICKS

- Do not miss out on this essential component of presurgical workup. It can help prevent many nail surgeries, other than pre-empting possible complications in the long-term.
- Onychoscopy is an important emerging tool which can help in many ways. It can help delineate the appropriate area from where nail biopsy needs to be taken, thus increasing the histopathologic diagnostic yield.

Nail Unit Anesthesia

Anesthesia of the nail unit is quite essential as finger tips and nails are richly innervated and sensitive structures. It has been sufficiently proven that 2% lignocaine with adrenaline (1:200,000) is safe and versatile anesthetic agent for digital anesthesia. The authors have been routinely using it for many years without any complications. Other than producing adequate and long-lasting anesthesia, it also decreases the arterial flow by 50%, which then returns to normal in 1 hour. This makes nail surgery easier, though most surgical procedures require a completely bloodless field for which tourniquet has to be invariably used. Using lignocaine without adrenaline has a relatively lower toxicity and quicker onset of action, though the anesthesia may wear off more quickly.[3]

The commonly used anesthetic techniques in nail surgery include proximal and distal digital blocks and discussed in detail. Other techniques like metatarsal block, ring block, matricial block, transthecal block and hyponychial block are not widely used by nail surgeons.

Proximal Digital Block

This is the most commonly resorted to technique of nail unit anesthesia.

Step-by-Step Procedure (Figs. 24.2A to D):

- The digit to be operated is thoroughly cleansed with surgical spirit and painted with betadine.

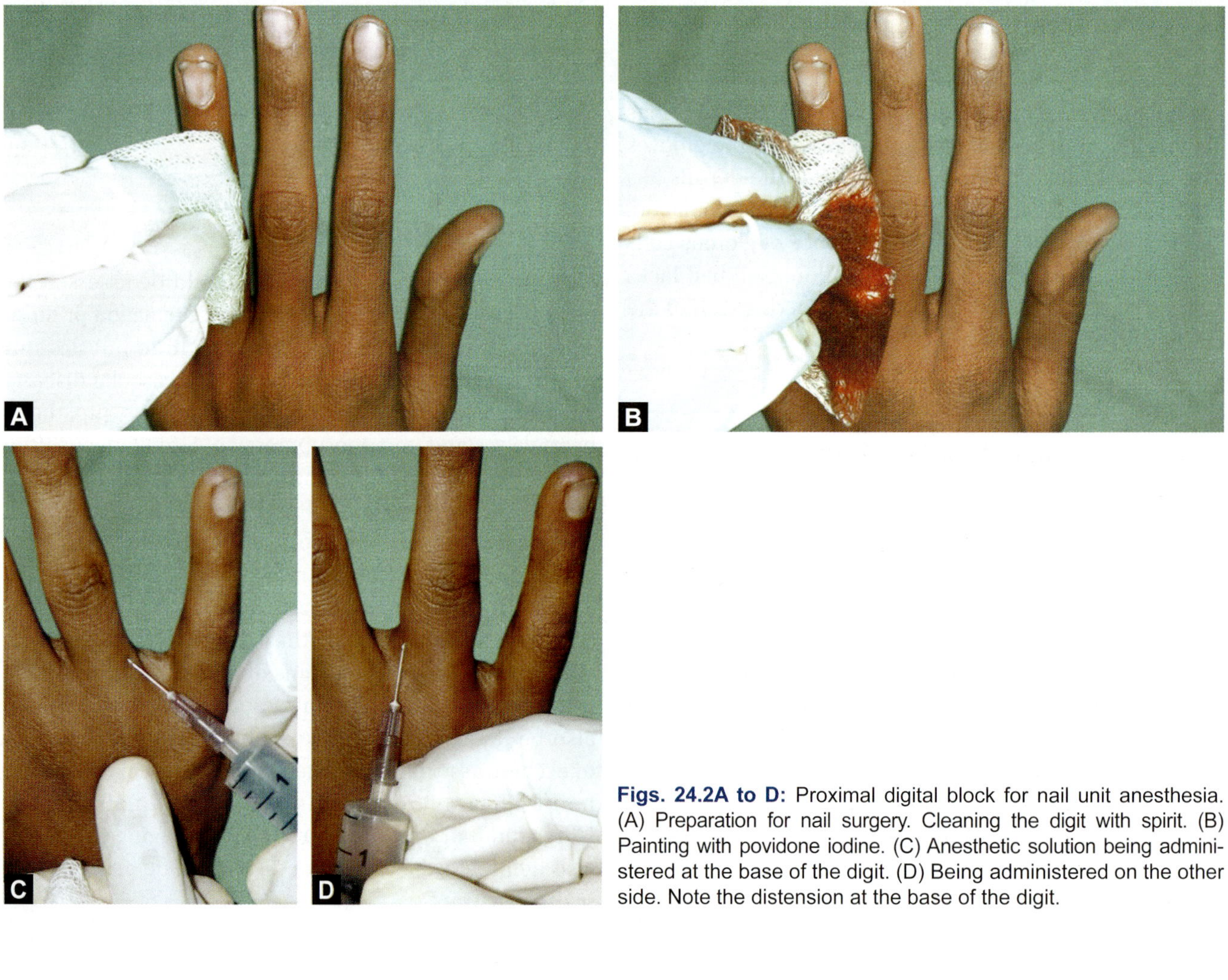

Figs. 24.2A to D: Proximal digital block for nail unit anesthesia. (A) Preparation for nail surgery. Cleaning the digit with spirit. (B) Painting with povidone iodine. (C) Anesthetic solution being administered at the base of the digit. (D) Being administered on the other side. Note the distension at the base of the digit.

- The anesthetic solution is administered with a hypodermic needle over each side of the base of finger/toe. This is done through the dorsal aspect of the finger/toe close to the metacarpophalangeal or metatarsophalangeal joint.
- The needle is advanced towards the ventral aspect of the digit till there is loss of initial resistance.
- The needle is slightly withdrawn to ensure that the digital vessels have not been entered. Then 0.5–1 mL of the anesthetic solution is injected in the loose tissue, close to the dorsal aspect of the digit.
- The same is repeated on the other side of the digit.
- A total of 4 mL is generally needed to adequately anesthetize the great toe and up to 2–2.5 mL for other digits.

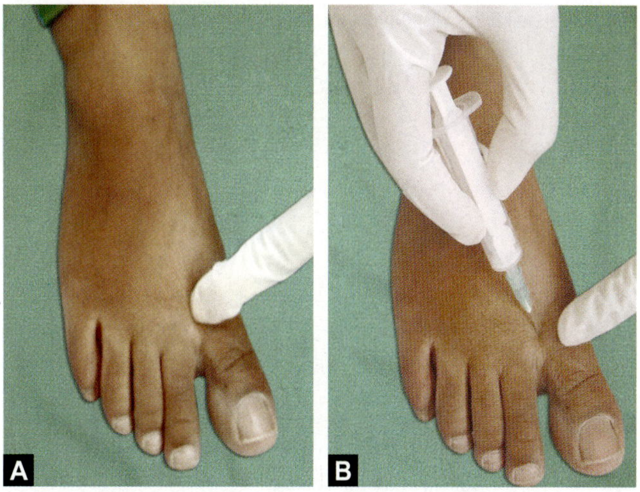

Figs. 24.3A and B: (A) Palpate for metatarsophalangeal joint. (B) Injecting just proximal to metatarsophalangeal joint.

Metatarsal Block: Step-by-Step Procedure

- The digit to be operated is thoroughly cleansed with surgical spirit and painted with betadine.
- The anesthetic solution is administered with a hypodermic needle over each side of the base of finger/toe. This point of injection is a little proximal at the level of metacarpo/metatarsophalangeal joint termed as metacarpal or metatarsal block carries relatively less risk of vascular injuries (Figs. 24.3A and B).[4]
- The same is repeated on the other side of the digit.
- Lignocaine without epinephrine preferred to prevent ischemic injury of digits.

TIPS AND TRICKS

- Always withdraw the plunger of the syringe before administering the nerve block as the nerves lie close to vascular structures in the digits.
- The block will have an onset over a few minutes. Hence, we have to wait before starting the procedure.

Distal Digital Block

This technique of nail unit anesthesia is extremely useful for smaller nail procedures as it has an immediate onset of action. It also known as Wing block (Fig. 24.4A).

Step-by-Step Procedure:

- The site of injection is 1 cm proximal and lateral to the junction of proximal nail fold (PNF) and lateral nail fold (LNF).
- The needle is directed at 45° angle, down up to the periosteum, and then withdrawn slightly, and 0.5 mL of the solution is injected distending and blanching both the folds.
- This is also known as 'wing block' as the area of blanching resembles a wing as the anesthetic solution diffuses distally.
- Anesthesia can also be injected into the lateral nail fold up to the hyponychium.

TIPS AND TRICKS

- This anesthesia can be more painful as they are being administered in the more sensitive part of the digit, which is also an area with much lesser loose tissue. Hence, both the injection as well as the infiltration is more painful.
- This technique anesthetizes only one half of the nail unit. Hence, it is of use, if the surgical intervention remains confined to a limited area. For most routine procedures, proximal block is preferred.

Other Techniques

These are required to be used under special circumstances.

Ring block: This involves injection of anesthesia all around the base of the digit thus producing a tourniquet effect. The procedure is more of a historical interest and not resorted to now.

Matricial block: This is identical to the intramatrix injections of steroids. It allows anesthesia to PNF, nail matrix and proximal half of nail bed (Fig. 24.4B).

Transthecal block: This technique involves injection of anesthetic solution into the flexor tendon sheath of the

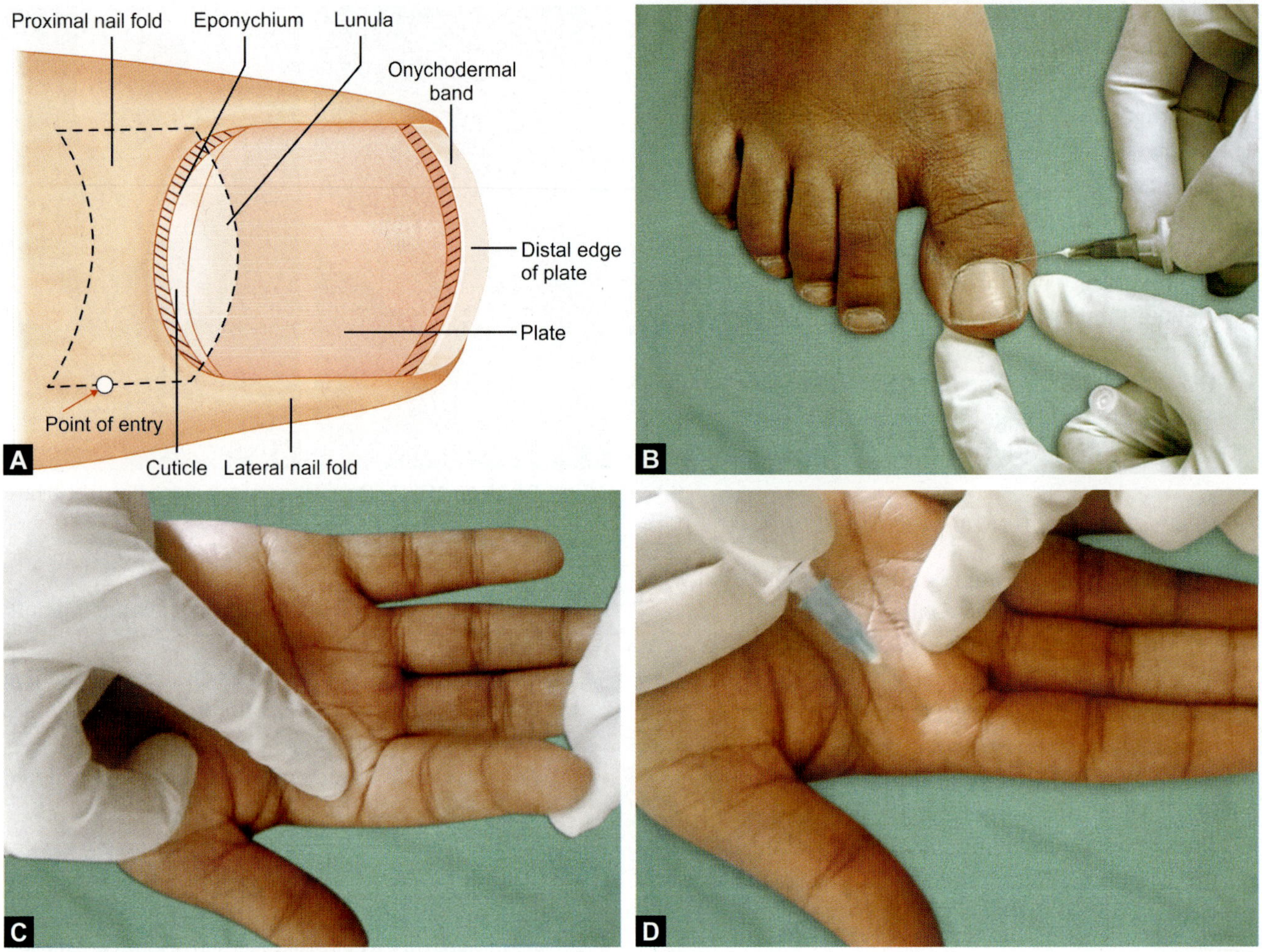

Figs. 24.4A to D: (A) Distal digital block. The point of entry is shown. It lies at approximately 1 cm proximal and lateral to the junction of the PNF and LNF. The red arrow shows the direction of needle entry. The needle enters at a 45° angle and goes down to the periosteum. (B) Intramatrix injection of anesthesia to PNF, nail matrix and proximal half of nail bed. (C) Palpate the flexor tendon by flexing the index finger. (D) Inject into the flexor tendon sheath.

digit, from the palmar aspect. It is useful only for procedures resorted to on the index, middle and ring fingers. Too much resistance while injecting indicates that the needle is probably inside the tendon and this should be avoided. The advantages offered are the rapid onset of anesthesia with little risk to adjacent neurovascular bundles (Figs. 24.4C and D).

Hyponychial block: It is an extremely painful block technique, to anesthetize the distal part of the nail bed.

Tips and tricks to decrease pain during anesthesia:[5]
- Inject slowly.
- Inject through the dorsal aspect of finger which has relatively thinner skin.
- Talk to the patient while injecting (Talkesthesia).
- Use thinner needles for injection and inject with the bevel side up.
- Topical anesthesia can be applied before injection.
- Exposure to icepacks or cold air prior to injection can help.
- Similarly, application of vibration or pressure at the injection site for 5 minutes prior to injection also helps.
- Alkalinization of lignocaine with sodium bicarbonate (in a ratio 9:1) can also be tried. However, it is not routinely encouraged as addition of too much sodium bicarbonate results in a milky solution due to flocculation; this has been associated with necrosis.
- Bring the anesthetic solution to body temperature prior to use.

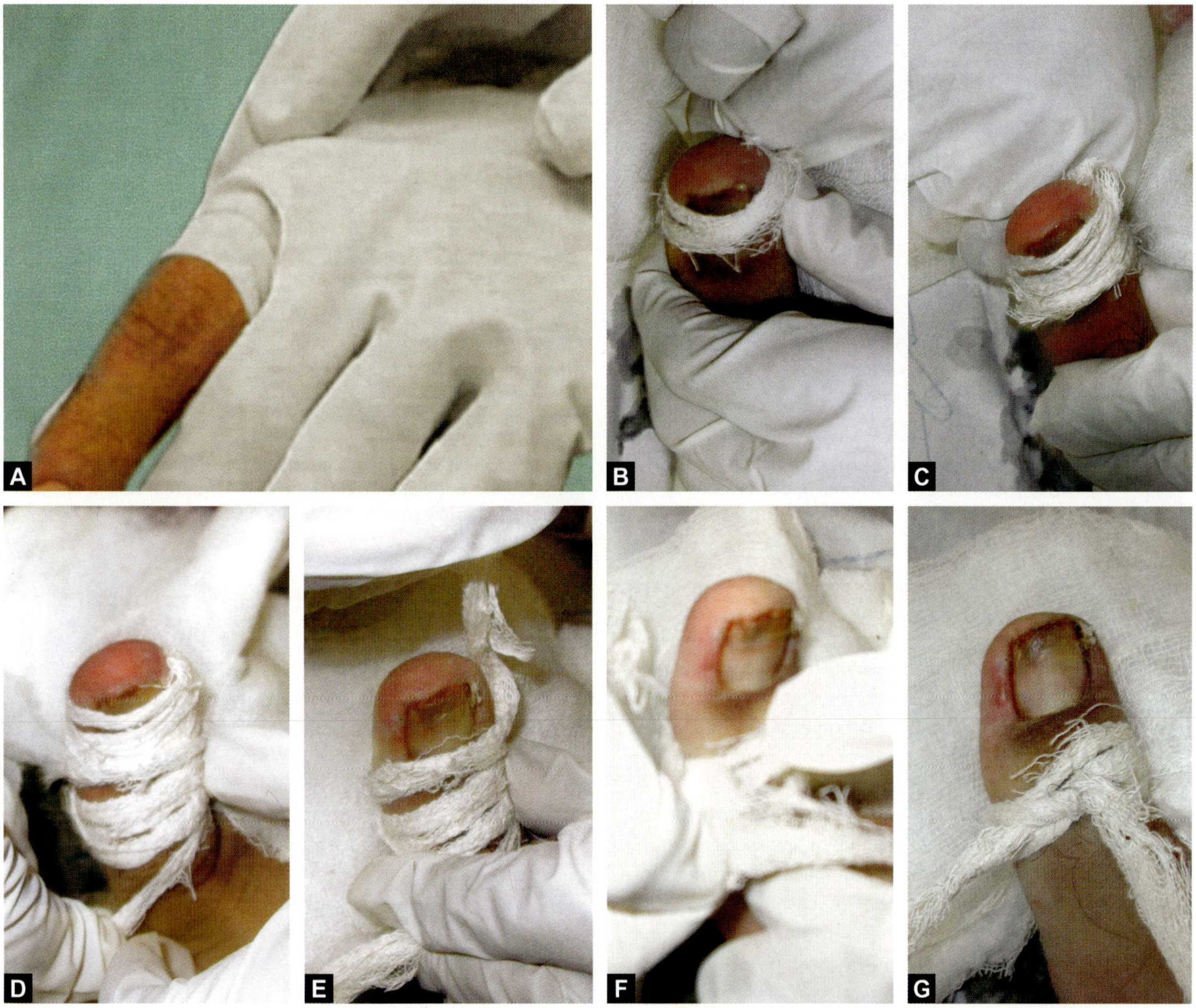

Figs. 24.5A to G: (A) Sterile glove being used as a tourniquet. The fingertip is cut and then rolled back. This serves the purpose of exsanguination and tourniquet. (B) Use of gauze strip tourniquet. The long gauze piece is tightly wound around the digit from the distal end to the proximal end, exsanguinating the digit (B and C). When we reach the base, we take an extra round (D). Then we start untying from the distal end to the proximal (E). The loose ends are then tied tightly at the base (F and G) to secure the tourniquet. Note the long gauze piece tied at the base of the finger as a tourniquet.

Exsanguination and Tourniquet

The nail unit being a very vascular structure, exsanguination and tourniquet is required to achieve hemostasis and visualization of structures clearly during the surgical procedure. Many types of tourniquet have been described in literature. These include:

- *Sterile glove tourniquet*: A sterile glove can be used as a tourniquet by cutting a finger of the glove and making a small opening at its tip. It is inserted into the digit on which the surgery is performed and rolled back proximally to exsanguinate the blood in the digit. The rolled glove piece is tightened and clamped with a straight artery forceps (Fig. 24.5A).
- *Gauze strip tourniquet*: A sterile gauze strip can also be used to exsanguinate the digit and apply a tight tourniquet at the base (Figs. 24.5 and 24.6).[6]
- *Others*: A sterile Penrose drain and Foley's catheter have also been described to be used for the same purpose.

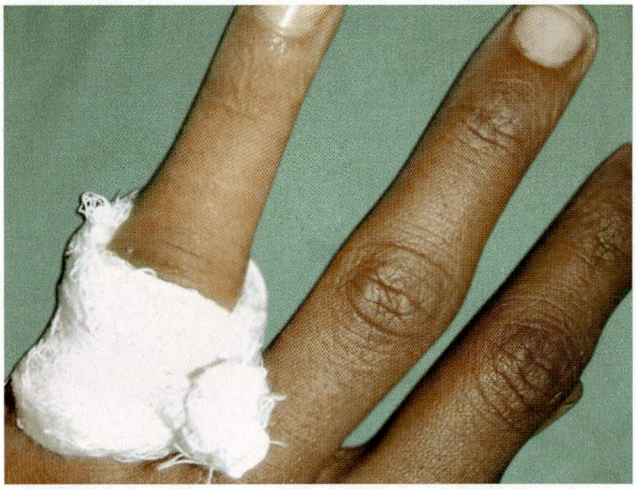

Fig. 24.6: The digit to be operated clearly appears blanched and less vascular than surrounding digits.

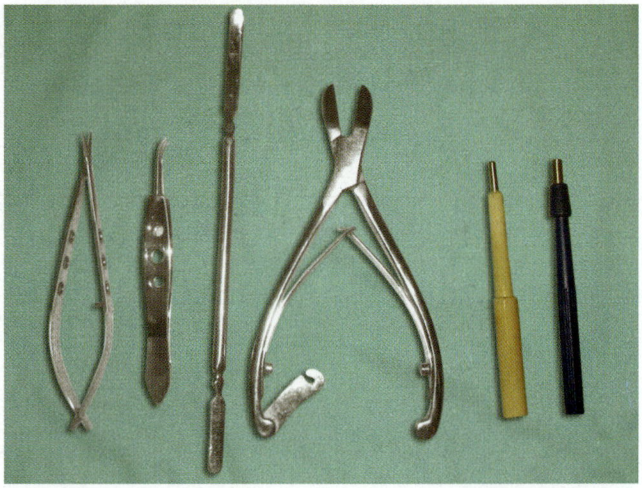

Fig. 24.7: Nail surgery instruments. (From left to right) Fine curved iris scissors, fine jeweller's forceps, nail spatula, nail splitter and disposable biopsy punches of various sizes.

TIPS AND TRICKS

- Use of tourniquet really enhances the ease of nail surgery. Even tightly pressing on the sides of the digit can produce the same effect as it compresses the lateral digital arteries.
- Many experts now believe that exsanguination is non-essential. However, in the author's opinion, it does help.
- Gauze strip tourniquet is a very practical tourniquet as sterile gauze piece is available in any surgical setup. There is no need to procure any special equipment for that. It is entirely disposable and practically cost-less. The same gauze piece is used to first exsanguinate the digit and then tie a tourniquet at the base. It also produces and evenly distributed pressure (because of its breadth), thus minimizing the possibility of damaging the vascular endothelium.[6]
- The tourniquet can be left in place for 10–12 minutes. If your surgery lasts longer than this, then it is highly advisable to release the tourniquet for 2–3 minutes and then re-apply it.

Instruments for Nail Surgery

The job of a nail surgeon is simplified by the use of certain special instruments. These include (Fig. 24.7):

- Nail splitter
- Nail spatula/Freer septum elevator
- No. 3 BP handle, with No.10 and15 blade
- Adson's plain and toothed forceps
- Fine curved iris scissors
- Fine jeweller's forceps
- Needle holder
- Gel foam.

TIPS AND TRICKS

- It is worthwhile investing to procure two important nail surgical instruments: the nail spatula and the nail splitter. Infact, both instruments should be procured in 2–3 different sizes and tips by any aspiring nail surgeon.
- The important feature of the nail spatula is the atraumatic tip. This helps to minimize damage to the nail bed.

Postoperative Care

The patient undergoing nail surgery needs to be advised specially regarding postoperative care. This starts with the initial preparation when the patient is forewarned about the functional compromise, be it the finger nail (inability to type, to write) or the toenail (inability to wear normal shoes, to cycle).

- The surgeon needs to ensure appropriate hemostasis as the nail bed being a very vascular structure, may continue to ooze for long. The staining of the dressing is likely to be very scary for the patient.
- Absorbent dressing (to absorb the extra drainage) with adequate padding (to prevent impact over the digital tips) needs to be given, unlike other operated areas. (Figs. 24.8A to C)

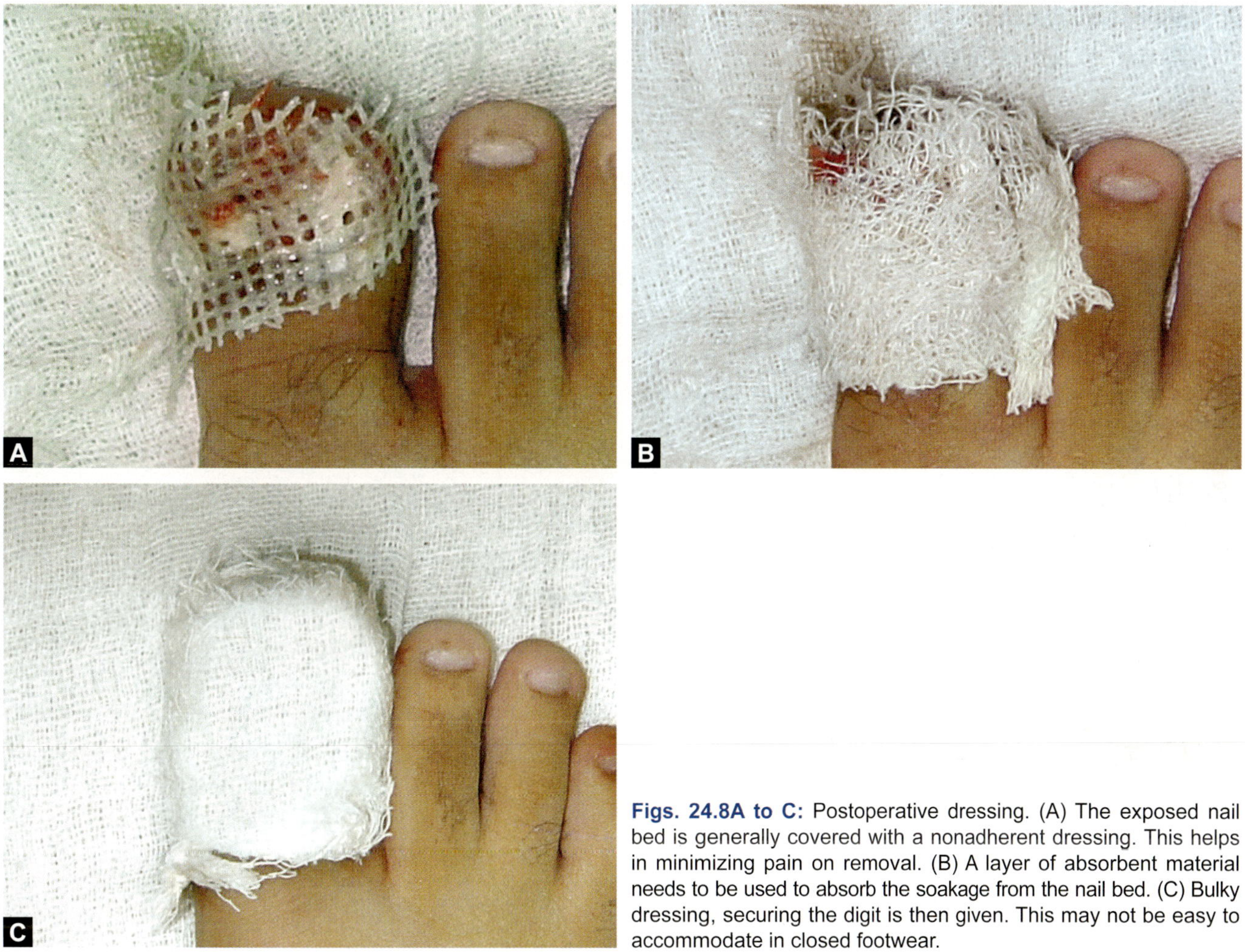

Figs. 24.8A to C: Postoperative dressing. (A) The exposed nail bed is generally covered with a nonadherent dressing. This helps in minimizing pain on removal. (B) A layer of absorbent material needs to be used to absorb the soakage from the nail bed. (C) Bulky dressing, securing the digit is then given. This may not be easy to accommodate in closed footwear.

- Serous drainage may continue for a long period of time, especially, if a chemical matricectomy has been done. The patient needs to be pre-warned as well as supported through the healing process.
- Analgesic cover for the initial 48–72 hours is an absolute must. Thereafter, it is dependent on variables like the type and extent of surgery and patient's tolerance.
- Elevation of the operated limb for the initial 24–48 hours is advised to avoid dependent edema in the operated area.
- Patients can resume peratively normal daily activities and office work 2–3 days postoperatively however, the handicap imposed by the bulky dressing as well as the pain needs to be kept in mind. There is a lot of individual to individual variation in this aspect.
- Appropriate footwear modification needs to be advised beforehand, so that the patient can comfortably leave the dermatologist's office.

TIPS AND TRICKS

- Ideal dressing in nail surgery should be absorbable, nonadherent.
- Use of antibiotic ointment and petrolatum soaked gauze allows easy painless removal of the dressing.
- The petrolatum gauze allows serous exudate to pass through to absorbent gauze dressing over it.
- Dressing is bulky and adequately secured to wrist or ankle.
- A dressing where the tip of the digit is visible is useful to track any occlusive changes. However, this may not be always possible as generally the tip is the area which has been operated.
- Specialized footwear ideally a sandal with velcro tapes above are most suited.
- Patients are best advised to keep the operated limb elevated to avoid aggravation of postoperative edema which can further tighten the dressing and precipitate tourniquet effect on the operated digit.
- Patients are advised to loosen/remove the dressing in case they feel any throbbing pain and to report to the operating dermatologist at the earliest.

COMMON NAIL SURGICAL PROCEDURES

This section covers some commonly resorted to nail surgical procedures.

Nail Avulsion

Nail avulsion implies separation of nail plate from its attachments. This can be achieved surgically or chemically with 40% urea applied over the nail plate for 3–7 days. However, surgical nail avulsion is a faster and a much more controlled procedure causing lesser patient discomfort and less lateral damage.

Principles

The nail plate can be separated from the nail bed both by using a distal approach (more commonly) or a proximal approach (less commonly used). Depending on the extent of nail removed, nail avulsion can also be classified as complete nail avulsion or partial nail avulsion. The third basis for classifying could be whether post-procedure the nail plate has been repositioned on the bed or not.

Types of Nail Avulsion[7]

Distal Nail Avulsion

Indications:

- Removal of dermatophytoma in totally dystrophic nails
- Exposure and removal of tumors of nail bed and matrix.

Step-by-Step Procedure (Figs. 24.9A to I):

- Nail unit anesthesia—Generally administered by proximal digital block (Fig. 24.9A).
- Exsanguination and tourniquet (Figs. 24.9B and C).
- Elevation of PNF—Nail spatula or Freer's septum elevator is inserted between PNF and proximal nail plate and extended to corners to elevate both LNF similarly (Fig. 24.9D).
- Undermining nail plate—Elevator is inserted in the gap between the distal nail plate and nail bed to separate the connections (Fig. 24.9E). The most adherent connection is between nail plate and nail bed at onychodermal band. Motion has to be longitudinal and parallel close to the nail plate. Side-side movements can injure the longitudinal ridges causing permanent onycholysis.
- Nail plate avulsion—Avulsion is performed by grasping the nail plate with artery forceps and twisting one lateral edge to free lateral horn (Fig. 24.9F). Same is repeated on other side to free the other horn and the nail plate is removed in rotating wrist movement (Fig. 24.9G).
- Cleansing—The remaining fragments and subungual hyperkeratotic tissue is curetted, excised or gently removed (Fig. 24.9H).
- Release of tourniquet and firm pressure dressing with antibiotic ointment.
- Phenol can be applied to the nail matrix as part of matricectomy (Fig. 24.9I).

TIPS AND TRICKS

- The tip of the spatula should be atraumatically inserted to avoid damage to nail plate.
- Shearing away the plate from bed by pulling with an artery forceps causes unnecessary damage to nail bed. It is better to separate the nail plate by side-ways movement of spatula and slowly lift it up.

Proximal Nail Avulsion

This procedure is uncommonly resorted to if the distal plane of cleavage between nail plate and nail bed is obliterated or difficult to penetrate. It may also be needed if the plate is to be removed only proximally.

Indications:

It is indicated when nail avulsion is required when

- Nail plate is firmly adhered to the nail bed
- Severe distal hyperkeratosis.

Step-by-Step Procedure (Figs. 24.10A to E):

- Nail unit anesthesia—Generally administered by proximal digital block.
- Exsanguination and tourniquet.
- Elevation of PNF.
- Undermining nail plate from proximal side—The elevator then is inserted under base of the nail plate where it is loosely attached to the matrix and the plane is cleaved distally.
- Nail plate avulsion—The nail plate is held with an artery forceps and remaining subungual attachments are freed with iris scissors to avulse the nail plate.
- Cleansing—The remaining fragments, subungual hyperkeratotic tissue curetted, excised or gently removed.
- Release of tourniquet and firm pressure dressing with antibiotic ointment.

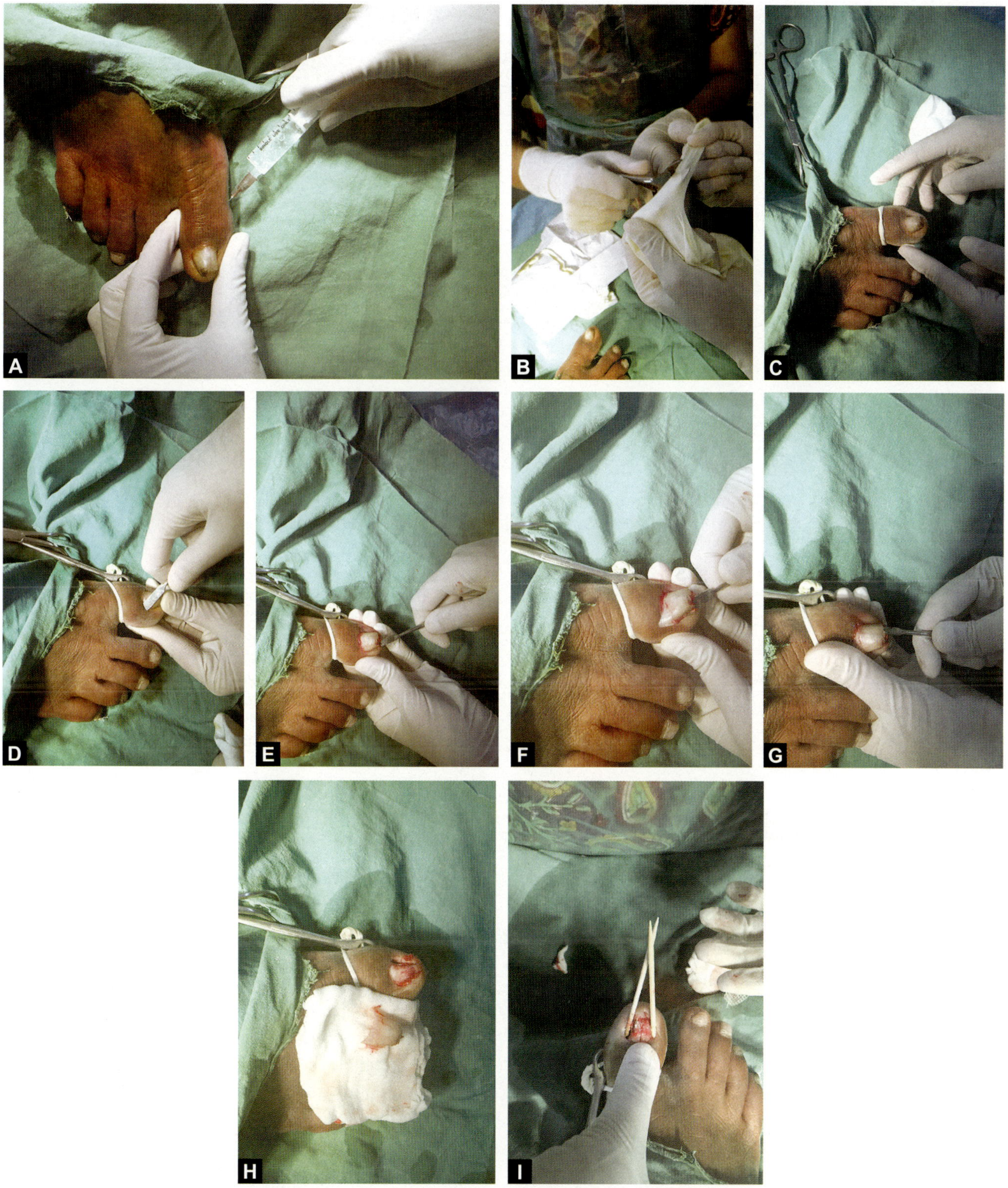

Figs. 24.9A to I: Technique of distal nail avulsion. (A to C) Anesthetized and exsanguinated digit with a tourniquet tied at the base. The aim of nail avulsion here is to assess the nail bed for longitudinal erythronychia. The direction of insertion of nail spatula is shown. (D and E) Separation of proximal nail fold from the nail plate by lateral sweeping movements of the spatula. (F and G) Separation of lateral nail folds. This is followed by separation of distal nail fold from nail plate. (H) Totally separated nail plate. (I) Application of phenol to the matrices.

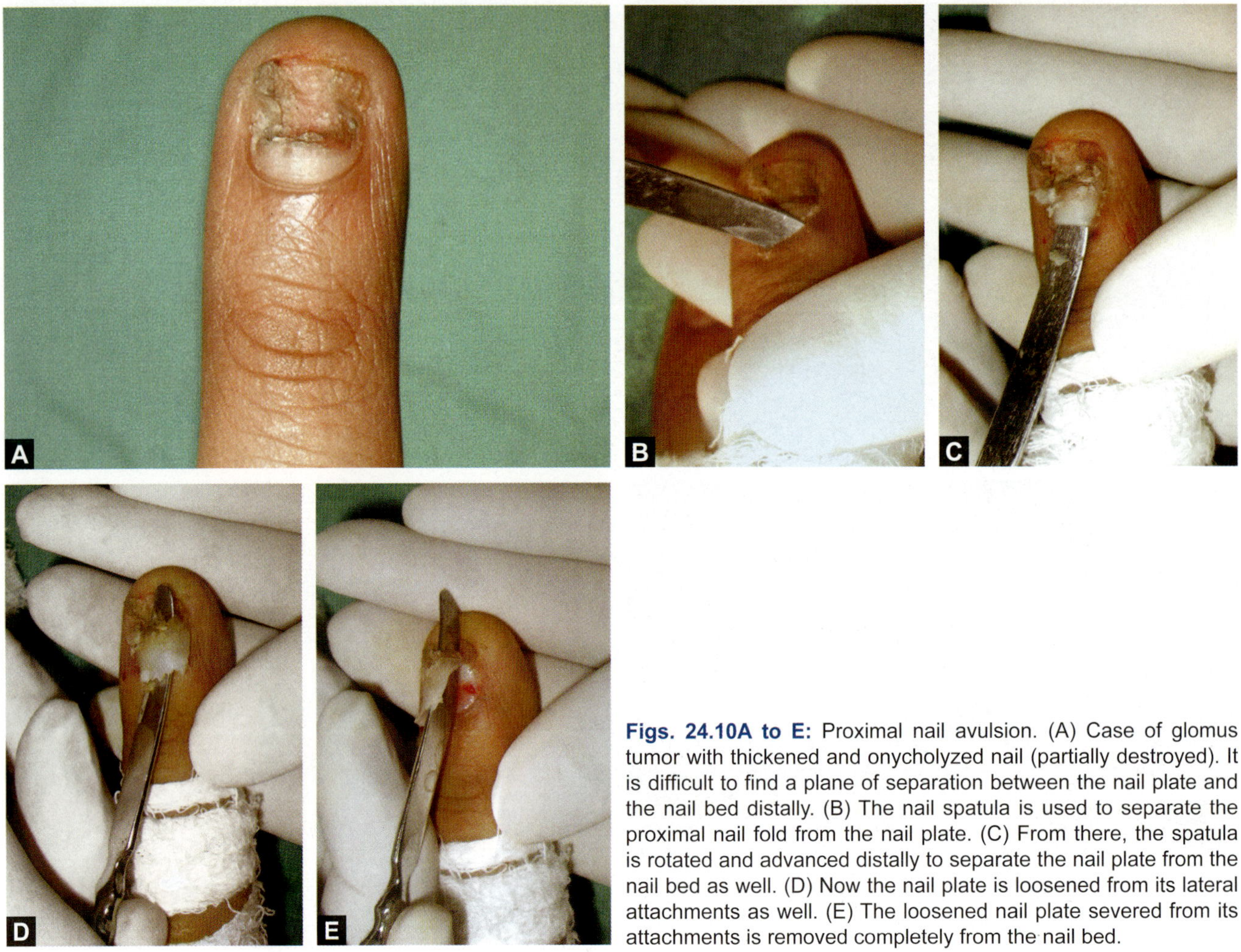

Figs. 24.10A to E: Proximal nail avulsion. (A) Case of glomus tumor with thickened and onycholyzed nail (partially destroyed). It is difficult to find a plane of separation between the nail plate and the nail bed distally. (B) The nail spatula is used to separate the proximal nail fold from the nail plate. (C) From there, the spatula is rotated and advanced distally to separate the nail plate from the nail bed as well. (D) Now the nail plate is loosened from its lateral attachments as well. (E) The loosened nail plate severed from its attachments is removed completely from the nail bed.

TIPS AND TRICKS

- Care should be taken to loosen the attachments from nail bed with the help of lateral sweeping motion of the nail spatula/elevator. Minimizing the extent of twisting and turning with an artery forceps will help preserve the integrity of nail bed, and in turn prevent complications. Similarly, minimizing the use of sharp instruments is also recommended.
- As far as possible (i.e if the primary indication for nail removal allows), the avulsed nail plate should be repositioned post-surgery. It may or may not be secured with sutures. Repositioning of the nail plate helps reduce the postoperative morbidity and hastens healing. The repositioned nail plate only acts as a biological dressing and is shed off in a week.

Partial Nail Avulsion

This happens to be the procedure of choice as far as possible, the advantage being limited traumatization and exposure of nail bed, ensuring faster postoperative recovery and lesser risk of infections.

Indications:

- As a part of surgical procedures such as partial matricectomy, acute paronychia treatment and longitudinal melanonychia evaluation.
- Treatment of onychomycosis with lateral nail disease.

Step-by-Step Procedure (Figs. 24.11A and B):

- Nail unit anesthesia—Generally administered by proximal digital block.
- Exsanguination and tourniquet.
- Elevation of PNF.
- Undermining the nail plate.
- Nail plate avulsion: The portion of nail plate to be avulsed is cut with a nail clipper from distal edge till PNF and using a straight scissors to cut the portion under PNF. Using a straight artery forceps, the nail plate is grasped and rotated through 180° medially to deliver the lateral horn.

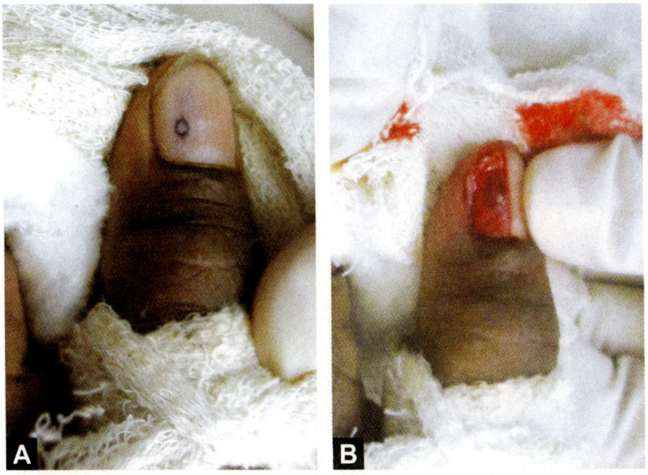

Figs. 24.11A and B: Partial nail avulsion. (A) Case of glomus tumor. The tumor location is marked beforehand. (B) Only lateral partial nail avulsion is done, just enough to expose the extent of the tumor.

- Cleansing: The remaining fragments and subungual hyperkeratotic tissue is curetted, excised or gently removed.
- Release of tourniquet and firm pressure dressing with antibiotic ointment.

TIPS AND TRICKS

- Partial nail plate avulsion may be lateral partial, proximal partial or distal partial. This entirely depends on the indication/pathology being dealt with
- Partial avulsion reduces the postoperative morbidity significantly.

Management of Ingrown Nail

Ingrown nail (commonly the great toe nail) is a commonly encountered dermatologic morbidity. Although, initial stages can be dealt with conservatively, most cases would sooner or later require surgical intervention.[8]

Principle

The surgical procedure involves removal of narrow strip of the lateral in-growing nail plate. A full length removal of this lateral in-growing nail strip is accompanied by permanent matricectomy of the lateral horn, to prevent growth of a broad nail plate and minimize recurrences. The permanent matricectomy can be attempted either chemically or surgically.

Lateral Nail Matrix Phenolization[9-12]

This is the most commonly resorted to procedure which has very low recurrence rate.

Step-by-Step Procedure (Figs. 24.12A to G):

- Nail unit anesthesia—Generally administered by proximal digital block.
- Exsanguination and tourniquet.
- Elevation of PNF—Nail spatula or Freer's septum elevator is inserted between PNF and proximal nail plate on the side of the ingrown toe nail
- Undermining nail plate—Elevator is inserted in the gap between the distal nail plate and the most lateral part of the nail bed on the side of ingrown nail to separate the connections by performing longitudinal motions.
- Nail plate avulsion—The narrow strip of nail plate to be avulsed is cut with a nail clipper from distal edge till PNF. A straight scissors is used to cut the portion under PNF. Using a straight artery forceps, the nail plate is grasped and rotated through 180° medially to deliver the lateral horn
- Nail matrix phenolization—Phenol is applied using a wooden stick dipped in pure liquefied phenol (BP 80% w/w, USP 89% w/w) in lateral nail matrix cavity and LNF groove for 3 times with a contact period of 1 minute each time. Then it has to be neutralized with alcohol or swab and remove excess phenol.
- Cleansing—The remaining fragments and subungual hyperkeratotic tissue is curetted, excised or gently removed.
- Release of tourniquet and firm pressure dressing with antibiotic ointment.

Modifications: Although the procedure for lateral nail avulsion remains the same, the technique of lateral horn matricectomy can vary. These include:

- *Surgical*: resection of matrix horn[13]
- *Chemical*: 88% phenol,[10,11] 10% sodium hydroxide[12,14] 100% trichloro acetic acid[15]
- *Laser*: CO_2 laser[16]
- *Electrical*: Electrocautery, radiosurgery coagulation

TIPS AND TRICKS

- Surgical resection may require incision at the junction of proximal and lateral nail fold to expose the underlying matrix. This is a more traumatic procedure with potentially more scarring. However, the chances of recurrence are the least.
- Chemical matricectomy being a blind procedure does carry a chance of recurrence, even though minor.
- Varying durations of application of chemical solution have been compared in literature. A one minute application time (by vigorous rubbing) has been found to be optimal.[10,12]
- Excess phenol has to be neutralized with alcohol or washed repeatedly with saline to avoid postoperative maceration of the treated area.

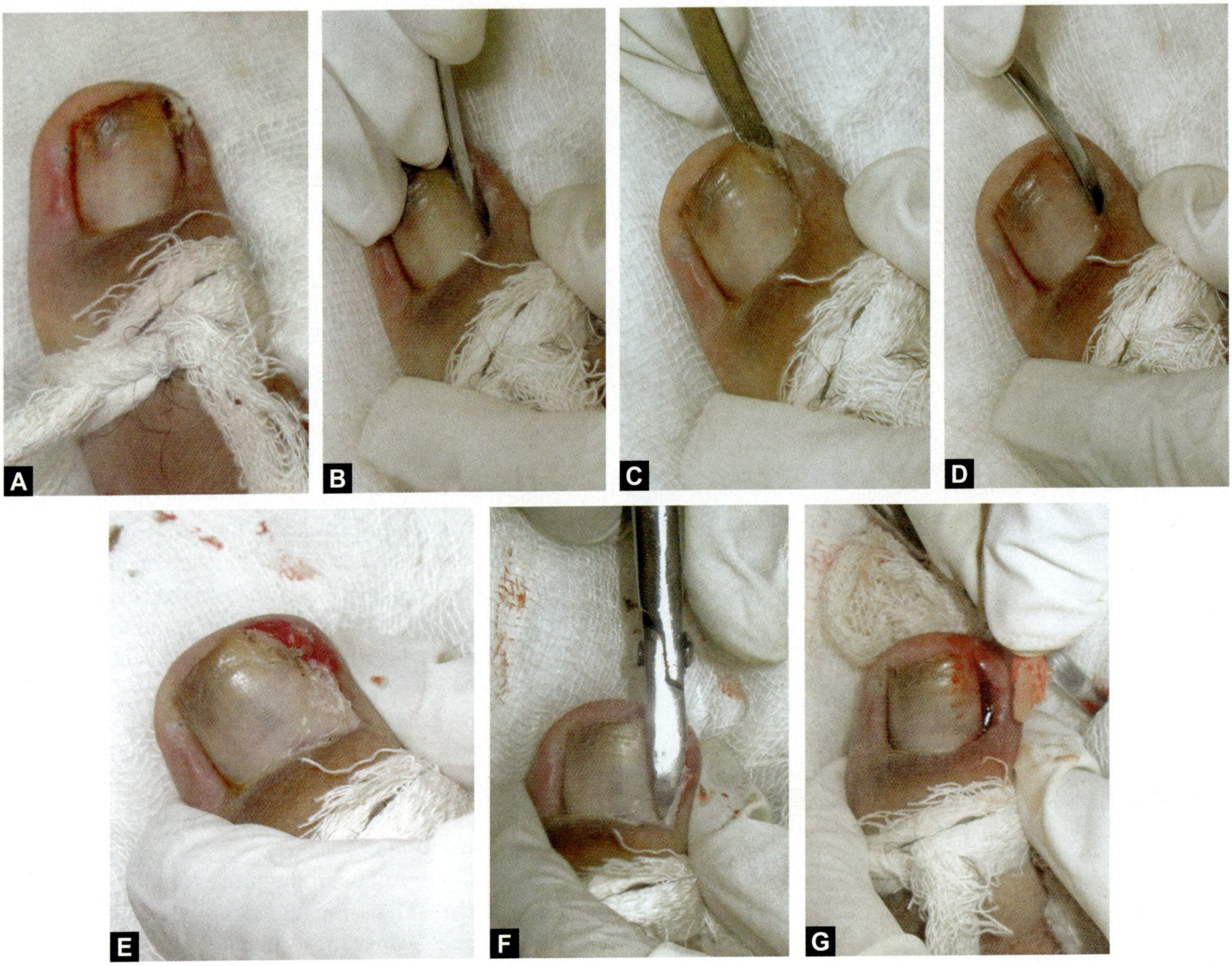

Figs. 24.12A to G: Lateral nail matrix phenolization. (A) Ingrown nail. The great toe has been anesthetized, exsanguinated and tourniquet tied. (B) Nail spatula used to separate nail plate from the lateral nail fold. (C) Nail spatula now being used to separate the lateral one-third of nail plate from the nail bed. The ingrown part of nail plate is clearly seen. (D) Nail spatula now being used to separate the nail plate from the lateral part of the proximal nail fold. (E) The separated one-third of the nail plate has been lifted up after being separated from its attachments. (F) Nail splitter is now used to atraumatically section the lateral nail plate. (G) The lateral nail gutter with overlying partial nail plate avulsion can be seen. Cotton tipped applicator is used to apply the solution (phenol/NaOH) on the lateral horn of the nail matrix as described previously.

Pincer Nail

Pincer nail is an increase in transverse curvature of nails that increases distally and occurring more frequently over toes. X-ray of the affected phalanx is important before surgery of pincer nail to rule out an osteophyte at the base of distal phalanx increasing the curvature of the nail plate. In the presence of osteophyte, matrix horn resection with nail bed plasty is performed. In most cases, selective matrix horn resection with chemical cautery results in release of pressure due to over curvature and alleviates pain after the surgery.[17,18]

Selective Matrix Horn Resection

Step-by-Step Procedure (Figs. 24.13A to E):

- Proximal digital block.
- Basal tourniquet.
- Partial nail avulsion of lateral strips of nail plate.
- Chemical cauterization of lateral horns of nail matrix.
- Application of povidone iodine wick in the lateral nail grooves including lateral nail horn.
- Cleansing—The remaining fragments and subungual hyperkeratotic tissue is curetted, excised or gently removed.

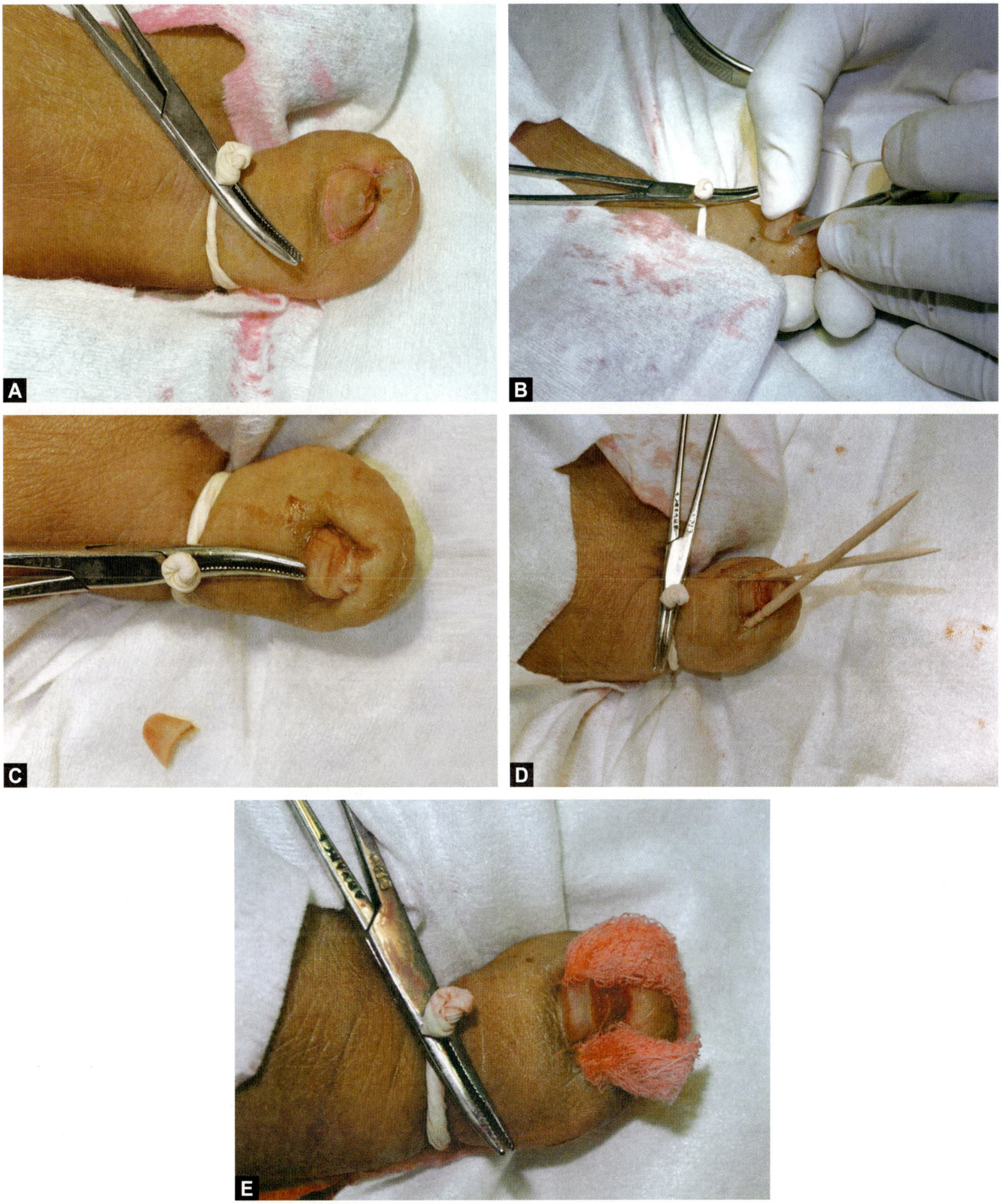

Figs. 24.13A to E: Pincer nail surgery. (A) Basal tourniquet with glove. (B) Undermining the nail plate. (C) Partial nail avulsion of lateral strips and distal half of nail plate. (D) Chemical cauterization of lateral horns of nail matrix. (E) Application of povidone iodine wick in the lateral nail grooves including lateral nail horn.

- Release of tourniquet and firm pressure dressing with antibiotic ointment leaving the tip of the digit visible to track any occlusive changes.

Matrix Horn Resection with Nail Bed Plasty

Step-by-Step Procedure:

- Proximal digital blck.
- Basal tourniquet.
- Partial nail avulsion of lateral strips of nail plate.
- Chemical cauterization of lateral horns of nail matrix.
- Distal two-thirds of the nail plate is avulsed transversely.
- Traction osteophyte is resected with a bone rongeur after exposing it with a reversed T incision.
- The two tongue flaps are spread laterally and sutured.
- Release of tourniquet and bulk dressing secured to the ankle.

Nail Biopsy[19,20]

Nail biopsy is a procedure not very commonly resorted to. However, many times, there may be no alternatives available and nail biopsy may be the only diagnostic clue left.

Indications

To demonstrate fungal organisms, nail plate deformity, to confirm the diagnosis of diseases confined to nail unit, to diagnose benign and malignant nail tumors.

Types of Nail Biopsy

Depending on the part of the nail unit being sampled, there are various types of nail biopsy procedures.

Nail Plate Biopsy

This procedure samples only the affected part of the nail plate. This can give valuable clues in the form of presence/ absence of fungal elements in routine hematoxylin and eosin (H and E) sections or Periodic acid-Sehitt (PAS) stained sections.[21]

Step-by-Step Procedure (Figs. 24.14A and B):

- Proximal digital block.
- Basal tourniquet.
- The biopsy technique is different with different sites of involvement of the nail plate.
- Distal involvement—Scissors/scalpel is used to remove a wedge of dystrophic nail with distal hyponychium.
- Proximal involvement—3 mm punch is driven into the nail plate up to the nail bed and the incised nail plate is lifted out with 26G needle.

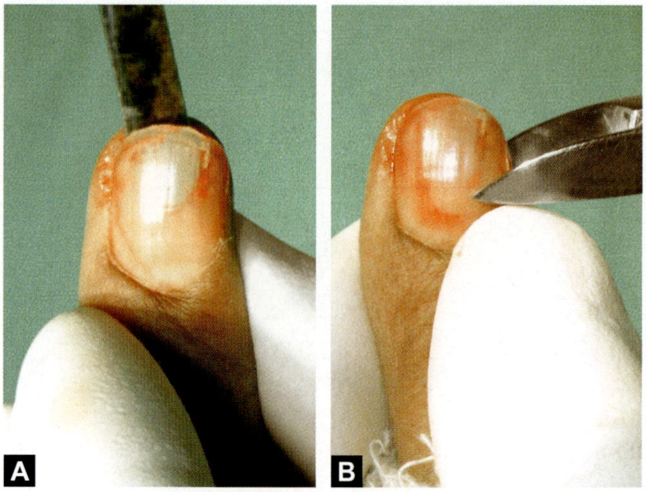

Figs. 24.14A and B: Nail plate biopsy. (A) Separation of nail plate from nail bed. (B) The distal part of the nail plate is removed with nail splitter and sent for histopathologic examination.

- Release of tourniquet and firm pressure dressing with antibiotic ointment.

TIPS AND TRICKS

- This is a very simple procedure which serves as gold standard for diagnosis for onychomycosis.
- If only distal, onycholyzed nail plate removal is required, then nail unit anesthesia may not even be needed.

Nail Bed Biopsy

This procedure is resorted to for identifying the cause of any painful lesion of the nail bed or for changes confined to the nail bed, e.g subungual hyperkeratosis, nail bed discoloration.[22,23]

Step-by-Step Procedure (Figs. 24.15A to D):

- Proximal digital block.
- Basal tourniquet.
- Types of nail bed biopsy:
  - *Single punch technique*: 3 mm punch driven down till periosteum distal to the lunula to avoid injury to nail matrix. The nail bed specimen is lifted out with 26G needle and cut with curved iris scissors.
  - *Two punch technique*: This technique uses a larger 4 mm punch to cut the nail plate and a smaller 3 mm punch is driven through the earlier created window down to periosteum. The technique is easier than single punch technique.
  - *Fusiform biopsy*: Partial or complete nail avulsion is carried out to visualize the nail bed. Fusiform excision

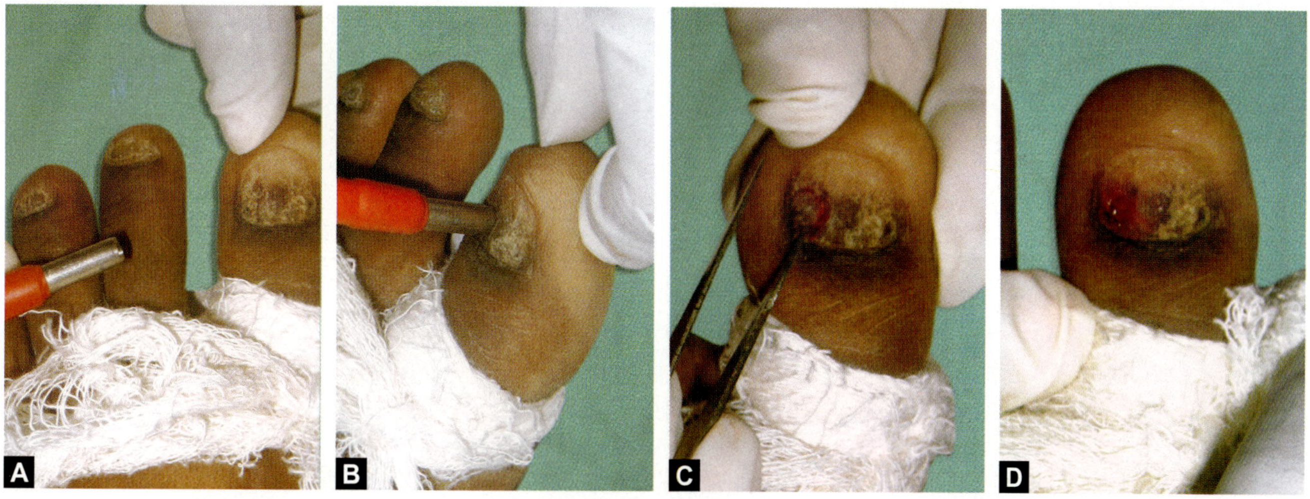

Figs. 24.15A to D: Nail bed biopsy. (A) Dystrophic nails with a partial loss of nail plate. The great toe has been anesthetized and tourniquet tied. (B) Sharp, disposable biopsy punch is used to define a cylindrical punch biopsy specimen. The punch is taken down to the periosteum. This step may require some force. (C) The tissue cylinder is then extracted with the help of jeweller's forceps and iris scissors. (D) The remaining defect which is the covered with a dressing and allowed to heal. With the growth of the nail plate, this defect slowly grows out. The risk of scarring is minimal to absent if the matrix has not been injured.

is directed longitudinally up to the periosteum and the wound is closed with 6-0 vicryl. Longitudinal relaxing incision at lateral edges of nail fold can help reduce wound tension.

- Release of tourniquet and firm pressure dressing with antibiotic ointment.

TIPS AND TRICKS

- The two punch technique or the fusiform technique are easier to perform but give incomplete histopathological results. This is because, the nail bed epithelium tends to peel off with the removed nail plate and what is left behind is the nail bed dermis. It requires an experienced pathologist to piece together the information form the avulsed nail plate and the underlying dermis. Also, the interface changes are very difficult to interpret.
- A newer nail biopsy punch driven by motor has been devised to ensure delivery of specimen from thick nails.[24]

Nail Matrix Biopsy

This type of biopsy is less routinely resorted to. It is needed in cases where the pathology is confined to the nail matrix, e.g. longitudinal melanonychia, nail pitting or onychorrhexis.

Step-by-Step Procedure (Figs. 24.16A to C):

- Proximal digital block.
- Basal tourniquet.
- Nail spatula is inserted between nail plate and PNF.
- Bilateral longitudinal incisions from junction of PNF and LNF is extended 6 mm proximally upwards.
- PNF is lifted with skin hooks.
- Nail plate may or may not be avulsed.
- 3 mm punch or transverse fusiform biopsy with distal edge of ellipse parallel to the curve of lunula from distal matrix with nonviolation of lunula edge.
- Punch allowed to heal with secondary intention while longitudinal and transverse incisions are closed with 6-0 vicryl.
- Reflected PNF returned to natural position and sutured with 6-0 prolene.
- Release of tourniquet and firm pressure dressing with antibiotic ointment.

TIPS AND TRICKS

- Nail matrix biopsy is the diagnostic gold standard for evaluation of longitudinal pigmented bands. This procedure is needed to rule out melanoma of the nail unit.

En Bloc Nail Unit Biopsy

This biopsy procedure is rarely, if ever, resorted to. It samples all the parts of the nail unit but is associated with a higher risk of scarring. The technique is based on a longitudinal resection to diagnose neoplastic conditions. Additionally, it can assist in providing the chronology of the pathological process.[25]

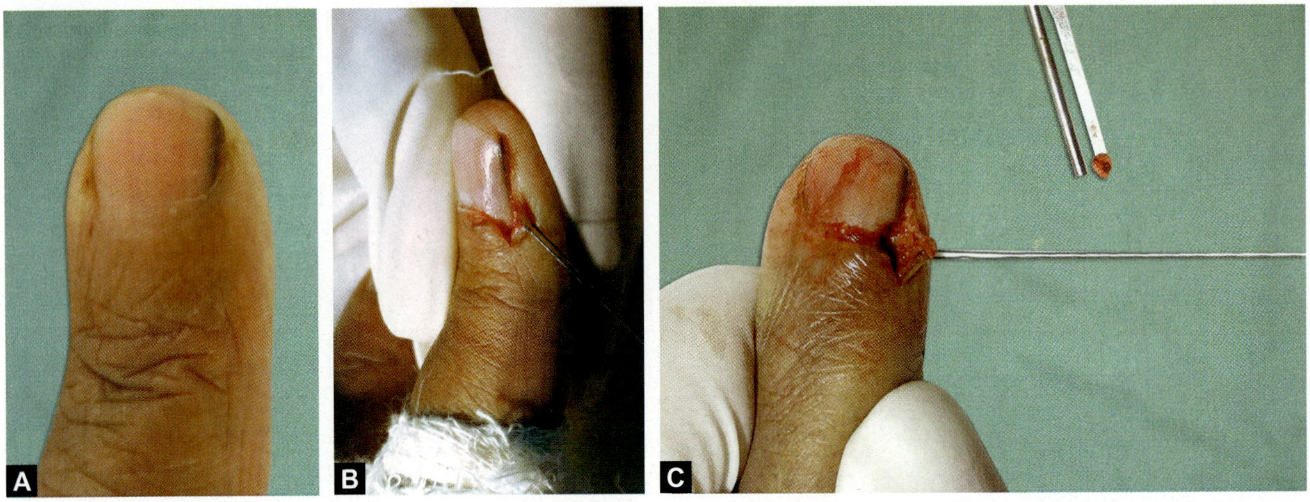

Figs. 24.16A to C: Nail matrix biopsy. (A) A recent onset longitudinal pigmented band with proximal spread of pigment. Matrix biopsy to be done from the point of origin of the pigment. (B) Anesthetized digit with tourniquet at the base. The nail fold is reflected to visualize the origin of the pigmented band. The reflected nail folds are held back with stay sutures. A skin hook can be used for the same purpose, if the band is more centrally placed. (C) punch biopsy specimen is taken from the origin of the band. The nail fold is reflected back and sutured into place.

Step-by-Step Procedure (Figs. 24.17A to C):

- Proximal digital block.
- Basal tourniquet.
- Longitudinal fusiform incision from PNF to tip of the finger which includes LNF, nail plate, nail matrix and nail bed.
- Width of the biopsy specimen should not be more than 3 mm and should not extend bone deep.
- Incised tissue excised with iris scissors.
- The defect is undermined, closed with 4-0 prolene.
- Release of tourniquet and firm pressure dressing with antibiotic ointment.
- Suture removal after 10 days.

TIPS AND TRICKS

- In routine practice, it is almost never necessary to resort to this type of biopsy. It has been of more or less academic interest only.

Surgical Management of Subungual Hematoma

Subungual hematomas mostly resolve spontaneously. However, a surgical decompression may be required for a large sized subungual hematoma.[22]

Step-by-Step Procedure:

- Proximal digital block.
- Basal tourniquet.
- Hematoma small (less than 25% of visible nail) and proximal—Opening made with No.11 blade/punch/electrocautery over nail plate.
- Hematoma small and distal—Hyponychium is incised with No.11 blade.
- Hematoma large (more than 25% of visible nail)—Fracture of disal phalanx has to be excluded. If no fracture, total nail avulsion and nail bed repair with 6-0 vicryl.
- Release of tourniquet and firm pressure dressing with antibiotic ointment.

TIPS AND TRICKS

- Any surgical intervention is reserved for acute subungual hematoma which is very symptomatic and progressing. More chronic hematomas or asymptomatic ones are better left to resolve on their own. They may however need to be evaluated more thoroughly with onychoscopy/biopsy in case a melanoma is suspected.
- A preoperative digital X-ray is needed to evaluate the underlying phalanx. A fractured phalanx is the most common cause of acute pain, rather than the hematoma itself.

Paronychial Surgery

The paronychium refers to the proximal and the lateral nail folds. These can be the seat of inflammatory as well as neoplastic processes. The surgical technique while dealing with the paronychial tissue is slightly different.

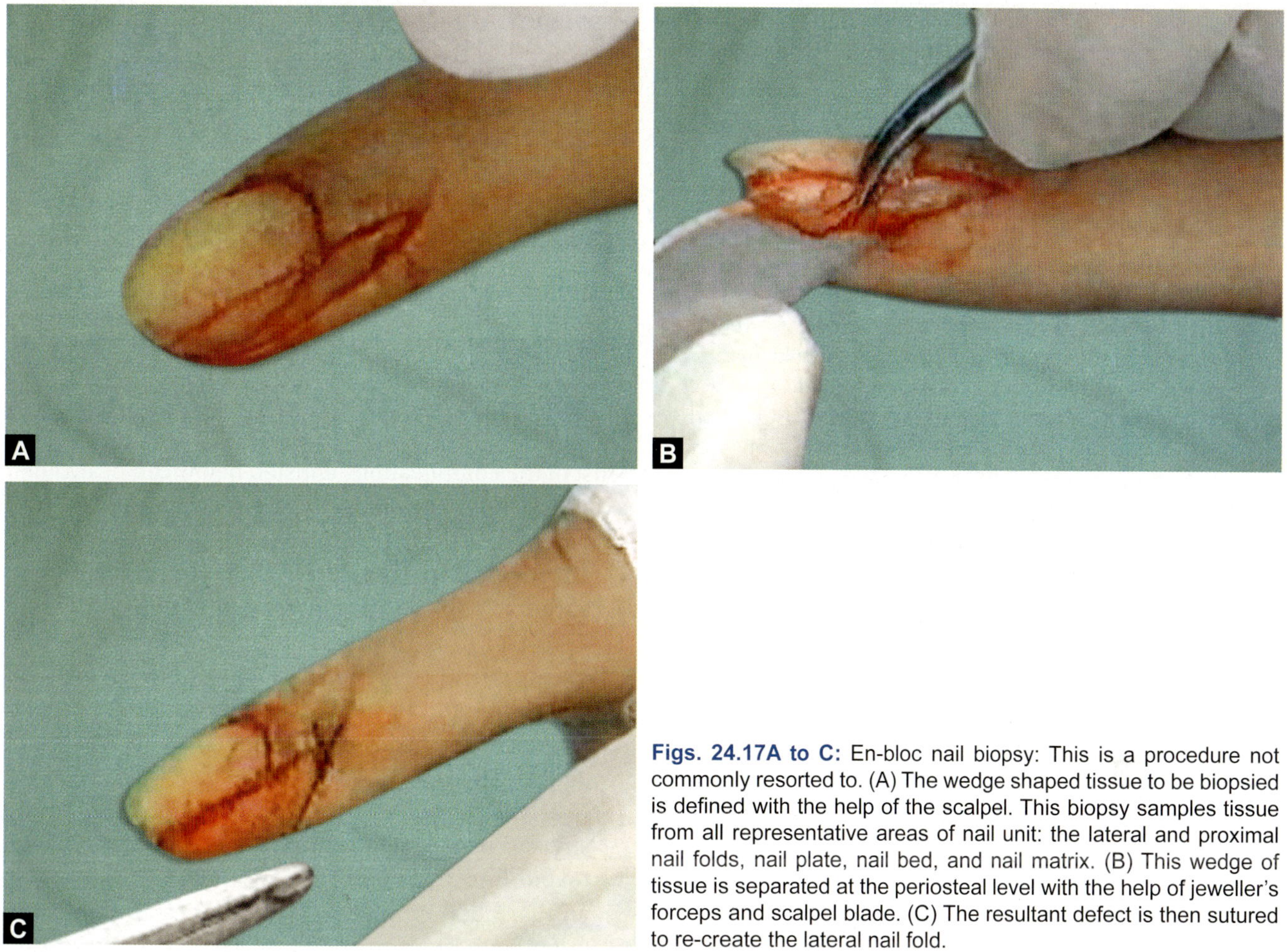

Figs. 24.17A to C: En-bloc nail biopsy: This is a procedure not commonly resorted to. (A) The wedge shaped tissue to be biopsied is defined with the help of the scalpel. This biopsy samples tissue from all representative areas of nail unit: the lateral and proximal nail folds, nail plate, nail bed, and nail matrix. (B) This wedge of tissue is separated at the periosteal level with the help of jeweller's forceps and scalpel blade. (C) The resultant defect is then sutured to re-create the lateral nail fold.

Acute Paronychia

Surgical management of acute paronychia is performed when antibiotics fail after 24 hours in children and 48 hours in adults.

Step-by-Step Procedure:

- Incision and drainage—No local anesthesia is usually required. Larger abscess requires digital block. No.21 G needle with bevel facing upwards is advanced parallel to lateral groove at the point of maximum fluctuation till its tip pierces the space with a feel of give away and free flow of pus. Pressure is given till the pus is squeezed out and blood stained fluid drains out. Pressure dressings are applied.
- Avulsion of proximal third of nail plate—Elevator is inserted under PNF which releases pus from cul-de-sac. Proximal avulsion starts at the edge of distal edge of lunula where the nail plate is loosely attached to the nail bed. The nail plate is split transversely by inserting a jaw of nail splitter under lateral side of nail plate.

TIPS AND TRICKS

- Surgical intervention is reserved for paronychia not responding to therapy or showing a pus point.
- It is required to rule out herpetic whitlow as a cause of acute inflammation.
- Patient needs to be maintained on antibiotic therapy for further 7–10 days.

Chronic Paronychia

Inflammation lasting more than 6 weeks is known as chronic paronychia. In the initial stages, it is amenable to medical therapy coupled with rigorous precautions. However, for cases fibrosis and rounding off of the edges of swollen PNF, surgical therapy is needed in addition.[26]

Step-by-Step Procedure:

- Proximal digital block.
- Basal tourniquet.
- Crescentic incision from one LNF to the other reaching its maximum width of 5 mm in the midline of PNF.

- Scalpel blade is held obliquely and a thin slice of the fibrotic tissue is excised down to the underlying nail plate.
- No suture is necessary.
- Release of tourniquet and hemostasis is achieved with pressure dressing or gel foam.
- Healing is by secondary intention.

TIPS AND TRICKS

- Crescentic excision of proximal nail fold is reserved for thickened , fibrotic, rounded proximal nail fold. In these cases, the response to medical therapy is unlikely as well as incomplete due to poor penetration of drugs, both topical and oral.
- Extra care should be taken to prevent damage to the underlying nail matrix.
- If the nail plate is highly dystrophic, it makes sense to avulse it in the same sitting. This should be however done only after crescentic excision has been done.

Glomus Tumor

These are benign vascular tumors, commonly seen to be arising in the subungual location. Owing to their symptomatic nature, surgical removal is warranted.[27,28]

Step-by-Step Procedure (Figs. 24.18A to G):

- Proximal digital block.
- Basal tourniquet.
- Creation of window with 6 mm punch or partial nail avulsion.
- Longitudinal incision, if the tumor is in the nail bed and transverse incision, if the tumor is in nail matrix.
- Tumor is enucleated and edges are approximated with 6-0 vicryl.
- If no tumor is found, with a 4 mm punch, the nail bed is incised up to periosteum and excised.
- Release of tourniquet and firm pressure dressing with antibiotic ointment.

Modification: After punch excision of nail bed, base and inner peripheral circular margin is electrocauterized.

TIPS AND TRICKS

- Depending on the location and size of the tumor, the approach (proximal or lateral) needs to be planned in advance.
- It is advised to attempt partial nail plate avulsion, as far as possible.
- Nail plate repositioning after the surgery is completed, helps improve the healing process.[27]

Periungual Fibroma

Step-by-Step Procedure (Figs. 24.19A to D):

- Proximal digital block.
- Basal tourniquet.
- Periungual fibroma beneath the proximal nail fold.
- A vertical incision put on the proximal nail fold.
- Proximal nail fold raised on either side to expose fibroma fully.
- Fibroma completely removed and proximal nail fold to be sutured back.

COMPLICATIONS IN NAIL SURGERY

Most of the complications enlisted below can be avoided by proper evaluation of the patient before the nail surgery.

- *Pain*: Pain can occur during the surgery and post-surgery. Though there is considerable individual variation in pain threshold, perioperative pain is mostly due to poor anesthesia. Preoperative sedation is also helpful. Post-surgical pain can be alleviated with adequate padding, elevation of operated site and analgesics.
- *Infection*: Infection risk can be decreased by following strict aseptic technique during the procedure. Tetanus toxoid injections are advised for bare foot walkers and farmers. Prophylactic antibiotics are indicated in patients with prosthetic valves and compromised circulation. Postoperative infection has to be treated promptly to avoid complications including cellulitis, lymphangitis and osteomyelitis.
- *Necrosis*: Necrosis of nail folds can be seen with the use of excessive sodium bicarbonate in the anesthetic solution. Necrosis also ensues when sutures are too tight and with overt infection.
- *Deformities*: Permanent residual nail deformities result from matrix involvement, crossing the lunula border, retained suture material and lateral deviation of the nail plate.
- *Pterygium*: In procedures on nail matrix, it is advisable to insert a tulle under PNF and sutured to LNF for 2 weeks to avoid adherence of naked matrix to ventral surface of PNF resulting in pterygium.
- *Permanent onycholysis*: Repeated lateral-to-lateral movement can result in permanent onycholysis due to injury to the longitudinal ridges.
- *Distal embedding*: Loss of nail plate after complete nail avulsion results in loss of counter pressure causes

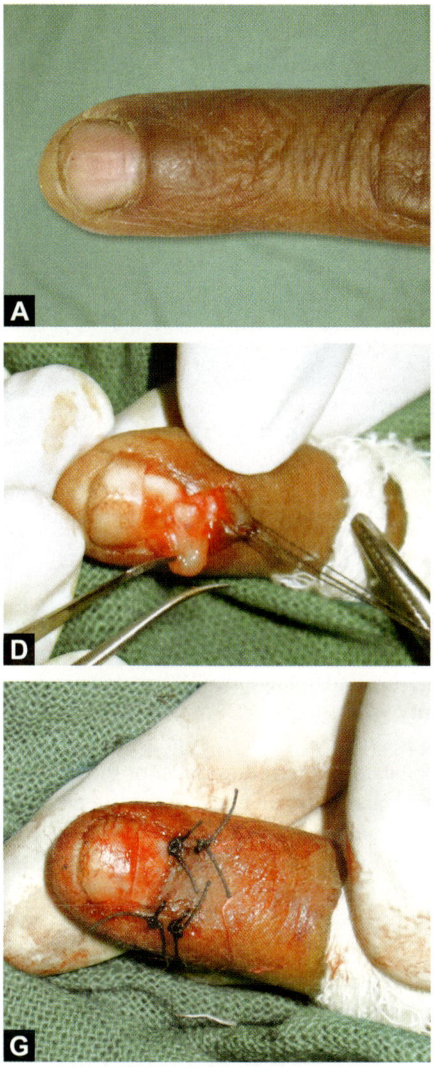

Figs. 24.18A to G: Glomus tumor excision. (A) Little finger showing a prominent fullness at the proximal nail fold, this swelling was intensely painful even on minor trauma and was cold sensitive as well. (B) The digit is anesthetized, exsanguinated and tourniquet tied. The proximal nail fold is reflected back by two linear incisions at the junction of proximal nail fold with the lateral nail folds. The retracted PNF is held back with stay sutures. Only proximal partial avulsion of nail plate is done to expose the underlying matrix. It reveals a prominent swelling in the matrix area. (C) Blunt dissection with fine forceps exposes the glomus tumor just underneath the matrix epithelium. (D) The tumor is excised in-toto with the help of blunt dissection, separating it from its base. (E) The excised tumor as well as the resultant defect is shown. (F) The retracted nail fold is released and allowed to fall back in place. The removed nail plate is shortened from all four sides and repositioned. (G) The proximal and lateral fold edges are sutured ensuring that the underlying plate and matrix are not injured. This is followed by absorbent dressing over the operated area. The sutures can be removed after 7–10 days.

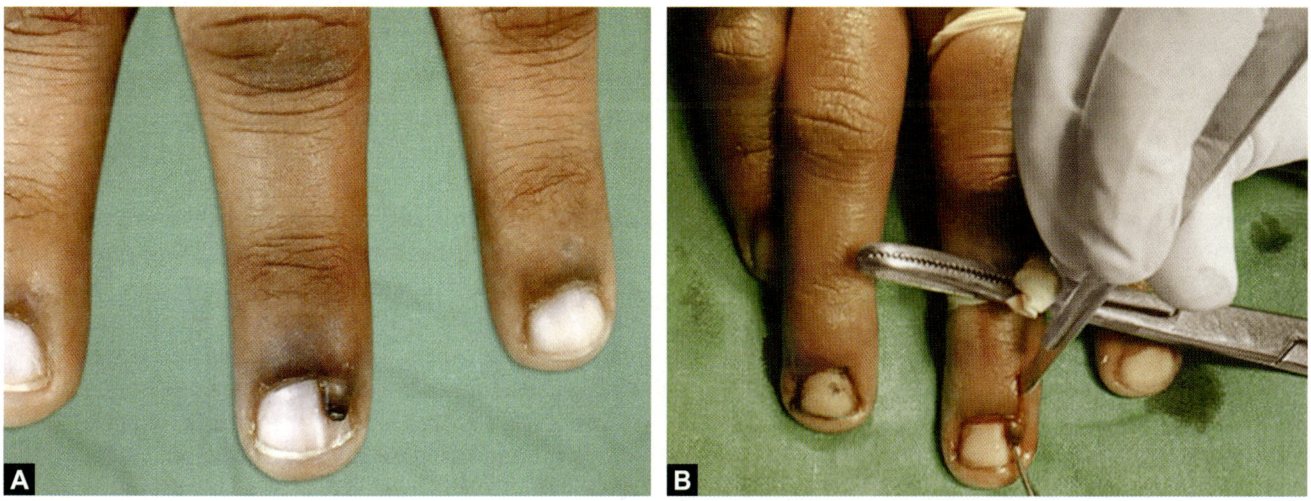

Figs. 24.19A and B: (A) Periungual fibroma beneath the proximal nail fold. (B) A vertical incision put on the proximal nail fold.

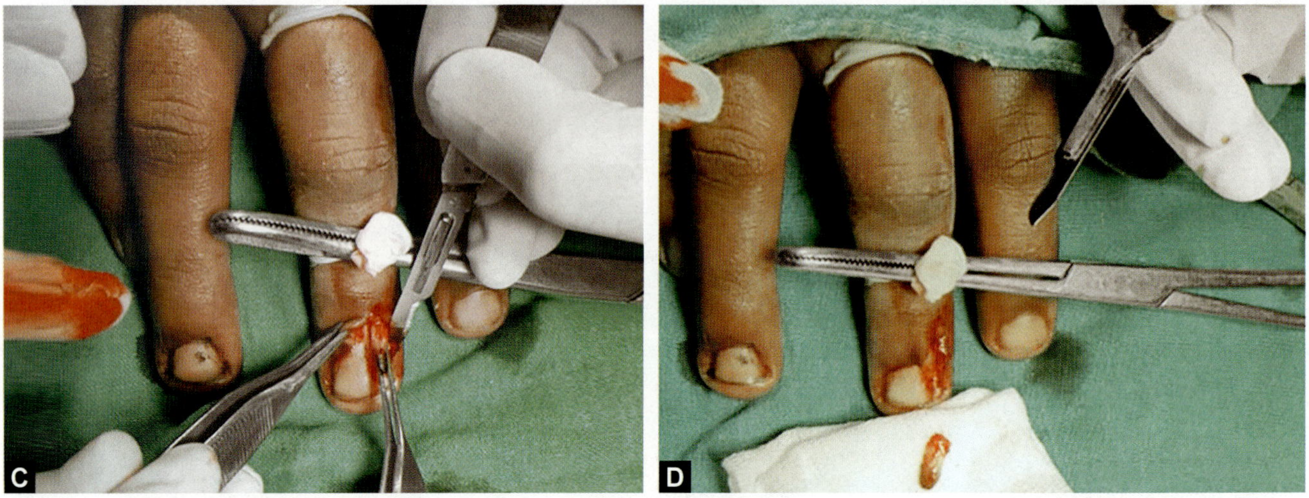

Figs. 24.19C and D: (C) Proximal nail fold raised on either side to expose fibroma fully. (D) Fibroma completely removed and proximal nail fold to be sutured back.

dislocation of distal pulp resulting in 'distal embedding'. It results in a subsequent hyperkeratotic reaction. This complication can be prevented by massaging in a distal-plantar direction, consistent taping, fixing an acrylic nail to new regrowing nail, replace the shed nail in place secured with adhesive tapes or stitches to the LNF. Stiches should be removed after 3 weeks. Nail should be kept in position as long as possible with adhesive tapes till new nail grows back.[29]

REFERENCES

1. Haneke E. Surgical anatomy of the nail apparatus. Dermatol Clin. 2006;24:291-6.
2. Thomas L, Zook EG, Rosio TJ, et al. Nail surgery and traumatic abnormalities In: Baran R, de Berker DA, Holzberg M, Thomas L (Eds). Diseases of the Nails and their Management 4th edition. UK: Blackwell Science Ltd; 2012. pp. 552-6.
3. Krunic AL, Wang LC, Soltani K, et al. Digital anesthesia with epinephrine: An old myth revisited. J Am Acad Dermatol. 2004;51:755-9.
4. Noel B. Anesthesia for ingrowing toenail surgery. Dermatol. Surg. 2010;36:1356-7.
5. Grover C, Nanda S, Nagi Reddy BS. Gauze strip tourniquet for nail surgery. J Cutan Aesthet Surg. 2014;7(3): 164-6.
6. Mutalik S. How to make local anesthesia less painful? J Cut Aesth Surg. 2008;1:37-8.
7. Pandhi D, Verma P. Nail avulsion: Indications and methods (surgical nail avulsion). Indian J Dermatol Venereol Leprol. 2012;78:299-308.
8. Khunger N, Kandhari R. Ingrown toenails. Indian J Dermatol Venereol Leprol. 2012;78:279-89.
9. Bostanci S, Ekmekçi P, Gürgey E. Chemical matricectomy with phenol for the treatment of ingrowing toenail: A review of the literature and follow-up of 172 treated patients. Acta Derm Venereol. 2001;81:181-3.
10. Tatlican S, Yamangöktürk B, Eren C, et al. Comparison of phenol applications of different durations for the cauterization of the germinal matrix: An efficacy and safety study. Acta Orthop Traumatol Turc. 2009;43:298-302.
11. Andreassi A, Grimaldi L, D'Anello C, et al. Segmental phenolization for the treatment of ingrowing toenails: A review of 6 years' experience. J Dermatologic Treat. 2004; 15:179-81.
12. Grover C, Khurana A, Bhattacharya SN, et al. Controlled trial comparing the efficacy of 88% phenol versus 10% sodium hydroxide for chemical matricectomy in the management of ingrown toenail.Indian J Dermatol Venereol Leprol. 2015;81(5):472-7.
13. Peyvandi H, Robati RM, Yegane RA, et al. Comparison of two surgical methods (winograd and sleeve method) in the treatment of ingrown toenail. Dermatol Surg. 2011;37:331-5.
14. Tatlican S, Eren C, Yamangokturk B, et al. Chemical matricectomy with 10% sodium hydroxide for the treatment of ingrown toenails in people with diabetes. Dermatol Surg. 2010;36:219-22.
15. Kim SH, Ko HC, Oh CK, et al. Trichloroacetic acid matricectomy in the treatment of ingrowing toenails. Dermatol Surg. 2009;35:973-9.
16. Serour F. Recurrent ingrown big toenails are efficiently treated by CO_2 laser. Dermatol Surg. 2002;28:509-12
17. Jellinek NJ. Nail surgery: Practical tips and treatment options. Dermatol Ther. 2007;20:68-74.
18. Baran R, Haneke E, Richert B. Pincer nails: Definition and surgical treatment. Dermatol Surg. 2001;27:261-6.
19. Grover C, Nanda S, Reddy BS, et al. Nail biopsy: assessment of indications and outcome. Dermatol Surg. 2005;31(2):190-4.

20. Grover C, Chaturvedi UK, Reddy BS. Role of nail biopsy as a diagnostic tool.Indian J Dermatol Venereol Leprol. 2012; 78(3):290-8.
21. Grover C, Reddy BS, Chaturvedi KU. Onychomycosis and the diagnostic significance of nail biopsy. J Dermatol. 2003; 30(2):116-22.
22. Savant SS. Nail surgery. In: Savant SS, (Ed). Textbook of Dermatosurgery and Cosmetology. 2nd edition. Mumbai, India: ASCAD; 2005. pp. 241-5.
23. Grover C, Reddy BS, Uma Chaturvedi K. Diagnosis of nail psoriasis: importance of biopsy and histopathology.Br J Dermatol. 2005;153(6):1153-8.
24. Gupta S, Jangra RS, Gupta S, et al. Saw-toothed power punch for effortless nail biopsy.J Am Acad Dermatol. 2016; 75(3):e109-11.
25. Grover C, Khandpur S, Reddy BS, et al. Longitudinal nail biopsy: utility in 20-nail dystrophy. Dermatol Surg. 2003; 29(11):1125-9.
26. Grover C, Bansal S, Nanda S, et al. En bloc excision of proximal nail fold for treatment of chronic paronychia. Dermatol Surg. 2006;32:393-8.
27. Grover C, Khurana A, Jain R, Rathi V. Transungual surgical excision of subungual glomus tumour. J Cutan Aesthet Surg. 2013;6(4):196-203.
28. Song M, Ko HC, Kwon KS, et al. Surgical treatment of subungual glomus tumor: A unique and simple method. Dermatol Surg. 2009;35:786-91.
29. Richert B. Surgery of the nail plate. In: Richert B, Di Chiacchio N, Haneke E (Eds). Nail Surgery. Informa Healthcare, New York; 2011. pp. 32-4.

CHAPTER 25

Hair Transplantation: Follicular Unit Transplantation

Vaishalee Kirane, Narendra Patwardhan, Venkataram Mysore

INTRODUCTION

Follicular unit transplant (FUT) is the gold standard method of hair transplantation. FUT is a procedure of transplantation of autologous hair in their naturally present follicular units to a bald area on the body. For a good success rate and high patient satisfaction, the art of giving a good cosmetic visual density to each individual's recipient area, is as important along with an up-to-date technical expertise.

PRINCIPLES OF FUT

Principle of donor dominance discovered in 1950s by the New York dermatologist, Norman Orentreich gave birth to hair restoration as we know today.[1] This established that hair follicles transplanted from their original location to another area will behave as they did in their original site. Thus hair roots harvested from the safe zone of occipital scalp when transplanted to bald frontal and mid-scalp areas of male pattern hair loss (MPHL), will grow similar to their original donor area which is resistant to the process of androgenetic alopecia.

HISTORY OF FUT

Shows a journey from earlier performed 4–5 mm punch grafts to macro/mini grafts in 1980's and then evolved to the modern advanced strip (follicular unit transplantation) in 1990's. Headington, in 1984 discovered the concept of follicular unit in which hair grow naturally in groups of 1–4 as a single unit.[2]

In 1996, the Choi implanters were developed to enable more proficient insertion of the grafts. Follicular unit extraction (FUE) was developed by Rassman in 2002's and 2010s got the Robotic surgery.[3]

RATIONALE AND FEATURES OF FUT

Follicular unit structure has tightly packed 1–4 hair with a smaller size and thus allows units to be placed in smaller holes and allows dense packing.

FUT is normally used for harvesting a strip of skin of width 1–1.5 cm from the safe donor area of the occipital scalp. Follicular unit extraction method (FUE) is harvesting follicular hair grafts one by one without excising any strip. This has made harvesting grafts from the body hairs like beard or chest area also possible along with the occipital scalp. This has increased the popularity and reach of the procedure to many indications of baldness.

INDICATIONS

- *Male pattern hair loss (MPHL)*: Primary and commonest indication for hair restoration surgery of giving hair density to frontal/mid-scalp/vertex areas of scalp affected by androgenetic alopecia.
- *Female pattern hair loss (FPHL)*: Widened hair partition, thinned out area on top of scalp.
- *Congenital* causes of hair loss.
- *Scarring alopecia:* Bald patches after injury or burns.
- *Burnt-out inflammatory alopecia:* Patches where sites could also be hair bearing area other than scalp like that of eyebrows, beard area, moustache, side locks, etc.

CASE SELECTION AND PLANNING

Patient selection by detailed consultation and examination is crucial for successful outcome of hair restoration surgery. Proper examination, evaluation of the recipient and donor sites of the patient's scalp and hair and recording of the findings in the preoperative notes is essential.[4]

Table 25.1: Major and minor factors that determine procedure planning.

Major factors	*Minor factors*
Classification	The amount of terminal hair that may remain in the bald area
Curl	The amount of vellus hair remaining in the bald area
Color	The color of the skin
Texture	
Caliber	
Density (amount of donor hair)	

- *The recipient area of the scalp* is thoroughly examined regarding:
  - The exact cause of thinning, extent of baldness and its classification. The classification of pattern baldness has always been the main key factor in determining the patient selection, but hair density and hair characteristics like caliber, curl and color also gain importance.
  - Any pathological findings of scalp or hair which may prove to be relative or absolute contraindications for surgery are also noted. For example inflammatory or infective lesions on scalp, any associated scarring, frizzy, fragile easily breakable hair shafts, etc.
  - Examination of previously transplanted hairs for favorable or poor results.
  - Supporting temporal hair density is also noted to plan the position of the frontal hairline and the density of the frontal region as a whole.
- *Donor area evaluation*[5] includes examination of the scalp skin from the occipital area for its elasticity, hair density, hair diameter and characteristics. Good elasticity of the donor scalp is important to get better wound scar and more number of available donor hairs. Norwood emphasizes six major factors and three minor donor hair characters (Table 25.1) to be taken into consideration when selecting patients and planning procedure for hair transplant.

Less the contrast between the hair and scalp color, more the natural look. Thick, curly frizzy hair will give an illusion of high visual perceived density.

Dr. Alejandro Camps Fresneda from Spain in his article added another factor of patient's age, which will determine a different approach for the same type of alopecia extent. A patient above 50 years of age may need a higher hairline in contrast to a younger patient.[6]

PREOPERATIVE COUNSELING

- *Primary aim of HRS* is to carefully tailor an optimal surgical approach to the patient's expressed concerns and particular regional hair deficit and to determine the surgical plan appropriate for his age and expected long term donor-recipient area ratio.
- *Counseling* prior to HRS is of utmost importance to educate the patient about the nature of the medical problem of hair loss as well as benefits and limitations of hair transplantation. A good rapport with the patient enables the physician to understand his concerns and requirements and then relay to him/her the objectives which can be realistically achieved by the surgery. Counseling can be done through brochures, presentations and videos.
- *Visual or cosmetic density* must be emphasized rather than the original hair density of the twenties.
- *Psychologically unfit patients*[7] and in some instances, those who exhibit symptoms of major depressive or body dysmorphic syndrome need to undergo specific counseling from professional psychiatrist before even contemplating HRS or are then not accepted for surgery at all.
- *Eliciting history of medicines.*
- *Previous use of cosmetic hair replacement and camouflage products.*
- Counseling regarding the use of FDA approved *Minoxidil and Finasteride* for the male and only Minoxidil for the female patient prior to and post HRS to retard further hair loss as well as to counter the unbearable, albeit temporary, telogen effluvium postoperatively.
- *Explanations regarding the progressive nature of hair fall,* and that HRS is not a one-time solution is essential.
- *Photodocumentation* of design of the area of hair reconstruction preoperatively.
- *Counsel regarding treating a large recipient area* in order of priority and addressing it in more than one session.

INFORMED CONSENT

Detailed consent form listing details about the procedure and possible complications should be signed by the patient. The consent form should specifically state the limitations of the procedure and should clearly mention if more procedures are needed for proper results. Patient should be provided with adequate opportunity to seek information through brochures, computer presentations, and personal discussions. Need for concomitant medical therapy should be emphasized. Patients should understand that proper hair growth can be expected after about 9 months after transplantation.

PREOPERATIVE ASSESSMENT

A detailed preoperative assessment is essential to decrease risk of untoward events, rule out any contraindications for HRS, carry out the subsequent surgery in a more efficient manner, leading to a more successful outcome. A preoperative instruction package is given to the patient which gives certain specific instructions prior to surgery making it more organized and systematic.

It should primarily contain:

- *Preoperative instruction checklist* (Table 25.2).
- *Laboratory investigation requisition form* (Table 25.3).
- *Consent form.*
- *Postoperative instructions sheet* can be given at the same time, so that the patient has time to review them adequately before surgery.
- *History for checking risk for bleeding during surgery* (Table 25.4).
- *List of over-the counter medications and herbal remedies (Table 25.5) List of prescription drugs* (Table 25.6) and *which need to be avoided or* discontinued prior to surgery so as to avoid any complications or drug interactions during HRS.

Scalp Laxity Exercises[8]

- Certain exercises of massaging the back and sides of scalp are advised about 1 month before surgery to increase the laxity of the skin of the posterior scalp from where the donor strip is excised.
- A loose scalp enables harvesting a longer donor strip and thus more number of grafts. The lesser wound tension would, in addition, help to give a better cosmetic scar.
- Palm of the hands being placed on the back/sides of the head with the fingers pointing upwards and thumbs pointing towards each other, the scalp skin is moved up and down over the bone as vigorously as possible using the palms and thumbs, with the fingers resting stationary on the top of the scalp. This exercise is performed for around 15 minutes daily.

Table 25.2: Preoperative instruction checklist.

S. no	*Time before surgery*	*Instruction*
1.	4 weeks	Start the scalp laxity exercises
2.	3 weeks	Notify any prescription or over the counter medications taken at least 3 weeks prior to surgery, so as to either discontinue or give alternative, if needed after final approval of a physician
3.	3 weeks	Stop taking vitamin E, fish oil or garlic supplements 3
4.	1 week	Stop taking any anticoagulants, clopidogrel, MAO inhibitors or aspirin (read the label of over-the-counter cold remedies to make sure they do not contain aspirin or acetylsalicylic acid)
5.	1 week	Stop drinking alcohol, smoking
6.	1 week	Stop minoxidil and resume 2 weeks after surgery in an effort to decrease the frequency and/or severity of any temporary hair loss caused by surgery in hair-bearing recipient areas and increase the growth potential of transplanted hairs too
7.	1 day	Stop taking ibuprofen or naproxen
8.	1 day	Shampoo and rinse hair well with an antibacterial shampoo
9.	1 day	Avoid heavy exercises till about 2 weeks after surgery
10.	1 day	Start the prescription given
11.	Night before	Get sufficient sleep
12.	Morning of surgery	Have a light breakfast In the rare case of need of intravenous sedation by the anesthesiologist, patient is advised not to eat anything after midnight the night before surgery and sips of water is permitted mostly till 6 hours prior.
13.	Morning of surgery	Wear any clothing that does not need to be pulled over the head to be removed and one with front buttons or zipper which opens completely. Patients can bring scarf or hat to cover the bandage of the donor area and cover the top of scalp while going home after surgery.
14.	Hair length and styling	Patients should ideally avoid getting their hair cut very short at least for two or three weeks before surgery for couple of reasons. First, for strip excision from the donor area we need to have hair at least 1 cm in length and not trimmed very short. Secondly, longer length of adjacent hair would help to cover the donor suture site and the recipient area by proper styling after surgery.

Table 25.3: Laboratory requisition form.

- Hemogram
- Urine: routine examination
- Blood sugar: fasting and postprandial
- Liver function tests: serum bilirubin, SGPT, SGOT, alkaline phosphatase, serum proteins
- Kidney function tests: blood urea, serum creatinine
- Bleeding time, clooting time, prothrombin time
- HBsAg, hepatitis C
- VDRL
- HIV
- ECG
- Xylocaine testing

Table 25.4: Bleeding checklist.

History of bleeding diasthesis	During previous injury or surgery
Over-the-counter medications	Vitamins or herbal remedies which increase tendency to bleed by inhibiting platelet aggregation as well as other coagulation factors, e.g. Ginkgo biloba, garlic, ginger, Vitamin E[9-11]
Alcohol	Impairs primary hemostasis as well as the platelet function.[12]
Nicotine	Infection, tendency for bleeding, decreases circulation.[13]
Anticoagulants	ASA, NSAID'S, clopidogrel, warfarin.

Table 25.5: Over-the-counter medicines and herbal remedies that theoretically prolong bleeding.[14]

Anise	Clove
Garlic	Saw palmetto
Ginkgo biloba	Vitamin E
Ginseng	Licorice root
Guggul	

Table 25.6: Medications that can increase bleeding.[15]

Aceclofenac acetylsalicylic acid (ASA)	Indomethacin
Clopidogrel	Ketoprofen
Dipyridamole	Naproxen
Escitalopram	Pentoxifylline
Enoxaparin	Piroxicam
Fluoxetine	Tranexamic acid
Ibuprofen	Warfarin

Preoperative Assessment to Achieve Good Hemostasis

A good intraoperative and postoperative hemostasis in HT is important to avoid the inconvenience and interference in the surgical procedure as well as other serious effects of excessive bleeding.

As HT requires hundreds of small incisions in highly vascular recipient area of the scalp, any excessive or prolonged bleeding during stage of graft insertion, especially in a scenario of close dense packing of very small grafts, may cause popping of the grafts, extra handling and increased risk of graft damage thus hampering their survival. Postoperative bleeding increases the risk of graft loss, infection, flap or graft necrosis, wound dehiscence, pain and scar formation.

Because ASA's effect on platelet function is irreversible and thus lasts for the lifetime of the platelet, it needs to be discontinued for 7 to 10 days before surgery.[16]

Warfarin by depleting vitamin K, interferes with the production of vitamin K dependent clotting factors 11, VII, IX, and X. It should not be discontinued without consulting the prescribing physician which is on an average 2–5 days before surgery.[17]

If warfarin is discontinued, then long-acting heparin is started six days prior to the date of surgery. The last dose of heparin is given on the morning of the day before surgery and restarted soon after surgery (as deemed fit by treating dermatologist and the patient's managing physician) which is usually 36 hours. Warfarin is restarted at the same time as the heparin is discontinued.

Clopidogrel bisulfate is an inhibitor of platelet aggregation and needs to be stopped 7–10 days before surgery and only with the agreement of the prescribing physician.

Preoperative Medications Used in Hair Restoration Surgery

Antibiotics[18]

Surgical site infection (SSI) in HRS is controlled by strict protocols for asepsis in the hospital or a daycare theatre, postoperative care of the donor and recipient sites and prophylactic antibiotics. For example, Anti-staphylococcal penicillins or first generation cephalosporins from 1 hour to 2 days before the procedure and postoperatively, ranging 5–7 days.[19,20]

Application of mupirocin ointment in the nose to treat the nasal colonization of Staphylococcus aureus and preoperative shampooing of scalp hair with use of chlorhexidine gluconate medicated soap is also advocated.[21]

Systemic Corticosteroids[22]

Systemic corticosteroids are given to patients during or after surgery, in an effort to decrease the possibility of severe postoperative facial edema, depending upon certain factors like amount of tumescent anesthesia injected into the frontal scalp. Steroid is also administered in the forehead (to prevent postoperative edema) and donor area to prevent postoperative pain due to edema. For vertex areas their requirement would not be as much.

Sedatives[23]

Sedatives can be given from night before surgery, in morning on day of surgery, to 1–2 days after, e.g. Tablet Alprazolam 0.25–0.5 mg. This helps to decrease the patient's anxiety and thus any risk of resultant rise in blood pressure and intraoperative bleeding.

Clonidine[24]

Being an alpha 2-adrenergic agonist, it exhibits sedative, anxiolytic, analgesic, and hemodynamic stabilizing properties. It can thus be prescribed at night before surgery.

Tranexamic acid[25]

It is an antifibrinolytic agent and thus helps to reduce excessive bleeding. It is taken orally a day before and morning of surgery. It is not safe to be given in patients with blood clots in the brain, eyes, legs or bleeding related to kidney problems.

PROCEDURE OF FUT

Steps mentioned in the preoperative checklist are followed preceding the main surgery.

- *Donor area marking* (Fig. 25.1) is done which is from the safe zone of the occipital scalp extending horizontally ear to ear, approximately 25 to 30 cm.[26]

  The width of the strip is preferred to be not more than 1.2 cm to facilitate wound closure with minimal tension, to avoid tissue ischemia and a wide unsightly scar. The strip is excised in 2 to 3 sections, if the entire length of 25 to 30 cm is required. Width should be lesser in mastoid area as skin has less laxity and higher risk of complications of wound closure.[27]

  If more than one session is needed, the wisest approach is to remove the older scar as part of the new strip.

  Hair in the donor area is clipped to a preferred length of 1 cm, so as to assess the angle and direction of the hair after insertion.

  Patient is placed in a lateral decubitus or prone position and special prone pillow is used to enhance patient comfort and allow better air circulation for breathing.

- *Antiseptic cleansing* of the donor area is done by isopropyl alcohol followed by betadine before infiltrating local anesthesia (Fig. 25.2).
- *Anesthesia (Table 25.7):*
  - Usually 2% Lignocaine or Bupivacaine or Sensorcaine agents are used (Fig. 25.3). To lengthen time

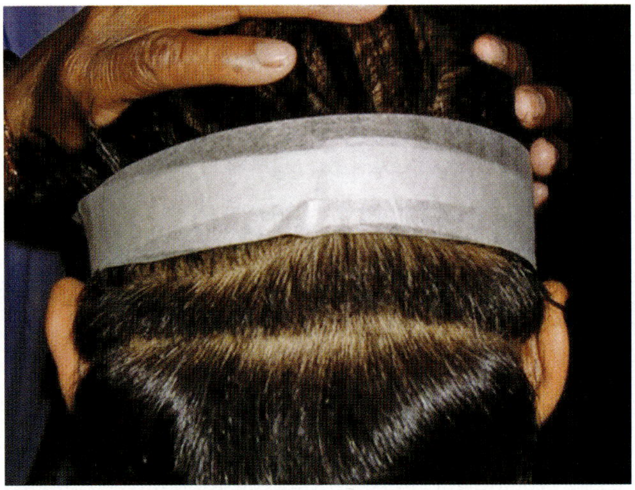

Fig. 25.1: Donor strip marking.
Courtesy: Trichotransform HT team, Pune, Maharashtra, India.

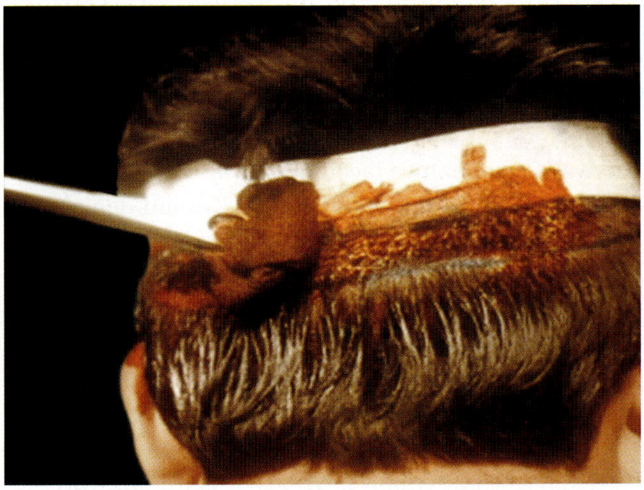

Fig. 25.2: Antiseptic cleansing of the donor area.

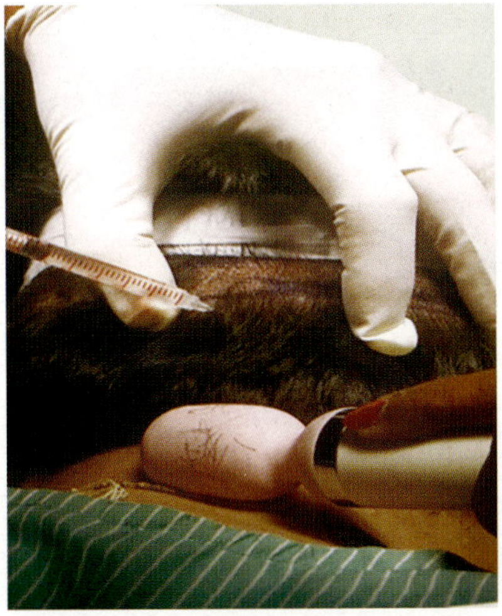

Fig. 25.3: Anesthesia of the donor area and use of vibratory device to distract the patient from the pain of needle pricks.

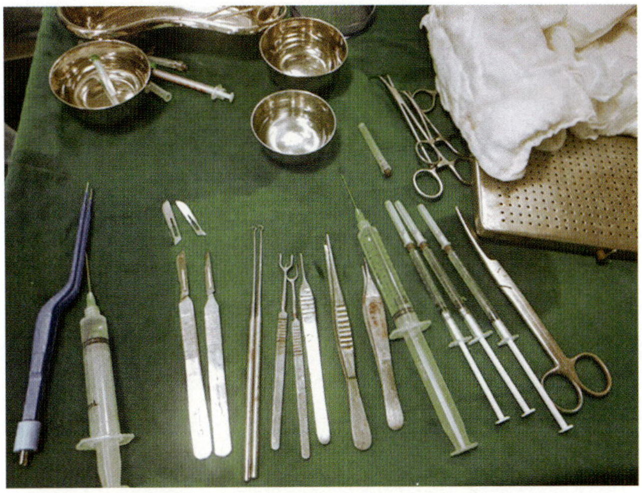

Fig. 25.4: Instruments for donor strip excision.
Courtesy: Dr. Narendra Patwardhan, Pune, Maharashtra, India

Table 25.7: Few tips to make anesthesia as comfortable to patient as possible.

- Addition of sodium bicarbonate alkaline solution to make it neutral and decrease the stinging sensation which occurs due to the acidic form of local anesthetic stock solution.
- Tapping forehead or using a vibratory device near injection site, distracts patient from the discomfort of the needle pricks and helps in pain relief.[28]
- Patient can listen to music with set of earphones to help distract from process.

Table 25.8: Methods of strip harvesting.

- Single blade scalpel
- Double, multiblade scalpel
- Hemostat technique
- Skin hook technique
- Spreader technique

of anesthesia and minimize intraoperative bleeding, epinephrine in concentration of 1/100,000 or 1/200,000 is added.
  - The donor and recipient areas are anesthetized using very small gauze needle of number 26 or 30 to inject the local anesthetic.
  - After the anesthesia, saline solution is infiltrated at the level of the deep dermis/subcutaneous tissue called as Tumescent anesthesia. This provides hemostasis by mechanical compression and also helps to lift up follicles from underlying tissue decreasing risk of transection.
- *Donor strip excision:* Meticulous and skillfully performed excision of the donor strip is important because it is the most surgically invasive part of hair transplant procedure, keeping with the goals to harvest the most permanent hair, to minimize hair transection and to leave a fine aesthetically undetectable scar. The instruments required for this are depicted in Figure 25.4.

Magnification of at least 2.5× lens is necessary to be worn by the surgeon for proper visualization. The demarcated strip is excised with a scalpel blade with incision made parallel to the direction of hair shafts to a depth of 5 to 6 mm, just deep to hair bulbs at level of subcutaneous fat.

In order to avoid the risk of follicular transection and injury to severe deep vessels and nerves, modifications have been done using different techniques as enumerated in Table 25.8.

  - *Hemostat technique:* Sandoval (Mexico) introduced this novel technique of 'Score and Spread'. This involved making a superficial scoring incision first along the edges of the strip with the scalpel blade to a depth of 1 to 2 mm only (Fig. 25.5). Then a hemostat was used to puncture the incision and then opened to force tissue to separate along a natural plane of dissection, leaving follicles intact with no transection.
  - *Skin hook technique:*[29] Pathomvanich (Thailand) introduced the skin hook technique at the same time, where the assistant and the surgeon use skin hooks to pull edges on opposite sides to produce traction (Fig. 25.6) and then perform the dissection in the natural

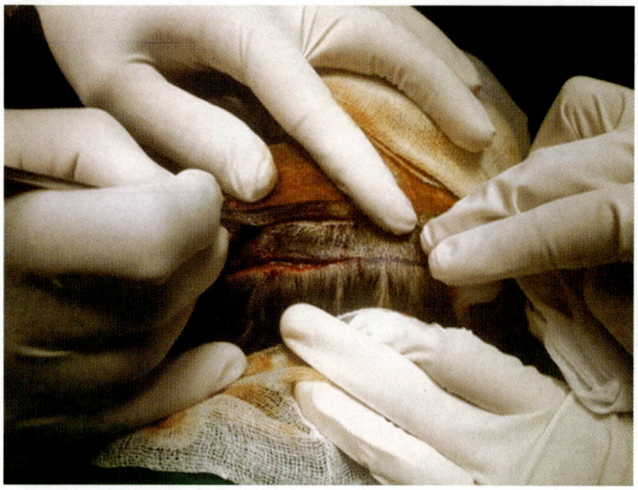

Fig. 25.5: Superficial scoring incision along the strip edges.

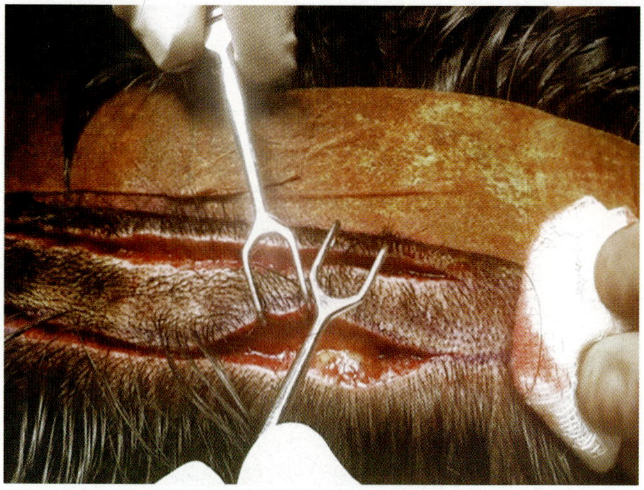

Fig. 25.6: Skin hooks used to give traction and spread the deeper tissue avoiding cutting.

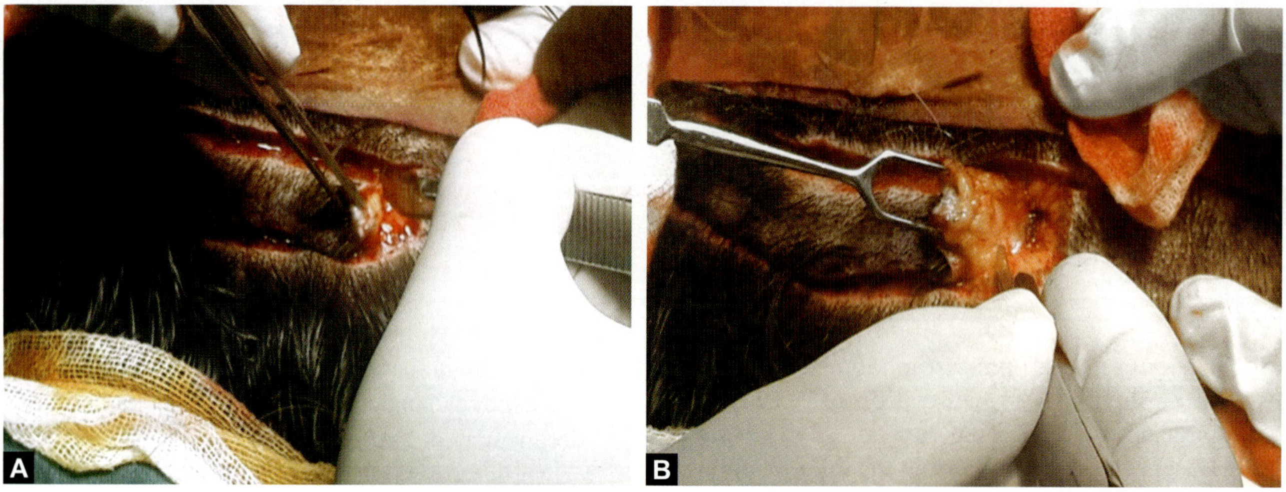

Figs. 25.7A and B : Dissection at level of subcutis below hair roots to excise the strip.

plane between follicular units, rather than cutting the tissue (Figs. 25.7A and B).

- *Spreader technique*:[30] After the first scoring incision is made, prongs of the spreader instrument separate the tissue horizontally when the spreader is opened. Good hemostasis is to be ensured (Fig. 25.8).

  Small gauze pieces can be roll-packed into the incision to soak blood to have clearer field for dissection. The strip is then released from the deeper tissue with scalpel taking care to avoid severing the deep vessels. Use of electrocautery is rarely needed for hemostasis.

- *Trichophytic closure method (Table 25.9):* [33,34] This technique involves the removal of the epidermal rim of one edge of the donor wound before it is closed using the single or double layer suture method. As the wound heals, hair grows out through the scar adding to its camouflage (Figs. 25.9A to C).
- *Donor wound closure:*[31,32] The wound can be closed with staples or a running single layered suture either non-absorbable or absorbable sutures- 4.0 nylon or vicryl rapid (depending on the preference of the surgeon) (Figs. 25.10A to D). Staples are inert and cause less damage but more discomfort than sutures. Main aim of donor wound closure is to obtain a fine, esthetically undetectable scar for which many modifications can be done as enumerated in Table 25.10 (Fig. 25.11).

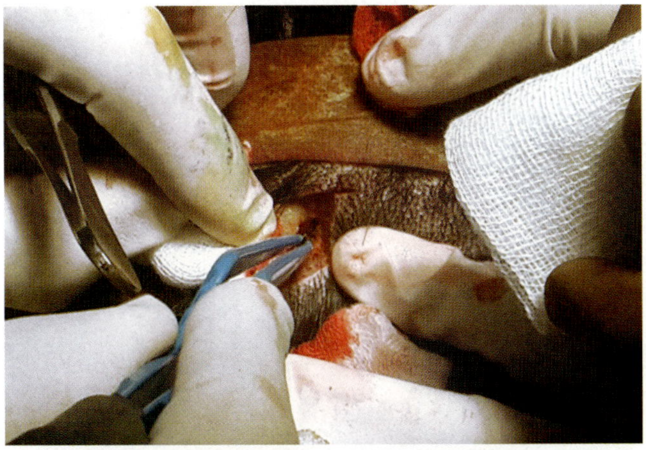

Fig. 25.8: Judicious use of cautery for hemostasis.

Table 25.9: Trichophytic closure.

- Avoid transection of follicles along the incisional edges.
- Removing epidermis along inferior edge of the wound rather than superior edge results in a cosmetically better scar.
- Depth and width of the cut epidermis must not exceed 1 mm.
- Avoid tension on the wound closure.

Table 25.10: Modifications to achieve a fine donor scar.

- Scalp laxity exercises done a month before surgery.
- Wound closed with minimal tension.
- Width of strip to be not more than 1 to 1.2 mm.
- Neurovascular structures to be better preserved.
- Two layered suturing with inner absorbable 3.0 vicryl for deeper galeal suturing and outer epidermal approximation by nonabsorbable 3.0 prolene.
- Using the trichophytic closure method.

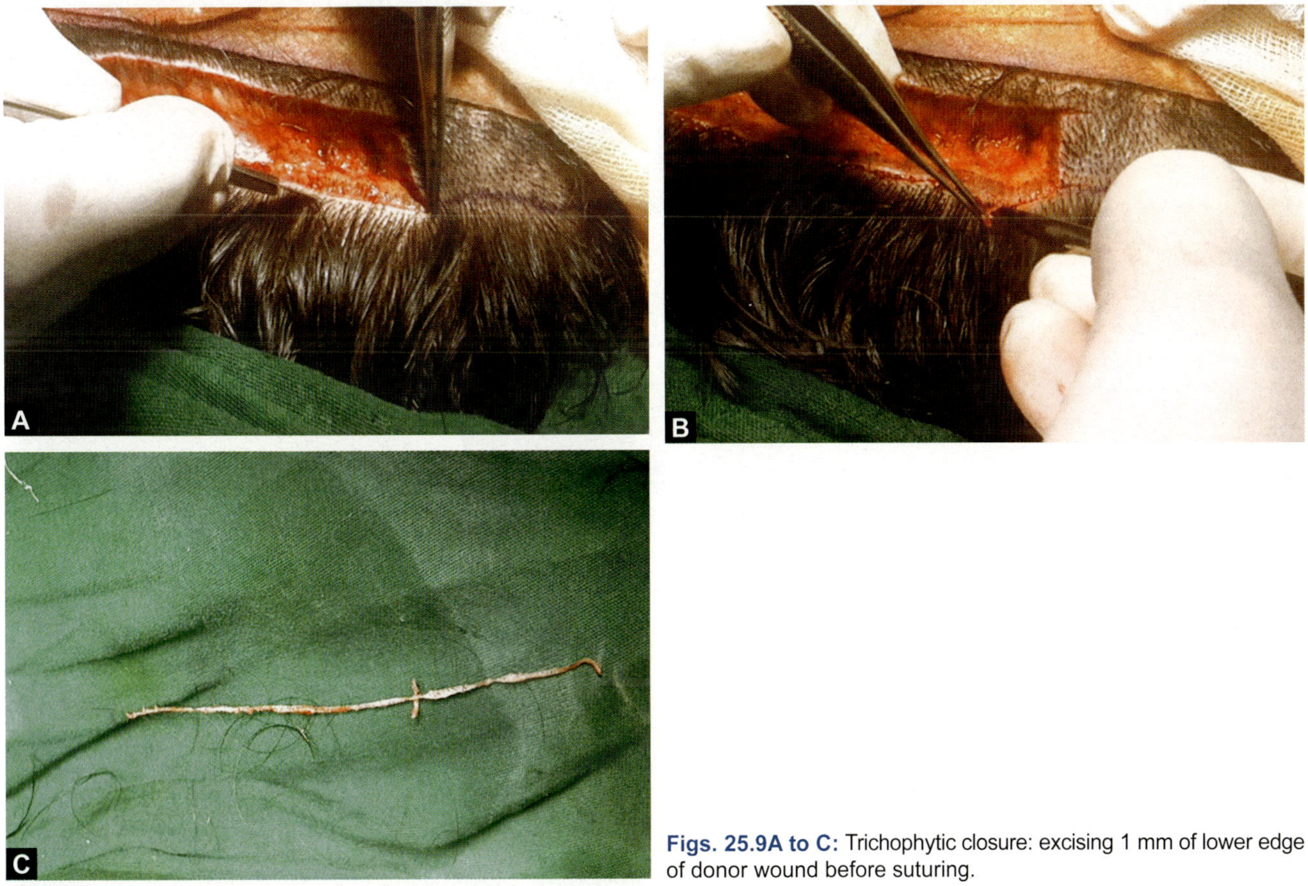

Figs. 25.9A to C: Trichophytic closure: excising 1 mm of lower edge of donor wound before suturing.

GRAFT PREPARATION[35,36]

Strip excision is followed by preparation of the follicular unit grafts taking care of two main factors of avoiding transection and dehydration, which will render tissue non-viable. Right from the time of harvesting till the grafts are inserted in the recipient holes, hydration has to be maintained by keeping them either in chilled normal saline, Ringers lactate or other holding solutions like platelet rich plasma. Saline spraying is done to keep grafts moist during the entire process of cutting.

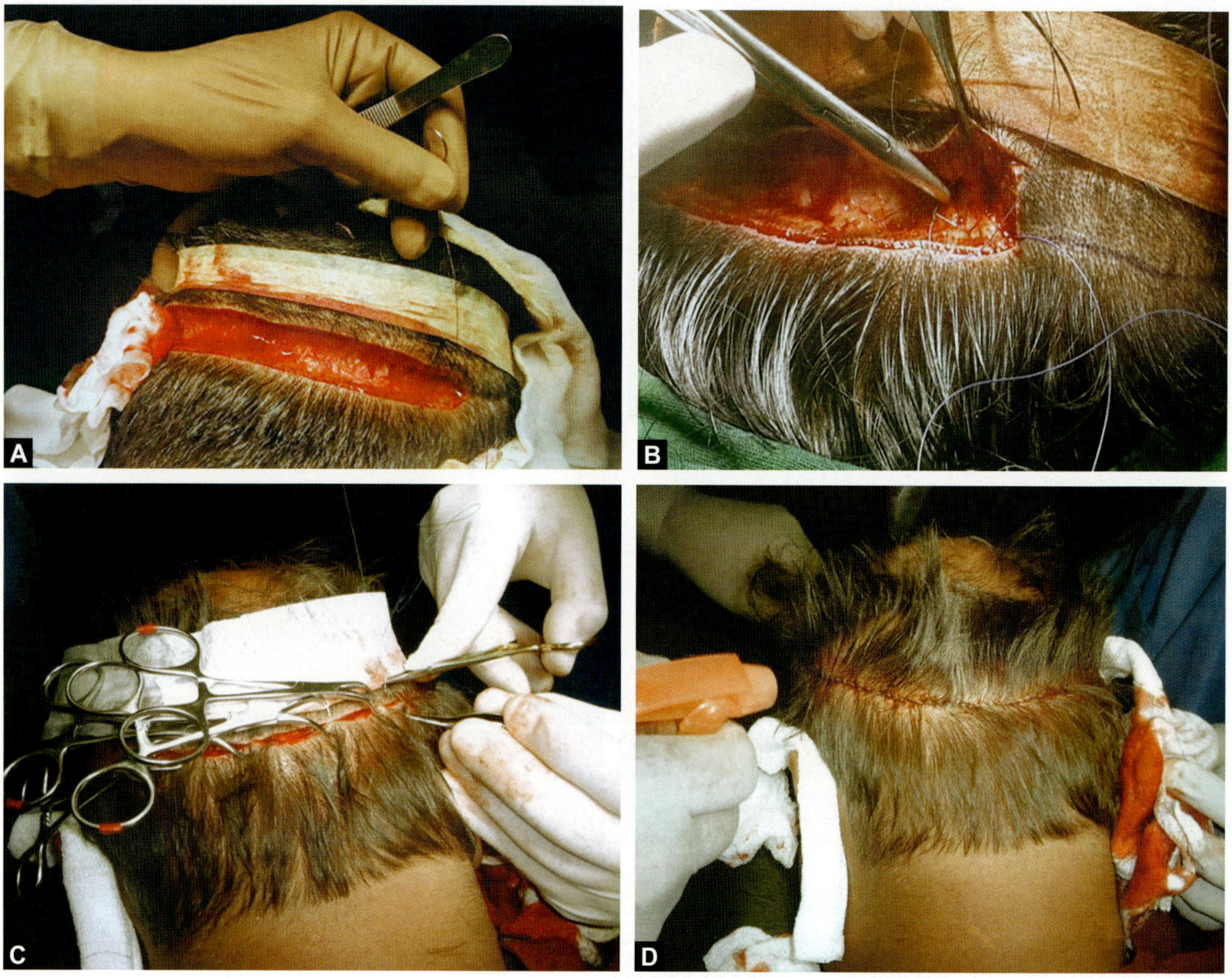

Figs. 25.10A to D: Donor wound closure.

- *Ergonomics:* Graft preparation involves application of many ergonomic factors for higher quality of work and better productivity with less fatigue.
  - Good body posture while sitting with back and neck straight, looking forward into the microscope while cutting grafts, instead of bending down. Hands and elbows should rest on table. This prevents fatigue and strain and increases productivity.
  - Optimal magnification of minimum 4–6×, appropriate focal distance which facilitates comfortable proper posture, reduces eye fatigue at the same time enables cutting with good average speed.
  - Good illumination using cool diffuse lights to avoid rise in temperature and graft dehydration.
  - Instruments (Table 25.11 and Figs. 25.12 to 25.16).

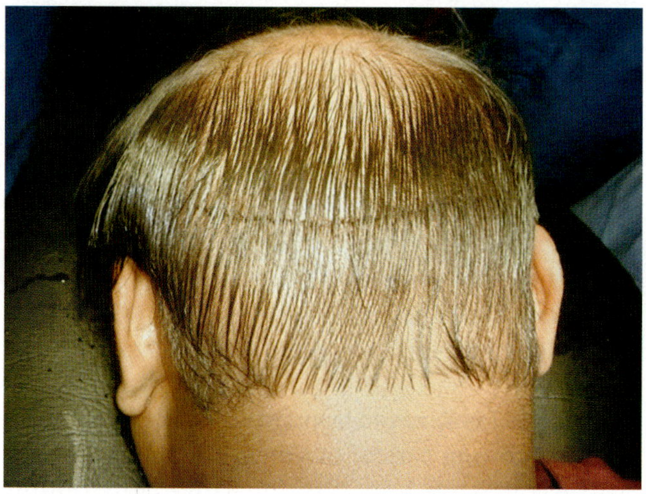

Fig. 25.11: Donor area scar after 4 weeks.

Table 25.11: Instruments for graft preparation.	
Cutting board	Needs to be sterile, nonslippery and translucent to enable transillumination. After testing various surfaces, a white or yellow, rough and polyethylene surface was found to be the best by the authors.
Silicone block or sterilized ice-cream stick and 25G hypodermic needles	To fix the strip during slivering.
Forceps	Tooth forceps like Jewellers forceps 5 needed to hold donor tissue and give lateral tension while cutting.
Cutting blade	No. 10, 15 Personna scalpel blades or regular razor blades mounted on special handles.
Graft containers	SS small bowls to hold slivers, petri-dishes containing gauze strips to place 1 and 2–3 FU's separately.

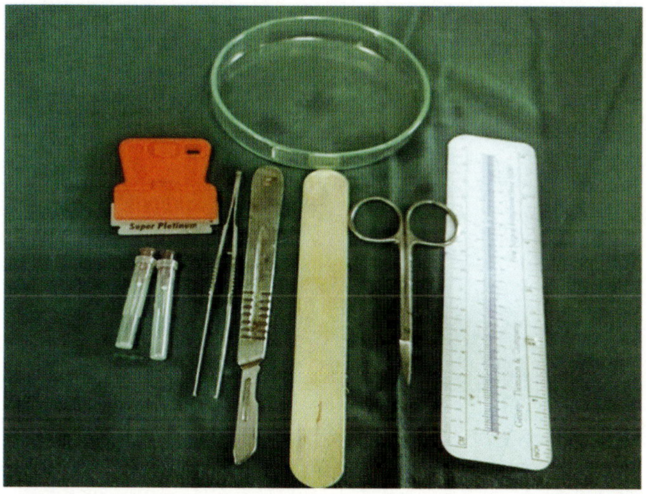

Fig. 25.12: Instruments for strip dissection into slivers and then grafts.
Courtesy: Dr. Narendra Patwardhan, Pune, Maharashtra, India

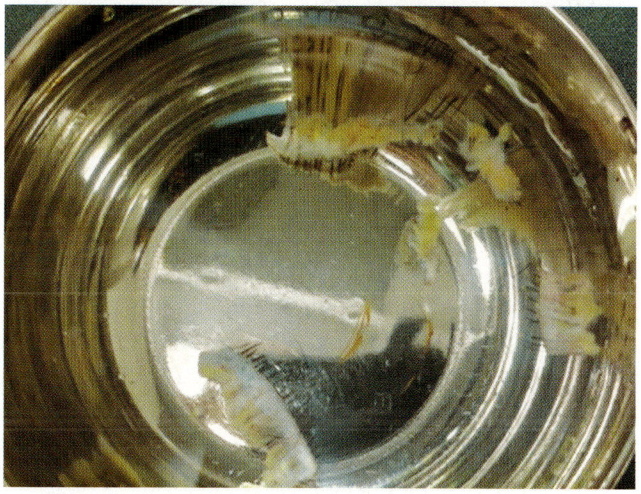

Fig. 25.13: SS Bowl containing the slivers in the holding solution, mostly chill RL solution.

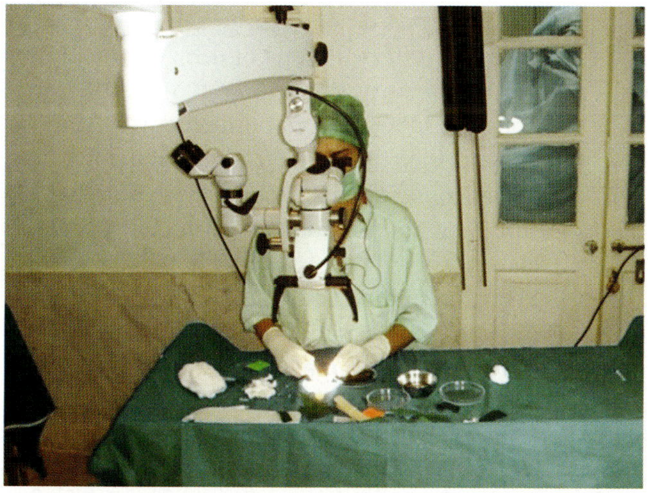

Fig. 25.14: Microscope for stereomicroscopic dissection of the strip into slivers.

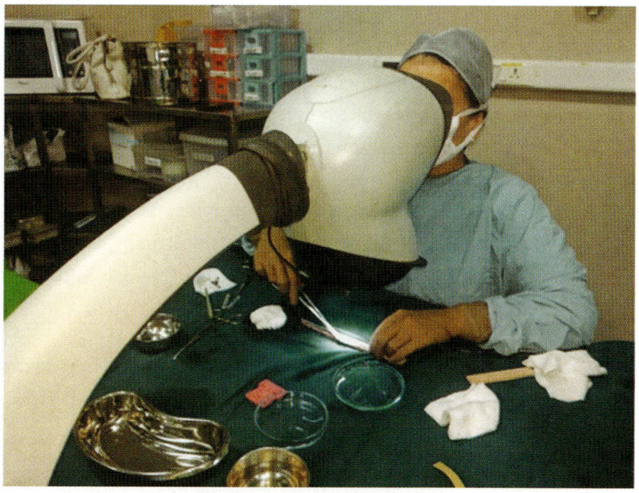

Fig. 25.15: Mantis microscope.
Courtesy: Dr. Narendra Patwardhan, Pune, Maharashtra, India

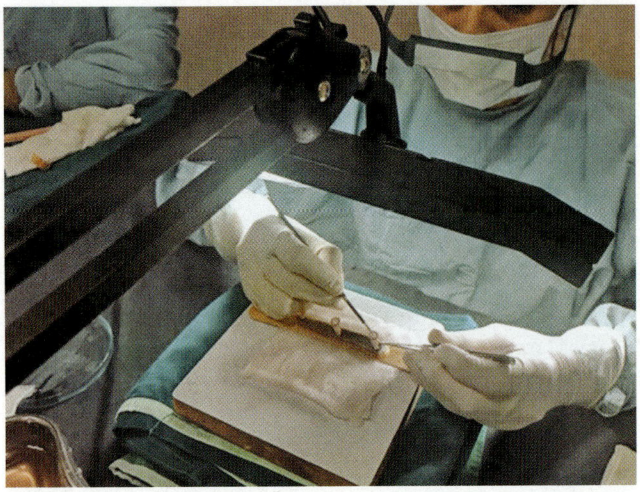

Fig. 25.16: Magnifying glass and loupe each 2.5X (give higher magnification when used together).

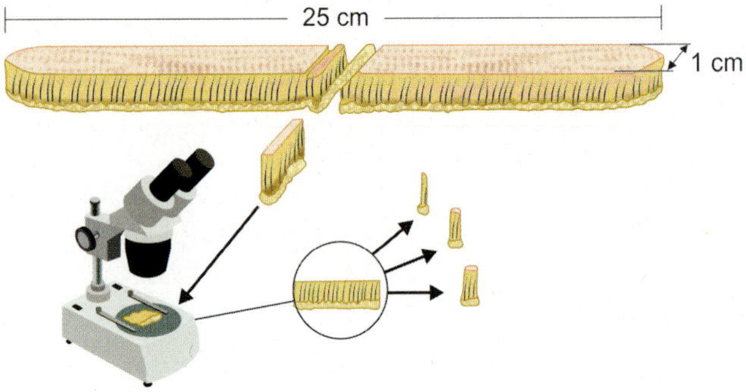

Fig. 25.17: Schematic diagram showing dissection of strip into slivers and then individual grafts.

- *Stages of graft dissection:*
  - *Slivering*: Division of the donor strip into thin sections or slivers which are one or two follicular units wide.

    Strip is washed in saline to scrub off any blood debris and then its length and width is measured. This number is multiplied by the hair density to get an estimate of potential grafts which is relayed to the physician working on recipient area. Donor strip is fixed or anchored to a silicone or tongue depressor with needles. Holding strip with forceps in left hand and giving gentle traction, razorblade is used to cut between and around FUs to tease apart one whole FU-wide slivers from the rest of the donor strip (Figs. 25.17 to 25.20).

TIPS AND TRICKS

- Strip is examined for channels which exist naturally between FUs, through which it becomes easier to cut with razor blade in between and around follicles decreasing risk of their transection.
- In order to minimize exposure outside the body and dehydration, it is preferred to dissect the strip in sections, which can be distributed to other 'Sliverers 'for greater efficiency.

  - *Graft preparation:*[37] Slivers are then dissected further to obtain the final individual grafts of different sizes as they are naturally present in 1 or 2–3 hair follicular units:

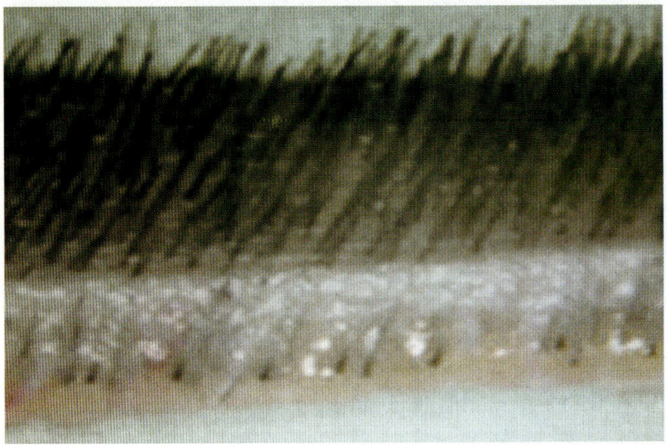

Fig. 25.18: Donor strip.

- Sliver is laid horizontally onto the tongue depressor or cutting board.
- Using Jewellers forceps and razor blade, cuts are made longitudinally from epidermal border to subcutaneous border between the FUs.
- They are then trimmed off any surplus epidermis, dermis and subcutaneous fat, keeping behind sufficient amount along with intact sebaceous glands.
- FU count and recording on a log sheet is done by each technician before putting them in bowls filled with cold Saline. They are placed separately as 1 and 2–3 hair FUs to be inserted later in frontal hair line and behind on the recipient scalp respectively (Figs. 25.21 to 25.23).

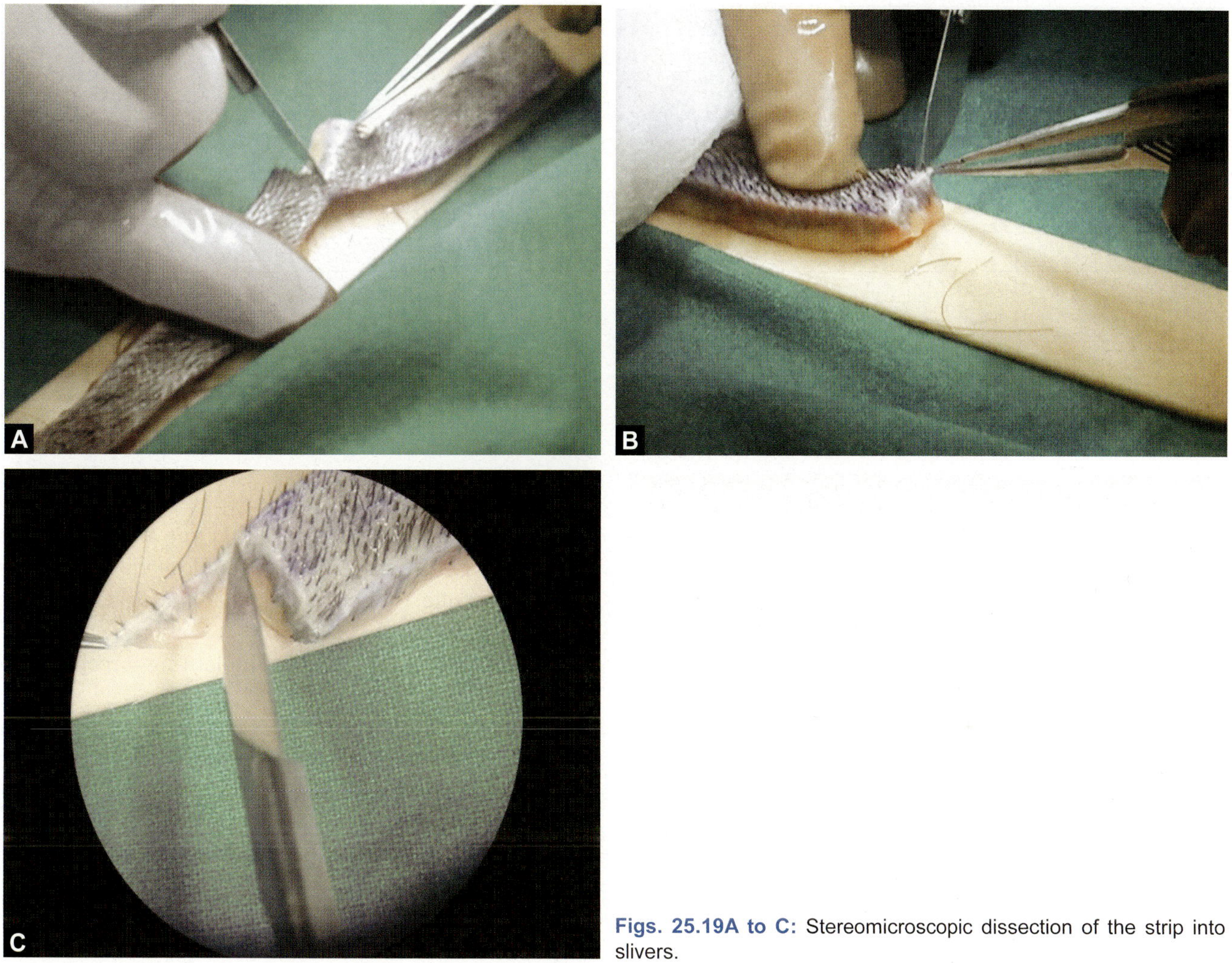

Figs. 25.19A to C: Stereomicroscopic dissection of the strip into slivers.

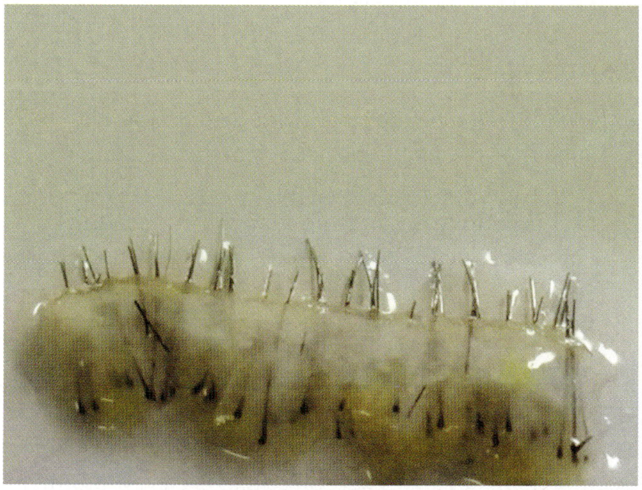

Fig. 25.20: Sliver.

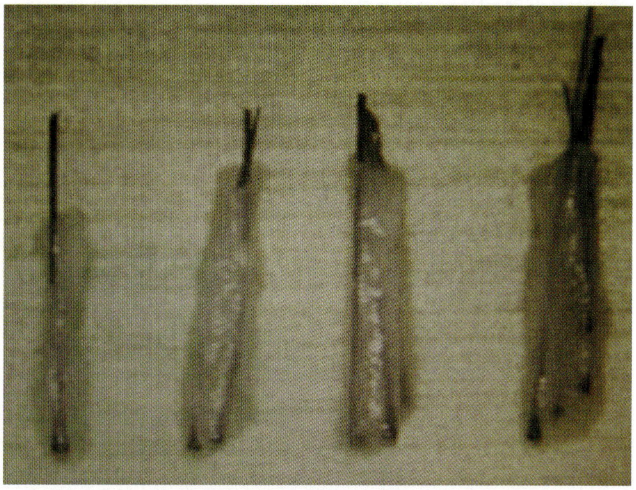

Fig. 25.21: Follicular unit grafts having 1, 2, 3 and 4 hairs.

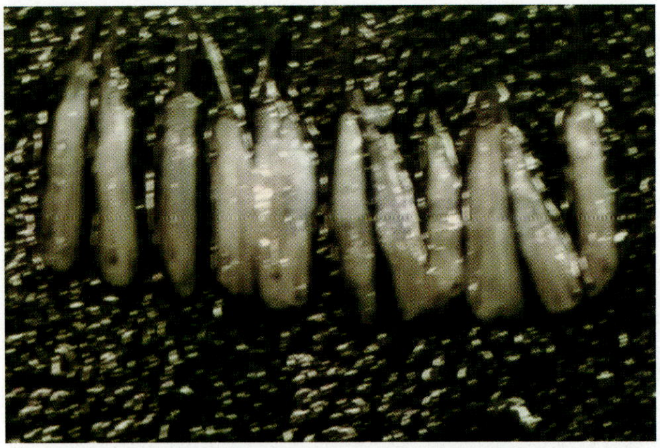

Fig. 25.22: 2–3 hair follicular unit grafts.

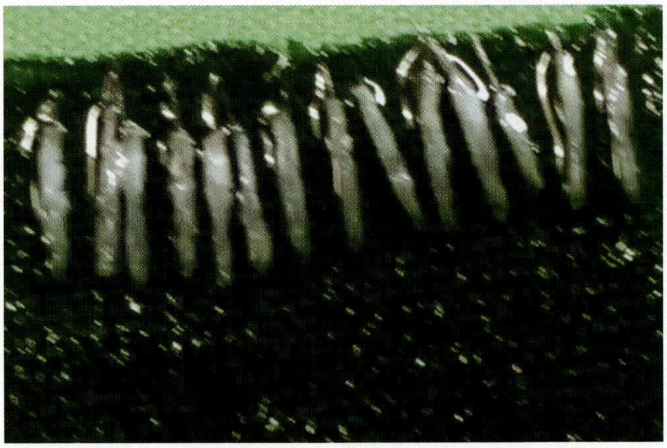

Fig. 25.23: Single hair grafts.

TIPS AND TRICKS

- Binocular stereo-microscopic dissection technique for donor strip dissection to obtain FUs was developed by Limmer.[38,39] It gives proper magnification from 2× to 20× for enhanced view of FU anatomy and powerful illumination, thus providing good quality grafts of consistent size and shape taking care to preserve sebaceous glands, dermal papilla and little surrounding perifollicular adipose tissue for better growth, thus avoiding 'naked grafts.' Too chubby grafts can 'pop out' during insertion risking drying and trauma while handling.
- Beginning the cut from the epidermal border inferiorly into the dermis is better, so that dermal portion can be teased apart to avoid transection.
- Traction given to strip by the forceps is needed to be optimal as excess force can 'stripaway' perifollicular fat and inadequate tension will not separate follicles enough for safe dissection.

RECIPIENT AREA

Anesthesia: Anesthesia can be induced by any of the methods, such as ring block, infiltration and nerve blocks (supraorbital, supratrochlear, auriculotemporal).

There are three methods of placement of grafts in recipient area, each with its own advantages and disadvantages:

- Slit and place technique
- Preformed slits
- Implanters.

IMPLANTATION (BY SLIT AND PLACE)

Here each slit is made followed immediately by placement of the graft. The graft is held in the right hand with a forceps and the slit is made with a blade or needle of appropriate size with the left hand. The procedure is as follows:

Instrumentation

- Hypodermic needles (19, 20, 21G one and a half inch long) or chisel blades which could be customized or Minde's knife. Choice of needle or blade size depends on the size of grafts.
- Angular, curved or straight implanting forceps—fine tipped
- Magnification in form of loupes/magnifying visors (good quality with at least 3× magnification).

Slit and place consists of following steps:

Creating incision:

- Insert the needle only up to the bevel to make a slit.

Grasping the Graft

- Grasp the graft at the subcutaneous tissue below the bulb or just lateral to it, or just above it gently (without crushing)—do not hold either over the bulb or higher up where bulge area resides)

Insertion of Graft

- Withdraw the needle slightly to visualize the slit
- Slide the graft along the bevel into the recipient site
- When the graft is three fourths inside withdraw the needle completely and simultaneously push the graft
- This step can also be performed by an assistant.

Adjusting Position of the Graft

- Push the graft inside the recipient site gently
- Make sure it is flush with skin or slightly above it.

This method has some advantages. As graft placement is immediate, it causes less bleeding, is easier to implant between hairs and variations are possible as the process progresses gradually. There is also total surgeon control as he is present throughout the surgery. It is particularly useful for a beginner. It is particularly useful for areas like eye brows, temporal angle where frequent change in direction is needed. It is also useful at the end of a preformed slit insertion process for skip areas. However, this method has the following disadvantages:

- During creating sites:
  - Lack of depth control for a beginner—it depends on the feel of surgeon's hand to judge depth
  - If site created is deep, there may be bleeding—hence immediate placement may be difficult-this is common with beginners
  - Creating sites in close proximity may lead to popping and hence dense packing may be difficult
  - Since each graft needs a different sized hole, frequent change of needles is necessary.
- During placement:
  - During placement, grafts may be crushed, squeezed, bent, destroyed or pushed too deep to produce pitting, particularly in the hands of a beginner
  - Overall, this procedure is slower and time consuming
  - Surgeon involvement is more as he has to be present throughout surgery

Again, it has to be pointed that all the challenges apply to beginners only.

PREFORMED SLITS AND PLACE

This method involves making all the slits at one time. It needs proper coordination between surgeon and dissecting team to avoid disparity in the number of slits made and final outcome of the number of grafts dissected. Likewise, it is a challenge to precisely make an estimate of the specific number of slits for one hair, two hair and three hair grafts beforehand. Therefore this method needs an experienced surgeon and an experienced team for proper execution.

Steps:

- *Tumescence*: The area is tumesced with normal saline as the surgeon progresses from one region to another. Saline is infiltrated in the superficial layer with a 26 g needle.
- *Making the slits*: Slits can be made with different types of blades or needles mounted on different types of handles. Designer blades of different sizes are available, but are costly. Customized blades can be prepared from ordinary shaving blades through a blade cutter (Fig. 25.24). Nokor needles have also been used. Ordinary needles of different sizes can be used for smaller holes. The slits are made in rows but the two rows do not lie parallel to each other—some zig zag configuration is necessary or else the transplant will look very unnatural, also the see through effect of parallel lying grafts will make the final density look much less. Precision is important in making uniform distribution of slits which needs experience- skip areas may occur.
- The slits are counted as they are made.
- *Staining the slits*: With time, identification of sites may become difficult—small slits may close, and hence some slits may be missed during implantation especially in dark skinned people. Methylene blue or gentian violet staining can be used to identify the slits (Fig. 25.25).
- Insertion of grafts is done by assistants 2-3 in number depending on the area. The technique is the same as

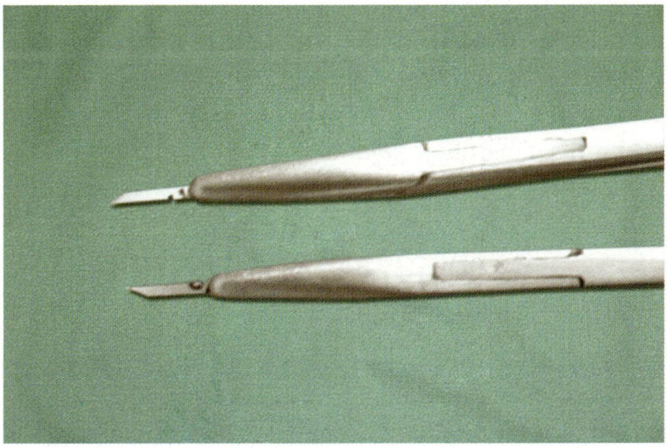

Fig. 25.24: Customized blades held by artery forceps. *Courtesy*: Dr. Venkataram Mysore, Bengaluru, Karnataka, India

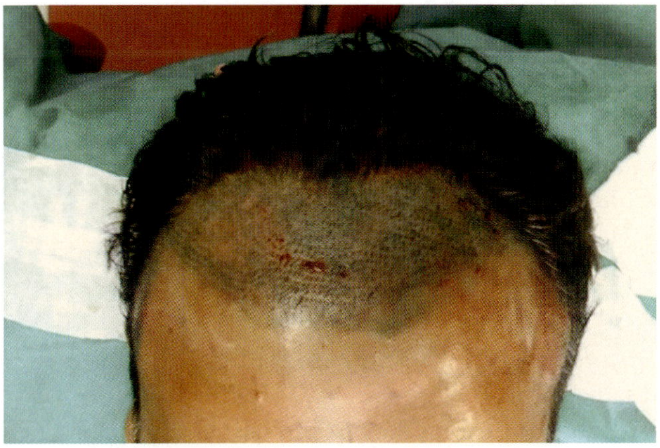

Fig. 25.25: Preformed slits stained with methylene blue. *Courtesy*: Dr. Venkataram Mysore, Bengaluru, Karnataka, India

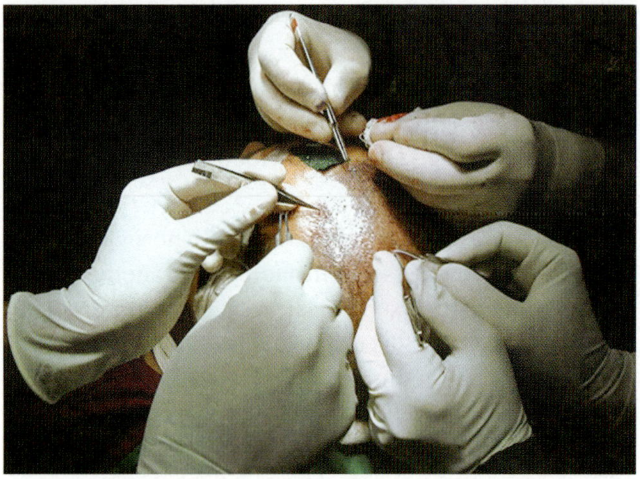

Fig. 25.26: Grafts insertion into the recipient holes.
Courtesy: Dr. Narendra Patwardhan, Pune, Maharashtra, India

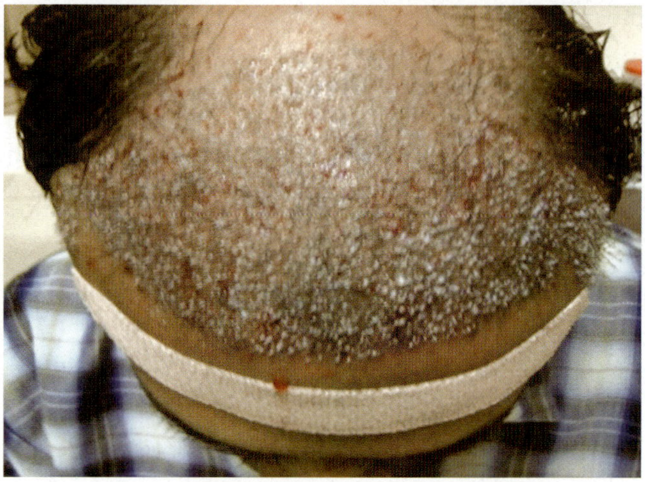

Fig. 25.27: Grafts in place after insertion.
Courtesy: Dr. Venkataram Mysore, Bengaluru, Karnataka, India

the one described above under slit and place technique (Figs. 25.26 and 25.27).

Popping may occur, if the slits are placed too close to each other and this needs to be avoided by proper technique of placing the grafts from behind forwards.

One of the disadvantages is that once slits are all made, then the job is entirely left to the assistants to implant the grafts. This can lead to lack of control, poor handling of grafts and poor communication with patients.

It has the advantages of speed and lesser surgeon involvement time. It allows overall planning and control for the surgeon as he can plan entire recipient session in one step. It also gives time for the surgeon to perform other tasks (as his task of making the slits gets over quickly) and perform other procedures.

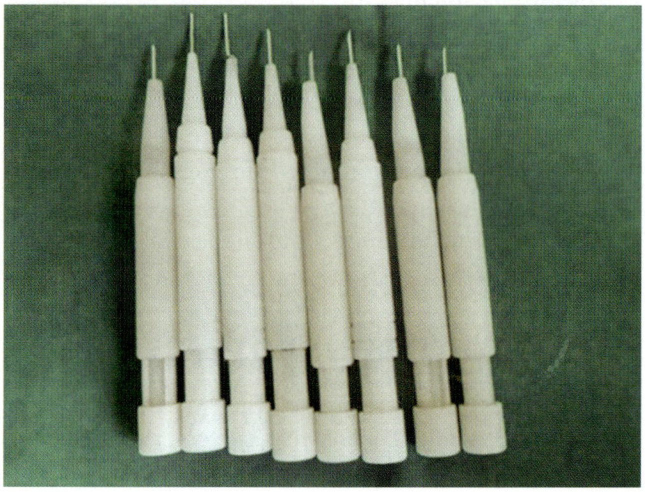

Fig. 25.28: KNU implanters.
Courtesy: Dr. Venkataram Mysore, Bengaluru, Karnataka, India

IMPLANTERS

Different types of implanters are available; such as Choi, KNU, Sava, etc (Fig. 25.28).

Implanters have some advantages:

- Implanters make handling of the graft minimal
- Implantation is quick
- It is easy to use in between existing hairs
- Implantation in different angles is possible
- Depth control is possible.

Disadvantages: The implanters have the following disadvantages:

- Additional cost as they are disposable
- Dissection needs to be precise as graft needs to be loaded into the slit on the needle of the implanter
- Loading the implanter with the graft needs training and additional staff
- Popping can occur in which case graft has to be place by the above other method.

Table 25.12 summarizes the features of each method.

Summary of Recommendations for Recipient Site Insertion

- Greatest advantage of premade slit and place is that surgeon involvement is least and takes least total surgical time. It allows surgeon to perform other tasks or even start another case. Its biggest disadvantages are that there could be miscalculations in the number and

Table 25.12: Advantages and disadvantages of each method of recipient insertion.

Features	*Preformed slit and graft placement*	*Slit and place*	*Implanters*
Description	All slits are performed in one go and grafts are placed by assistants, one by one after all slits are made	Each slit is performed followed by placement of each graft	Slit and placement in one step using a device
Speed	Quick	Slower	Quick
Staff	2–3 staff can perform at the same time	Usually 1 person	Usually 1 person
Surgeon dependency	Surgeon can make the slits and then assistants can place grafts—less surgeon time	Surgeon dependent	Surgeon dependent
Accuracy	Calculations may go wrong in inexperienced grafts	Accurate	Accurate
Placement	Some slits may be missed, some slits may close	Accurate	Accurate
Bleeding	Bleeding may occur during initial place	Bleeding while making slit making graft placement difficult	Bleeding may push the graft out
Identification of slits	May be difficult with time	Not a problem	Not a problem
Grafting in between existing hairs	Difficult	Easy	Very easy
Angulation, precision of placement	May vary since done by assistants	Accurate	Accurate
Cost	Cheap	Cheap	Cost of devices

errors in orientation as it is assistant dependent. So it is a method for teams lead by experienced surgeon and an experienced team. It still needs additional implantation by slit and place at the end for any skip areas.

- The greatest advantages of stick and place are its control and accuracy due to its near total surgeon involvement. It is also suitable for hairy areas. However, it gives little time for the surgeon to do other tasks. It is also more time consuming. It is a method of choice for beginners.
- The greatest advantages of implanter method are its speed, accuracy and near total surgeon control and utility in hairy areas. The disadvantages are expense of devices, more precise dissection for placement in the implanter and the need for additional staff to load implanters.

A surgeon should be proficient in all methods, so that he can use the right method for the right patient in the right situation.

POSTOPERATIVE CARE

Proper postoperative care is very much essential for a successful outcome of surgery and an instruction sheet enumerating all the instructions in detail are given to the patient in preoperative phase itself (Table 25.13).

COMPLICATIONS

Complications in hair transplantation can be due to general reasons or those specific for HT, most of which are infrequent, minor and can be avoided by proper techniques.

- General complications (Table 25.14)[40-42]
- Donor site complications[43-51]

As the strip technique involves excision of a strip of skin followed by suturing and needs proper surgical expertise, this step is associated with most problems (Table 25.15).

- *Recipient area complications:*
  - *Poor hair line:* A proper hairline in HRS is very important to give a natural frame to the face as onlookers visualize a person mainly from the front and to create a natural-appearing, soft hairline to establish the illusion of density.[52]

    Several problems can occur due to improper frontal hair line like (Table 25.16).
  - *Low perceived cosmetic density and unnatural coverage* of the bald area reflect errors in surgical and esthetic judgment. Failure to consider the possibility of progressive hair loss in young patient and calculation of sufficient projected donor hair to cover future hair loss is also the reason.

Table 25.13: Instruction sheet for patients postoperative.

Take care not to bang the head	While getting in and out of car, overhead shelves, etc. as the anesthesia given to the scalp makes it numb for few more hours.
Keep recipient area moist by spraying saline every 2 hours for the first day	Drying of the grafts in situ postoperatively can also increase chance of graft loss and viability.
Pain, discomfort	Painkillers are prescribed in the prescription.
Bleeding	To apply firm continuous pressure for 10 to 20 mins. till it stops. Apply cold compresses, if necessary.
Swelling	Swelling can occur from 2nd to 5th day, on forehead and even around the eyes. So let the sticking tape on the forehead be in place for 5 days and sleep as directed with head elevated at 45° on 2 pillows or on the side. Apply ice packs.
Donor bandage	Donor bandage applied on the back of scalp is removed on the 3rd day. Antibiotic cream is applied on the sutured area twice a day.
Head wash	Head wash is done from the 3rd day onwards daily till crusts/scabs fall off: • *Recipient area*: Apply shampoo on the scalp, gently spread on the grafts site, let it remain for 5 mins. Care taken to not rub and have no direct shower jet pressure but to just let warm water flow gently on scalp • For the suture area on back of scalp, gently scrub and remove the shampoo.
Combing	Dab scalp gently with a towel and comb with wide toothed comb only, not touching scalp directly.
Smoking/alcohol	To be avoided for 2 weeks.
Exercise	Avoid upper body exercises or any neck stretches till sutures are removed. Lower body exercises after 1 week.
Suture removal	After 10 to 15 days.

Table 25.14: Complications and management.

Cause	*Management*
Adverse systemic reactions to local anesthetics.	Prior testing of local anesthetic.
Drug induced gastritis to analgesics and antibiotics.	Administration of antacids and H2 blockers.
Tachycardia due to adrenaline in tumescent fluid, more risk in a cardiac compromised patient.	Do an ECG and physician assessment above 40 years.
Syncope can occur at the end of a long surgery, either due to pain, postural hypotension or xylocaine toxicity.	Avoided by: • Proper anesthesia and analgesia. • Making the patient sit before he gets up. • Minimizing xylocaine usage by completing surgery quickly. • Proper water, electrolytes and nutrition balance. • Preoperative administration of clonidine 0.5 mg helps by its anticholinergic and analgesic activity.
Pain due to wide strip, bleeding, wound tension, large sessions with inadequate anesthesia.	• Proper surgical technique and use of analgesics. • Postoperative administration of prednisolone which reduces wound edema.

Correction and repair of hair transplants require great skill and judgment. Transplanting additional follicular units using FUE method either from the scalp occiput or body hairs is done to give further density.[53,54]

- *Recipient area edema*:
  - This is common on 3–5th day of surgery, starting on the forehead and gradually spreading on to eyelids and nose. Several factors thought to be responsible are large quantity of tumescent anesthetic fluid, gravity which pulls the fluid down and lymphatic drainage of frontal scalp. This untoward effect can be reduced by sticking an elastoplast band on the forehead at the end of surgery, reclining position for 24 hours postsurgery, ice packs or manual massage to push fluids to the sides.[55]
- *Postoperative pustules*: They occur 1–3 months after surgery are related to presence of poorly dissected grafts and improper graft dissection technique. They are sterile, usually heal by itself and may need drainage of pus (Fig. 25.30).
- *Central scalp necrosis:* can occur after large sessions or in elderly with vascular compromise. It is characterized by a dusky red discoloration of scalp followed by extensive crusting and heals with scarring

Table 25.15: Donor site complications.

Bleeding	• Tumescence to raise hair follicles away from underlying neurovascular plane. • Anxiolytics and sedatives are prescribed the night before and morning of surgery to allay anxiety and lower blood pressure, e.g. Clonidine • Removing the strip in parts and not in one piece • Monitoring blood pressure • Avoiding deep incision. To first score superficially and then stretch the wound edges by a Haber spreader or skin hooks • Once bleeding occurs, it needs to be controlled by pressure, using an artery forceps or electrocautery used, if really necessary.
Pits	Proper suturing technique
Infection may occur due to nonadherence to aseptic norms of surgery or lowered patient resistance.	• Prophylactic antibiotics.[43] • If infection occurs, appropriate antibiotics after sensitivity testing is necessary.[44] • Lower risk of infections has been reported by treating nasal colonization of Staphylococcus aureus by the application of mupirocin ointment and preoperative shampooing of scalp hair with use of Chlorhexidine gluconate medicated soap the night before and the morning of surgery.[45,46]
Wound dehiscence or necrosis of the donor wound site is a very unusual complication and mostly due to excessive tissue removal of width more than 1.5 cm, wound closure under extreme tension, overzealous use of cautery and malnourished patients.[47]	• Restrict width of the strip excised less than 1.5 cm. • Proper wound care, dressings, antibiotics
Numbness usually transient, can occur because of transection of superficial sensory branches during donor strip excision.	
Pain can result especially, if donor wound is closed under extreme tension or due to damage to the underlying neurovascular supply.	Prevented by injecting sufficient tumescent solution of saline with 0.5% Lidocaine/ Bupivacaine and 1: 50,000 epinephrine to raise the donor tissues and enabling cutting above the plane of the deeper neurovascular structures.[48]
Persistent pain possibly to development of neuropraxia and neuromas.	Gabapentin, intralesional steroid injection
Suture extrusion	
Hypertrophic scar (Figs. 25.29A and B)	
Donor hair effluvium or shock loss	Temporary, reassure the patient.
Donor site scarring occurs in all techniques used in HRS with the scars ranging from imperceptible to noticeable and very unsightly and disfiguring. In strip excision technique of graft harvesting, a wide linear donor scar is the most feared consequence of modern HRS. This mainly results due to an increased tension on the donor wound closure in the occipital scalp area and mainly determined by the laxity of the occipital scalp skin.	Various preventive and corrective steps to avoid a wide unsightly donor scar are:[49] *Scalp laxity exercises started 4 weeks prior to the surgery. *Not extending the width of the donor strip to more than 1–1.5 cm, and closing the donor wound using sound surgical principles. *Double layer suturing *Trichophytic closure method. *Minimizing the use of electrocautery to stop bleeding and instead applying compression for minimum 5–6 mins. *Corticosteroid like 3.33 mg/ml solution of Triamcinolone acetonide mixed with Bupivacaine 0.5% (prolongs the anesthetic effect) in dose of 5 to 6 ml is injected intralesional inferior to the closed wound immediately after.s *Oral steroids has also shown to decrease edema and wound tension.

Table 25.16: Improper frontal hairline.

Asymmetry: Unnatural straight line hairline with poor temporal angles is very common and reflect poor technique. Female hairlines appear more rounded without the bitemporal recession occurring in males. *Cornrow plugs* resulted in the time of the old punch grafting technique and can still occur when larger units are used for hair line.	FHL is designed two-dimensionally with the help of mirror and three-dimensionally when the hairline is examined straight on. Ruler and laser guiding system help additionally.

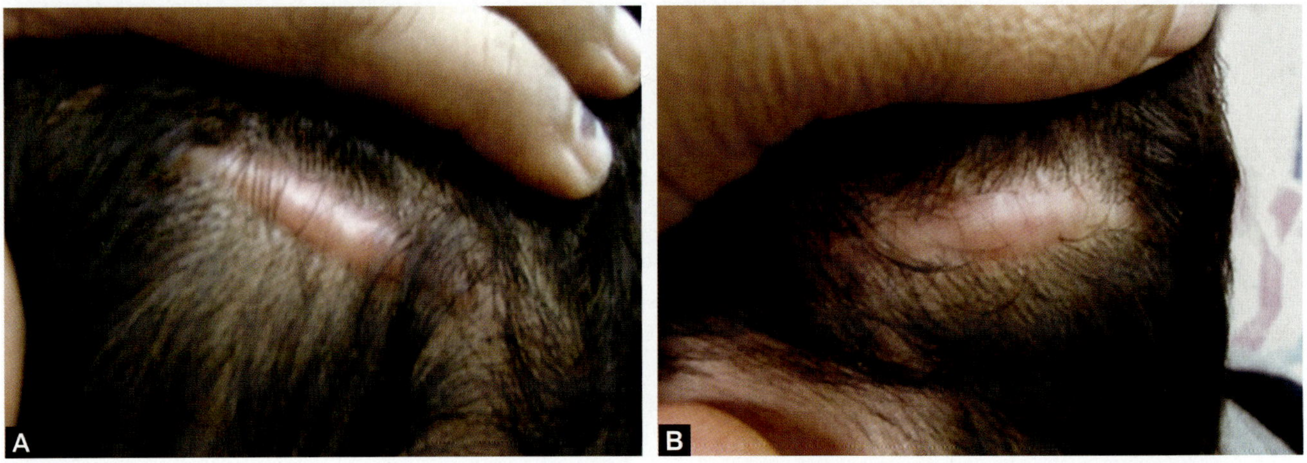

Figs. 25.29A and B: Hypertrophic scar at donor area.

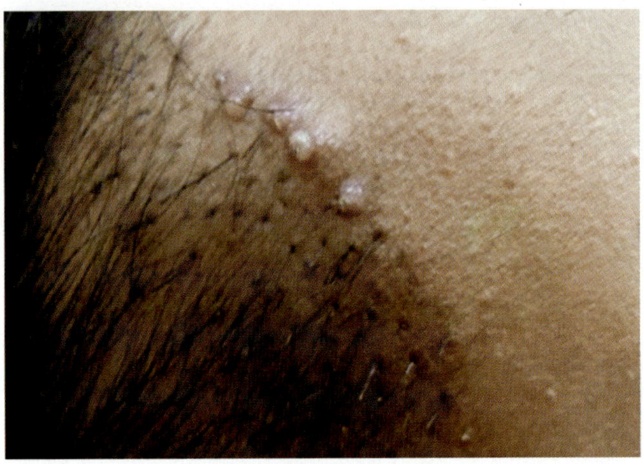

Fig. 25.30: Folliculitis.
Courtesy: Dr. Narendra Patwardhan, Pune, Maharashtra, India

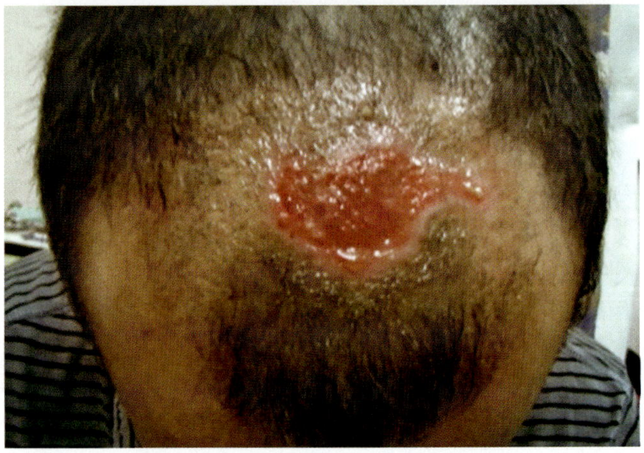

Fig. 25.31: Necrosis in recipient area.
Courtesy: Dr. Narendra Patwardhan, Pune, Maharashtra, India

(Figs. 25.31 to 25.33). While the exact cause is not known, it is postulated to the fact that central scalp receives comparatively less blood supply. Smoking, diabetes, actinic damage may predispose to the condition.[56]

- *Poor hair growth:* can occur due to following reasons:
  - Trauma to the hair grafts either during dissection or placement.
  - Desiccation of the grafts.
  - Poor quality donor hair like vellus telogen hair.
  - Heavy smoking, diabetes.

Counseling is done regarding the shedding of the transplanted hairs at around 6 weeks and the onset of new growth from 10 to 12 weeks with full growth achieved at 10–12 months.

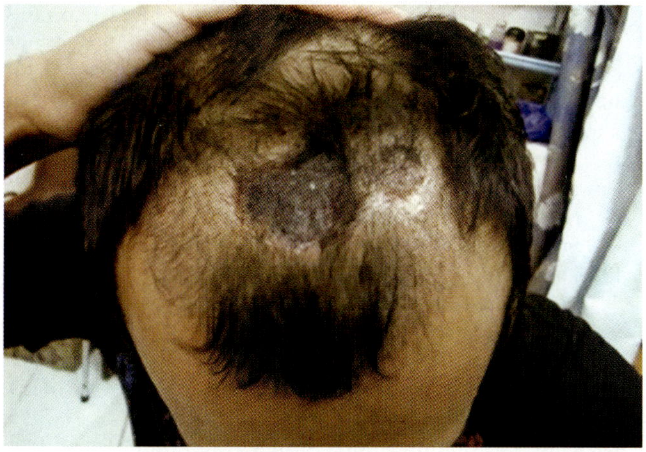

Fig. 25.32: Eschar formed after necrosis.

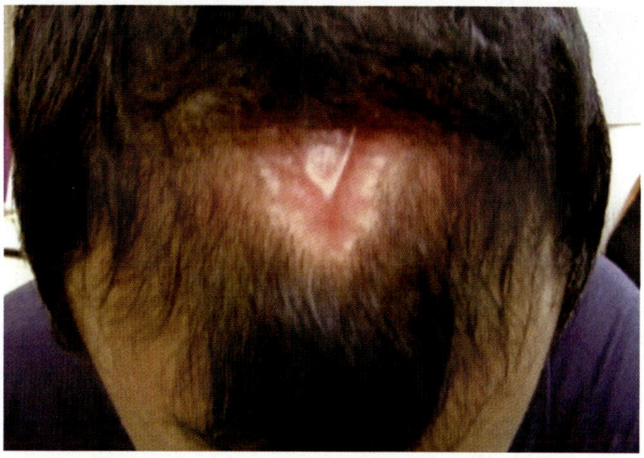

Fig. 25.33: Scar resulting from necrotic area.

- *Temporary hair loss:* called as shock loss is a kind of telogen effluvium of the surrounding hairs occurring due to the trauma of the surgery in 10–15% of males and more number in females. The patient can be forewarned about its possibility to alleviate anxiety or alarm. Use of topical Minoxidil in males and females and oral Finasteride only in males, for at least 4–6 months prior to surgery can help to minimize this hair loss.
- *Arteriovenous fistula* can occur but is extremely rare (Figs. 25.30 to 25.33).[57]

TIPS AND TRICKS

- Reoperative counseling regarding the benefits, limitations and risks of hair restoration surgery and recording in the medical chart goes a long way in preventing complications.
- Selection of a suitable candidate for surgery, thorough preoperative assessment and surgical planning of the recipient area is very essential.
- Good design of transplanted hair uses sound surgical skills and techniques combined with artistry for hairline reconstruction and for high perceived mid-scalp or vertex cosmetic density.
- Avoid complications by proper postoperative management.
- Quality control for every step of the surgery should be on a continuous basis, improving whenever and wherever possible.

REFERENCES

1. Orentreich N. Autografts in alopecia and other dermatological conditions. Ann NY Acad Sci. 1959;83:463.
2. Headington JT. Transverse microscopic anatomy of the human scalp. Arch Dermatol. 1984;120:449-56.
3. Shin JW, Kwon SH, Kim JY, et al. Characteristics of robotically harvested hair follicles in Koreans. J Am Acad Dermatol. 2015;72(1):146-50.
4. Konior RJ, Simmons C. Patient selection, candidacy, and treatment planning for hair restoration surgery. Facial Plast Surg Clin North Am. 2013;21(3):343-50.
5. Norwood OT. Patient selection, hair transplant design, and hairstyle. J Dermatol Surg Oncol. 1992;18(5):386-94.
6. Camps-Fresneda A. Age and patient selection in planning hair transplantation procedures. J Dermatol Surg Oncol. 1994;20(3):221.
7. Mowlavi A, Bass MJ, Khurshid KA, et al. Psychological sequelae of failed scalp replantation. Plast Reconstr Surg. 2004;113(6):1573-9.
8. Mayer M, Pauls T. Scalp elasticity scale. Hair Transplant Forum Int. 2005;15:122-3.
9. Chang LK, Whitaker DC. The impact of herbal medicines on dermatologic surgery. Dermatol Surg. 2001;27:759-63.
10. Cox AC, Rao GHR, Gerrard JM, et al. The influence of vitamin E quinone on platelet structure, function, and biochemistry. Blood. 1980;55:907-14.
11. Burnham B. Garlic as a possible risk for postoperative bleeding. Plast Reconstr Surg. 1995;95:213.
12. Elrner O, Goransson G, Zoucas E. Impairment of primary hemostasis and platelet function after alcohol ingestion in man. Haemostasis. 1984;14(2):223-8.
13. Kadimpati S, Nolan M, Warner DO. Attitudes, beliefs, and practices regarding electronic nicotine delivery systems in patients scheduled for elective surgery. Mayo Clin Proc. 2015;90(1):71-6.
14. Unger WP, Shapiro R, Unger R, et al. Hair Transplantation, 5th edition. London: Informa Healthcare;2010. p. 224.
15. Table compiled from WFH (World Federation of Hemophilia): Drugs that can cause bleeding.
16. Lawrence C, Sabruntabhai A, Tiling-Gross S. Effect of aspirin and non-steroidal anti-inflammatory drug therapy on bleeding complications in dermatologic surgery patients. J Am Acad Dermatol. 1994;31:988-92.

17. Goldsmith S, Leshin B, Owen J. Management of patients taking anticoagulants and platelet inhibitors prior to dermatologic surgery. J Dermatol Surg Oncol. 1993;19: 578-81.
18. Whitaker DC, Grande DJ, Johnson SS. Wound infection rate in dermatologic surgery. J Dermatol Surg Oncol. 1988;14(5):525-8.
19. Bencini PL, Galimberti M, Signorini M, et al. Antibiotic prophylaxis of wound infections in skin surgery. Arch Dermatol. 1991;127(9):1357-60.
20. Kaiser AB. Antimicrobial prophylaxis in surgery. N Engl J Med. 1986;315(18):1129-38.
21. Van Rijn MM, Bode LG, Baak DA, et al. Reduced costs for Staphylococcus aureus carriers treated prophylactically with mupirocin and chlorhexidine in cardiothoracic and orthopaedic surgery. PLoSOne. 2012;7(8):e43066. Epub 2012 Aug 14.
22. Willemoot G, Knight KR, Ayad M, et al. The beneficial anti-inflammatory effect of dexamethasone administration prior to reperfusion on the viability of cold-stored skin flaps. Int J Tissue React. 1999;21(3):71-8.
23. De Witte JL, Alegret C, Sessler DI, et al. Preoperative alprazolam reduces anxiety in ambulatory surgery patients: a comparison with oral midazolam. Anesth Analg. 2002; 95(6):1601-6.
24. Bischoff P, Kochs E. Alpha 2-agonists in anesthesia and intensive medicine. Anasthesiol Intensivmed Notfallmed Schmerzther. 1993;28(1):2-12.
25. Coetzee MJ. The use of topical crushed tranexamic acid tablets to control bleeding after dental surgery and from skin ulcers in haemophilia. Haemophilia. 2007;13(4):443-4.
26. Unger W, Solish N, Giguere D, et al. Delineating the "safe" donor area for hair transplanting. Am J Cosm Surg. 1994; 11:239-43.
27. Mohebi P, Pak J, Rassman W. How to assess scalp laxity? Hair Transplant Forum Intl. 2008;18:167.
28. Smith KC, Comite SL, Balasubramanian S, et al. Vibration anesthesia: a non-invasive method of reducing discomfort prior to dermatological procedures. Dermatol Online J. 2004;10:1-19.
29. Pathomvanich D. Donor harvesting, a new approach to minimise transection of hair follicles. Hair Transplant Forum Int. 1998;8(5):4-5.
30. Haber R. The spreader technique and indications. In: W Unger, R Shapiro, Unger R, et al (Eds). Hair Transplantation. 5th edition. Informa Healthcare. 2011:279-81.
31. Seery G. Hair transplantation: management of the donor area. Dermatol Surg. 2002;28:136-42.
32. Unger W, Cole J. Donor Harvesting. Hair Transplantation, 4th ed. New York: Marcel Dekker. 2004:301-37.
33. Marzola M. Trichophytic closure of the donor area. Hair Transplant Forum Int. 2005;15:113-6.
34. Rose P. The ledge closure. Hair Transplant Forum Int. 2005;15:113-6.
35. Rassman WR, Bernstein RM, McClellan R, et al. Follicular unit extraction: minimally invasive surgery for hair transplantation. Dermatol Surg. 2002;28:720-8.
36. Blugerman G, Schavelzon D. Graft Preparation and Storage. Hair Transplantation, 5th edition. 2010;309-12.
37. Seager D. Classic microscope dissection of follicular units. In: Unger W, Shapiro R (Eds). Hair Transplantation, 4th ed, Revised and Expanded. New York: Marcel Decker. 2004. p. 361.
38. Limmer B. Bob, Limmer does it all one hair at a time. Hair Transplant Forum Int. 1991;2:8-9.
39. Bernstein RM, Rassman WR. Dissecting microscope versus magnifying loupes with transillumination in the preparation of follicular unit grafts. A bilateral controlled study. Dermatol Sur. 1998;24:875-80.
40. Loganathan E, Sarvajnamurthy S, Gorur D, et al. Complications of hair restoration surgery: a retrospective analysis. Int J Trichology. 2014;6(4):168-72.
41. Salanitri S, Gonçalves AJ, Helene A Jr, et al. Surgical complications in hair transplantation: a series of 533 procedures. Aesthet Surg J. 2009;29(1):72-6.
42. Lam SM. Complications in hair restoration. Facial Plast Surg Clin North Am. 2013;21:675-80.
43. Kaiser AB. Antimicrobial prophylaxis in surgery. N Engl J Med. 1986;315(18):1129-38.
44. Zoumalan RA, Rosenberg DB. Methicillin-resistant Staphylococcus aureus: positive surgical site infections in face-lift surgery. Arch Facial Plast Surg. 2008;10(2):116-23.
45. Van Rijn MM, Bode LG, Baak DA, et al. Reduced costs for Staphylococcus aureus carriers treated prophylactically with mupirocin and chlorhexidine in cardiothoracic and orthopaedic surgery. PLoS One. 2012;7(8).
46. Farjo N. Infection control and policy development in hair restoration. Hair Transplant Forum Int. 2008;18:141-4.
47. Karaçal N, Uraloğlu M, Dindar T, et al. Necrosis of the donor site after hair restoration with follicular unit extraction (FUE): a case report. J Plast Reconstr Aesthet Surg. 2012;65(4):e87-9.
48. Wesley CK, Unger RH, Rosenberg M, et al. Factors influencing postoperative hyperesthesia in hair restoration surgery. J Cosmet Dermatol. 2011;10(4):301-6.
49. Unger WP. Correction of cosmetic problems secondary to hair transplantation. In: Unger WP, Shapiro R (Eds). Hair T transplantation, 4th ed. New York: Marcel Decker. 2004:372-9,475-80.
50. Donovan J. Lichen planopilaris after hair transplantation: report of 17 cases. Dermatol Surg. 2012;38(12):1998-2004.
51. Chiang YZ, Tosti A, Chaudhry IH, et al. Lichen planopilaris following hair transplantation and face-lift surgery. Br J Dermatol. 2012;166(3):666-70.
52. Shapiro R. Principles and techniques used to create a natural hairline in surgical hair restoration. Facial Plast Surg Clin North Am. 2004;12(2):201-17.
53. Bernstein RM, Rassman WR, Rashid N, et al. The art of repair in surgical hair restoration part I: basic repair strategies. Dermatol Surg. 2002;28(9):783-94.
54. Vogel JE. Correcting problems in hair restoration surgery: an update. Facial Plast Surg Clin North Am. 2004;12(2):263-78.
55. Gholamali A, Sepideh P, Susan E. Hair Transplantation: preventing postoperative edema. J Cutan Aesthet Surg. 2010;3(2):87-9.
56. Yildiz H, Ercan E, Alhan D, et al. Recipient site necrosis after tumescent infiltration with adrenaline in hair transplantation. Acta Dermatovenerol Croat. 2015;23(3):233-4.
57. Unger W. Re: Arteriovenous fistula following hair transplantation. Dermatol Surg. 2011;37(12):1816-7.

CHAPTER 26

Hair Transplantation: Follicular Unit Extraction

Aman Dua, Venkataram Mysore, Nirav V Desai

INTRODUCTION

Follicular unit extraction (FUE) is one of the most important advances in the last decade and has rapidly established its place in hair transplantation because of its safety, less scarring, ease and rapid healing.

DEFINITION

Follicular unit extraction (FUE) was first described in 2002 by Dr Bill Rassmann and Dr Bob Bernstein as *"the removal of individual clusters of follicles from the donor area using a sharp dissecting punch or trephine".*[1]

FUE is some times called follicular isolation technique (FIT) because

- An extracted graft might not have all the follicles of a follicular unit.
- At times it may have follicles from more than one follicular unit.

PRINCIPLE

It is based on the principle that the site of attachment of arrector muscle to the follicular unit is the tightest and narrowest zone. Once this is made loose and separated from the surrounding dermis, the inferior segment can be extracted easily. This is also the narrowest zone and hence a small punch less than 1 mm is enough to release the hold of arrectores (Fig. 26.1). Once the hold of the arrectores is released, the unit comes out easily.[2]

- In FUE, the grafts are extracted as individual follicular units; however the method of implantation remains the same as in the traditional FUT.
- As the follicular unit is narrowest at the surface, small micro punches of size 0.6 to 0.8 mm are used and therefore the resulting scar is too small to be easily recognized (Figs. 26.2A and B).

Follicle Depth

Defined by the distance from the surface of the skin to the full length of the follicle below the hair bulb.

Time Out of Body

This is the time between the removal of the graft from the donor area with forceps or suction and the reinsertion of the graft into the recipient area, i.e. the time that the grafts spends outside the body between extraction and implantation. The graft may be kept in a holding solution before transplantation or it may be immediately placed into a recipient site (called direct hair transplantation).[3]

Follicular Transection Rate

- The number of grafts transected for every 100 grafts is called as follicular transection rate (FTR).
- The number of partially transected grafts per 100 extracted grafts is called the partial transection rate (PTR).[4]

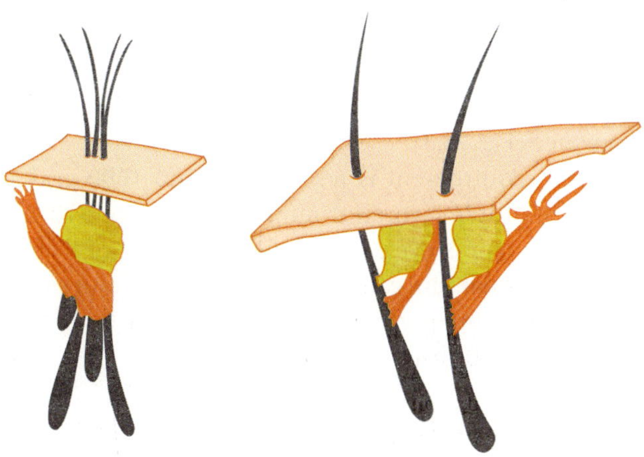

Fig. 26.1: Anatomy of the hair follicular unit and attachment of arrector pili muscle.

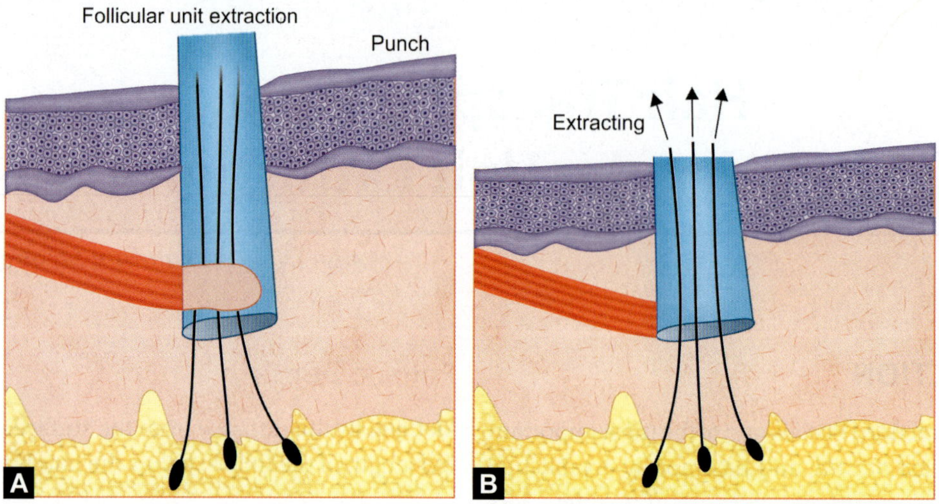

Figs. 26.2A and B: (A) Dissection of FU by insertion of the punch. (B) Removal of the follicular unit.

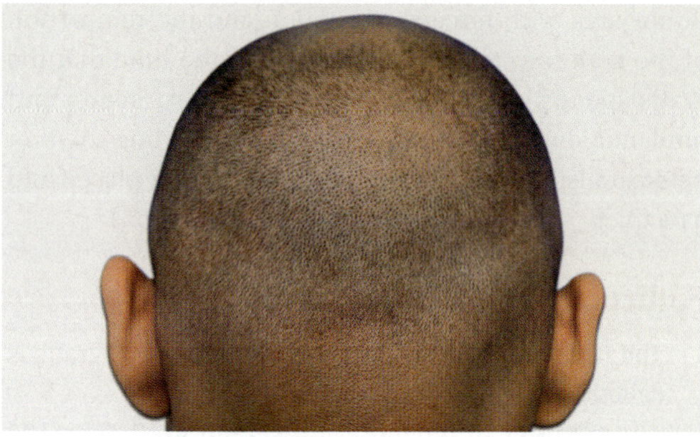

Fig. 26.3: Full trim of the donor area.

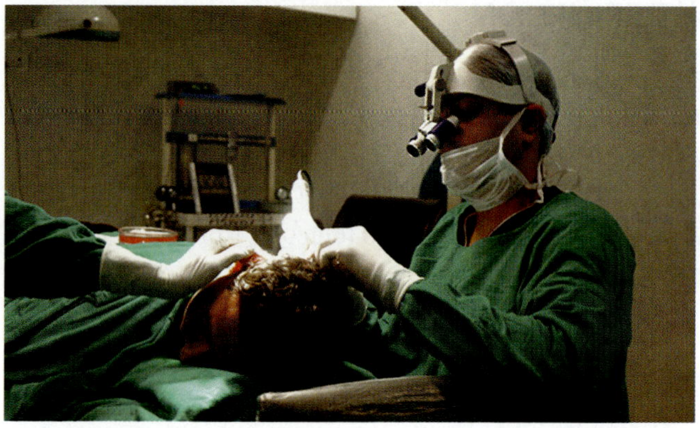

Fig. 26.4: Patient in prone position and surgeon in sitting position.

PROCEDURE[5]

Step 1: Preparation of the Donor Area

Trimming is usually done on the day of surgery. A typical case, for example of 2000 grafts requires full trimming of the donor area (Fig. 26.3).

- If the requirement is less, i.e. around 1000 grafts, then multiple layered trimming can be done; if the requirement is even less, i.e. around 500 grafts only, then a partial trim can be done; and in very rare cases, no- trim technique in which no trimming of donor hair is done can be used.

Step 2: Position of the Patient

Make the patient lie down in the prone position. The head may be turned to one side or be face down depending on the area from where extraction is being done. Some surgeons prefer to do the surgery in the sitting position but may switch to the standing position depending upon the alignment of the grafts and the ease of extraction (Fig. 26.4). A prone chair may also be used.

Step 3: Donor Area Preparation and Local Anesthesia

- Donor area needs to be cleaned with betadine—all aseptic precautions are to be followed as per standard protocols.
- Anesthesia needs to be given slowly. Use occipital block (Figs. 26.5A and B) (1 mL of 2% lignocaine with 1:100,000 adrenaline is given each side of midline) to anesthetize the donor area. Then give a field block

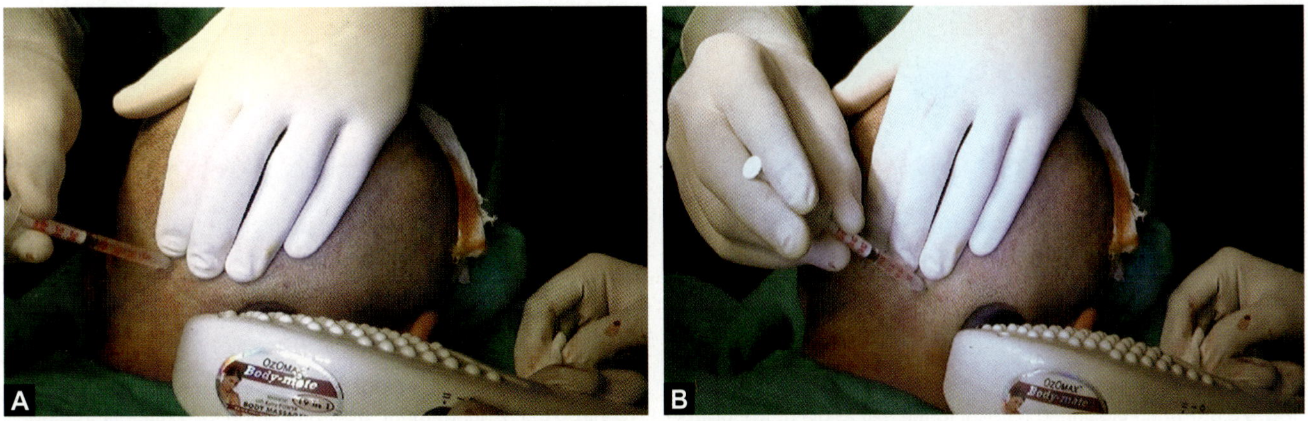

Figs. 26.5A and B: Demonstration of occipital block (LHS): The middle finger is placed on the occipital protuberance. Anesthesia is given around 2 cm lateral and inferior to the protuberance. (B) Demonstration of occipital block (RHS).

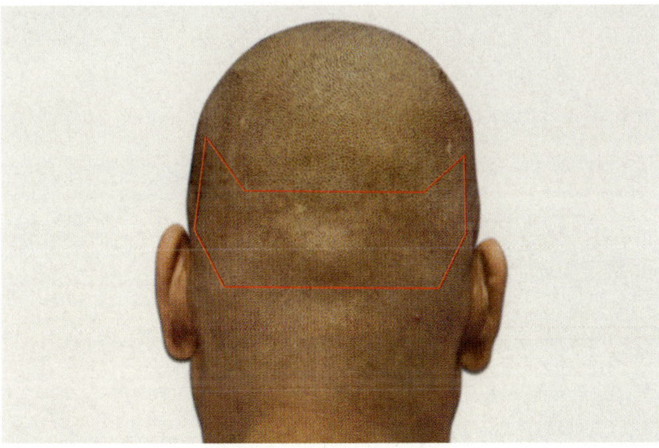

Fig. 26.6: Direction of filed block to anesthetize the donor area.

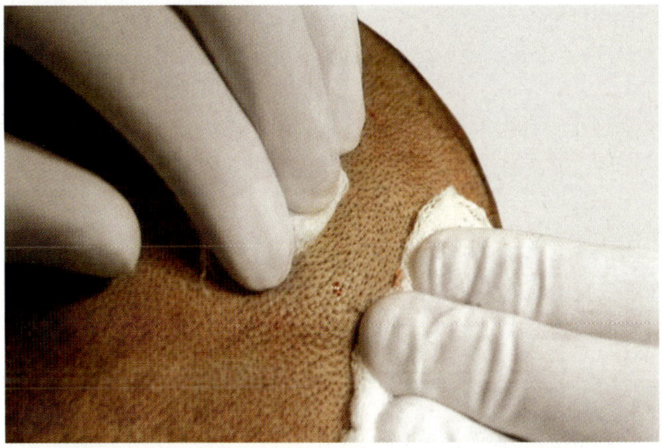

Fig. 26.7: Demonstration of traction and countertraction.

(Fig. 26.6) at the base using lignocaine 1% with 1:100,000 adrenaline. In rest of the donor area, plain lignocaine 1% is injected in a serial manner (Figs. 26.5 and 26.6).

Tumescent infiltration: Tumescence helps to make the area firm and facilitates extraction. Infiltrate around 1 mL of normal saline per 1 to 2 cm^2 of the donor area in a serial manner. Too much amount of fluid may alter the exit angle making alignment difficult.

Step 4: Extraction has Two Steps—Punching and Extraction

Only the motorized process is described here as manual technique has become almost obsolete. The motor has to be chosen carefully and should have variable speed and torque.

- Set the motor at the minimum possible speed (usually between 1000 to 2000 rpm for the dull punch and between 500 to 700 rpm for the semi-sharp punch), which is good enough to penetrate the epithelium with maximum possible control.

Traction-Countertraction

Traction is vital to ensure smooth FUE.

- Hold the handpiece in the dominant hand while sitting/standing on the left side or the head end of the patient and apply traction towards the head end with the nondominant hand. The assistant standing on the other side applies countertraction towards the foot end. This helps to stabilize the skin and decreases the exit angle of the hair which facilitates the entry of the punch into the skin (Fig. 26.7).

Punching has several steps: alignment, engagement, advancement and withdrawal.

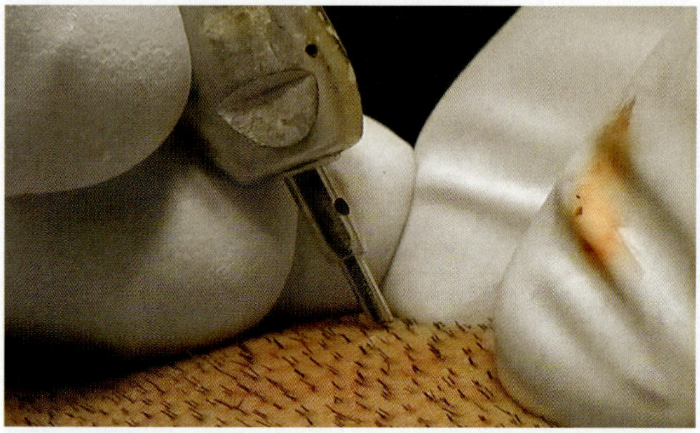

Fig. 26.8: Punch is aligned parallel to the exit angle of the graft.

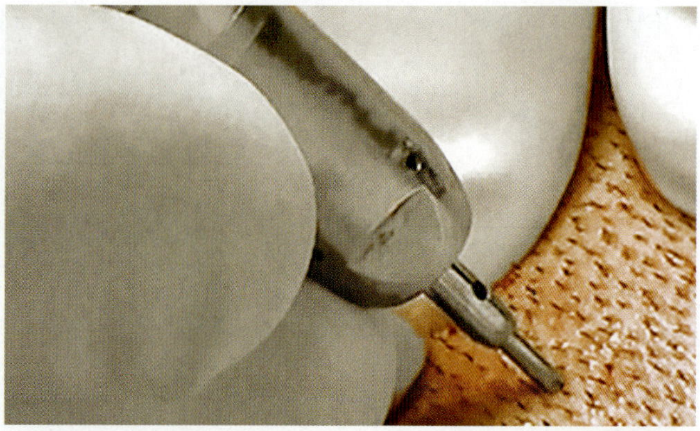

Fig. 26.9: Engagement: the point when the cutting surface comes in contact with the epithelium.

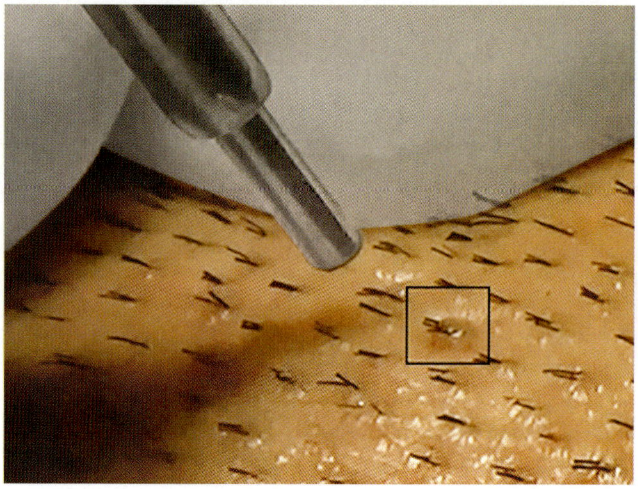

Fig. 26.10: The targeted hair is in the center of the impression by engagement of the punch on the scalp.

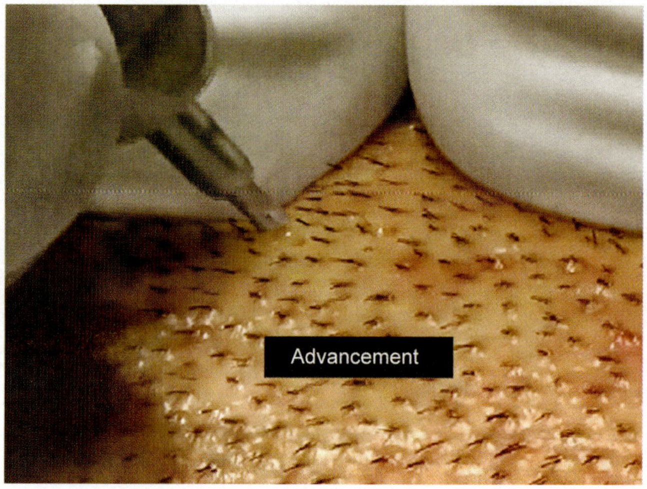

Fig. 26.11: Advancement: when the punch is pushed through the epithelium.

Alignment

- Alignment means placing the shaft of the punch parallel to the targeted hair emerging from the scalp. The direction of the hair and the exit angle of the hair change every few centimeters, as a result of which, the alignment changes accordingly.[4] However the straight dark hairs of South Asians are relatively easier to visualize as compared to the Caucasians making alignment comparatively easier (Fig. 26.8).[6]

Engagement

Engagement refers to the process when the tip of the punch touches the epithelium around the targeted hairs. It is one of the most important steps in the entier surgery. The targeted hair is either in the center of the circular impression of the punch or in the superior part. If the hair is in the inferior part, then the graft will be transected while advancing the punch (Figs. 26.9 and 26.10).

Advancement

Advancement refers to the process of downward movement of the punch parallel to the hair shaft, up to the level of arrectores (Fig. 26.11). Take out five test grafts from the middle of the donor area to know the average length of the hairs (from the epithelium to the inferior surface of the hair bulb); to see the health of the grafts (whether the follicles are strong or weak, whether they are loosely or firmly attached) and to judge the laxity of the scalp, so as to select the right type of punch for the patient.

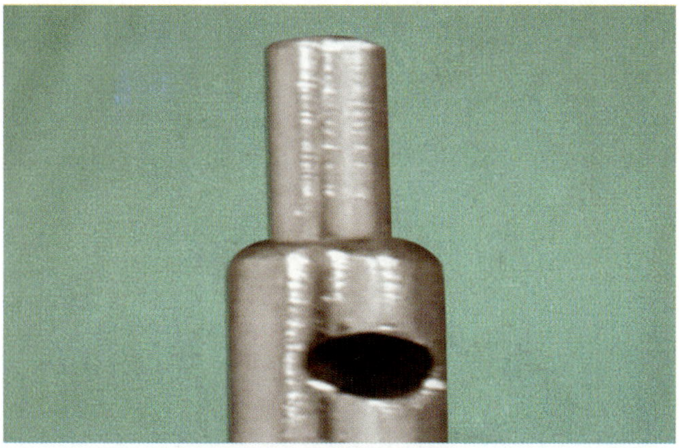

Fig. 26.12: Blunt punch.

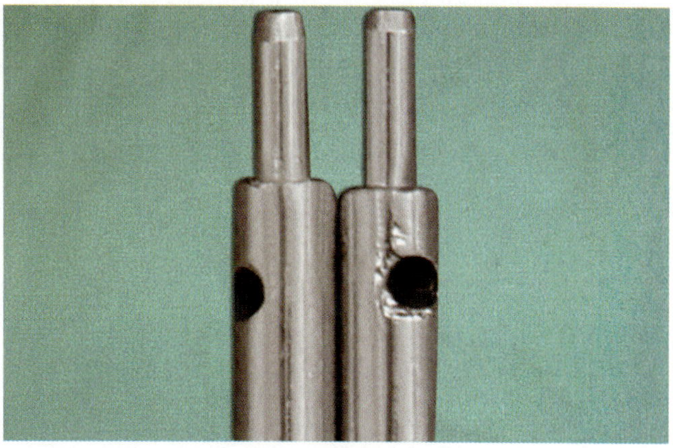

Fig. 26.13: Sharp punch.

Selection of the punch: Type of cutting surface, the diameter of the punch and the length of the shaft of the punch are all important for a smooth FUE.

- Both blunt and sharp punches have their advantages and disadvantages.
- *Blunt punch*: The amount of force which is required to advance a blunt punch (Fig. 26.12) into the skin is more as compared to the sharp punch (Fig. 26.13), but the complete transection of the grafts is very low (less than 2%). In case, more force is required, then the speed of the motor is increased to facilitate the advancement. Only when the skin is very firm, which is sometimes the case in patients of South India (Fitzpatrick type IV-VI), then use a semi-sharp punch.
- *Sharp punch:* The process is quicker, but the control is less and transection may be more in untrained hands.
- Whenever the surgeon uses a sharp punch, a general dictum is to stay as superficial as possible to loosen the pilosebaceous unit otherwise it will cause transection. However while working with the dull punch, one has the liberty of going deeper because of less chances of transection.
- It is important for the surgeon to gain proper experience and use the punches according the area of surgery.
- Smaller punch size is used for Asians (0.8 mm or 0.9 mm inner diameter) because of relatively less number of hairs per follicular unit (1.9) as compared to 0.9 to 1.0 mm in Caucasians. The smaller punch has the additional benefit of reducing the wound size. As the average hair per follicular units is less than 2, 0.8 mm punch would be the best one to use but some prefer the 0.9 mm punch as it not only facilitates the increase in the number of hair per grafts but also leads to the increase in the perifollicular tissue which comes in handy while delivering a good result in FUE surgery (Figs. 26.14A to C).[7]

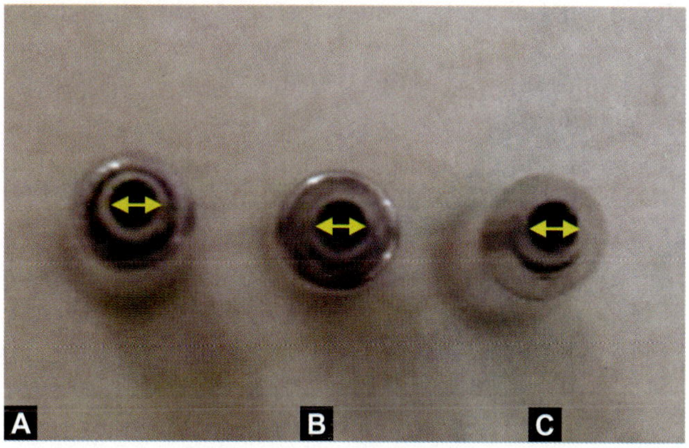

Figs. 26.14A to C: Punches with different diameter. (A) Blunt punch 0.8 mm. (B) Blunt punch 0.9 mm. (C) Sharp punch 0.8 mm.

- The average length of the hair follicle in Indians is between 5 to 5.5 mm.[3] In the unusual cases of length more than 6 mm, select a punch whose length of the shaft is around 1 mm less than the average length of the grafts. For example if the average length of the grafts is 5.5 mm, then use a punch of 4.5 mm length. In the unusual cases of length more than 6 mm, use a 5 mm punch (Figs. 26.15 and 26.16).

However, it is important to understand that the entire punch does not have to be introduced as the objective is to release the arrectors. The deeper the punch, greater the transection as hairs diverge at their lower ends.

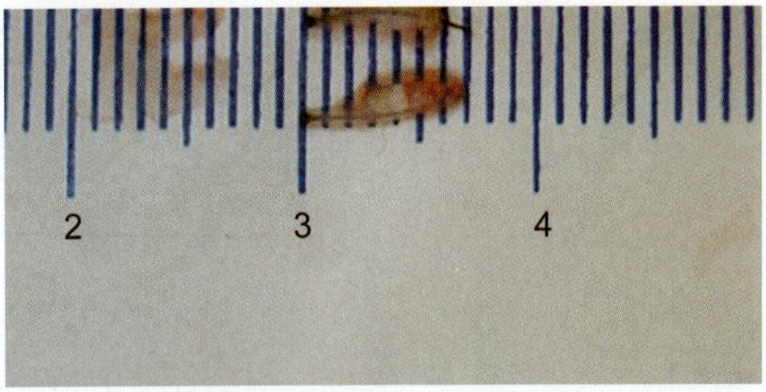

Fig. 26.15: Graft length 6 mm.

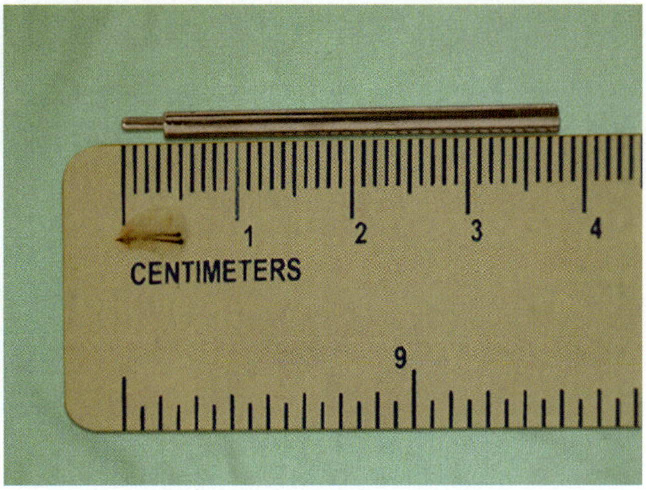

Fig. 26.16: Shaft length of the punch.

Different Methodologies of Manual Graft Extraction

These methods relate the steps that need to be applied, with a punch or other cutting tool, to release the graft from the surrounding tissue.

- *One-step method*: Uses an extraction punch that is inserted to the desired depth in a single incision using a rotational force, oscillating force, axial force, or combination of rotation and oscillation forces.
- *Two-step method*: Uses a sharp punch to first score the skin using a rotational, oscillating, or axial action. Then either the same sharp punch or a different punch is inserted through the epidermis via the same incision to the desired depth using a rotating or oscillating action. The second punch may be a different sharp punch or a dull punch.
- *Three-step method*: Uses a sharp punch to score the skin followed by a sharp or unsharpened punch to penetrate as in the two-step method. Then a needle or other sharp device is used to cut the graft free at the base while traction is applied with a forceps to remove the graft.

These steps have been rendered somewhat obsolete by the use of the automation.

Removal of grafts: There are different techniques for removal of grafts. One-forceps and two-forceps methods.

Different Techniques of FUE

Cole Isolation Technique (CIT)[8]

- Incorporates a variety of highly sharpened thin wall punches along with a precise depth control mechanism.
- Minimize follicular transection rate by varying the punch diameter, limiting depth, modifying punch geometry, altering tangential forces (Fig. 26.17).

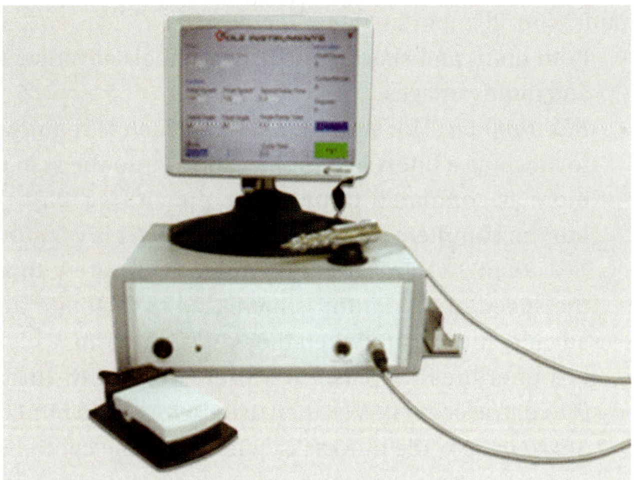

Fig. 26.17: Cole isolation device.

Harris Safe Technique[9]

- Initially using a sharp punch to score the dermis of the skin followed by deeper dissection with an unsharpened dull or blunt punch. After this the graft is removed with a pair of forceps.
- With the motorized version, the unsharpened punch is attached to a rotating drill, so the procedure can be done in a single step.
- *Simultaneous extraction*: The assistant removes the grafts using his dominant hand only with wrist movement in a downward direction. The assistant holds the grafts just underneath of the epithelium so as not to damage the stem cells (Fig. 26.18).

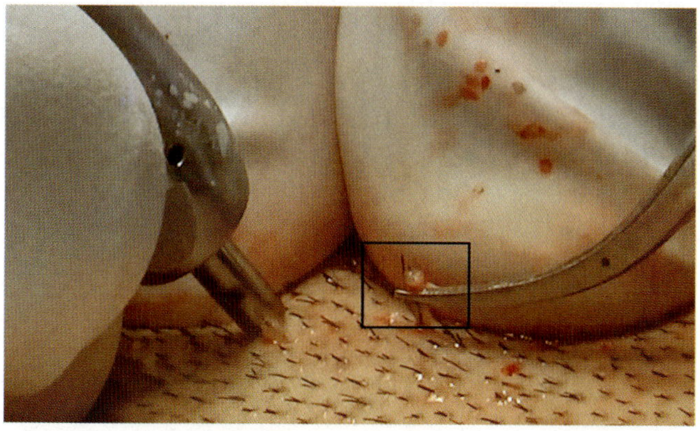

Fig. 26.18: The graft being removed simultaneously.

Out of Body Time of Grafts[10]

- Apart from the above mentioned points related to extraction, make the slits before starting extraction so that the grafts can be put back into the body immediately after the extraction is over. In difficult cases, also break up the surgery into two or three sessions to decrease the out of body time for grafts.

Some Important Issues in FUE

1. ***How are FUE grafts different from FUT grafts?***
   The FUT grafts can be chubbier and have more tissue cover compared to that of FUE. FUE grafts are more vulnerable to desiccation and need extra care while handling. FUE grafts may also be more susceptible to injury during extraction and due to the rotating effect of the punch in motorized machines. Neighboring hairs may undergo hidden transection while making punch holes particularly for hairs which emerge at acute angles.
2. ***What is the normal transection rate?***
   The term transection implies any microscopic or visible breakage of a follicle anywhere along its entire length. A graft can be a completely transected graft when all of the follicles are cut transversely or a partially transected graft when one or more follicles are cut leaving one or more intact follicle. The number of grafts transected for every 100 grafts extracted is called as the follicular transection rate (FTR) and number of partially transected grafts per 100 extracted graft is called the partial transection rate (PTR). This can be quite frustrating for the beginners as they are not able to harvest adequate number of grafts. Thus, it is best to start off with small cases (requiring around 500 grafts) so that the beginner can spend adequate time for extraction of grafts and minimize the transection of grafts.
   Transected grafts not only affect the results in the transplanted area, but also the donor area too, as the transected hair follicles left behind, may or may not grow back. This leads to depletion of donor area.
   The objective is to keep the FTR (Complete transection) to less than 1%- though this may not be possible in all cases and in all areas.
3. **How to minimize transection?**
   The following steps are offered as tips:
   - Depth control when punch produces incision
   - Proper position of operating surgeons and patients
   - Prone position for occipital area FUE and lateral decubitus position for temporoparietal area
   - Traction and countertraction over donor area
   - Use of tensioners or spreaders especially in tight scalp
   - Adequate lighting and proper magnification are essential
   - Insertion of punch at the proper angle during FUE
   - Repeated checking of grafts during procedure
   - Anterior or lateral traction over donor area while collecting punched grafts.

POSTOPERATIVE DRESSING AND HEALING

A detailed postoperative instruction sheet needs to be provided so those above events do not come as a surprise to the patient. It is in fact preferable to handover this sheet before surgery, so that the patient is prepared to face the issue and make appropriate plans for his travel, return to work, etc.

Bandaging

Bandaging is preferred by others as it prevents postoperative oozing.While it is true that FUE wounds close very early, still a bandage is preferred as small bleeding points and staining over pillow cover may cause anxiety to patients. Since the area here is large it is preferable to use thick rectangular pad. An antibiotic cream can also be used, if felt necessary and it will prevent adherence of the pad to the raw area. The bandage is removed next day.

Return to Work and Travelling

Purely from a medical view point, patients can return to work with a cap the next day. Patient should understand that FUE area remain noticeable for at least a couple of weeks hence those in whom where a cap is not an option, such as teachers, may need to apply for leave for 7 to 10 days. Doctors can manage by using a surgical cap at work. Travelling is allowed the next day.

Exercise

Follicular unit extraction patients can start all exercises and yoga the very next day.

COMPARISON WITH STRIP

The most common reasons why many patients choose FUE method for hair transplant is because there are no stitches involved and therefore does not leave any linear stitch mark in the donor area. A linear mark although is easy to hide under long hair in most cases, but some people, particularly younger patients like to keep their hair short or wish to experiment with different hair styles at different times. Such patients who use their freedom to wear short hair style feel uncomfortable with a strip scar. A significant number of patients may develop wide linear scar:due to tight scalp, wide strip, late removal of stitches, improper technique, early resumption of activities like Gym, sports, etc. or due to inherent scaring tendencies.

BODY HAIR TRANSPLANT[11]

- Donor follicles are harvested from any region of the body except the traditional scalp donor area.
- Body hair includes all hair inferior to and inclusive of the neck and beard.
- Yield is unpredictable and variable.
- Beard hair has higher mean yield and faster rate of growth compared to the other sources of body hair.

ROBOTIC HAIR TRANSPLANT: ARTAS® ROBOTIC SYSTEM[12]

- This is a computerized image-guided robotic system that scores the follicular units with image-guided motorized punch. It is a physician-controlled and computer-assisted system.

COMPLICATIONS[13,14]

The complications encountered in FUE cases can be discussed under the following headings:

General Postoperative Complaints

FUE is a relatively noninvasive and safe cosmetic surgery. Some of the common postoperative complaints that patients have are:

- Postoperative discomfort
- Oozing
- Numbness/ hypoesthesia
- Pruritus
- Vasovagal episodes.
- *Postoperative discomfort*: The postoperative pain and discomfort is minimal. This may occur on the evening of the surgery and disappear in the next couple of days. Analgesics like paracetamol, NSAIDs are given to avoid pain, especially for the first 1 week.
- *Oozing*: Postoperative oozing can occur from the donor site, although this is mild. This occurs when the patient lies supine on the surface, because of the pressure on the donor area. We advise the patient to keep a towel on the pillow to avoid any soiling of the bed sheet. The patients are also advised to apply firm pressure with gauze pieces for a few minutes when it occurs.
- *Numbness/paresthesia*: There is hardly any numbness or paresthesia in the donor area after FUE, although rarely reported.
- *Pruritus*: Some patients experience itching in the donor area, when the healing starts. Most of the times, it gets relieved after patient takes proper head bath and cleans the area appropriately. One can apply aloevera gel or steroid lotions if itching is severe.

Complications Specific to FUE in the Donor Area

- *Pinpoint white scars in the donor area*: Many people have a misconception that FUE is a scarless procedure, however in truth it is not so. FUE donor site usually heals as contracted circular scars which are hairless, depigmented, fibrotic, and palpable to the touch. Finally they appear as pinpoint atrophic white macules (Figs. 26.19A and B).
- *Moth-eaten or pseudosyphilitic appearance*: FUE also has a risk of clinically apparent depletion of hair from the donor region similar to strip cases. This can result in moth-eaten or pseudosyphilitic appearance (Fig. 26.20).
- *Postoperative effluvium*: Donor hair effluvium can occur after surgery, but it is relatively less common compared

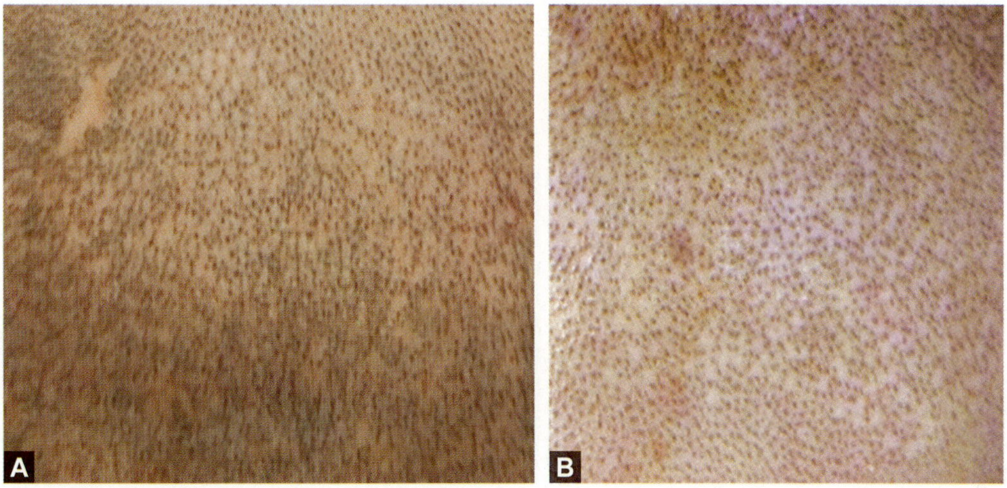

Figs. 26.19A and B: (A) Greater contrast of scar in Indian patient. (B) Less contrast in Caucasian patient.

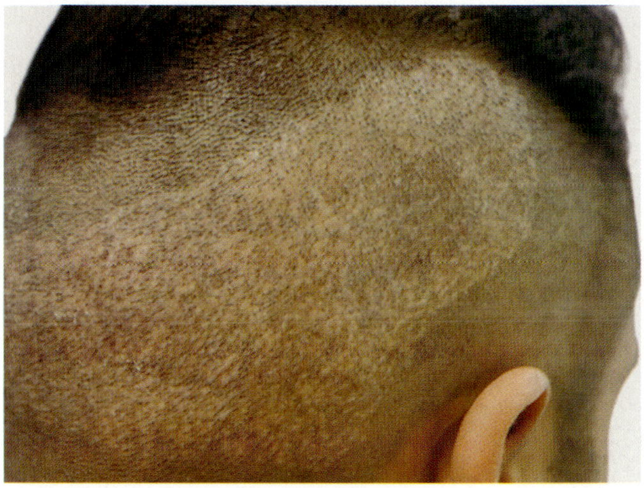

Fig. 26.20: Moth-eaten or pseudosyphilitic appearance.

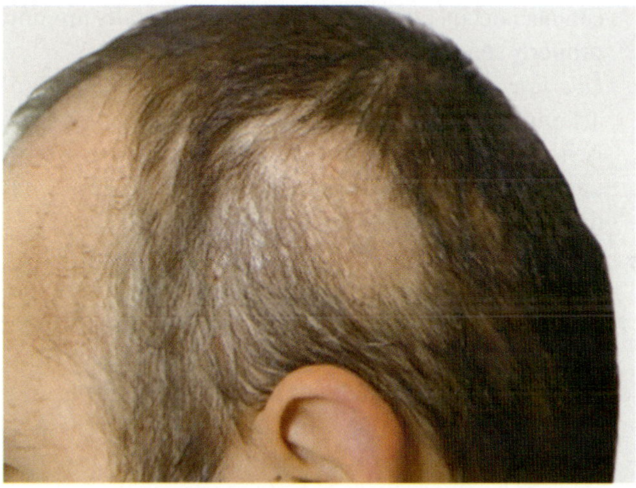

Fig. 26.21: Postoperative effluvium.

to the recipient hair effluvium. It presents mostly as diffuse hair loss after FUE, around 6 weeks after surgery and is temporary resolving over a period of 3 to 4 months (Fig. 26.21). Some of the reasons could be interrupted blood supply and overharvesting.

- *Buried grafts and epithelial cysts (pic)*: This is usually seen with dull punches. During extraction, when the punch is advanced into the dermis, the follicle is not in center of the punch; the follicle is pushed inside the dermis and gets embedded (subluxation). These buried grafts should be taken out simultaneously along with extraction by the assistant, failing which it gets embedded in the dermis and leads to cyst formation (usually multiple and painless) (Fig. 26.22).

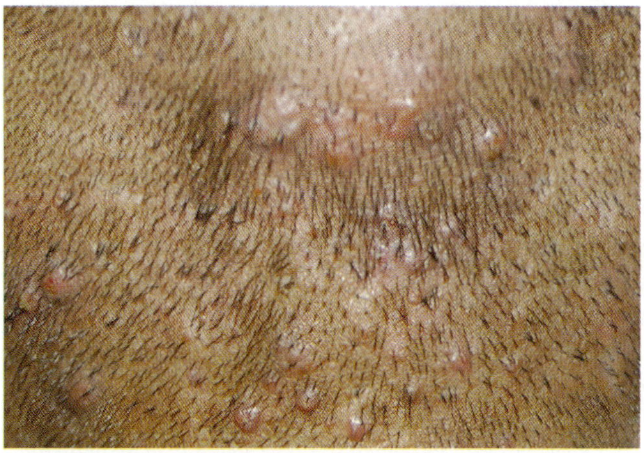

Fig. 26.22: Pseudofolliculitis and cyst due to buried grafts.

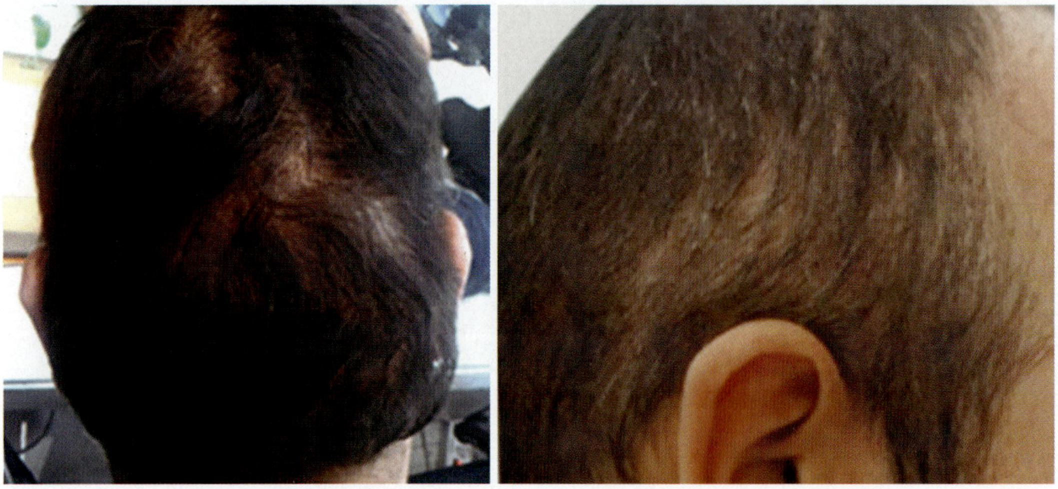

Fig. 26.23: Patchy area of thinning due to overharvesting from those sites.

- *Necrosis of the donor area*: Necrosis of the donor area can also occur rarely if the extraction of grafts are not properly spaced out.
- *Overharvesting of the donor area*: Sometimes in an attempt to perform large sessions, the donor area is harvested beyond their safe limits resulting in permanent damage. This can lead to visible thinning on these areas and patches of hair loss (Fig. 26.23).
- *Harvesting of grafts which are at an increased risk of future loss*: When grafts are harvested from outside the safe zones, especially in younger patients with ongoing process of hair loss, these grafts can later fall off. This usually occurs when grafts are taken from the upper and lower posterior occiput.
- *Temporary or long-term numbness*: It can occur over the posterior scalp similar to strip donor sites as mentioned above.
- *Folliculitis*: Folliculitis can occur on the donor area if the grafts are not taken out completely and part of them remains buried in the dermis.

CONCLUSION

FUE has established itself as a minimally invasive technique of hair transplantation because it is less invasive, less painful, heals quickly and removes the fear of surgery from patient's mind. The goal should be to keep FTR and PTR at the minimum (0-5%).

REFERENCES

1. Rassman WR, Bernstein RM, McClellan R, et al. Follicular unit extraction: minimally invasive surgery for hair transplantation. Dermatol Surg. 2002;28:720-8.
2. Poblet E, Jimenez F, Ortega F. The contribution of the arrcetor pili muscle and sebaceous glands to the follicular unit structure. J Am Acad Dermatol. 2004;51:217-22.
3. Sethi P, Bansal A. Direct hair transplantation: a modified follicular unit extraction technique. J Cutan Aesthet Surg. 2013;6:100-5.
4. Saxena K. Follicular unit extraction: technique and instrumentation. In: Venkataram M, Sattur S, Garg A, Dua K (Eds). Hair Transplantation. New Delhi: Jaypee Brothers Medical Publishers (P) Ltd. 2016;193.
5. Dua K, Dua A, Chahar M. Dos and dont's of follicular unit extraction. In: Venkataram M, Sattur S, Garg A, Dua K (Eds). Hair Transplantation. New Delhi: Jaypee Brothers Medical Publishers (P) Ltd. 2016;209-10.
6. Pathomvanich D, Imagawa K. Asian hair: knowing the differences. In: Pathomvanich D, Imagawa K (Eds). Hair Restoration Surgery in Asians. New York: Springer. 2010; pp.17-9.
7. Donor area harvesting. In: Unger W, Shapiro R (Eds). Hair Transplantation, 5th edition. New York: Informa Healthcare. 2011;292.
8. Cole J. Harvesting the fallows. ISHRS meeting, San Diego, California. 2006.
9. Harris JA. New methodology and instrumentation for follicular candidacy. Dermatol Surg. 2006;32:56-62.
10. Bernstein RM, Rassman WR. Pre-making recipient sites to increase graft survival in manual and robotic FUE procedures. Hair Transplant Forum Intl. 2012;4:128-31.
11. Cole J. Body to scalp. In: Unger W, Shapiro R (Eds). Hair Transplantation, 5th ed. New York: Informa Healthcare. 2011;304-6.
12. Wasserbauer SM. Robotic-assisted harvest of follicular unit. The ISHRS 19th annual scientific meeting, Anchorage. 2011.
13. Avram MR, Rogers N, Watkins S. Side-effects from follicular unit extraction in hair transplantation. J Cutan Aesthet Surg. 2014;7:177-9.
14. Dua K, Dua A, Kothottil R. Follicular unit extraction: mega and giga session. In: Venkataram M, Sattur S, Garg A, Dua K (Eds). Hair Transplantation. New Delhi: Jaypee Brothers Medical Publishers (P) Ltd. 2016;217.

CHAPTER 27

Hair Transplantation: Modifications for Other Uses

Madura C, Shilpa K

INTRODUCTION

Follicular unit extraction (FUF) technique can be employed in various situations to improve either cosmetic appearance or treating certain dermatological conditions. These include scarring and nonscarring alopecia, moustache, beard, side lock reconstruction, eyebrow reconstruction, eyelash transplantation and vitiliginous patches in hairy areas. Follicular unit extraction in above conditions has been explained in detail in this chapter.

SCARRING/CICATRICIAL ALOPECIA

Introduction

Scarring/cicatricial alopecia is characterized by permanent hair follicular destruction. It can be primary or secondary. The etiology of primary cicatricial alopecia is not known and is characterized by follicular unit inflammation that destroys the hair follicles. Based on histopathological examination of inflammatory infiltrate, they are classified as neutrophilic, lymphocytic and mixed cicatricial alopecia (Table 27.1). In secondary cicatricial alopecia, there is indirect destruction of hair follicles, either by trauma or inflammation of the skin. The common causes of secondary scarring alopecia are physical trauma, burns, irritant application in alopecia areata and postsurgical scars.[1,2]

Clinically, both varieties of cicatricial alopecia shows less follicular ostia. The differentiation of primary from secondary is by: Clinical history (trauma, known inflammatory conditions and acute or chronic onset history needs to be elicited). On examination, scars secondary to trauma or burns are often thick unlike flat, atrophic scars of primary cicatricial alopecia. In primary scarring alopecia there are other tale tell signs which has to be thoroughly looked in, that aids in diagnosis and also to assess the stability. Dermoscopy is a valuable tool to diagnose

Table 27.1: Classification of cicatricial alopecia[1,2–4]

Primary cicatricial alopecia	*Secondary cicatricial alopecia*
Lymphocytic	**Trauma**
• Chronic cutaneous lupus erythematosus	• Burns
• Lichen planopilaris (LPP)	• Radiation-induced alopecia
– Classic LPP	• Prior hair transplantation
– Frontal fibrosing alopecia	• Prior rhytidectomies and brow lifts
– Graham Little syndrome	• Traction alopecia
• Classic pseudopelade	• Trichotillomania
• Alopecia mucinosa	• Pressure alopecia
• Central centrifugal cicatricial alopecia[6]	
• Keratosis follicularis spinulosa decalvans	
Neutrophilic	**Congenital[5,6]**
• Folliculitis decalvans	• Aplasia cutis congenital
• Dissecting cellulitis	• Generalized atrophic benign epidermolysis bullosa
	• Incontinentia pigmenti
	• Cleft lip surgery scar
Mixed	**Others**
• Acne keloidalis	• Infections
• Acne necrotica	• Metastatic primary neoplasm
• Erosive pustular dermatosis	• Graft-versus-host disease

various primary scarring alopecias. Biopsy is a definitive tool to confirm the diagnosis, and always a deep biopsy from active area is preferred. The diagnostic markers of cicatricial alopecia are loss of follicular ostia and histopathological destruction of hair follicles.[7-10]

The treatment of primary scarring alopecia is timely management of active stages and stabilize the progression followed by surgical management for the end stage/ burnt out scarring alopecia.[11] The secondary scarring alopecia scars must be at least 6 months old and pliable and not hypertrophied. The surgical strategies depends mainly on size of the scar: it can be simple excision of scar, scar reduction by serial excision, reconstruction by tissue expansion, hair transplantation or scar reduction followed by hair transplantation and hair camouflage if scar is extensive. [12,13] This chapter will be limited to a discussion on hair transplantation.

Ideal Candidate for Surgery

- The disease must be stable (no disease activity). The duration of stability must be at least 1 year.[4]
- The secondary scarring alopecias must be at least 6 months old and scars should be pliable and not hypertrophied.
- Candidate to have suitable donor area (in extensive patchy disease, it is difficult to choose area for harvest, such cases are ideally deferred).[4]
- To have realistic expectations and understand that graft survival and cosmetic outcome are varied in scar transplants.

Factors Affecting Choice of Surgery in Cicatricial Alopecia[4]

- *Time of surgery:* According to Rose and Shapiro, it has been recommended that hair transplantation in scarred tissue be delayed until there are no signs of active disease for approximately 1 year. Always do a test session, in all patients with primary cicatricial alopecias before committing to a larger procedure.[4]
- *Availability of donor hair:* It must match the donor supply and recipient need. In extensive cases of alopecias, it could be difficult to harvest required number of grafts. Always take associated patterned hair loss also into consideration.[4]
- *The patient's inherent wound healing capacity:* Few patients heal with scar hypertrophy post-transplantation, therefore case selection is important.
- *Vascular supply:* The vascularity is less in scar and is prone for infection, tissue ischemia and necrosis after surgery.[14,15]

Preoperative Consultation

Every patient considered for hair transplantation in scar should be asked a proper history, subjected to a detailed examination and involved in a discussion on the pros and cons of having hair transplant and viable alternative methods of resolving the patient's problem. The patient should be able to state the problem that how scar occurred, and how long it has been there and any previous attempts to correct the problem should also be explored. Explore the patient's past history and family history for associated comorbidities and patient's medication history. After definitive diagnosis and stability of condition, the scars are evaluated for (1) size (to decide on treatment plan and number of grafts required), (2) thickness and skin texture (to know of hypertrophic scar/atrophic scar/ideal scar that helps to decide on time of surgery and also need for adjuvant therapies). Photo- documentation is mandatory.

Measures to Make Scar Bed Viable for Hair Transplantation

The ideal scar is soft, pliable and flat. If it is thick and hypertrophied, make it soft, flat and pliable before taking patient for surgery. Intralesional triamcinolone acetonide (TAC) 10 to 20 mg/mL is given every 3 weeks till it becomes less fibrous and pliable for surgery. CO_2 ablation can debulk the thick scars. Author uses combination treatment of CO_2 laser and TAC 10 mg/mL to debulk the thick small scars. Alternatively fractional CO_2 can be used for priming the scars especially: the atrophic scars, for a faster wound healing and a better cosmetically accepted result. It improves the skin texture, pliability and vascularity of scars by neovascularization and release of growth factors and cytokines during wound healing process which can increase graft uptake. If scar is very thin, there is risk of tear, so it must be handled gently with adequate density. Some authors recommend use of topical minoxidil solution (2–5%) on the recipient area for two weeks before and 12 weeks after surgery. Preoperative pentoxyphylline 400 mg three times a day can be given 2 weeks before surgery to increase oxygenation of the tissue.[4,15-18]

Selection of Donor Area[4]

If the scar is on eyebrow, select the postauricular grafts. If scar on moustache, can choose either beard or scalp hair. If scar is extensive on scalp, choose the donor area carefully, as disease process must have affected the remaining scalp. Therefore patient must have sufficient donor supply. It is important to consider associated patterned baldness while choosing the donor site. In males, the best donor area is the middle of the densest region of hair and these areas are usually on the occipital, parietal, and posterior temporal regions. In females, the donor areas are the occipital and posteroparietal areas.[19]

Test Grafting

Always do a test graft area of (1.5–2 cm^2) to assess the graft uptake 8 to 12 months before main surgery. A small area is selected, measured, photographed and 20 FU/sq cm^2 are implanted and monitored for uptake and subsequent growth.

Procedural Steps (Figs. 27.1A to D)

- The recipient site is marked, measured and number of grafts are planned with density based on vascularity, site and type of scar.
- Vascularity can be checked by anesthetizing small area with 2% lidocaine without epinephrine. Make several pricks with hypodermic needle and look for bleeding: based on this density can be decided. Regions with less blood supply should have density at most of 15 to 20 FU/cm^2. For the regions with better perfusion it is generally safe to increase the concentration of follicles to as high as 20 to 30 FU/cm^2.[15]

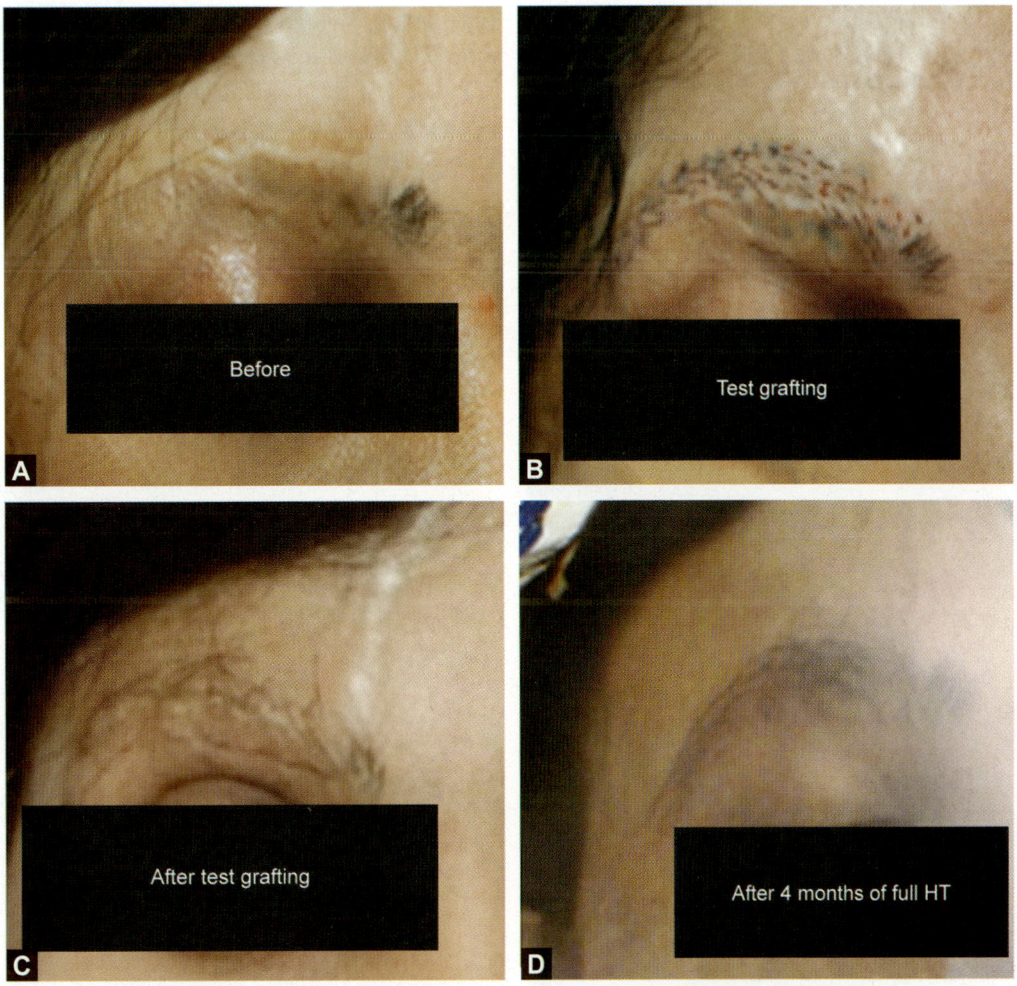

Figs. 27.1A to D: Steps of hair transplantation in cicatricial alopecia (250 grafts).
Courtesy: Cutis Academy, Bengaluru, Karnataka, India

- The donor area is selected and prepared with 2 mm trimming for FUE and 3 mm trimming for FUT.
- *Local anesthesia:* Avoid or minimize use of adrenaline with lignocaine for anesthesia as it affects the blood supply. Tumescent anesthesia is injected to raise the scar from the bed. This avoids damage to the under-lying structures and also ensures more acute creation of slits.
- Follicular unit extraction is preferred over strip technique due to the presence of subsequent scar in the latter. [11,14,15] The FUE grafts are harvested from donor zone after anesthesia. Some prefer to use small grafts than bulky ones. Authors prefer to harvest graft with 0.8 mm motorized punches, similar to any FUE. The grafts are stored in cold Ringer lactate and bulky grafts are pared to single and double units. It is important to minimize the amount of epidermis remaining on the grafts.
- *Implantation:* Though either method of implantation can be chosen, author prefers premade slit technique over stick and place method. Some of the rules to be followed during implantation are as follows:[20,21]
  - Higher FU densities are not recommended. The grafts must not be densely packed and educate on need for multiple sessions. Second session should be planned at 8 to 12 months interval.[4]
  - The recipient area holes can be made with minute punch, miniature blades (0.9, 1 mm), different sorts of needles (21G for 1 hair follicle, 20G -2HF and 19G-thick and MFUs) or CO_2 or Er:YAG lasers. [22]
  - Use smaller or same size slit in tissues with greater laxity or very little dermal recoil, as it has advantage of less "popping". However, if the tissue is tight and fibrotic, there may be difficulty in implantation: hence, the incision must be made larger to avoid excessive handling of the graft.
  - The general rule is to make slits slightly deeper and bigger compare to normal recipient scalp.
  - The angle of the incision, should be in a direction parallel to the existing hair and is more acute in areas like eyebrow, the temporal regions, and the hairline in supra-auricular and preauricular regions.
  - The grafts are implanted with 2 forceps technique without damaging the follicles and the grafts are fixed.
- The donor area is dressed with antibiotic ointment and open dressing is preferred for recipient site.

Postoperative Instructions

The grafts are hydrated for fixed 48 hours with normal saline sprays. The routine preoperative antibiotics are started, anti-inflammatory drugs will take care of the pain. 2 to 5% topical minoxidil is started at second week. Complete recovery is expected in 6 to 9 months (Figs. 27.2 and 27.3).

Complications[3,4]

- Graft failure
- Hypertrophic scar
- Crooked hair
- Misdirection of hair

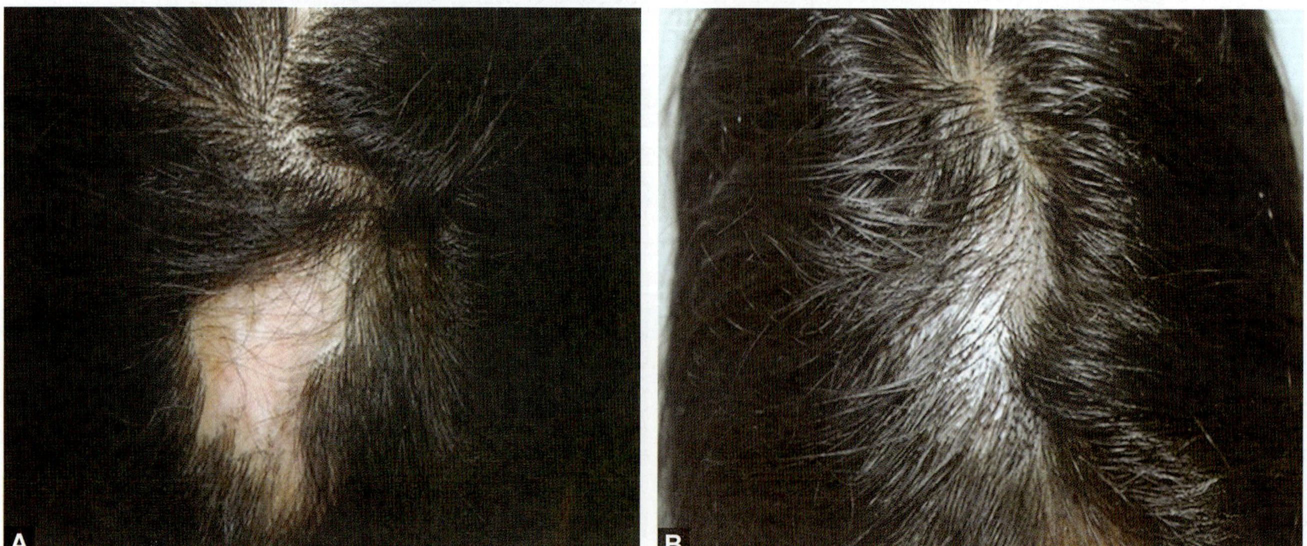

Figs. 27.2A and B: Hair transplantation in primary cicatricial alopecia (LPP), 300 grafts.
Courtesy: Cutis Academy, Bengaluru, Karnataka, India

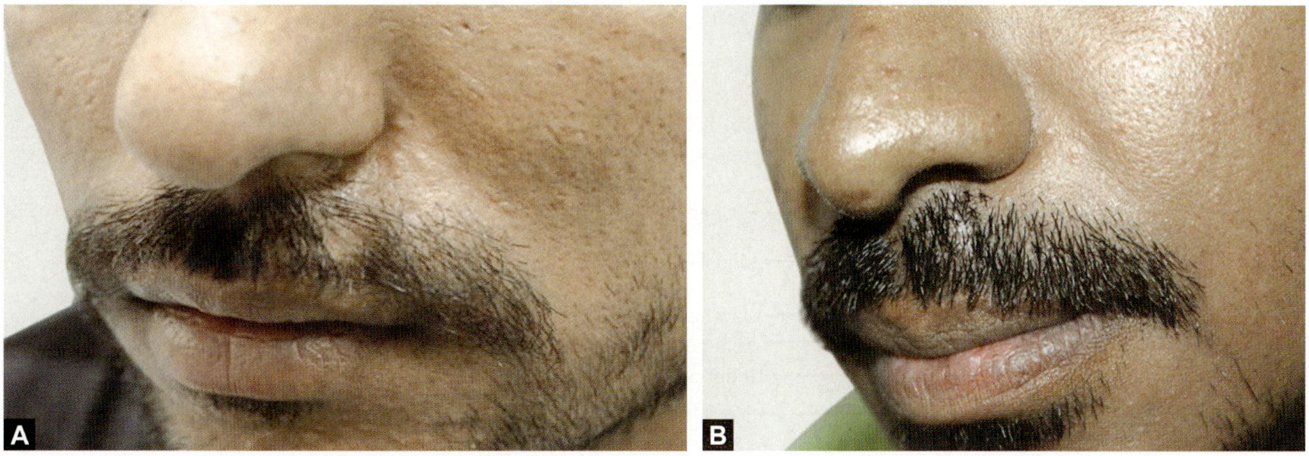

Figs. 27.3A and B: Moustache hair transplantation for post-traumatic scar, 80 to 100 grafts.
Courtesy: Cutis Academy, Bengaluru, Karnataka, India

- Infection
- Necrosis
- Postoperative hypo or hyperesthesia.

Tips to Optimize Results

- Do not do procedure when disease is unstable.
- Prepare the scar before transplantation.
- Use minimal adrenaline.
- Use less bulky grafts.
- Use large and longer slits.
- Low density packing.
- Planning in multiple sessions.
- Use 5% minoxidil solution one week before and after surgery.
- Pentoxifylline 400 mg thrice a day for 2 weeks can increase vascularity.

To conclude the management of patients of cicatricial alopecias is more satisfying as the patients accept even a little bit of hair growth as a good successful procedure. The proper case selection, timely surgical intervention and good technical skills will give gratifying results in cicatricial alopecias.

MOUSTACHE, BEARD AND SIDEBURN TRANSPLANTATION

The beard and moustache symbolizes masculinity and pride amongst men. There are different patterns of beard styles in this era with men having thick facial hair. Less density or loss of facial hair can be a source of stress and most of them seek medical help that often mandates treatment. There is increased popularity of facial hair restoration. The ISHRS 2013 Practice Census states, amongst 7% of nonscalp hair transplant surgeries more than 90% were the facial area (eyebrow is followed by beard, moustache and sideburns).[23]

The beard and moustache hair start appearing after puberty and increases up to third decade. The parts of beard on lateral aspect include the sideburns, cheek beard, jawline beard, and the submandibular beard area. The frontal view includes moustache and goatee (chin and infralabial beard) which marks the prominent feature. The cheek beard is cosmetically the most important (Fig. 27.4). The moustache and chin has 30 to 45 FU/cm^2 of density and beard has 25 to 30 FU/cm^2 of density.[24,25] Moustache is an area on face that occupies upper lip region. The moustache hairs are single, thick and coarser than beard hair. The beard is the area below the line joining the tragus and the angle of mouth and extends upto submandibular and submental region. The diameter of beard is thicker than scalp. Beard hair is also typically more elliptical in shape compared to the circular or oval shape of scalp hair. The anagen phase of beard is 12 weeks and telogen phase is 16 weeks.[24,25] Density of beard and moustache varies amongst various ethnic groups: it is higher in Indians and Caucasians.

Sideburn/side lock zone occupies the lateral part of face; it is 1.5 cm in width and extends from temple to the tragus. It has anterior and posterior border, posterior border is 2 cm in front of the tragus. Most of time anterior border is connected with beard and moustache. The Asian men will have longer and wider sideburn. The hair texture is softer than beard with low density and has mixture of

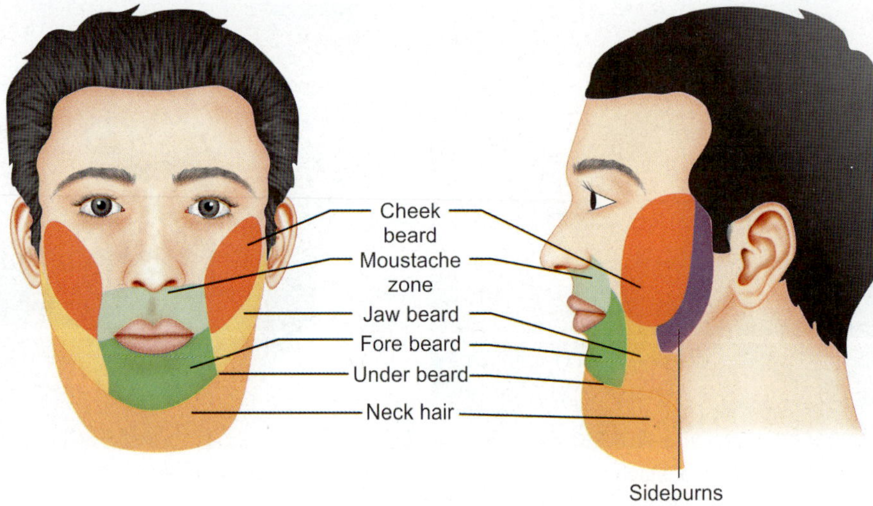

Fig. 27.4: Anatomy of beard.

1 or 2 hair follicles.[25] The technical aspects of hair transplantation in these areas are similar, only salient features will be discussed.

Indications[23,25]

- Complete reconstruction in absence or decreased density of beard and moustache hair (congenital hypotrichia/atrichia).
- To cover the areas of scarring alopecia (secondary to trauma/burns/surgery/cleft lip repair). Most of the beard are designed based on two fixed points: side lock and moustache. So any hair loss in these areas.
- Traction alopecia in Sikh population.
- Postfolliculitis scarring.
- Chronic stable nonresponding alopecia areata.
- Some men want cosmetic enhancement in certain areas or simply to increase density to adapt certain styles, this group must be handled cautiously as they may not have realistic expectations.

Preoperative Consultation

Organized consultation confirms the indication for which the patient has sought medical help. Rule out associated comorbidities. Examine the whole face and calculate the required number of grafts. The smaller areas like moustache scar may require only 20 to 100 grafts depending on size of patch, whereas with congenital hypotrichia or atrichia may need as many as 2,500 grafts to construct all of the beard and the moustache.[23] Donor area examination is equally important. Patient must have realistic expectation. They must understand to expect results by the end of 1 year and look more natural over a period of time.

Important Surgical Considerations[23,25-27]

- The anatomic variations of hair direction and density to be considered while designing.
- The donor area chosen is parietal rather than mid-occipital part of scalp and if it is for moustache or small beard zone, beard area (under chin) itself can be a site for donor harvest if the patient is willing.
- Choice of graft harvest technique can be strip for larger reconstructions and FUE for smaller number of harvest. Whatever may be number of grafts most of the patients desire FUE technique.
- The important areas are sideburns and the cheek in the lateral view. The total number of grafts for sideburn is 150 to 200 per side. The margin must have single hair and end of side lock must be broad in men and pointed like tail in women. Density 40 to 44 FU/cm^2 in males and 20 to 30 FU/cm^2 in females. The density must be more in upper part of the sideburn as it will have overlapping effect inferiorly and better coverage.
- In the cheek, the slits are directed laterally and downward, the borders are restored with less density with single-hair grafts to give hazy margins. The center of cheek must have good density with 1 and 2 HF units. It requires 500 to 600 grafts on each side. The jawline beard is constructed similar to sideburns, with more density on top to cover the inferior zones.

- The moustache and goatee requires a higher number of grafts compared to the lateral aspects. The moustache needs 400 to 500 grafts, with around 35 to 40 FU/cm^2 of density. The hairs are directed downward, sagittal slits are preferred with slightly higher density in the upper part to have overlapping effect on lower part, so that it can be packed with lesser density. The goatee requires 600 to 700 grafts. The slits are directed inferiorly.

Procedural Steps

- Marking must always be done in sitting position. Ensure symmetry and approval from patient. Most of the beards are designed based on two fixed points, side lock and moustache.
- Donor site selection, marking and preparation. Trim the donor hair, 1 cm for FUE harvest or 2 cm for strip harvest (for large beard and moustache reconstruction).[25]
- Anesthesia: Lignocaine 1% with adrenaline is given as local infiltration for smaller areas or facial blocks are preferred in large areas of transplantation, to ensure painless surgery.
- Tumescence: The advantage of tumescence anesthesia is hemostasis and to keep area taut. Intradermal tumescence is injected in insulin syringes 10 to 15 minutes before surgery. Adequate stretching with plain saline can taut the lax facial tissue and ease the surgery.[23]
- Graft harvest and preparation: Donor anesthesia, techniques of graft harvest, storage of grafts is similar to FUE/strip technique. Strip size is calculated based on number of grafts required; the dissected grafts must be slim grafts with minimal epidermis. The FUE grafts must be parred if they are multifollicular units to have single and 2 FU grafts.
- The density must be 40 to 45 grafts with upper margin of beard to be reconstructed with only single hairs and dense pack in the center to simulate the natural beard. Direction of implantation must follow the direction of existing hair or inferior posteriorly at more acute angle. In moustache, dense packing at center and around philtrum is desired.
- Stick and place method or premade slits can be employed. Author prefers premade slits for larger areas and sticks and place method for smaller areas and also in areas like sideburns and margins. Select 21G hypodermic needle for single follicle and 20G for 2 hairs.
- The needle held in left hand is pierced at acute angle to a depth of 3 to 4 mm and grafts are held with a traumatic jewellers forceps to insert grafts by stick and place method.
- In premade slit, select 1 mm slit and make acute angle slits with 40 to 45 FU/sq cm^2 of density. The grafts are inserted by 2 jeweller forceps method by authors no touch technique. The slits are dilated with left hand forceps and grafts held at the epidermis in right hand forceps are slided into slits without touching bulb or bulge of follicle.
- The grafts are fixed and author prefers open dressings.

Postoperative Measures

- The patient sprays the normal saline for 48 hours every 2 to 4 hours. Few authors suggest closed dressing with antibiotic application which has to be removed on day 3. This avoids accidental removal of grafts by scratching. This is followed by washing with a less harsh low-pH liquid soap and cold water.
- The broad spectrum antibiotics and anti-inflammatory drugs are given.
- The patient must take soft liquid diet to avoid pain and graft displacement.
- Avoid brushing and can use fingers rolled in gauze piece for cleaning the teeth and mouthwash rinse for 48 hours.
- Postsurgery minoxidil should be started after 2 weeks.

Results

Results from beard and moustache transplantation (Figs. 27.5 to 27.7) can be seen in as little as 3 months and complete results at the end of 1 year.

Complications

- Graft dislodgement.
- Esthetic complications like variation in angle and directions, tenting or bumpy look and mismatch of hairs.
- Infection and poor results.

Tips to Optimize Results

- Remember the anatomic considerations of beard hair and other facial hair.
- In mobile areas popping can be more; immobility is established by keeping gauze on inner aspect of lips.
- The grafts must be slim and distribute singles on borders for more natural look and 2 hair follicular units and dense packing in the center of moustache.

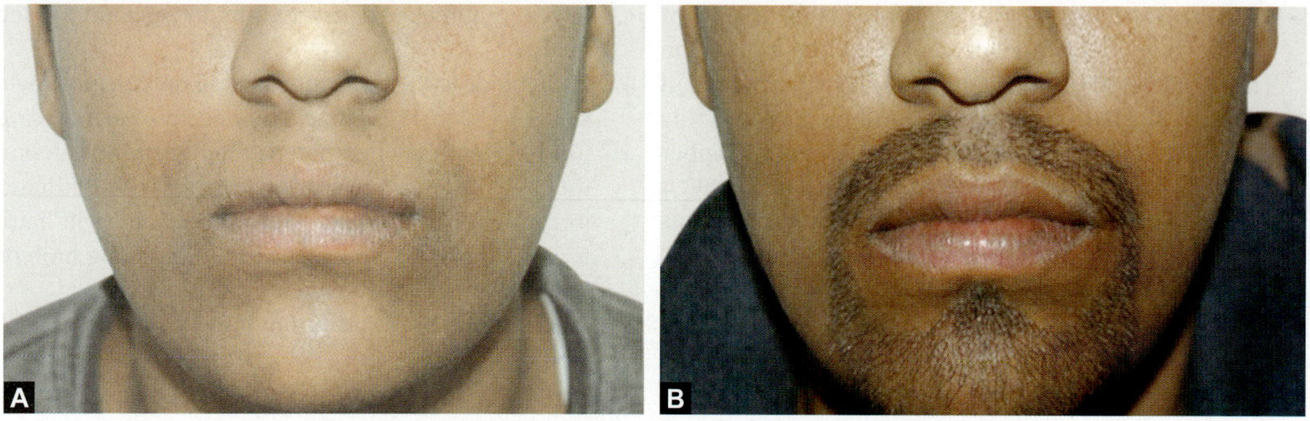

Figs. 27.5A and B: Complete beard and moustache reconstruction with 2125 grafts.
Courtesy: Cutis Academy, Bengaluru, Karnataka, India

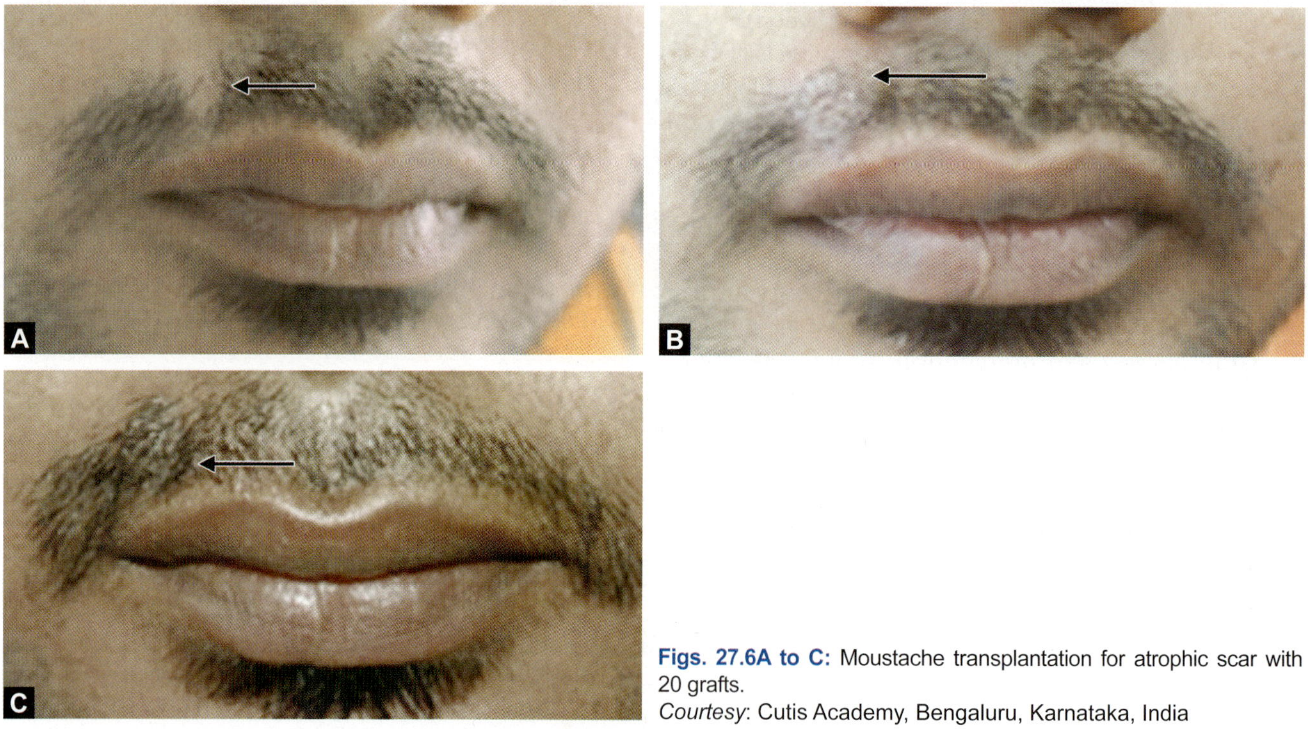

Figs. 27.6A to C: Moustache transplantation for atrophic scar with 20 grafts.
Courtesy: Cutis Academy, Bengaluru, Karnataka, India

- Place the grafts more parallel along direction of existing hairs.
- Use lesser gauge hypodermic needle while placing grafts at more acute angle, the needle can be bent slightly to ease the job of slit making at more acute angle.
- Use single hair grafts on margins and 1- or 2-hair grafts over the other areas, and 2 and 3 at the center. If the diameter of the scalp hair is much thinner than the beard hair, then it is highly recommended to transplant 2-hair FU grafts or paired FU.
- Author prefers lower densities in areas of cicatricial alopecia.

EYEBROW TRANSPLANTATION

Eyebrow Anatomy

The outcome of eyebrow transplantation depends on the knowledge about the anatomy of the eyebrow and ability of the surgeon to maintain the direction, angle of hair

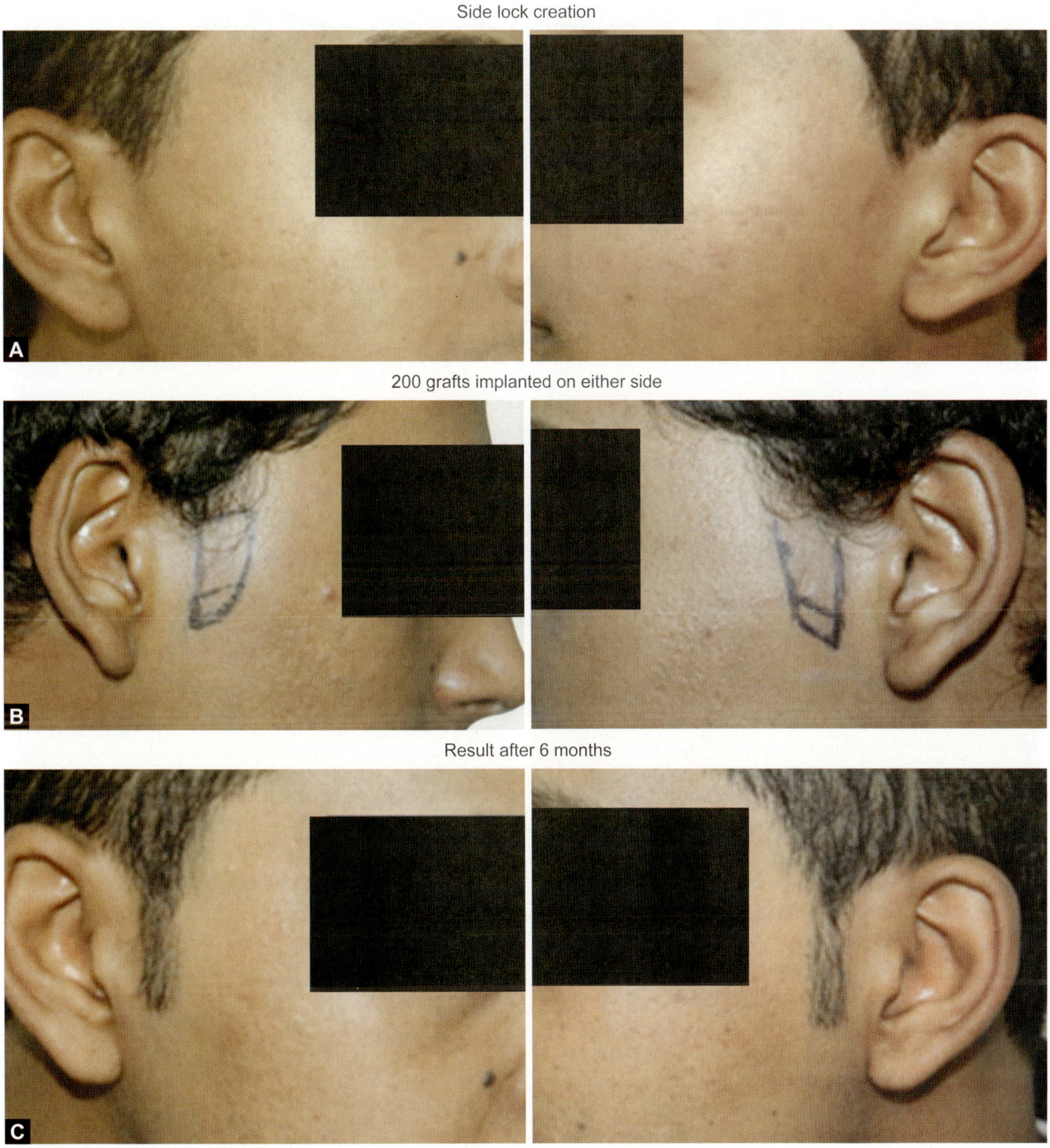

Figs. 27.7A to C: Side lock creation.
Courtesy: Cutis Academy, Bengaluru, Karnataka, India

to give a more natural look.[28] The shape of the eyebrow in Asian men and women are not much different. Men appear to have wider eyebrows than women.[28a] Women's eyebrows are located little higher over the orbital rim and arch into a C shape, while men's eyebrows are at slightly lower position, are straighter, and have a T shape as in Figures 27.8A and B.

While subtle variations occur between men and women certain generalities may be made about size and shape. Each eyebrow measures about 4.5 to 5.5 cm. Each

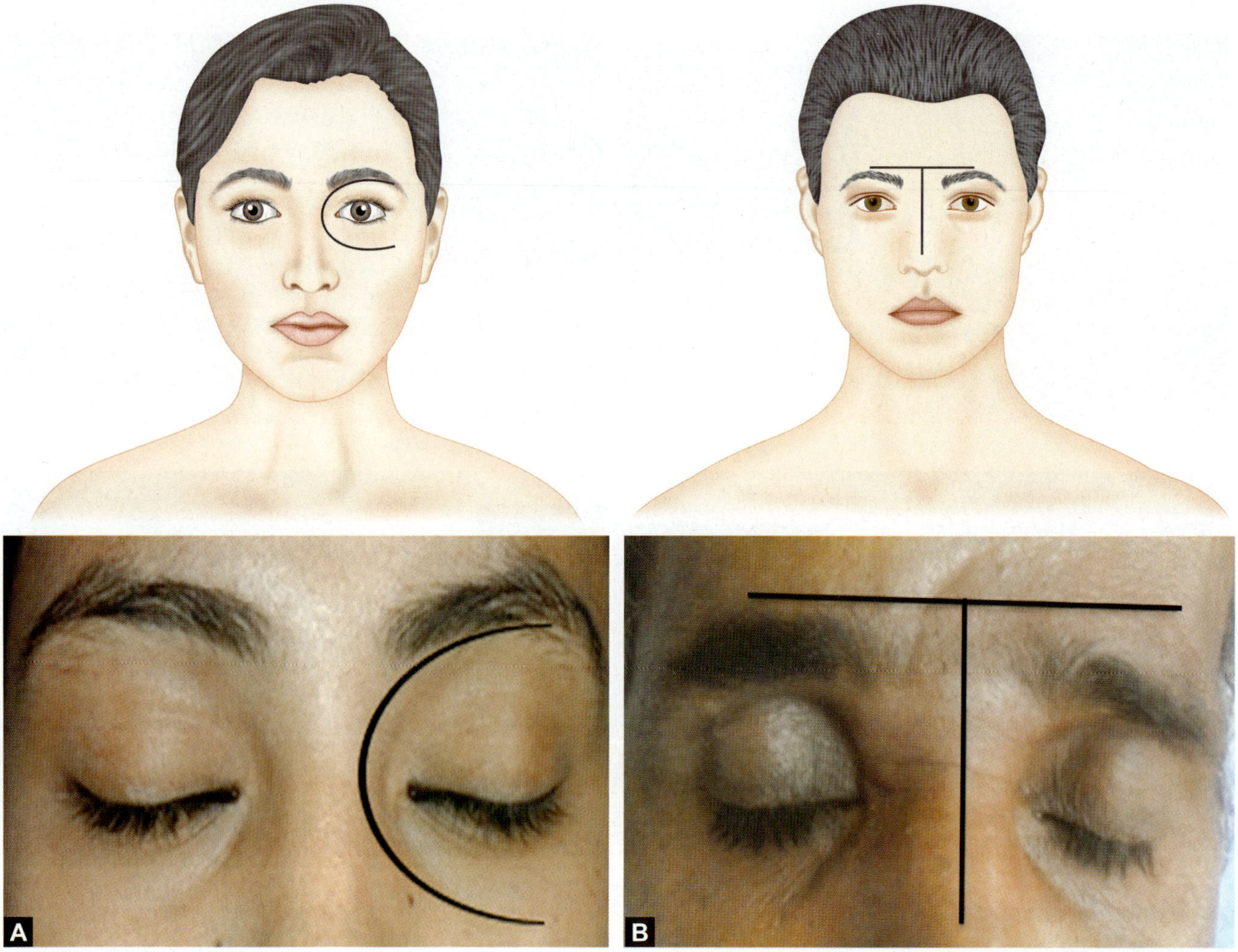

Figs. 27.8A and B: C shape arched female eyebrow placed little higher and staighter male eyebrow placed at little lower level.

eyebrow is divided into three parts—(a) medial head, (b) middle body, and (c) lateral tail (Fig. 27.9).

Medial head: Head part measures about 0.5 to 1 cm in length and is located 1 to 1.5 cm lateral and cephalic to the central glabella. It generally has vertical or rounded medial border.

Middle body: It is approximately 2.5 cm. It is the area of maximum density. Being the widest part of the eyebrow it gives prominent appearance to eyebrows. It has a flat lower border in the medial part which then changes in cephalic direction to give an arch. At the same time it narrows in the lateral part which is more pronounced in females than in males. In some males this narrowing may not happen and it may remain as the widest part of the eyebrow.

Lateral tail: It is approximately 1 cm long, it extends laterally and downwards caudally as it descends down from peak of arch. It is the narrowest part and has the lowest density of hair.

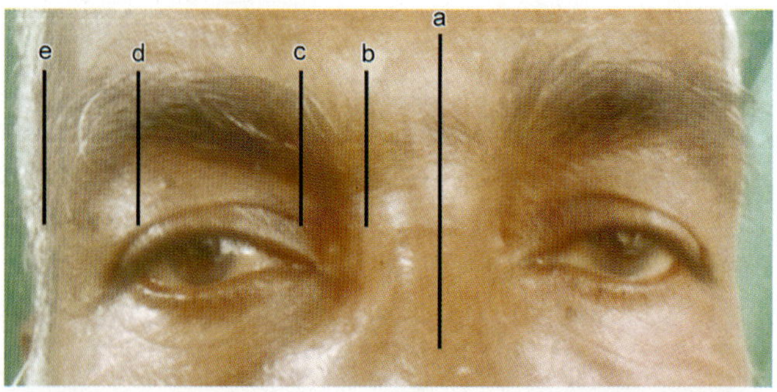

Fig. 27.9: Parts of eyebrow: (a) Central glabella line. (b and c) Medial head. (c and d) Middle body. (d and e) Lateral body.

Indications for Eyebrow Transplantation

The patients seek eyebrow transplantation mainly for the following reasons:[30]

- Scar due to various causes like trauma, surgical wound, acid burns, fire accidents, self inflicted, radiotherapy, etc.

- Madarosis due to various dermatological conditions like Hansen's disease.
- Having uneven eyebrow from lack of lateral third or medial portion of the brow.
- Having congenital absence of eyebrow.
- Those who have normal eyebrow may seek transplantation to get thicker esthetically better eyebrow.

Counseling

Counseling is very important in eyebrow transplantation like any other dermatosurgical procedure. Apart from the general complications patients should be counseled about the necessity of the trimming of the hair as the transplanted hair will continue to grow. After a few years, hair transplants adapt to the recipient site by a mechanism that we call "field effect," as in pubic restoration.[31] The patient must also be informed that the aim of eyebrow restoration is to improve his or her appearance and it is impossible to perfectly reproduce a new natural eyebrow.[29] The patients should also be counseled that they may require two to three sessions to achieve good density as too dense packing transplant to be completed in one session may be technically difficult when transplanting in very acute angle.[29]

The outcome of eyebrow transplantation depends on four important aspects:

- Shape
- Symmetry
- Direction
- Angle.

Perfect shape and symmetry can be achieved with proper planning an eyebrow design.

Planning an eyebrow design when there is complete absence of eyebrow (Fig. 27.10).[29]

While planning a design patient should be placed in sitting position. First point, the midglabellar point is marked. The second point is marked just below the superomedial orbital rim approximately 4 mm medial to the medial canthus. This marks the medial most part of the eyebrow. The third point marked at about 1 cm above the orbital rim between the lateral limbus and lateral canthus. This marks the apex of the eyebrow. The fourth point is the lateral end which is lateral to the rim in the same horizontal plane of the medial brow. The last three points are then joined and then the shape and size of the brow is drawn as described in anatomy section. The average length of each eyebrow to be maintained is at around 5.5 cm. Patient's

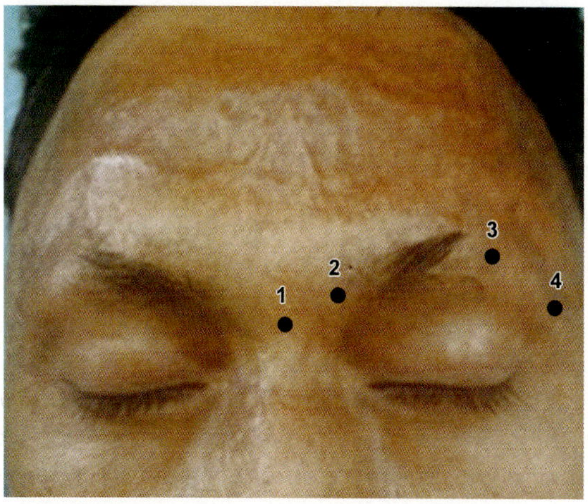

Fig. 27.10: Planning an eyebrow transplant: Point 1—The midglabellar point, Point 2—Just below the superomedial orbital rim approximately 4 mm medial to the medial canthus, Point 3—One cm above the orbital rim between the lateral limbus and lateral canthus, Point 4—Lateral end which is lateral to the rim in the same horizontal plane of the medial brow.

assistance may be taken while marking for better patient satisfaction.

These points must be marked simultaneously on both sides to achieve symmetry.

However when loss of eyebrow is unilateral and incomplete, perfect symmetry can be obtained by drawing the eyebrow on transparent paper, which is then used as a template for the design of a perfectly symmetrical contra-lateral eyebrow.[31]

Donor Area

The donor hair is the scalp, in the occipital area. Sanusi Umar in his case report has suggested that leg hairs can be an alternate donor area in eyebrow transplantation as the leg hair width after transplantation generally approximates eyebrow hair caliber. He also states that this gives better match than traditional head donor-sourced hair because of its finer quality and shorter length and reduced frequency of trimming. The same author has also used forearm, and nape of the neck as donor areas.[32] Leg donor areas were pretreated with 5% minoxidil for 3 months before surgery to induce anagen phase and then shaved 10 days before surgery to better identify late-phase anagen hair.

Extraction

In scalp follicular unit extraction is performed under tumescent anesthesia. However for leg the author has done under local anesthesia using subcutaneous injections of epinephrine (1:100,000) and lidocaine 1%, and bupivacaine hydrochloride 0.25%, without tumescence.

Grafts are obtained using 0.8 mm titanium punches in a FUE micromotor machine. Grafts should be extracted with minimal damage and micrografts of single hair are dissected using magnifying loupes.

Implantation

The micrografts prepared so are transplanted microsurgically into an incision prepared for it by using of a needle bayonet of 18/19G. This needle is extremely handy. Though preformed slits using various instruments are used by various dermatosurgeons the author prefers prick and place method using 18G needle as it simplifies and speeds up the creation of the microincision.

It overcomes the main difficulty of reproducing the very acute angle between the hair-stem and the skin.[31]

This needle can be inserted virtually flat to the skin easily, mimicking the original anatomy at the same time shortening the operative time. On average, 100 to 300 follicular unit grafts are transplanted microsurgically.

Direction of Implantation (Figs. 27.11A and B)

In the medial most part of the eyebrow the hairs remain vertical. In this area follicles are placed sparsely in a fanning fashion to reproduce natural look and as we move laterally they tend to become parallel to the long axis of the eyebrow. In the middle part hairs are implanted in a converging pattern so that the hairs in the upper part are directed downwards and laterally and lower part of hair directed upwards and laterally so together they form a crisscross pattern. Middle part of the eyebrow is packed densely to give prominent eyebrow. In the lateral most part finer hairs are implanted in a progressively sparse density. Lower lateral part is feathered to give natural soft appearance.

Postoperative Care

- Routine antibiotics and analgesics to be given.
- Saline sprays to be continued every 2 hours to prevent drying of follicles and to prevent crust formation.
- Protective glasses are recommended for the first night to prevent dislodging of grafts, especially during sleep.[33]
- Careful washing of face can be recommended after 3 days.

Complications

Bruise, crusting and swelling usually last for 3 to 4 days.

Course

Bruise edema will subside by 3 to 5 days. Crusts will fall off by a week. Most of the eyebrow transplants do not shed and continued to grow in contrast to the scalp hairs and need trimming once a week. About 90 to 94% of transplanted hairs will grow back with high patient satisfaction.

Tips

- When transplantation is planned for dermatological conditions like alopecia areata, trichotillomania, the disease must be quiescent for at least six months (authors preference), as the active disease may interfere with follicle uptake.
- If partial eyebrow transplantation is planned for scarred area, pretreatment with intralesional steroids is required

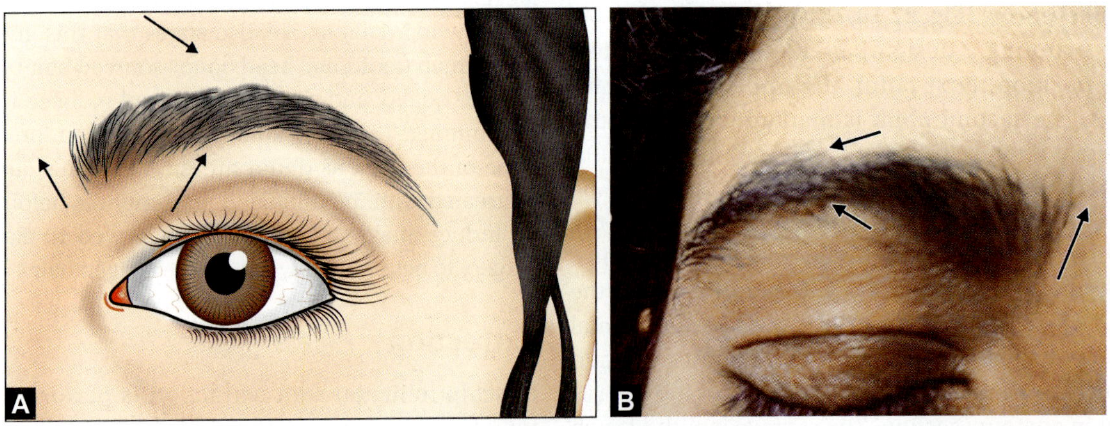

Figs. 27.11A and B: Showing direction of hair. In the medial part hairs remain vertical, in the middle they become parallel to long axis and arranged in crisscross pattern, lateral part has progressively sparse density.

for hypertrophic scars if any. Pretransplant platelet-rich plasma for scar may improve scar bed and improve graft survival.

- Proper designing with due attention given to symmetry, shape direction and angle of the hair enhances natural appearance.
- While planning subtle variation between male and female eyebrow to be kept in mind.
- The patient should be allowed to look in the mirror upon completion to see if adjustment is needed and consent can be taken for the same.
- If the patient has already tattooed it can be retained to give additional camouflage effect.
- Around 300 to 400 follicles may be needed for each eyebrow.
- Single follicles dissected should be transplanted.
- Transplanted follicles should match the quality of eyebrow as much as possible. Nape of the neck or retroauricular area may be the preferred site.
- Follicles should be handled gently during the procedure with jewellers forceps. Alternatively implanters can be used.
- Postoperative care as described earlier should be strictly followed for maximum benefit.

Results

Results of eyebrow transplantation is shown in Figures 27.12 to 27.14.

EYELASH TRANSPLANTATION

Eyelid anatomy in relation to eyelash transplantation (Fig. 27.15)

The lid margin is about 2 mm broad and is divided into two parts by punctum. The medial, lacrimal portion is rounded and devoid of lashes or glands. The lateral, ciliary portion consist of rounded anterior border, a sharp posterior border and an intermarginal strip. Eyelashes are present in this intermarginal strip. A normal upper eyelid contains about 100 lashes, the lower eyelid about 60 lashes.

Indications

Loss of eyelash due to any of the following causes:

- Alopecia areata
- Trichotillomania
- Lupus erythematosus
- Trauma.
- Blepharitis
- Eyelid surgery
- Thyroid disease
- Ectodermal dysplasia
- Radiation/chemotherapy
- Sparse eyelashes for cosmetic enhancement
- Vitiligo with leukotrichia of eyelashes.[34]

Counseling

As in eyebrow transplantation patient should be counseled about need for continuous trimming of lashes and during

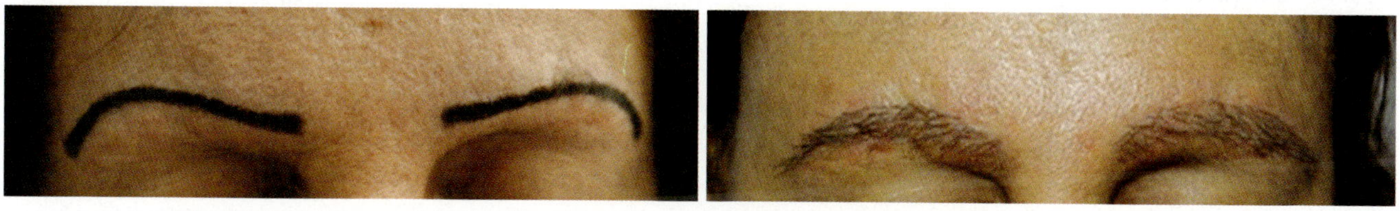

Fig. 27.12: A 22-year-old lady after complete reconstruction of eyebrow with 250 grafts on each side.
Courtesy: Cutis Academy, Bengaluru, Karnataka, India

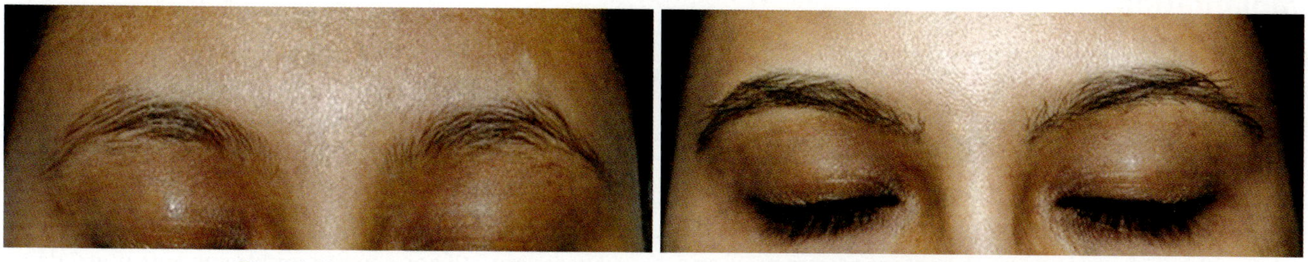

Fig. 27.13: Complete cosmetic enhancement of eyebrow with 150 grafts on each side.
Courtesy: Cutis Academy, Bengaluru, Karnataka, India

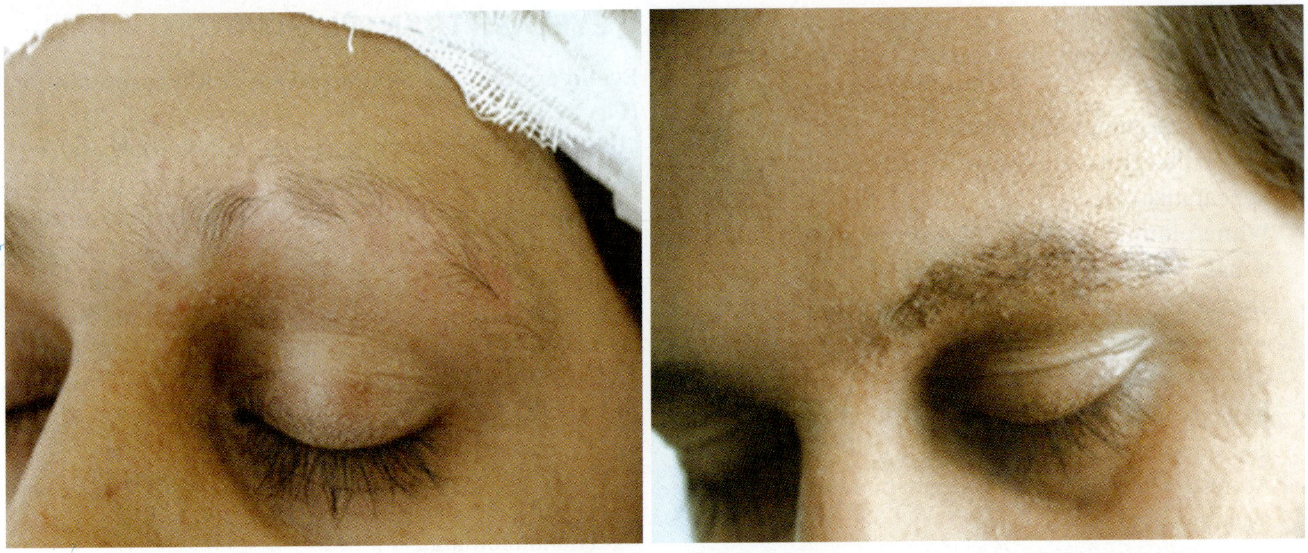

Fig. 27.14: A 25-year-old-male, chronic alopecia areata, after eyebrow transplant by strip harvest with 200 grafts. *Courtesy*: Cutis Academy, Bengaluru, Karnataka, India

the growing period lashes should be curled and directed upwards using eyelash curlers.

Preoperative Evaluation

Apart from the routine investigations done for all surgery, evaluation that are specific to eyelash transplantation include thyroid levels, psychiatric evaluation to rule out body dysmorphic disorders especially when eyelash transplantation is done for cosmetic enhancement. Any active disease like vitiligo, trichotillomania, alopecia areata must be stabilized before surgery.

Donor Area

Occipital area of the scalp is the preferred donor site. Umer has used leg hair as the donor site for eyelash transplantation. As in eyebrow it requires less frequent trimming of lashes when leg is the donor site.[35] Extraction and harvesting is similar to eyebrow transplantation.

Implantation

Cornea is anesthetized using topical lignocaine preparation followed by application of corneal shield. The micrografts (single hair) prepared are implanted in a fanning pattern using stick and place method with 20G needle and jewellers forceps (Figs. 27.16A to D). Some surgeons prefer to use suturing needle with follicle passed into the eye of needle to insert the grafts.[36] However, the author prefers prick and place technique.

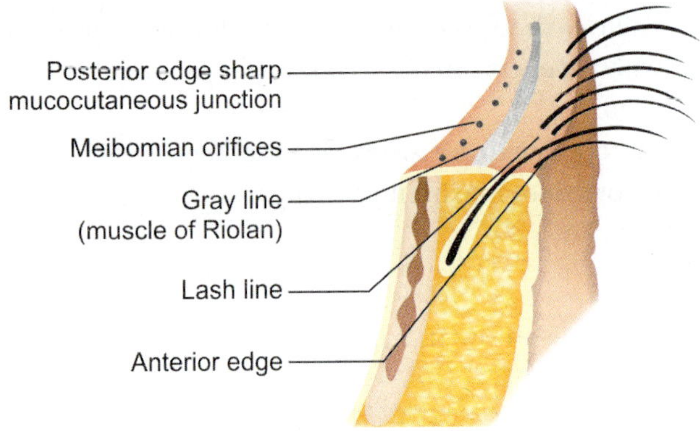

Fig. 27.15: Eyelid anatomy.

Postoperative Care

- Antibiotics, analgesics and steroid (to reduce lid edema) to be.
- Regular saline spray every two hours to prevent drying of grafts and crust formation for first 2 to 3 days. Thin layer of ophthalmic eye ointment can be applied in the night.[37]
- Protective goggles may be worn while sleeping for the first 2 nights to prevent dislodging of grafts.[38]
- Gentle facewash can be started after 48 hours. But care should be taken not to rub the follicles which may dislodge the follicle. Gently pat dry. Regular washing can be started after 7 days.
- Avoid contact lens use for a week.
- Excess crust, if any can be gently wiped off after 7 days.
- Eyelash make up can be used only after 2 weeks.

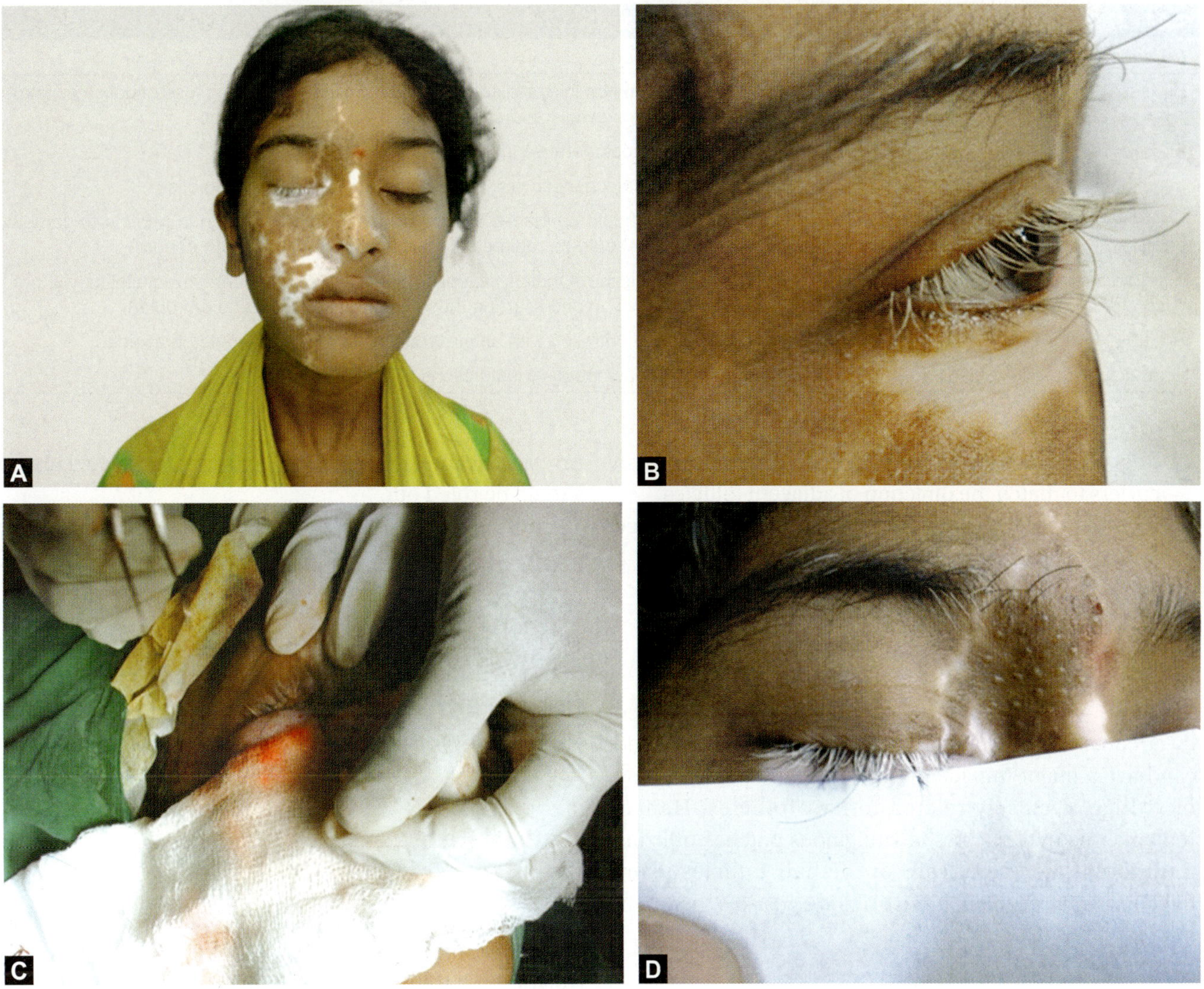

Figs. 27.16A to D: Eyelash transplantation for leukotrichia correction showing prick and place technique.

Complications

Complications and to tips to avoid has been tabulated below (Table 27.2).

Course

The transplanted hair may fall off in next to 2 to 3 weeks. And they grow back normally in next 3 to 4 months. Around 90% of the transplanted hair will regrow if done meticulously.

Tips for Eyelash Transplantation

- When transplantation is planned for dermatological conditions like vitiligo, alopecia areata, trichotillomania, the disease activity must be controlled as the active disease may compromise the outcome.
- Around 60 follicles may be needed for each eyelid.
- Single follicles dissected should be transplanted.
- Transplanted follicles should match the quality of eyelashes as much as possible. Postauricular area may be the preferred site.
- Follicles should be handled gently during the procedure with jewellers forceps. Alternatively implanters can be used.
- Care should be taken to avoid chlorhexidine antiseptics as it can damage cornea.[36]
- Postoperative care as described earlier should be strictly followed for maximum benefit.

Table 27.2: Complications and tips to avoid in eyelash transplantation.

Complications	*Prevention*
Bruise	Very common in eyelid surgeries. Gentle tissue handling, use of delicate instruments like jewellers forceps, avoid using toothed forceps
Edema	Use of postoperative steroids will prevent edema
Infection or stye	Follow strict aseptic precautions and postoperative antibiotics
Formation, trichiasis,[39] corneal punctate epitheliopathy[40]	Grafts should be placed in proper location and direction in relation to cornea. Lashes should be redirected using curlers during growth period
Ectropion, entropion	Gentle tissue handling, aseptic precautions postoperative antibiotics will prevent infection and scarring thus avoiding ectropion and entropion
Pruritus	Can be controlled with antihistamines. Scratching should be avoided
Graft displacement	Follow postoperative instructions given previously in text

- Regrowing lashes should be curled using eyelash curlers to match the direction of adjacent follicles.
- Intervention in the inferior eyelid is not recommended due to a high incidence of postoperative trichiasis.[36]

FOLLICULAR UNIT EXTRACTION (FUE) FOR VITILIGO

Vitiligo is an acquired, idiopathic disorder characterized by circumscribed depigmented macules and patches and can have a major impact on personality. Repigmentation of vitiligo is closely related to hair follicles. Hence, replenishing melanocytes in vitiliginous patches utilizing undifferentiated stem cells of the hair follicles using follicular unit transplantation (FUT) is a possible treatment option.[41]

Principle

Vitiligo causes a partial or total destruction of melanocytes, initially only of the epidermis and later even of the hair follicles known as leukotrichia. Repigmentation can be achieved by either activating the existing melanocyte reservoir or providing a melanocyte reservoir as a source for pigmentation. This forms the underlying principle for various treatment modalities available today. Follicular unit transplantation (FUT) is one such surgical technique that relies on providing a reservoir of undifferentiated stem cells to the depigmented lesional skin.[42]

Procedure

As with any procedure detailed history about the disease such as the site of onset, duration, progression, stability of the disease, and history of medication should be taken. Any significant medical illness contraindicated for surgery should be ruled out.

Follicular Unit Extraction

Occipital area is the preferred donor site. Extraction will be done under tumescent anesthesia using 0.8 to 1 mm motorized punches. The hair follicles so extracted are stored in Petri dish with cold normal saline or Ringer lactate solution till the transplantation was complete. The hair follicles are transplanted intact as follicular units.

Transplantation

Implantation is done under local anesthesia. The follicles so extracted are transplanted using Kolkata slits/18G needle/ SAVA ®transplanter (Vasa Surgiart Pvt. Ltd., Ahmedabad, Gujarat, India) to create slits in the recipient area and the hair follicle was gently inserted using a jeweller's forceps into the created slits.

Postoperative Care

Recipient area is left open with saline spray every hour for first 3 days to prevent drying of follicles. Phototherapy is advised after 10 days to stimulate pigment spread.

Practical Tips

- Careful selection of patient with stable vitiligo for 12 months.
- This technique is preferred in hairy areas like beard, eyelash, pubic area, extremities, chest in males, etc.
- Number of grafts depends on the area and follicles are transplanted at the gap of 3 to 5 mm.

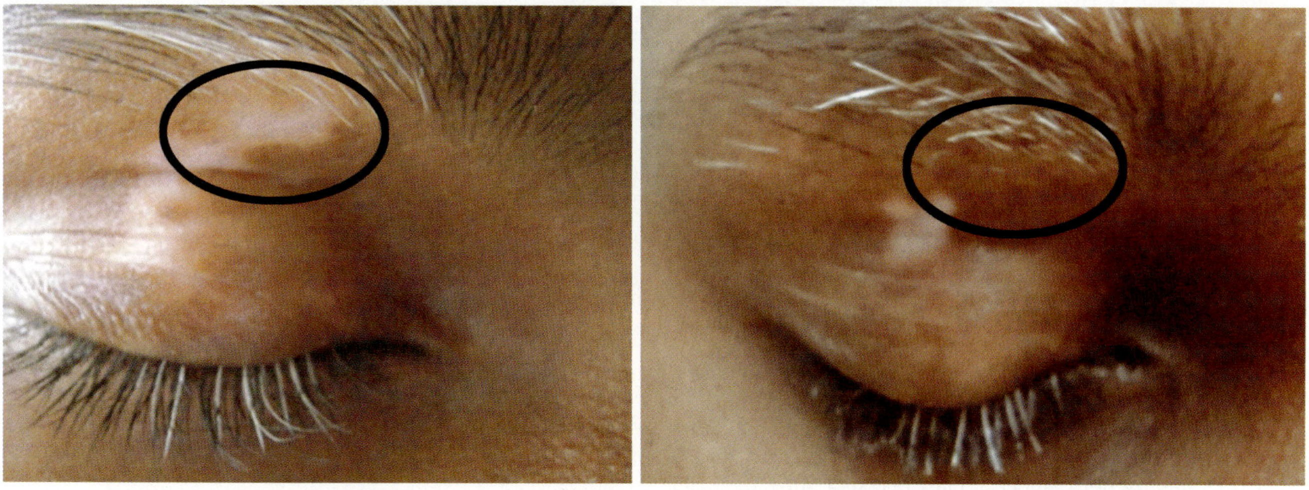

Fig. 27.17: Follicular unit extraction for hairy areas of eyebrow vitiligo.

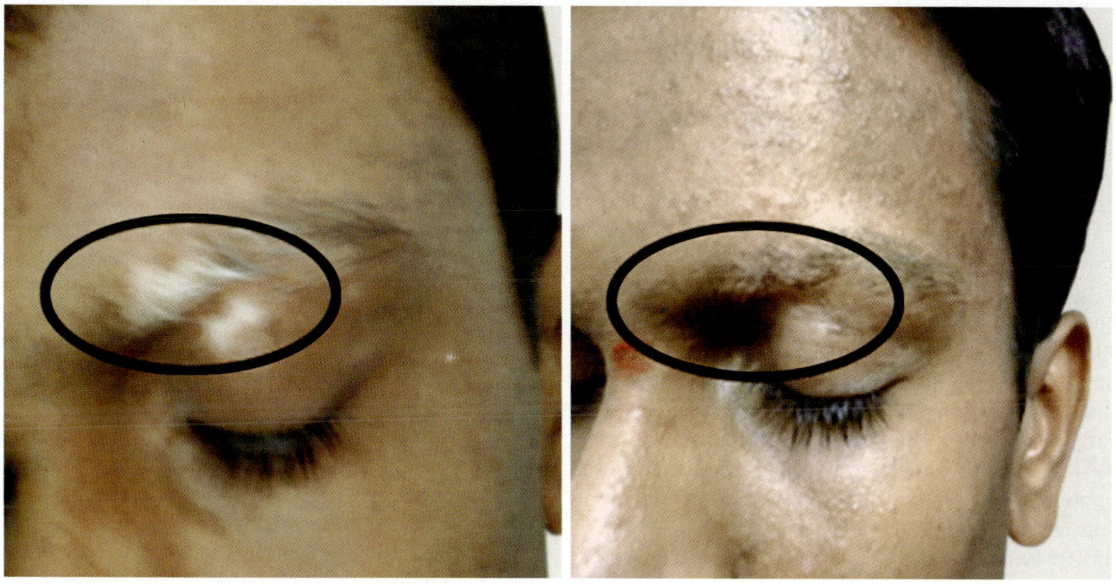

Fig. 27.18: Follicular unit extraction for eyebrow vitiligo.

- Follicles should be stored in cold saline or Ringer lactate solution till completion. Follicles should be handled gently.
- Phototherapy should be started after 10 days of procedure.

Results of FUE for vitiligo in hairy areas are shown in Figures 27.17 and 27.18.

CONCLUSION

To conclude, the number of nonscalp transplantations are increasing. Proper case selection and counseling before can have satisfied results.

REFERENCES

1. Somani N, Bergfeld WF. Cicatricial alopecia: Classification and histopathology. Dermatol Ther. 2008;21(4):221-37.
2. Ross EK, Tan E, Shapiro J. Update on primary cicatricial alopecias. J Am Acad Dermatol. 2005;53:1-37.
3. Kutlubay Z, Kucuktas M, Engin B. Hair transplantation in the cicatricial alopecias. Hair Ther Transplant. 2013;3:109.
4. Rose P, Shapiro R. Transplanting into scar tissue and areas of cicatricial alopecia. In: Unger WP, Shapiro R, (Eds). Hair Transplantation, 4th edn. New York: Marcel Dekker. 2004;606-9.
5. Callender VD, Lawson CN, Onwudiwe OC. Hair transplantation in the surgical treatment of central centrifugal cicatricial alopecia. Dermatol Surg. 2014;40(10):1125-31.

6. Reed ML, Grayson BH. Single follicular unit hair transplantation to correct cleft lip moustache alopecia. Cleft Palate Craniofac J. 2001;38:538-40.
7. Sellheyer KBW. Histopathologic evaluation of alopecias. Am J Dermatopathol. 2006;28:236-59.
8. Headington JT. Cicatricial alopecia. In: Whiting DA (Ed.) Update on Hair Disorders. Philadelphia. Saunders: 1996; 773-82.
9. Harries MJ, Sinclair RD, Macdonald-Hull S, Whiting DA, Griffiths CE, et al. Management of primary cicatricial alopecias: options for treatment. Br J Dermatol. 2008;159:1-22.
10. Kabaker S, Kidel R, Krugman N, Swensen R. Tissue expansion in the treatment of alopecia. Arch Otolaryngol. 1986; 112:720.
11. Barrera A. The use of micrografts and minigrafts for the treatment of burn alopecia. Plast Reconstr Surg. 1999;103: 581-84.
12. Wang SC, Chen FL, Li JY. Soft tissue expansion in the treatment of scar alopecia in preschool children. Chin Med J. 1991;104:164-7.
13. Unger W, Unger R, Wesley C. The surgical treatment of cicatricial alopecia. Dermatol Therapy. 2008;21:295-311.
14. Otberg N, Finner A, Shapiro J. Cicatricial alopecia. In: Avram MR, Rogers NE (Eds). Hair Transplantation. Cambridge Medicine. 2010;53-71.
15. Kwon OS, Kim MH, Park SH, Chung JH, Eun HC et al. Staged hair transplantation in cicatricial alopecia after carbon dioxide laser-assisted scar tissue remodeling. Arch Dermatol. 2007;143:457-60.
16. Unger W, Unger R, Wesley C. The surgical treatment of cicatricial alopecia. Dermatol Ther. 2008;21:295-311.
17. Tyagi V, Singh PK. A new approach to treating scarring alopecia by hair transplantation and topical minoxidil. Indian J Dermatol Venereol Leprol. 2010;76:215.
18. Avram MR, Cole JP, Gandelman M, Haber R, Knudsen R et al. The potential role of minoxidil in the hair transplantation setting. Dermatol Surg. 2002;28:894-900.
19. Capon A, Mordon S. Can thermal lasers promote skin wound healing? Am J Clin Dermatol. 2003;4:1-12.
20. Unger WP. Delineating the "safe" donor area in hair transplanting. J Am Acad Cosmet Surg. 1994;239-43.
21. Cooley J. Complications of hair transplantation. In: Unger WP, Shapiro R (Eds). Hair Transplantation, 4th ed. New York: Marcel Dekker. 2004;573.
22. Moser K, Hugeneck J, Rohrbacher W, Moser C. The pairing technique of the Moser Medical Group. Hair Transpl Forum Int. 2005;15:41-6.
23. Bernstein RB. Follicular unit hair transplantation. In: Robinson JK, Hanke CW, Siegel DM, Fratila A (Eds.). Surgery of the Skin Procedural Dermatology, (2nd edn.), Edinburgh: Mosby Elsevier. 2010;485-512.
24. Dua K, Dua A, Kothottil R. Facial Hair Transplantation in ISHRS Practice Census. 2015;25(4):139-42.
25. Vogt A, McElwee KJ, Blume-Peytavi U. Biology of the hair follicle. In: Blume-Peytavi U, et al. (Eds.). Hair Growth and Disorders. 1.8.7 Duration of the Hair Cycle. Table 1.5, page 13.
26. Pathomvanich D, Imagawa K. Hair restoration surgery in Asians. Part XII. Special procedures in hair restoration surgery: Sideburn transplant and moustache transplant.
27. Gandelman M, Epstein JS. Reconstruction of the sideburn, moustache, and beard. Facial Plast Surg Clin N Am. 2004; 12:253-61.
28. Kulahci M. Moustache and beard hair transplanting. In: Unger W, Shapiro R, (Eds.). Hair Transplantation, 5th edn. New York. 2011;465.
28a. Laorwong K, Pathomvanich D, Bunagan K. Eyebrow transplantation in Asians. Dermatol Surg. 2009;35:496-503.
29. Pathomvanich D. Anatomical restoration surgery of the eyebrow in Asian. The THAI Journal of SURGERY. 2004;25:47-52.
30. Gandelman IM. Patient selection in hair transplantation. Ann Braz Symp Facial Contour. Sao Paulo: Brazil. 1983.
31. Toscani M. Monarca C, Rizzo MI, et al. Eyebrow reconstruction: technical strategies. Aesth Plast Surg. 2011;35: 1189-91.
32. Umar S. Eyebrow transplantation: alternative body sites as a donor source. J Am Acad Dermatol. 2014;71:140-1.
33. Gandelman M. Eyebrow and eyelash transplantation. In: Unger WP, Shapiro R. (Eds.). Hair transplantation. New York:Marcel Dekker Inc. 1995;294-308.
34. Chatterjee M, Neema S, Vasudevan B, Dabbas D. Eyelash transplantation for the treatment of vitiligo associated eyelash leucotrichia. J Cutan Aesthet Surg. 2016;9:97-100.
35. Umar S. Eyelash transplantation using leg hair by follicular unit extraction. Plast Reconstr Surg Glob Open: 2015;3(3) e324.
36. Gandelman M. A technique for reconstruction of eyebrows and eyelashes. Semin Plast Surg. 2005;19(2):154-58.
37. Gandelman M, Epstein JS. Hair transplantation to the eyebrow, eyelashes, and other parts of the body. In: Epstein JS (Ed). Facial Plastic Surgery Clinics of North America. Philadelphia: Elsevier Saunders. 2004;253-61.
38. Gandelman M. Eyebrow and eyelash transplantation. In: Unger WP, Shapiro R (Eds.). Hair Transplantation. New York: Marcel Dekker Inc. 1995;294-308.
39. Murchison AP, Wojno TH. Trichiasis after eyelash augmentation with hair follicle transplantation. Ophthal Plast Re-constr Surg. 2007;23(4):323-4.
40. Chaudhry NL, Chaturvedi R, Maino A. Corneal punctate epitheliopathy secondary to trichiasis following eyelash transplantation. Can J Ophthalmol. 2012;47(6):e37.
41. Sacchidanand S, Thakur P, Purohit V, et al. Follicular unit extraction as a therapeutic option for vitiligo. J Cutan Aesthet Surg. 2013;6(4):229-31.
42. Thakur P, Sacchidanand S, Nataraj HV, et al. A study of hair follicular transplantation as a treatment option for vitiligo. J Cutan Aesthet Surg. 2015;8(4):211-7.

CHAPTER 28

Eyelash Transplantation

Manas Chatterjee, Shekhar Neema

INTRODUCTION

Leukotrichia of eyelash is a disfiguring disease and is commonly associated with segmental vitiligo. Surgical management of vitiligo leads to repigmentation only of the cutaneous lesions. Eyelash leukotrichia does not respond to medical or usual surgical therapies done. Eyelash transplantation is a therapeutic option for eyelash leukotrichia and loss of eyelash due to other causes.

Eyelash transplantation is a procedure in which hair follicle from scalp is implanted on eyelids. It can be done to correct leukotrichic lashes or to provide lost eyelashes due to various causes.

ANATOMICAL CONSIDERATIONS

Eyelashes number about 100 in upper eyelid and 50–60 in the lower eyelids. The eyelash follicles lie in a space between the pretarsal orbicularis and the muscle of Riolan, which lie in front of tarsal plates and seen as 'grey line'. Sebaceous glands of Zeis empty into each eyelash follicle. Apocrine glands of Moll empty into the lumen of each follicle, into a sebaceous gland, or onto the eyelid margin proper. The cilia emerge from the skin at angles. The angle of the original eyelashes is important in planning the angle of the transplanted lashes.

INDICATIONS

- Loss of eyelashes due to injury, trichotillomania, alopecia areata.
- Leucotrichia of eyelashes.

CONTRAINDICATIONS

- Alopecia areata (active disease)
- Active blepharitis
- Untreated trichotillomania.

TYPES

- *Reconstructive*: For correction of loss due to injury, disease, iatrogenic alopecia, congenital atrichia, tricho-tillomania, alopecia areata (2 years postremission)
- *Aesthetic*: For leucotrichia of eyelash.

TECHNIQUES

There are different techniques which have been utilized by various authors for eyelash transplantation. These techniques are as below:[1-5]

- Follicular unit grafting
- Double follicular unit grafting
- Single hair micrografting using the 'sewing technique' or 'Choi/KNU implanter'
- Single hair micrografting using eyebrow hair.

PROCEDURE

Steps which are utilized for management of eyelash transplant are as follows:

- *Mild sedation*: Using tab diazepam 10 mg per oral half an hour prior to starting of procedure.
- Local anesthesia is administered in donor and recipient site with 1% lignocaine with adrenaline (Fig. 28.1).
- *Donor site*: Temporal area is prepared by clipping of hairs.
- Strip is harvested and single hair follicles are chosen for transplant, alternatively one can use FUE motor and using 0.8 mm punch, harvest single unit follicle as desired.
- Infiltration anesthesia is administered in donor area using 2% lignocaine with adrenaline.
- The involved eyelashes are removed with 20 gauge needle similar to creation of chambers for hair transplantation of the scalp (Figs. 28.2 and 28.3).
- Black hair obtained from the temporal scalp of the patient was harvested as in hair replacement surgery

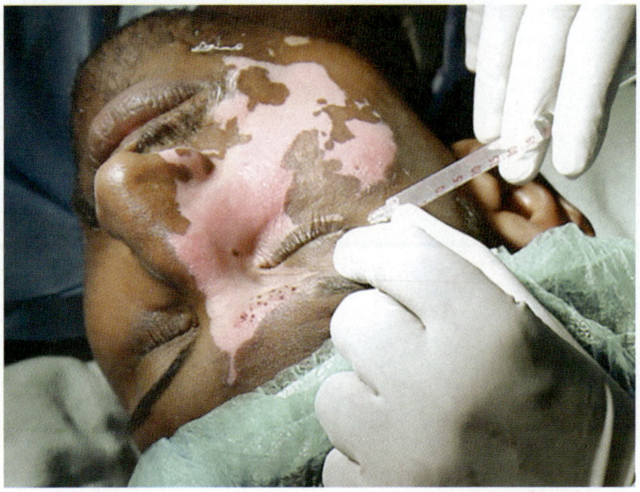

Fig. 28.1: Infiltration anesthesia in donor area using 2% xylocaine and adrenaline.

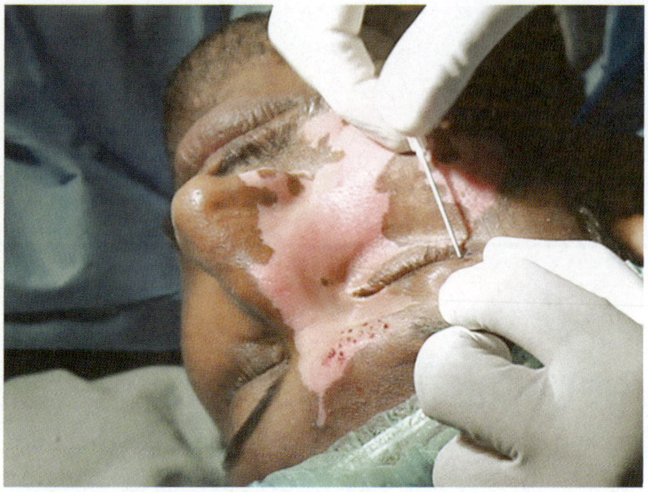

Fig. 28.2: Chamber creation and removal of leukotrichic eyelashes using 20G needle.

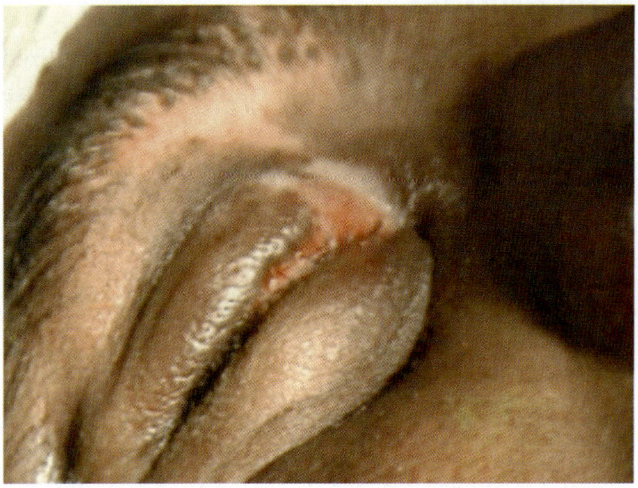

Fig. 28.3: Empty chambers ready for transplantation of eyelash.

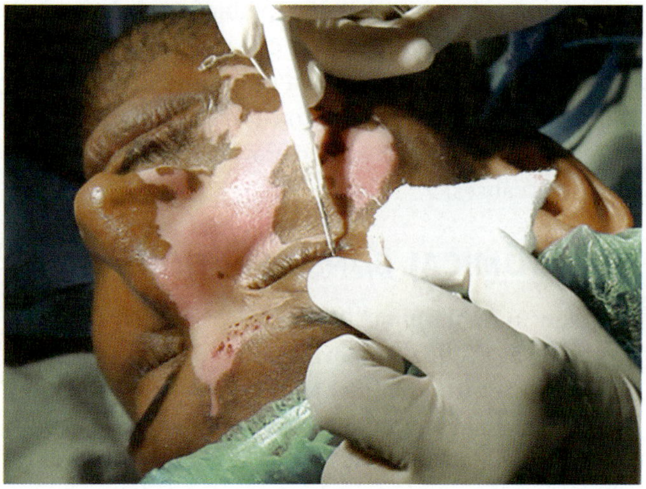

Fig. 28.4: Implantation of hair in empty chambers using Choi implanter.

and single hair grafted onto the chambers created, using fine Jeweler's forceps or implanter can be used, which is relatively faster (Figs. 28.4 and 28.5).

- Implantation done in one row in a fan-shaped manner.
- 15–20 hair per lash is transplanted in one sitting.
- Lower lid is comparatively more difficult in terms of making chambers/pockets.
- Donor lash trimmed to size of other lashes.
- Thereafter, a pad and bandage applied to the affected eye for a week.
- Follow-up after 3 months.
- Another session can be done once one is comfortable (earliest 2 weeks).

POST-PROCEDURE CARE

- Patient should be informed regarding the transplanted hair initially falling off, before regrowing. Complete results are seen in ten months.
- Prophylactic antibiotics and painkillers should be administered.
- Transplanted scalp hair over eyelashes would require trimming as they grow at a much faster pace of 0.39 mm/day and have a prolonged anagen.
- Maintain curvature with mascara or curling device every 4–6 weeks.
- Protective goggles should be worn while sleeping for several nights.

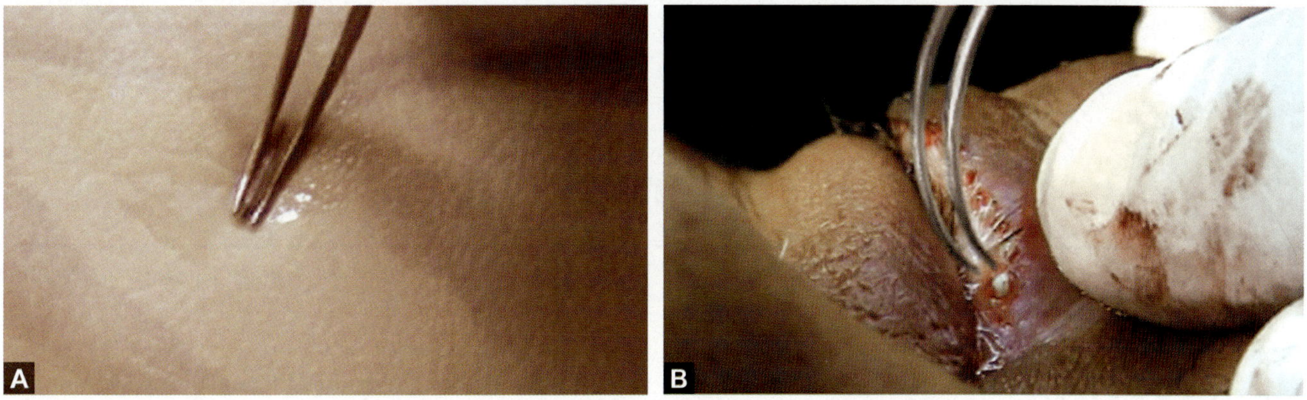

Figs. 28.5A and B: Implantation of eyelashes using forceps.

- Throw away present makeup and purchase new makeup for postoperative use as old makeup harbors bacteria and may lead to postoperative infection.

COMPLICATIONS

- Bruising and swelling may last 1–2 weeks
- Dislodging of grafts due to scratching
- Infection and entropion
- Stye (hordeolum), chalazion cysts
- Penetration and damage to tarsal plate
- Damage to glands of Zeis and Moll
- Damage to marginal artery
- Corneal punctate epitheliopathy.

CONCLUSION

Replacement of the vitiliginous eyelashes involved with leucotrichia with single hair from the patient's scalp seems to be a good therapeutic option in the management of vitiligo involving the eyelashes. Procedure has a steep learning curve and may take about two to three hours.

REFERENCES

1. Gandelman M, Epstein JS. Hair transplantation to the eyebrow, eyelashes, and other parts of the body. Facial Plast Surg Clin North Am. 2004;12:253-61.
2. Straub PM. Replacing facial hair. Facial Plast Surg. 2008; 24:446-52.
3. Caputy GG, Flowers RS. The "pluck and sew" technique of individual hair follicle placement. Plast Reconstr Surg. 1994;93:615-20.
4. Choi YC, Kim JC. Single hair transplantation using the Choi hair transplanter. J Dermatol Surg Oncol. 1992;18:945-8.
5. Kasai K. Eyelash reconstruction with strip composite eyebrow graft. Ann Plast Surg. 2008;60:649-51.

CHAPTER 29

Blepharoplasty

Tolong K, Shekhar Neema

INTRODUCTION

Blepharoplasty is a surgical procedure for reconstruction of the eyelids for functional or cosmetic indications. It is one of the most commonly performed facial surgeries.

INDICATIONS

Usual indications for upper eyelid blepharoplasty are dermatochalasis (loose upper eyelid skin in an older patient) and blepharochalasis (overhanging skin in younger patient). Double eyelid blepharoplasty or Asian blepharoplasty is the commonest upper eyelid blepharoplasty requested in Asia. It is, as the name suggests, the creation of an eyelid crease in a person who does not have a crease, or has an insufficient crease, or unequal height of folds between the two sides (Figs. 29.1A and B). Lower eyelid blepharoplasty is done to correct loose, lax skin below the eyelids and under eye bags.

Symptoms, such as tired looking eyes, excess skin, droopy eyelids, or circles around the eyes may benefit from blepharoplasty.[1]

SURGICAL ANATOMY[2,3]

A sagittal cross-section of the eyelid gives a clear picture of the various tissue layers at different levels. The upper and lower lids are considered analogous structures, with some differences in the arrangement of the eyelid retractor muscles.

For practical purposes, the upper and lower eyelid layers may be divided into the anterior, middle and posterior lamellae. The anterior lamella consists of skin and underlying orbicularis oculi muscle. The orbital septum along with the preaponeurotic fat pad forms the middle lamella, separating the true orbit from the eyelid. The posterior lamella is composed of the tarsal plate, eyelid retractor muscles (levator palpebrae superioris or LPS in the upper eyelid and capsulopalpebral fascia in the lower eyelid) and conjunctiva.

Upper Eyelid Anatomy (Fig. 29.2)

The layers of the upper eyelid from anterior to posterior are:

- *Lower part*: Skin, orbicularis muscle, tarsal plate, conjunctiva.
- *Upper part (above approximately 10 mm)*: Skin, orbicularis, orbital septum, preaponeurotic fat, levator aponeurosis, Muller's muscle, conjunctiva.

The Muller's muscle which lies deeper to the LPS is supplied by the sympathetic nervous system. The orbital septum is a membranous sheet that acts as the anterior boundary of the orbit. It extends from the superior orbital rim to the eyelids and lies beneath the orbicularis. Orbital

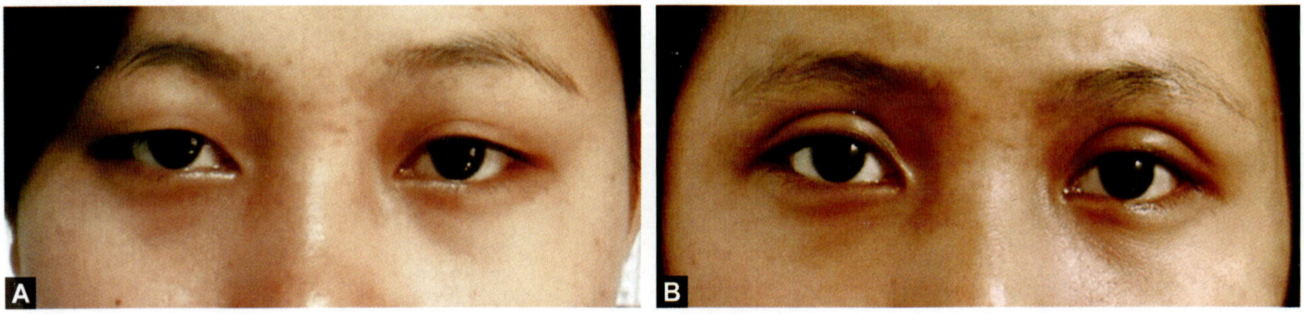

Figs. 29.1A and B: (A) Upper eyelid without crease; (B) Upper eyelid with crease, after double eyelid blepharoplasty or Asian blepharoplasty.

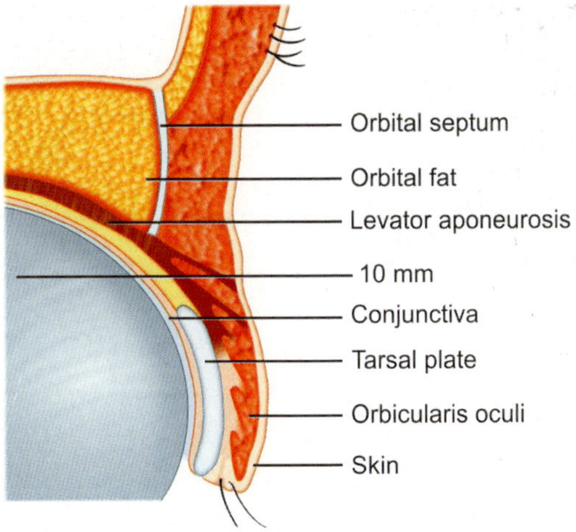

Fig. 29.2: Sagittal cross-section of the upper eyelid depicting the layers at various levels.

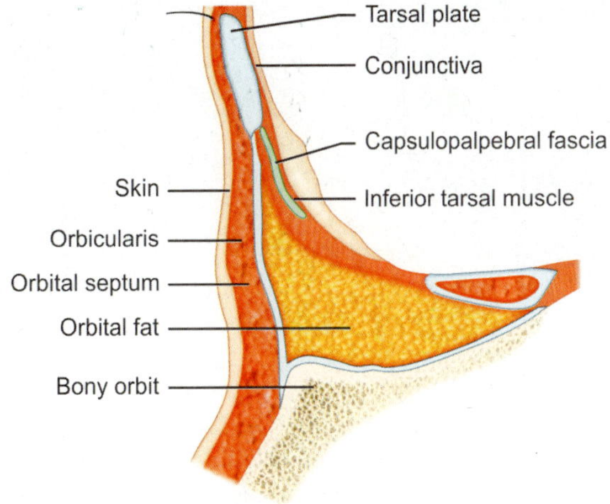

Fig. 29.3: Lower eyelid anatomy depicting various layers at different levels.

septum may weaken with age and allow orbital fat pad to prolapse forward. Tarsal plates are approximately 30 mm long and 10 mm wide centrally in upper eyelid and 5 mm wide in lower eyelid. Conjunctiva covers the sclera and reflects back on inner surface of eyelids, and are firmly adherent to the tarsal plates.

Lower Eyelid Anatomy (Fig. 29.3)

The layers of the lower eyelid encountered form anterior to the posterior are:

- *Upper part*: Skin, orbicularis muscle, lower tarsal plate and the conjunctiva.
- *Lower part*: Skin, orbicularis muscle, orbital septum, orbital fat, capsulopalpebral fascia and finally, the conjunctiva.

PREOPERATIVE CONSULTATION

- *Motivations and expectations of the patient*: This is important as blepharoplasty is often a cosmetic indication. Unrealistic expectations may result in an unhappy patient in spite of a perfect surgery.
- History should be taken regarding current medications (e.g. anticoagulants), major illnesses, past surgery or trauma in the facial area.
- Documentation of informed consent for surgery is essential.
- A thorough examination to rule out asymmetry and laxity of the eyelids as it may affect the outcome of the surgery.
- Ophthalmologic consultation to rule out any visual problem.
- Medical consultation to rule out any underlying systemic disorders like diabetes, hypertension and bleeding disorders.
- Preoperative photographs are important as in any cosmetic procedure.

INSTRUMENTS FOR BLEPHAROPLASTY

Diffent types of instruments used for blepharoplasty are shown in Figure 29.4.

UPPER EYELID BLEPHAROPLASTY[7-9]

Steps in Upper Eyelid Blepharoplasty

- *Marking of eyelids* (Fig. 29.5): Marking of skin redundancy and the incision sites is carried out with the patient sitting upright with eyes in neutral position, at the same level as the surgeon. The first line is the lower aspect of the incision. It usually follows the upper lid crease, 8 to 12 mm above the lid margin at the mid- pupillary line. Upper limit of excision should be at least 10 mm from the superior orbital margin.

  The second line denotes the area of skin that will be resected above eyelid crease. A pair of forceps is used to estimate the amount of skin that can be excised in the medial, central, and lateral eyelid. These points are joined and fused with the previously traced line. The amount and shape of skin excision can be determined by the skin pinch test.[4,5] In this test, the excess upper eyelid skin is grasped by a forceps. The amount or extent of the skin grasped in the forceps is slowly increased

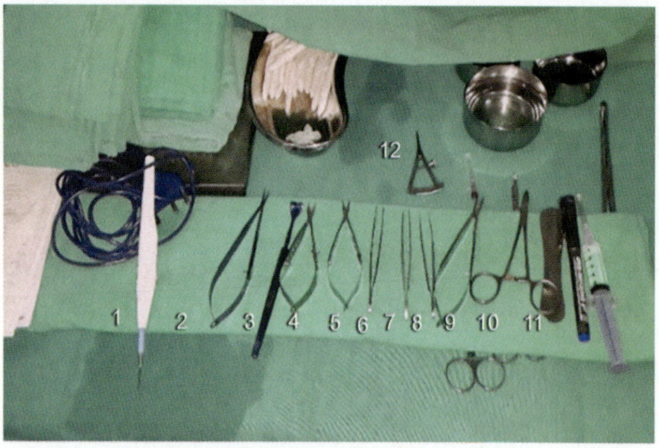

Fig. 29.4: Instruments for Blepharoplasty: 1. Cautery; 2. Barraquer needle holder; 3. Desmarres retractor; 4. and 5. Corneal spring scissors; 6, 7 and 8. Adson forceps—fine teeth; 9. Needle holder; 10. Artery forceps; 11. Lid spatula; 12. Callipers.

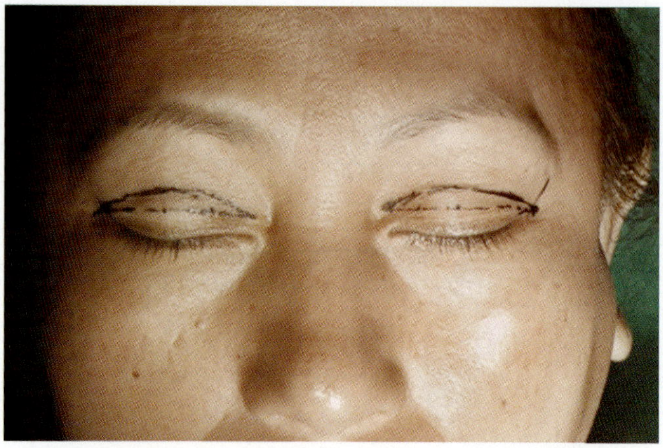

Fig. 29.5: Marking of incision lines with a marking pen.

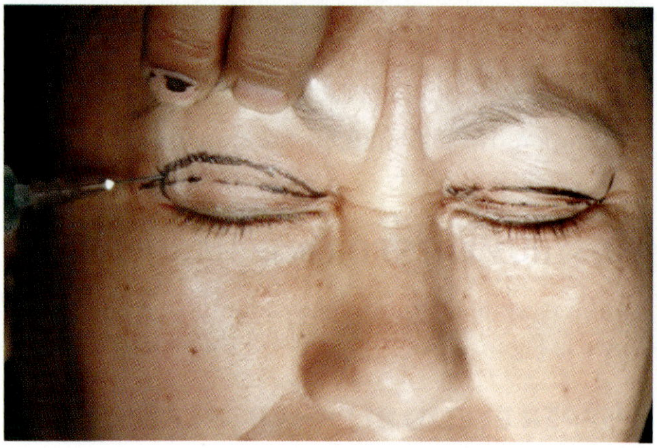

Fig. 29.6: Local anesthesia of upper eyelid.

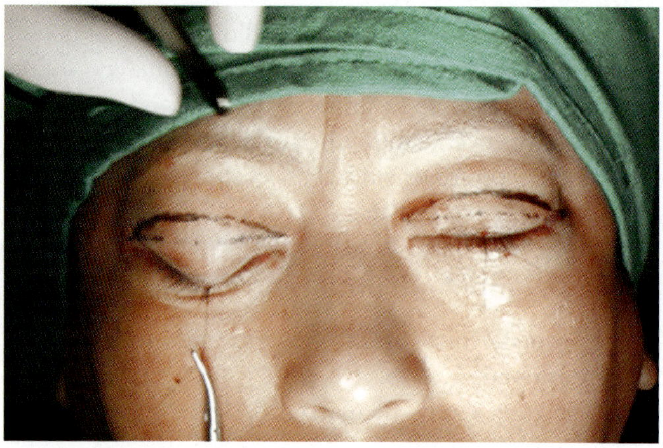

Fig. 29.7: Stay suture held by artery forceps.

till the upper lid margin slightly everts. This amount of skin grasped is then the extent of skin to be excised. A minimum of 20 mm of residual vertical lid height is essential for normal eye closure.[6]

It is important to maintain symmetry in the fold of the eyelid crease. Skin marking should show a gentle medial and lateral upturn. Laterally, the marking is extended to approximately 5 mm above the lateral canthus and then upturned to hide the lateral incision along a skin crease. Incisions should not extend beyond the lateral orbital rim to lessen scarring.

- *Local anesthesia* (Fig. 29.6): After cleaning with povidone-iodine paint, 2–3 mL of xylocaine 2% with epinephrine 1:100,000 should be injected superficially and slowly by a 26 gauge needle.
- *Incision*: Stay sutures (Fig. 29.7) help to stabilize the eyelid while operating. A 4-0 silk suture is taken a few mm away from eyelid margins and the ends are held with artery forceps to stabilize the eyelid during the procedure. Corneal shield (Fig. 29.8)/lid spatula should be used to protect the eye during the surgery.

  Skin incisions can be made either with a no. 15 blade (Fig. 29.9) or the tip of monopolar cautery. Redundant skin is excised using scissor (Fig. 29.10A) or electrocautery. Next we excise a small strip of muscle. Any bleed should be promptly cauterized to reduce bruising and hematoma (Fig. 29.10B).
- *Orbital fat removal* (*not done in all cases*) (Fig. 29.11): By gentle pressure on the globe, the orbital fat is made to protrude, which helps in identifying the septum. Excessive fat, if present can be removed. The septum is incised along its entire length to allow the fat to prolapse. It is then clamped with artery forceps and excised with the help of monopolar cautery.

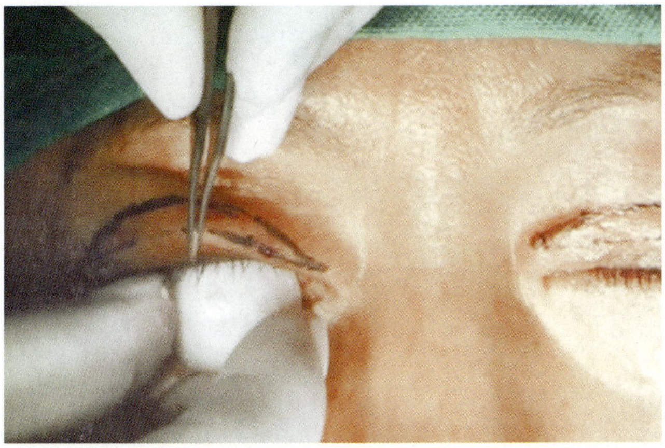

Fig. 29.8: Corneal shield is lubricated with antibiotic ointment and put over the eyeball.

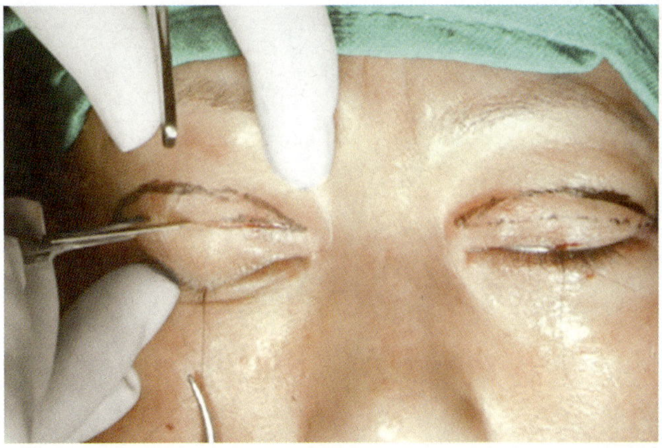

Fig. 29.9: Incision with blade.

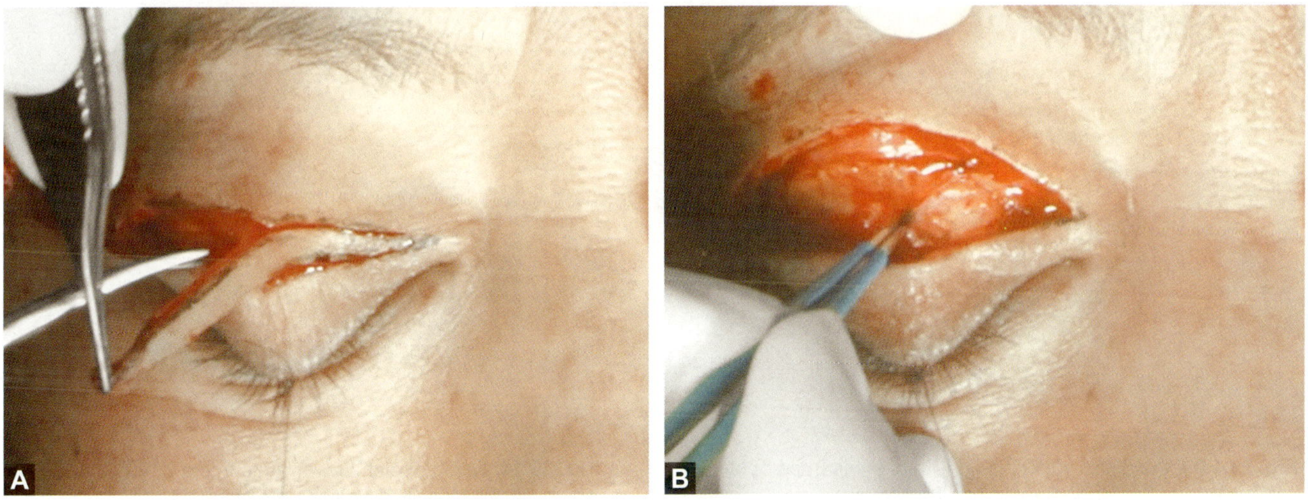

Figs. 29.10A and B: (A) Redundant skin is excised with scissors; (B) Cautery for bleeding points.

- *Suturing*: The skin is closed with 6-0 silk interrupted sutures (Figs. 29.12A and B). Sutures should be removed after five to seven days.

Points for Consideration

- Asymmetry in the upper eyelids is common and should be recognized preoperatively, as also dry eyes, since these symptoms may worsen after upper eyelid blepharoplasty.
- Preoperative evaluation of ptosis of the eyebrows and upper eyelids is also important in order to assess the need for an eyebrow lift or ptosis repair instead of, or in addition to, upper eyelid blepharoplasty.

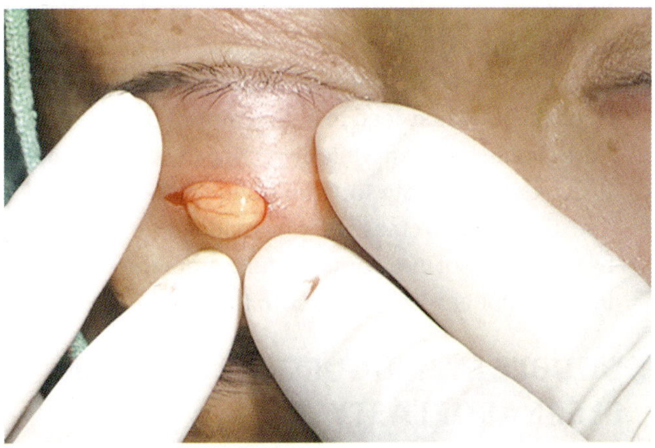

Fig. 29.11: Orbital fat removal.

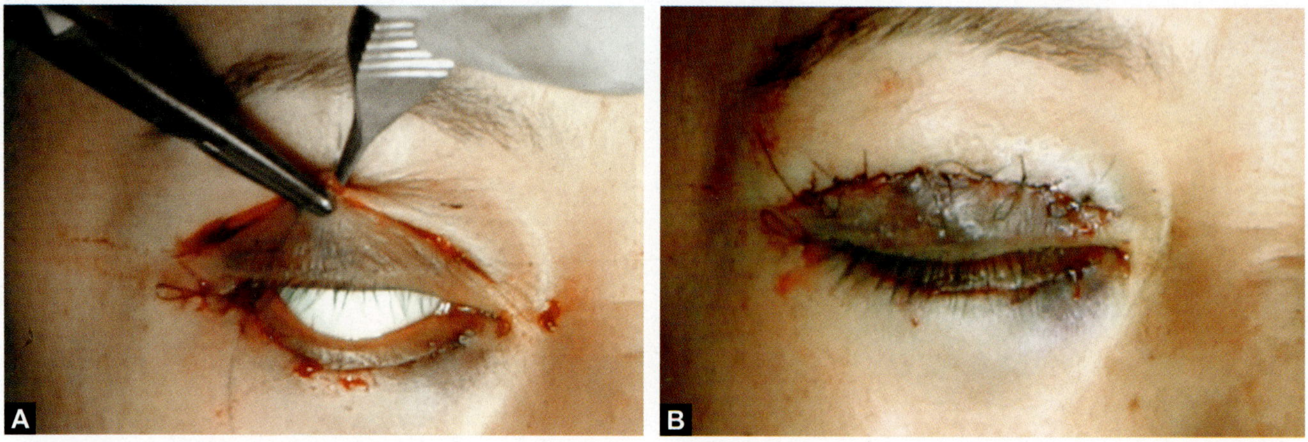

Figs. 29.12A and B: (A) Skin suture; (B) Completed skin suture. Upper eyelid incision has been closed with interrupted sutures.

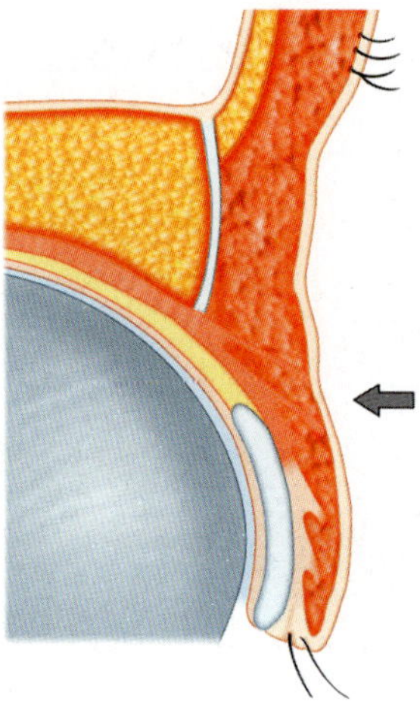

Fig. 29.13: Caucasian upper eyelid with high insertion of levator aponeurosis into the skin.

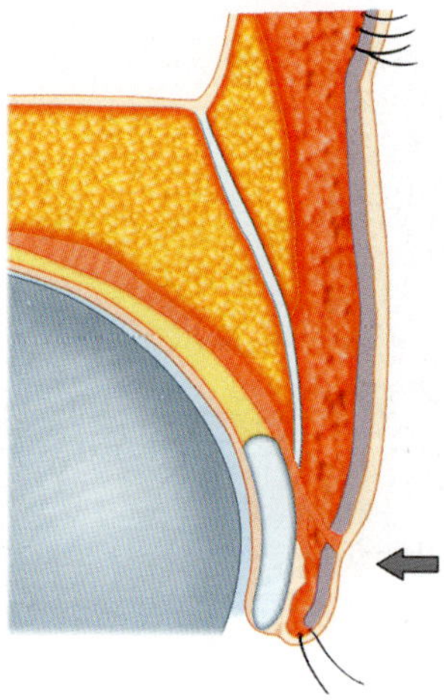

Fig. 29.14: Asian eyelid: Lower attachment of the levator aponeurosis to the skin.

- In anxious patients some sedation (e.g. Tab. Clonazepam 0.5 mg) can be prescribed before the surgery.
- Orbital fat excision should be conservative as excessive removal of fat may lead to hollowness of the orbit.
- Care should be taken while dissecting the medial fat pad to avoid injury to the superior oblique tendon.
- The upper eyelid crease may be made more prominent by placement of interrupted sutures from the skin to the levator aponeurosis and back to the skin.

DOUBLE EYELID SURGERY OR ASIAN BLEPHAROPLASTY[7-9]

Double eyelid surgery or Asian blepharoplasty is the commonest upper lid blepharoplasty surgery requested and done in Asia. This also holds true for North east India. It is estimated that 50% of Asians have single eyelids and double eyelid surgery makes the eyes look larger and brighter. It allows greater ease in the application of cosmetics, which is a major area of concern for females.

In the Caucasian eye, there is higher insertion of the levator aponeurosis to the skin which creates a high and prominent eyelid fold in the upper eyelid (Fig. 29.13). In contrast, in the Asian eye the lower insertion of the levator aponeurosis into the skin creates an insignificant or a small upper eyelid fold (Fig. 29.14).

Principle of Surgery

A suture from skin to levator aponeurosis or tarsal plate and back to the skin is taken to create an attachment between the levator/tarsus to the skin. This mimics the attachment

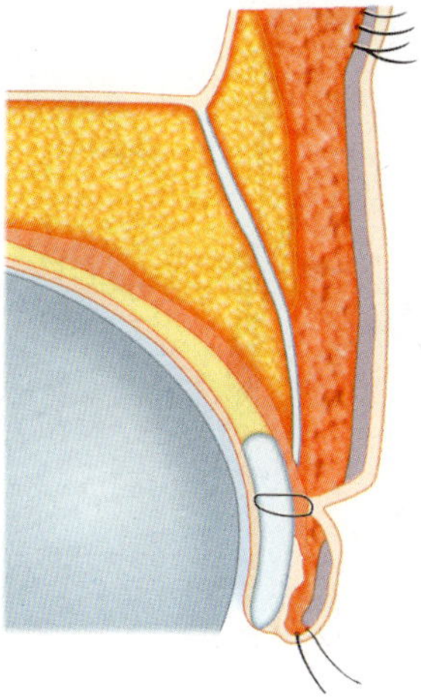

Fig. 29.15: Double eyelid surgery or Asian blepharoplasty: Site of attachment of the levator aponeurosis to the skin.

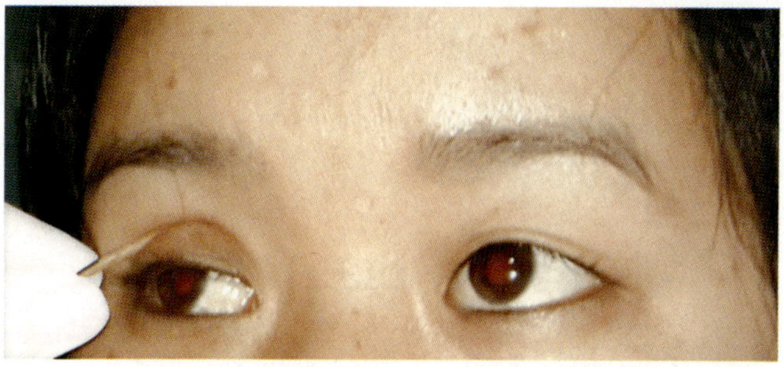

Fig. 29.16: Determining height of new eyelid crease with toothpick.

in the Caucasian eyelid or an Asian eyelid with a prominent eyelid crease.

The principle of double eyelid blepharoplasty is the creation of an attachment of skin to the levator aponeurosis at a higher level (Fig. 29.15). It can be performed with two techniques, open and closed.

Closed Technique (Suturing Technique)

It is not preferred as the results are temporary. This simple procedure involves placing intradermal sutures to anchor the subcutaneous tissue or orbicularis muscle to the aponeurosis or tarsal plate. This creates an adherence and gives the impression of a supratarsal crease as the aponeurosis exerts traction to open the upper eyelid.

Open Technique

The conventional open technique of the double eyelid surgery is similar to upper eyelid blepharoplasty described earlier with few major differences. The steps are:

- The markings for blepharoplasty in Caucasians and Orientals are different. In Caucasian eyes, the pre-existing eyelid fold can serve as a guide. In Oriental eyes, there are no such fold, and the surgeon has to create an entirely new supratarsal fold in an aesthetically pleasant location. A toothpick is gently pressed over the eyelid at a height desired by the patient (Fig. 29.16). A mirror held by the patient will help to discuss the size, style and appearance of the lid crease after surgery.

  In general, the desired location of the new eyelid fold in Orientals is 6 to 10 mm superior to the eyelid margin. The new location of the eyelid crease is measured from the center of the eyelid margin at a chosen distance. Alternatively, the tarsal height may be measured with the callipers over the central portion after everting the eyelid. The measured tarsal height is the transcribed onto the skin in the central part of the eyelid skin. This will serve as a guide in marking the incision line. The line for the new eyelid fold is drawn equidistant from the lash line resulting in a parallel crease.

  Slight variations like nasal tapering crease or temporal flare crease may be drawn depending on the wish of the patient.

  A strip of skin may be removed in some cases where there is redundant skin. Then a second line is drawn parallel and above the crease line and the ends are curved down to merge at the ends of the first line.
- *Local anesthesia*: Same as upper eyelid blepharoplasty.
- Skin is incised with blade or cautery (Fig. 29.17).
- Orbicularis muscle is separated with scissors.
- The orbital septum is identified and opened all along the length of the incision (Fig. 29.18).
- Beneath the orbital septum lies the orbital fat which may be removed in puffy eyes.
- Levator aponeurosis is identified as a silver white glistening fascia (Fig. 29.19). Dissection should stop here as deeper dissection into the levator muscle may cause bleeding and beyond it lies the conjunctiva. Tarsal plate (Fig. 29.20) is identified as a firm plate like structure inferior to the levator muscle.
- The new upper eyelid crease is created by placement of interrupted 6-0 silk sutures from the skin to the levator aponeurosis or tarsal plate and back to the skin. Three such sutures are made, one each in the medial, the middle and the lateral part of the eyelid. Subdermal 6-0 prolene buried sutures anchoring the

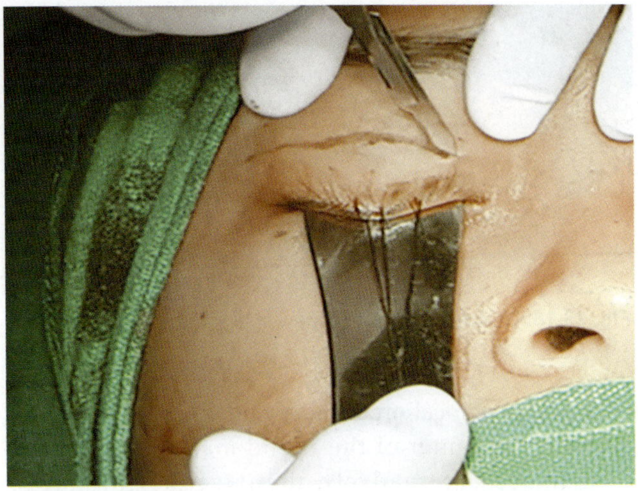

Fig. 29.17: Incision with blade along line of marking for the new crease for the creation of the double fold.

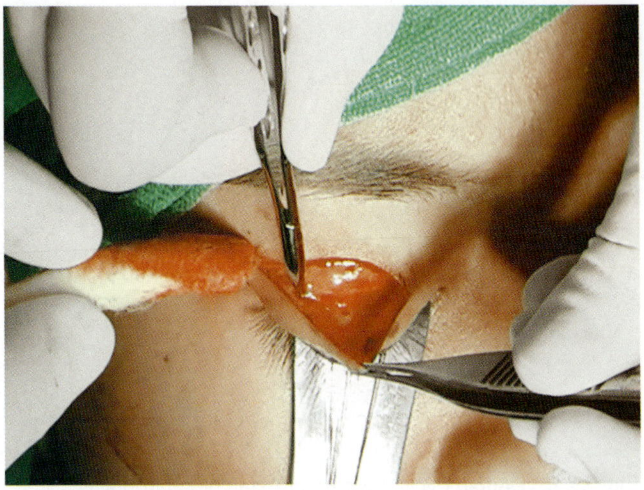

Fig. 29.18: Exposure of the orbital septum with the underlying orbital fat.

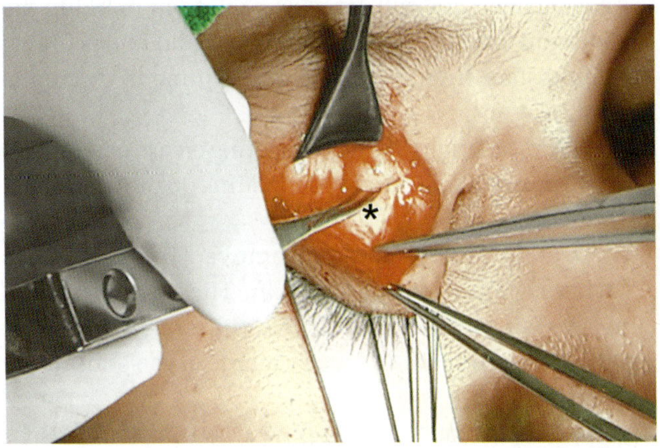

Fig. 29.19: Identification of the levator aponeurosis as the silver white glistening fascia (black asterisk) beneath the orbital fat.

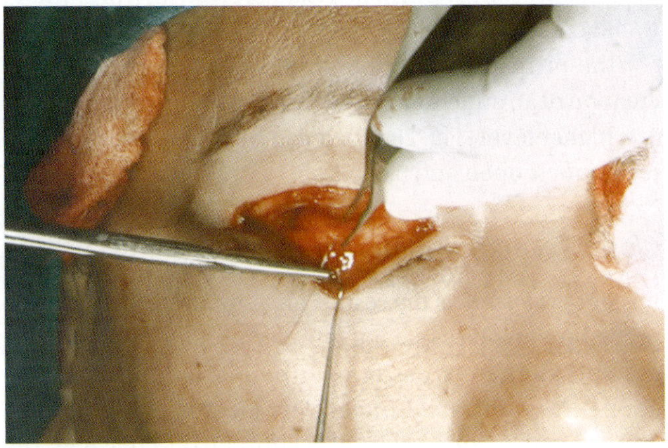

Fig. 29.20: Grasping the tarsal plate with the forceps and placing a suture from the tarsal plate to the skin.

subdermal tissue to the levator aponeurosis are left to ensure permanency of the new eyelid crease.

Modifications of this technique exist where the incision line vary from a few mm (short incision technique) to the whole length of the eyelid crease.

Postoperative Care

Ice packs on the surgical site after surgery are advised in order to minimize postoperative swelling and ecchymosis. Avoidance of bending over and heavy lifting or straining is advised and sleeping with the head elevated is encouraged. Oral and topical antibiotic ointments are given. Analgesics are given for a few days to reduce pain, discomfort and swelling.

Complications

Though major complications after upper eyelid blepharoplasty are rare and include retrobulbar or orbital hemorrhage with loss of vision or even blindness as a result, the most commonly encountered problem is a dissatisfied patient. Proper counseling may help prevent this. Some minor and often temporary complications are diplopia, dry eye syndrome, exposure keratopathy, corneal abrasion, lagophthalmos, epiphora, chemosis, subconjunctival hemorrhage, blepharoptosis, lid crease asymmetry, wound dehiscence, visible or excessive scarring, hypoesthesias, suture abscesses, cysts or granulomas, ecchymosis or hematoma and wound infections.[10]

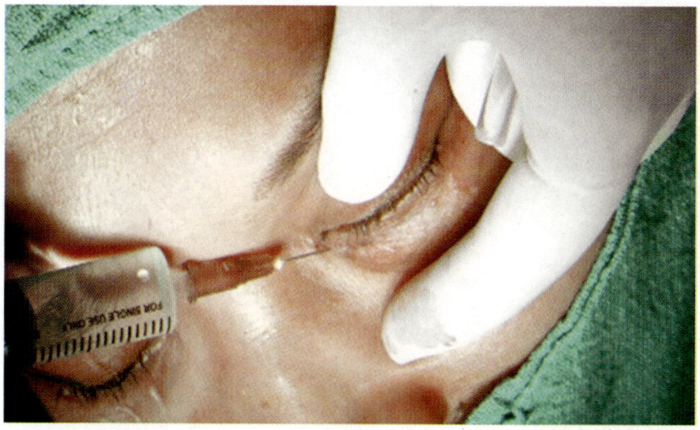

Fig. 29.21: Local anesthesia for lower eyelid.

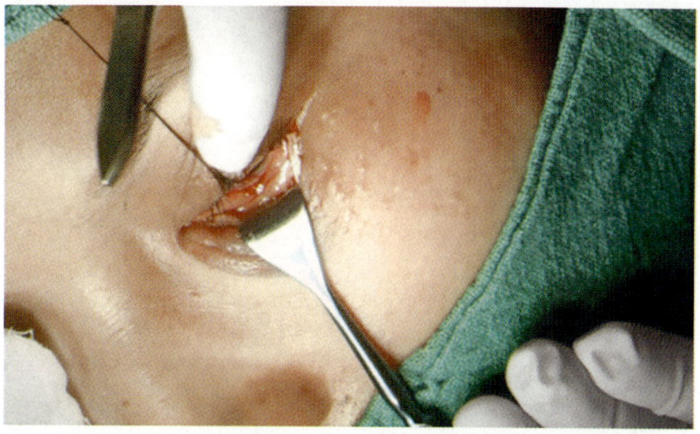

Fig. 29.22: Retraction of lower eyelid central portion.

LOWER BLEPHAROPLASTY[11,12]

Lower eyelid blepharoplasty is done to correct loose lax skin below the eyelids and the under eye bags which appear or worsen with ageing. Lower eyelid blepharoplasty rejuvenates and restores youthful appearance to the eyes. Basic principles are to reduce excess skin with or without fat, reduce tissue laxity and there should be no scleral show inferiorly.

Depending on the site of incision it may be classified into transconjunctival and transcutaneous.

Transconjunctival blepharoplasty is best suited for young patients with baggy eyes, puffiness and dark circles under eyes with minimal or no skin wrinkles. It is the most direct approach to the inferior orbital fat, located posteriorly to the orbital septum.[13]

Steps in Transconjunctival Lower Blepharoplasty

- It is performed under local anesthesia, which is injected subcutaneously into fat pad and subconjunctival area (Fig. 29.21).
- The central portion of the lower eyelid is retracted with a Desmarres retractor (Fig. 29.22). The eyeball is protected with an orbital metallic strip or corneal shield or conjunctiva (Fig. 29.23), which is pulled over the eyeball with a suture.
- To exteriorize inferior orbital fat over the edge of the inferior orbital surface, slight pressure is given over the eyeball. The incision can be performed with scalpel (number 11 or number 15 blade) or monopolar cautery.

  The incision is made 5 mm below the tarsal plate, between the lower border of tarsal plate and inferior fornix (Figs. 29.24A and B). The incision should be made at a distance from the fornix to avoid synechia or wounding of the inferior oblique muscle. Once the conjunctiva is incised, there is direct access to the inferior orbital fat without breaching the septum.

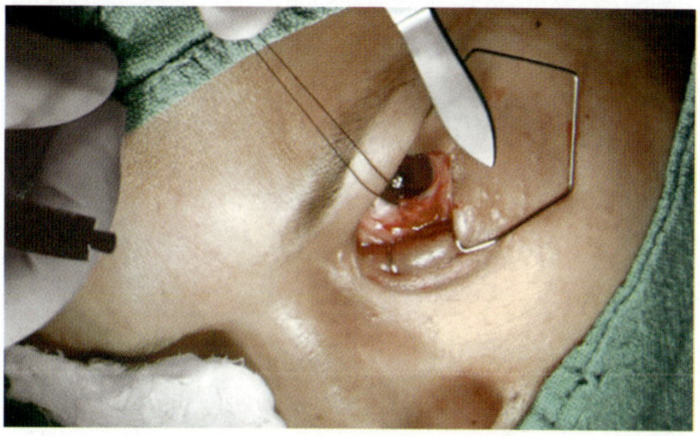

Fig. 29.23: Protection for eyeball.

- By a gentle pressure on the globe, the fat is made to herniate. Septum is opened in each compartment. Excision of the fat is done carefully keeping a watch on the external contour (Fig. 29.25). Care must be taken to avoid injury to the inferior oblique muscle which lies between the central and medial fat pads.
- Conjunctiva is approximated with 6-0 vicryl sutures (Fig. 29.26).

Transcutaneous Lower Lid Blepharoplasty

This is indicated in older patients where there is laxity of skin along with bulging of the lower eyelid.

- Local anesthesia is given along the lower eyelid (Fig. 29.27).
- A subciliary incision (Figs. 29.28A and B) is made approximately 1.5–2 mm below the lid margin, starting

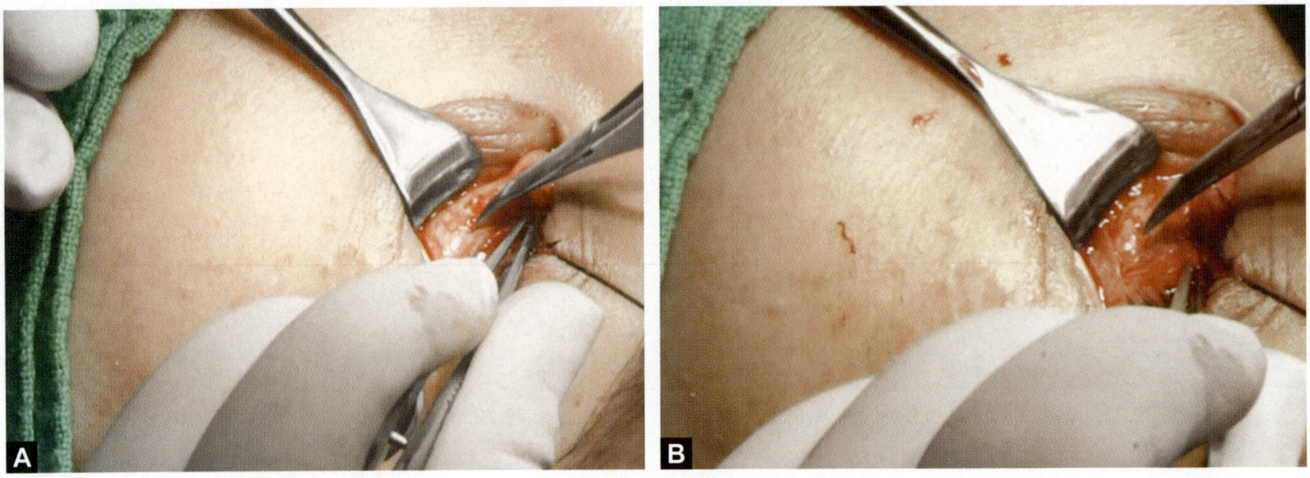

Figs. 29.24A and B: (A) Starting the incision of conjunctiva; (B) Completed incision of the conjunctiva. Underlying fat can be seen.

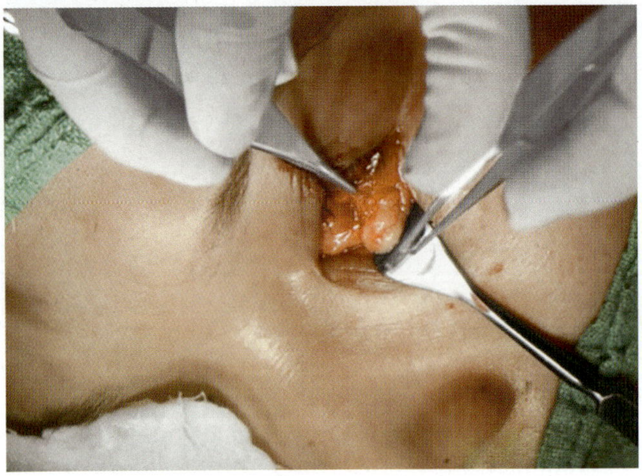

Fig. 29.25: Exposure and excision of fat.

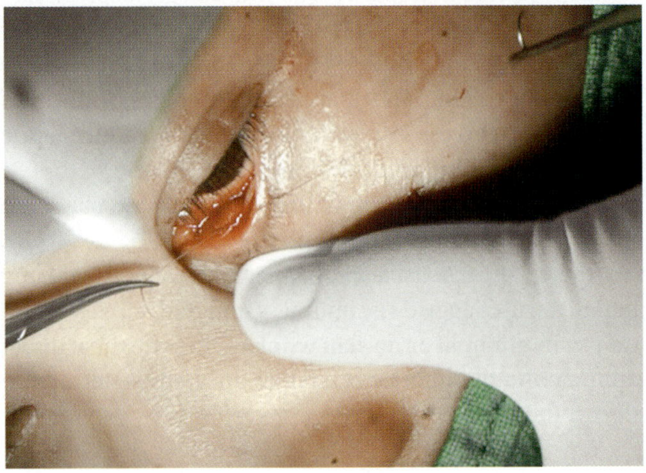

Fig. 29.26: Suturing the conjunctiva.

below the lacrimal punctum to lateral canthus and beyond downward along the lines of facial expression.

The amount of tissue to be excised is determined by undermining the skin from the orbicularis for a distance of 6–7 mm (Fig. 29.29). Then the skin along with the orbicularis is raised creating a myocutaneous flap which is then pulled upward and laterally over the incision line. A triangular myocutaneous flap is then excised starting from the lateral extent of the subciliary incision (Figs. 29.30A and B). The incision is adjusted by making the cut along the lateral facial lines.

- *Fat excision:*[14] Retracting the skin and muscle flap, gentle pressure is placed on the globe to herniate the orbital fat. The orbital septum is then opened along its entire length exposing the orbital fat (Fig. 29.31A). The excess amount

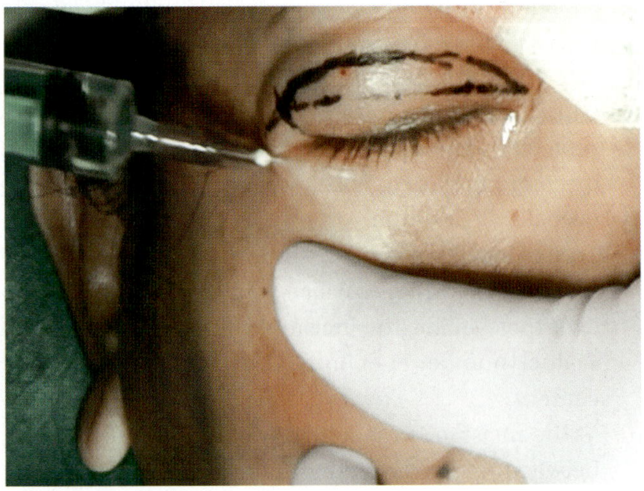

Fig. 29.27: Local anesthesia of the lower eyelid.

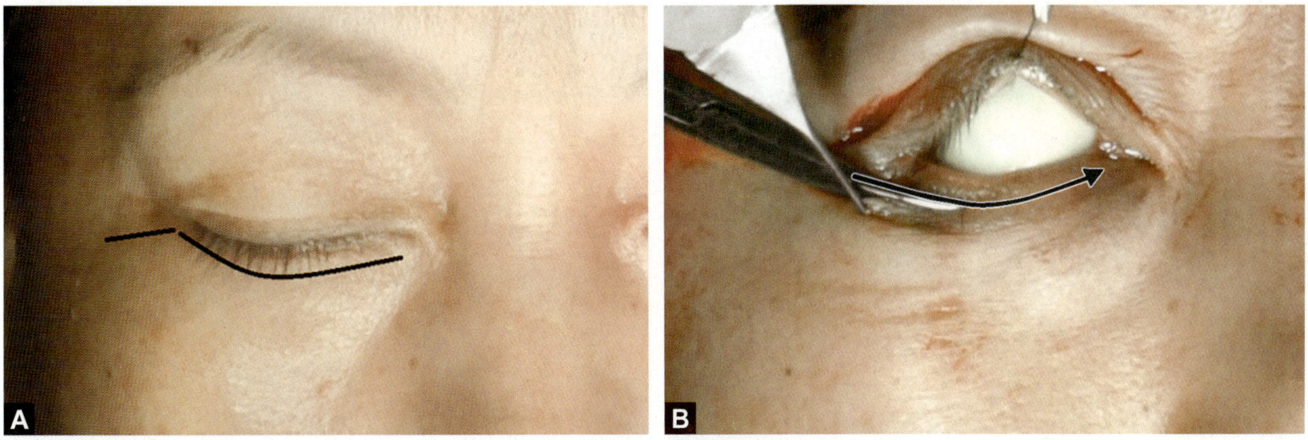

Figs. 29.28A and B: (A) Subciliary incision; (B) Subciliary incision (curved black arrow).

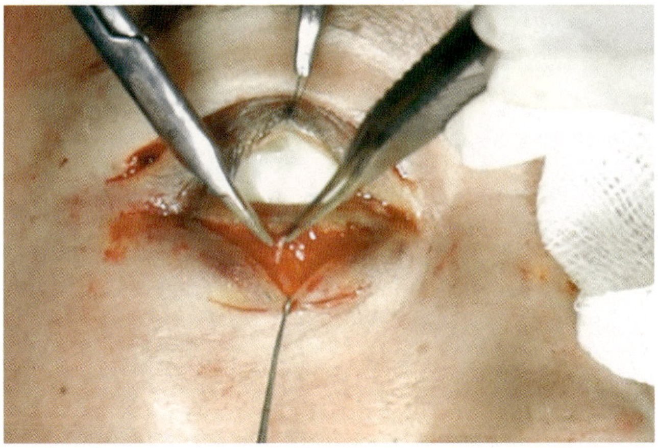

Fig. 29.29: Undermining of skin.

of fat is trimmed using a cautery to avoid retraction of the bleeders (Fig. 29.31B).

- *Suturing*: The wound is closed with 6-0 nonabsorbable suture by a running or subcuticular suture (Figs. 29.32A and B).

Postoperative Care

It is the same as in upper eyelid blepharoplasty. A six weeks wait is required for the swelling to resolve before judging the final outcome.

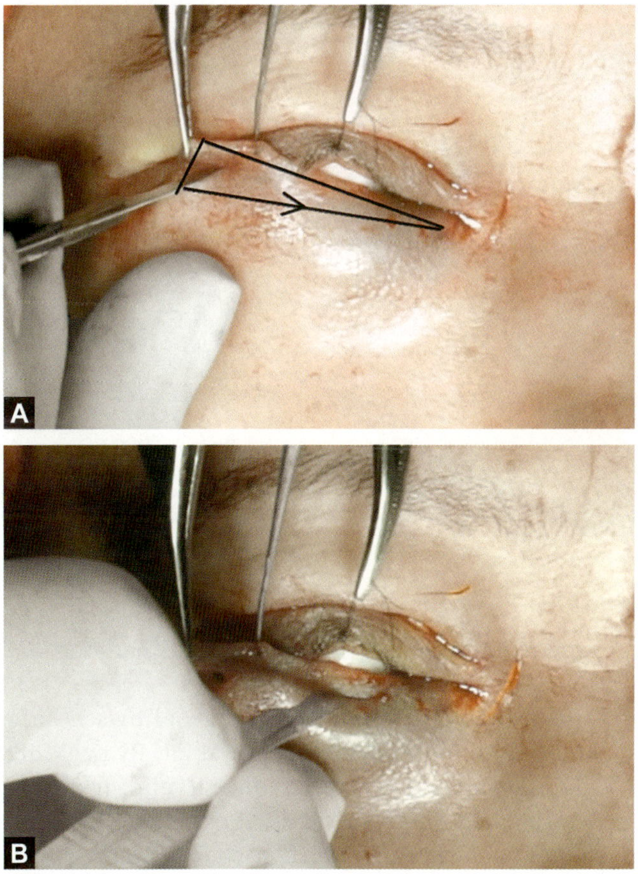

Figs. 29.30A and B: (A) Triangular myocutaneous flap is excised (black triangle) with apex just below lacrimal punctum. Incision is made along the black arrow; (B) Extending the incision.

Points to Consider

- Lower eyelid blepharoplasty is very efficient for the correction of orbital bags. Transcutaneous and transconjunctival approaches have similar success rates.
- Postoperative hemorrhage is very rare but must be identified early. If the patient complains of severe pain, the vision must be closely monitored. To reduce this incidence, intraoperative hemostasis must be very meticulous. Closing with a single suture enables the

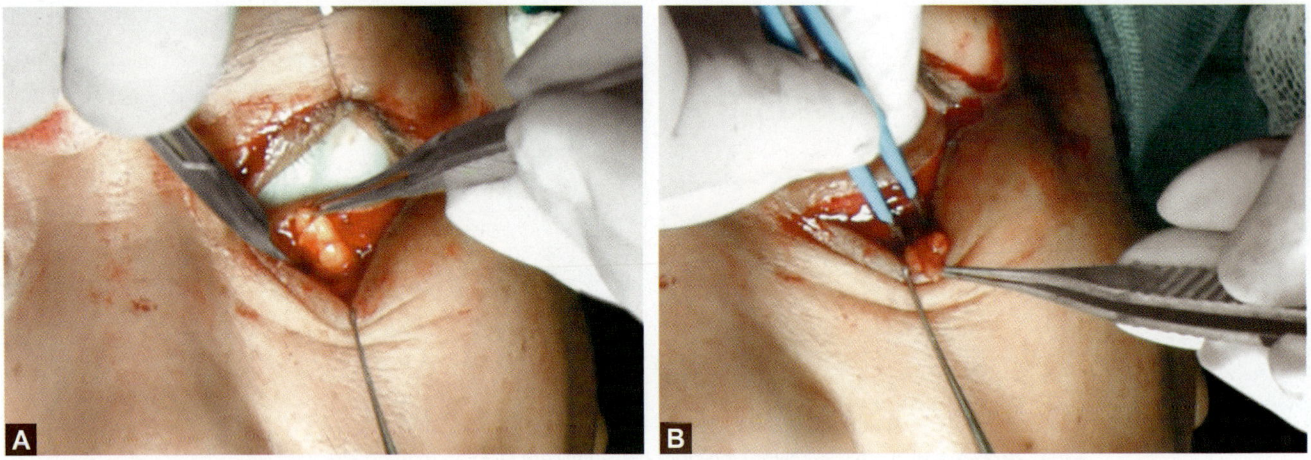

Figs. 29.31A and B: (A) Exposing orbital fat; (B) Trimming of excess fat with cautery.

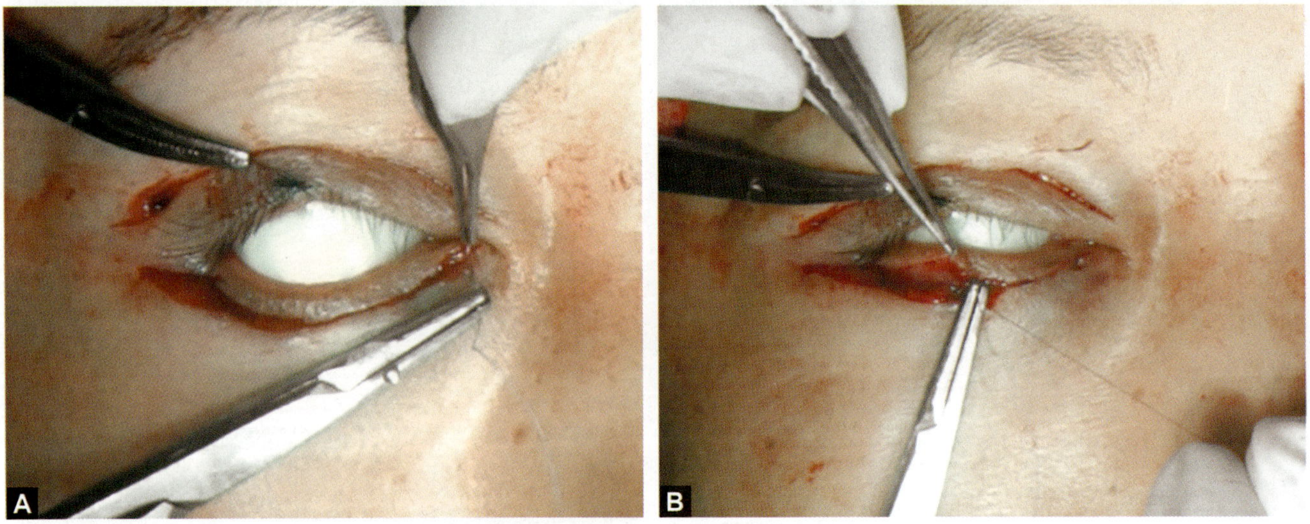

Figs. 29.32A and B: (A) Skin closure; (B) Subcuticular suture.

evacuation of hemorrhage and avoids early orbital hematoma in the event of hemorrhage.

- The transconjunctival approach allows a safe and quantified excision of orbital fat. By avoiding the anterior planes of the lower eyelid, it avoids scarring and reduces the risk of retraction. Classical complications are rarer with transconjunctival than with transcutaneous blepharoplasty (ectropion, entropion, fat over-resection, inferior oblique muscle palsy).
- If excess skin is noted in older patients, minimal cutaneous excision can be performed in association with the transconjunctival approach to preserve the septum.
- Wrinkles of the lower eyelid can persist after surgery for up to three months. After three months the wrinkles can be treated with laser or chemical peeling.

Few results of blepharoplasty are provided in Figures 29.33 to 29.37

Complications[15-18]

Bruising and edema of the lower eyelid is common. Excessive fat removal can lead to sunken eyes. On the contrary, insufficient fat resection can lead to under correction of the eye bags. The minor and common complications are the same as upper eyelid blepharoplasty (Fig. 29.38).

CONCLUSION

Chemical peels, botox, fillers and energy based devices have made minimally invasive rejuvenation of the

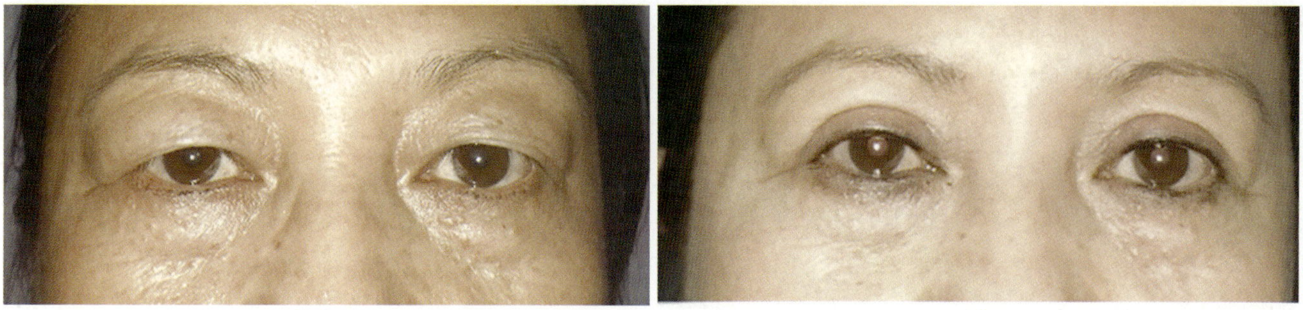

Before After

Fig. 29.33: Upper eyelid blepharoplasty for dermatochalasis—before and after.

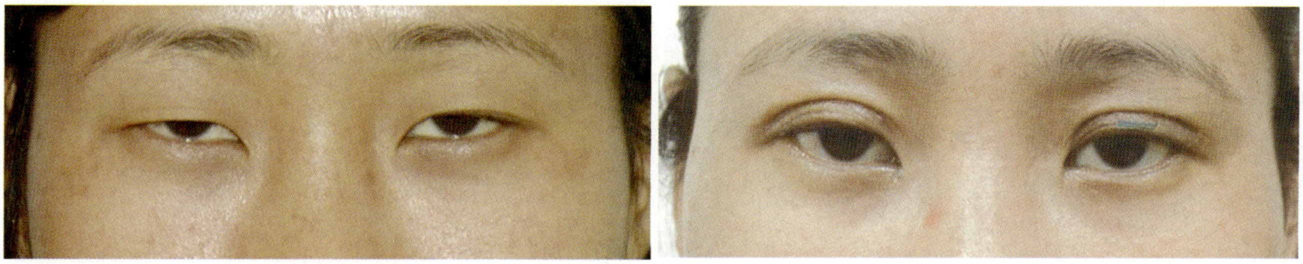

Before After

Fig. 29.34: Asian blepharoplasty—before and after.

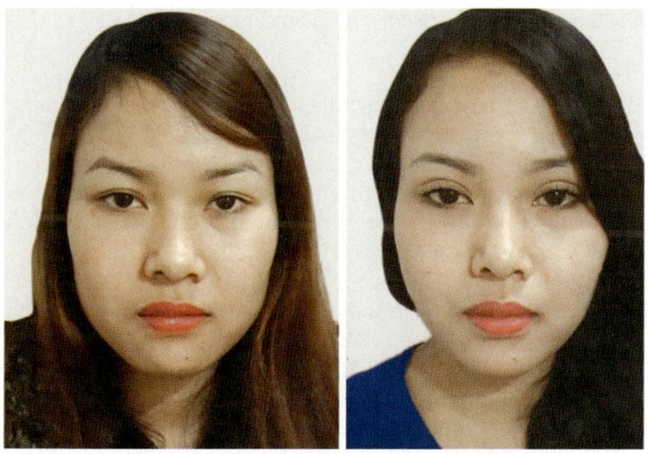

Before After

Fig. 29.35: Asian blepharoplasty as a part of facial rejuvenation. Before and after. Filler injection for mid face and botox for masseters.

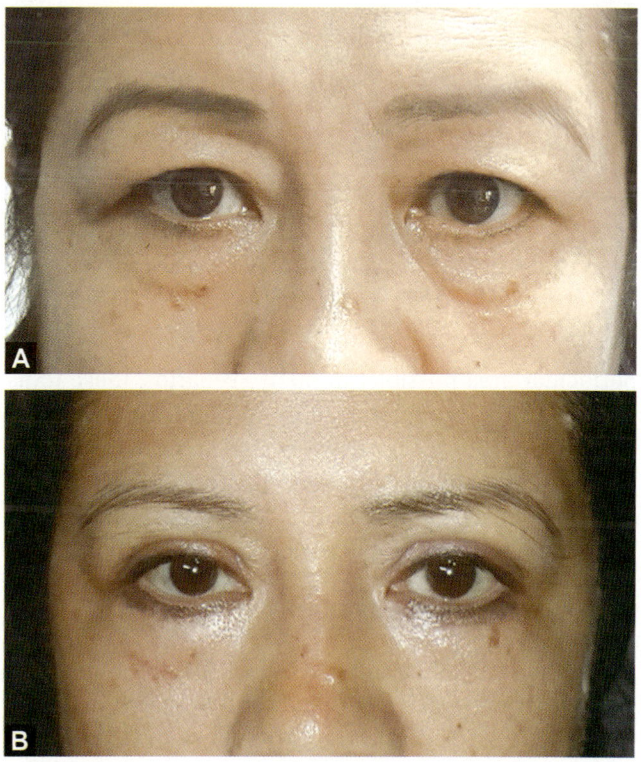

Figs. 29.36A and B: (A) Lower eyelid blepharoplasty: transcutaneous (upper eyelid blepharoplasty has also been done); (B) After lower eyelid blepharoplasty: transcutaneous (upper eyelid blepharoplasty has also been done).

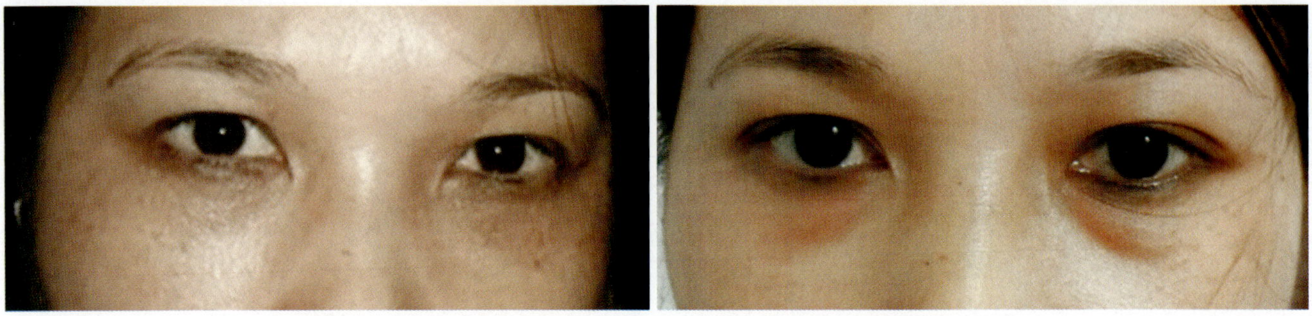

Before After

Fig. 29.37: Lower eyelid blepharoplasty—transconjunctival.

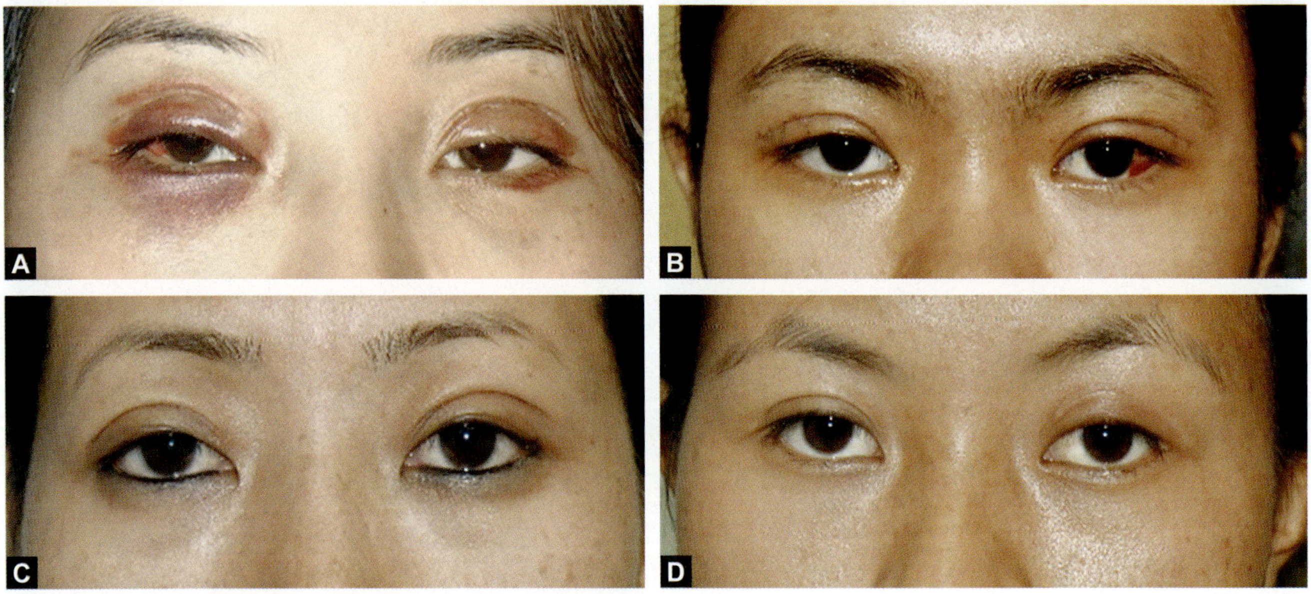

Figs. 29.38A to D: Complications. (A) Bruising and edema; (B) Subconjunctival hemorrhage; (C) Asymmetry of the eyelid crease after Asian blepharoplasty; (D) Loss of double eyelid crease on the left side. Needs revision surgery.

periocular area possible. In many scenarios, these tools available to a dermatologist are not enough to make a meaningful difference. There is also an ever increasing demand for double eyelid surgery in the north eastern part of India. Thus, blepharoplasty is a valuable skill set for a dermatologist interested in periocular rejuvenation.

ACKNOWLEDGMENT

Images and videos contributed by Dr Kh. Palin Singh, Shija Cosmetic Centre, Shija Hospitals and Research Institute, Imphal.

REFERENCES

1. Subramanian N. Blepharoplasty. Indian J Plast Surg. 2008; 41(Suppl):S88-S92.
2. Weng CJ. Oriental upper blepharoplasty. Semin Plast Surg. 2009;23(1):5-15.
3. Matsuo T, Takeda Y, Ohtsuka A. Stereoscopic three-dimensional images of an anatomical dissection of the eyeball and orbit for educational purposes. Acta Med Okayama. 2013;67(2):87-91.
4. Zimbler MS, Prendiville S, Thomas JR. The "pinch and slide" blepharoplasty: safe and predictable aesthetic results. Arch Facial Plastic Surgery. 2004;6:348-50.
5. Maegawa J, Kobayashi S, Yabuki Y, et al. Blepharoplasty in senile blepharoptosis: preoperative measurements and design for skin excision. Aesthet Surg J. 2012;32(4):441-6.
6. Flowers RS. Blepharoplasty. In: Courtiss EH (Ed). Male Aesthetic Surgery. St. Louis, MO: Mosby; 1982.
7. Boo-Chai K. Plastic construction of the superior palpebral fold. Plast Reconstr Surg. 1963;31(1):74-8.
8. Mutou Y, Mutou H. Intradermal double eyelid operation and its follow-up results. Br J Plast Surg. 1972;25:285-91.

9. Uchida JI. A surgical procedure for blepharoptosis vera and for pseudo-blepharoptosis orientalis. Br J Plast Surg. 1962;15:271-6.
10. Oestreicher J, Mehta S. Complications of blepharoplasty: prevention and management. Plast Surg Int. 2012;2012:252-368.
11. Yousif NJ, Sonderman P, Dzwierzynski WW, et al. Anatomic considerations in transconjunctival blepharoplasty. Plast Reconstr Surg. 1995;96(6):1271-6.
12. Netscher DT, Patrinely JR, Peltier M, et al. Transconjunctival versus transcutaneous lower eyelid blepharoplasty: a prospective study. Plast Reconstr Surg. 1995;96(5):1053-60.
13. Schwarz F, Randall P. Conjunctival incision for herniated orbital fat. Ophthalmic Surg. 1980;11:276-9.
14. Rosenberg GJ. Correction of saddlebag deformity of the lower eyelids by superficial suction lipectomy. Plast Reconstr Surg. 1995;96:1061-5.
15. Palmer FR, Rice DH, Churukian MM. Transconjunctival blepharoplasty. Complications and their avoidance: a retrospective analysis and review of the literature. Arch Otolaryngol Head Neck Surg. 1993;119(9):993-9.
16. McCord CD Jr, Shore JW. Avoidance of complications in lower lid blepharoplasty. Ophthalmology. 1983;90(9):1039-46.
17. Baylis HI, Long JA, Groth MJ. Transconjunctival lower eyelid blepharoplasty. Technique and complications. Ophthalmology. 1989;96(7):1027-32.
18. Palmer FR 3rd, Rice DH, Churukian MM. Transconjunctival blepharoplasty. Complications and their avoidance: a retrospective analysis and review of the literature. Arch Otolaryngol Head Neck Surg. 1993;119(9):993-9.

CHAPTER 30

Dimple Creation

Salim T, Laila Achampat

INTRODUCTION

Cheek dimples are considered as attractive features among various facial features. They enhance facial beauty and the expression. It occurs in males and females with equal prevalence, and present unilaterally or bilaterally. Bilateral cheek dimples are much more common than unilateral ones. They are inherited in an autosomal dominant fashion on the chromosome 16, with variable penetrance.[1,2]

Dimples are also considered as sign of good luck and prosperity among some cultures and it brightens up and adds character to a beautiful smile. Recently, there has been an increased demand for creation of facial dimples, and lot of people seek expertise of cosmetic and dermatologic surgeons to get facial dimple creation done. This chapter will explain technique of dimple creation and this can be easily done by a dermatologic surgeon.

ANATOMY OF DIMPLE

Anatomically, dimples are mainly caused by the insertion of the fibers of the double or bifid zygomaticus major muscle into the skin. This dermocutaneous insertion causes dermal tethering effect.[3]

PRINCIPLE

The surgery is aimed at creating a scar in the dermis which then adheres to underlying buccinator muscle, becoming a natural dynamic dimple. This can be achieved with either transcutaneous sutures or by open technique that is performed intra-orally, which would not show scarring.

POSITIONING OF DIMPLE

The position of dimple is marked by patient in front of mirror.

While positioning a dimple, the ideal location is the area where less obvious faint dimple is already present with smiling; thus pre-existing dimple is made much more prominent. The patient is then asked to create negative suction and suck cheeks inside. The site of maximum depression is then marked as site of the dimple.

If one of the cheeks has a dimple, ideal location for other dimple is marked at corresponding site on the other cheek that would create symmetry on face.

If pre-existing dimple is not naturally present, as per cosmetic viewpoint, ideal location would be intersection between horizontal line from angle of mouth and vertical line from lateral canthus of eye (Fig. 30.1A).[4]

The position of dimple marked by this earlier method might be too low. The point of intersection of two lines: a perpendicular one dropping down from the outer canthus and a horizontal one coming from the higher most point on the Cupid's bow on the lateral aspect may be a better choice (Fig. 30.1B).[5]

SURGICAL TECHNIQUE

Instruments required for dimple creation are as given in Figure 30.2.

Dimple surgery can be performed by a skilled dermatologic surgeon under local anesthesia, after obtaining an informed consent. After cleansing the face and intraoral space, 1.5–2.5 mL 0.5% lignocaine with adrenaline is administered into mucosa from the skin side. The procedure is done after about 10 min of administering the anesthesia. A needle is passed from the skin surface through the point marked on the skin into the buccal cavity so as to act as a guide (Fig. 30.3). A 6 mm punch is used to remove the tissue in full depth keeping the needle as a guide. Care should be taken not to injure and cut the skin including the dermal tissue. The soft tissue cylindrical fragment consisting of the mucosa, a small portion of the buccinator muscle, and a part of the fat pad is removed using scissors, leaving the skin with dermis intact. The defect is widened by scraping

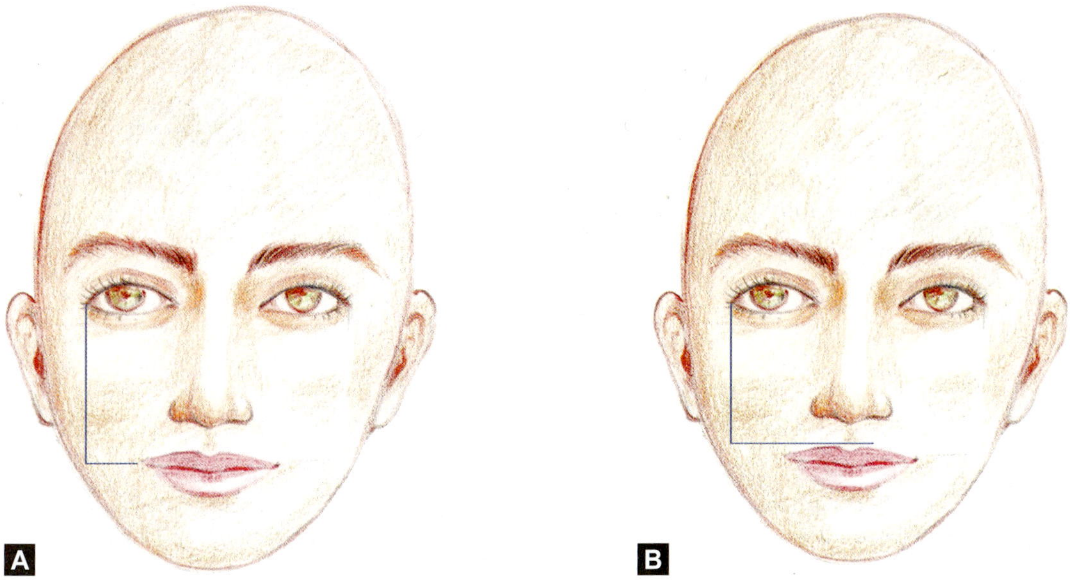

Figs. 30.1A and B: Positioning of the dimple. Intersection between a horizontal line from the angle of the mouth and a vertical line from the lateral canthus of the eye.

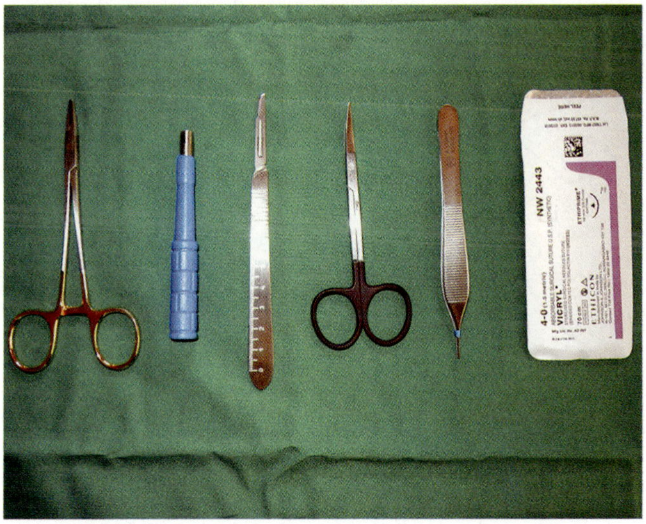

Fig. 30.2: Instruments required for dimple creation.

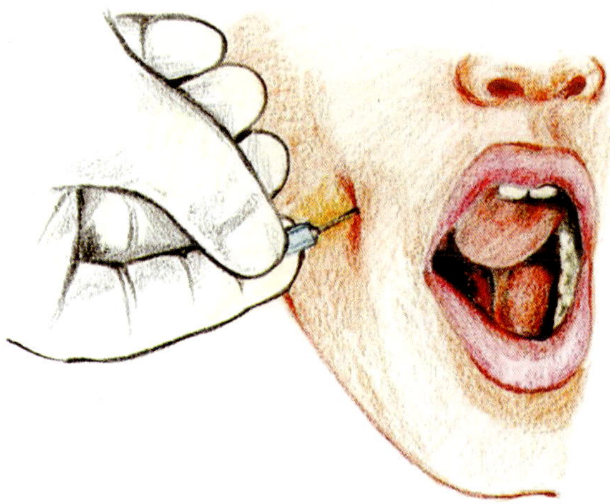

Fig. 30.3: Needle passed from the skin surface through the point marked for dimple creation.

with no. 15 blade and separating the muco-muscular attachments (Figs. 30.4 to 30.7).

Alternatively a no.15 blade can be used instead of a punch to make a stab incision followed by separation of the mucomuscular attachments. To create a wider dimple, wider area has to be removed, so that both the dermal and mucosal raw areas can be both created. These raw areas will then oppose and stick together resulting in the dimple. Depending on the size of dimple required, smaller or bigger areas can be created or scaled down. Confirmation can be done by bimanual palpation of an indentation at site of the dimple creation. This can be then used to either upscale or downscale the size.

Maintenance of the defect is the next important issue. For this the defect created is closed with 30 Vicryl absorbable suture usually which traverses through the cheek mucosa, muscle, and then the fat pad on the first side and then through the dermis, fat pad, buccinators and oral

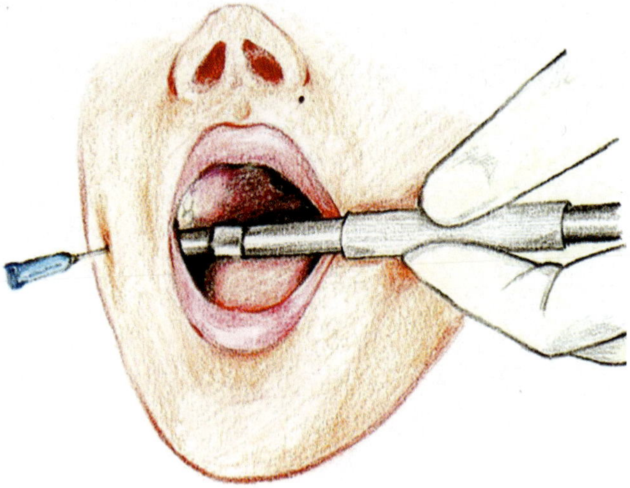

Fig. 30.4: A 6 mm punch placed at the buccal surface keeping the needle as a guide.

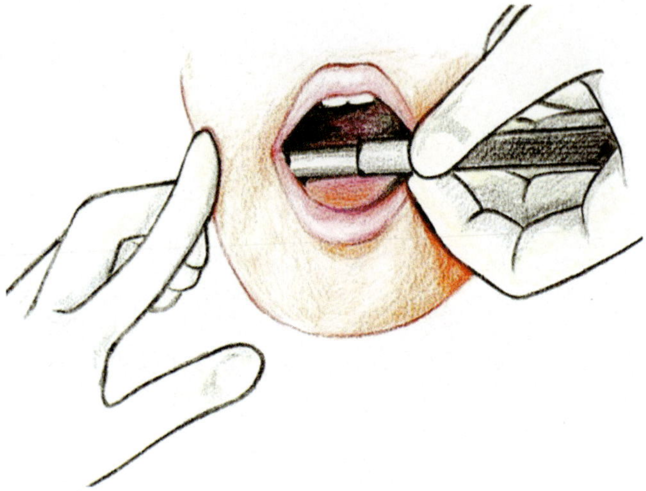

Fig. 30.5: The needle is removed and the punch is used to remove the tissue in full depth without injuring the skin including the dermal tissue.

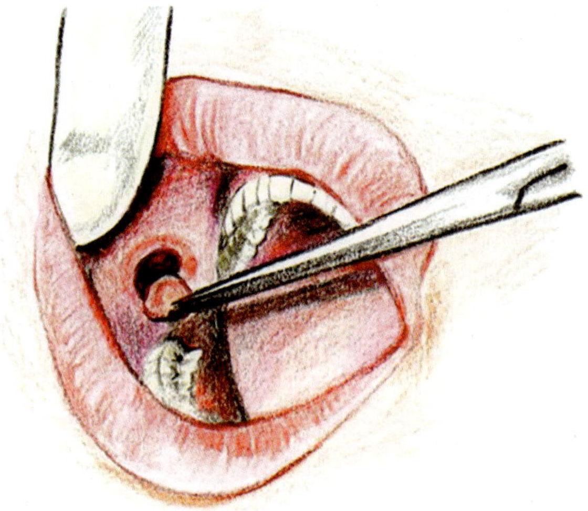

Fig. 30.6: The soft tissue cylindrical fragment consisting of the mucosa, a small portion of the buccinator muscle, and a part of the fat pad is removed using scissors.

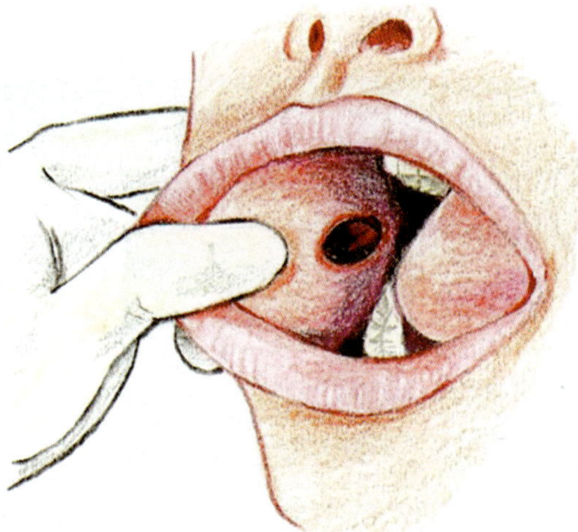

Fig. 30.7: The defect is widened by scraping with a No. 15 blade and separating the mucomuscular attachments.

mucosa on the second side (Fig. 30.8). The resultant knot is then tied, and dimple is thereby created (Fig. 30.9).

POSTOPERATIVE CARE

The patient can be discharged immediately with prescription of antibiotics and analgesics. Patient is also instructed to maintain a good oral hygiene with frequent mouthwash and oral rinsing in immediate postoperative period. It is advised not to fully smile during first 2 weeks.

Initially, there is static dimple which then deepens on animation, but gradually there is only hint of a dimple when static which accentuates on animation. It resembles natural dimple (appears only on smiling) within 4–6 weeks (Figs. 30.10 and 30.11).

Complications of dimple surgery are given in Table 30.1.

DISCUSSION

Literature reveals various techniques used by different authors for dimple creation.

- Khoo et al. Here nonabsorbable suture was used as a sling between skin and buccinator simulating integumentary insertion of muscle.[4]

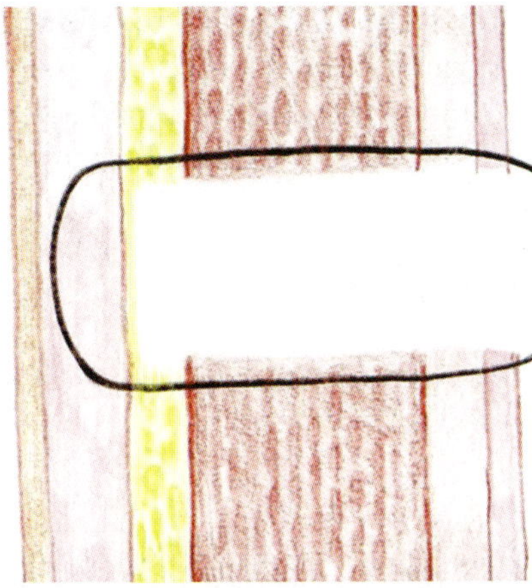

Fig. 30.8: The suture passed through the cheek mucosa, muscle, and the fat pad on one side of the defect; then through the dermis layer of the skin; and finally, through the fat pad, the buccinator muscle, and the mucosa on the other side of the defect.

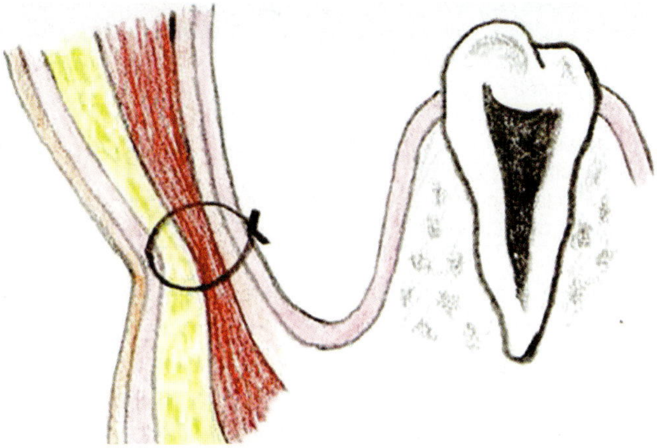

Fig. 30.9: The knot is tied, and the dimple is created.

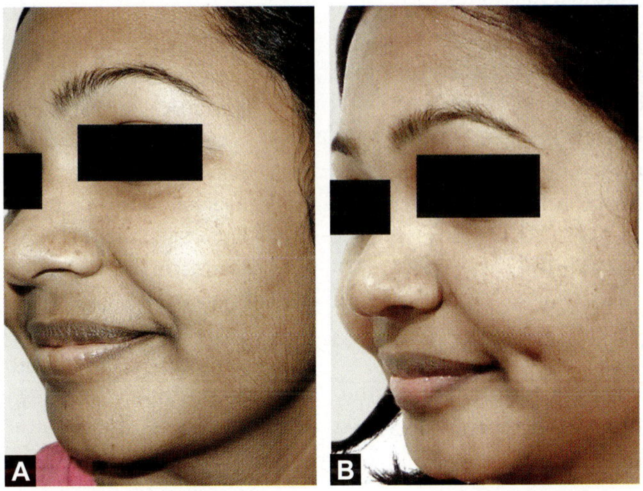

Figs. 30.10A and B: Before and after 6 months while smiling.

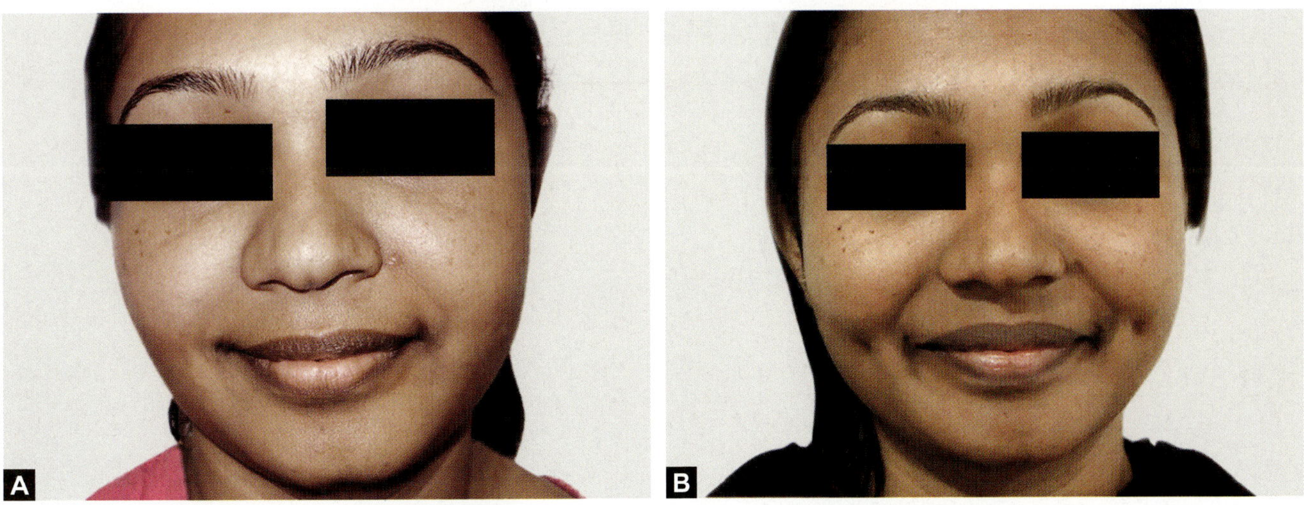

Figs. 30.11A and B: Before and after 6 months while smiling.

Table 30.1: Complications of dimple surgery.

- Sudden disappearance of the dimple
- Asymmetry
- Foreign body reaction
- Infection
- Bleeding
- Injury to a nerve (buccal branch of the facial nerve) or salivary gland duct (Stensen duct)

- Shiwei et al. used syringe needle to guide monofilament nylon suture through the dermis and buccinator muscle. This sling was formed between skin and the buccinator muscle and a knot was thereby tied to create the dimple.[5]
- Saraf et al. used punch biopsy and an intraoral approach to create dimple.[6]
- Thomas et al. described an open technique which actually replicated the anatomy of natural dimple. This did not require additional removal of soft tissue.[7]
- Lari AR et al. passed a transcutaneous bolster stitch following the after scraping of dermis of mucomuscular attachments and created the dimple.[8]

We feel that method described here is simple, safe method and therefore can be done by dermatologic surgeon as daycare procedure. The simple and open procedure herein described for placing facial dimple provides predictable outcome with expected minimal morbidity.

CONCLUSION

Dimples are attractive because they accentuate the smile. Unfortunately, not everyone possesses dimples. The above given simple techniques can be used to create beautiful dimples. Good knowledge of anatomy (especially vascularity and shape of face) are important to deliver a good outcome. The procedure is safe and gives good cosmetic satisfaction to the recipient.

ACKNOWLEDGMENT

The author thanks Ms. Heba J, final year medical student, VIMS, Wayanad, Kerala for the drawings.

REFERENCES

1. Argamaso RV. Facial dimple: Its formation by a simple technique. Plast Reconstr Surg. 1971;48:40–3.
2. Pentozos Daponte A, Vienna A, Brant L, et al. Cheek dimples in Greek children and adolescents. Int J Anthropol; 2004;19:289–95.
3. Pessa JE, Zadoo VP, Garza PA, et al: Double or bifid zygomaticus major muscle: Anatomy, incidence, and clinical correlation. Clin Anat. 1998;11:310.
4. Khoo BC. The facial dimple: Clinical study and operative technique. Plast Reconstr Surg. 1962;30:281-8.
5. Bao S, Zhou C, Li S, et al. A new simple technique for making facial dimples. Aesthetic Plast Surg. 2007;31:380-3.
6. Saraf S, Pillutia R. Complication of dimple creation. Indian Dermatol Online J. 2010;1:42-3.
7. Thomas M, Menon H, D'Silva J. Improved surgical access for facial dimple creation. Aesthet Surg J. 2010;30:798-801.
8. Lari AR, Panse N. Anatomical basis of dimple creation—A new technique: Our experience of 100 cases. Indian J Plast Surg. 2012;45:89-93.

CHAPTER 31

Lipobodysculpting

Nilesh Goyal

INTRODUCTION

Lipobodysculpting is a process wherein subcutaneous fat is removed into a receptacle with a cannula under the effect of local anesthesia using a suction machine or syringe. The procedure is a combination of the following techniques: lipodissection, lipolysis, lipocurettage and liposuction.

Lipodissection is the separation of adipocytes within the fat compartment with excess amounts of fluid, i.e. hydrodissection. This can also be done with the movement of cannula within the fat compartment. Lipolysis is the destruction of adipocytes with mechanical movement of cannula under the effect of vacuum within the fat compartment. Lipocurettage is thc scraping of the separated and dead adipocytes into the cannula under vacuum. Liposuction tends to be the final step of aspirating the curetting into a receptacle.[1]

Fat that is in excess over certain areas of the body can often be the cause for low self-esteem and social issues. This fat can be easily got rid of in a few hours with lipobodysculpting. This procedure where fat is removed in a scientific and artistic manner is akin to the work of a sculptor who works diligently on the body till the desired shape is achieved. It has to be very well understood that this procedure is not for those who seek weight reduction, but for those who are unable to get the fat deposits reduced despite good efforts.

The aim here is to introduce dermatosurgeons to this procedure and encourage them to take this up in their daily practice. It will be another tool in our armamentarium of procedures that can be offered to the cosmetically inclined patients.

HISTORY

Dr Arpad Fischer of Rome invented liposuction in early 1970s with suction cannulas.[2] The procedure underwent lot of modification in mid-1970s and early 1980s with Prof Illouz (Gynecologist) and Prof Fournier of Paris (Plastic Surgeon). They developed the concepts of blunt cannulas and syringe liposuction.[3-5] Prof Lawrence Field (dermatosurgeon) of California was the first dermatologist to learn the technique from his old buddy, Prof Fournier. Many dermatologic surgeons from USA who together with other cosmetic surgeons formed the American Society of Liposuction Surgery also mastered this. This was the first society to offer live courses to dermatologists and other physicians.[6] Dr Jeffrey Klein, a pharmacologist and dermatologist, invented Tumescent local anesthesia for liposuction that reduced the bleeding during this procedure making it very safe.[7] With the advent of Tumescent local anesthesia, the procedure soon got adopted into the core curriculum for training of dermatologists across many institutes in USA since 1990s. Today despite many dermatologists doing this procedure across the globe, it is still not part of the core curriculum for training of dermatologists in most countries. In fact in many countries, dermatologists are legally prohibited from doing it.

PROCEDURE

Patient Selection

Achieving successful fat removal from the deposits depends a lot upon patient selection. An ideal patient is one who has body weight near or a little above the ideal body weight for his/her height. The body mass index (BMI) should ideally be less than 30. The patient should have no medical illnesses needing long-term medications.

History Taking

A full medical history should be taken including list of medications taken regularly and even infrequently. This also includes any alternative medication list, i.e. homeopathy and ayurvedic treatments/supplements. It is of vital significance, as there are a whole host of medications that

Table 31.1: Common drugs that affect lidocaine metabolism via cytochrome P 450 enzyme inhibition or stimulation.

Antifungal	**Macrolide antibiotics**	**Miscellaneous**
Fluconazole	Erythromycin	Anastrozole
Itraconazole	Clarithromycin	Caffeine
Ketoconazole		Cimetidine
Miconazole	**Protease inhibitors**	Ciprofloxacin
	Indinavir	Isoniazid
Benzodiazepines	Nelfinavir	Norfloxacin
Alprazolam	Ritonavir	Omeprazole
Diazepam	Saquinavir	Acetazolamide
Flurazepam		Cyclosporine
Midazolam	**Selective serotonin reuptake**	Danazol
	inhibitors (SSRI)	Metronidazole
Calcium channel blockers	Fluoxetine	Grapefruit juice
Amiodarone	Paroxetine	Quinidine
Diltiazem	Sertraline	Troglitazone
Felodipine	Nefazodone	Zafirlukast
Nicardipine	Fluvoxamine	
Nifedipine		
Verapamil		

Source: Adapted from Klein JA. Tumescent Anesthesia.

inhibit or stimulate the cytochrome P450 enzyme system that incidentally also metabolizes lidocaine (Table 31.1).[8] This has a direct bearing on dose of lidocaine that can be administered for tumescent anesthesia on the day of surgery.

Examination

A thorough physical examination of the patient has to be done during the preoperative consultation that lays particular stress on cardiovascular fitness and exclusion of abdominal and inguinal hernias. When considering working on lower limbs it is essential to rule out presence of varicose veins. An extensive skin examination has to be carried out of the areas that are to be worked upon. This will include preexisting scars, indentations and bulges, asymmetry of areas, cellulite and dimples. Taking photos graphs of these anomalies pre operatively often prevents future disagreements.

Plan

The dermatosurgeon and the patient should discuss and demarcate areas that can be treated with lipobodysculpting. In case of patient wanting many areas to be done, then a realistic idea has to be given regarding multiple sessions required to treat all areas. A session of photography can be done during preoperative consultation.

Investigations

Patients have to undergo blood tests to determine their fitness for the procedure. These include a complete hemogram, liver function tests, serum creatinine and blood urea nitrogen levels, prothrombin time and activated partial thromboplastin time. Microcannular lipobodysculpting should preferably be avoided on patients with communicable blood borne viral diseases like human immunodeficiency virus (HIV), Hepatitis B, Hepatitis C and syphilis. These have to be ruled out prior to posting the patient for surgery. One of the proposed reasons for this is that the microcannulae cannot be used for other patients once they have been used on a patient with any of these diseases.[9] These days one time use disposable microcannulae are available in the international market to avoid such delicate situations (Fig. 31.1). Diabetic patients tend to be poor healers. Avoid diabetics due to higher risk of postoperative complications.[9] However, this is by no means an absolute contraindication during selection of patient. Further appropriate blood tests have to be conducted as per medical history of the patient, viz. thyroid illness requiring tests to ascertain euthyroid status. Any concurrent medical illnesses have to be corrected with or without treatment prior to taking up the patient. It goes without stating that this procedure cannot be performed on patients with bleeding disorders and in those on blood thinners or platelet inhibitors.

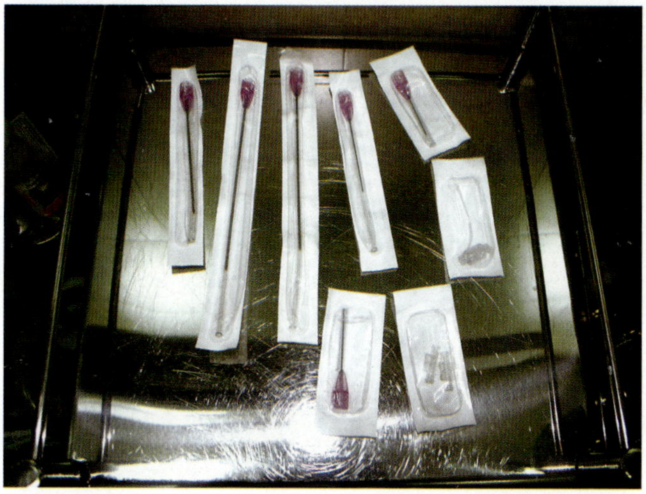

Fig. 31.1: Disposable cannula kit for liposuction and fat transfer. *Courtesy*: Tulip Medical Inc., San Diego, CA, USA

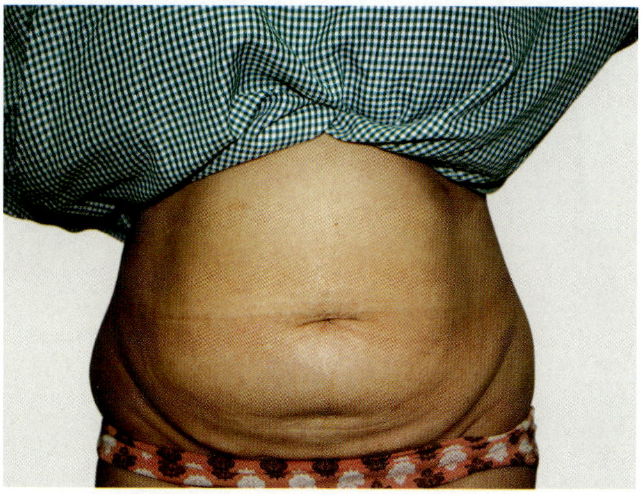

Fig. 31.2: Front view of abdomen of a 31-year-old lady on the day of lipobodysculpting to upper and lower abdomen.

Consent

A detailed consent form has to be signed by the patient. Ideally this should include details of the procedure, areas to be treated on the day of surgery, current and maximum body weight of patient, list of potential side effects of the procedure and medications and a postprocedure care sheet. The patient can be given this information at the preoperative check-up when they come with their blood workup.

Preoperative

Many dermatosurgeons and plastic surgeons prefer to start the patient on preoperative oral antibiotics with the idea to prevent a possible infection of the incisions that are made for cannula entry. However, risk of infection in a lipobodysculpting procedure done with proper aseptic precautions is very low (less than 1 in 2,000 cases).[10,11] The patient can be spared the risk of antibiotic allergies and drug reactions. I definitely start postoperative antibiotics to avoid any infection of the adits.

Day of Surgery

On the day of surgery, patient's current body weight has to be recorded on the anesthetic chart. A record of maximum nonpregnant body weight should also be recorded, as it will help in deciding the total dose of lidocaine for anesthesia. The dermatosurgeon or a trained staff takes clinical photos of the areas that are to be treated (Fig. 31.2). Proper guidelines have to be followed regarding patient confidentiality and protecting modesty.

Steps of Procedure

Marking Area

The dermatosurgeon then proceeds toward marking the areas on the patient's body. Special markers that do not get washed away easily during the procedure are preferred for the marking. The patient is standing in front of the dermatosurgeon who is seated on a height adjustable stool. It is preferable to have the dermatosurgeon have his eyes at the same level as the area to be marked. Marking of the areas helps in determining boundaries for anesthesia and also fat aspiration. They work as guide in preventing the dermatosurgeon from going into the non-anesthetized areas while aspirating. During marking, the dermatosurgeon delineates the mounds of fat with special attention to preexisting scars and pigmented marks. Encircling the mounds helps in administering tumescent anesthesia in multiple layers. Proper tumescence of the mounds enables better fat aspiration and consequently betters result. The marking is done by first circling the fat mounds and then dividing the entire area into grids (Fig. 31.3). The adits are also marked during marking phase. These are the entry points for the infiltration and aspiration. The sites are usually gravitationally dependent so that the excess fluid infiltrated and collections post operatively come out when pressure dressing is applied.

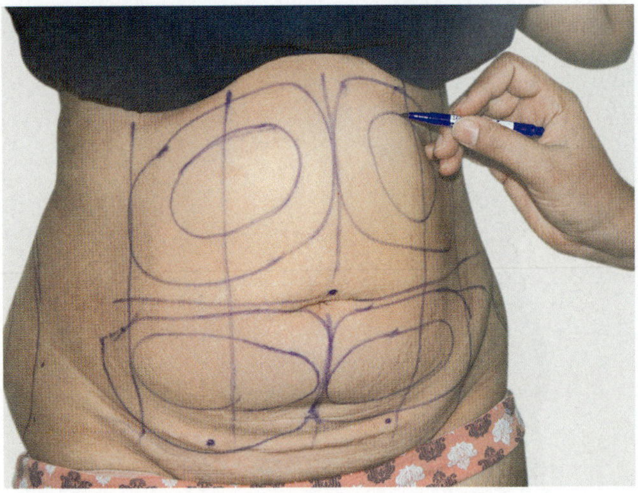

Fig. 31.3: Marking of upper and lower abdomen showing delineation of mounds of fat and division of the area into smaller quadrants.

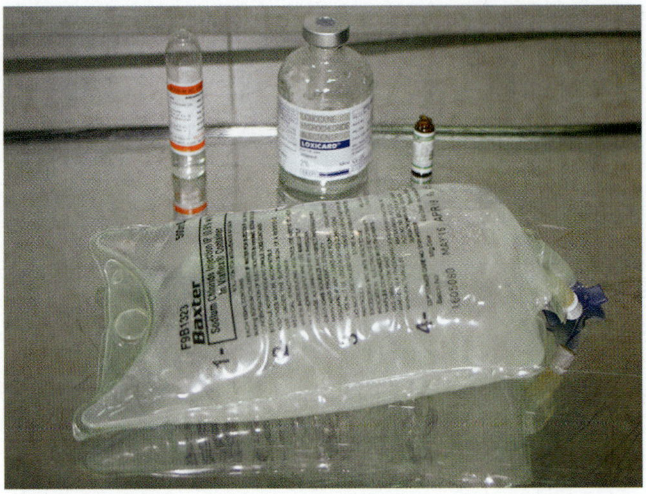

Fig. 31.4: Ingredients for making of Kleins' tumescent anesthesia solution.

Clean and Prepare

The next step is to cleanse and prepare the surgical area. The usual areas that patients seek for lipobodysculpting are around the abdomen, waist, thighs, chest (males), arms and back. In all cases, it is easier to get them prepared in the standing position. A mixture of povidone Iodine scrub and povidone iodine solution in equal proportions is preferred for scrubbing the areas to be worked upon. In addition, the areas adjacent to the surgical areas are also cleaned so as to create a sterile field for the surgery. The areas are then washed with saline soaked gauzes. A final coat of spirit follows this on to the entire surgical field. The patient is then asked to lie on the surgical table and draped with sterile clothes or disposable drapes creating a window for working. A sterile drape or sheet is placed on the operating table prior to the patient lying on it.

Anesthesia

Whilst the dermatosurgeon and/or staff are preparing the patient, one of the trained staff is given written instructions for preparing the tumescent anesthesia solution. This is prepared as per Klein's formula by mixing lidocaine (2%; as is easily available in India), Adrenaline (1:100000) and Sodium Bicarbonate 8.4 mEq/L in 1 liter of 0.9% normal saline (Fig. 31.4). The dose of lidocaine to be used depends upon the body weight and gender of patient. Usual maximum doses employed are between 45–55 mg/kg body weight.[12] A 55 mg/kg dose can be safely employed in an obese female patient who has more subcutaneous fat while a 45 mg/kg dose can be used for a leaner patient, i.e. male. Lidocaine has been chosen as the drug of choice for tumescent anesthesia due to its high affinity for fat and its slow release into the systemic circulation from the subcutaneous space. In addition, it is rapidly metabolized in the liver by the cytochrome P450 enzymes forming its metabolites, monoethylglycinexylidide and glycine xylidide. These in turn also exert a local anesthetic effect. Adrenaline in the mixture serves the primary purpose of vasoconstriction that reduces blood lost during the procedure. In addition, vasoconstriction reduces the rate of absorption of lidocaine from subcutaneous space, which prolongs anesthetic effect of the mixture. Sodium bicarbonate helps in lowering pH of the solution as lidocaine has an acidic pH that causes stinging during injection. Once the total dose of lidocaine has been calculated, it is then divided into number of bags of normal saline that would be required for anesthetizing the areas to be treated. The amount of lidocaine, adrenaline and sodium bicarbonate can be varied as per the area of body that is to be treated. This is because fat in certain areas of body can be more fibrous requiring higher concentration of drug to achieve adequate anesthesia. The doses of each of the three drugs to be added in 1 liter of normal saline when working on different areas of the body are illustrated in the adjoining table (Table 31.2).[13] These doses can be halved when using 500 mL normal saline bags. Each bag that is prepared for infiltration has to be labeled in detail with exact dosages of all three ingredients added to it.

Table 31.2: Variation in composition of tumescent anesthesia solution as per area of body to be treated (dose of sodium bicarbonate remains 10 mL/L of tumescent solution).

Areas	*Lidocaine (mg/L)*	*Epinephrine (mg/L)*
Hips; lateral, medial and anterior thighs; knees	700–750	0.65
Back; male flanks; arms	1000	0.65–1.0
Female abdomen (medial)	1000–1250	1.0
Male abdomen (medial); Male breasts	1250	1.0
Abdomen lateral	750	0.65
Female breasts; chin; cheek and jowls	1500	1.5

Source: Adapted from Klein JA. Tumescent Anaesthesia.

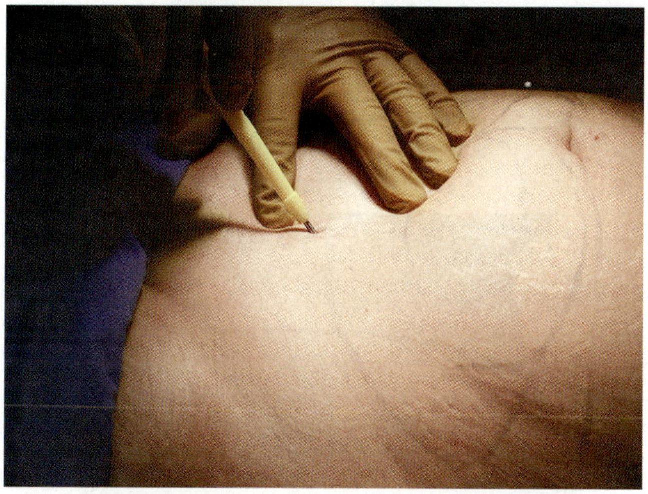

Fig. 31.5: Making of adits with 2 mm skin punch.

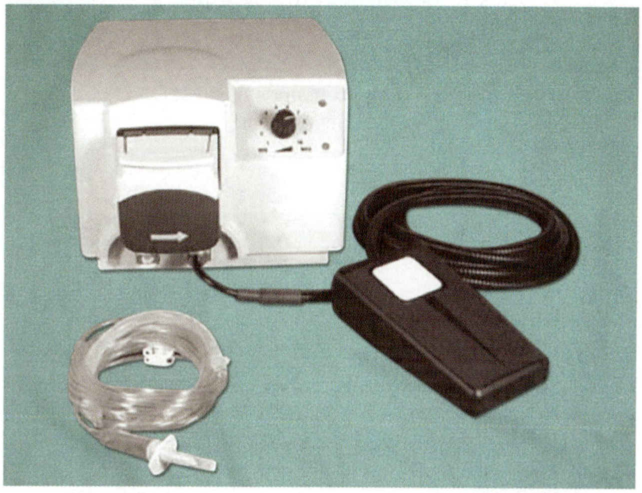

Fig. 31.6: Infiltration pump with foot pedal and specialized rubber tubing.

Meanwhile, the cleaned and prepped patient is made to lie on the operating table. A ready mix of lidocaine and adrenaline solution (available in India as 2% lidocaine plus adrenaline 1:200000) is injected into the spots demarcated as adits. Around 2 mL is injected into the intradermal and subcutaneous spaces at each of the marked spots. With a 1.5 or 2 mm sterile skin biopsy punch, circular holes are made at each of the spots and the skin excised is discarded making sure that it does not get deposited into the fat compartment (Fig. 31.5). A round entry point has the advantage of lessening the damage caused by to and fro motion of the round cannula. In addition, a round hole does not close immediately post operatively under the effect of compression bandaging thus permitting drainage of the blood stained discharge and avoiding subcutaneous collections.

The success of lipobodysculpting under total local anesthesia is completely dependent upon achieving perfection in tumescence of the tissues. This prerequisites the use of an infiltration pump that has a peristaltic flow. The pump works by pushing the fluid into the subcutaneous space till adequate tissue pressure is achieved (Fig. 31.6). The flow stops once this pressure is reached. The infiltration cannula is then moved into a different area so as to continue with infiltration. An ideal tissue infiltration causes uniform swelling of the entire subcutaneous space. During infiltration care has to be taken to start infiltration of the deeper planes prior to going into the superficial planes of fat. Here the marking of the mounds preoperatively helps in determining the areas with fat in deep and superficial planes. The infiltration cannula is inserted through the adit with the sensory or nondominant hand holding the fat in a firm grip between the thumb and all four fingers and pulling it in an outward direction. The cannula gets directed into the deeper planes as a consequence (Fig. 31.7). After the deeper planes are done with, the fat in superficial planes is then infiltrated in a similar manner. Here the grip of the sensory hand is less firm causing limited lifting of the superficial tissues. In

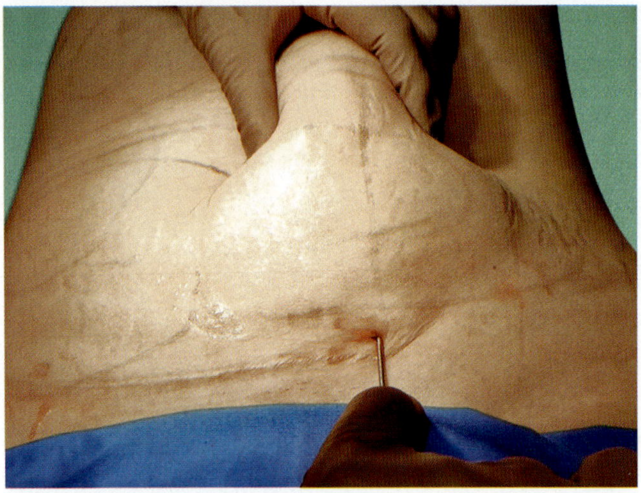

Fig. 31.7: Infiltration of tumescent anesthesia solution beginning in the deeper plane.

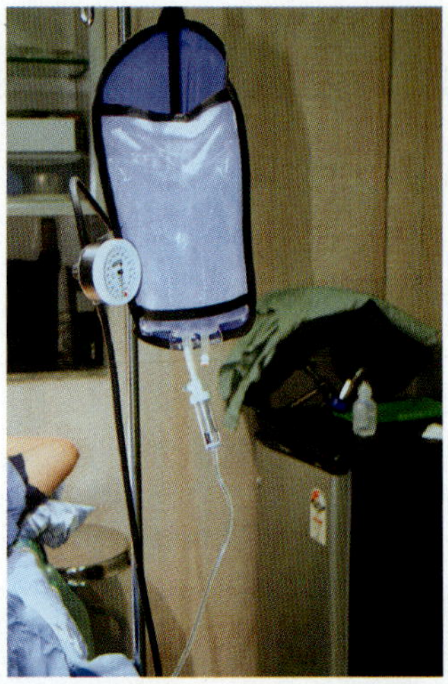

Fig. 31.8: Pressure infusion bag.

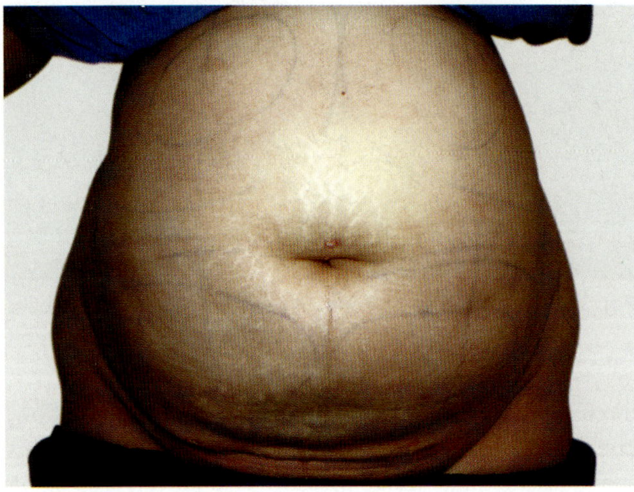

Fig. 31.9: Area to be treated (upper and lower abdomen) immediately after infiltration of tumescent anesthesia solution.

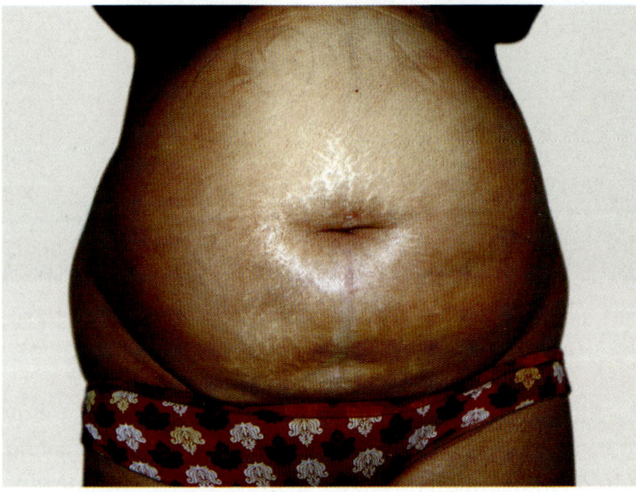

Fig. 31.10: Area (upper and lower abdomen) infiltrated showing detumescence after settling time.

certain cases where the patient is very apprehensive or in patient undergoing repeat Lipobodysculpting and whilst working on the breast, upper abdomen and other areas with very fibrous fat, it is advisable to start infiltrating all areas with a long spinal needle no. 23 or 20. This needle is much thinner and sharper at the tip than a 2 mm internal diameter infiltration cannula. By initiating infiltration with a spinal needle, all areas begin to get anesthetized without much initial stretch pain to the patient. After finishing use of spinal needle through all adits, full infiltration is continued using a standard infiltration cannula as described above. Infiltration can also be done using a pressure infusion bag, which is easily available in India (Fig. 31.8). The area infiltrated grows two to three times the original volume (Fig. 31.9).

The full effect of tumescent anesthesia with lidocaine is evident only when the treated tissue is allowed to detumesce for up to an hour before suctioning is initiated (Fig. 31.10). During this waiting time, lidocaine binds with the adipose tissue cells. The anesthetic effect starts due to the numbing of the nerves in the subcutaneous tissue. The pressure of the fluid molecules causes adipose cells to separate from one another thus weakening their intercellular adhesive bonds. The adrenaline in the solution causes constriction of blood vessels helping in further reducing absorption of lidocaine into systemic circulation. It is estimated that less than 30% of lidocaine gets absorbed into systemic circulation at any given time and hence, there is very little that gets degraded by liver enzymes. The local anesthetic effect is enhanced and prolonged which serves ideal to perform a lipobodysculpting.[12] The volume of tumesced tissue reduces a little, as there is a loss of some of the infiltrated solution. This is part due to absorption into systemic circulation and part due to loss from adits as they are open.

Intraoperative Monitoring

The patient's vital parameters including pulse, blood pressure, oxygen saturation and cardiac leads are constantly monitored before and during the entire procedure. A trained staff nurse keeps recording these parameters and entering them into the anesthetic chart at frequent intervals, i.e. every 30 minutes. The operating dermatosurgeon is made aware of all readings, especially any abnormal ones, as soon as they have been recorded. The patient is awake during the entire procedure, which helps the dermatosurgeon to ensure that the patient is comfortable at all times. The speed and direction of the infiltration and suctioning of fat can be changed as per the patient comfort levels. In addition, the air conditioning temperature and fan speeds also have to be conducive to patient's comforts. The trained staff is entrusted with maintaining a strict record of times of start and end of infiltration.

Once sufficient time has elapsed after the infiltration, the patient is again prepped for the surgery. The cleansing solution remains the same, i.e. an equal mixture of povidone iodine solution and povidone iodine scrub. This is washed off with normal saline solution and then finally followed by a coat of spirit solution to the entire surgical area. It is easier to access all areas with the patient in a standing position. After prepping, the patient is made to lie on a sterile surgical drape spread on the operating table. Sterile drapes are then placed on the patient and secured with sterile clips to create a sterile surgical field. All staff including the dermatosurgeon wears fresh sets of sterile gloves. In some cases, the dermatosurgeon may have to wear two sets of gloves as during suctioning they get torn due to friction with the cannulas and its handle. Some dermatosurgeons prefer two sets of gloves as it helps to have a firm grip of the cannula handle during aspiration and a good grip on the skin with the nondominant hand.

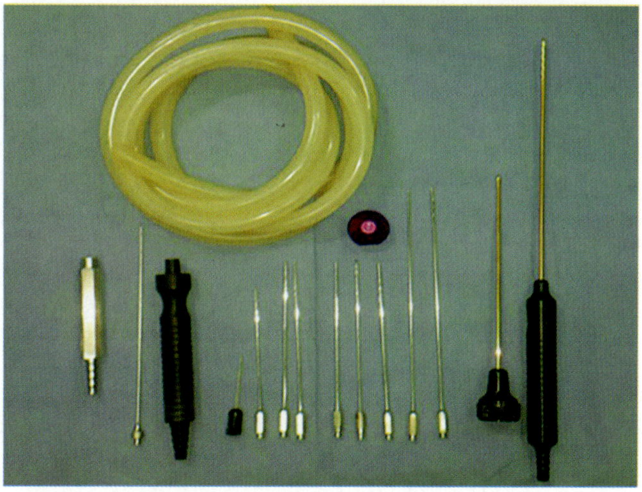

Fig. 31.11: Lipobodysculpting and fat transfer kit showing cannulas of varying diameters and lengths, silicon tubing and decant stand.

Fat Aspiration

Aspiration/suctioning of fat is done using microcannulae in a serially increasing diameter size (Fig. 31.11). Once the patient is positioned on table a 16 G (1.2 mm internal diameter) cannula attached to a handle and suction tube (noncollapsible silicon rubber tubing that is attached to a suction pump) is inserted through the adit. The nondominant hand works as a guide for the cannula tip. It is used to pinch and lift the skin along with superficial fat so as to facilitate the passage of cannula into the deeper planes. This would also have been the plane of initial tumescence. The dominant hand grasps the cannula handle in the palm. The thumb is placed onto the suction hole and index finger tip is placed onto the front of hub of cannula (Fig. 31.12). This helps is reducing damage to skin around adit. The cannula is moved in a horizontal plane in and out of the adit keeping the cannula holes inside the subcutaneous space at all times. The usual dictum that is followed is a rule of three, i.e. three movements are done in a direction with the cannula. After every three strokes, the cannula is partially withdrawn and inserted in a different direction in the same horizontal plane for another three strokes. The strokes cover all areas from an adit in a radial fashion, i.e. "spoke wheel" aspiration.[13] Further strokes are done using a 14 G (1.6 mm internal diameter) and 12G (2.1 mm internal diameter) cannulae in a similar manner through all adits. In certain areas, a 10 G (2.7 mm internal diameter) cannula is employed to help remove larger quantities of fat. At all times, it is mandatory to ensure comfort of the patient.

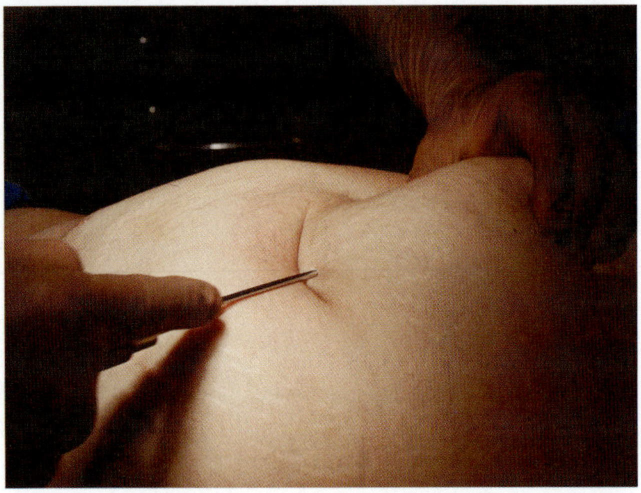

Fig. 31.12: Fat aspiration: note placement of thumb on the handle hole controlling suction, index finger on upper end of hub of cannula and left hand grasping the skin and superficial fat in a firm grip.

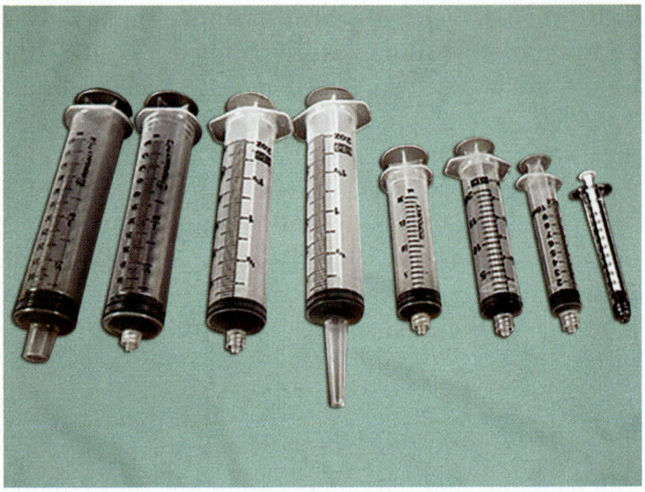

Fig. 31.13: Large volume Toomey syringes used for fat aspiration.

A close eye is kept on the vital parameters at all times during aspiration.

Aspiration can also be done using the Syringe method (devised by Prof Pierre Fournier, Paris, Inventor of Liposuction in 1975) wherein the cannula is attached to specially designed large volume syringes (50 mL/60 mL)[4] (Fig. 31.13). Once the syringe fills up, fat aspirated is discarded into a measuring jar for record keeping. Cannulas of different sizes can be attached to the syringes and fat can be aspirated in a similar manner as that done using suction machine. An easy way could be to use a Luer Lock syringe. Specially designed cannulas are available that go with the specific syringe hubs for attachment.

Fat close to and under the adits can be tackled by using multiple adits for suctioning. Microcannular lipobodysculpting works on the premise of taking out small quantities of fat from each area by using multiple entry points which leads to near equal removal of fat leading to a smooth natural feel postoperatively.

Special mention of fat in the superficial plane is a must, as this space tends to have the blood vessels and nerves traversing through it. Prof Illouz of Paris has categorically stated that it is mandatory to leave the upper 5 mm of fat in the subdermal plane to achieve a smooth natural feel postoperatively.[14] However, Carlo Gasperoni and Paolo Gasperoni of Rome, promoters of Superficial Subdermal Liposuction (SSL), advocate removal of this fat to get rid of cellulite or indentations caused by disease or iatrogenically.[15] It is recommended that fresh starters of liposuction should refrain from very superficial liposuction

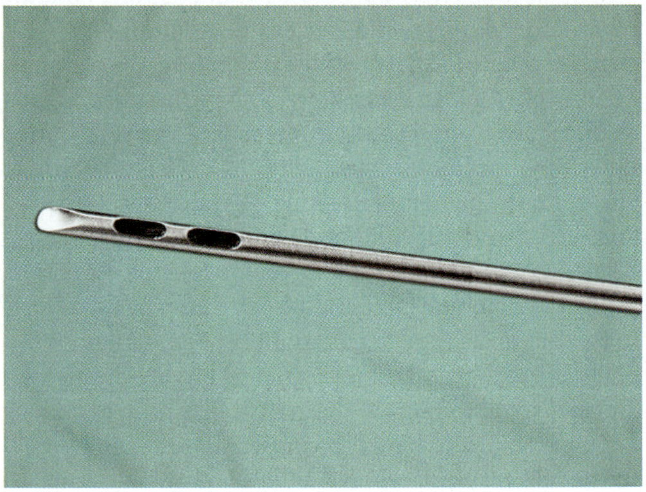

Fig. 31.14: Finesse cannula with aspiration apertures on the bottom surface of cannula near the tip.

as the limited experience clouds their judgment of thickness of subdermal fat layer.[13] Fat in the superficial planes is removed by using thinner cannulas specially designed for such use.[14] These cannulas have holes only on the under surface of the cannula (Fig. 31.14).[16] This prevents scraping under surface of the dermis, which could lead to complications postoperatively. When the cannula is under the surface of skin, the nondominant hand is placed flat on the surface guiding and determining position of tip of cannula. Fat comes out in small aliquots but this works as a finishing touch to the procedure. The suctioning of fat very close to the under surface of dermis is thought to stimulate deposition of collagen and elastin fibers leading to a tightening effect.[14] This takes care of the first query that

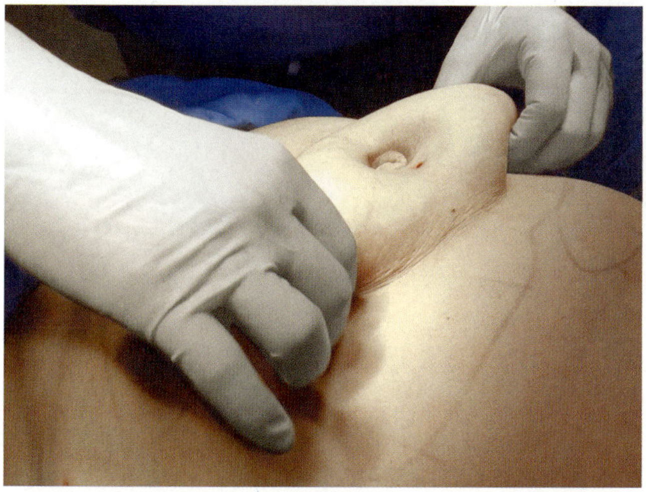

Fig. 31.15: Pinch test to ascertain adequacy of aspiration of fat; it is advisable to compare the two sides to avoid uneven appearance.

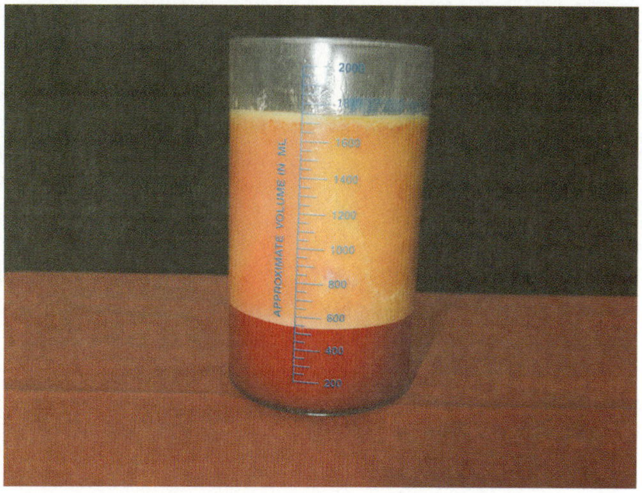

Fig. 31.16: Suction machine canister showing aspirated material with fat in the upper part separated from the blood tinged solution at the bottom.

a patient would ask prior to operation, i.e. is this procedure going to leave me with loose skin once the fat is removed?

The nondominant hand serves as the guide for the entire procedure as it helps in determining the position of the tip of the cannula and guides the cannula into the appropriate plane. In effect, it acts as sense organ for the surgeon. It helps in determining the depth of the cannula. The thumb and the medial border of palm help in relaying cannula tip position to the surgeon. It also helps in feeding the lysed fat lobules into the cannula holes under the effect of suction. An effective fat removal can be achieved only by firm immobilization of the fat by the nondominant hand. By lifting the superficial layers it helps in protecting the surgeon from doing very superficial liposuction. At no time should this hand touch the tip of cannula.[17]

Adequate suctioning of fat is determined by pinching of skin over each of the treated areas and comparing by viewing from end of table. This is an easy way of ensuring symmetry of appearance postoperatively (Fig. 31.15). It also helps in deciding adequacy of fat removal from each half of the body. It is essential that the dermatosurgeon does not leave areas of depression arising from excess localized fat removal, i.e. *lipotrops* or areas of bulge due to inadequate fat removal, i.e. *liponots.*[17]

Fat removed during the procedure is either in a suction canister or a plain canister. The quantity of total aspirate is measured along with quantity of infranatant blood tinged fluid and that of supranatant fat (Fig. 31.16). This is recorded in the patient's notes. The total aspirate after measuring is discarded as a bio waste material in accordance with the local laws.

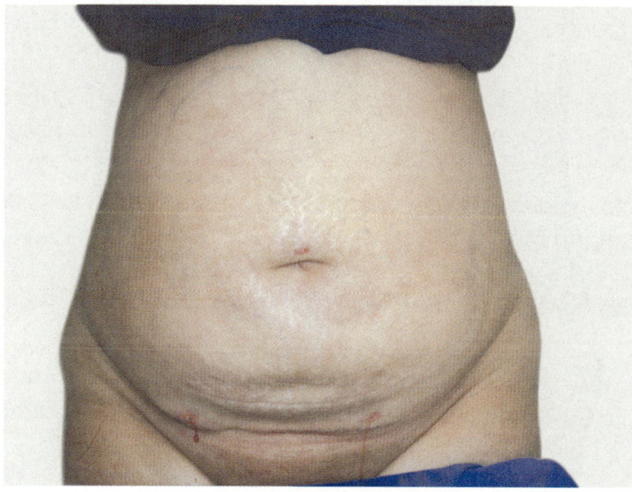

Fig. 31.17: Immediate intraoperative photograph showing treated area (upper and lower abdomen).

Once it is ascertained that adequate removal has been achieved and further aspiration is either painful or causing more blood than fat to come into the suction tube then the patient is asked to stand. A visual confirmation of adequacy of fat removal is done. A photograph is taken of the treated areas (Fig. 31.17).

Dressing

Postoperative dressing of the patient plays a vital role in preventing immediate complications. The patient is cleaned

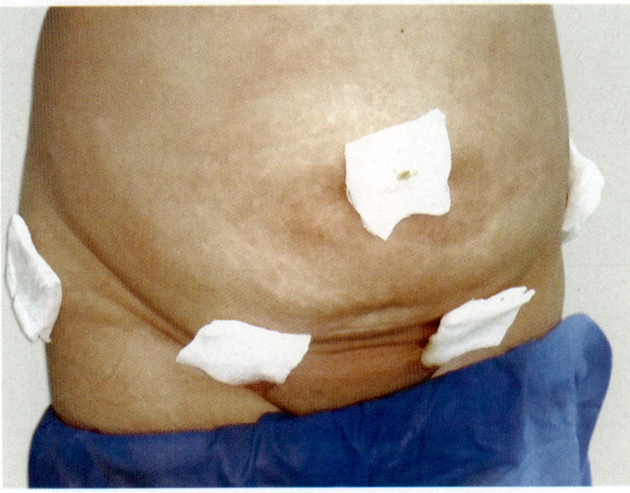

Fig. 31.18: Adits covered with antiseptic ointment and gauze swabs.

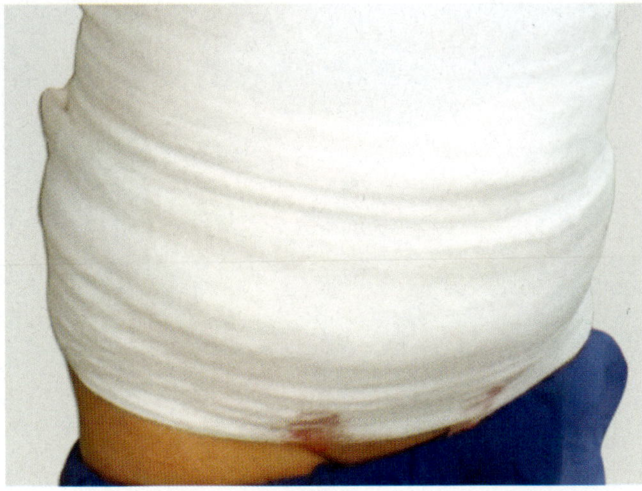

Fig. 31.19: Gamjee roll dressing to cover treated area over the gauze swabs.

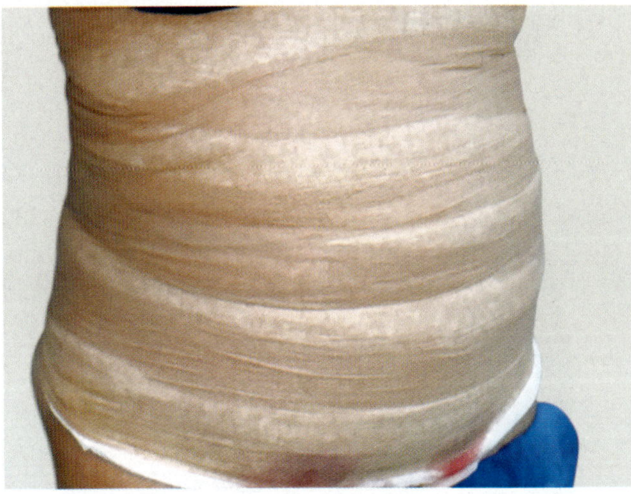

Fig. 31.20: Coban dressing over Gamjee roll dressing to exert maximal pressure onto the treated area.

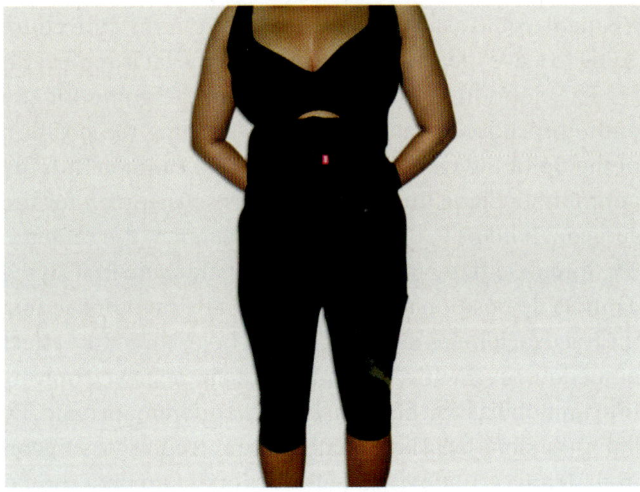

Fig. 31.21: Final layer of bimodal compression dressing with compression garment.

using sterile gauze pads of the blood-tinged fluid draining from all the open adits. Small gauze/Gamjee pads are placed at each of the adits (Fig. 31.18). The entire area is covered with a 6" Gamjee roll dressing (Fig. 31.19). This is then compressed using Coban™ (3M Healthcare, USA) (Fig. 31.20). It helps to increase pressure onto the treated area squeezing out any fluid that is left behind after suctioning and effectively preventing any free space for collections to form. Coban dressing has a self-adhesive surface that tends to stick to the underlying layers keeping the entire dressing in place. It can be further secured using sticking plaster making sure that the plaster does not come in direct contact with the skin surface. A better way to ensure nonslippage of dressing is by using a net dressing over the Gamjee and Coban dressings. Finally the area is then dressed with a tight compression garment specially measured and fitted for the patient (Fig. 31.21). The author finds garments made of synthetic stretchy material to be more helpful than those made of cotton. These are easy to clean leaving no blood stains behind and also dry sooner than cotton garments. This further helps to secure the multilayer dressing. The patient is asked to stay indoors for up to 24 hours till the drainage stops. Once the drainage stops, the garment and all dressing material can be removed. The patient is encouraged to take a clean wash with soap and water in particular the treated area. He/she is to apply an antibiotic ointment to each of the adits and wear the compression garment daily for two weeks. In addition, a prescription for oral antibiotics (cephalosporin or penicillin group) and pain killers (paracetamol preferred) is given to the patient. Once it is ensured that the vital parameters postoperatively are within normal limits then the patient is sent home with an accompanying person. The patient is also handed a Postoperative Instruction Sheet (Addendum 2) that mentions all the advice about care of treated areas and what to expect after procedure. In particular, there are phone numbers provided which the patient can call in case of emergency. Symptoms of lidocaine toxicity that can arise after 12 to 24 hours later are listed. It is customary for the clinic staff to call upon the patient after 24 hours to ensure smooth postoperative recovery. The patient is generally called back to clinic on 2nd postoperative day to check for early signs of any complications like bruising, bleeding, hematoma formation, excessive pain due to possible infection, fever, etc. At this time a photo is taken of the treated areas and added to the records.

Postoperative Advise

The patient is advised not to indulge in heavy exercise and swimming for at least two weeks till the treated areas have healed and cause no pain at movement. They are advised to wear the compression garment for the whole of two weeks at least. This helps in reducing the chances of collection within the treated fat compartment and also relieves pain by giving a constant and firm support to the treated area.

The patient is seen in clinic postoperatively at 1 week, 2 weeks, 6 weeks and 3 months. At each of these visits photos are taken for record keeping. Patient is advised to follow sensible dietary restrictions and a regular exercise schedule daily.

Modifications for Site

Fat is distributed across the body in the subcutaneous plane. However, in certain areas it tends to be densely packed and has more fibrous bands traversing through it. This can make it difficult to achieve complete anesthesia and separation of adipocytes. To make this possible, a variation in the amount of lidocaine and adrenaline in the tumescent solution helps. Dr Jeffery Klein has suggested these doses after years of extensive work in this field (*see* Table 31.2).

On a similar note, tumescent anesthesia is administered with spinal needles initially when working on an area with fibrous fat or in patients who are undergoing a repeat procedure. Similarly, the suction cannula size also would need to smaller in certain areas like breast (male/ female), upper abdomen, inner thighs, medial knees, chin, cheeks and jowls.

Female breast reduction requires a multiple adit approach much more than what are required for other areas. The entire breast is divided in to conical zones that are then individually anesthetized using spinal needle only. Also, during suctioning, the cannula size should not exceed more than 14 G (1.6 mm internal diameter) in any of the zones. It has to be ensured that the fat removed makes the nipple lift upwards and outwards (superiorly and laterally) and both breasts have near equal amount of fat left after the procedure.

Complications

The very mention of *Liposuction* for fat removal and body shaping evokes negative responses from most patients who come to the clinic seeking solutions for their body weight and abnormal shape. This is because of the very bad reputation it has in the layman's world, as it is fraught with multiple complications including death in many cases. However, since the invention and inculcation of tumescent anesthesia with lidocaine for performing this procedure there is a significant reduction in the incidence of complications. To add to this, till date there has not been single death reported worldwide when lipobodysculpting is performed adhering to the principles of tumescent anesthesia and microcannulae for suctioning.

The untoward effects following lipobodysculpting can be broadly divided into immediate effects, late effects and those due to excessive liposuction.

Immediate Effects

These are effects that occur within the first 2 weeks following lipobodysculpting.

- On the day of the procedure, after the patient is dressed with bimodal compression, there can be *discharge of copious amounts of blood-tinged fluid* from all the adits that was used for fat removal. This usually subsides within 18 to 24 hours following the procedure. At this stage, the patient is advised to take off all the dressings and garment and have a wash making sure all adits are cleaned well with soap and water.
- During this dressing removal, some patients can report of *dizziness or "morning-after-Liposuction" syncope* that is temporary and can be easily corrected by lying down.

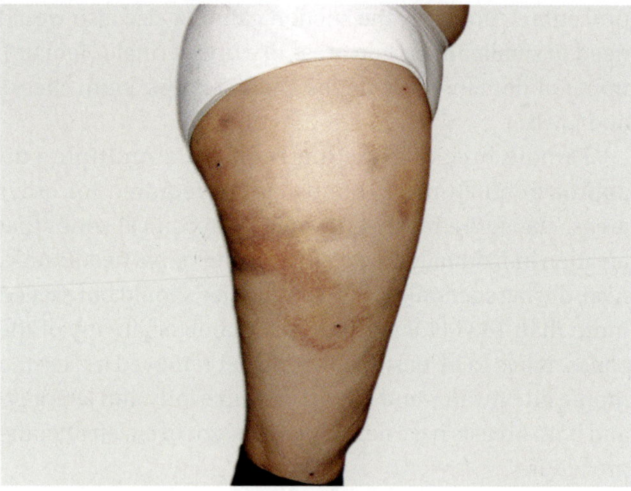

Fig. 31.22: Significant bruising seen 2nd day after lipobodysculpting done to saddle bags in a young lady.

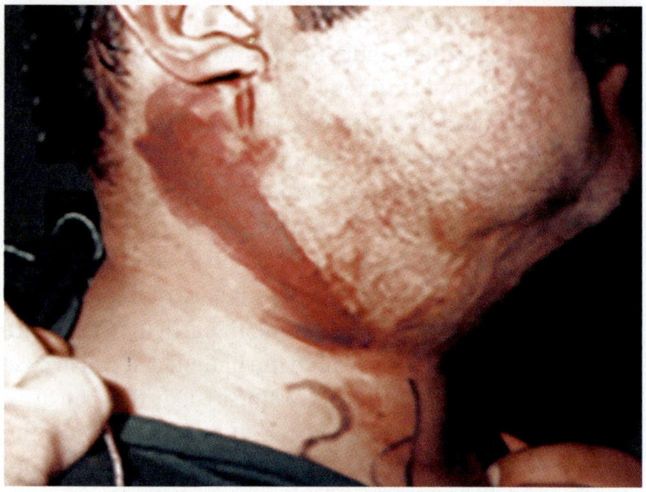

Fig. 31.23: Hematoma formation after liposuction of neck tracking into the posterior triangle.
Courtesy: Prof Lawrence M Field, USA.

Just seeing blood colored stains on the dressing that is removed can also bring it about. A few patients could also have syncope during the procedure but this is not so pronounced as the patient is lying on the table. It is wise to keep an ampoule of atropine close to hand at such times.

- It is absolutely essential for the dermatosurgeon to be aware of the potential effects of lidocaine absorption. These show onset within 12–24 hours of administration. They can present as drowsiness, tinnitus, dysgeusia, dizziness and twitching. These are mainly due to central nervous system (CNS) stimulation. Further absorption can lead to onset of seizures, coma, respiratory failure and arrest. Drug levels beyond these lead to cardiovascular depression and death.[18]
- *Pain* or an aching sensation can be experienced in the areas that have undergone the procedure. A generous dose of non-nonsteroidal antiinflammatory drug (NSAID)-based drug (i.e. Acetaminophen or Paracetamol) can help with this. The pain usually starts at first dressing change and gradually gets worse over the next 5–7 days after which it starts to settle down. This is because the fat compartment has been injured badly during the procedure and healing takes place as per the stages of inflammation. It is very important during the preprocedure consultation that the patient is made aware of intensity and duration of pain that is to be expected in the postoperative period. Often pain postoperatively is the first question raised by the patient when they come for first consultation.
- *Bruising and swelling* of the treated areas can be seen from the third day postoperative. These primarily occur when adequate compression is not applied to the treated areas. It is the direct result of aggressive liposuction causing damage to blood vessels and accumulation of blood in the treated fat compartment (Figs. 31.22 and 31.23).
- *Facial flushing and temperature elevation* can occur in some individuals. These are probably secondary to the inflammation and settle easily with regular Paracetamol and rest.
- *Edema* has been reported in many cases postoperatively distal to the treated areas. This can be due to destruction of the natural lymphatic drainage within the treated area, excess anesthesia fluid infiltration and added compression of the area. It usually settles with rest and elevation within a week. In rare cases, there is a need for making further adits in the dependent areas to release the collection. This could be required in case of severe edema of the genitals following lower abdomen lipobodysculpting.
- *Prolonged numbness of the skin* overlying the treated fat deposits can become an issue in some patients. It occurs due to damage to the superficial sensory nerves that traverse within the fat compartment. It is often reported when the patient first comes for a one week check-up and can be reported up to three months by when it usually resolves.
- *Itching* specially at the sites of entry is common. This is part of the wound healing process and settles very well with regular moisturizing of the skin.

- *Post-liposuction panniculitis* is a problem that can happen when the adits are closed with sutures thus entrapping the blood-tinged solution within the fat compartment. It can lead to formation of microseromas that present with increased redness, tenderness, swelling and warmth of skin on the treated area. It warrants bacterial culture and sensitivity testing. The treatment is initially with oral antibiotics and then a short course of oral steroids to take care of the inflammation.[19]

Delayed Effects

- *Irregularity of skin* over the treated fat areas can be a result of excess superficial liposuction. This can be because of uneven fat removal from the superficial plane resulting in lumpy feel and wrinkling of skin. Some of this appearance gets corrected when the skin contracts and firms up by 3 months.
- *Scars* at adits can be hypopigmented or more so hyperpigmented in dark skinned individuals. Trauma to the dermoepidermal junction during the procedure with to and fro movement of the cannula and constant hitting of the cannula hub to the adit skin can result in pigment alteration and scarring. These can be minimized by making adequate sized incisions as adits, using small bore cannulas that are effective, making sure to keep the finger at the tip of the hub while moving cannula to and fro, making enough number of adits to treat all the areas, moving cannula in the horizontal plane with minimal friction during entry and exit from adit and also avoiding suturing the adits postprocedure. One way to avoid bad scarring is by lifting the skin near the adit and then passing the cannula through the adit. Pigmentation can be taken care of by use of depigmenting creams. Fractional lasers can be employed in case of unsightly scars that can start as early as 2 weeks postprocedure.
- *Allergic contact dermatitis* can occur to prolonged use of topical antibiotics ointment applications to the adits. Care has to be taken not to apply any sticking plasters directly to the skin during fixing of the compression dressings. Some patients can be sensitive to the adhesive in the tape. Also due to altered sensation on the skin in some patients, it is wise to avoid contact of sticking plasters of any kind to skin.
- *Lipotrops* are formed as a result of excess unequal fat suctioning (Fig. 31.24).
- *Liponots* form due to inadequate suctioning of fat from certain areas. Both these can be a cause of dissatisfied patient and can be avoided by regular skin pinch checks during the procedure. However, the patient should be made aware of a temporary lumpiness or heaviness in the area treated which can last from 2 to 6 weeks postoperative. This is due to the inflammatory processes occurring in the fat compartment following the procedure.

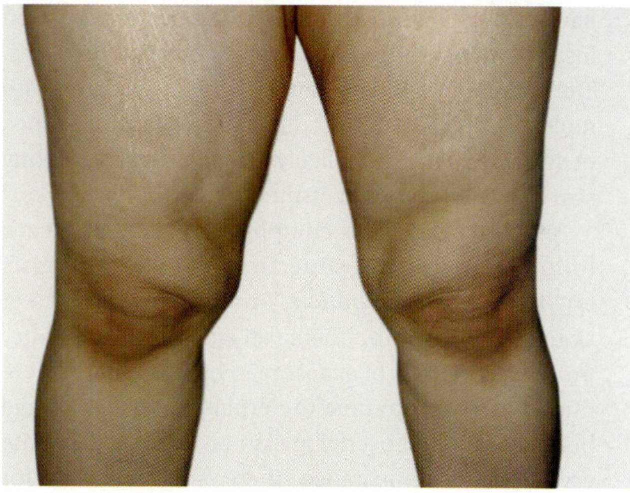

Fig. 31.24: Excessive lipobodysculpting above knees showing areas of depression.
Courtesy: Prof Lawrence M Field, USA.

- An unusual problem that is often reported is *irregularity of the menstrual cycle* in females after the procedure. This is of no significance once the pregnancy tests are negative. The cycles return to normal rhythm within the next 2 months postoperatively.
- *Fascial and muscular injury* can occur during deep suctioning for prolonged periods. This happens more so when larger bore cannulas are employed for suctioning. The patient, being awake, is more likely to make the surgeon aware of this injury during the procedure. This prevents further deep suctioning and internal damage.
- *Excessive liposuction:* Excessive liposuction or lipobodysculpting can in essence mean excessive superficial fat suctioning that leads to various complications. Large bore sharp holed cannulas used for superficial fat suctioning can cause damage to the neurovascular bundle that runs in the subdermal fat layer. This can lead to vascular compromise of the overlying dermis and epidermis, which can result in *overlying skin necrosis.* This is a dreaded complication occurring in a shape enhancing procedure that can lead to legal complaints. However, with the advent of microcannular lipobodysculpting these complications

have reduced in their occurrence. The treatment of skin loss will depend upon the extent and the body area. The patient may end up having to be hospitalized with multiple skin grafting procedures and prolonged periods of dressings. Finally it is likely to heal with an unsightly scar that would warrant further cosmetic procedures.

Another permanent complication that can occur following excessive superficial fat suctioning is *erythema ab lipoaspiration*. This is an appearance of skin very similar to erythema ab igne that is seen after prolonged periods of exposure to heat. Similarly, here due to excessive trauma to dermal vessels by a large bore cannula the overlying skin takes on a reticulate erythematous appearance. There is no treatment for this skin appearance and it also does not get better with time. *Seromas* are formed as result of damage to the connective tissues network after excessive fat suctioning. This results in destruction of the lymphatic channels and formation of a subcutaneous cavity that becomes the site of collection. They are usually noticed within a few days of the procedure (Fig. 31.25). The usual incriminating factors for formation of seromas are use of large bore cannulas, aggressive and excessive cannula movement in the fat compartment, inadequate hemostasis due to inadequate tumescence, use of Ultrasonic waves for fat destruction and recent use of NSAIDs. Seromas can be avoided by using microcannulae for lipoaspiration and multiple adits creating criss-cross movements of cannulae helping drainage of all subcutaneous collections.

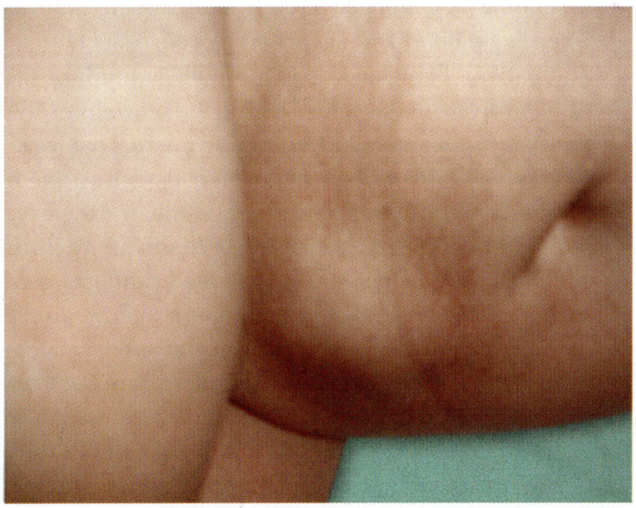

Fig. 31.25: Seroma formation on lower abdomen.
Courtesy: Dr Ioannis Peros, Greece.

- An *increased risk of thromboembolic events* has been reported with the use of systemic anesthesia for liposuction. Prolonged periods of immobilization following large area liposuction and consequent pain increase the risk of deep vein thrombosis (DVT) and pulmonary embolism (PE). In addition, hypothermia and intravenous fluid administration add to the risk of hypercoagulability. This leads to overall increase in risk of DVT and PE.
- *Postliposuction edema* is the appearance of edema of treated areas within 24 to 72 hours after extensive liposuction surgery. This can also spread to involve distant areas when it is labeled as amplified liposuction edema (ALE). The collection is the result of excess fluid collection in the subcutaneous space postoperatively due to the obstruction plus destruction of lymphatic drainage system and excessive capillary filtration into the treated area. The fluid collected in the subcutaneous space has higher osmotic pressure due to large protein molecules that leak into this space postoperatively. This attracts greater amount of intravascular fluid further increasing the collection. The problem can be avoided or reduced by adopting open drainage and bimodal compression postoperatively. Open drainage allows maximum removal of the fluid from the subcutaneous space after the surgery. Bimodal compression involves a high grade compression immediate after surgery to press out as much fluid as possible followed by a low grade compression with a compression garment for up to two weeks to gradually allow the subcutaneous edema to drain via the lymphatic channels by increasing the interstitial hydrostatic pressure.
- *Infection* following a lipobodysculpting procedure can be a doomsday scenario for the dermatosurgeon. However, the risk of infection is very low when all the steps are followed aseptically. Measures to prevent infections include profound tumescent anesthesia with open drainage and bimodal compression to reduce postoperative edema, hematomas and seromas. Use of lidocaine, which is bactericidal, helps in reducing the growth in the subcutaneous space. By not suturing the adits, adequate drainage of the infiltrated fluid occurs which prevents infections.

Patients are encouraged to take daily showers and clean all adits with soap and water. Further they are advised to apply an antibiotic ointment daily to all adits. Apart from low-grade cutaneous infection of the adits, the more serious infections that can occur are necrotizing fasciitis, toxic shock syndrome, cellulitis and rarely atypical mycobacterial infections. *Necrotizing fasciitis* is the most serious complication of liposuction surgery that occurs due to infection spreading from subcutaneous fat to the dermis. It can occur because of perforation of abdominal organ or poor sterilization techniques or even direct contamination of the entry points after surgery. It has to be diagnosed clinically without any waste of time, as it is a life threatening condition.

- One has to mention here regarding *injury to internal organs* during liposuction. There have been reports of liver tear and pleural punctures during liposuction of the abdomen and breast areas. These have occurred with use of large bore cannulas with excessive force while the procedure is performed under systemic anesthesia. They have resulted in major complications requiring prolonged hospital admissions and even surgical correction. This is yet to occur with the correct use of microcannulae for liposuction under tumescent anesthesia. One major advantage of working with an awake patient is that any movement of cannula into the unanesthetized area can be alerted immediately and damage to internal organs avoided. The microcannulae cannot be used with great force, as they would not be able to withstand it. This helps in preventing any internal injury.

ACKNOWLEDGMENTS

The author has learnt the art of lipobodysculpting and autologous fat transfer from Dr Jeffrey Klein, doyen of tumescent Anesthesia. He is forever indebted toward his teacher for introducing him to a whole new world of fat removal. He is also grateful to Prof Pierrre Fournier, inventor of liposuction and Prof Lawrence M Field, first dermatologist to learn liposuction, for always encouraging and inspiring him to teach and spread awareness about liposuction and fat transfer amongst all dermatologists. He also extends his gratitude toward Prof Field, Father of Dermatosurgery, Dr Ioannis Peros, Dermatologist from Greece and Prof Kee Yan Chung, Dermatologist and Mohs Surgeon from South Korea for sharing their photographs for this chapter.

REFERENCES

1. Collins PS. The methodology of liposuction surgery. Dermatol Clin. 1990;8(3):395-400.
2. Fischer A, Fischer G. First surgical treatment for molding body's cellulite with three 5 mm incisions. Bull Int Acad Cosmet Surg. 1976;3:35.
3. Illouz YG. Body contouring by lipolysis: a 5-year experience with over 3000 cases. Plast Reconstr Surg. 1983;72(5):591-7.
4. Fournier PF. Reduction syringe liposculpturing. Dermatol Clin. 1990;8(3):539-51.
5. Fournier PF, Otteni FM. Lipodissection in body sculpting: the dry procedure. Plast Reconstr Surg. 1983;72(5):598-601.
6. Coleman WP 3rd. The history of dermatologic liposuction. Dermatol Clin. 1990;8(3):381-3.
7. Klein JA. Tumescent technique for liposuction surgery. Am J Cosm Surg. 1987;4:263-7.
8. Klein JA. Cytochrome P450 3A4 and lidocaine metabolism. In: Klein JA (Ed). Tumescent Technique. St. Louis: Mosby Inc.; 2000.
9. Klein JA. Personal communication. 2011.
10. Culver DH, Horan TC, Gaynes RP, et al. Surgical wound infection rates by wound class, operative procedure and patient risk index. Am J Med. 1991;91(Suppl 3B):152S-157S.
11. Klein JA. Infections. In: Klein JA (Ed). Tumescent Technique. St. Louis: Mosby Inc.; 2000.
12. Klein JA. Pharmacokinetics of tumescent lidocaine. In: Klein JA (Ed). Tumescent Technique. St. Louis: Mosby Inc.; 2000.
13. Klein JA. Clinical pharmacology. In: Klein JA (Ed). Tumescent Technique. St Louis: Mosby Inc.; 2000.
14. Illouz YG. History and current concepts of lipoplasty. Clin Plast Surg. 1996;23(4):721-30.
15. Gasperoni C, Gasperoni P. Subdermal liposuction: long term experience. Clin Plast Surg. 2006;33(1):63-73.
16. Klein JA. Microcannulas. In: Klein JA (Ed). Tumescent Technique. St. Louis: Mosby Inc.; 2000.
17. Klein JA. Surgical technique: microcannular tumescent liposuction. In: Klein JA (Ed). Tumescent Technique. St. Louis: Mosby Inc.; 2000.
18. Catterall WA, Mackie K. Local anesthetics. In: Brunton L, Chabner B, Knollman B (Eds). Goodman & Gilman's The Pharmacological Basis if Therapeutics. 12th edition. New York: McGraw-Hill; 2011.
19. Klein JA. Miscellaneous complications. In: Klein JA (Ed). Tumescent Technique. St. Louis: Mosby Inc.; 2000.

CHAPTER 32

Autologous Fat Transfer

Nilesh Goyal, Nitin Barde

INTRODUCTION

Dermatologists are the worldwide experts when it comes to using fillers for facial rejuvenation. As the understanding of science of ageng face has increased, so is the need for using large quantities of fillers for achieving a youthful look. This has a huge impact on costs involved, which in many cases forbids patients from undertaking the procedure. On the other hand, fat that is present in abundance around the waist and thighs can be utilized for this purpose. The process of acquiring fat from one area of body and injecting it into other area as a filler material is called as autologous fat transfer or fat grafting. Fat is a live organ with multiple adipocytes interspersed with stem cells, endothelial cells, smooth muscle cells, fibroblasts and even immune cells that makes it a much better material for filling a wrinkle or lifting a scar. There are studies, which prove fat as a far superior material for facial rejuvenation and scar remodeling than hyaluronic acid fillers.[1]

INDICATIONS[2]

- Cosmetic
  - Facial
    - Aging changes
    - Melolabial grooves
    - Central cheek depressions
    - Subcommissural depressions
    - Flattened upper lip
    - Glabella
    - Diffuse age-related lipoatrophy.
  - Augmentation
    - Lip augmentation
    - Chin augmentation
    - Malar augmentation.
  - Scars
    - Traumatic
    - Lipoatrophy, acne
    - Idiopathic lipodystrophy
    - Facial hemiatrophy.
  - Nonfacial
    - Rejuvenation of the hands
    - Body contour defects
    - Depressions, liposuction induced
    - Breast enlargement
    - Traumatic scars.
- Congenital defects
  - Hemifacial atrophy
  - Soft-tissue defects of the body.
- Noncosmetic
  - Migraine headaches
  - Clival chordoma surgery
  - Congenital short palate
  - Vocal cord paralysis
  - Lumbar laminectomy
  - Sulcus vocalis
  - Vocal cord scar
  - Hemifacial atrophy
  - Myringoplasty
  - Eye socket reconstruction
  - Frontal sinus fracture
  - Temporomandibular joint reconstruction.

PRINCIPLES OF FAT TRANSFER

- *Fat harvesting*: This should be as atraumatic as possible, to preserve the maximum number of viable adipocytes.
  - *Donor site selection*: The choice of donor site depends upon the ease of access and safety. There is no true consensus as to donor site selection.[3] The retention rates of abdominal and non-abdominal fat are same, though fat from lower abdominal areas and inner thigh may have high concentration of stem cells.[4,5]

- *Tumescent solution*: A large volume of fluid with diluted amount of a local anesthetic (LA) and a vasoconstrictor is called as tumescent solution. It reduces pain and bleeding and facilitates liposuction. Fat grafting can be performed under general, epidural, or local anesthesia with or without sedation. All local anesthetics impair adipocyte differentiation, when used for harvesting.[6] However with the doses used, their effects are minimal. The most commonly used LA is lignocaine. It is used in doses of 35 mL/kg, with some studies reporting maximum dose up to 55 mL/kg.[7]

  No differences were observed between adipocyte samples harvested with or without tumescent solution.[8] The infiltration should be performed very gently and slowly and the amount of fluid infiltrated is in the ratio of 1:1 to the aspirated fat.
- *Selection of the harvesting cannula*: There are multiple cannulas having variable diameter with one or more either blunt or sharp openings through which the fat is aspirated. However, the most commonly used cannulas are the ones which have blunt openings. The aspiration of fat with larger diameter cannula has greater viable fat cells and have better survival.[9,10] In general, 3 mm aspiration cannula is used with blunt openings.
- *Liposuction*: The various methods used to aspirate fat are handheld syringe aspiration and vacuum-assisted, water assisted, or ultrasound-assisted lipectomy. There is evidence to suggest that no difference exists in cell viability between syringe aspiration and liposuction pump aspiration.[11] A low pressure aspiration system, usually by syringe, using a blunt harvesting cannula is the generally accepted norm. The pressure generated with 10 cc syringe is about 0.37 atm.

• *Fat processing techniques*: There are various fat processing techniques like centrifugation, washing, filtering, sedimentation and telfa rolling. These fat processing techniques have important roles in graft survival.[12] They are intended to isolate the fat tissue aspirated from the oil, blood, and debris and other unwanted components of the tumescence solution. This is important for the viability and retention of the fat graft.[7]
  - *Centrifugation*: When this method is used the speed of processing should not be more than 3000 rpm (1200 g), as the speed above this damages the adipocytes.[7] After centrifugation, three levels can be observed in the syringe. The lower level is made up of blood and debris, water, and components of the tumescence solution; the middle layer consists of the fat to be injected; and the top layer is formed by the oil resulting from the broken down fatty acids.
  - *Washing and filtration*: In this method, fat aspirated is washed and filtered with normal saline.
  - *Telfa rolling*: This procedure consists of pouring the aspirated fat onto large pieces of Telfa nonadherent dressings, which is gently rolled and kneaded around the gauze and then transferred back again into the syringes for use. One study has shown that telfa/mesh processed fat results in equivalent results without a costly and time-consuming centrifuge.[13]

• *Fat injections*: Injections may be done in multiple passes, in multiple tissue planes, and in multiple directions, injecting small volumes in each pass. For injection in normal areas, blunt cannulae are most commonly used. However, needles can be used when fat transfer is done in scar or fibrosed areas to release their adherence. There is evidence to support that fat should be injected soon after harvesting.[14]

  Glycerol-3-phosphate dehydrogenase activity, which is a measure of adipocyte destruction, increases linearly until 4 hours. So aspirated fat should be injected as soon as possible. The process of injection should be very slow, so as to avoid shear stress to fat cells. There is evidence to show that low shear stress increases fat cells survival.[15,16]

  The fat should be injected at the time of withdrawing, i.e. retrograde injection technique, depositing small aliquots of fat at each site. Presently, overcorrection to obtain better graft survival seems to lack scientific support. Compressive bandages or massages on the grafted area should be avoided.[7]

BASIS/RATIONALE OF FAT TRANSFER

Autologous fat transfer should be considered in patients who need a large quantity of filler for deep filling for facial rejuvenation or a large depressed scar. Fat can be considered as a replacement for soft tissue lost due to atrophy secondary to inflammation or injury, e.g. morphea, depressed scars, etc.

After fat transfer, nearly 50% of fat transferred gets resorbed within 2–3 months leading to recurrence of depression or wrinkling. But the amount that stays behind encourages laying down of new collagen and elastin. It becomes the framework underneath the tissues on which further fat can be deposited. Studies have proved that fat injected intramuscularly is viable for many years post-injection and also tends to grow as the area fattens up.[17] Fat injection has to be repeated usually at three monthly intervals till the desired cosmetic result is achieved. The results then tend to last for many years.[18] One important observation to be noted here is that the skin overlying the injected area tends to get a glow and looks much younger and livelier. It is often observed that pigmented depressed scars get lighter following fat injection under them. Patients have to be counseled regarding the pros and cons of fat grafting vis-à-vis dermal filler injection.

PREPROCEDURE

Investigations

Patients are required to undergo blood tests to determine fitness for the procedure. These are as for lipobodysculpting, i.e. a complete blood count, liver function tests, creatinine, clotting parameters like prothrombin time and activated partial thromboplastin time. In addition, the viral markers for human immunodeficiency virus (HIV), Hepatitis B and Hepatitis C have to be done to rule out their presence.

PROCEDURE

Anesthesia

The tumescent solution required for anesthetizing the donor area is prepared just prior to the procedure. Here the concentration of lidocaine is kept at half compared with that in the Klein's formula used for normal lipobodysculpting. To explain this further, if one were to add 400 mg lidocaine to a 500 mL bag of normal saline as per Klein's formulation then the amount added would be 200 mg in 500 mL for a case of fat transfer. The reason behind this is that lidocaine has high affinity for adipocytes. Fat transfer is a procedure requiring healthy adipocytes that are deposited into the new site. Lidocaine afflicted adipocytes would be toxic and not have a long life. The concentration of adrenaline and sodium bicarbonate tends to be the same as in Klein's formula.[18] Usually the amount of tumescent solution required for fat harvesting is very small (up to 250 mL). Using an infiltration cannula the tumescent solution is injected under the skin with the help of a pressure bag or infiltration pump or even with a large (20 mL/50 mL) Luer Lock syringe. Adequate time has to be given as for lipobodysculpting for the tumescent anesthesia to act. This is about 45–60 minutes depending upon the extent of the donor area.

Preparation

On the day of the procedure, the patient is asked to have a light meal prior to the procedure. The area of fat harvesting is marked with a surgical marker. It is cleansed with Povidone Iodine solution and then with surgical grade spirit. The patient is then shifted onto the operating table and draped to demarcate the sterile surgical field. An entry point for the cannula, i.e. adit is marked. This is infiltrated with 2% lidocaine and 1:200,000 adrenaline mixture solution (usually up to 2 mL is required) (Fig. 32.1). A 1.5 mm/2.0 mm skin punch is used to make a precise circular hole within the anesthetized area (Figs. 32.2 and 32.3).

Fat Harvesting

The first step for fat transfer is the acquisition of fat, i.e. fat harvesting. The best areas for this are the lateral thigh, lower buttocks, lower abdomen and waist. The fat in these areas is less fibrous, can be acquired without much difficulty and in addition is found to have stem cells. This is determined following examination during pre-procedure consultation. Also, the amount of fat to be harvested can have a bearing on the area from which it is acquired. It is prudent to determine the amount of fat that will be required to fill the wrinkles or scar prior to starting the procedure. This can be done by injection of normal saline into the treatment area. This

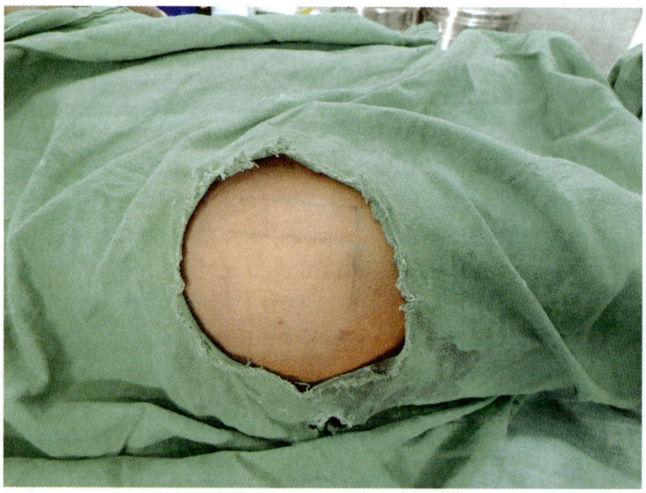

Fig. 32.1: Donor area of fat is infiltrated with tumescent anesthesia.

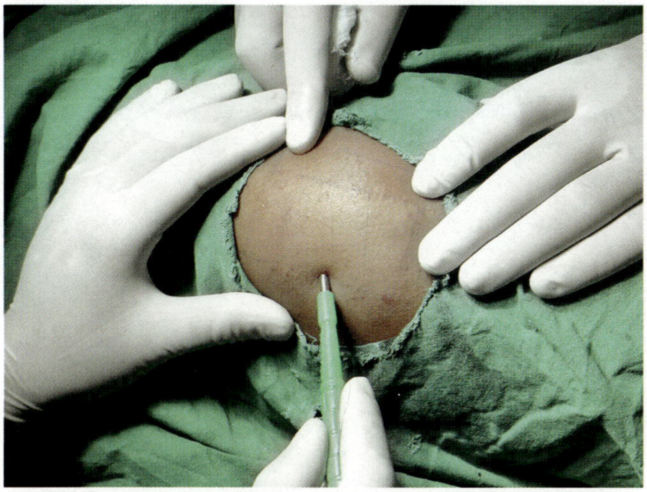

Fig. 32.2: A circular punch is used to make point of entry for aspiration cannula.

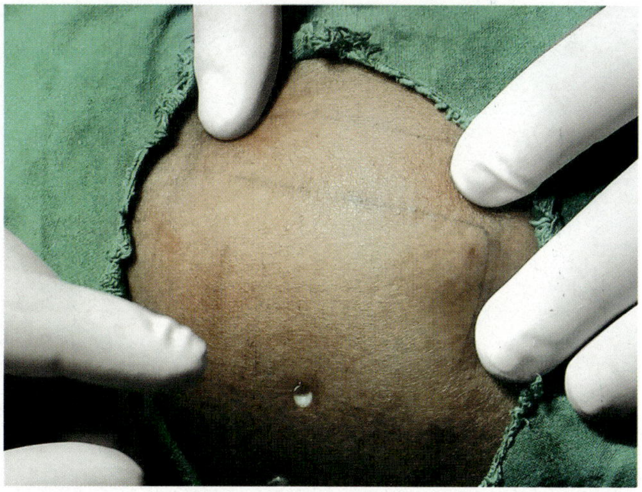

Fig. 32.3: A circular hole seen in skin as point of entry.

also helps in giving the patient an idea about how the area will appear after filling. The author recommends extracting three times the quantity of fat that will be injected in one sitting. The extra aspirated fat can be stored in deep freezer for future injections.

Adequate clinical photographs of the area of fat harvesting and fat injection have to be taken. The patient is explained the procedure during the clinic visit. As the whole procedure is done under local anesthesia there are no fasting requirements prior to the procedure. A thorough medical history has to be taken including history of previous herpes infection, diabetes and regular medications.

Steps of Procedure (Fig. 32.4A)

- Once the anesthesia time has elapsed, using 12 G/10 G, 8–15 cm length cannula attached to a 10 mL Luer Lock syringe, fat harvesting can be commenced (Fig. 32.4B). A higher gauge cannula is preferred so as to cause less damage to the adipocytes. The Fat aspirated will have more complete fat cells that will increase their survival in the recipient area.
- The syringe method works by inserting the cannula tip under the skin till all the holes are inside the fat compartment. Then pulling the piston of the syringe and holding it by abutting the thumb in-between base of syringe and the piston, creates a vacuum (Fig. 32.4C).
- To and fro movements of this vacuum created syringe cannula system within the fat compartment with the nondominant hand guiding the fat lobules into the cannula helps in collecting good quality fat for grafting (Fig. 32.5). The vacuum created in the syringe should be kept at a low pressure, as this will cause lesser damage to the adipocytes during aspiration. This is usually called as gentle suctioning (in contrast to fat suctioning for lipobodysculpting where higher vacuum pressures are applied to get more fat per stroke).
- The syringe with aspirate thus obtained is then made to stand upside down in a test tube stand after detaching the cannula (Fig. 32.6A). This causes a separation of the fat and fluid components (hydrohematic component) within the syringe (Fig. 32.6B). Fat being lighter in weight and density tends to float up and the fluid tends to gravitate downwards.
- The separated blood tinged fluid is drained off from the syringe (Fig. 32.7A). This process is repeated till all fluid is drained off and only fat remains in the syringe (Fig. 32.7B).
- Further this aspirate is passed through a filter paper kept on a small bowl. This filter paper without lint (fat for injection cannot have any nonviable elements) is obtained by separating a facemask used in operating theatres. The fat stays on top of the paper and any remaining fluid gets filtered into the bowl.
- This fat can be filled into Luer Lock syringes of 1 mL with the help of a spoon. Such 1 mL syringes filled with only fat are kept ready for injection.
- Some proponents of fat transfer suggest breaking of the bonds between fat cells by passing it from one syringe to another syringe using a connector. This can be done in cases where the fat aspirated is to be injected into the periorbital area, which would look bad cosmetically if the fat is lumpy.

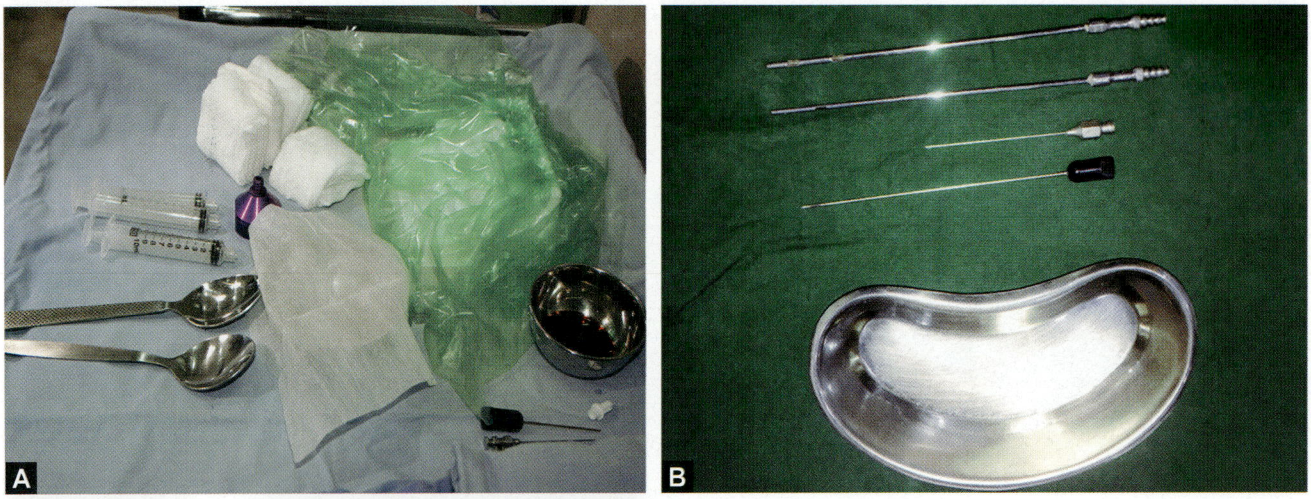

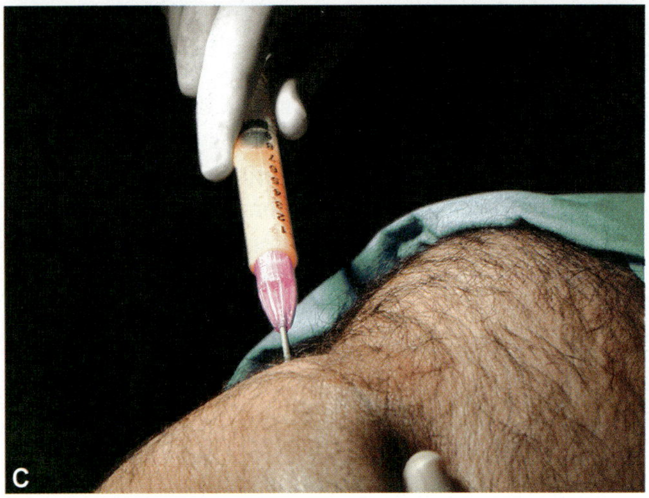

Figs. 32.4A to C: (A) Trolley prepared for fat transfer showing tube stand, decant stand, Luer Lock syringes with spoon and filter paper. (B) Tumescent anesthesia solution and cannulas for fat aspiration and fat transfer. (C) Fat harvesting using broad cannula attached to 10 mL Luer Lock syringe assisted by low vacuum.

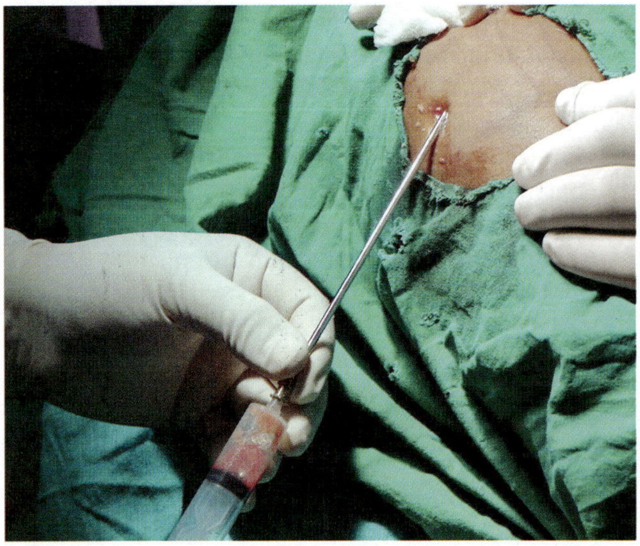

Fig. 32.5: Low pressure 10 mL syringe suction method showing collected fat in syringe.

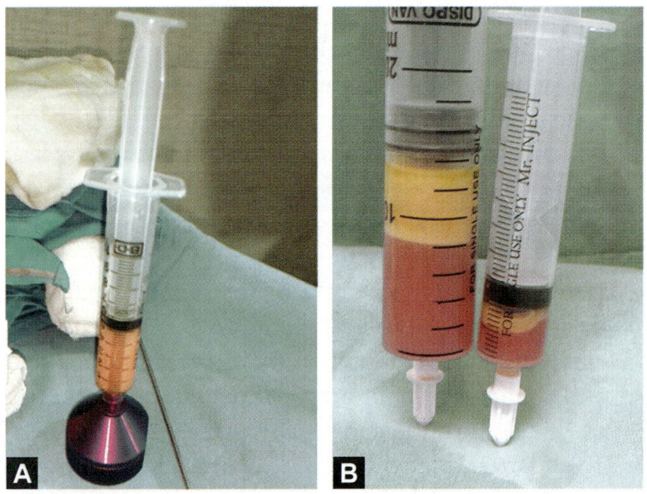

Figs. 32.6A and B: (A) Aspirated fat filled syringe attached to decant stand to separate the hydrohematic components. (B) Showing separation of fat from blood tinged solution after making stand syringe for a while.

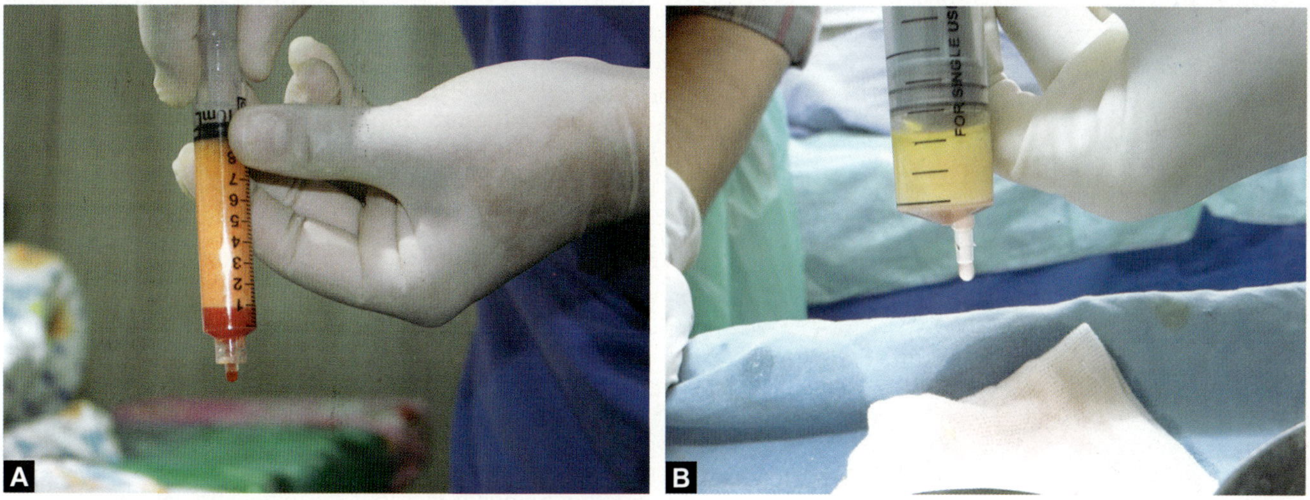

Figs. 32.7A and B: (A) Draining of the separated blood tinged fluid from bottom of the syringe in a drop-by-drop manner. (B) Draining of separated blood tinged fluid from the syringe.

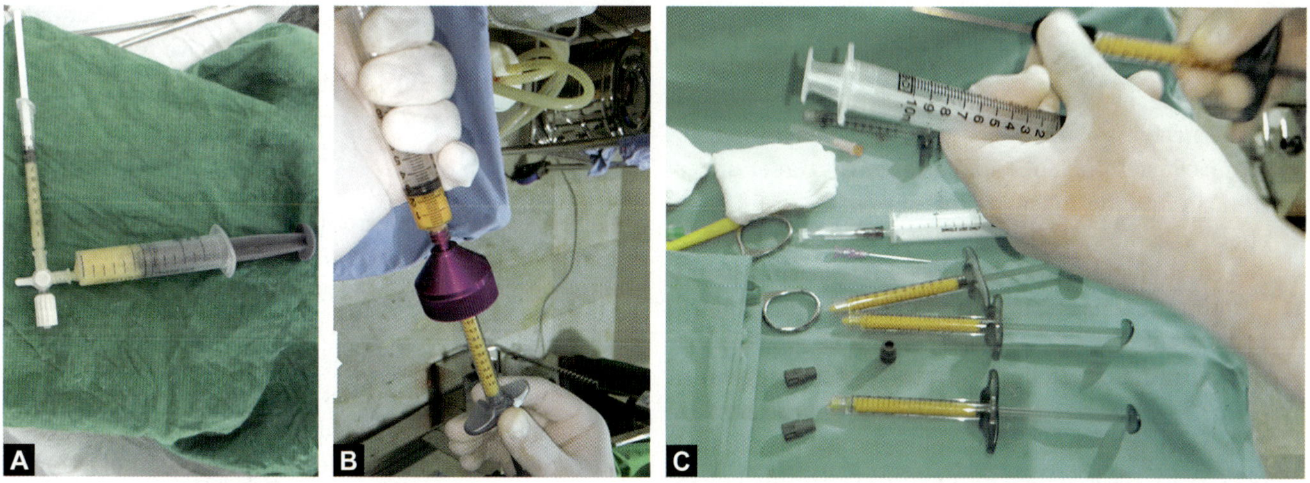

Figs. 32.8A to C: (A) Filling of 1 mL syringe from 10 mL syringe containing fat with the heip of 3-way cannula. (B) Transfer of harvested fat from 10 mL Luer Lock syringe to 1 mL Luer Lock syringe via the decant stand cum connector. (C) 1 mL Luer Lock syringe prepared for injection of fat into recipient area.

- Multiple 10 mL Luer Lock syringes can be filled with fat aspirate. The amount used at the first session can be separated and filled into 1 mL syringes with the help of 3-way cannula (Figs. 32.8A to C).
- The remaining syringes with the aspirate can be similarly drained off the fluid and then stored in a sterile container in a deep freezer at around –20°C.
- Once enough fat has been aspirated, the donor area is cleansed and the adit is covered with a gauze dressing and taped.
- The recipient areas are marked using a surgical marker pen as before. If work is to be done for facial rejuvenation, marking is preferably done in the sitting position. This helps in understanding the effect of gravity on facial curves and the depth of the wrinkles. Marking of the areas also gives an idea about the amount of fat required for filling.
- The recipient area is prepared similarly with Povidone Iodine solution followed by surgical spirit. Sterile drapes are placed to demarcate the surgical field.
- Local anesthesia (2% lidocaine plus adrenaline) is used for nerve blocks to reduce the pain during fat injection. In case of scars on the face or body, a ring block may be used to get the area numb.

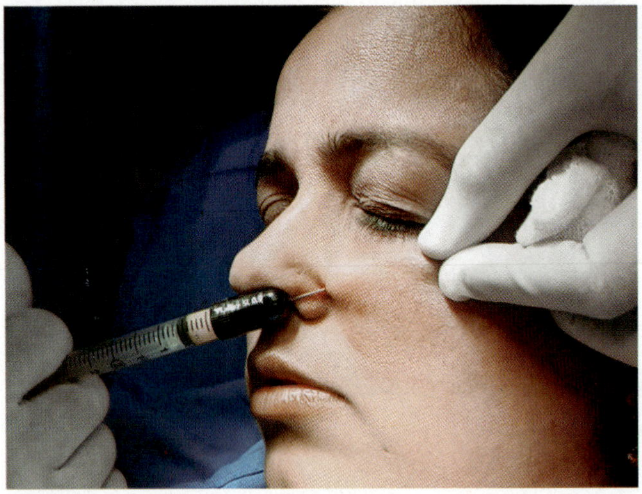

Fig. 32.9: Injection of fat into periorbital area through an entry close to alae nasi. Note fingers of other hand guide the tip of cannula. They also prevent the cannula from entering the orbit.

- The entry point for the injection cannula is marked and often a small amount of local anesthesia is placed underneath it.
- A 18 G needle is used to make an entry at the site marked. This facilitates the blunt tipped cannula to enter under the skin into the subcutaneous space. This cannula is attached to the fat filled 1 mL Luer Lock syringe.
- The cannula is gently inserted through the entry point with the nondominant hand fingers guiding the tip of the cannula and restricting it from overshooting the boundaries of the marked area for injection (Fig. 32.9). During insertion care is noted to keep the cannula in the subcutaneous plane. When deep filling of tissues is desired then the cannula can be pushed to the periosteal plane and filling can be done at this level.
- Filling of fat on the face is to be done in a similar manner to that of dermal fillers except that here it is mandatory to use a thicker cannula or needle compared to the one used for fillers. Small aliquots are placed under the skin and molded repeatedly. This spreads the deposited fat evenly under the skin preventing formation of lumps. Fat is placed in layers under the skin in the entire area.
- Over correction is usually avoided especially when filling in the periorbital region. Here the skin is very thin with minimal supportive structures underneath.
- When filling under scars, one should look out for adhered areas that may cause the injected fat to diffuse into the surrounding skin rather than under the scar. These firmly stuck areas of scar can be released with a Nokor Needle (BD Corporation, USA). Injection of fat can be commenced once the scar has been released from its underlying structures.
- Once adequate filling has been done, the area is cleansed using Povidone Iodine solution and an antibiotic ointment is applied to the entry point.
- The patient is given prophylactic oral antibiotics of the cephalosporin or penicillin group along with pain killers for 5 days.
- It is advised not to massage the treated area or apply any hot fomentation in case of excess pain. These measures can have a deleterious effect on injected fat and overlying skin, which can have alteration of sensation following the injection.
- It is a known fact that up to 25–50% fat cells survive after 3 months of injection. Hence, repeat sessions have to be performed to get the desired cosmetic effect.
- Fat that is stored in deep freezer has to be gradually thawed using water baths at successive temperatures from 0°C till 37°C. A laboratory thermometer that measures from 0°C upwards is utilized for this purpose. A gradual thaw prevents damage to cells due to sudden change in temperatures.[19]
- Again, the treatment area is photographed, marked and prepared for injection. While working on the face it is preferable to keep the patient in the semi recumbent or near sitting position to help in accommodating the gravity induced effects. It is always good clinical practice while doing filler injection to have a mirror in the hand of the patient while the injection is being done. The patient can help in deciding the extent of filling of fat. Both the treating surgeon and patient can jointly assess the fat filling and achieve a satisfactory result.

COMPLICATIONS

As with any procedure, fat transfer is fraught with risks of edema, infection, bruising, pain and poor results.

- Edema of the fat filled areas is not much of a complication as much as it is a desirable event, post fat filling. This is a reactive phase swelling following trauma of the procedure. It settles within three day.[18]
- It is of utmost importance that the sterile chain for aspirated fat is maintained during the procedure and also during storage. This will ensure least chances of infection postoperatively (Figs. 32.10 and 32.11). Fat stored at subzero temperatures can be amenable to growing bacteria that propagate at low temperatures

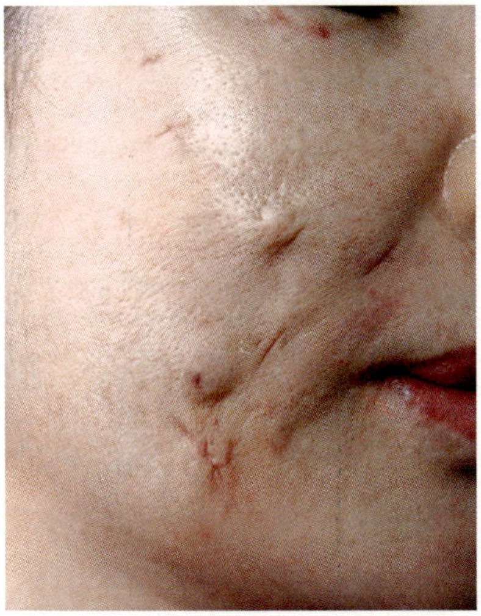

Fig. 32.10: Scarring secondary to infection following fat transfer to cheeks.
Courtesy: Prof Kee Yang Chung, South Korea.

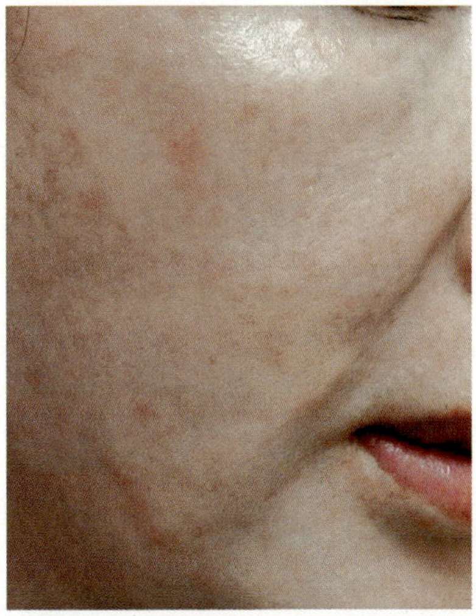

Fig. 32.11: Healing of scars in above patient after further fat transfer under the scars.
Courtesy: Prof Kee Yang Chung, South Korea.

such as Listeria and Yersinia. These get destroyed when adequate thawing is done bringing the fat to room temperature in a slow graduated manner using water baths. Also the anesthetic and blood tinged fluid that is aspirated along with fat should be drained as much as possible before the fat is put into deep freezer. Postoperative antibiotics are a must to prevent any possible infections. Fat is injected through micro incisions made with large bore needles. These are the entry point for the cannulas and can also be the site of entry of organisms. They have to be dressed with topical antibiotic ointments till they seal adequately.

- Bruising and sometimes ecchymoses around the sites of fat aspiration and injections are common. These happen due to damage to superficial vessels and friction while working through a small hole.
- Pain can occur especially while injecting fat. Giving nerve blocks wherever possible and at least giving adequate local anesthetic prior to making holes for cannula entry can alleviate this. Pain can also be a complaint when too much filling has been done. This is due to sudden stretching of the skin overlying a scar.
- Injecting fat into the recipient area in larger quantities can lead to irregular contours and consequently a poor finish (Fig. 32.12).
- Over filling of fat in large aliquots can lead to increased destruction of fat cells and poor survival rates.

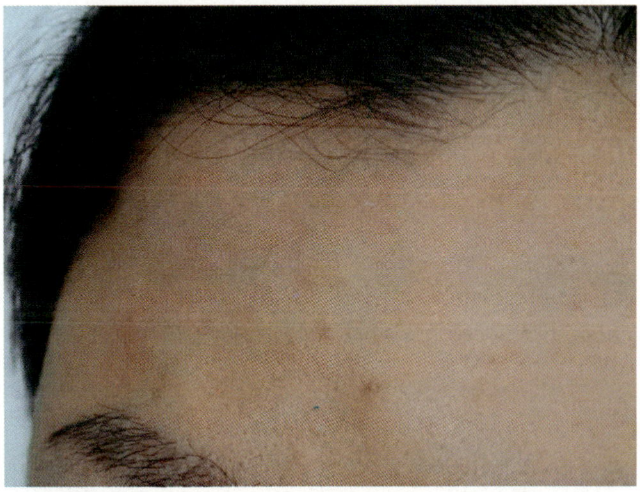

Fig. 32.12: Irregular contour secondary to large aliquots of fat deposited during fat injection into forehead for wrinkle reduction.
Courtesy: Prof. Kee Yang Chung, South Korea.

- Accidental injection of fat into the venous or arterial system can lead to sudden onset of thromboembolic complications. This can be avoided by using blunt cannulas for injection and aspirating every time before injecting fat.
- There is report of a patient upon injection of fat into the glabellar frown lines complained of pain and loss of vision in one eye. There was central retinal artery thrombosis, probably secondary to fat particle embolism.[20]
- Adipose derived stem cells have the potential like bone marrow derived stem cells to differentiate into

bone cells or cells of other tissues. Multiple sessions of fat filling can potentially predispose to formation of unwanted tissues under the skin.[1] This is yet to be proven but can be a cause of concern for the dermatosurgeon.

CONCLUSION

Autologous fat transfer is a versatile procedure. If carried out in the correct manner it has an effective and long-lasting result. It has been a very successful filler in the facial area and is cost effective.

Key Message

Lipobodysculpting and autologous fat transfer are recently inducted procedures in Dermato-Cosmetology field. Both these procedures can be performed in a dermatologists' clinic with access to sterile surgical theater. They are effective in bringing about a permanent change in the patients appearance. Body shaping with fat removal helps in restoring confidence. Fat acquired under local anesthesia is a live organ that can be used to restore skin qualities tonear normal when placed under scars. These procedures increase the domain of dermatosurgery.

Below are before and after photographs of patients who have undergone lipobodysculpting (Figs. 32.13 and 32.14) and autologous fat transfer (Figs. 32.15 and 32.16) at the author's clinic.

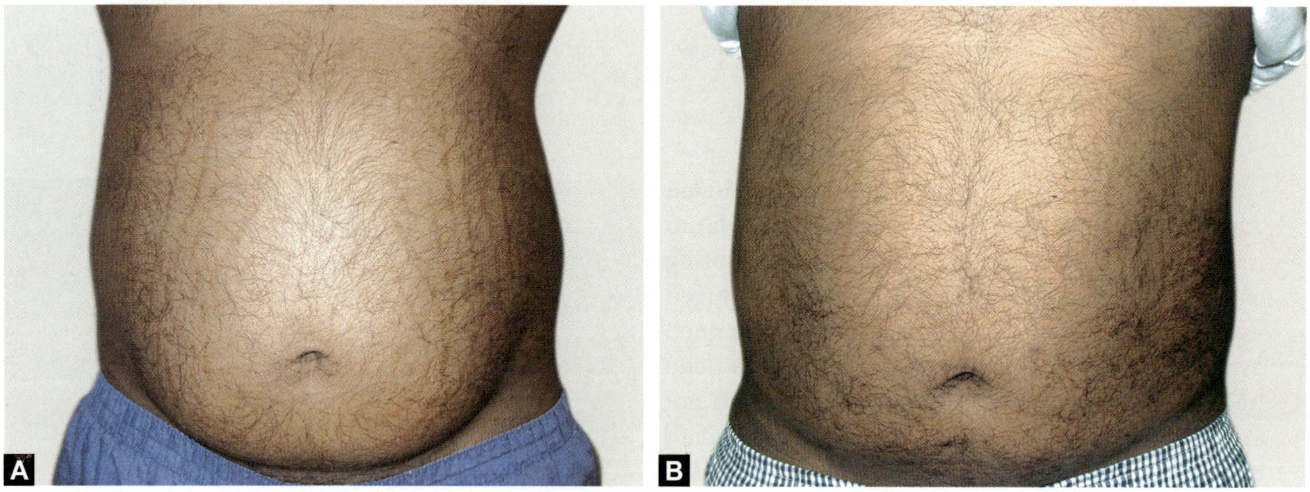

Figs. 32.13A and B: A 30-year-old male before and 3 months after lipobodysculpting to lower abdomen. Note the level of retraction following the procedure.

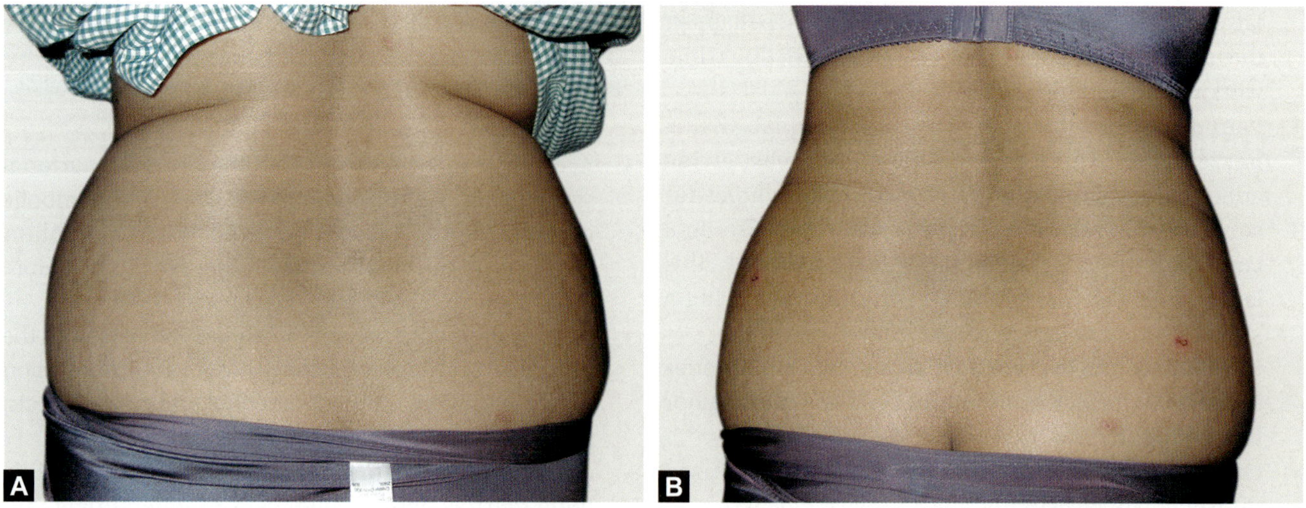

Figs. 32.14A and B: A 39-year-old female who underwent lipobodysculpting to waist and flanks. Note the absence of fold on flank in the 1 week after photograph.

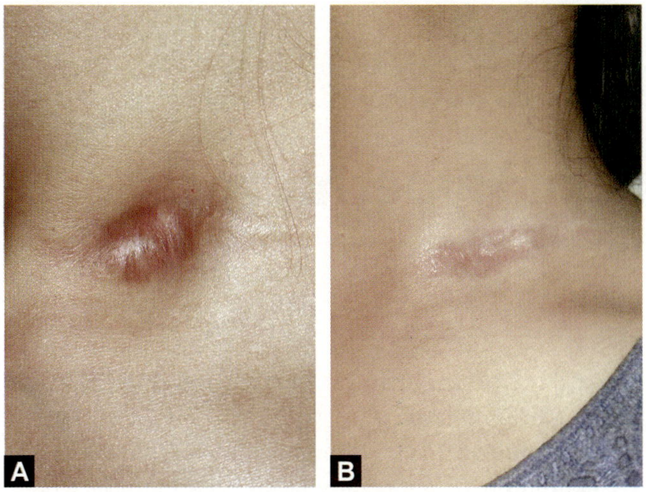

Figs. 32.15A and B: Postsurgical depressed scar in between two tendons of sternocleidomastoid. The scar was treated with three session of Fat injection at 3 monthly intervals with fractional CO_2 laser treatments in between. Note reduction in pigmentation along with improvement of texture of overlying skin.

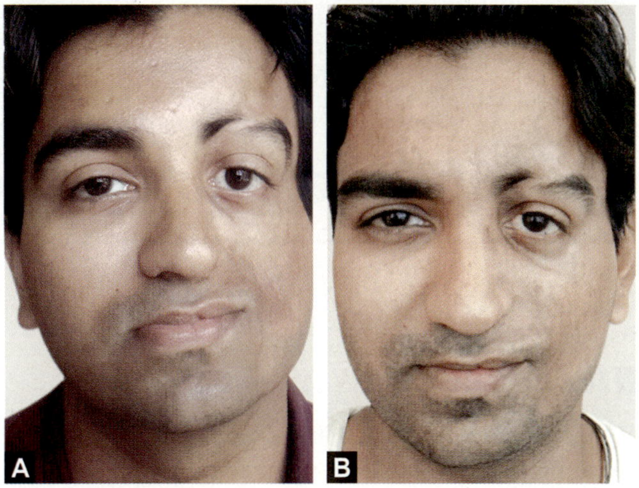

Figs. 32.16A and B: A 24-year-old with morphea affecting left forehead and cheek since the age of 7 years. Fat transfer done to the entire affected areas. Patient underwent 5 sessions over 2 years. Note the change in skin color and texture. There is fullness noticed over left cheek extending up to the left temple. The forehead depression is filled up very well with no contour defect.

ACKNOWLEDGMENTS

Dr Jeffrey Klein, Prof Pierrre Fournier and Prof Lawrence M Field for inspiring and teaching. Prof Field, Dr Ioannis Peros, Prof Kee Yan Chung, for sharing their photographs for this chapter.

REFERENCES

1. Tholpady S, Llull R, Ogle R, et al. Adipose tissue: stem cells and beyond. Clin Plast Surg. 2006;33(1):55-62.
2. Shiffman MA. Principles of Autologous Fat Transplantation. In: Shiffman MA (Ed.), Autologous Fat Transfer. Berlin: Springer; 2010, p. 13-15.
3. Li K, Gao J, Zhang Z, et al. Selection of donor site for fat grafting and cell isolation. Aesthetic Plast Surg. 2013;37:153-8.
4. Small K, Choi M, Petruolo O, et al. Is there an ideal donor site of fat for secondary breast reconstruction? Aesthet Surg J. 2014;34:545-50.
5. Padoin AV, Braga-Silva J, Martins P, et al. Sources of processed lipoaspirate cells: influence of donor site on cell concentration. Plast Reconstr Surg. 2008;122:614-8.
6. Keck M, Zeyda M, Gollinger K, et al. Local anesthetics have a major impact on viability of preadipocytes and their differentiation into adipocytes. Plast Reconstr Surg. 2010;126:1500-5.
7. Liposuction in practise. Shiffman MA. Principles of Autologous Fat Transplantation. In: Shiffman MA (Ed.), Autologous Fat Transfer. Berlin: Springer; 2010, p. 12.
8. Agostini T, Lazzeri D, Pini A, et al. Wet and dry techniques for structural fat graft harvesting. Plast Reconstr Surg. 2012;130:331e-9.
9. Özsoy Z, Kul Z, Bilir A. The role of cannula diameter in improved adipocyte viability: a quantitative analysis. Aesthet Surg J. 2006;26:287-9.
10. Kirkham JC, Lee JH, Medina MA, et al. The impact of liposuction cannula size on adipocyte viability. Ann Plast Surg. 2012;69:479-81.
11. Smith P, Adams WP Jr, Lipschitz AH, et al. Autologous human fat grafting: effect of harvesting and preparation techniques on adipocyte graft survival. Plast Reconstr Surg. 2006;117:1836-44.
12. Shiffman MA, Mirrafati S. Fat transfer techniques: the effect of harvest and transfer methods on adipocyte viability and review of the literature. Dermatol Surg. 2001;27(9):819-26.
13. Salinas HM, Broelsch F, Fernandes J, et al. Abstract 136: Centrifugation compared to a combined mesh/telfa technique for fat grafting: mechanism, outcomes and effect on ADSCs. Plast Reconstr Surg. 2014;133(3 Suppl):152.
14. Matsumoto D, Shigeura T, Sato K, et al. Influences of preservation at various temperatures on liposuction aspirates. Plast Reconstr Surg. 2007;120:1510-7.
15. Atashroo D, Raphel J, Chung MT, et al. Studies in fat grafting: Part II. Effects of injection mechanics on material properties of fat. Plast Reconstr Surg. 2014;134:39-46.
16. Chung MT, Paik KJ, Atashroo DA, et al. Studies in fat grafting: Part I. Effects of injection technique on in vitro fat viability and in vivo volume retention. Plast Reconstr Surg. 2014;134:29-38.
17. Aygit AC, Sarikaya A, Doganay L, et al. The fate of intramuscularly injected fat autografts: an experimental study in rabbits. Aesthetic Plast Surg. 2004;28(5):334-9.
18. Fournier PF. Facial recontouring with fat grafting. Dermatol Clin. 1990;8(3):523-37.
19. Moore JH, Kolaczynski JW, Morales LM, et al. Viability of fat obtained by syringe suction lipectomy: effects of local anesthesia with lidocaine. Aesthetic Plast Surg 1995;19:335-9.
20. Teimourian B. Blindness following fat injections. Plast Reconstr Surg. 1988;82(2):361.

CHAPTER 33

Surgical Management of Hyperhidrosis

Leelavathy B, Eswari L

INTRODUCTION

Hyperhidrosis is described as the condition where sweating occurs more than the amount that is required to maintain the body temperature. Sweating may be either idiopathic, i.e primary hyperhidrosis or it could be secondary to underlying causes like hyperthyroidism, heart diseases, pheochromocytomas, carcinoid tumors, obesity, structural lesions of autonomous nervous system, tumors of brain, peripheral vascular diseases (Raynaud's disease, erythromelalgia, acrocyanosis, etc.) or few spinal cord diseases.[1]

Primary hyperhidrosis may involve axilla, palms and soles and the craniofacial region. It can affect both the sexes. It can be severely disabling and socially distressing.

Table 33.1 shows different management options for hyperhidrosis.

Table 33.1: Different management options for hyperhidrosis.

Palliative management	*Surgical management*
Topical application • Aluminum hexachloride (2%) • Glutaraldehyde (10%) • Tannic acid (2–5%) • Potassium permanganate	**Nerve surgeries** • Thoracic sympathectomy • Endoscopic thoracic sympathectomy • CT-guided percutaneous sympathicolysis
Systemic anticholinergic drugs • Oxybutynin • Glycopyrrolate • Probanthine hydrochloride	**Excision surgeries** • Extensive en-bloc resection of axillary skin (Skoog procedure) • Partial skin excision with subsequent surrounding curettage (Shelly's procedure)
Iontophoresis	**Minimally invasive procedures** • Subcutaneous Liposuction • Subcutaneous curettage • Combined Liposuction and curettage
Intradermal injection • Botulinum toxin A • Botulinum toxin B	**Others** • VASER • Nd:YAG laser • Microwave device

Surgical procedures that will be discussed in detail in this chapter are as follows:

- Botulinum toxin for palmoplantar hyperhidrosis
- Botulinum toxin for craniofacial hyperhidrosis
- Botulinum toxin for axillary hyperhidrosis
- Subcutaneous curettage of sweat glands for axillary hyperhidrosis.

Patient evaluation and analysis of sweating.

Patient history

- Age of onset
- Location and symmetry of sweating
- Aggravating and alleviating factors
- Previous treatment
- Family history
- Current medications

Surgical risks

- Antiplatelet therapies
- Bleeding diathesis
- Significant arthritis/injury of shoulder area

Variety of methods have been used for analysis of sweating.

Quantitative assessment	*Nonvolumetric assessment*	*Subjective assessment*
Gravimetry test	Minor's starch iodine test	To quantify the intensity of sweat production using a visual analog scale (VAS) (1 to 100)
Resistance hygrometry	Digital image analysis of Ninhydrin-stained sheets	Individual satisfaction with an hydrotic effect on a semiquantitative scale (worse, unchanged, mild improvement, moderate improvement, marked improvement)
	Evaporimeter	Hyperhidrosis disease severity scale (HDSS).

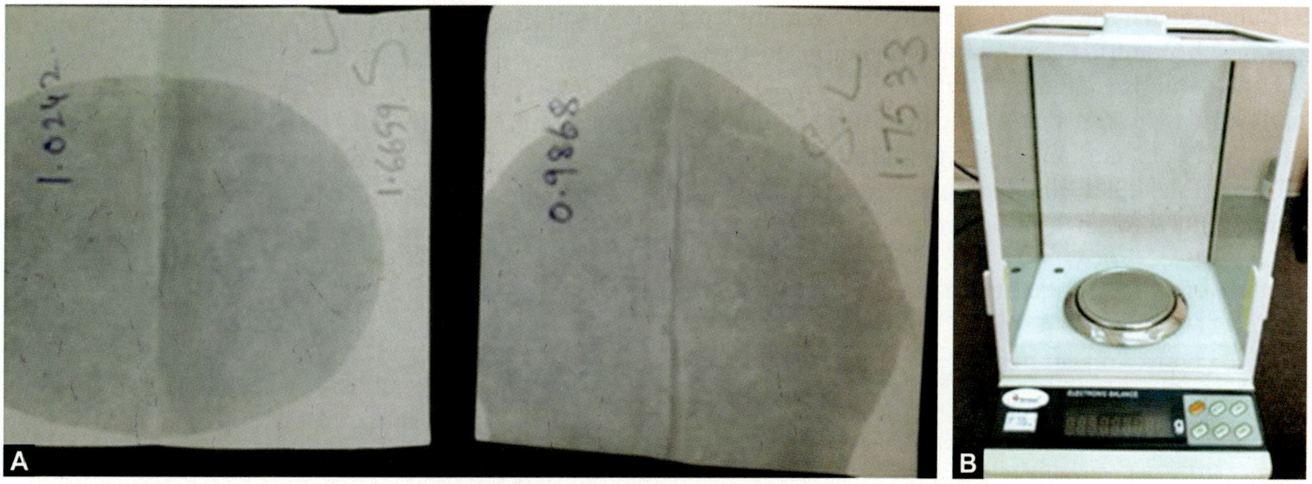

Figs. 33.1A and B: Gravimetry test.

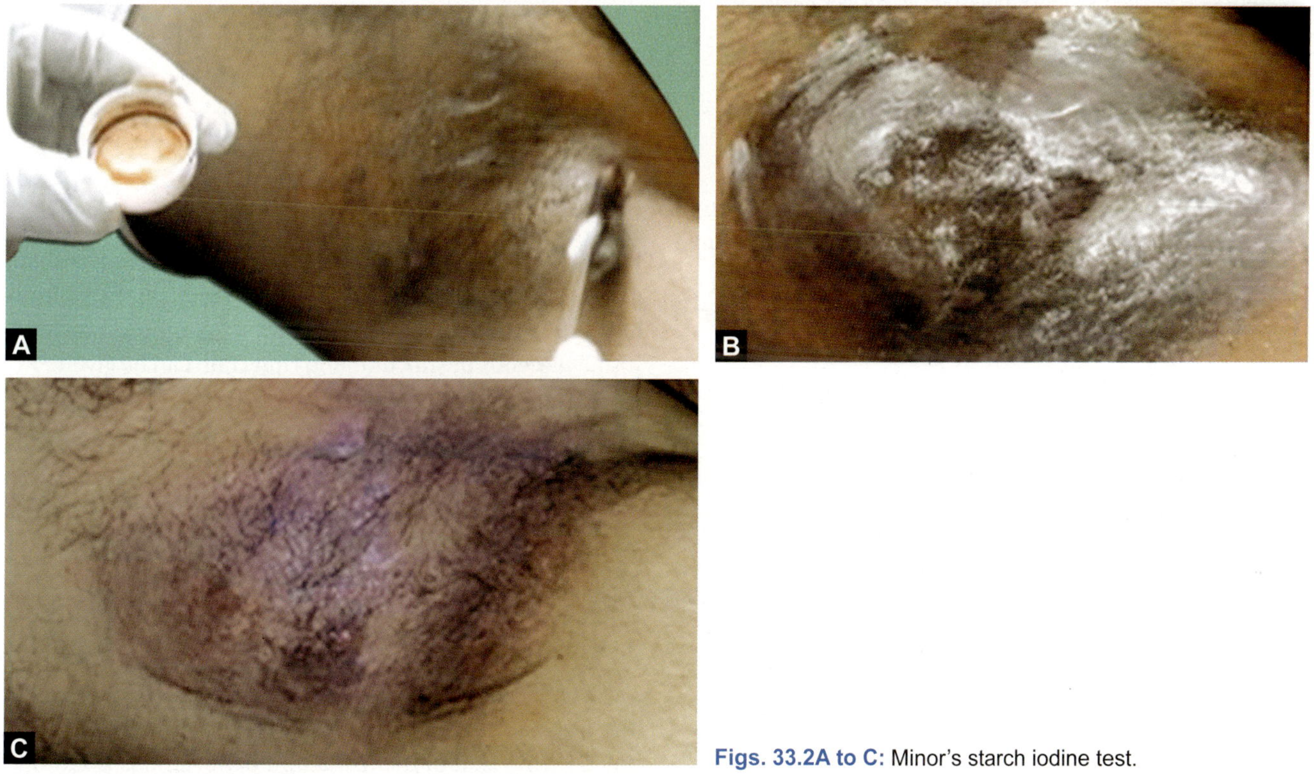

Figs. 33.2A to C: Minor's starch iodine test.

Gravimetry Test[2] (Figs. 33.1A and B)

A 10 × 10 cm filter paper is normally weighed on high precision laboratory scale and weight is recorded. This paper is placed under axilla for about 5 min and re-weighed. The difference of weight between the two is taken as sweat produced in mg over 5 minutes. Only patients with the baseline gravimetric measurement of accurate spontaneous resting sweat production amounting to at least 50 mg/axilla/5 min are normally included for the surgical procedures.

Minor's Starch Iodine Test[3] (Figs. 33.2A to C)

For starch test, Lugol's solution (iodine - 1.0 g; potassium iodide - 2.0 g; distilled water - 100.0 mL) is used. First axilla is dried, then painted with the iodine tincture, then air dried and finally starch powder is smeared. When sweat produced reacts with iodine in the moist starch, a blue to violet color is visible. The size of the area of the changed color can be outlined on a transparent plastic foil using standardized grids (0.5 × 0.5 cm) and the hyperhidrotic area can be measured in square cm.[4] Measurement is done about 1 minute after the starch powder smearing.

Hyperhidrosis disease severity scale[5]	
Severity of hyperhidrosis	*Score*
Underarm sweating is never noticeable and it never interferes with my daily activities.	1
Underarm sweating is tolerable but it sometimes interferes with my daily activities.	2
Underarm sweating is barely tolerable and it frequently interferes with my daily activities.s	3
Underarm sweating is intolerable and it always interferes with my daily activities.	4

INDICATIONS FOR THE PROCEDURAL MANAGEMENT

- Severe hyperhidrosis resistant to all conventional treatment (anticholinergic drugs, astringents, local antiperspirants containing mainly aluminum salts).
- Patients who are socially handicapped by condition and who ask for such surgeries.

PROCEDURES

Botulinum Toxin A Injections

Botulinum A toxin has a very potent inhibitory effect on the cholinergically innervated sweat glands. Local intracutaneous is the preferred route of administration for cases of focal hyperhidrosis though subcutaneous inj can also be given.

Inclusion Criteria

- Patients not responding to topical antiperspirants and systemic anticholinergics.
- Patients willing to spend for the procedure
- Patients not willing to undergo surgical procedures.

Exclusion Criteria[6]

- Treatment with
  - Anticholinergics
  - Aminoglycoside antibiotics
  - Calcium channel blockers

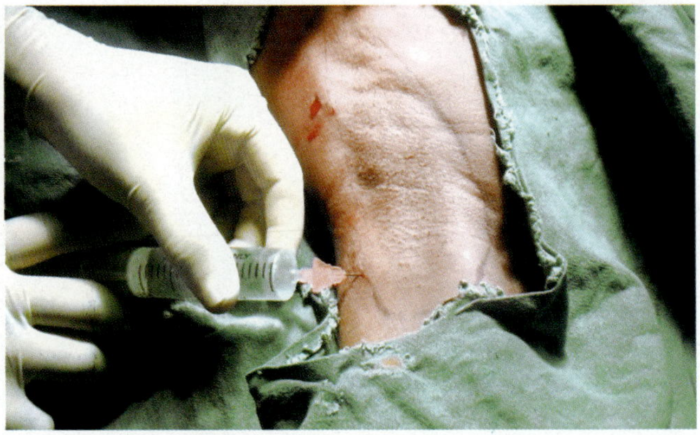

Fig. 33.3: Field block.

- Allergy to
  - Iodine
  - Castor oil
  - Starch
- Pregnancy or nursing mothers
- Presence of neuromuscular disease
- Infection at the injection site.

Anesthesia

Pain during the injection of the palms and soles is a main disadvantages of use. Injection is aimed at junction of dermis and subcutaneous tissue where sweat glands are located. Intracutaneous or subcutaneous injection can be given:

- Without anesthesia
- With ice packs
- Topical anesthesia-Topical EMLA.[7]

Reconstitution with lignocaine:[8] Botulinum toxin A can be reconstituted in 5 mL of 2% lignocaine. This does not alter efficacy of botulinum toxin in reducing sweat production. It is associated with significantly reduced pain during injections.

Field block (Fig. 33.3): This is preferred method for axilla. The area is marked 1 cm peripheral to the region of the hair bearing skin of the axilla and lignocaine is infiltrated all around.

Regional Blockade of Median and Ulnar Nerves[9]

Nerve Block of Palm

Analgesia of palm is achieved with median and occasionally the ulnar nerve block. Radial nerve blocks could be considered for fingertip injections.

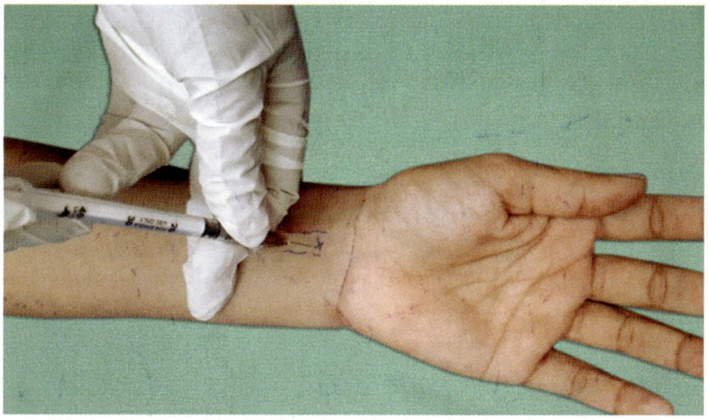

Fig. 33.4: Median nerve block.

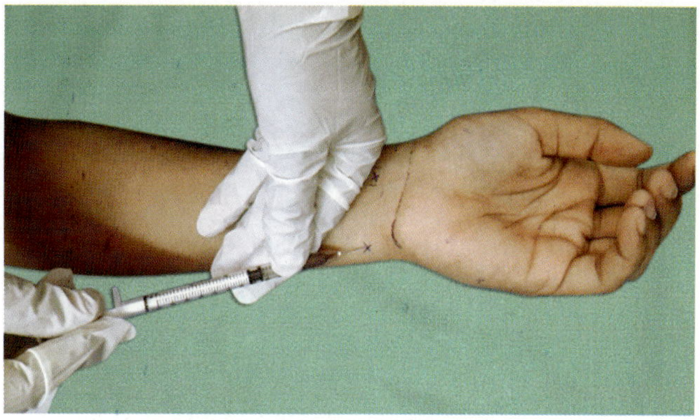

Fig. 33.5: Ulnar nerve block.

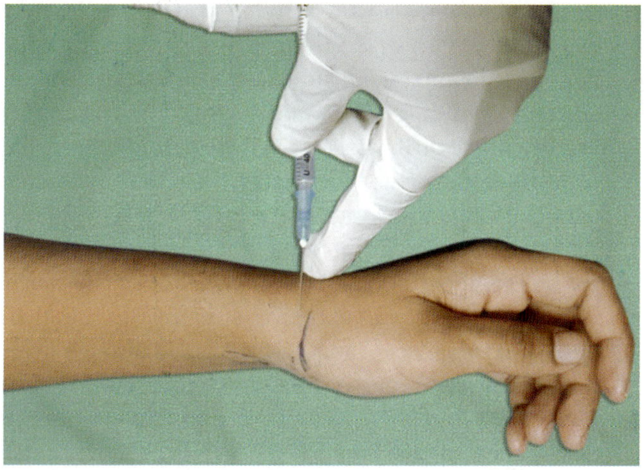

Fig. 33.6: Radial nerve block.

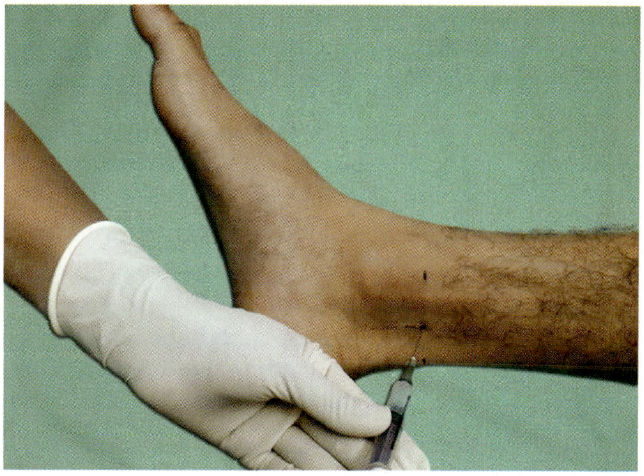

Fig. 33.7: Posterior tibial nerve block.

Median nerve block (Fig. 33.4): This is done on the wrist. First the palmaris longus and flexor carpi radialis tendons are identified during wrist flexion. The needle is inserted 1 cm proximal to the wrist crease between the two tendons. The needle is introduced perpendicularly into the deep fascia and the local anesthetic is administered.

Ulnar nerve block (Fig. 33.5): First the ulnar artery is palpated, and then the flexor calparis is identified. The needle is introduced between these two structures: 1 cm proximal to the crease of the wrist, with a direction aimed at the styloid process of the ulna. Then the local anesthetic is administered.

Radial nerve block (Fig. 33.6): This nerve is blocked by injecting the local anesthetic subcutaneously at the wrist crease anteriorly to posteriorly on the lateral aspect.

Nerve Block to the Soles[9]

Block the posterior tibial and sural nerves.

Posterior tibial nerve Block (Fig. 33.7): In the lateral or prone position of the patient, needle is introduced at the level of the superior border of medial malleolus, posterior to the posterior tibial artery, midway between the medial malleolus and the Achilles tendon. The needle is advanced perpendicularly until bone is encountered and then the local anesthetic is injected.

Sural nerve Block (Fig. 33.8): The sural nerve is anesthetized midway between the Achilles tendon and the superior border of the lateral malleolus and by directing the needle perpendicular to the skin until bone is felt. Local anesthetic, 6 to 7 mL, is injected in a fanning technique to partially fill the groove between the lateral malleolus and calcaneus.

Drawbacks of nerve blocks:

- Vascular puncture
- Impaired dexterity of the hand
- Repeated injuries can cause scarring of the nerves
- Difficult in sites like axilla.

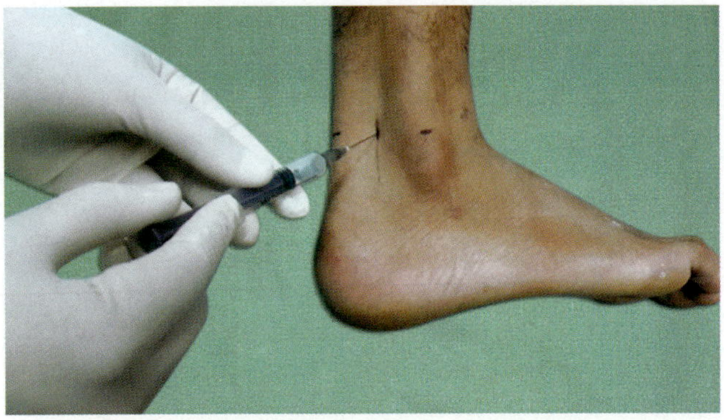

Fig. 33.8: Sural nerve block.

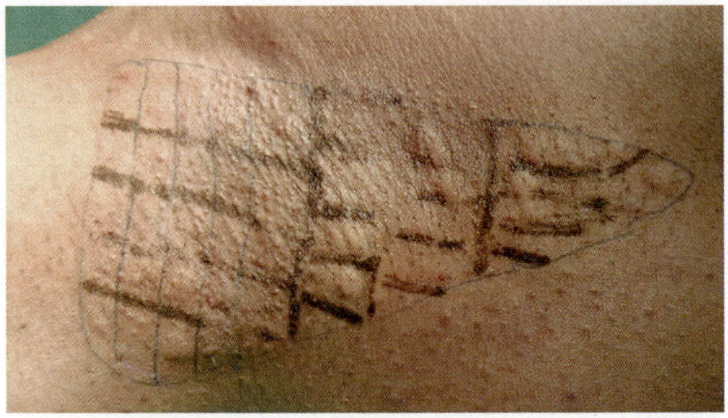

Fig. 33.9: Grid pattern for injection of Botulinum toxin A into axilla.

Reconstitution of Botulinum Toxin A

Injection Syringes[10]

- *Dilution*: 2.5 mL/100 units (5 insulin syringes—entire bottle). Each syringe—0.5 mL.
- The 30-gauge insulin syringe needle is swaged directly into chamber of syringe, thus eliminating the usual dead space that may occur with the routine needles. This also minimizes wastage of the toxin.
- After removing the metal cap and rubber stopper, the botulinum toxin is aspirated into the syringe directly. This minimizes loss of sharpness of the needle which may occur when the needle passes through the stopper.

Injection Technique

- Each syringe = 0.5 mL solution (20 U)
- It thus becomes easy to give the requisite 2–4 units (0.05–0.1 mL) as the markings on syringe are clearly outlined in single digits. Each syringe can be used to administer 10–12 injections.

Technique of Botulinum Toxin A Administration in Axilla

Reconstitution

One vial of Botulinum toxin A (100 units) is usually diluted with 5 mL of the normal saline solution, resulting in concentration of 2 units/0.1 mL. Using small 26-gauge needle 2–2.5 mL = 40–50 units is then administered by 20–25 intradermal injections into area of each axilla.

Technique

- *Spiral pattern*: 50 U of Botulinum toxin A is injected in 0.05 mL to 0.01 mL (2 to 4 U) amounts intradermally raising tiny wheals which are spaced approximately 1.5 to 2.0 cm apart, beginning at periphery of hair-bearing skin and circling into center of axillary vault.
- *Grid pattern*[11] (Figs. 33.9 and 33.10): More commonly used method is to draw grid of 1 cm^2 and to administer the toxin at central point of each pattern of grid. This method, although found to be useful, is however time consuming.
- *Tips*: A template grid can then be made from a flexible silicon sheet with multiple holes punched at 1 cm distance. After defining area of excessive sweating, grid is then positioned on affected area. Site is marked through holes in grid with skin marker pen. This takes few seconds. Marked spots are then used as injection sites for the even distribution of botulinum toxin. This grid is very quick to make and quite easy to use, saves physicians' time.
- The skin being rather thin in this area, care is taken to avoid injecting the material subcutaneously where it could go beyond the targeted glands.
- Keeping the needle bevel up and more parallel to the skin surface and advancing the needle 2 mm before injecting helps prevent backflow of the Botulinum toxin A from the injection tract, which minimizes any loss of the toxin.
- Procedure can be performed quickly with minimal discomfort and virtually no sequelae.

Adverse Events

No side effects except for occasional transient minimal bruising.

Technique of Botulinum Toxin A Administration in Palms and Soles

- The technique for injection in palms is similar, but here, injections must be spaced much closer together because of smaller zone of the radial diffusion produced in the palmar skin.

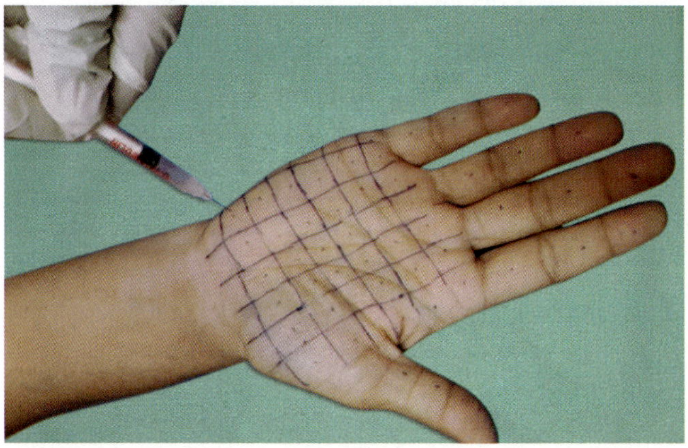

Fig. 33.10: Grid pattern for injection of Botulinum toxin A for palmar hyperhidrosis.

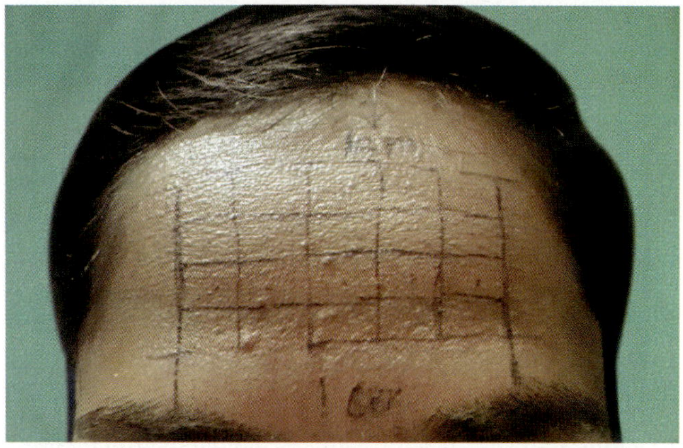

Fig. 33.11: Injection of Botulinum toxin A for facial hyperhidrosis.

- Palms and soles are then divided into squares of 1.5 × 1.5 cm with pen.
- Needle should enter palmar skin at an oblique angle, if needle enters perpendicular to skin surface, there is then a significant amount of backflow of material which leaks out of injection tract. Since volumes of Botulinum toxin A are typically less, this backflow will significantly impact the effectiveness of injections.
- Mechanical needle flanges also can be used, which provide support for assisting depth of the injection.[12]
- In the axilla however, the individual injections are so placed as to produce separate wheals. This is not possible in the tighter palmar skin, however a zone of blanching can be used as marker of material administered into the deep dermis.
- Backflow of material can be avoided by removing the pressure from the plunger and letting a pause of few seconds before withdrawing needle from the injection site.
- Injections on palms are usually placed approx every 1.5 cm.
- On fingers, individual injections are placed on the volar pads of each phalanx.
- Fingertips are administered 2 injections: one in mid finger pad and another at the tip of the finger as these are high sweat volume areas.
- Extra injections in rows are administered into the dominant/writing hand on the ulnar aspect midway between the dorsal and palmar surfaces to cater for maximum dryness.
- These patterns give adequate coverage for entire palm by diffusion.
- Subcutaneous injection should be appropriately minimized because these increase the likelihood of the diffusion of drug into intrinsic muscles of hand.
- Injection of soles of feet follows same technique and same pattern as palms.
- Sole has a much larger surface area, so the doses usually exceed those of palms.

Side Effects

- Small hematomas.
- Slight transient weakness of small muscles due to diffusion of the toxin.
- Pain at the injection sites (not seen when nerve blocks are given).

Technique of Botulinum Toxin A Administration for Forehead (Fig. 33.11)

There are usually 10 injection points which are evenly distributed over forehead to cover the area:[13]

- *Inferior forehead area*: Imaginary line 1 cm above eyebrows
- *Superior area*: Imaginary line 1 cm below hairline
- *Sides*: 2 imaginary lines vertically across pupils.

This is to provide safety against events like drooping of eyelids and muscular paralysis.

After cooling the area with frozen cold packs, 20 units of botulinum toxin are then injected intracutaneously using the 2 units of botulinum toxin A, per injection. The distance between each injection is 2 cm usually.

Side Effect

Inability of the patient to frown after injection; as a result of weakness of the forehead muscles.

Duration of Effects

- *Axilla*: Response times for the duration of anhidrosis in axillae ranges from 4 months to 10 months mainly depending on the dosage and technique.[14]
- *Forehead*: Similar responses can be seen as in treatment of forehead sweating.[15]
- *Palms and soles*: Responses to the palmar treatmentvaries from 3 to 12 months.[16] Interestingly, effect does not seem to last as long as it is with the axillary hyperhidrosis. Speculative reasons for this could be the problem with backflow, smaller diffusion distance in the thicker palmar skin, higher number of cholinergic nerve endings in palmar skin, or differential recovery-rate between nerves of palm and those in axillary skin.

Adverse Events

- Burning sensation/Painful injections
- Temporary muscle weakness
- Muscle soreness
- Injection site hematomas
- Bruising
- Local numbness.

SURGICAL PROCEDURES

Thoracic Sympathectomies

This is beyond the scope of this book and dermatologists but a brief note about the procedure is as follows:[17]

- History:
  - First sympathectomies via the endoscopy were performed in late 1940s.
  - 1990s—development of the video-assisted thoracic sympathectomy.
- Selection of patients for sympathectomy:
  - Patients having severe hyperhidrosis which do not improve with clinical treatment.
- Surgical technique:
  - Patients are placed under the general anesthesia by using simple or a double-lumen endotracheal tube.
  - Patient is then positioned in dorsal decubitus (semi-seated position) with arms abducted at 90° and also supported on operating table arm-support. Trunk is elevated to about 45°.
  - 2 incisions of approximately 3–10 mm are then made to carry out sympathetic chain thermoablation.
- Extent of the resection or thermoablation:
  - Extent of resection or thermoablation depends on clinical condition being treated.
  - For palmar hyperhidrosis, thermoablation of third or fourth ganglion is also recommended. For axillary hyperhidrosis, the thermoablation of fourth ganglion is indicated and also for craniofacial hyperhidrosis, thermoablation of second ganglion is done.
- Complications:
  - Most important complication is the compensatory hyperhidrosis, which is present in almost all patients who are submitted to sympathectomy in different grades.

Surgical options for the treatment of hyperhidrosis include: direct axillary sweat gland excision or a curettage that are preferred to the sympathectomy in few cases because of lesser systemic effects.

LOCAL SURGICAL PROCEDURES

- Excision of skin and glandular tissues [radical skin excision (RSE) and limited skin excision (LSE)]
- Curettage or liposuction procedures to remove subcutaneous glands
- A combination of limited skin excision with glandular tissue removal.

Goals

- Permanent long lasting solution
- Minimally invasive
- Cost-effective
- Minimal side effects and down time.

Excision

Radical Excision of Skin and Glandular Tissue[18]

- With Z-plasty or Y-plasty closure
- For wound closure, 3-0 subcutaneous interrupted sutures and 4-0 interrupted vertical mattress sutures
- Subcutaneous drain left in situ for 2 days.

Side Effects

- Hematoma formation
- Paresthesia

- Focal alopecia
- Skin infection
- Scarring and skin retraction
- Decreased range of motion of shoulder
- Long recovery time.

Limited Skin Excision with Glandular Tissue Removal

Modified Shelley's procedure[19]

- A central elliptical excision of axillary skin 4 cm × 1 cm.
- Subsequent undermining of the surrounding axillary skin with Metzenbaum scissors.
- The undermined skin is turned over to visualize sweat glands.
- The glands are then snipped off with scissors.
- The wound is closed with 4-0 subcutaneous interrupted sutures and 4-0 interrupted vertical mattress sutures.
- A figure of 8 dressing for 10 days or compression bandage for 24 hours.

Side Effects

- Hematoma formation
- Paresthesia
- Focal alopecia
- Seroma formation
- Fibrotic bridles
- Skin erosion
- Skin infection
- Hypertrophic scarring
- Flap necrosis.

LIPOSUCTION

Liposuction has become worldwide one of the most demanded of the cosmetic procedures. Liposuction has also proven to be of great interest in any noncosmetic conditions. Search for less invasive procedures has resulted in use of liposuction which is suction assisted removal of the sweat glands subdermally. Liposuction was carried out under general anesthesia, until a dermatological surgeon first reported the liposuction with "tumescent anesthesia".[20]

Tumescent Anesthesia

This involves use of large volumes of very dilute anesthesia along with adrenaline that induces profound vasoconstriction while also delivering good anesthesia over very large areas without causing any systemic lignocaine toxicity.[21] The firmness of tissue following infiltration of the tumescent anesthetic allows for more controlled technique for the removal of glands, with great potential for lessened contour irregularities. The ability to carry out liposuction in outpatient setting under the tumescent anesthetic, is much more advantageous when compared with cosmetic liposuction under the general anesthesia as an inpatient, like:

- Reduced risk of the general anesthesia
- Greatly reduced cost of the hospitalization
- Lower infection rate
- Lesser down time
- Lesser blood loss during the liposuction.

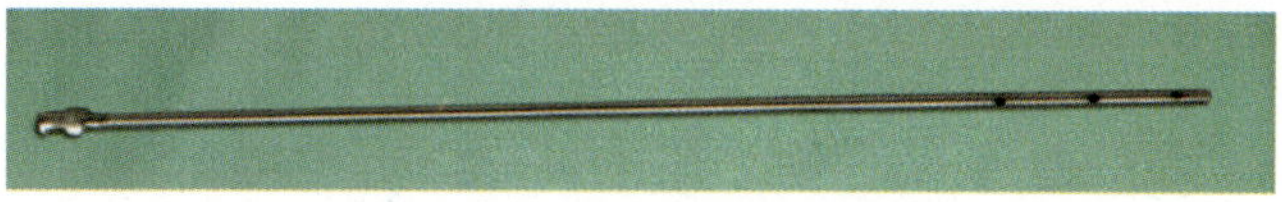

Fig. 33.12: Liposuction cannula.

Instruments

- *Cannula*: In the literature, a variety of instruments for suction curettage have been recommended. In a comparative trial, a sharp suction curettage cannula was more effective than liposuction cannulas with either one or three holes to reduce axillary sweating.[22] A rasping-type cannula is somewhat more effective than a suction curettage cannula with sharpened holes, only that the aggressiveness of curettage of the deep dermis has a strong impact on the outcome of the operation. For successful surgery it is mandatory that the curettage at the dermal/subcutaneous interface is performed in a way that only a full-thickness skin graft is left. This is the cannula used by the authors (Fig. 33.12).
- Infusion cannulas
- Syringes.

Tumescent solution composition:[23] 1,000 mL of normal saline, 1 mL of 1:1,000 epinephrine, 500 mg of 2% lidocaine, 15 mL of 8.4% sodium bicarbonate, and 1 mL of 10 mg/mL triamcinolone.

Procedure

- Patient is asked to shave area a day before surgery. Shaving on the day of surgery makes identification of borders of hair-bearing area more difficult, especially in the light-haired individuals.
- 1 hour before surgery, the patients receive single dose of oral antibiotic as infection prophylaxis.

- Surgical field is then prepared and draped, with sterile towels.
- Iodine-starch test is thereby not required to define area of maximal sweating because this area closely corresponds to hair-bearing area of axillae.
- Area 1 cm beyond perimeter of hair-bearing area defines targeted area for treatment and the borders are marked with methylene blue.
- Procedure is performed under local anesthesia.

Tumescent Anesthesia[23]

The patients are placed in a supine position with the arms abducted approximately 90°.

- The hair-bearing area of bilateral axillae is marked and infiltrated throughout the marked field and at least 1 cm beyond the marked field.
- A short 16-gauge or 18-gauge infusion cannula is used. The small-diameter infusion cannula is important for the comfort of the patient.
- Alternately 5 mL syringes can be used to infiltrate.
- A total of 300–400 mL is infiltrated in each marked axillary region.
- It is important to use sufficient volumes of infiltrate as the infiltrate dissipated rapidly in the axillae.
- The vasoconstriction from the epinephrine at 1:500,000 concentration is sufficient after 8–10 min, but the numbing effect of the lidocaine can take an additional 5 min to be sufficient.

Liposuction and Subcutaneous Curettage

Tsai and Lin[24] reported that tumescent liposuction combined with curettage is preferred over simple tumescent liposuction alone. Superficial liposuction could remove only the subcutaneous fat and could not remove the dermal tissue containing the eccrine and apocrine glands, so treatment by liposuction, combined with curettage,[25] excision, or ultrasound[26] has been developed and reported to be effective and safe.

After the steps performed as described above, two or three tiny stab incisions (3 or 4 mm) are made at the anterior and distal border of each axilla. Liposuction cannula is inserted through them, and subcutaneous tunnels are made by it. The cannula was invented and introduced into the treatment of hyperhidrosis by Dr Fatemi in Germany in 1999. It is 3 mm in diameter and 20 cm long with one blunted end; the other end is connected to a suction device which has three suction holes on the upside and four on both sides, which has characteristic sharp edges enabling effective and synchronous dermal curettage and suction of deep dermis and upper subcutaneous fat, including eccrine and apocrine glands, without damage to the underlying tissue. The suction apparatus, with a negative pressure of 18 mm Hg, is used during the procedure of tumescent infiltration and suction curettage.

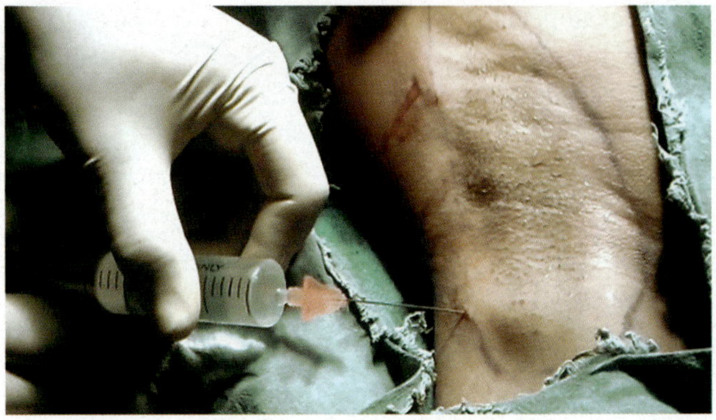

Fig. 33.13: Tumescent anesthesia.

Subcutaneous Curettage

Procedure:

- Prepare and give the tumescent anesthesia (Fig. 33.13) as described above.
- The site for incision is chosen so as to lie within the natural axillary crease at anterosuperior border of axillary hairline or on inferior outer border.
- Small stab incision (Figs. 33.14A and B) (0.5 cm) is made with #11 blade.
- The liposuction cannula which is used for curettage has blunt tip and 3 large sharp-edged openings on upper side, which helps in effective dermal curettage of the sweat glands and subcutaneous fat tissue without any damage to underlying tissue.
- Placing cannula in subcutaneous tunnels with 3 holes turned upward to face subdermis, a back-and-forth movement is then performed in crisscross pattern which is aided by other hand to compress skin for effective subdermal scraping (Figs. 33.15A and B).
- End point is when axillary skin becomes thin and can then be pinched up easily like a piece of cloth.
- Curettage is stopped when overlying skin starts to show slightly violaceous color, indicating relevant damage to dermal vascular plexus.
- 5 intraoperative, clinical clues which indicate sufficient Liposuction-curettage.[27]

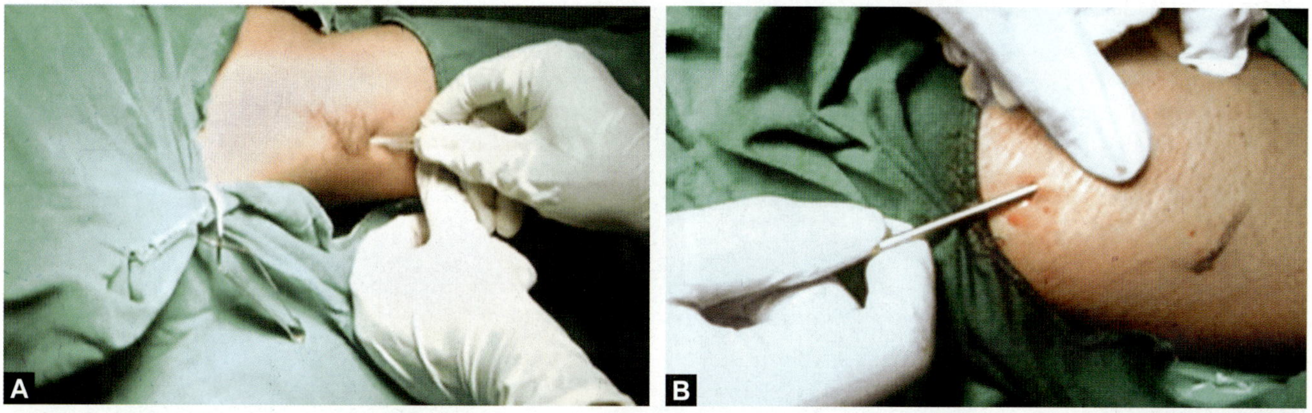

Figs. 33.14A and B: Stab incision to introduce liposuction cannula.

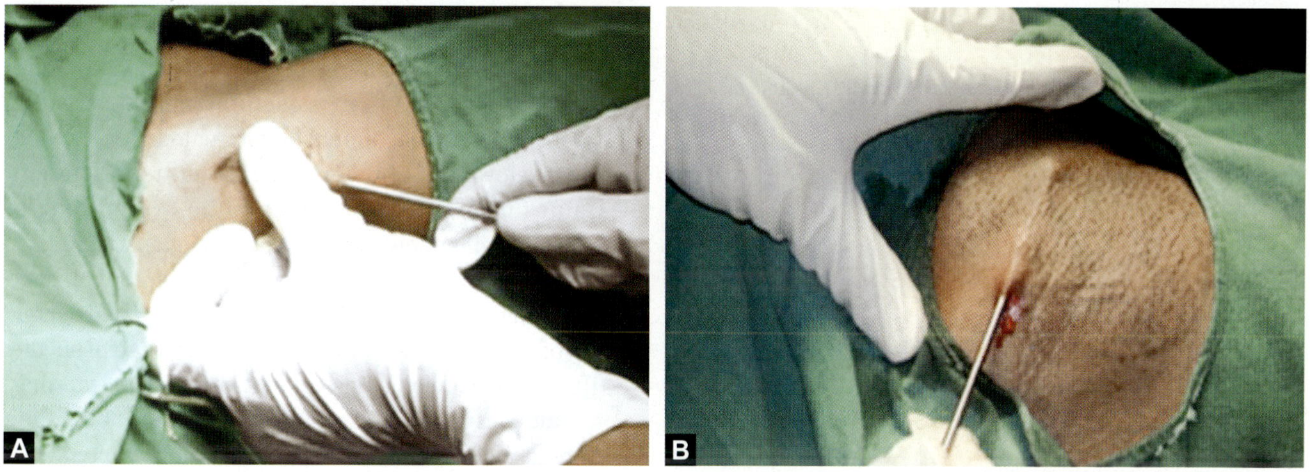

Figs. 33.15A and B: Subcutaneous curettage.

  - Complete elevation of the axillary skin from the subcutaneous fat
  - Slight lividity of the axillary skin
  - "Skin to skin" rolling which shows no more fat which is adhering to dermis
  - Palpable hair follicles present during the "skin to skin" rolling
  - "Sipping" sounds caused by cannula due to axillary "cavity" caused by the complete dissection of the fat and dermis
- Procedure in one axilla will take about 15 to 20 minutes.
- Aspirate should be sent for histological identification of sweat glands.
- Incision sites may be closed with 3-0 prolene sutures; however, authors prefer to leave them not sutured for easy drainage.
- Bulky compressive dressings (Figs. 33.16A and B) are then applied to axillae and patient is instructed to keep arm down.

Postoperative care and instructions:
- Patient should return in next 24 hours to have wound inspected.
- Tumescent anesthesia lasts for 2–3 days and patients might feel some discomfort in axilla from Day 3.
- Patients are allowed to then resume daily activities without restrictions, though hard labor and severe abduction are prohibited for at least 2 weeks.
- Prophylactic oral antibiotics and oral analgesia are prescribed as usual.
- Compression dressings should be continued for a week.

Follow-up

At each visit the following data are recorded:
- Patient's postoperative assessment for level of sweat, odor, pain, and satisfaction
- Hyperhidrosis questionnaire to assess impact on lifestyle
- Surgeon's assessment for complications and pain.

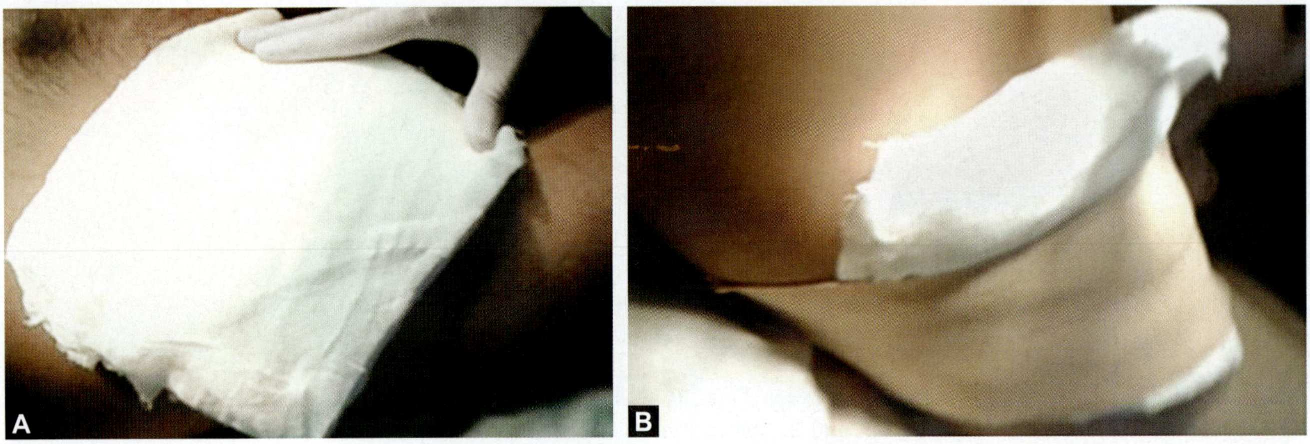

Figs. 33.16A and B: Compression dressing.

Complications[28]

- Detectable scars
- Induration
- Bridle formation
- Ecchymoses
- Pain
- Paresthesia
- Pigmentation
- Partial alopecia
- Skin ulceration
- Seroma
- Incomplete shoulder elevation
- Refractory hyperhidrosis[29]—3 patterns: crescent, circular or spot-like pattern.

Nd:YAG

Pulsed 1,064 nm Nd:YAG system[30]

- *Principle*: Laser–tissue interaction. Compared to other techniques, luminous energy acts directly on anatomical location of sudoriferous glands. Acting subdermally, the laser reaches its target directly, without necessity of the transdermal energy conduction. The way in which energy is transmitted to tissue, through a micro-spinal needle, offers surgeon direct and the complete knowledge of where laser beam is thereby acting and thus decreases possibility of cutaneous lesions.
- Laser energy is then conducted to subcutaneous tissue through 300 mm fiberoptic cable delivered through 18-gauge epidural needle (disposable).
- 100 ms pulsed laser with 40 Hz frequency and 15 mJ energy (working at 6 W) is used for all patients.
- Total accumulated energy used for each axilla ranges from 7,000–20,000 J/cm^2 depending on the sweating intensity, skin type, dimension of treated area.
- Most relevant parameter which could represent end point for laser action seems to be overcoming of resistance of needle in its movement against tissue.
- Other important parameters are dimension of affected area, intensity of sweating, and total accumulated energy.
- Tip of fiberoptic is extended 2 mm beyond end of needle.
- This epidural needle has smooth curve in its extremity to guide laser beam in an angle of approx 30°, aiming at reaching dermal/subdermal junction where sweat glands are located.
- For visualization purposes, Helium-Neon laser source is combined into beam path providing exact view of where laser is working because positioning of cannula is highlighted via transillumination by red guiding beam.
- A crisscross manner most probably optimizes complete laser action in affected area.

VASER[31]

- VASER system (Sound Surgical Technologies, Louisville, CO) is third-generation ultrasound system which is cleared by FDA for soft-tissue emulsification/aspiration and for body-contouring surgery.
- VASER system provides a much more precise control of ultrasonic energy at tip of probe than he earlier generation of ultrasound-assisted lipoplasty (UAL) devices. Primary author postulated that VASER system could be used more effectively and safely for treatment of soft tissues associated with axillary hyperhidrosis/bromidrosis.

MICROWAVE DEVICE[32]

Microwave devices, although not commonly used in dermatology, can be optimized to focus heat at the interface between the skin and subcutaneous tissue and cause irreversible thermolysis of apocrine and eccrine sweat glands that reside at that interface. The microwave-based device included integrated vacuum and cooling.

REFERENCES

1. Macía I, Moya J, Ramos R, et al. Primary hyperhidrosis. Current status of surgical treatment. Cirugía Española (English Edition). 2010;88(3):146-51.
2. Darabaneanu S, Darabaneanu HA, Niederberger U, et al. Long-term efficacy of subcutaneous sweat gland suction curettage for axillary hyperhidrosis: a prospective gravimetrically controlled study. Dermatologic Surgery. 2008;34(9):1170-7.
3. Minor V. Einneues Verfahrenzu der klinischen Untersuchung der Schwei Xabsonderung. Dtsch Z Nervenheilkd. 1927;101:301-6.
4. Bechara FG, Sand M, Sand D, et al. Focal hyperhidrosis of the anal fold: a simple technique for diagnosis and evaluation of therapy. Br J Dermatol. 2006;155:858.
5. Glaser DA, Coleman WP, 3rd, Fan LK, et al. A randomized, blinded clinical evaluation of a novel microwave device for treating axillary hyperhidrosis: the dermatologic reduction in underarm perspiration study. Dermatol Surg. 2012;38:185-91.
6. Basciani M, Rienzo FD, Bizzarrini M, et al. Efficacy of botulinum toxin type B for the treatment of primary palmar hyperhidrosis: a prospective, open, single-blind, multi-centre study. Archives of Dermatological Research. 2014;306(5):497-503.
7. O'Riordan JM, Fitzgerald E, Gowing C, et al. Topical local anaesthetic (tetracaine) reduces pain from botulinum toxin injections for axillary hyperhidrosis. Br J Surg. 2006;93(6):713-4.
8. Vadoud-Seyedi J, Simonart T. Treatment of axillary hyperhidrosis with botulinum toxin type A reconstituted in lidocaine or in normal saline: a randomized, side-by-side, double-blind study. Br J Dermatol. 2007;156(5):986-9.
9. Fujita M, Mann T, Mann O, et al. Surgical pearl: use of nerve blocks for botulinum toxin treatment of palmar-plantar hyperhidrosis. J Am Acad Dermatol. 2001;45(4):587-9.
10. Doft MA, Hardy KL, Ascherman JA. Treatment of hyperhidrosis with botulinum toxin. Aesthet Surg J. 2012;32(2):238-44.
11. Lam DGK, Choudhary S. Use of a grid to simplify botulinum toxin injection for axillary hyperhidrosis. Plast Reconstr Surg. 2003;112:1741-2.
12. de Almeida A, Kadunc B, de Olivieria EM. Improving botulinum toxin therapy for palmar hyperhidrosis: wrist block and technical considerations. Dermatol Surg. 2001;27:34-6.
13. Santana-Rodríguez N, Clavo-Varas B, Ponce-GonzÁlez MÁ, et al. Primary frontal hyperhidrosis successfully treated with low doses of botulinum toxin A as a useful alternative to surgical treatment. J Dermatolog Treat. 2012;23(1):49-51.
14. Bushara KO, Park DM, Jones JC, et al. Botulinum toxin: a possible new treatment for axillary hyperhidrosis. Clin Exp Dermatol. 1996;21:276-8.
15. Boger A, Herath H, Rompel R, et al. Botulinum toxin for treatment of craniofacial hyperhidrosis. J Neurol. 2000;247:857.
16. Schnider P, Binder M, Auff E, et al. Double-blind trial of botulinum A toxin for the treatment of focal hyperhidrosis of the palms. Br J Dermatol. 1997;136:548.
17. Wolosker N, Krutman M, Kauffman P, et al. Review of the surgical technique for the treatment of hyperhidrosis. Expert Rev Dermatol. 2012;7(6):529-38.
18. Bechara FG, Sand M, Hoffmann K, et al. Histological and clinical findings in different surgical strategies for focal axillary hyperhidrosis: histologic and clinical findings. Dermatol Surg. 2008;34(8):1001-9.
19. Wollina U, Köstler E, Schönlebe J, et al. Tumescent suction curettage versus minimal skin resection with subcutaneous curettage of sweat glands in axillary hyperhidrosis. Dermatol Surg. 2008;34(5):709-16
20. Swinehart JM. Treatment of axillary hyperhidrosis: combination of the starch-iodine test with the tumescent liposuction technique. Dermatol Surg. 2000;26(4):392-6.
21. Bechara FG, Sand M, Tomi NS, et al. Repeat liposuction-curettage treatment of axillary hyperhidrosis is safe and effective. Br J Dermatol. 2007;157(4):739-43.
22. Bechara FG, Sand M, Sand D, et al. Surgical treatment of axillary hyperhidrosis: a study comparing liposuction cannulas with a suction-curettage cannula. Ann PlastSurg. 2006; 56:654-7.
23. Lee D, Cho SH, Kim YC, et al. Tumescent liposuction with dermal curettage for treatment of axillary osmidrosis and hyperhidrosis. Dermatologic Surgery. 2006;32(4):505-11.
24. Tsai RY, Lin JY. Experience of tumescent liposuction in the treatment of osmidrosis. Dermatol Surg. 2001;27:446-8.
25. Rompel R, Scholz S. Subcutaneous curettage vs. injection of botulinum toxin A for treatment of axillary hyperhidrosis. J Eur Acad Dermatol Venereol. 2001;15(3):207-11.
26. Lee MR, Ryman WJ. Liposuction for axillary hyperhidrosis. Australas J Dermatol. 2005;46(2):76-9.
27. Bechara FG, Sand M, Tomi NS, et al. Repeat liposuction-curettage treatment of axillary hyperhidrosis is safe and effective. Br J Dermatol. 2007;157:739-43.
28. Glaser DA, Coleman WP, Fan LK, et al. A randomized, blinded clinical evaluation of a novel microwave device for treating axillary hyperhidrosis: the dermatologic reduction in underarm perspiration study. Dermatologic Surgery. 2012;38(2):185-91.
29. Bechara FG, Sand M, Altmeyer P. Characteristics of refractory sweating areas following minimally invasive surgery for axillary hyperhidrosis. Aesthet Plast Surg. 2009;33(3):308-11.
30. Goldman A, Wollina UW. Subdermal Nd-YAG laser for axillary hyperhidrosis. Dermatol Surg. 2008;34(6):756-62.
31. Commons GW, Lim AF. Treatment of axillary hyperhidrosis/bromidrosis using VASER ultrasound. Aesthet Plast Surg. 2009;33(3):312-23.
32. Glaser DA, Coleman WP, Fan LK, et al. A randomized, blinded clinical evaluation of a novel microwave device for treating axillary hyperhidrosis: the dermatologic reduction in underarm perspiration study. Dermatol Surg. 2012;38(2):185-91.

CHAPTER 34

Treatment of Hidradenitis Suppurativa

Shekhar Neema, Kumaresan M

INTRODUCTION

Hidradenitis suppurativa (HS) is a chronic, relapsing disorder of apocrine gland bearing skin of axilla, perineal and perianal region. It is characterized by tender subcutaneous nodules, painful abscesses, draining sinus and double ended comedones.[1,2] These abscesses heal producing fibrosis and bridging scars. HS generally starts after puberty in second to third decade of life. It is more common in females, obese individuals and in smokers.[3]

CLINICAL FEATURES, DIAGNOSIS AND DISEASE STAGING

Hidradenitis suppurative is insidious in onset and presents with tender subcutaneous nodules, abscess which rupture resulting in foul smelling discharge and ulceration. Chronic HS results in fibrosis, induration and bridging scars in affected area. Body areas most commonly involved are axillae, perianal, perineal, mammary and submammary regions.

Diagnosis of HS is clinical. However, differential diagnosis which needs to be considered are furuncles, carbuncles, actinomycosis, Crohn's disease, granuloma inguinale, slymphogranuloma venereum, nocardiosis, pilonidal sinus, tuberculosis and ischiorectal abscess.[4]

Clinical staging is very important for deciding treatment as well as knowing the effect of treatment in trials. Two most commonly used staging systems are Hurley staging system and Sartorius system. Hurley staging system is simpler and more widely used staging system in clinical practice.

Hurley Staging System[5]

Stage I: Abscess formation (single or multiple) without sinus tracts and cicatrization.

Stage II: Recurrent abscess with sinus tract and scar formation

Stage III: Multiple interconnected tracts and abscess.

Sartorius Staging System[6]

It is a more objective staging system in which numerical scoring is done in following manner:

- Anatomical regions involved—axilla, groin, gluteal (Left or right—3 points per region
- Number and scores of lesions—nodules -2, fistula -4, scars 1, others 1
- Distance between two relevant lesions—<5 cm -2; <10 cm, 4; > 10 cm, 8
- Are lesions clearly separated by normal skin? In each region (yes 0/ no 6).

Dermatology Life Quality Index (DLQI) can also be added to this Sartorius staging system.

TREATMENT

Treatment modalities for HS are varied and are not uniformly effective. It consists of medical and surgical therapy.

Medical therapy consists of topical antibiotics like clindamycin, oral antibiotics like rifampicin, clindamycin, dapsone; retinoids like isotretinoin, antiandrogens like finasteride and cyproterone acetate, TNF alpha-blockers like infliximab and adalimumab. Other treatment modalities which have been used for treatment of HS are radiotherapy, botulinum toxin, photodynamic therapy, cryosurgery, ablative carbon dioxide laser and nonablative laser and radiofrequency device.[7-13]

Surgical Therapy

Surgical therapy is considered as curative therapy in treatment of HS. It can be used as monotherapy or in combination with other medical therapy like antibiotics and TNF alpha-blockers. Individuals with Hurley stage II or III benefit most from surgical treatment. HS in extra axillary sites is a premalignant condition and should be treated by surgical excision and not by conservative medical management.[14,15] Surgical treatment options available for management of HS are as follows:

- Incision and drainage
- Deroofing
- Wide excision
  - With healing by secondary intention
  - Primary closure
  - Split thickness skin graft or flap.

Incision and Drainage

It can be done if patient presents with extremely painful fluctuant abscess. However, this procedure has high recurrence rate and should be avoided.[16] A modified technique for abscess drainage has been described by Haoxiang et al. which included administration of antibiotics for 5–7 days before surgery and sinuses were washed with gentamicin containing saline daily. Blunt probe is inserted in sinus discharging purulent exudate and unroofing of sinus is done and floor is left to heal by secondary intention. Sinuses are washed with hydrogen peroxide and saline containing gentamicin. Petrolatum gauze is pushed into drained sinuses till they healed completely. This modified technique was found to be very effective for management of HS.[17]

Deroofing

Deroofing of the abscess cavity and sinuses followed by marsupialization is another minimally invasive procedure for management of HS. Deroofing of the cavity can be done using scissors, radiofrequency or electrosurgical cutting or carbon dioxide laser. Wound is left open for secondary intention healing. Marsupialization is a procedure in which abscess or sinus is slit and edges are sutured, so that interior and exterior surface forms a continuous surface and contents can drain freely.[18]

Wide Excision

- Surgical excision of the diseased tissue is the only curative treatment for HS. Excision can be localized or wide local excision. Limited local excision can be done for limited disease, however the risk for recurrence with limited local excision is higher as compared to wide radical excision.
- Wide radical excision involves removal of entire diseased skin along with 2 cm of normal skin. Excision involves skin, subcutaneous tissue down to the level of fascia (Figs. 34.1 to 34.4). Reconstruction after wide radical excision is extremely important to maintain functionality, prevention of contracture and good aesthetic outcome.
- Reconstruction can be done with primary closure, secondary intention healing, split skin grafting, flaps and vacuum assisted closure.
- Primary closure can be attempted only when excised area is small. There are many studies which suggest that primary closure results in higher chances of recurrence.[19]
- Secondary intention healing can be used for reconstruction. However, it requires long postoperative recovery period and meticulous wound care for 8–30 weeks depending on size of the wound.[20]
- Split skin grafting is most widely used technique for reconstruction of surgical wound in HS. It results in low recurrence rate and rapid wound healing. Split skin grafting can be performed either immediately or

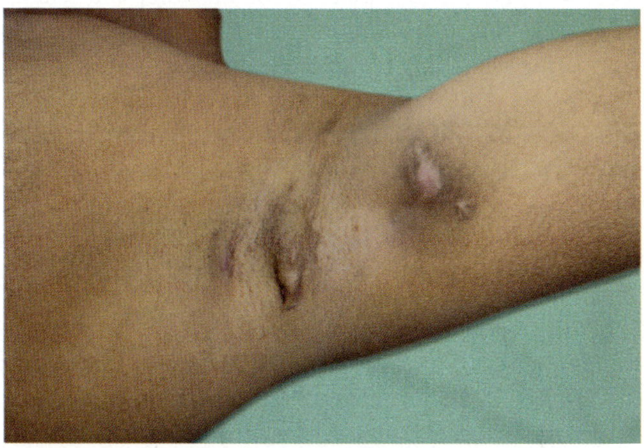

Fig. 34.1: Case of hidradenitis suppurativa: left axillary involvement.

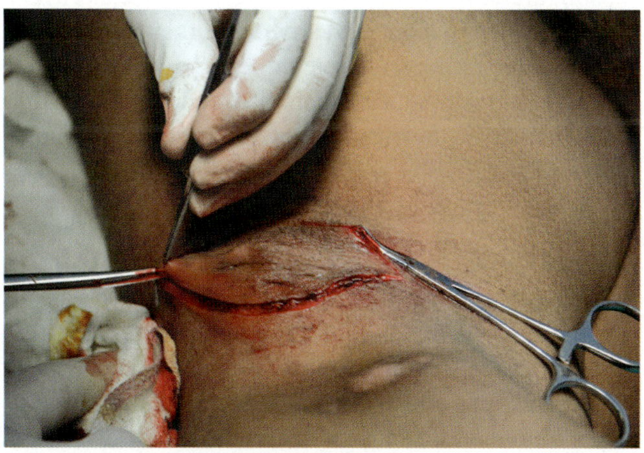

Fig. 34.2: Excision of skin and subcutaneous tissue till the level of fascia.

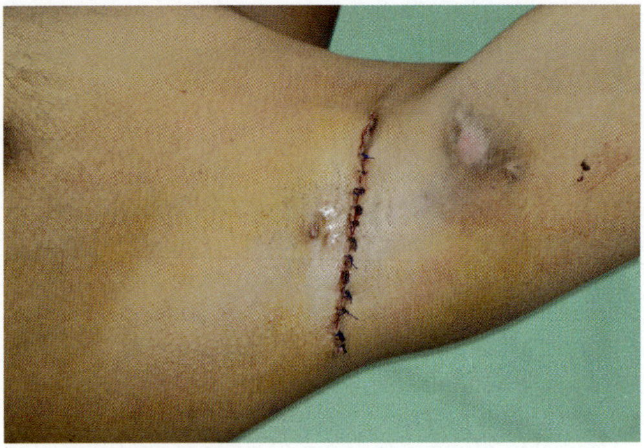

Fig. 34.3: Suturing of the resulting wound.

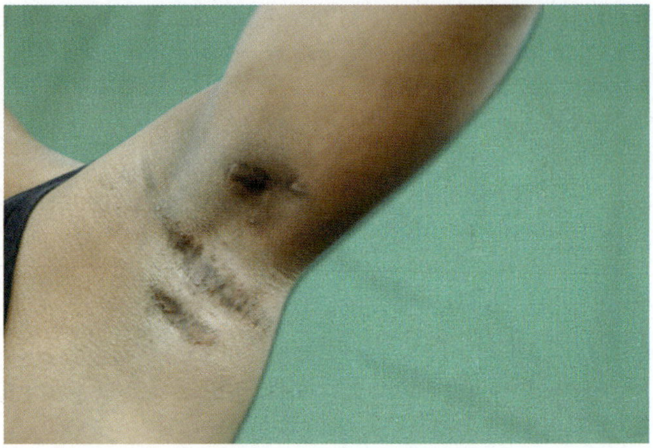

Fig. 34.4: Post-surgical scar.

as a delayed procedure once wound contraction has taken place. It can be combined with negative pressure dressing for faster healing. Vacuum assisted closure, either alone or in combination with split skin grafting promotes angiogenesis and secure the graft in place for faster uptake. Meshing of graft can be done to cover larger defect.

- Split skin grafting has some disadvantages like poor aesthetic results and additional wound at donor site. However, it is most preferred procedure for reconstruction because it is technically easier as compared to flaps, leads to faster wound healing and aesthetics are not a major concern in HS affected area.[21,22]
- Flaps can be used for reconstruction of defect created by wide radical excision. Flap can be random cutaneous flaps, fasciocutaneous or musculocutaneous flap. Fasciocutaneous flaps are those which includes skin, subcutaneous tissue and underlying fascia. Fascial plexus and fasciocutaneous perforators supply this flap. Musculocutaneous flap includes underlying muscle apart from skin, subcutaneous tissue and fascia and they are named on the muscles they are based like latissimus dorsi flaps.[23]

Which Method to Choose?

There are several reviews which have compared various surgical modalities for management of hidradenitis suppurativa. This comparison is done on basis of ease of performance of surgery, aesthetic and functional outcome, time required for healing and recurrence of the disease.

Surgical modality of treatment improves the quality of life and Kohorst et al. conducted a study which concluded that patient who underwent surgical treatment were more satisfied with medical treatment and had significant improvement in quality of life postsurgery.[24]

Incision and drainage provides rapid relief of symptoms, however it is associated with high risk of recurrence as compared to surgical excision. Deroofing had recurrence risk similar to excision and risk of recurrence increases in patients who have involvement of multiple sites.[25] Recurrence rate after primary closure has been reported to be approximately 50–60%, while approximately 15% with use of grafts and flaps by Mandal and Watson in their cohort.[19] Few studies have had minimal recurrence with primary closure, while general consensus is that risk of recurrence is high in patient who undergo primary closure of defect.

Secondary intention healing is a good option for reconstruction of surgical site. Secondary intention healing takes more time as compared to graft, however in a study comparing secondary intention healing and graft, patients have preferred secondary intention healing over graft because of ease of use of limb and lack of painful donor site.[26]

Lasers and Light-based Devices for HS

The usage of lasers and light-based devices is increasing for HS. Laser treatment is an adjunctive therapy in HS, to reduce the frequency of painful flares. Lasers act by decreasing the number of hair follicles, sebaceous glands, bacteria in affected areas, and ablative laser by debulking chronic,

Table 34.1: Parameters for Nd:YAG laser in HS.[28,29]

Skin type	*Fluence J/cm²*	*Pulse duration (ms)*	*Spot size (mm)*
I-III	40–50	20	10
IV-VI	35–50	35	10

(Nd:YAG: Neodymium-doped yttrium aluminum garnet; HS: Hidradenitis suppurativa).

problematic lesions. Neodymium-doped yttrium aluminum garnet (Nd:YAG) and CO_2 laser vaporization and excision of sinus tracts are commonly employed in HS.

Nd:YAG Laser

Nd:YAG laser acts by selectively destroying the hair follicles and secondarily destroying the sebaceous glands.The longer wavelength of Nd:YAG is suitable for destroying the hair follicle located in the mid reticular dermis and the subcutaneous tissue. Inguinal and axillar lesions respond better than the inframammary lesions.[27] First week after Nd:YAG treatment, neutrophilic inflammation predominates leading to rupture of nodules and discharge from the lesions. This subsequently transitions to granulomatous inflammation, followed by scarring and fibrosis 1 to 2 months later.[28,29] Nodules are typically treated with double pulsing, while background skin is treated with a single pulse. Scarring in stage III impairs the efficacy of Nd:YAG by limiting the penetration of the laser. Recommended parameters are displayed in Table 34.1.

CO_2 Laser[30]

CO_2 laser is an effective alternative to the cold steel surgery in HS due to good hemostasis, better operative field visualization, minimal tissue removal and improved wound healing. CO_2 laser is suitable for treatment in outpatient setting. CO_2 laser can be used to deroof the sinus tract, vaporize until no affected tissue is visibly present, or completely excise the affected area along with perilesional skin. The wounds secondary to CO_2 laser is allowed to heal by secondary intention or split skin grafting. In general, patients who undergo CO_2 surgery report better scores for pain, scarring, and overall satisfaction compared to those undergoing traditional surgery. The residual scarring secondary to HS can be treated with fractional CO_2 laser. [31]

Other Devices[32]

Other hair reduction lasers (i.e. the 800 nm diode laser, intense pulsed light therapy, and Q-switched ruby laser have also been used with success in small case series for the treatment of HS and related follicular occlusion conditions.

Intralesional Corticosteroids (ILS)

Injection of triamcinolone into inflamed nodules and abscesses of patients with HS is beneficial in the short-term management of disease flares. The usual dosage is 10 mg/mL of triamcinolone acetonide. It can be employed as a monotherapy for acute disease flares or adjuvant of systemic therapies. In cases of acute flares the ILS reduces the pain after 1 day and signs of inflammation approximately 7 days later. This therapy is contraindicated in the presence of local infection. The complications are atrophy, depigmentation and telangiectasia.

REFERENCES

1. Slade DE, Powell BW, Mortimer PS. Hidradenitis suppurativa: pathogenesis and management. Br J Plast Surg. 2003;56:451-61.
2. Mortimer PS, Lunniss PJ. Hidradenitis suppurativa. J R Soc Med. 2000;93:420-2.
3. Wiseman MC. Hidradenitis suppurativa: a review. Dermatol Ther. 2004;17:50-4.
4. Gordon SW. Hidradenitis suppurativa: a closer look. J Natl Med Assoc. 1978;70:339-43.
5. Hurley H. Dermatologic Surgery, Principles and Practice. New York: Marcel Dekker; 1989.
6. Sartorius K, Lapins J, Emtestam L, et al. Suggestions for uniform outcome variables when reporting treatment effects in hidradenitis suppurativa. Br J Dermatol. 2003; 149(1):211-3.
7. Clemmensen OJ. Topical treatment of hidradenitis suppurativa with clindamycin. Int J Dermatol. 1983;22:325-8.
8. Mendonca CO, Griffiths CE. Clindamycin and rifampicin combination therapy for hidradenitis suppurativa. Br J Dermatol. 2006;154:977-8.
9. Mortimer PS, Dawber RP, Gales MA, et al. A double blind controlled cross-over trial of cyproterone acetate in females with hidradenitis suppurativa. Br J Dermatol. 1986;115: 263-8.
10. Fernandez-Vozmediano JM, Armario-Hita JC. Infliximab for the treatment of hidradenitis suppurativa. Dermatology. 2007;215:41-4.
11. Bong JL, Shalders K, Saihan E. Treatment of persistent painful nodules of hidradenitis suppurativa with cryotherapy. Clin Exp Dermatol. 2003;28:241-4.
12. Dalrymple JC, Monaghan JM. Treatment of hidradenitis suppurativa with the carbon dioxide laser. Br J Surg. 1987;74:420.
13. Strauss RM, Pollock B, Stables GI, et al. Photodynamic therapy using aminolaevulinic acid does not lead to clinical improvement in hidradenitis suppurativa. Br J Dermatol. 2005;152:803-4.

14. Lavogiez C, Delaporte E, Darras-Vercambre S, et al. Clinicopathological study of 13 cases of squamous cell carcinoma complicating hidradenitis suppurativa. Dermatology. 2010;220:147-53.
15. Constantinou C, Widom K, Desantis J, et al. Hidradenitis suppurativa complicated by squamous cell carcinoma. Am Surg. 2008;74:1177-81.
16. Ritz JP, Runkel N, Haier J, et al. Extent of surgery and recurrence rate of hidradenitis suppurativa. Int J Colorectal Dis. 1998;13:164-8.
17. Haoxiang X, Chengrang L, Baoxi W, et al. Modified abscess drainage in treatment of eight cases with hidradenitis suppurativa in China. Dermatol Surg. 2013;39(5):779-83.
18. Danby FW. Commentary: unroofing for hidradenitis suppurativa, why and how. J Am Acad Dermatol. 2010;63: 481-e1.
19. Mandal A, Watson J. Experience with different treatment modules in hidradenitis suppuritiva: a study of 106 cases. Surgeon. 2005;3:23-6.
20. Ather S, Chan DS, Leaper DJ, et al. Surgical treatment of hidradenitis suppurativa: case series and reviewof the literature. Int Wound J. 2006;3:159-69.
21. Broadwater JR, Bryant RL, Petrino RA, et al. Advanced hidradenitis suppurativa. Review of surgical treatment in 23 patients. Am J Surg. 1982;144:668-70.
22. Walls B, Mohammad S, Campbell J, et al. Negative pressure dressings for severe hidradenitis suppurativa (acneinversa): a case report. J Wound Care. 2010;19:457-60.
23. Blanc D, Tropet Y, Balmat P. Surgical treatment of suppurative axillary hidradenitis: value of amusculocutaneous island flap of the latissimus dorsi. Apropos of 3 cases. Ann Dermatol Venereol. 1990;117:277-81.
24. Kohorst JJ, Baum CL, Otley CC, et al. Patient satisfaction and quality of life following surgery for hidradenitis suppurativa. Dermatol Surg. 2017;43(1):125-33.
25. Kohorst JJ, Baum CL, Otley CC, et al. Surgical management of hidradenitis suppurativa: outcomes of 590 consecutive patients. Dermatol Surg. 2016;42(9):s1030-40.
26. Morgan WP, Harding KG, Hughes LE. A comparison of skin grafting and healing by granulation, following axillary excision for hidradenitis suppurativa. Ann R Coll Surg Engl. 1983;65:235-6.
27. Tierney E, Mahmoud BH, Hexsel C, et al. Randomized control trial for the treatment of hidradenitis suppurativa with a neodymium-doped yttrium aluminium garnet laser. Dermatol Surg. 2009;35:1188-98.
28. Xu LY, Wright DR, Mahmoud BH, et al. Histopathologic study of hidradenitis suppurativa following long-pulsed 1064-nm Nd:YAG laser treatment. Arch Dermatol. 2011;147:21-8.
29. Mahmoud BH, Tierney E, Hexsel CL, et al. Prospective controlled clinical and histopathologic study of hidradenitis suppurativa treated with the long-pulsed neodymium:yttriumaluminium-garnet laser. J Am Acad Dermatol. 2010;62:637-45.
30. Hamzavi IH, Griffith JL, Riyaz F, et al. Laser and light-based treatment options for hidradenitis suppurativa. J Am Acad Dermatol. 2015;73(5 Suppl 1):S78-81.
31. Krakowski AC, Admani S, Uebelhoer NS, et al . Residual scarring from hidradenitis suppurativa: fractionated CO_2 laser as a novel and noninvasive approach. Pediatrics. 2014;133(1):e248-51.
32. Riis PT, Boer J, Prens EP, et al. Intralesional triamcinolone for flares of hidradenitis suppurativa (HS): a case series. J Am Acad Dermatol. 2016;75(6):1151-5.

CHAPTER 35

Surgeries of Oral Mucosa

Raghunatha Reddy, BM Shashikumar, Savitha AS

INTRODUCTION

The lips are graceful structures that symmetrically occupy the lower third of the facial profile. Lips represent the anterior border of the mouth. The skin of the lips contains hair, sebaceous glands, and eccrine glands. In the male, the entire upper lip and central portion of the lower lip are hair-bearing. The vermilion border is the mucocutaneous junction between the skin and the dry mucosa of lip, red in color because of a lack of keratinization and the underlying capillary plexus. Sebaceous glands are found in normal vermilion tissue 50% of the time, although no hair follicles are seen. The dry vermilion becomes a wet mucous membrane proximally in the oral cavity. The bulk of the tissue comprising the lips consists of striated muscle, primarily the orbicularis oris. The vasculature of the lips consists mainly of the inferior and superior labial arteries, which are the main branches of the facial artery (Figs. 35.1 and 35.2).[1]

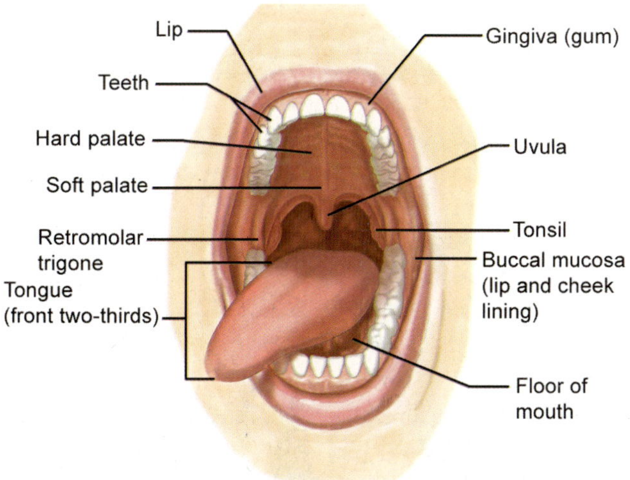

Fig. 35.1: Anatomy of the oral cavity.

COMMONLY PERFORMED PROCEDURES ON ORAL MUCOSA (TABLE 35.1)

Table 35.1: Commonly performed procedures on oral mucosa.

Conditions	*Surgical methods*
Lip vitiligo	• Mini punch grafting • Suction blister grafts • Simple excision and closure • Ultrathin split skin graft • Mucosal advancement flap • Noncultured epidermal cell suspension
Mucous cyst	• Simple excision • Radiofrequency • Deroofing and removal • Sclerotherapy
Benign lesions, premalignant and malignant lesions	• Simple excision and closure • Shave excision • Flap surgery
Lip enhancement surgery	• Autologous fat graft • Dermal graft • Vermilion advancement • Lip implants • Surgical lip lift

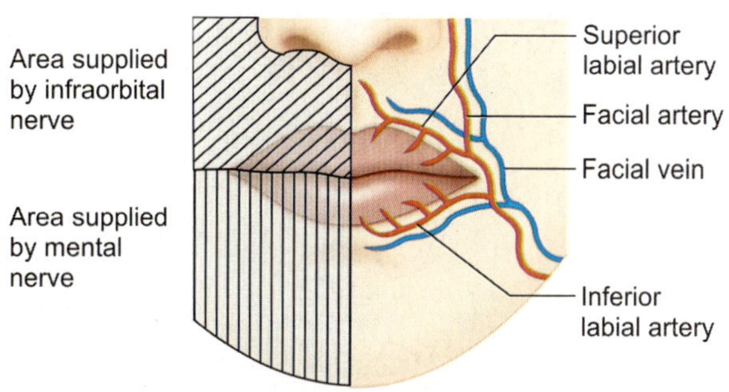

Fig. 35.2: Blood supply and nerve supply of lips.

PRINCIPLES OF PROCEDURES (TABLE 35.2)

- The vermilion border is very important structure for esthetic appearance of lips and it should not be distorted. In an inevitable situation, if violated, it must be precisely reconstructed surgically to preserve normal lip symmetry. Every attempt should be made to retain the normal contours, with the philtrum and Cupid's bow (Fig. 35.3).
- Undermining in the philtral area has to be done superficial to underlying muscle, and may be more difficult. Care should be taken to avoid damage to subdermal hair bulbs (upper lip and midline lower lip skin) in male patients.
- Incisions around lips should follow skin tension lines (Fig. 35.4). Incisions should be made at the junction of natural boundaries to hide their placement, (i.e. vermilion border, nasolabial fold, and chin horizontal crease).
- Defects involving up to one-third of the upper or lower lip can be closed primarily in a layered fashion. Larger defects may require local or pedicle flap closure.
- Nonirritating suture materials are preferred over the mucosa. A comparative study of suture material over mucosa showed faster wound healing with polyglactin 910 (Vicryl rapid) compared to polyglycolic acid and catgut.[2]

ANESTHESIA

Nerve block anesthesia is better tolerated by patients. Infraorbital nerve supplies the upper lip and the mental nerve supplies the lower lip (*see* Fig. 35.1). Local infiltration may then be added for hemostasis.

- Mental nerve block (Figs. 35.5 to 35.7).
- Infraorbital nerve block (Figs. 35.8 to 35.10).

TIPS AND TRICKS

- Marking lip margins with marker pen, methylene blue, 7-0 silk suture (Fig. 35.11), or with scalpel nicks prior to administering local anesthesia can help identify the border during closure.
- For excision of smaller lesions use of chalazion ring forceps helps to stabilize the lesion on the lip/tongue during biopsy/excision. The ring of the forceps also helps to achieve circumferential pressure and hemostasis providing a bloodless field during surgery. As the instrument is self retaining, need of the assistant is eliminated (Fig. 35.12).

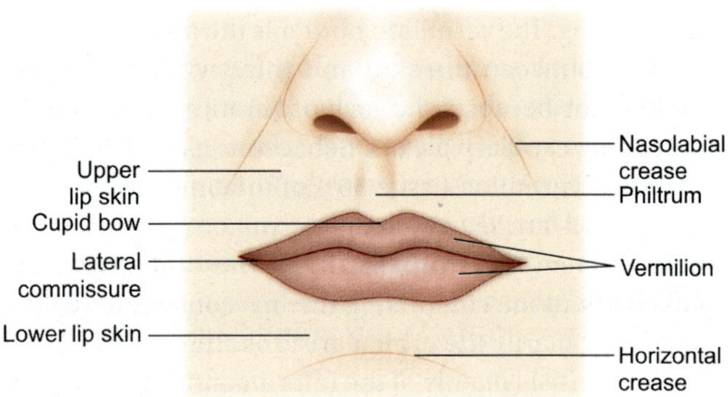

Fig. 35.3: Topical anatomy of the lips.

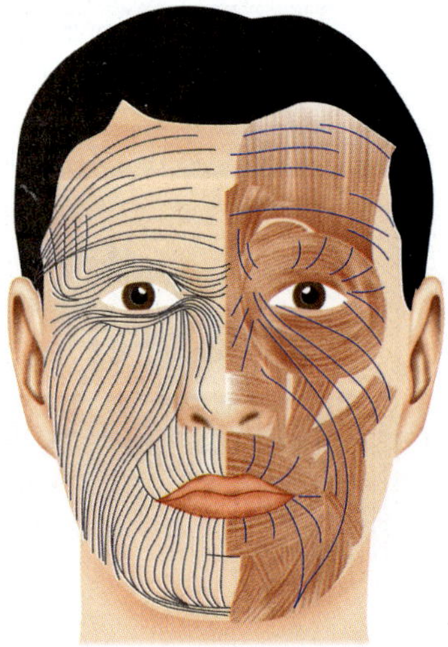

Fig. 35.4: Relaxed skin tension lines around the lips. Incisions should be vertical all around except at the commissures.

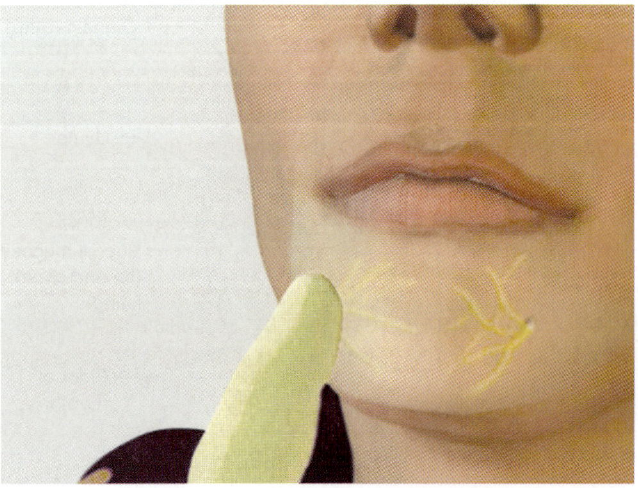

Fig. 35.5: Palpate the mental foramen with the index finger of nondominant hand.

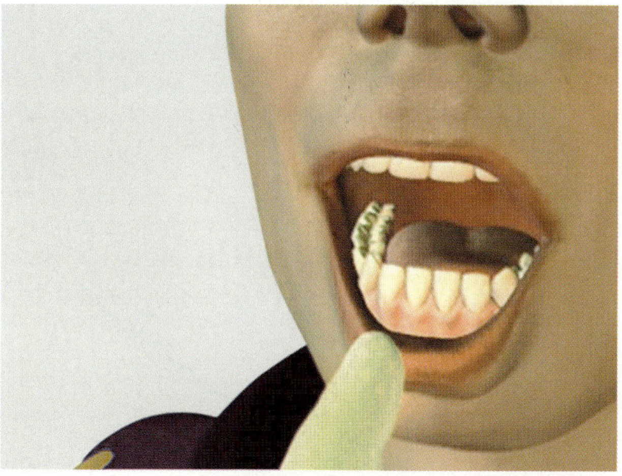

Fig. 35.6: Retract the lower lip with nondominant hand.

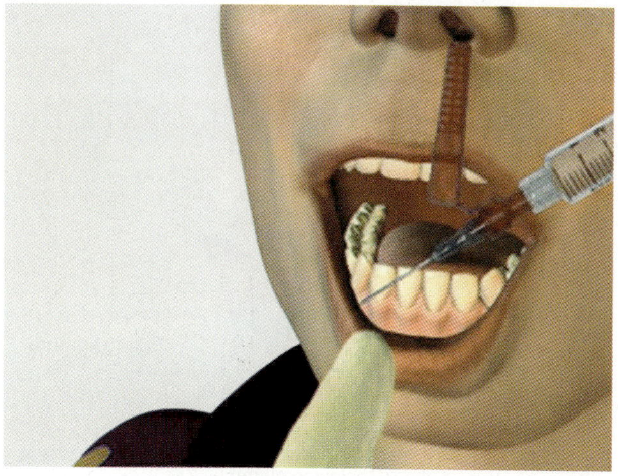

Fig. 35.7: Insert the needle 5 mm inferior to the 2nd bicuspid apex, aspirate and inject the anesthetic slowly.

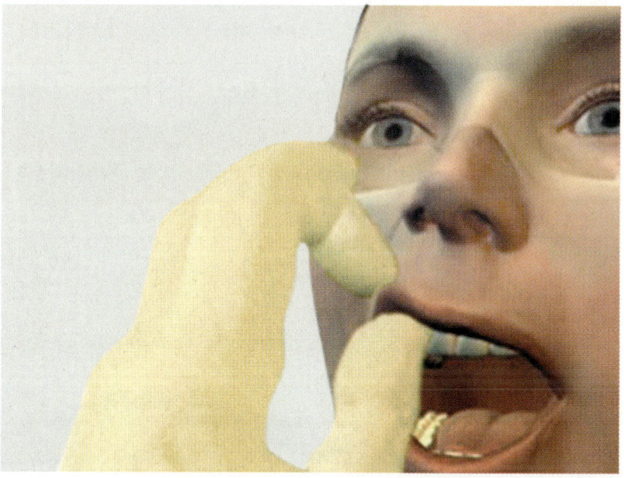

Fig. 35.8: Use the middle finger of nondominant hand to palpate infraorbital foramen, and the thumb and index finger to grasp the upper lip.

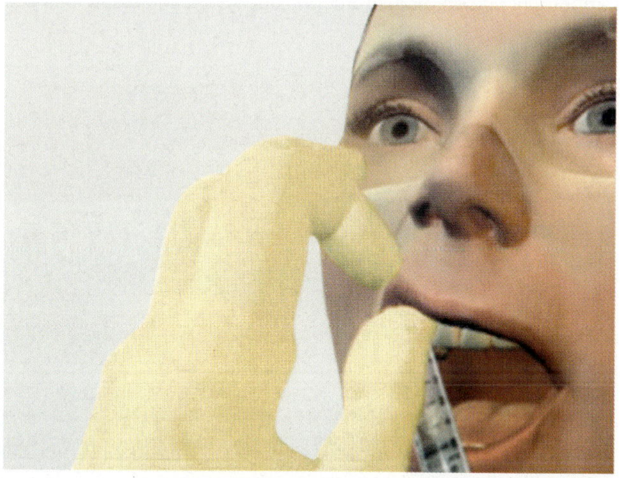

Fig. 35.9: Insert the needle over the canine tooth into the buccal mucosa recess and direct it towards the infraorbital foramen.

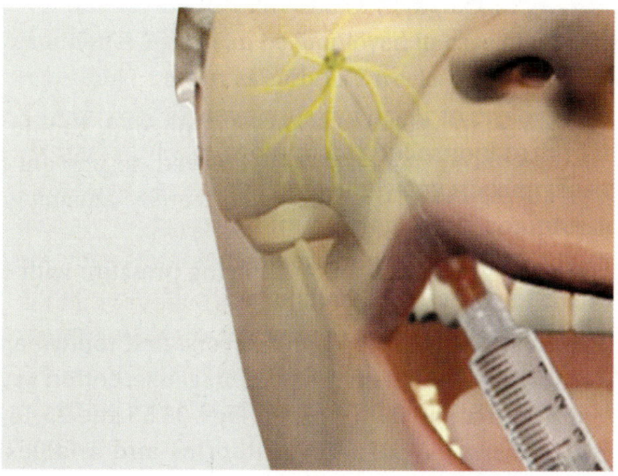

Fig. 35.10: Aspirate and place 2–3 mL of anesthetic in the region of infraorbital foramen.

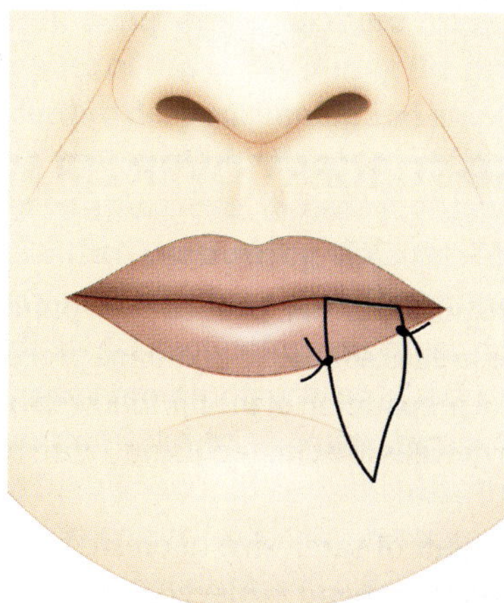

Fig. 35.11: Preanesthesia marking of the vermilion border with 7–0 silk suture prior to local infiltration can allow exact recreation of the border.

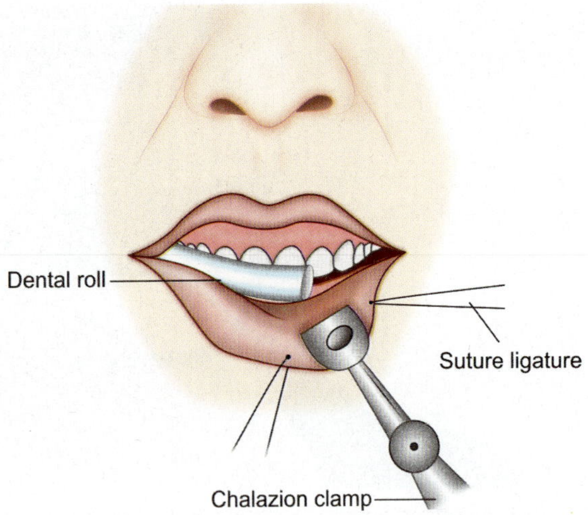

Fig. 35.12: Stabilization of the lip may be achieved with dental rolls (or rolled gauze) between the lip and gums, suture ligatures temporarily placed, or instruments, such as a chalazion clamp.

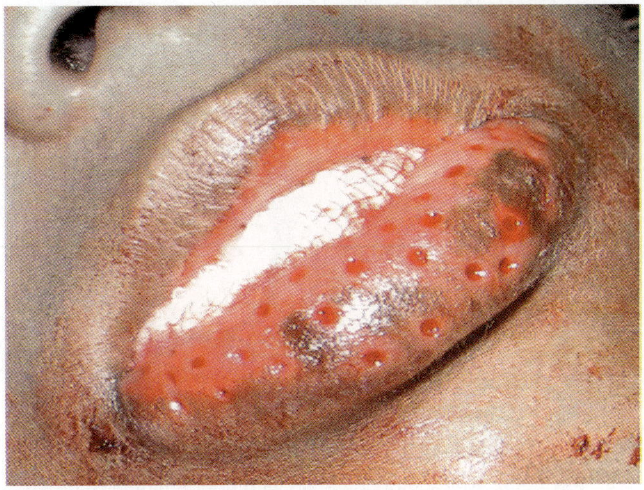

Fig. 35.13: Uniform wells created using 1 mm punches.

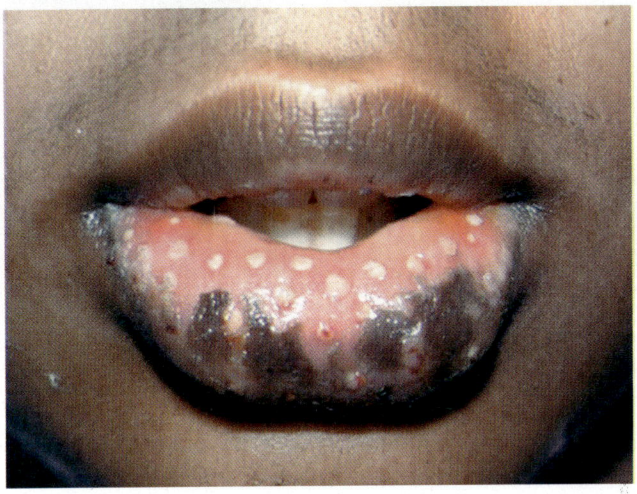

Fig. 35.14: Donor graft placed in the recipient site with dermal side down.

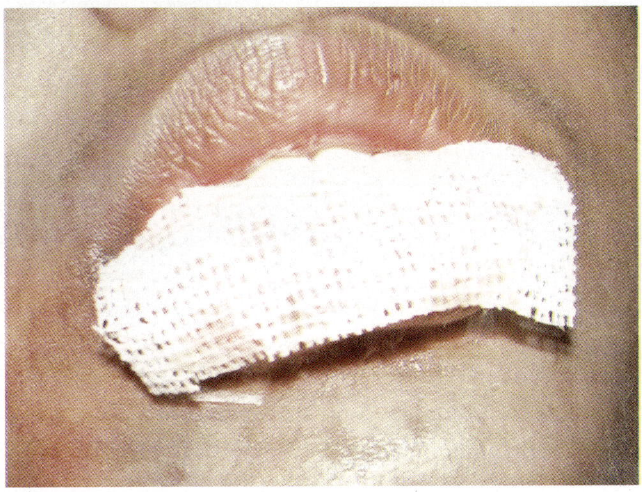

Fig. 35.15: Paraffin gauze dressing.

VITILIGO SURGERY OVER LIP MUCOSA

Procedures

- **Miniature punch grafts:** Extraction of punch grafts from the donor area is similar to standard procedure.
  - Surgical preparation of the lip, followed by anesthesia.
  - Uniform wells are created using 1 mm punches (Fig. 35.13).
  - Donor graft of same size harvested either from the inner thigh or hand is placed in the lip with dermal side down (Fig. 35.14).
- Application of glue is optional, if needed, should be applied after hemostasis is achieved, to prevent the glue gaining entry to the punch thereby causing graft rejection.
- Bleeding is controlled by applying pressure with wet gauze.
- Dressing is to be applied in layers, first topical antibiotic followed by sterile paraffin gauze, cotton gauze and cotton pad in that order (Figs. 35.15 and 35.16).
- *Postoperative period*: Antibiotics and analgesics are prescribed for 5-7 days. Patient is advised

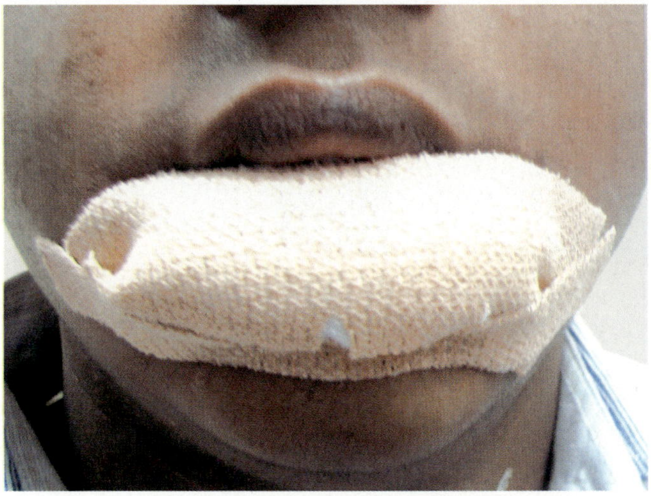

Fig. 35.16: Compression dressing.

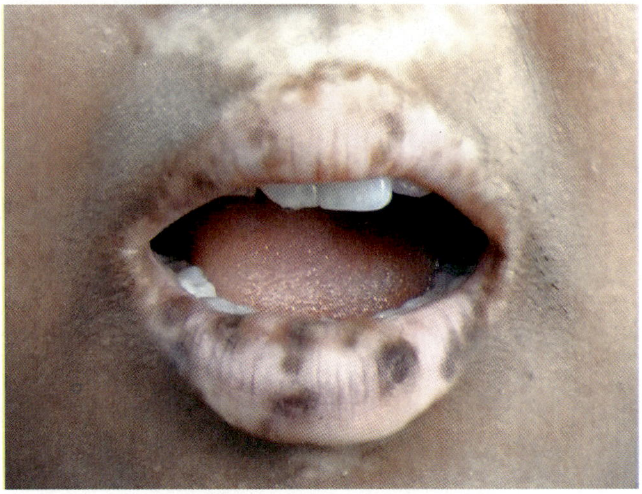

Fig. 35.17: Presurgical photo of lip vitiligo.

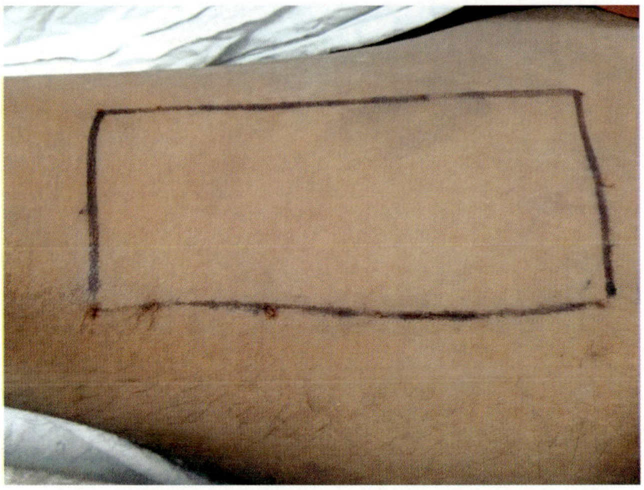

Fig. 35.18: Surgical preparation of donor area, i.e. thigh. The area is marked and anesthesia infiltrated along the borders.

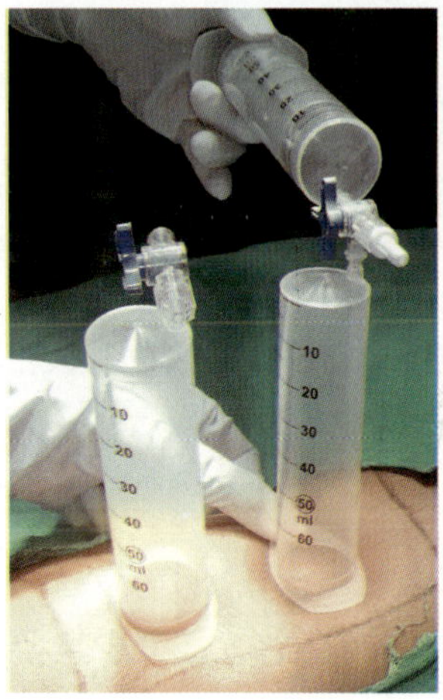

Fig. 35.19: The donor skin is stretched and syringe connected to 3 way cannula is placed on it. Negative pressure is created by withdrawing air through the 3 way cannula in unlock position.

liquid diet on the day of procedure followed by soft food to be taken for few days carefully with a spoon and liquids with a straw to prevent wetting of the dressing. Dressing to be changed once in 2 to 3 days after surgery and may be left open after 7 days depending on the healing. Phototherapy is advised once the dressing is removed.

- **Suction blister graft:** Induction of blister and removal of graft from donor area is similar to standard procedure of harvesting suction blister grafts (Figs. 35.17 to 35.25).
  - The lip as a recipient bed has to be anesthetized and prepared (Fig. 35.26). It can be done either with radiofrequency, erbium YAG or carbon dioxide laser by superficially de-epithelializing the tough epidermal layer followed by superficial dermabrasion by either manual or motor dermabrader (Figs. 35.27 and 35.28).
  - The graft is then gently placed on the lip (Figs. 35.29 to 35.33].
  - Patients are advised soft diet for 3 to 5 days. Dressing is changed on day 3, and removed 3 to 5 days later.
- **Excision and closure for small depigmented areas**
  - Mark the borders of the area to be excised before infiltrating the lesion or giving the block.

  This procedure is ideal only for smaller/linear lesions which can be excised and sutured without distorting the shape of the lip (Figs. 35.34 and 35.35)

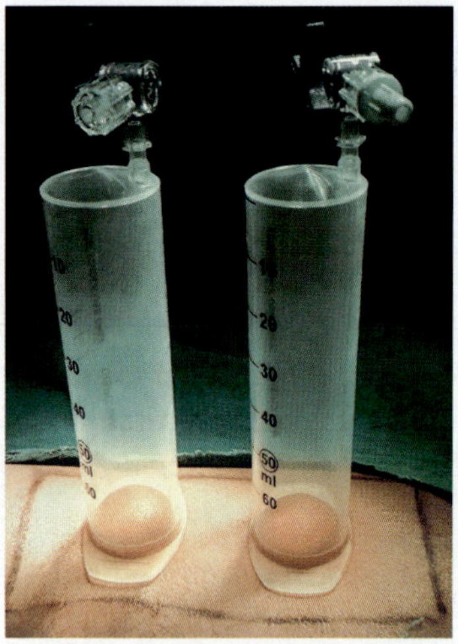

Fig. 35.20: Syringe under suction with approximately 0.5 cm rise of skin from basal rim.

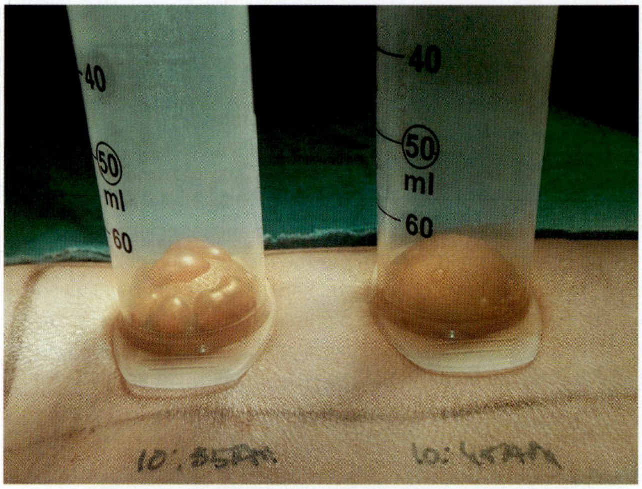

Fig. 35.21: Appearance of multiple blisters which coalesce to form a single blister.

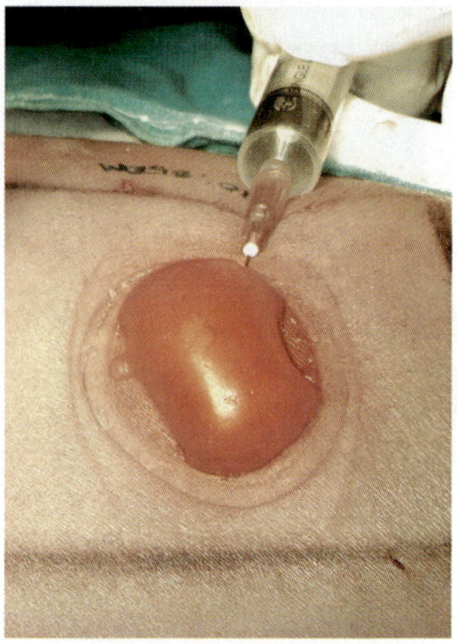

Fig. 35.22: Injection of normal saline into the blister cavity through the needle inserted via the base of the blister, helps in faster formation of blister and coalescing the smaller blisters into a single large one.

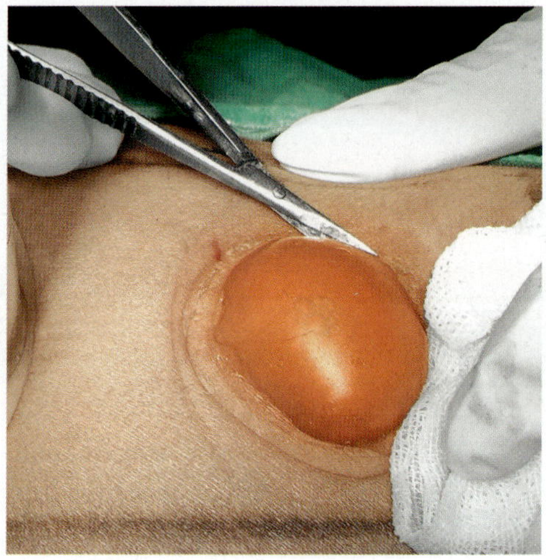

Fig. 35.23: Removal of the blister with small scissors.

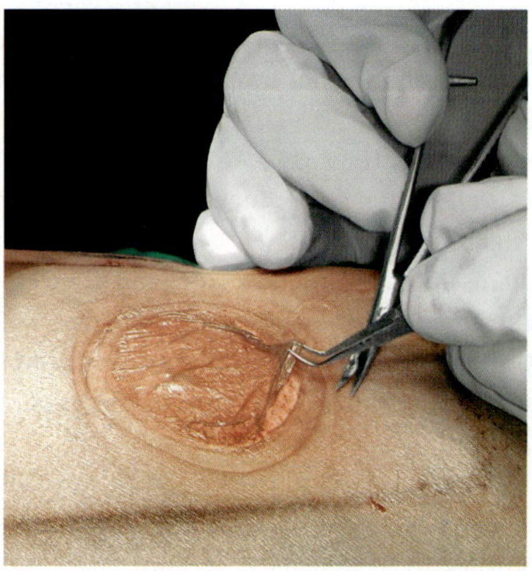

Fig. 35.24: The blister graft is gently separated circumferentially.

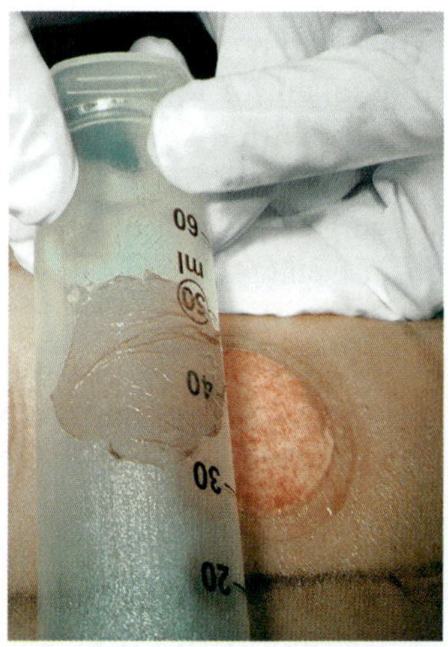

Fig. 35.25: The graft is rolled on to a 50 mL syringe. By this procedure it can be ensured that the dermal side is placed easily on the graft bed.

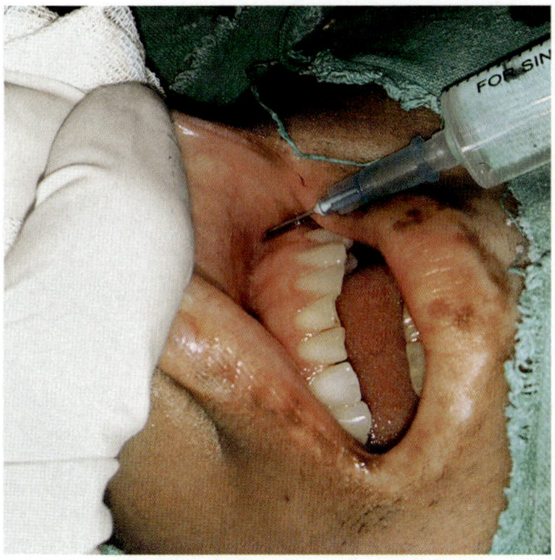

Fig. 35.26: Mental nerve block.

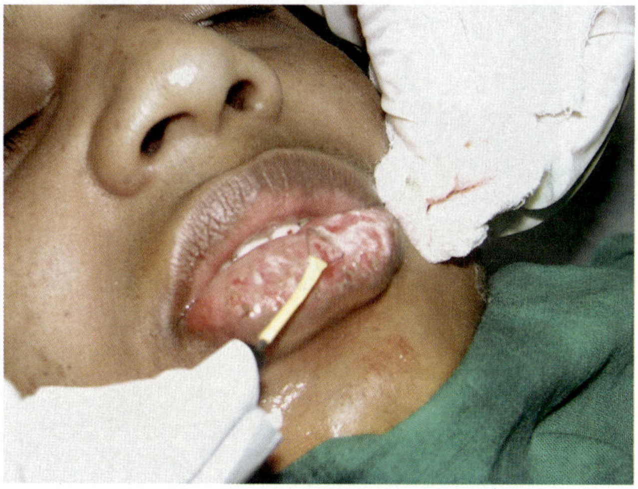

Fig. 35.27: Superficial de-epithelialization by triangular RF probe done under 'cut-coagulation' mode with low energy.

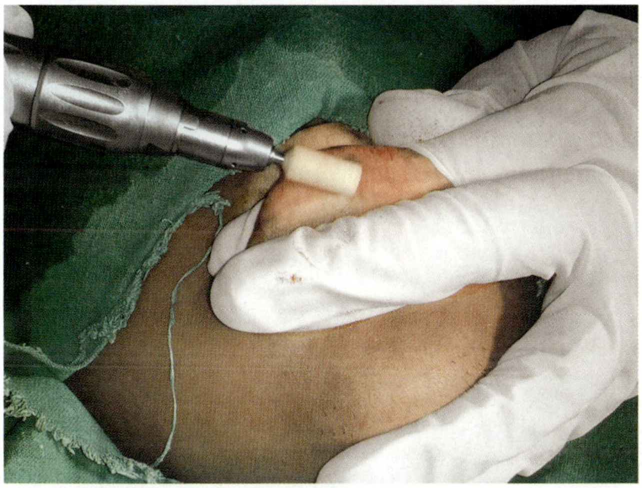

Fig. 35.28: Dermabrasion should always be superficial and optimal for graft uptake, to prevent possibility of hematoma formation and for faster healing.

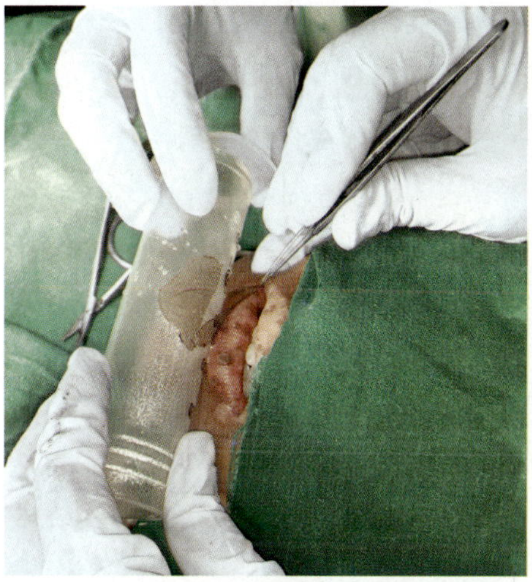

Fig. 35.29: The graft is gently placed on the dermabraded lip with dermal side down.

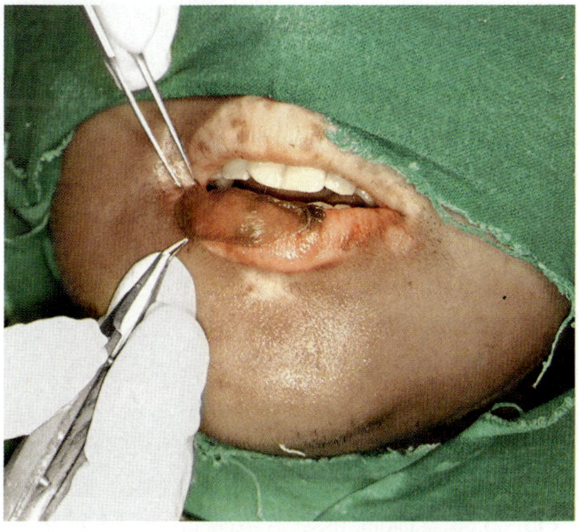

Fig. 35.30: The edges of the graft are smoothened out to avoid folds and incurving at borders.

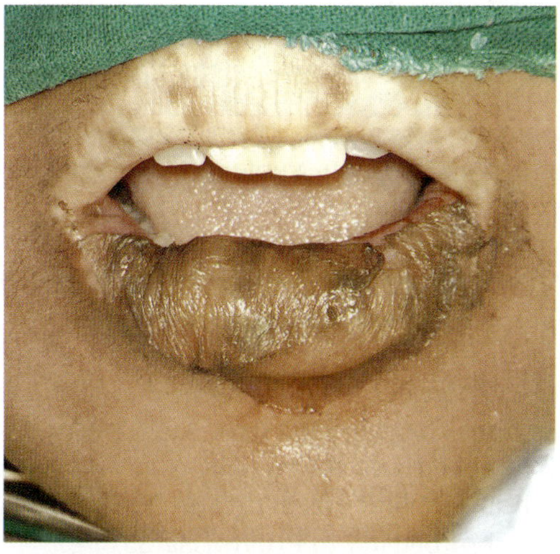

Fig. 35.31: The lower lip area is covered with the graft.

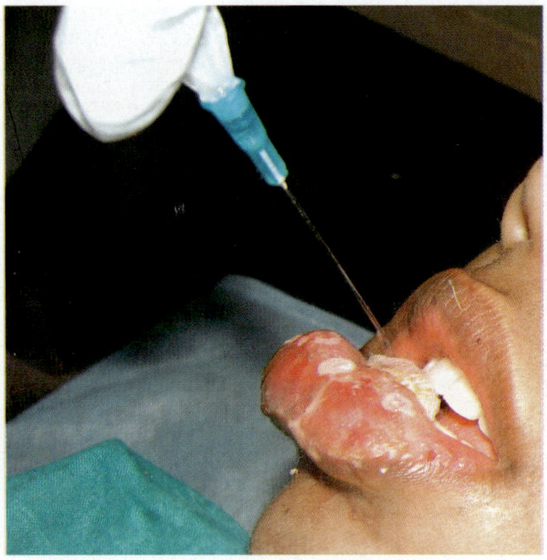

Fig. 35.32: Stay sutures can be applied to the edges, or glue can be applied carefully without touching the graft.

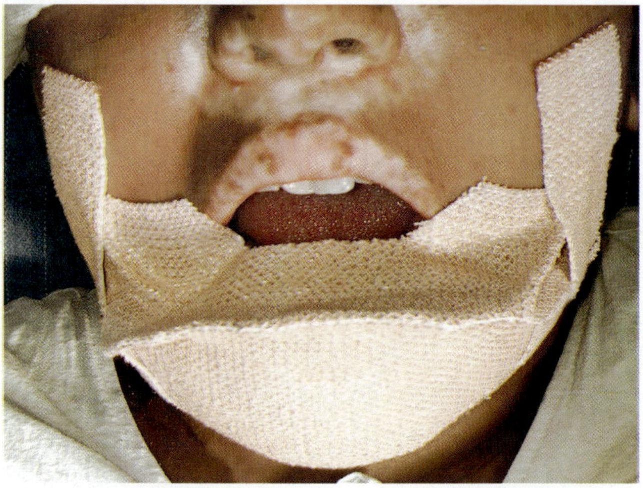

Fig. 35.33: Vaseline gauze followed by pressure dressing is done.

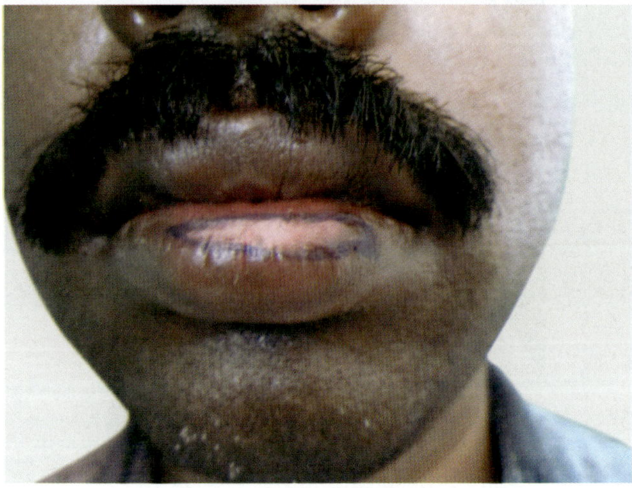

Fig. 35.34: Marking of the area before infiltration.

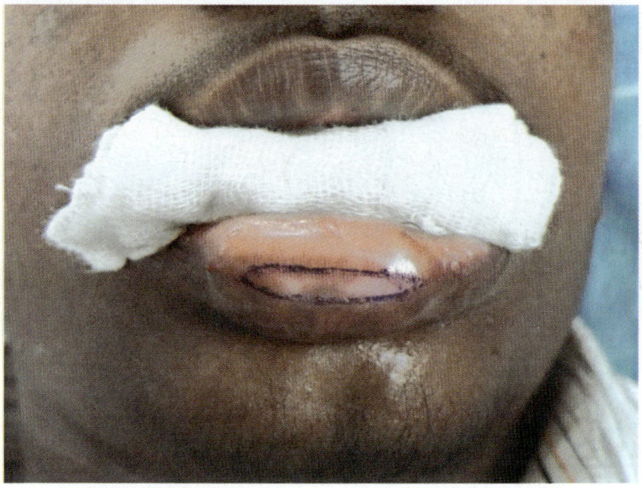

Fig. 35.35: Infiltration of the lip with local anesthesia.

- A sponge holding forceps can be used to achieve homeostasis during the procedure.
- Incision is put along the premarked lines and the vitiliginous area excised (Fig. 35.36).
- Wound edges are approximated with running sutures or percutaneous interrupted sutures. Caution to be exercised to prevent lip inversion or distortion of the shape by undermining (Figs. 35.37 and 35.38).
- After applying topical antibiotic, paraffin dressing, followed by sterile gauze dressing is done.
- Postoperatively, patients are put on antibiotics and analgesics, advised a soft diet and to avoid vigorous chewing for 3 days. After 3 days dressing is removed and the patient is advised to apply topical antibiotic cream for 1 week. Suture material gets absorbed in 7 to 10 days (Fig. 35.39).

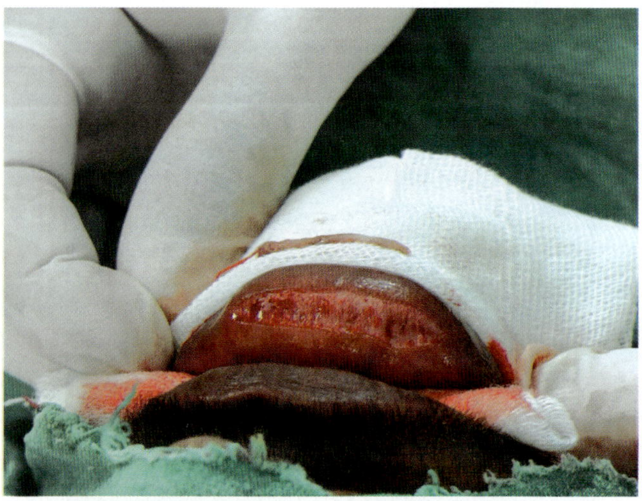

Fig. 35.36: Vitiliginous area excised, superficially.

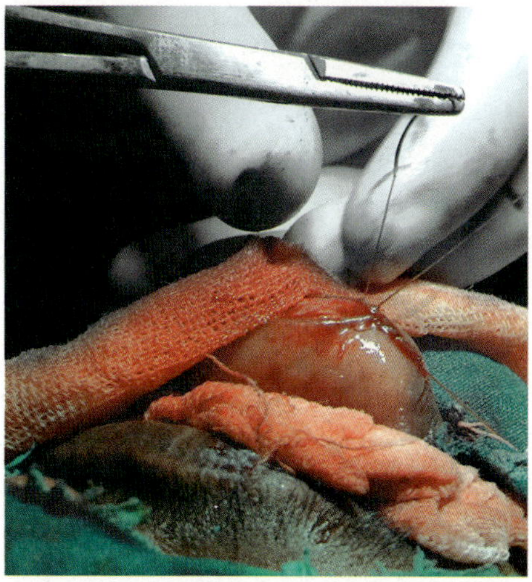

Fig. 35.37: Wound edges approximated using chromic catgut.

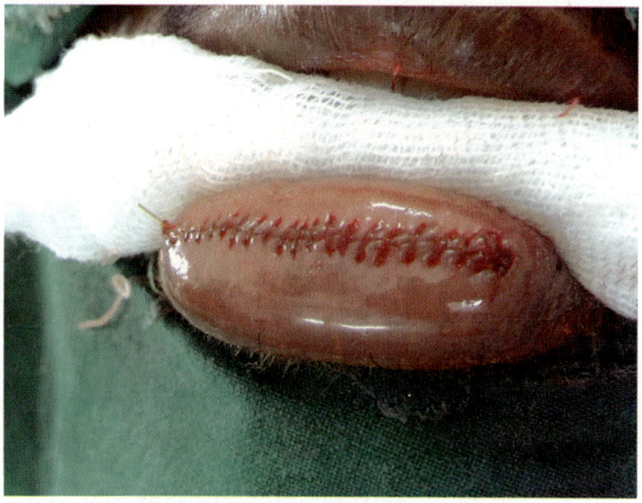

Fig. 35.38: Immediate postoperative period.

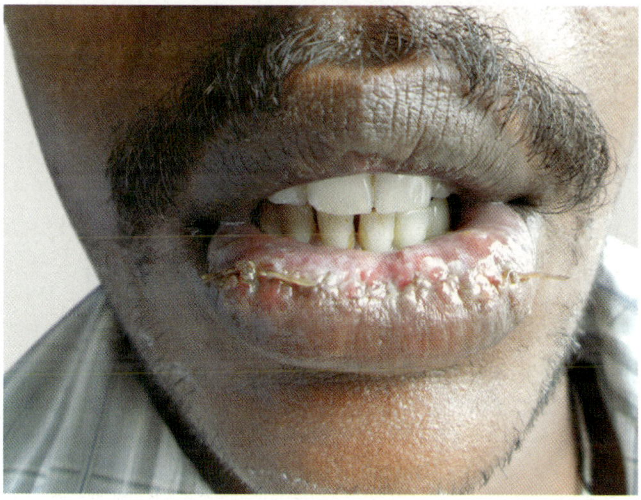

Fig. 35.39: Day 5, suture material is almost absorbed.

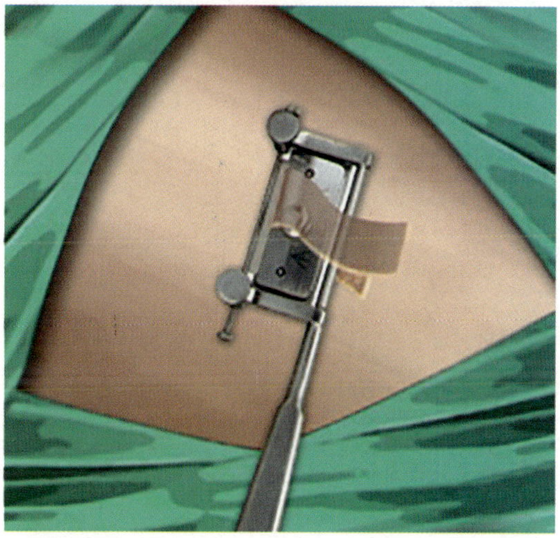

Fig. 35.40: Ultrathin split thickness graft obtained from the upper thigh.

- **Ultrathin graft:** Conventional thin split thickness skin grafting technique continues to be the most commonly practiced and also the most successful amongst all methods of vitiligo surgery.[3] Ultrathin grafts taken without any dermal component, gives excellent results at both the recipient as well as donor sites (Fig. 35.40). Ultrathin grafts are harvested either with a dermatome or Silver's knife. It needs a properly trained person to do the procedure. The quality of the grafts can be gauged by means of their translucent nature and by their ability to float on the isotonic saline solution and the edges should not roll upon themselves.[4] The graft placement and follow-up are similar to that of suction blister grafting, however the graft has to be fixed with sutures, preferably 5-0 absorbable.
- **Mucosal advancement flap**[5]
  - The principle of mucosal advancement flap is shown in Figure 35.41.
  - Two perpendicular lines are drawn from the lateral edges of the depigmented lesion over the lower lip, extending downward up to 1 cm above the junction of gingivolabial sulcus. Burrows triangles are marked on either side at the lower end of the marking, 2 cm above the anterior sulcus (Fig. 35.42).
  - The area is infiltrated with 2% xylocaine hydrochloride, and an incision is made along the markings. Depigmented mucosa is excised (Figs. 35.43 and 35.44).

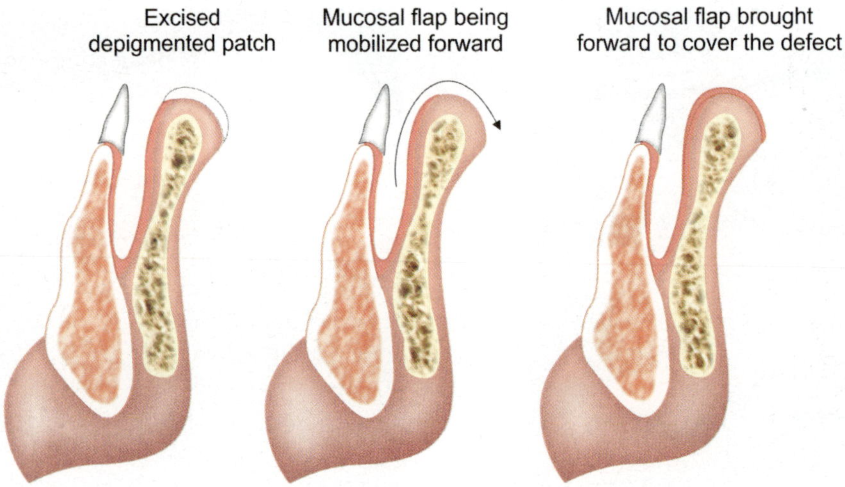

Fig. 35.41: Principle of mucosal advancement flap.

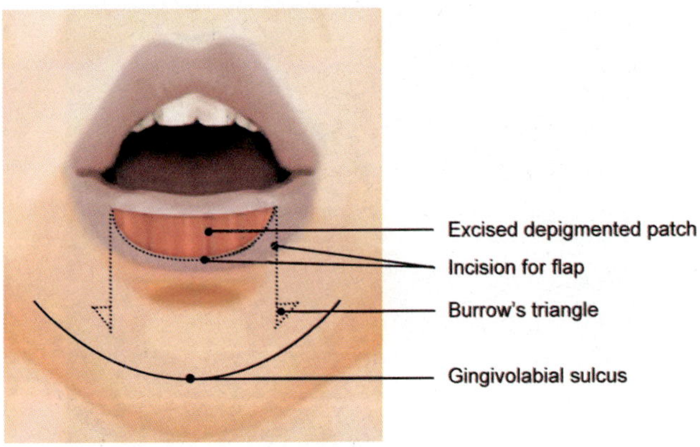

Fig. 35.42: Surgical markings for mucosal advancement flap inside the oral cavity.

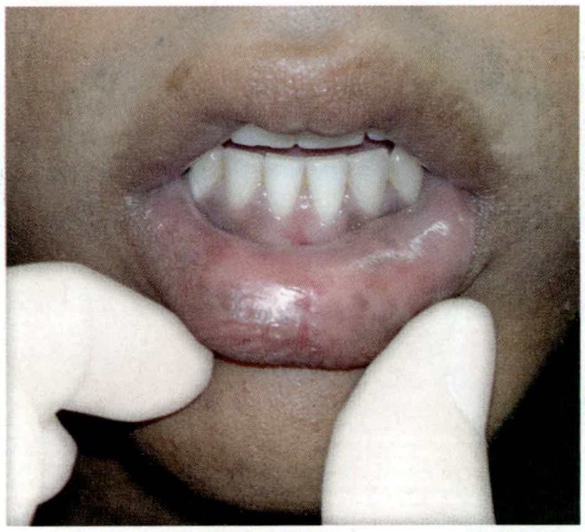

Fig. 35.43: Vitiligo patch on lower lip mucosa.

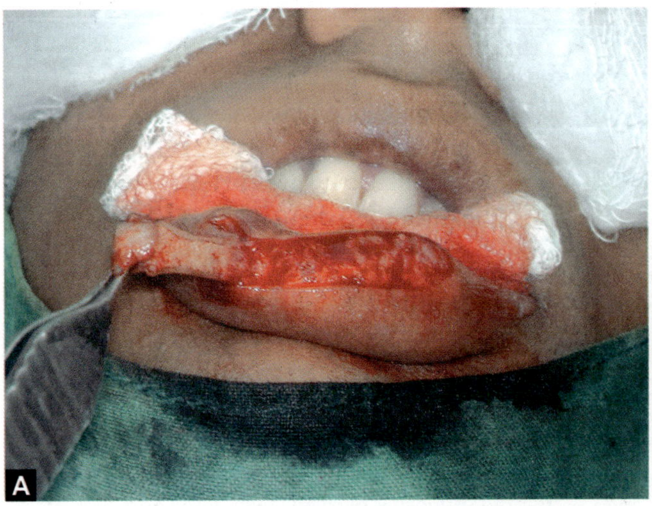

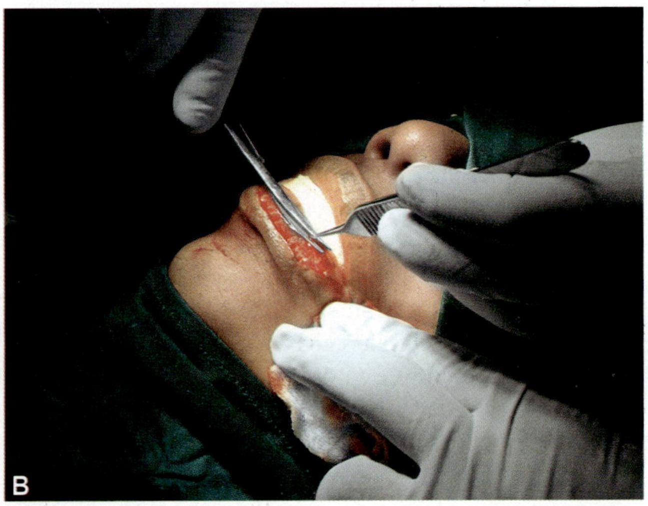

Figs. 35.44A and B: Excision of depigmented mucosa (vitiliginous patch).

- The flap is dissected in the submucosal plane up to 2 cm above the gingivolabial sulcus.

Burrows triangle is excised to prevent possible dog ear deformity which may occur as a result of mucosal advancement. The dissected mucosal flap with the intact attachment at the lower end is advanced and mobilized forward to cover the excised defect (Figs. 35.45 and 35.46).

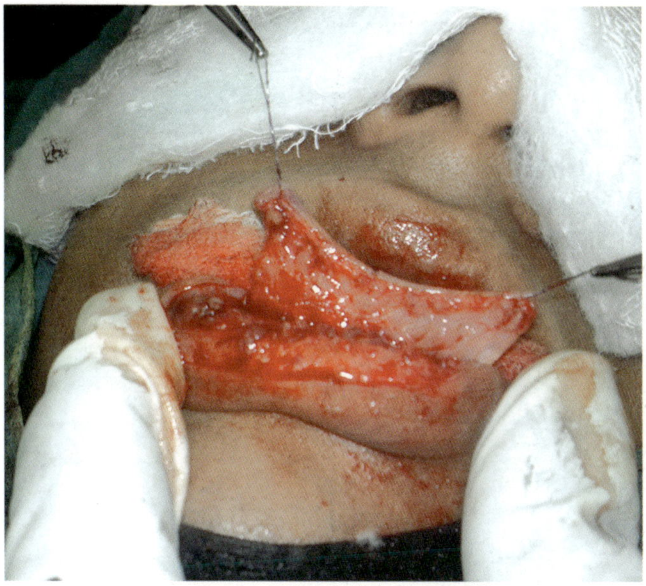

Fig. 35.45: Mobilized mucosal flap in submucosal plane from within the oral cavity to cover the defect.

- Routine postoperative procedures are followed. Almost complete healing can be noticed within a week (Figs. 35.47 and 35.48).

All relevant procedures for lip vitiligo surgery are discussed in Table 35.3.

PROCEDURES FOR MUCOUS CYST

Mucous cyst arises either due to extravasation of mucus from the damaged salivary gland duct or due to obstruction of the duct. Lower lip is the most common site for mucous cyst. High rate of recurrences are common as feeding mucous glands are left behind. Modalities of treatment include:

- **Method A: Excision and closure**
  - Mark the margins and infiltrate the surrounding skin with lignocaine 1% with adrenaline.
  - Fix the mucocele with chalazion forceps (optional).
  - Deroof the cyst with scissors and remove the contents.
  - Electrofulgurate the base.
  - Remove chalazion forceps.
  - The wound is left open and will heal by secondary intention.
- **Method B: Simple excision and closure (better method)**
  - Mark the margins and infiltrate the surrounding skin with lignocaine 1% and adrenaline (Fig. 35.49).

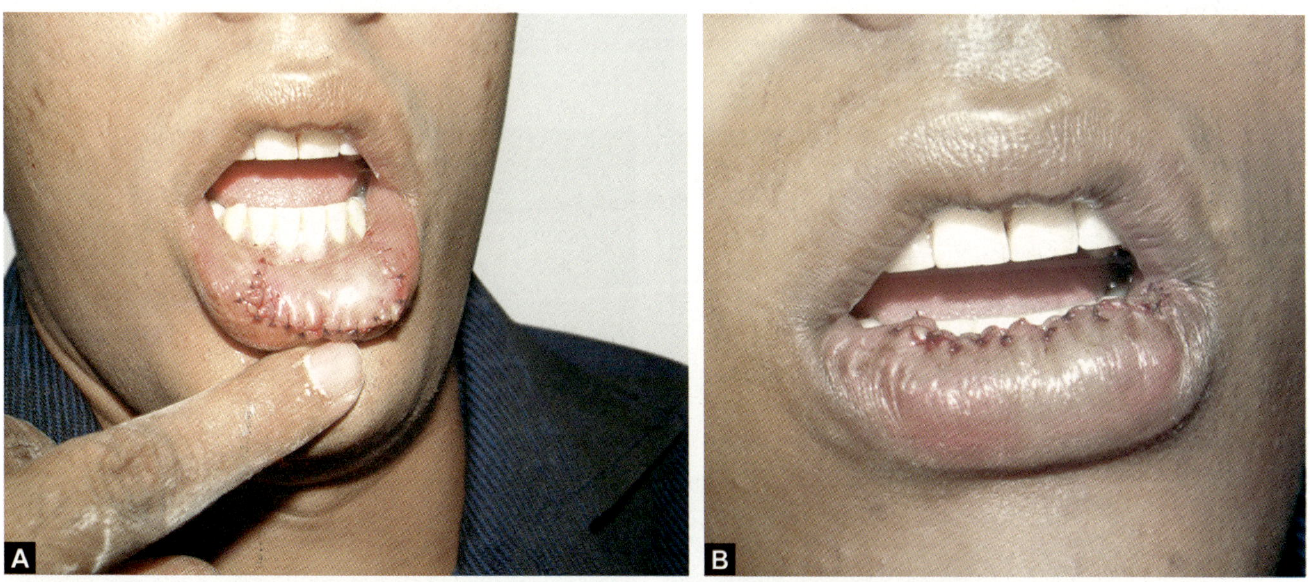

Figs. 35.46A and B: The defect is sutured with 5–0 Vicryl interrupted sutures along the incision and to the incised margin of the lip.

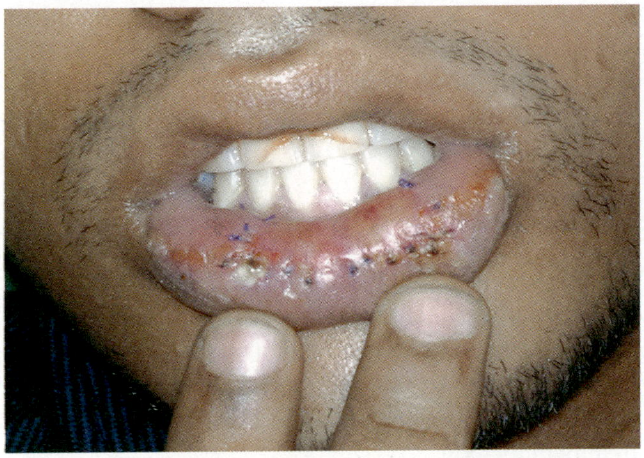

Fig. 35.47: Almost complete recovery within a week.

- A linear or elliptical incision is placed over the cyst superficially taking care not to rupture the cyst preferably. When the mucosa is incised, the cyst pops out (Fig. 35.50), or else dissect it carefully to excise it in total. If the cyst ruptures, remove the cyst wall and sack in total (Fig. 35.51).
- The mucosa sutured with prolene 5- 0 with simple interrupted sutures or with absorbable sutures (Fig. 35.52).
- Healing is complete in a week without any scar (Fig. 35.53).

- **Method C: Complete excision (Figs. 35.54 to 35.57):** Postoperative follow-up is like other procedures mentioned above.

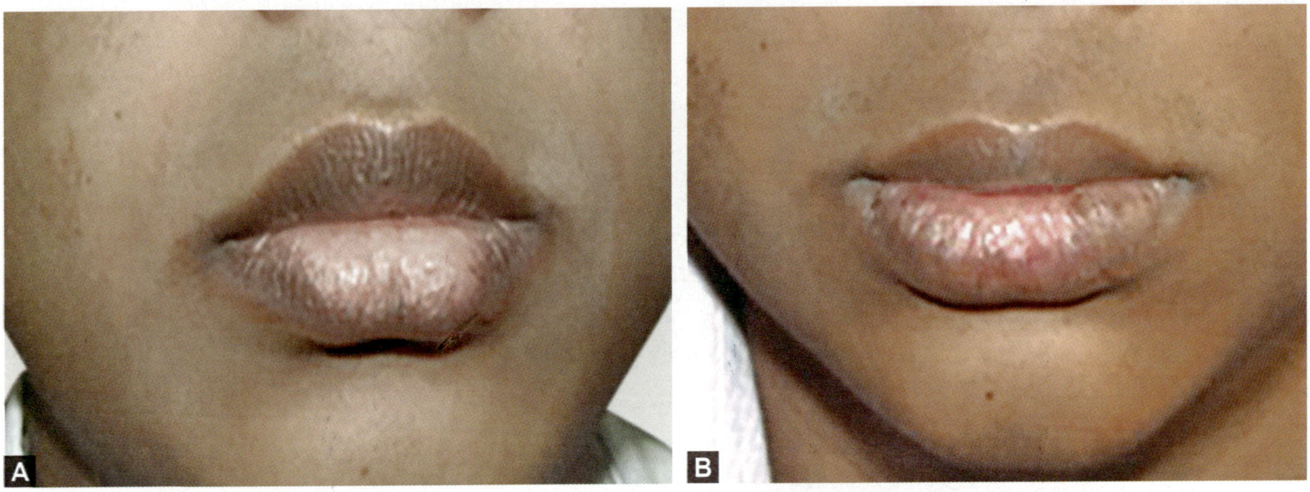

Figs. 35.48A and B: Resolved lesion, without scar or pigmentation of another patient.

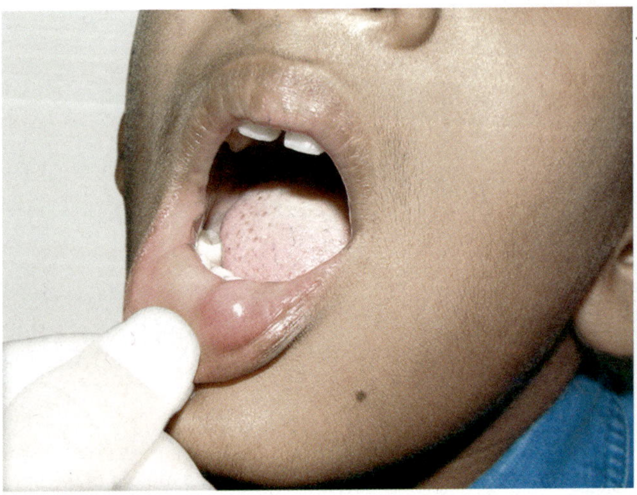

Fig. 35.49: Mucus cyst over the lower lip.

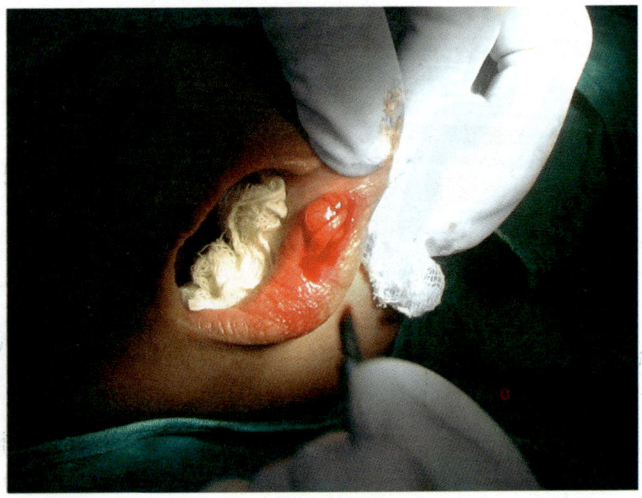

Fig. 35.50: The cyst pops out when the mucosa is incised.

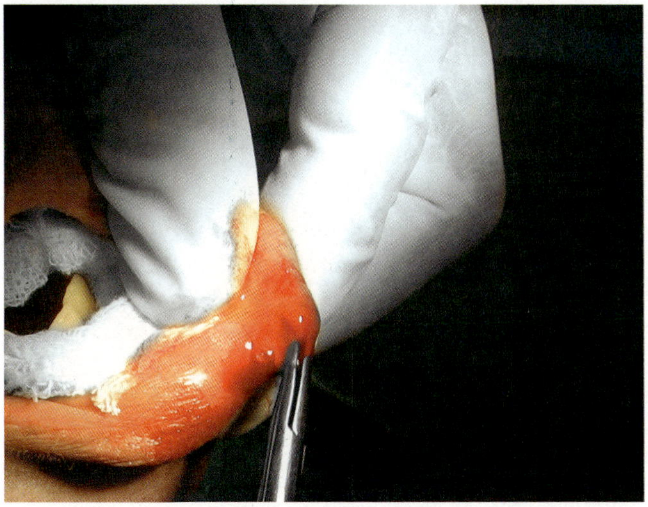

Fig. 35.51: If the cyst ruptures remove the cyst wall and sack in total.

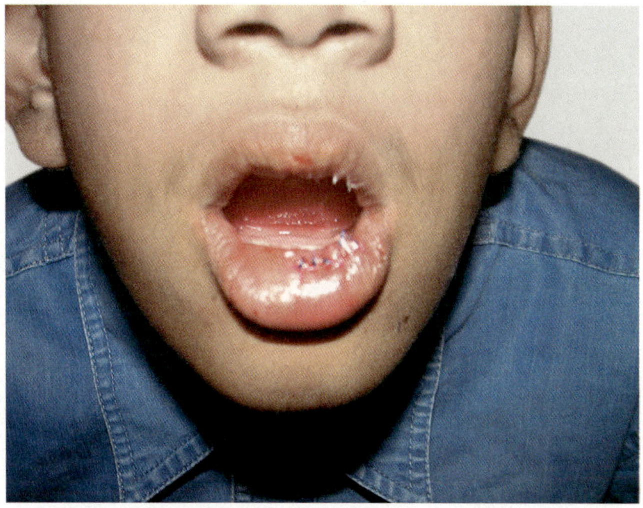

Fig. 35.52: The cyst is removed and mucosa sutured with prolene 5–0 with simple interrupted sutures or with absorbable sutures.

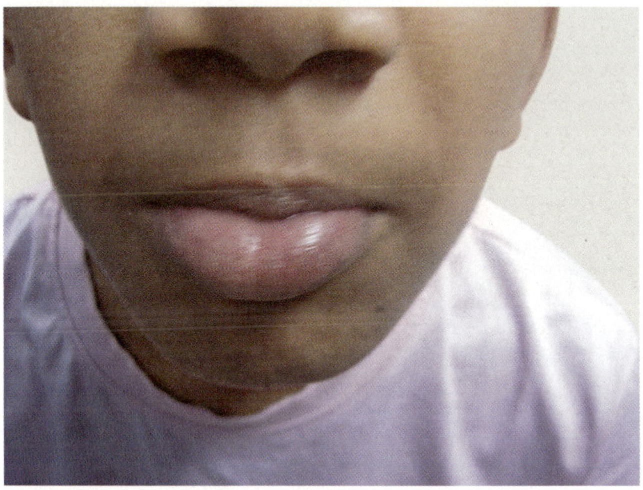

Fig. 35.53: Healing is complete in a week without any scar.

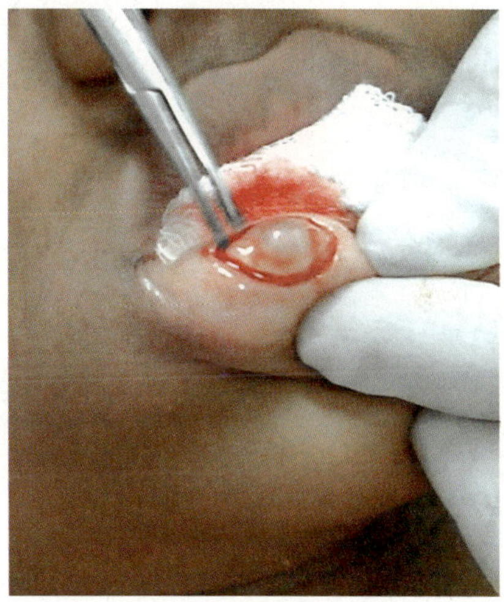

Fig. 35.54: After anesthesia, elliptical incision is placed around the mucus cyst.

- **Application of caustic chemicals**: Caustic agents like phenol can be used to treat mucoceles. No local anesthesia is required. Under aseptic precautions a very small quantity of 88% phenol is injected into the cyst cavity using insulin syringes. No dressing is given afterwards. Patients are given analgesics post procedure for 1 day (Fig. 35.58).[6]
- **Sclerotherapy**: Sclerosing agents like polidocanol or sodium tetradecyl sulfate can also be injected into the mucous cysts. The minimum concentration required to produce desired results with least complications is 1.5%. In those patients who show partial response in initial sittings, concentration can be increased to 2%. Common complications include pain on injection, erythema and healing with postinflammatory hyperpigmentation (Figs. 35.59 and 35.60).

REMOVAL OF SUPERFICIAL GROWTHS

Small superficial lesions around the lip which are removed by shave excision with a #15 blade heal well by secondary intention with excellent cosmetic results. Small excision or punch biopsy also will heal satisfactorily by secondary intention but may heal more rapidly by simple primary closure (Figs. 35.61 to 35.63).

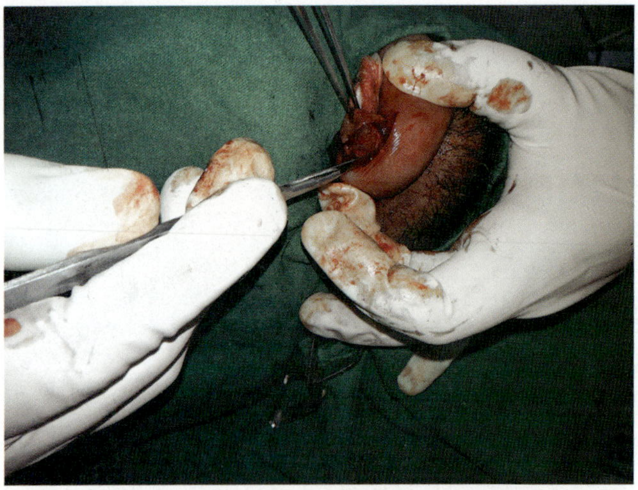

Fig. 35.55: The cyst is dissected from the surrounding tissue.

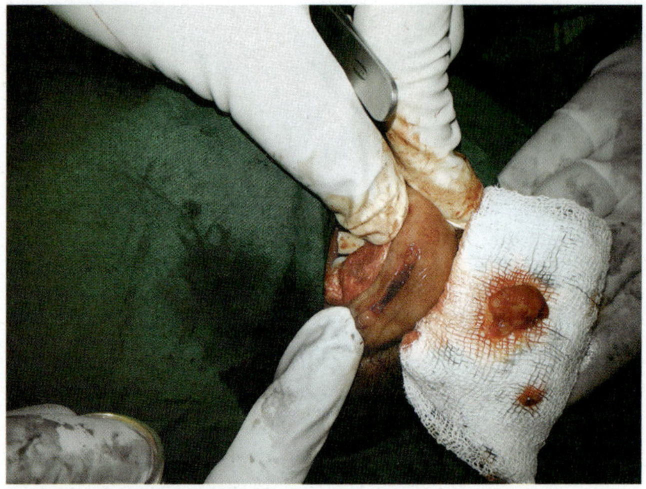

Fig. 35.56: The cyst is removed in total.

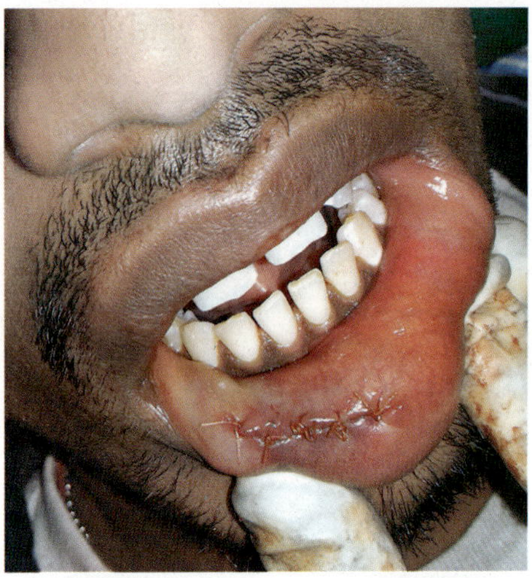

Fig. 35.57: After achieving hemostasis by compression, sutures are placed.

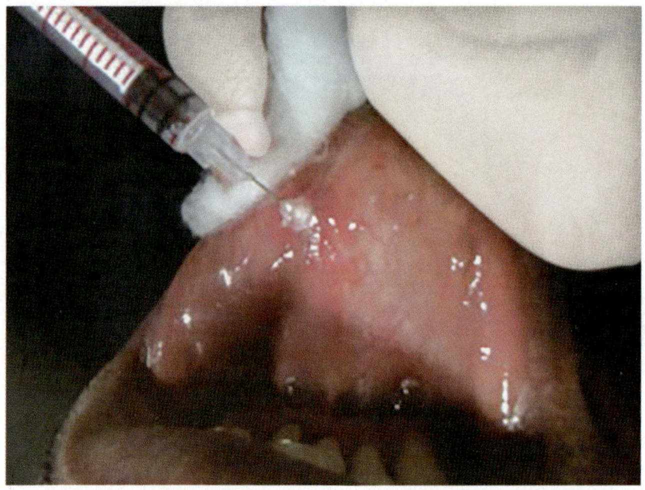

Fig. 35.58: Injection of phenol into the mucus cyst.

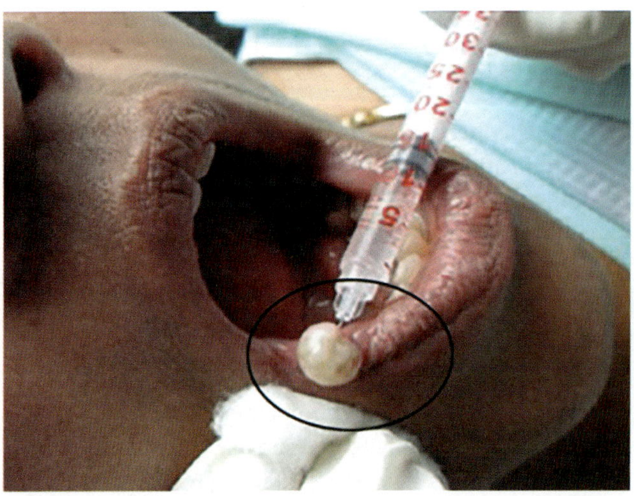

Fig. 35.59: Blanching of the mucous cyst on sclerosant injection.

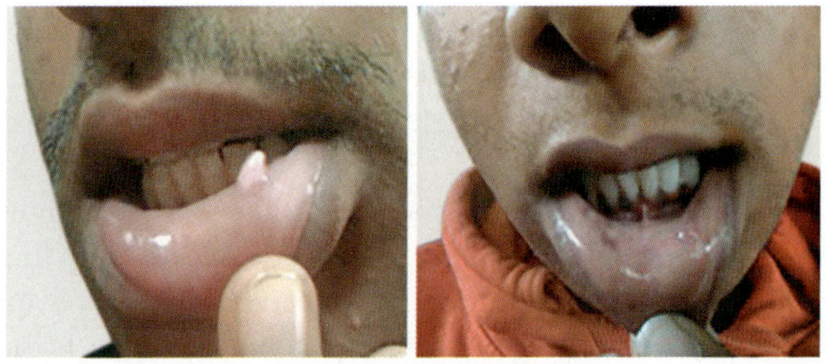

Fig. 35.60: Before and one week after sclerosant injection.

SOME IMPORTANT CONSIDERATIONS IN ORAL MUCOSAL SURGERY (TABLE 35.2)

Postoperative Management and Care

- For small lesions of the lip, no dressing is needed.
- Infections are rare with minor lip and oral cavity procedures. They must be looked for and treated appropriately.
- Postoperative care in most cases includes gentle rinsing with mouthwash or saline solution several times a day.
- Soft diets are encouraged.
- Movement should be decreased initially to avoid bleeding and wound edge separation. Minimize talking.
- The use of dentures may need to be restricted accompanied by dietary management.
- Dressings should be adherent and moisture-resistant and must not interfere with underlying circulation.

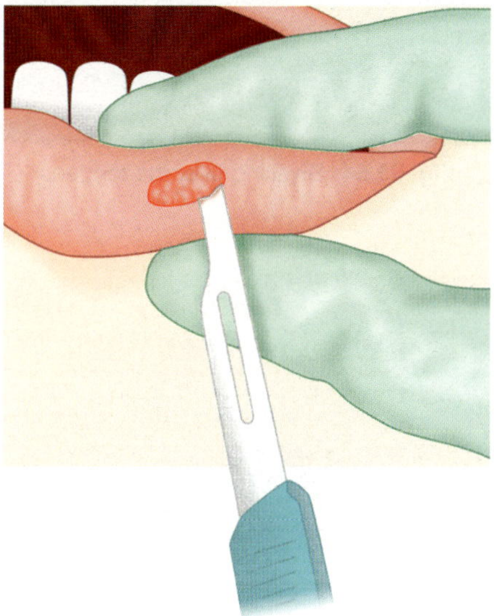

Fig. 35.61: Schematic diagram of shave excision.

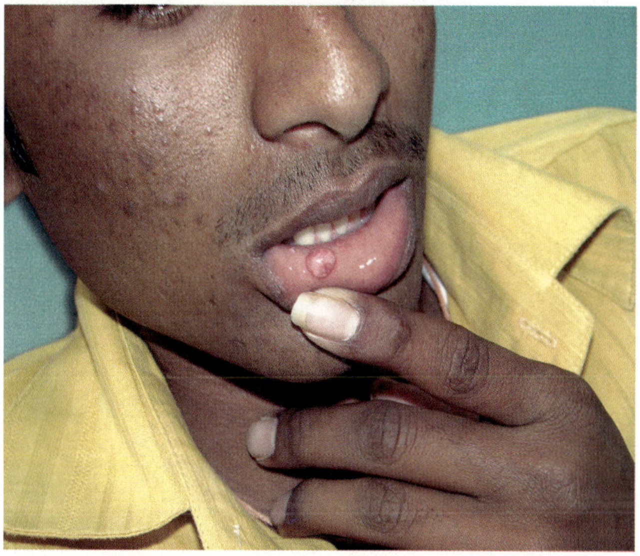

Fig. 35.62: Benign growth on the lip.

Table 35.2: Principles of surgery of oral mucosa.

Anatomic considerations	Stenson's duct is the opening of the parotid duct into the oral cavity located opposite the upper second molar tooth. Wharton's duct in the anterior floor of the mouth empties the submandibular gland. The orifices of these ducts should be avoided if possible during surgical procedures.
Airway	Airway maintenance is of utmost importance both during and after surgical procedures. Postoperative edema may impair the airway.
Surgical field visualization	Direct visualization and exposure is essential and may be different from most cutaneous procedures. Headlights, proper instrumentation, traction sutures, and a suction apparatus must be available.
Sutures	Primary closure can be accomplished in most cases and offers less morbidity than other techniques. Primary closure can be accomplished with nonirritating sutures, which can be removed in three to five days in most cases. Interrupted 3-0 or 4-0 silk/Ethilon/prolene or absorbabale sutures can be used for closure. Interrupted suturing provides a margin of safety over running suture as constant intraoral movement may loosen a suture. Interrupted sutures always have an advantage in the event of postoperative hematoma and for its evacuation. Silk is a soft braided material, which is more comfortable to the patient (Figs. 35.64 to 35.66).
Hemostasis	Removal of oral lesions often causes brisk bleeding from the wound edges because of the excellent vascularization of the mouth. Electrocautery and direct pressure with gauze can be used for hemostasis prior to wound closure. Alternatively, sutures can be placed under the lesion as desired in number before excision, so as to enable closure immediately and conveniently without much bleeding (Figs. 35.64 to 35.66).

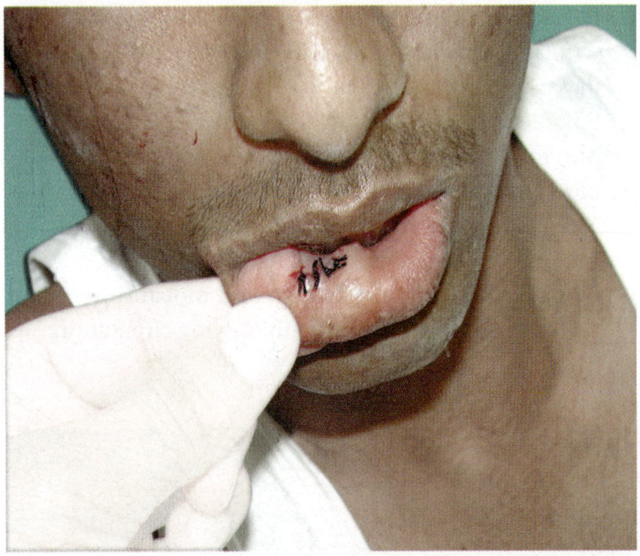

Fig. 35.63: Primary excision and suture of the growth and suture.

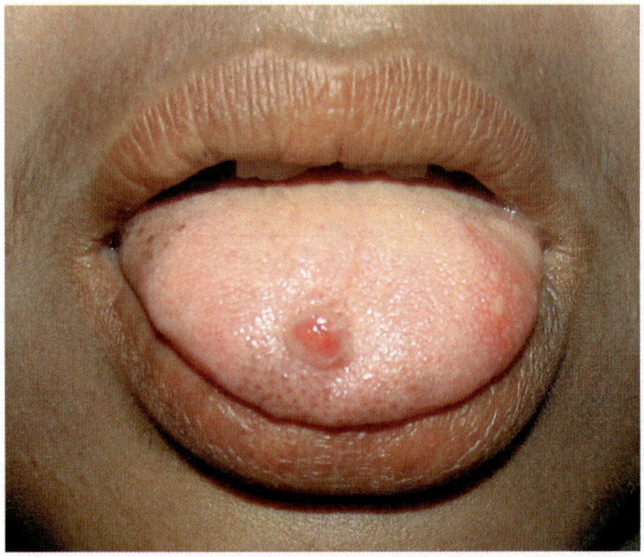

Fig. 35.64: Swelling over the tongue.

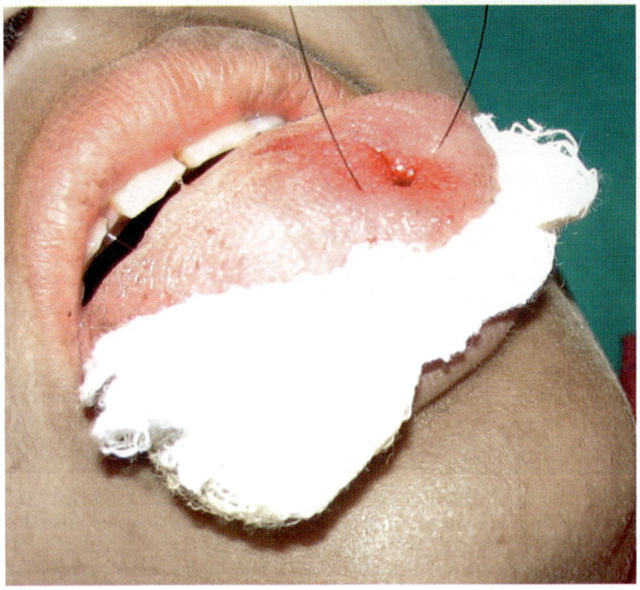

Fig. 35.65: Sutures taken before the incision to enable closure without much bleeding.

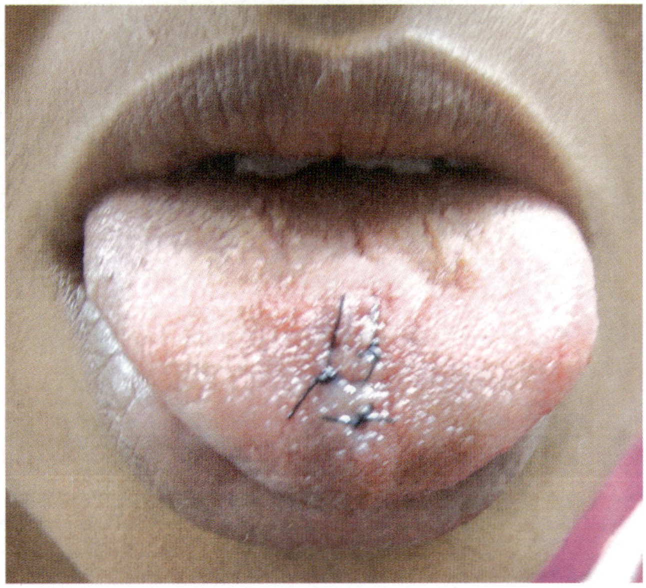

Fig. 35.66: Closed with simple interrupted sutures either absorbable or removable.

- Dehiscence and notching of the lip can occur because of the high mobility of the area. If this occurs, conservative management may be all that is necessary; but notch formation will require surgical revision.
- Lip contracture with elevation of the vermilion border may be simply corrected and, if due to scar contracture, may require a Z-plasty.
- In females, the use of lip color may provide the finishing touch to conceal scars and a more pleasing appearance.

ACKNOWLEDGMENTS

Figures 35.17 to 35.26 and 35.28 to 35.31, 35.59 and 35.60 are courtesy of Dr Shruthi C, Department of Dermatology, BMCRI, Bengaluru, Karnataka, India.

Table 35.3: List of transplantation procedures commonly used for lip vitiligo with their advantages, disadvantages, and outcome in various studies.[7]

Type of grafts for lip leukoderma	*Advantages*	*Disadvantages*	*Summary of the outcome of literature analysis for surgical treatment of lip vitiligo. [Successful/total (%)]*
Thin and ultrathin split thickness skin grafts (STSG)	High success rates with immediate results, but not a best choice	Color and texture mismatch, donor area scarring, recipient area contracture, occurrence of dermatological diseases, such as psoriasis, malignant transformation, expertise skill needed. Lip may look heavy with stuck on appearance	2/2 (100%)
Suction blister grafting (SBG)	The ease of procedure, the high success rate, and the excellent cosmetic results. No scarring at donor site as the graft consists of only epidermis	Time-consuming, hyperpigmentation at the recipient site and donor site, unsuitable for larger areas. Lip should not be covered partially. Even if the lesion is small grafting should be done for the entire lip to have uniformity in color	40/45 (88.88%)
Miniature punch grafting	Easy to perform and can take care of a relatively larger vitiligo area	Cobblestone appearance, polka dot appearance, depigmentation of the grafts, perigraft halo, graft rejection, hypertrophic scarring, and variegated appearance with color mismatch at the recipient sites, scarring at the donor site. Usually requires post-surgical medical management	102/132 (77.21%)
Noncultured melanocyte grafting of epidermal suspensions	Larger area can be treated with a smaller size of donor graft. Excellent color match	Time-consuming, need for specialized equipment (such as, centrifuge, incubator), and reagents, training and experience to obtain standardized uniform results and, hence, there is an initial learning curve. The Epidermal cell suspension may run away and produce irregular pigmentation. Not a best procedure for the lip compared to other sites	6/14 (42.9%)
Cultured "pure" melanocytes (CM) and epithelial grafts (CE)	Large area can be treated in a single session	Time-consuming and labor intensive technique, requires a sophisticated laboratory setup for cell culture	Not available at all places except in specialized centers
Micropigmentation	Relatively inexpensive, simple office procedure with instant results	Difficult to adjust or homogenize tone of skin color, pigment migration, bluish discoloration due to Tyndall effect. Is almost an obsolete procedure	100%. However the authors experience does not recommend this since the long-term results are very bad with undesirable results due to color change of pigmentation and many complications. It should be discouraged as much as possible due to availability of much better procedures
Mucosal advancement flap	Single case report. Best and suitable graft to replace the excised mucosa due to various causes, since it is a natural replacement of lip mucosa with oral mucosal tissue	If performed in a suitable case where the patch is small, the results are excellent with complete natural appearance and function. Is a skilled procedure and requires surgical expertise	Though a single case report in published literature, authors' experience is good with 8 cases performed in a situation where other grafting techniques have failed

REFERENCES

1. Hubert T Greenway. The Lips and Oral Cavity. In:Randal K, editor. Current Techniques in Dermatologic Surgery. 3rd ed. New York: Informa Health Care; 2007.p. 231-45.
2. Mirković S, Durdević-Mirković T, Branislav B, Sarcev I. Choice of surgical suture material used in oral cavity-clinical study. Med Pregl. 2010;63(7-8):497-501.
3. Khunger N. Recent advances in the surgical treatment of vitiligo. In: Ghosh S (Ed). Recent advances in dermatology, Vol 2. India. Jaypee Brothers Medical Publishers (P) Ltd New Delhi:2007;319-40.
4. Majid I, Imran S. Ultrathin split-thickness skin grafting followed by narrowband UVB therapy for stable vitiligo: An effective and cosmetically satisfying treatment option. Indian J Dermatol Venereol Leprol. 2012;78:159-64.
5. Raghunatha R Reddy, Shashikumar M Basavapura, Girish A. Chandramouli. Mucosal Advancement Flap: An Innovative Surgical Technique for Treatment of Lip Vitiligo. Dermatol Surg 2012;1-4.
6. Sacchidanand S, Sujaya SN, Venkatesh Purohit. Phenolisation as a Mode of Treatment of Mucosal Cysts. Journal of Cutaneous and Aesthetic Surgery. Jul-Sep 2012, Volume 5, Issue 3.
7. Kanathur S, Sacchidanand S, Savitha S, et al. A study of the outcome of primary excision and closure technique in the management of lip Leukoderma in 30 patients. J Cutan Aesthet Surg. 2016;9:20-6.

CHAPTER 36

Surgeries of Genitalia

Revathi TN, Lakshmi DV, Divya Gorur

INTRODUCTION

Anogenital dermatology encompasses a wide spectrum of disorders: venereal and nonvenereal conditions to benign and malignant diseases. Surgical intervention in dermatology set-up pertaining to genital conditions is often limited to basic dermatosurgical procedures comprising of electrocautery, cryotherapy or excisional surgeries but, nowadays with improved skills, a section of genital surgeries like circumcision, frenulectomy and preputioplasty can also be performed. This chapter includes these procedures and also highlights briefly surgeries on vaginal mucosa which is still a new and less performed entity in the dermatosurgery arena.

ANATOMY OF MALE EXTERNAL GENITALIA

Penis

Penis comprises of three main components: root, body and glans. Root is the attached part of penis, which consists of the bulb in the middle and the crus, one on either side of the bulb. The root lies within the superficial perineal pouch. The body of penis has two surfaces: dorsal (posterosuperior in an erect penis) and ventral or urethral (facing downwards and backwards in a flaccid penis). The shaft of penis consists of 3 erectile columns, the two corpora cavernosa and the corpus spongiosum, along with enveloping fascial layers, blood vessels, lymphatics, and nerves, all covered by skin. Glans penis is a conical shaped end part of corpus spongiosum. The urethra ends with the external urethral orifice at the tip of glans.

The prepuce consists of an inner leaf and an outer leaf, and covers the glans of a flaccid penis. The foreskin serves as a reserve skin and stretches during erection. The frenulum is located at the ventral side of glans and attaches the prepuce to glans. The epithelium here is nonkeratinized which becomes keratinized after circumcision.

Blood supply and nerve innervations: The blood supply of penis is mainly derived from pudendal artery (a branch of internal iliac artery). The pudendal artery becomes penile artery at the root of penis and gives rise to 4 main branches: dorsal artery, cavernosal artery, bulbar artery and urethral artery. The venous drainage occurs through superficial dorsal vein into pudendal branches of saphenous vein and also through dorsal vein, cavernosal veins and crural vein into internal iliac veins.

Penis is innervated by the somatic and the autonomic nerves. Somatic nerve supplies sensory fibers and to perineal motor fibers. The penis is also innervated by both sympathetic and parasymphathetic nervous system. Parasymphathetic innervation results in erection, while symphathetic innervation is involved in ejaculation (also refer penile anesthesia).

Scrotum

This is an external sac of skin, which is divided into two compartments, and each compartment contains one epididymis and one testis. Scrotum is continuous with the skin of lower abdomen. It is located directly behind the penis and in front of the anus. Scrotal wall is a thin layer of skin and lined with smooth muscle tissue (dartos fascia). The scrotal skin is more pigmented than surrounding areas and also has many sebaceous and sweat glands.

Layers of Scrotal Skin

- *Skin*: Thin, pigmented, wrinkled with rugosities.
- *Superficial fascia*: It is continuous with the fatty and the membranous layers of fascia of the anterior abdominal wall. The fatty layer in this region is replaced by the dartos muscle (smooth muscle innervated by sympathetic nerve fibers). The membranous layer of fascia in the scrotal region is known as Colle's fascia, this is continuous in front with the Scarpa's fascia.

- *Spermatic fascia*: This lies beneath the superficial fascia and is derived from three layers of anterior abdominal wall (external spermatic fascia, cremasteric fascia and internal spermatic fascia).
- *Tunica vaginalis*: It lies within the three spermatic fascias, covering anterior, medial and lateral surfaces of testis.

Blood supply and nerve supply: Anterior and posterior scrotal nerves, perineal branches of posterior femoral cutaneous nerve and genital branch of genitofemoral nerve supply the scrotum. Blood supply is from the anterior scrotal artery (a branch of the deep external pudendal artery) and the posterior scrotal artery (a branch of internal pudendal artery). Venous drainage is through the testicular veins into the inferior vena cava.

ANESTHESIA

Local anesthesia and regional block are performed in genital area. For simpler procedures like biopsy and excision of small tumors: infiltration of local anesthetic is sufficient, whereas regional blocks are ideal for circumcision or larger procedures.

Penile Anesthesia[1]

The two dorsal penile nerves located on top and sides of penis, at the 11 o'clock and 1 o'clock position near the base of penis fan out toward the glans. They emerge from underneath symphysis pubis bone and innervate entire dorsal surface of penis. The superficial nerves also innervate the ventral penile surface and frenulum. In surgical procedures involving penis, local anesthesia is preferable, since it is less risky and less expensive. Lidocaine with epinephrine is avoided due to the risk of vasoconstriction of blood vessels, which can lead to gangrene.

There are two techniques for local penile anesthesia: the penile nerve block and the ring block.

Penile Block

Patient is made to lie in supine position. Palpate the inferior aspect of symphysis pubis bone and the base of penis at 2 o'clock and 10 o'clock positions. To anesthetize the dorsal penile nerve, insert a 27 gauge 3–4 cm length needle superior to the 2 o'clock site over the inferior portion of the symphysis pubis. Advance the needle until it reaches the bone, then walk the needle in a caudal fashion off the pubis. A popping sensation is noted as the needle goes through superficial fascia, which is inferior to pubis. At this site, inject 5 cc of 1% lidocaine or 0.25% bupivacaine without epinephrine. Repeat the procedure at the 10 o'clock site to anesthetize the right dorsal penile nerve. The needle should be inserted to hit the symphysis pubis and then directed below it through the fascia into the space where the local anesthetic is deposited to block the dorsal nerve of the penis.

Ring Block Technique

Using a fine (23-gauge) needle, inject about 0.1 mL of anesthetic subcutaneously at the 11 o'clock position. Then, advance it into the subdermal space without withdrawing the needle, which should be freely mobile. At this point, inject 2–3 mL of the anesthetic to block both the dorsal penile nerves. Then the same needle is advanced subcutaneously around the side of the penis and an additional 1 mL of anesthetic is injected. Withdraw the needle and repeat the procedure, starting at the 1 o'clock position so as to complete a ring of anesthetic infiltration. After the injection, the base of penis is massaged for 10–20 seconds to increase the diffusion of anesthetic into surrounding tissues. Gently pinch the foreskin with an artery forceps after 3–4 minutes to confirm anesthesia of infiltrated area.

TIPS AND TRICKS

- Before injecting any anesthetic, aspirate to make sure no blood enters the syringe to avoid intravascular injection.
- For anesthesia, an alternative is a mixture of 5 mL of 1% lignocaine and 5 mL of 0.25% plain bupivacaine can be used, as it gives a longer duration of action (4–5 hrs).

Anesthesia of Female External Genitalia

The female external genitalia is supplied by ilioinguinal and genitofemoral nerves majorly and also branch of pudendal nerve (dorsal nerve of the clitoris, perineal nerve and inferior rectal nerve).

Pudendal Block

The needle is directed through the wall of the vagina toward the ischial spine and lidocaine is injected around the pudendal nerve as it enters the ischiorectal fossa here.

SIMPLE SURGICAL TECHNIQUES OVER GENITALIA

1. ***Biopsy*:** A punch or snip technique is usually adequate for sampling biopsy. For smaller lesions, it can also be useful as therapeutic option. Using a punch biopsy on the genital skin and subcutaneous tissue, the distortion of the overlying epidermis or mucosa is minimal due to the rugosities and redundant skin. Absorbable sutures should be placed perpendicular to the skin tension lines. In the penis, this should be perpendicular to the long axis to prevent traction during erection.[2] Snip excision is a good technique for removal of cystic or papillomatous lesions when histologic examination is desired. With this technique, traction is placed on the lesion with forceps, and scissors are used to gently dissect beneath the lesion and then check for hemostasis. The superficial wounds heal by second intention.
2. ***Excision and primary closure*:** It is a simple and easy procedure done routinely. The various indications of the technique are as given in Table 36.1.
3. ***Mohs micrographic surgery*:**[2] Mohs micrographic surgery is an excellent option for those with locally invasive, non-metastatic disease given the spectrum of benign and malignant conditions like HPV associated diseases over genitalia, Bowens disease, erythroplasia of Queyrat, extramammary Paget's disease, basal cell carcinoma. Surgical excision is the treatment of choice for SCCs of the genitalia, and close follow-up of all genital SCCs is a must. Penectomy and en bloc vulvectomy may be required in more extensive lesions.

In genital melanomas, depth, ulceration, and lymph node status are significant prognostic indicators, hence depth and extent of the disease should be assessed aptly prior to surgery. In men with thin (less than 1 mm) melanomas, wide local excision or distal amputation may be sufficient and penile melanoma less than 1 mm thick, five-year survival rates are greater than 90%. Treatment for women with vulvar melanoma is similarly based on depth and lymph node status. However, survival of women is ranges from 23% to 63% at five years. In addition to surgery, adjuvant therapies including radiotherapy, interferon-alpha and cytotoxic chemotherapy also play a role in a multimodal approach.

Table 36.1: Indications for excision and primary closure.

	Characteristics	*Note*
Benign cysts	Epidermoid cyst and median raphe cyst are commonest	In Bartholin's cyst, excision is not recommended because the function of the gland is lost. Better treatment options include carbon dioxide laser vaporization
Syringomas	These are benign tumors of eccrine sweat gland origin, may be multiple, also occurring over vulva with an exacerbation during menses	Excision provides definitive treatment. Carbon dioxide laser vaporization is also effective
Papillary hidradenoma (hidradenoma papilliferum)	Benign tumor of apocrine sweat gland origin that presents as a flesh-colored to reddish papule or nodule on the vulva	Excision provides definitive treatment
Genital leiomyomas	Solitary, smooth muscle tumors that arise from the dartos muscle of the scrotum and vulva	Excision
Idiopathic calcinosis cutis	Asymptomatic calcified dermal nodule with chalky white discharge can affect the scrotum or vulva	Excision provides definitive treatment
Vascular lesions	• Angiokeratoma of Fordyce, hemangioma, glomus tumor occur commonly over genitalia	When benign vascular lesions of the genitalia are asymptomatic, observation and follow-up are sufficient. Lasers may provide better cosmetic and functional results
	• Lymphangiomas	Small lesions can be treated with electrosurgery or carbon dioxide laser ablation

4. ***Management of steatocystoma multiplex***:[3] Steatocystoma multiplex is a disorder of pilosebaceous unit characterized by multiple sebum containing dermal cysts. It could be hereditary (AD) or sporadic in nature. It occurs in adolescence/early adult life over trunk, proximal extremities and scrotum.

Surgical procedures advocated (Table 36.2):

- Cryosurgery
- Aspiration
- Surgical excision
- Incision with surgical blade
- Radiocautery
- Expression of cyst contents
- Forceps associated removal of cyst wall
- Carbon dioxide laser ablation.

CIRCUMCISION

Circumcision (derived from Latin "circumcidere" - to cut around) is the excision of the preputial skin (foreskin) that covers the glans of penis. Globally around 25% of men are circumcized for religious, cultural, or medical reasons.[8]

It is found that following circumcision there is reduced risk of sexually transmitted infections (STIs), especially ulcerative diseases, such as chancroid, syphilis, HIV, it also reduces urinary tract infections in childhood, decreases inflammation of the glans (balanitis) and the foreskin (posthitis), phimosis, paraphimosis and decreases the incidence of penile cancer.

Indications

- Religious grounds among Muslims and Jews[9]
- Phimosis and paraphimosis
- Chronic inflammatory or infective conditions: Balanoposthitis, recurrent herpes genitalis
- Benign and pseudo-malignant conditions: Giant condyloma acuminata
- Premalignant and malignant lesions: Bowens, erythroplasia of Queyrat, leukoplakia, balanitis xerotica-obliterans, squamous cell carcinoma.

Requirements

Equipment and instruments required for the procedure are enlisted in Table 36.3.

Procedure[1]

- *Mark the line of circumcision (Fig. 36.1):* With the foreskin returned to a natural "resting" position, the intended line of the incision is marked with a marker pen/gentian violet corresponding with the corona.
- *Preparation of the skin*: Prepare the skin with povidone iodine antiseptic solution, starting with the glans and the shaft of the penis, and moving out to the periphery to include scrotum, adjacent areas of the thighs and suprapubic area. Retract the foreskin and clean the glans.
- *Anesthesia: Penile block (Refer above) (Fig. 36.2).*
- *Retraction of foreskin:* The foreskin should be fully retracted, if the opening of the foreskin is tight, dilate it with a pair of artery forceps. The aperture of the foreskin only must be stretched and the forceps should not be pushed in too far, because there is a risk of injury to the urethra and glans. Once the foreskin has been retracted, separate any adhesions by gentle traction or using a blunt probe, such as a pair of closed artery forceps.

Table 36.2: Various procedures for management of steatocystoma multiplex.

Procedure	*Side effects and modifications*	
Cryosurgery	Not suitable for genital lesions	Side effects: Pain, blistering, residual scarring and postinflammatory hypo/hyperpigmentation
Aspiration[4]	Simple aspiration is done with 18G needle. Not suitable for bigger and calcified cysts and have a higher rate of recurrence	Modified method: Insertion and gentle extirpation of cyst contents without removing cyst wall
Excision[5-7]	Elliptical excision can be done. Its time consuming and has risk of scarring	Modification: 1. Punch excision followed by cyst removal can be done. 2. Incision with sharp tipped cautery and expression of cyst wall contents, later forceps assisted removal of cyst wall. 3. Mini – incision with no 11 surgical blade/RF probes/phlebectomy hook followed by expression of cyst contents and exochleation of cyst wall using 1 mm curette
CO_2 laser	Preferred for multiple lesions in single treatment session and gives good cosmesis	Side effects include scarring and postinflammatory hyperpigmentation

TIPS AND TRICKS

If foreskin is lax, apply artery forceps at the 3 and 9 o'clock positions in the resting position. This helps to apply a little tension to the foreskin before marking the circumcision line.

- *Technique:* Three methods are widely used
  - The forceps guided method
  - The dorsal slit method
  - Sleeve resection method.

Method	Advantages	Disadvantages
Forceps guided method	Simple, suitable for clinical setting without a surgical assistant	Here, 0.5 and 1.0 cm of mucosal skin proximal to the corona is left behind
Dorsal slit method	Can be done in emergency situations Simple technique	Requires more surgical skill than the forceps guided method. There is a risk that more skin is cut away from one side than the other, giving an asymmetric result
Sleeve resection method	The cosmetic results are better than with the other two techniques, there is more room for surgical error, either by cutting too deep when making the two circular incisions or cutting too deep when dissecting the skin flap free	It is better suited to a hospital rather than a clinic setting, requires an assistant

Table 36.3: Equipment and instruments for circumcision.

- Instrument tray wrapped with sterile drape
- "O" drape (80 cm × 80 cm, with ~5 cm hole)
- Gallipot for antiseptic solution, i.e. povidone iodine (50 mL of 10% solution)
- Injection needles (18- or 21-gauge)

Forceps and scissors:
- Dissecting forceps (finely toothed)
- Artery forceps (2 straight, 2 curved)
- Sponge-holding forceps
- Stitch scissors
- Curved Metzenbaum's scissors
- Mayo's needle holder
- Scalpel knife handle and blades

Anesthesia:
- 15 mL of 1% plain lidocaine (without epinephrine) anesthetic solution

Dressing:
- Plain gauze swabs (10 × 10 cm; 10 for the procedure, 5 for dressing)
- Petroleum-jelly-impregnated gauze (5 × 5 cm or 5 × 10 cm) (*tulle gras*) and sticking plaster

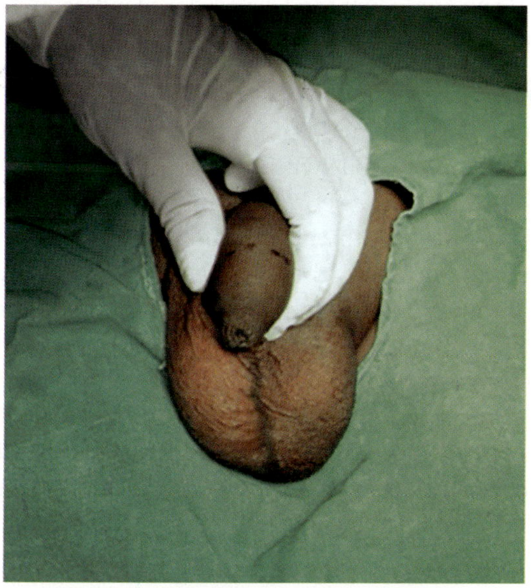

Fig. 36.1: Marking the line of circumcision.

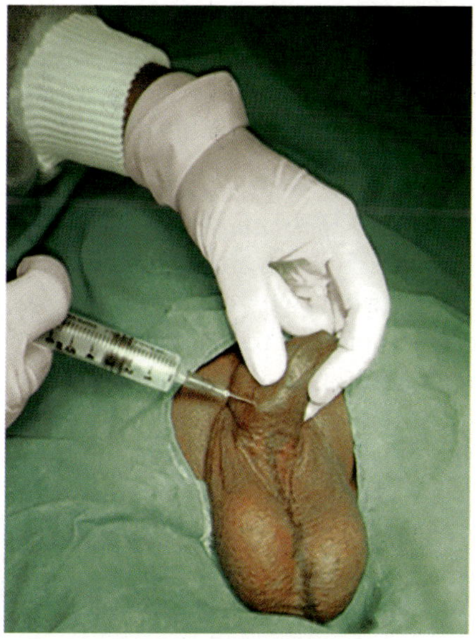

Fig. 36.2: Penile block.

Forceps-guided method: The foreskin is grasped at the 3 o'clock and 9 o'clock positions with two artery forceps (Fig. 36.3). Place both these forceps on the apex of foreskin, in such a way as to put equal tension on inside and outside surfaces of the foreskin. Pull the previously made mark to just beyond the glans by putting sufficient tension on the foreskin. Then apply a long straight forceps across the foreskin, just proximal to the mark, with the long axis of the forceps going from the 6 o'clock to the 12 o'clock position (taking the frenulum as the 6 o'clock position). After the forceps is in position, feel the glans all around to check that it has not been accidentally caught in the forceps. Now, using a scalpel, cut away the foreskin flush along the outer aspect of the forceps. Pull back the skin to expose the raw area.

For maintaining hemostasis: Clip any bleeding vessels with artery forceps. Tie each vessel or under-run with a suture and tie off taking care not to injure urethra and not to place deep hemostatic sutures. Place a horizontal mattress suture at the frenulum. When placing the frenulum suture, take care to align the midline skin raphe with the line of the frenulum. Place a vertical mattress suture opposite the frenulum, in the 12 o'clock position. The suture should be placed so that there is an equal amount of skin on each side of the penis between the 12 and 6 o'clock positions. Place two further vertical mattress stitches in the 3 o'clock and 9 o'clock positions. It is helpful to leave a long end of the horizontal mattress suture at the frenulum (at 6 o'clock position) and on the vertical mattress suture placed opposite (at 12 o'clock position). The long ends of these sutures can be held by an assistant with artery forceps to stabilize the penis during suturing. After placement of sutures at 6, 12, 3 and 9 o'clock positions, place two or more simple sutures in the gaps between each of them. Once the procedure is finished, check for bleeding. If there is none, apply a dressing.

Dorsal slit method of circumcision:

- Grasp the foreskin with artery forceps at 3 o'clock and 9 o'clock positions with equal tension on inner and outer aspects of the foreskin. Place two artery forceps on the foreskin at 11 o'clock and 1 o'clock positions. Check that the inside blades of the two artery forceps are lying between the glans and foreskin, and have not been inadvertently passed up the urethral meatus.
- Between the two artery forceps, at the 12 o'clock position, use a dissection scissors to make a cut (the dorsal slit) up to but not beyond the previously marked incision line.

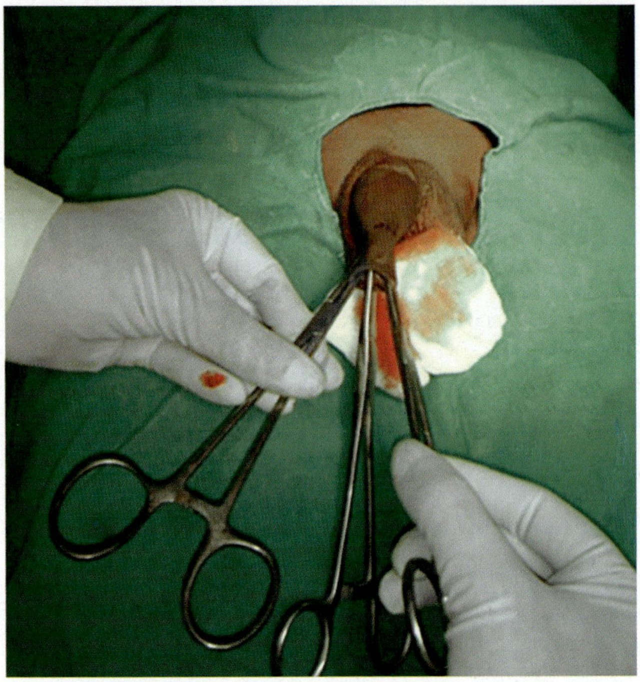

Fig. 36.3: Grasping of foreskin by multiple forceps.

- Using dissection scissors, cut the foreskin free, following the previously marked circumcision line.
- Any skin tags on inner edge of foreskin can be trimmed to leave approximately 5 mm of skin proximal to corona. Care must be taken to trim only the skin and not to cut deeper tissue.
- Achieve hemostasis and suture, as described in the forceps-guided method. Check for bleeding. If there is none, apply a dressing.

Sleeve resection method of circumcision:

- Mark the intended outer line of incision, with a V shape, on the underside (ventral aspect) of penis and pointed toward the frenulum. The apex of V should correspond with the midline raphe. Retract the foreskin and mark the inner (mucosal) incision line, 1–2 mm proximal to the corona. At the frenulum, the incision line should cross horizontally.
- Using a scalpel, make further incisions along these marked lines, taking care to cut through skin till the subcutaneous tissue but not deeper. As the incision is made, an assistant should retract the skin with a moist gauze swab. Any bleeding vessels should be clipped with an artery forceps and hemostasis should be achieved by tying or securing with an under-running suture.

- Then cut the skin between the distal and proximal incisions with scissors.
- Now hold the sleeve of foreskin under tension with two artery forceps, and dissect the skin from the shaft of penis, using dissection scissors.
- Tie off any bleeding vessels with under-running sutures. Stop any bleeding and achieve hemostasis with suturing, as described in steps 7–10 of the forceps-guided method. Once the wound has been sutured, check for bleeding. If there is none, apply a dressing.

Dressing: A standard penile dressing technique is used. Check that there is no bleeding. Place a piece of gauze impregnated with petroleum-jelly around the wound. Then, place a sterile dry gauze overthis, and secure them in position with an adhesive tape, but not too tightly as it could restrict blood supply and cause necrosis of the glans. This dressing should be left in position for 48 hours. It is important not to disrupt the wound healing by pulling at a dressing that has dried and stuck to the wound, rather dab with antiseptic solution until it softens and then remove.

Variations in Technique[1]

Phimosis

Phimosis is the scarring of the aperture of foreskin to such an extent that the foreskin cannot be retracted. Often the tip of foreskin will appear white because of the scar tissue. If the scar tissue is extensive, then a clinic-based circumcision is not preferred. The first step is to mark the foreskin with the line of incision. If the sleeve resection method is used, the phimosis will prevent retraction of foreskin and line of incision near the corona cannot be marked. In such a case, a small dorsal slit should be made, that is just long enough to allow the foreskin to be retracted. Once retracted, any adhesions must be divided and any debris under the foreskin needs to be cleaned with a swab soaked in cetrimide or povidone iodine. Once all adhesions have been divided, the second line of incision on the foreskin near the corona has to be marked and the circumcision operation can proceed as usual.

In either of the forceps-guided or dorsal slit methods, line of incision is marked on outer aspect of foreskin in the normal manner. However, with minor degrees of phimosis, it will be necessary to make a small dorsal slit to allow full retraction and cleaning under the foreskin before proceeding with the operation. The forceps-guided method should not be used, if there is evidence of extensive scarring.

Tight or Scarred Frenulum

All males have a band of tissue (the frenulum) on ventral side of penis, just below the glans. Usually, frenulum does not interfere with retraction of foreskin. During early sexual experiences, the frenulum may be stretched as the foreskin is retracted, and minor tears are a frequent problem. Such tears can heal, leaving in elastic scar tissue, which tightens and makes further tearing and scarring more likely. This problem can be noted when the foreskin is retracted during physical examination, instead of the normal pink frenulum, a tight band of white tissue will be evident. This restrictive frenular band can be easily corrected during circumcision. Foreskin is spread open and retracted ventrally to put the frenular band under tension. Using dissection scissors, snip this band at its center, taking care not to injure the urethra (which is just under the frenulum). Any bleeding from the frenular artery should be controlled by careful tying or under-running. After the frenulum has been cut, there will be an inverted V-shaped defect.

The circumcision can then be performed as usual. In this case, however, do not suture the penile skin up to the edge of the foreskin defect, since this will cause increased tension on the ventral side. This tension may cause curvature of the penis or possibly make erection or coitus uncomfortable. Instead, close the V-shaped defect by placing the frenular suture 1–2 cm (depending on age and penis size) back from the apex of the V, taking both sides of the defect. The V incision is thus converted into an inverted T. Suture the rest of the skin as in a normal circumcision procedure.

Postoperative monitoring:

- Monitor the patient for at least 30 minutes after surgery.
- Advise that he should avoid masturbation and sexual intercourse for 4–6 weeks after the procedure, so as to allow the wound to heal.
- A condom should be used to protect the surgical wound during every act of sexual intercourse for at least the next six months. Thereafter condoms should always be used to prevent sexually transmitted infections, HIV or unwanted pregnancy.
- The dressing applied during surgery should be removed 24–48 hours later, provided that there is no bleeding or

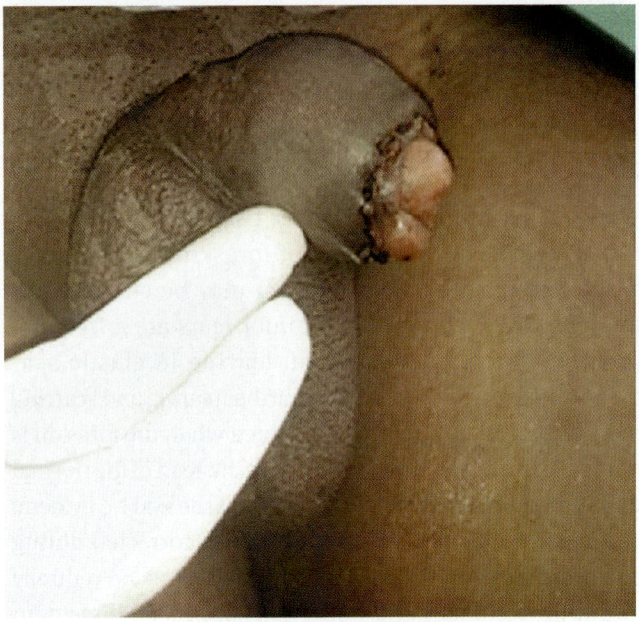

Fig. 36.4: Removal of dressing.

oozing (Fig. 36.4). If there is any oozing or bleeding, then a new dressing may be applied for a further 24–48 hours, and then checked again. Once the bleeding has stopped, no further dressing is necessary but the patient should be instructed to wear freshly laundered, loose-fitting underwear. Underwear should be changed each day. After the dressing has been removed, patient can take bath and should gently wash the genital area with mild soap (baby soap) and water.

Complications[10,11]

Early Complications

- Pain
- Bleeding

Bleeding from the frenular artery: If there is excessive bleeding from the frenular artery, an under-running hemostatic stitch should be used to occlude the artery. Urethra is near to the surface skin and care should be taken as it can be easily damaged.

- Hematomas are best left alone, unless they are very large or there is continuous bleeding.
- Wound dehiscence is unusual in the first few days, but if the disruption occurs within 48 hours of the operation, explore and resuture; otherwise depending on the skin edges, it can be left alone to heal by secondary intention.
- Infection: Occurs after 2–3 days, appropriate antibiotic is given.
- Fournier's gangrene.

Late Complications

Decreased/over sensitivity of the glans; unsightly circumcision wounds, ragged scars, persistent adhesions at the corona and inclusion cysts can occur. Discomfort during erection from scrotal skin being pulled up the shaft of penis and a tight scrotal sac can result from removal of too much skin during circumcision. These problems can be avoided with careful preoperative marking of incision lines. Torsion (misalignment) of skin of penile shaft can be avoided by taking care during the operation to align the midline raphe with the frenulum.

Circumcision in Infants[12]

Here devices such as the Gomco clamp, Plastibell (Hollister plastibell), and Mogen clamp are commonly used. The amount of foreskin to be removed is estimated. The foreskin is opened via the preputial orifice to reveal the glans underneath and ensure it is normal. The inner lining of foreskin (preputial epithelium) is bluntly separated from its attachment to glans. The device is placed and it remains there until blood flow has stopped. Finally, the foreskin is removed.

FRENULECTOMY/FRENULOPLASTY[13,14]

Frenulectomy is a surgical procedure for cutting and removal of the frenulum of the prepuce of the penis. It is simple office procedure which can avoid circumcision in short frenulum.

Indications

Frenulum breve (short frenulum): It prevents the full retraction of the foreskin with and without an erection.

Procedure

- Procedure is carried out under local anesthesia with prior consent and counseling. Subcutaneous or ring block anesthesia, circumferentially at the base of the penis is given.
- Prepuce is retracted and normal saline is injected on either side of the median raphe at the base of the frenulum (Ballooning).

- Two small mosquito forceps are applied along median raphe on either side of the frenulum and a two point traction is applied on either side.
- An incision is made on the frenulum, then it is stretched to lengthen the frenulum and stitch closed. Incision can be Z shaped, Y shaped or a single horizontal cut. When transverse incision is made on the stretched frenulum, a diamond slit is formed which stretches longitudinally with its long axis along ventral median raphe due to traction.
- The frenular mucosal surfaces are opposed longitudinally along direction of ventral raphe with interrupted sutures (plain catgut 3-0).
- After hemostasis is achieved, antibiotic ointment is applied over suture and prepuce pulled over back to its position.
- Postoperatively oral and topical antibiotics and analgesics are prescribed for 7 days.
- Once healed, it effectively elongates the frenulum, allowing normal function.

TIPS AND TRICKS

Transverse incisions can be extended downwards depending on lengthening to be achieved. These stitches in the frenulum are generally more painful, but heal faster. And usually no dressing is required.

PREPUTIOPLASTY[14]

Preputioplasty or prepuce plasty also known as "limited dorsal slit with transverse closure", is performed to widen a narrow nonretractile foreskin which cannot comfortably be drawn back off the head of penis in erection because of a stenosis which either has not relaxed during the childhood and adolescence or has narrowed after sexual maturity. It is advantageous over circumcision as it is a conservative, nontraumatic and less invasive procedure and can be performed on an outpatient department under local anesthesia, and also the healing is quicker with good cosmesis.

Indications

Phimosis

Procedure: It may be performed by Y plasty or Z plasty and also by techniques used in plastic surgery to loosen constricting scar tissue following traumatic scars. It comprises of one or more very short longitudinal incisions, which release the stenosis: the constricting ring of tissue in foreskin is closed transversely. If incisions are placed on the sides of phimotic ring, cosmesis is better. It is also recommended to undermine the subcutaneous tissue to ensure better cosmetic result.

The opening will be wide enough for foreskin to be easily retracted. It is also slightly shorter (by half the length of the longitudinal incisions which are now closed transversely) as the widening of the phimotic ring takes up some foreskin.

Dorsal Slitting

This is a simple procedure and indicated as an emergency in phagedena or phimosis with growth or ulcerative lesion in the preputial sacs, which needs proper visualization for the purpose of biopsy and treatment. In phagedena there is phimosis and impending gangrenous balanoposthitis.[14]

Procedure

- A ring block is given at the base of the penis.
- The preputial sac is stretched by applying traction along the free margin of the prepuce at 3 o'clock and 6 o'clock with artery forceps—two point traction.
- The swollen preputial sac is then slit in the mid dorsal line creating two small flaps from the free preputial edge up to but immediately distal to the base of the glans. In phagedena, there is an immediate letting off of the accumulated purulent discharge.
- The mucosa of individual flap is sutured with interrupted plain 3-0 catgut after thorough cleaning of glans and inner lining of the preputial sac.
- Antibiotics and analgesics are prescribed post procedure.
- Post operatively once edema and inflammation subsides, and skin returns to normal, the preputial sac is then examined for any growth, ulcers which are treatment. After necessary treatment or investigation, this is followed by circumcision.

Management of Paraphimosis[14]

Paraphimosis occurs as a result of a tight prepuce which is forcibly retracted behind the corona and remains there as a constricting ring. The inner layer of the prepuce forms an edematous collar, which prevents pulling down of the prepuce over the glans. Immediate treatment is to be done as this is an emergency situation, by either manipulative or operative reduction to prevent gangrene and sloughing. Circumcision may be performed at a later date to prevent recurrence.

Manipulative Reduction:

- Consent, premedication with analgesics and anti-inflammatory drugs.
- Constriction prepuce is drawn further up toward base of the penis as far as possible.
- Swollen mucosa along with distal shaft and glans is gently squeezed for 3–5 minutes.
- Surgical lubrication jelly is the applied around the constricting ring and over the distal end.
- Gradual upward traction with minimum force is applied to the retracted preputial skin.
- The prepuce is gradually reduced and slipped over the glans.

Operative Reduction:

- Circumferential ring block at base of the penis to be given first.
- A longitudinal incision is made on the dorsal aspect of the constricting ring, which causes reduction of swelling and prepuce which can be drawn over the glans.
- Incise wound heals gradually by secondary intention.
- Postoperatively antibiotics, analgesics, anti-inflammatory drugs are prescribed for 5–7 days.

LOCAL SKIN FLAPS FOR PENILE/ GENITAL SKIN LOSS[15]

Penile skin loss can be surgically managed by skin grafting. Full-thickness skin grafts (FTSG) provide superior results to their split thickness counterpart since they heal with less contractures, they maintain elasticity of skin better and therefore preserve the physiological girth and length expansion during erection. Split-thickness skin graft is used in numerous reports successfully, but the tight scarring and consequent contracture of the skin graft may restrict the filling of the corpus spongiosa.

A scrotal fascio-myocutaneous flap for the management of a large or circumferential penile skin loss can also be used.[16] The skin of scrotum is soft, thin, and extensible, and due to the multiorigin blood supply system to this skin, ischemic necrosis seldom occurs. The membranous superficial fascia has no adipose layer. The feeding arteries of a scrotal flap course in the Dartos fascia of scrotum. This makes the scrotal flap an axial fascio-myo-cutaneous flap. Compared with a skin graft, this flap provides better skin laxity for erection and durability for sexual intercourse, along with superior skin color match. As a single stage procedure, general or spinal anesthesia with antibiotic prophylaxis is given. Debridement of necrotic tissue is done initially, followed by the separation of suspensory ligament at the root of penis to counteract the wound contraction. Scrotal myocutaneous flap is designed to match the size of defect. The flap pedicle width can range between 2.5 and 4 cm at the neck of scrotum while flap length can vary between 8 and 12 cm. The flap should include the Dartos myo-fascial layer but not the tunica vaginalis. The donor site is closed primarily. From the 2nd day on, 5 mg diazepam is given 30 minutes before sleep for 5 days to reduce painful nocturnal erections. Patient can be advised to do laser hair ablation of their new penile skin if hair growth occurs.

FEMALE GENITALIA SURGERIES

Vaginoplasty

In vaginoplasty, portions of mucosa is excised from the vaginal fornices by scalpel, needle or RF electrode, scissors, or laser. It consists of an anterior colporrhaphy, high posterior colporrhaphy, excision of lateral vaginal mucosa, or a combination of the above, which tightens the upper vagina.

Vulvo-vaginal rejuvenation and vaginal skin tightening: Various noninvasive and invasive procedures are available for vaginal tightening. The noninvasive methods are Kegel exercises, hormonal creams and sprays. But these have to be used for longer duration to see any visible effects which may not be long lasting once the treatment is stopped. Though surgical vaginoplasties offer better and long lasting results, the risk of operating in this sensitive area outweighs the benefit. Ablative lasers such as fractionalCO_2 (10600 nm) and the Er:YAG (2940 nm) are nonreconstructive methods aimed at restoring the muscle tone of the vagina by tightening the supportive structures of the vulvovaginal complex.[17] Transcutaneous temperature-controlled radiofrequency therapy at the vulvovaginal region is another modality, which has shown promising results in restoration of vaginal elasticity and tightness.[18]

CONCLUSION

The decision of surgical management in genital area should be finalized only after a complete evaluation of the presenting dermatological condition and then validate need for surgery. It is essential to understand the anatomical considerations during genital surgeries and then plan the procedures accordingly with better therapeutic outcome and also cosmesis.

REFERENCES

1. Manual for male circumcision under local anaesthesia: WHO manual Version 3.1(Dec 09). (http://www.who.int/hiv/mediacentre/news68/en/index.html).
2. Rochelle T. The genitalia. In: Roegnik's Dermatologic Surgery: Current Techniques in Procedural Dermatology, 3rd edition. New York: Informa; 2007. pp. 289-97.
3. Sanjiv C, Sankha K, Atul S. A modified surgical technique for steatocystoma multiplex. J Cutan Aesthetic. Surg. 2010;3(1): 25-8.
4. Sato K, Shibuya K, Taguchi H. Aspiration therapy in steatocystoma multiplex. Arch Dermatol. 1993;129:35-7.
5. Schmook T, Burg G, Hafner J. Surgical pearl: mini incisions for the extraction of steatocystoma multiplex. J Am AcadDermatol. 2001;44:1041-2.
6. Kaya TI, Ikizoglu G, Kokturk A, et al. A simple surgical technique for the treatment of steatocystoma multiplex. Int J Dermatol. 2001;40:785-8.
7. Lee SJ, Choe YS, Park BC, et al. The vein hook successfully used for eradication of steatocystoma multiplex. Dermatol Surg. 2008;33:82-4.
8. Moses S, Bailey RC, Ronald AR. Male circumcision: assessment of health benefits and risks. Sex Transm Inf. 1998;74:368-73.
9. Rizvi SA, Naqvi SA, Hussain M. Religious circumcision: a Muslim view. BJU Int. 1999;83:13-6.
10. Kaplan GW. Complications of circumcision. Urol Clin North Am. 1983;10(3)543-9.
11. Williams N, Kapila L. Complications of circumcision. Br J Surg. 1993;80:1231-6.
12. Fowler C. The urethra and penis. In: Williams NS, Bulstrode CJK, O'Connell PR (Eds). Bailey and Love's Short Practice of Surgery, 25th edition. London: Edward Arnold Publishers; 2008. pp. 1371-3.
13. Brown JS. Miscellaneous minor surgical procedures. In: Brown JS, Das S (Eds). Minor Surgery. Calcutta; 1988. pp. 191-8.
14. Satish S Savant. Dermatosurgery for male genitalia. In: Satish Savant S (Ed). Textbook of Dermatosurgery and Cosmetology, 2nd edition. Mumbai: ASCAD 2011. p. 280.
15. Cosmetic and plastic penile surgery. In: Daniel Yachia (Ed). Text Atlas of Penile Surgery. UK: Informa Healthcare; 2007. pp. 203-18.
16. Tolba AM, Azab AA, Nasr AM, et al. Dartos fascio-myo-cutaneous flap for penile skin loss: A simple flap with an immense potential. Surgical Science. 2014;5:6-9.
17. Lee MS. Treatment of vaginal relaxation syndrome with an erbium: YAG laser using 90° and 360° scanning scopes: a pilot study & short-term results. Laser Ther. 2014;23(2): 129-38.
18. Magon N, Alison R. Thermi Va. The revolutionary technology for vulvovaginal rejuvenation and noninvasive management of female SUI. J Obster Gynaecol. 2016;66(4):300-2.

CHAPTER 37

Moh's Micrographic Surgery

Vandana Chatrath

INTRODUCTION

Moh's micrographic surgery is a specialized surgical procedure developed in circa 1930 to primarily treat nonmelanoma skin cancers like basal cell carcinoma and squamous cell carcinoma. The procedure involves resection of the tumor in a staged manner followed by evaluation of the resected materials as frozen sections until complete clearance of the tumor is achieved. The technique over the years has evolved and is now being used to treat many other cutaneous malignancies besides nonmelanoma skin cancer. The uniqueness of Moh's surgery lies in the fact that the technique allows most effective removal of tumor with maximum tissue sparing.

HISTORY

Moh's surgery, as the name suggests, was first developed by Dr. Frederic Moh's in 1938.[1] His original technique involved the use of 20% zinc chloride paste as a fixative and was at that time known as Moh's chemosurgery. This was modified in 1953 by Dr. Moh's himself where in the fixative was abandoned and fresh frozen sections were used making it an even simpler, less time consuming yet effective surgical technique.[2] Although the methodology over the ensuing years has undergone technological advancements like the use of confocal microscopy and dermoscopy to assist the standard surgical procedure, frozen sectioning and evaluation remain the 'gold standard' for the treatment of nonmelanoma skin cancers.[3]

INDICATIONS

A wide variety of cutaneous malignancies are now being treated with Moh's micrographic surgery.[4,5] These include:

- Basal cell carcinoma:
  - With poorly defined clinical margins
  - High risk sites on the face (central face, eyelids, eyebrows, periorbital area, nose, lips, chin, mandible, temple, ears and pre- and postauricular areas)
  - Aggressive histopathological types (morpheaform, infiltrative, micronodular, basosquamous)
  - Perineural/perivascular/periappendageal invasion
  - Recurrence
  - Arising on previously irradiated skin
  - Over areas requiring tissue conservation like face and genitals.
- Squamous cell carcinoma:
  - Mucocutaneous lesions
  - Recurrence
  - Tumor in high risk areas
  - Aggressive histopathological types
  - Perineural invasion.
- Malignant melanoma in situ (lentigo maligna)
- Large keratoacanthoma
- Extra-mammary Paget's disease
- Appendageal tumors like:
  - Dermatofibrosarcoma protuberans
  - Sebaceous cell carcinoma
  - Malignant fibrohistiocytoma
  - Atypical fibroxanthoma.
- Merkel cell carcinoma
- All cutaneous malignancies >1 cm on the face and >2 cm on the trunk and extremities.[6]

Moh's micrographic surgery can be used for treatment of any malignancy that fulfils two criteria:

- Tumors in locations that require sparing of adjacent tissue
- Tumors with high recurrence rate.

TECHNIQUE

Once a lesion is suspected to be malignant on clinical examination, the diagnosis has to be confirmed histopathologically with a biopsy. The histopathological features and the type of malignancy determine the treatment of choice. If Moh's micrographic surgery is to be undertaken, the procedure should be discussed with the patient in detail and the consent obtained.

- The site of residual tumor is identified and cleaned with alcohol (Fig. 37.1). It is then delineated with a skin marking pen keeping a margin of 1–2 mm of normal skin around the tumor (Fig. 37.2).
- Local anesthesia is then administered (1% lidocaine with epinephrine except in sites with end arteries like the nose and digits).
- The lesion is then debulked with a curette to give an idea of the horizontal and vertical extent of tumor (Fig. 37.2).
- Using a blade holder with no. 15 blade the first layer of tissue is excised keeping the blade at a 45° angle to produce a saucer-shaped specimen with beveled edges to allow proper placement of the tissue on the cryostat for proper sectioning (Figs. 37.3 and 37.4).
- For optimal orientation of the tissue hash marks are made with the blade both on the tissue being excised and the surrounding skin in accordance with clock positions (12 o'clock double hash and 6 o'clock single hash) (Fig. 37.5).
- The tissue with the hash marks is placed on a piece of paper (Fig. 37.6). A paper drawing of the specimen is made keeping the orientation in mind. The residual defect called the Moh's defect is then cauterized to obtain hemostasis and covered with a temporary dressing (Fig. 37.7).

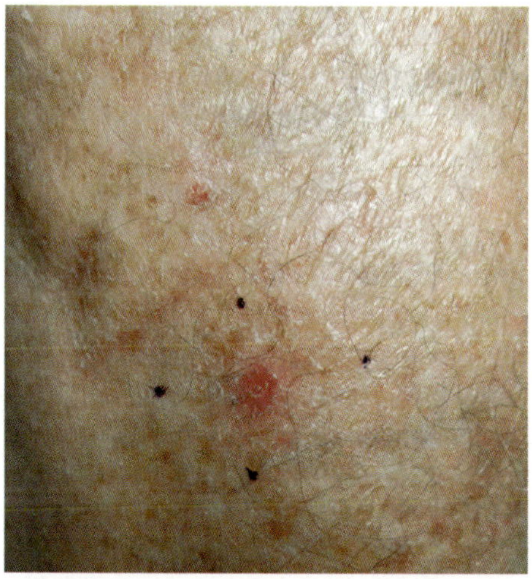

Fig. 37.1: Site of residual tumor postbiopsy.

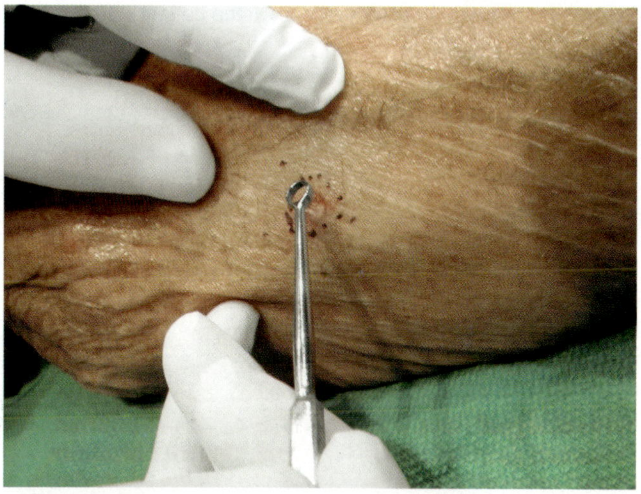

Fig. 37.2: Site marked and lesion being curetted to know extent of tumor.

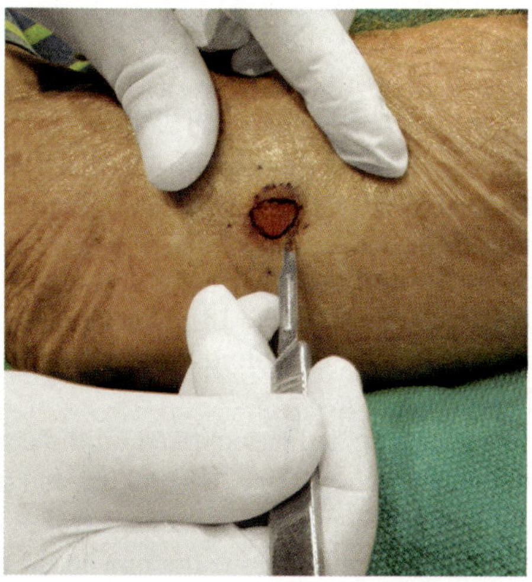

Fig. 37.3: Tissue being resected using a no.15 blade held at a 45° angle.

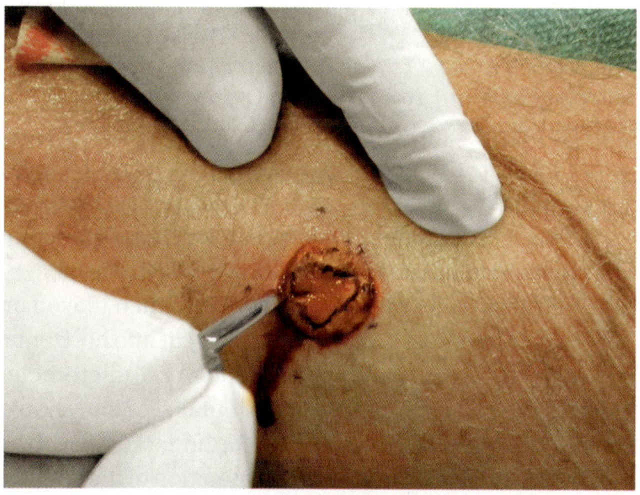

Fig. 37.4: The tissue is excised in the shape of a saucer with epidermis all around.

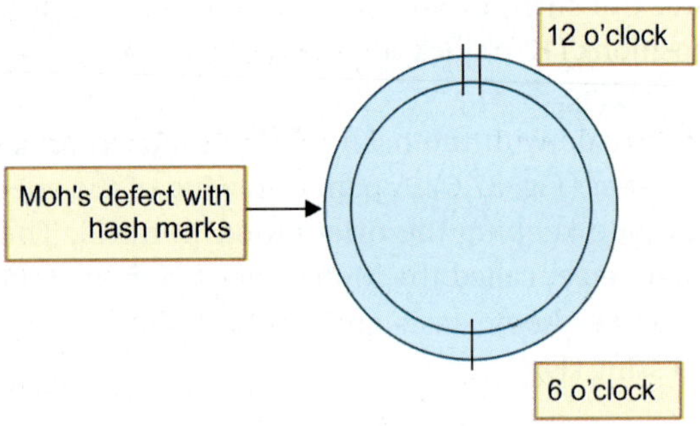

Fig. 37.5: Drawing of the specimen on the paper for proper orientation with respect to the patient.

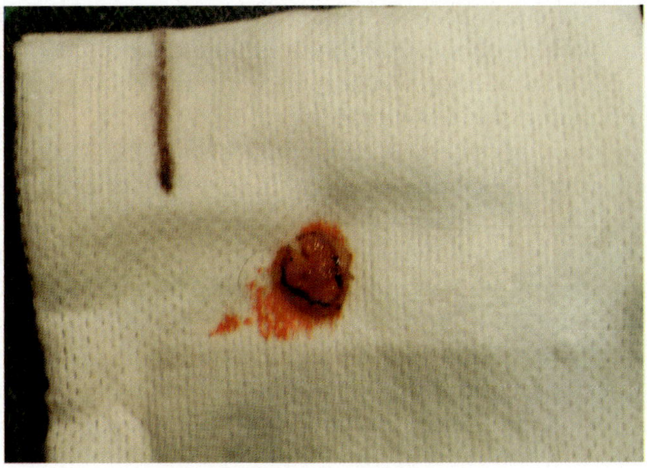

Fig. 37.6: The excised tissue with hash mark at 12 o'clock position for orientation.

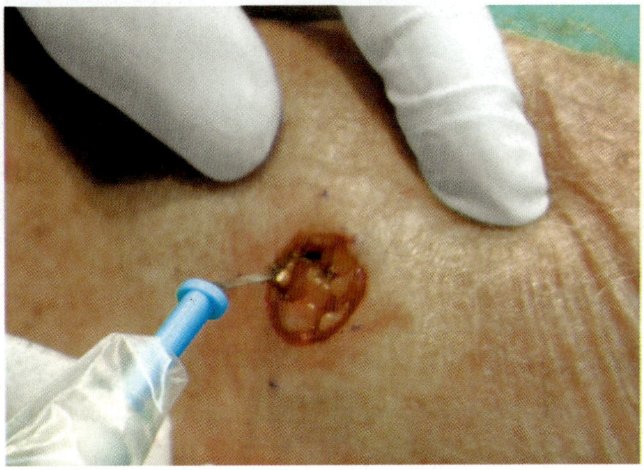

Fig. 37.7: The Moh's defect is cauterized for hemostasis.

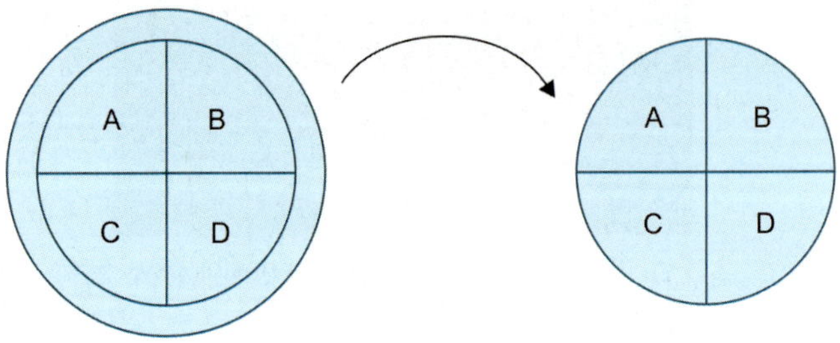

Fig. 37.8: The resected tissue is inked and cut into sections small enough to fit onto glass slides.

- The resected tissue is divided into quadrants or sections small enough for each section/quadrant to fit onto the glass slide (Fig. 37.8). Each of these sections/quadrants are inked with different colored dyes and the corresponding colors marked on the paper for proper orientation (Figs. 37.9 and 37.10).
- Each section is flattened, inverted and then placed on the cryostat (Figs. 37.11 to 37.14) to be cut into horizontal sections with an average thickness of 5 micrometer (Fig. 37.15). Each of these horizontal sections should include the epidermis as well as the under surface of the tissue. This allows complete examination of the surgical margins offering a distinct advantage over the 'bread-loafing' method used to section the paraffin-embedded tissue in routine histopathology (Fig. 37.16).
- These thin sections are carefully transferred onto the glass slide (Fig. 37.17) that are then stained with hematoxylin and eosin either manually or with an automated stainer (Fig. 37.18), The slide is now ready to be viewed under the microscope for the presence of residual tumor (Fig. 37.19).
- If a tumor is identified it is marked on the corresponding section of the paper drawing and handed over to the surgeon. The surgeon then goes back to the patient to excise a second layer of tissue but only in the quadrant/section that showed residual tumor in the frozen section.

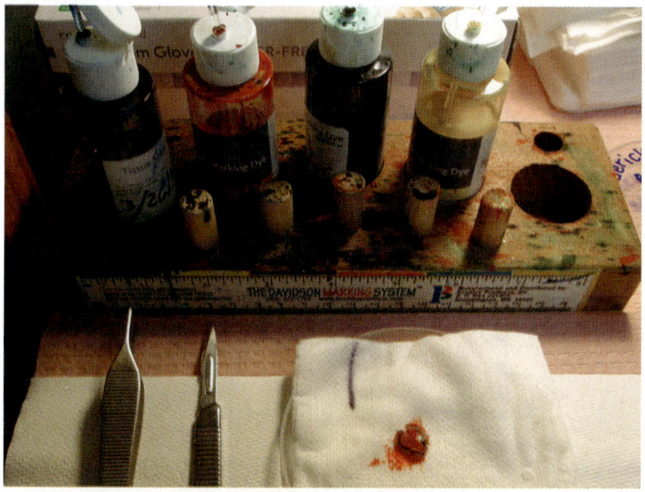

Fig. 37.9: The specimen is being prepared for cutting into sections and inking.

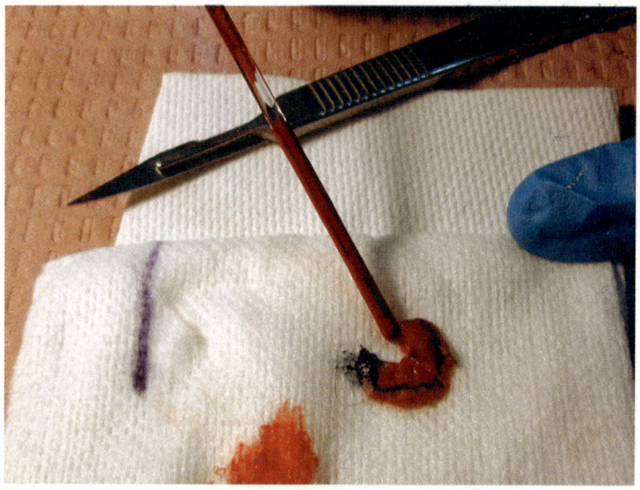

Fig. 37.10: The specimen is cut and the margins inked with different colored ink.

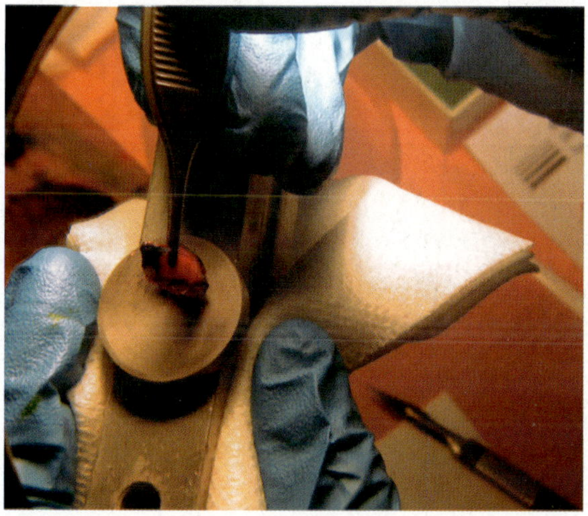

Fig. 37.11: The specimen is being placed on the cryostat to cut horizontal sections.

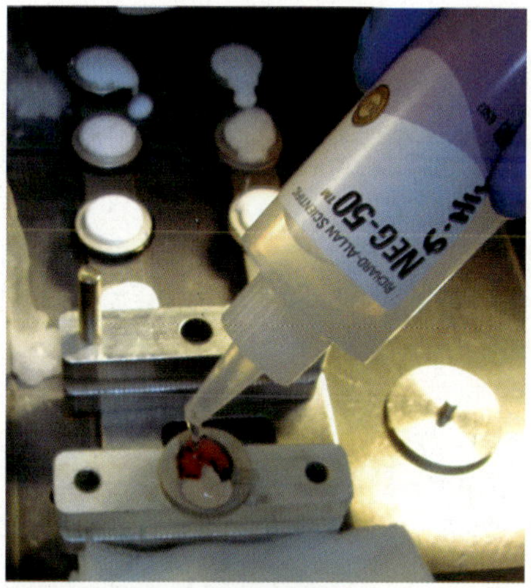

Fig. 37.12: Tissue being immersed in the compound to prepare the frozen section.

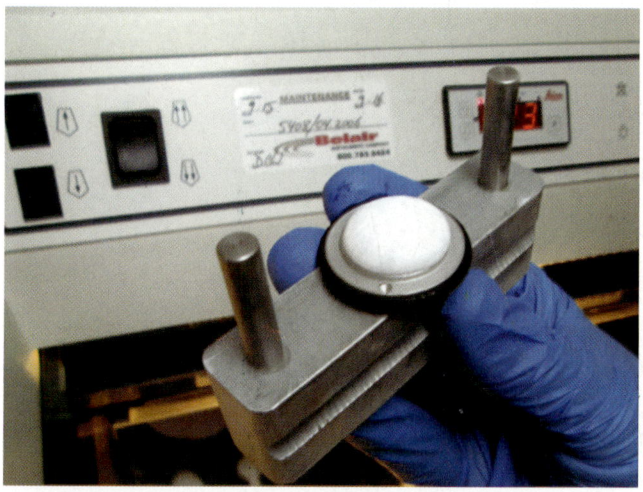

Fig. 37.13: Frozen section being placed on the cryostat for horizontal sectioning.

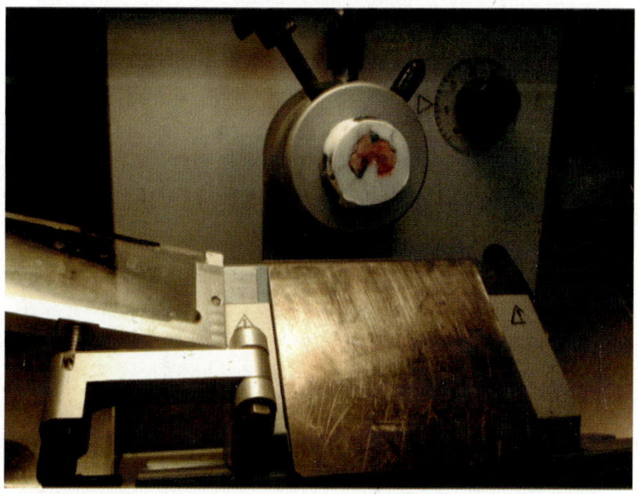

Fig. 37.14: Frozen tissue of which sections are being taken.

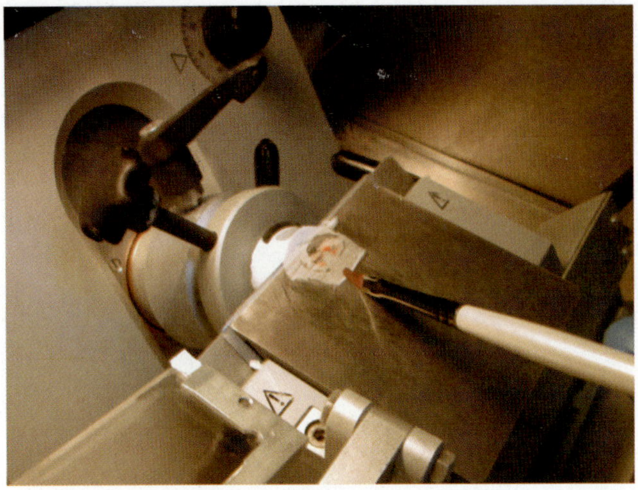

Fig. 37.15: Percentage micrometer thick horizontal sections are obtained.

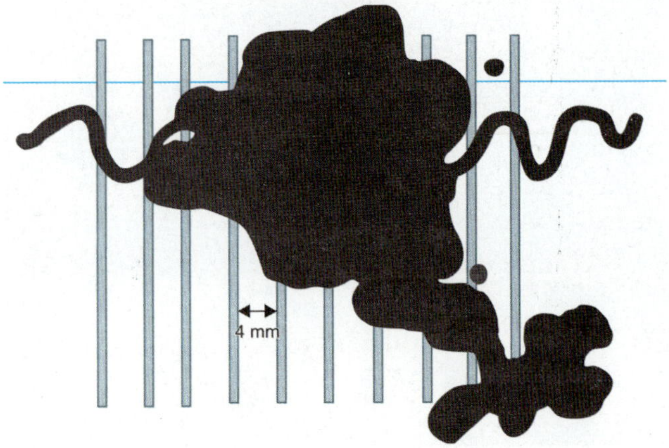

Fig. 37.16: The tumour (black) can be missed when 'bread loafing' technique is used to section the resected tissue at 4 mm intervals giving false-negative results.

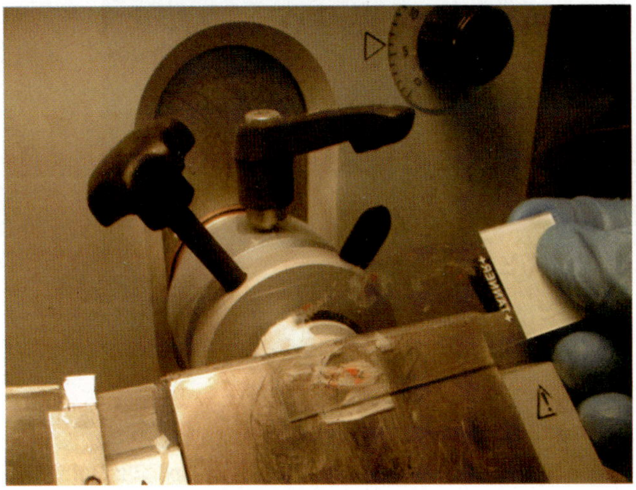

Fig. 37.17: Horizontal frozen sections being transferred carefully onto a glass slide.

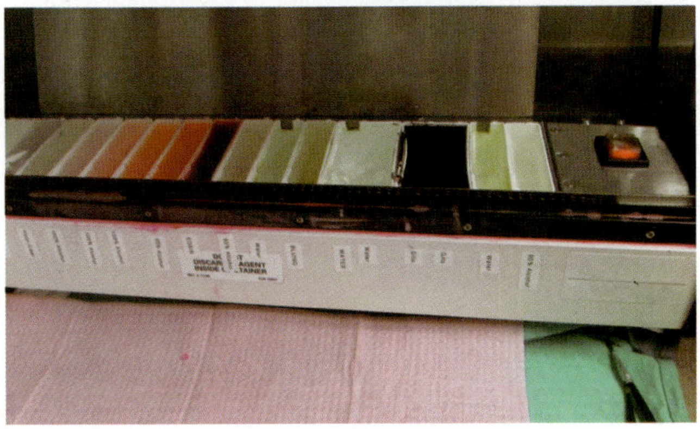

Fig. 37.18: Staining of the glass slides with an automated stainer after horizontal sections have been placed on them.

- This process is repeated until 100% clearance of both the peripheral and deep margins is achieved.

TISSUE RECONSTRUCTION

Depending on the size of the resultant Moh's defect one of the following methods of reconstruction are chosen.

- Healing by secondary intention
- Simple primary closure
- Flaps
- Grafts

The factors influencing the final choice of repair are:

- Site of the defect
- Laxity of the surrounding tissue
- Morbidity involved in repair

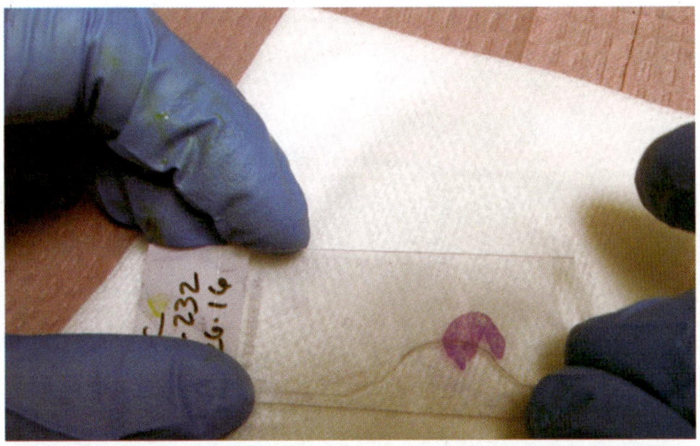

Fig. 37.19: Hematoxylin and eosin stained frozen section slide ready to be evaluated for residual tumor.

- Cosmetic units involved
- Esthetically superior scar.

Healing by Secondary Intention

This method is chosen, if the Moh's defect is small and is overlying a concave surface with enough surrounding tissue mobility, such as concha of the ear, medial canthus, alar groove and postauricular area.

Primary Closure

This type of repair mimics that of a simple linear closure where in the circular Moh's defect of made into an ellipse (width to length ratio 1:3) to allow a linear scar without any 'dog ears'. The ellipse is oriented along the natural skin tension lines to achieve an esthetic surgical scar. One must be mindful of the cosmetic units and avoid their distortion at any cost (examples include eyelid, lip etc.). Lastly, the surgeon should ensure that there is not too much tension on the sutures to ensure fast and adequate healing (Fig. 37.20).

Flaps

A flap is the movement of surrounding skin with its vascular supply over the surgical defect. Flaps can be of the following types:

- Rotational
- Advancement (Figs. 37.21 to 37.23).
- Transposition.

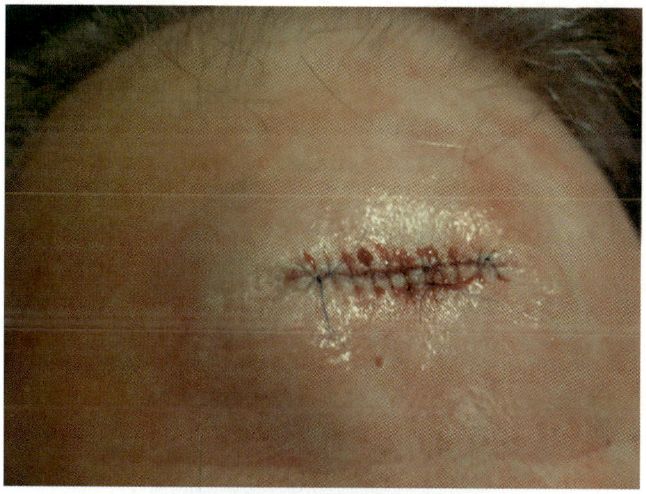

Fig. 37.20: Complex linear closure of the Moh's defect.

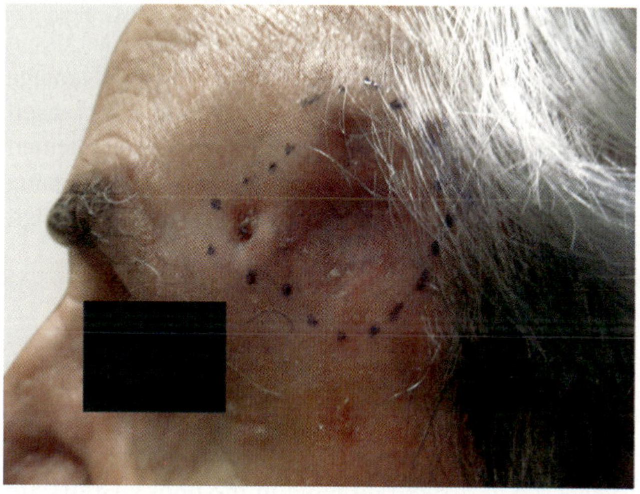

Fig. 37.21: Large basal cell carcinoma (biopsy proven) on the temple.

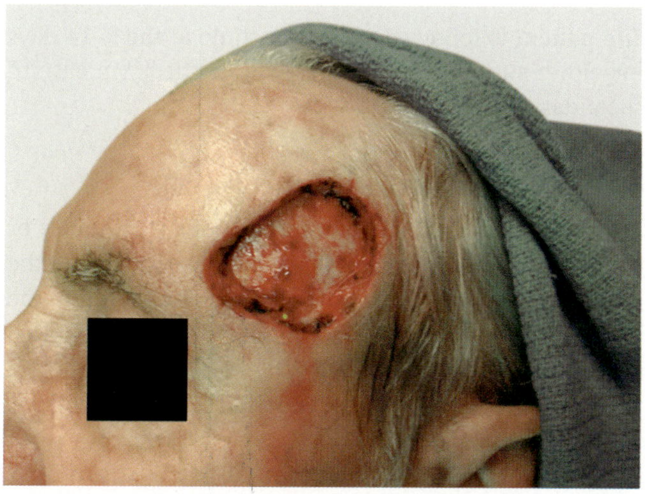

Fig. 37.22: Removal of the tumor with Moh's micrographic surgery.

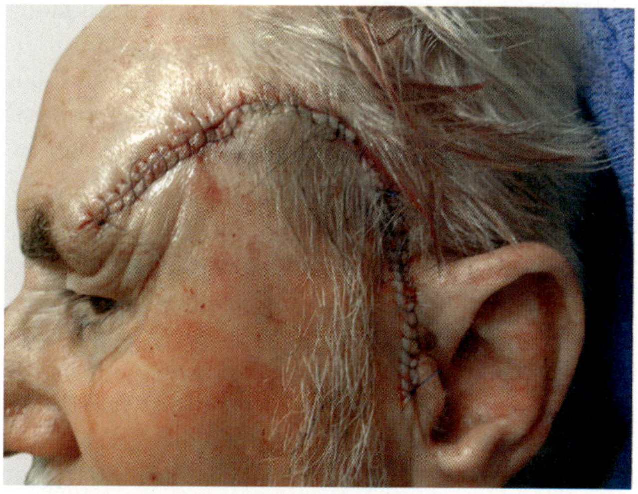

Fig. 37.23: Repair of the Moh's defect with an advancement flap (repair of choice due to the availability and laxity of the neighboring tissue).

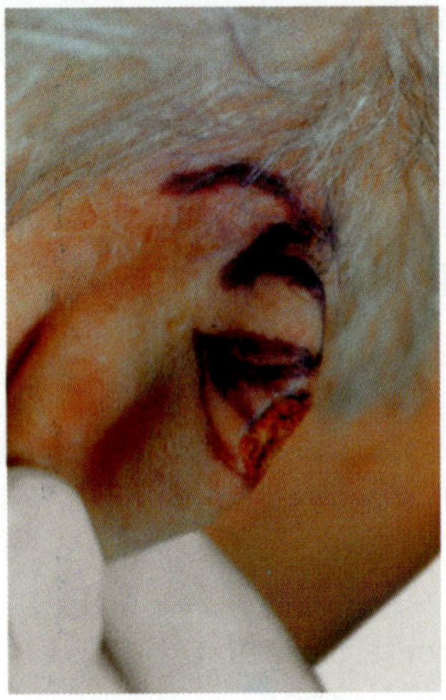

Fig. 37.24: Planning a bilobed flap for repair of Moh's defect on the rim of the ear.

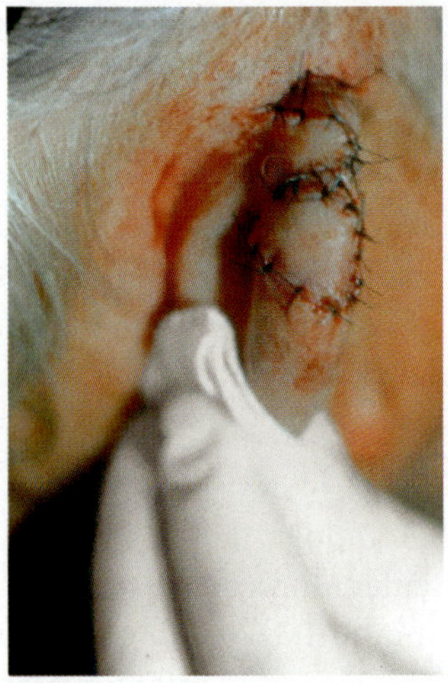

Fig. 37.25: Well-executed bilobed flap with no tension on the sutures.

Flaps have the advantage of providing an exact tissue match when compared to grafts but have the disadvantage of requiring greater skill of the surgeon and increased morbidity and longer healing time. If flaps are not planned and executed correctly, they have the risk of undergoing necrosis resulting in cosmetically unacceptable scars (Figs. 37.24 and 37.25).

Grafts

Grafts are movements of tissue from a distant site without its own vascular supply. These can be of different types namely, split-thickness, full-thickness and composite (discussed as a separate topic in the book). Grafts are generally performed as a method of repair post Moh's surgery when primary closure or use of flaps is not possible due to lack of enough tissue laxity or morbidity surrounding the surgical defect (Fig. 37.26).

All these repairs can be done by the Moh's surgeon but sometimes demand the expertise of a reconstructive surgeon for a functionally and cosmetically adequate final result.

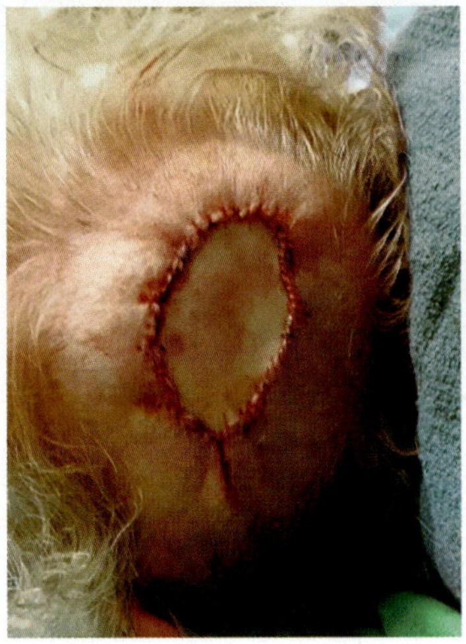

Fig. 37.26: Full thickness skin graft on the scalp. The size of the Moh's defect and the location.

POSTOPERATIVE CARE

The Moh's defect once repaired and cleaned is covered with a pressure dressing. The surgical site should be kept out of contact with water for 24–48 hours (depending on the type of repair). The patient is advised to remove the dressing after 24–48 hours and clean the wound with alcohol, cover with an antibacterial ointment (mupirocin) and replace the dressing. Oral antibiotics are usually not administered, if a sterile surgical setting is maintained. The patient is followed up in the clinic at the 7–14 days for either suture removal or a wound check (in case of secondary intention).

COMPLICATIONS

Although the incidence of complications (temporary or permanent) is low, the incidence largely depends on the method of repair, the skill of the Moh's surgeon and the presence of comorbidities in the patient being operated such as diabetes mellitus.

Some of the complications reported in the literature are:

- Hematoma
- Wound infection
- Wound dehiscence

- Flap necrosis
- Graft rejection
- Cosmetically unacceptable scars (hypertrophic/keloid)
- Distortion of cosmetic unit junctions
- Nerve damage (temporary causing paraesthesia/ permanent causing loss of sensation).

ADVANTAGES

- Moh's micrographic surgery provides the lowest recurrence rates and maximum tissue sparing when compared to all surgical modalities available for the treatment of basal cell carcinoma. The 5-year recurrence rate for primary basal cell carcinoma for the head and neck is 1.4% and 4% for recurrent basal cell carcinoma.[7] Comparatively, surgical excision with the recommended 4 mm margin for basal cell carcinomas mm has a recurrence rate of 3.2%; 6–9 mm a rate of 8% and >9 mm a rate of 9%. Similarly, electrodessication and curettage of basal cell carcinomas of the head and neck had a recurrence rate of 5% for lesions < 6 mm and 18% for >6 mm.[8] There is a significant difference in the cure rates achieved with Moh's surgery. Basal Cell carcinomas with aggressive growth type on histopathology and perineural invasion have shown to exhibit extensive spread (not visible clinically) and thus are most appropriately treated with this modality.[9]
- The cost of Moh's micrographic surgery is comparable to the cost of conventional surgical excision with permanent-section margin control when performed in a clinic setting under local anesthesia, but lower when the surgical excisions are performed in a hospital.[10] Additionally, fewer recurrences and therefore, reduced need for repeat treatments reinforces the cost-effectiveness of the procedure.[11]
- The goal of treating most cutaneous malignancies especially, nonmelanoma skin cancers (as they mostly occur in cosmetically sensitive areas) is to completely remove the tumor while achieving maximum tissue conservation and cosmesis. This is particularly applicable to all tumors occurring on the face. When availability of surrounding tissue is sparse, such as the nose and eyelids or the ear, Moh's micrographic surgery offers the advantage of minimal tissue resection with complete tumor removal.
- When standard surgical excision is performed, the specimen sent for histopathological evaluation is embedded in paraffin and processed to make permanent sections that are then read by the pathologist to rule out any residual tumor. With this traditional sectioning of the tissue (bread-loafing) less than 1% of the surgical margin is analyzed increasing the risk of missing the residual tumor by many folds. In contrast, when the tumor is resected using the Moh's technique, the tissue is frozen and sectioned in a way that enables 100% examination of the surgical margins of the resected tissue. This ensures that there is minimal to no risk of missing the detection of residual tumor.[12]

DISADVANTAGES

- Moh's micrographic surgery is a highly-specialized procedure that requires specific training and skill development by the operating physician/dermatologist.
- A proper clinic set-up wherein the operating room and the cryostat (where the frozen sections are prepared) and the histopathology lab are in close proximity, if not adjacent.
- A histopathology technician who is technically sound to produce high quality and uniform frozen sections is key to the success of the Moh's procedure.
- The morphology of the cells in frozen sections is distorted and the cellular details are not as well-delineated as in paraffin embedded sections making the interpretation of the tumor cells difficult. Thus, the operating surgeon and/or the dermatopathologist should be skilled in evaluating frozen sections for the presence of tumor in the resected tissue.
- As Moh's micrographic surgery is a staged procedure it is more time consuming than a routine surgical excision. Lastly, the surgical defect may require complex closure necessitating the expertise of a reconstructive surgeon.

CONCLUSION

Moh's micrographic surgery is considered the 'gold standard' for the treatment of nonmelanoma skin cancer and wide variety of other cutaneous tumors. This technique ensures highest cure rates compared to the other modalities available for treating these tumors. Moh's surgery offers the unique advantage of tissue conservation, a prerequisite for removing tumors from cosmetically sensitive areas. With lowest recurrence rates, minimal morbidity and maximum tissue preservation, Moh's surgery is a 'one of its kind' surgical technique in the armamentarium of a dermatologic surgeon.

REFERENCES

1. Brodland DG, Amonette R, Hanke CW, et al. The history and evolution of Moh's micrographic surgery. Dermatol Surg. 2000;26(4):303-7.
2. Skin Cancer Recognition and management. Robert A Schwartz, Robert A Contributor 2008. Hoboken: Wiley 2nd Ed 2008.
3. Longo C, Ragazzi M, Gardini S, et al. Ex vivo fluorescence confocal microscopy in conjunction with Moh's micrographic surgery for cutaneous squamous cell carcinoma. J Am Acad Dermatol. 2015;73(2):321-2.
4. Miller SJ, Alam M, Andersen J, et al. Basal cell and squamous cell skin cancers. J Natl Compr Canc Netw. 2010;8(8):836-64.
5. Connolly SM, Baker DR, Coldiron BM, et al. Ad Hoc Task Force. AAD/ACMA/ASDSA/ASMA 2012. Appropriate use criteria for Moh's micrographic surgery: a report of the American Academy of Dermatology, American college of Moh's surgery, American society of Dermatologic Surgery Association, and the American Society for Moh's Surgery. J Am Acad Dermatol. 2012;67(4):531-50.
6. Shriner DL, McCoy DK, Goldberg DJ, et al. Moh's Micrographic Surgery. J Am Acad Dermatol. 1998;39:79-97.
7. Leibovitch I, Huilgol SC, Selva D, et al. Basal cell carcinoma treated with Moh's surgery in Australia II. Outcome at 5-year follow-up. J Am Acad Dermatol. 2005;53(3):452-7.
8. Marzuka AG, Book SE. Basal cell carcinoma: Pathogenesis, epidemiology, clinical features, diagnosis, histopathology and management. Yale J Biol Med. 2015;88(2):167-79.
9. Batra RS, Kelley LC. Predictors of extensive subclinical spread in non-melanoma skin cancers treated with Moh's micrographic surgery. Arch Dermatol. 2012;138(8): 1043-51.
10. Cook J, Zitelli JA. Moh's micrographic surgery: a cost analysis. J Am Acad Dermatol. 1995;33(2 Pt 1):271-8.
11. Chatrath V, Rohrer TE. Moh's micrographic surgery. Atlas Office Procedures. 2002;5:243-61.
12. Grekin RC. Moh's micrographic surgery. In: Robinson JK, Arndt KA, LeBoit PE, Wintroub BJ (Eds). Atlas of Cutaneous Surgery. Philadelphia: WB Saunders;1996;211-7.

CHAPTER 38

Sclerotherapy

S Sacchidanand, Sujala S Aradhya, Nagesh TS

INTRODUCTION

Sclerotherapy remains defined as targeted eradication of varicose veins, small vessels, and vascular anomalies by injecting a sclerosant into them.[1]

Aim of sclerotherapy is to damage vessel walls and convert them into fibrous cords that cannot be recanalized. Sclerotherapy is a simple, efficacious, cost-effective, and a more aesthetically acceptable modality for therapeutic as well asaesthetic purposes.[1]

Sclerotherapy has still not become a widely practiced procedure in our country. This is a simple but conservative procedure, which also helps to reduce morbidity and also cost associated with a surgery.

MECHANISM OF ACTION

The sclerosants can cause sufficient damage to endothelium of vessels and, sometimes possibly, to the entire vascular wall. Eventually a local thrombus that remains attached to vessel wall is generated. Finally, the vessel is transformed into a fibrous cord, i.e. it gets sclerosed.[2]

INDICATIONS

Sclerotherapy is a well-known technique used for treatment of telangiectasias, varicose veins, symptomatic hemangiomas, low-flow vascular malformations, and benign vascular tumors (Table 38.1).

However, sclerotherapy is not effective for the treatment of flat portwine stains, high-flow lesions like arteriovenous (AV) fistulas and large varicose veins with incompetent sapheno-femoral junction.

CONTRAINDICATIONS

Sclerotherapy is contraindicated in an immobile patient because ambulation post-procedure is important to minimize the risks of thrombosis. While in diabetes and edema, there is compromised circulation and prolonged healing (Table 38.2).[3]

SCLEROSANTS

There are 3 main classes of sclerosing agents:[4,5]

Detergents	*Osmotic agents*	*Chemical irritants*
These agents act by *protein theft mechanism*. These agents cause vascular injury by altering the surface tension around the endothelial cells. • Sodium tetradecyl sulfate (STS) • Polidocanol (POL) • Sodium morrhuate • Ethanolamine oleate	These agents cause endothelial cell damage through *dehydration*. • Hypertonic sodium chloride solution • Sodium chloride solution with dextrose	These agents cause endothelial cell damage by their *direct corrosive action*. • Chromated glycerin • Polyiodinated iodine • Alcoholic solution of Zein • OK 432 (Picibanil) • Bleomycin

Comparison of various sclerosing agents are listed in Table 38.3.

Calculation of dilution volume is as given below:[7]

$$C_f = C_i[V_s/(V_s + V_d)]$$

C_f - final concentration (in %) of sclerosant

C_i - initial concentration (in %) of sclerosant

V_s - initial volume (in mL) of undiluted sclerosant

V_d - diluent volume (in mL) of 0.9% saline solution

PREPROCEDURE WORK UP

History

- Detailed medical history which includes general condition, lifestyle activities, physical activity, use of oral contraceptives, hormone replacement therapy or any other drugs routinely, habits like intake of alcohol and smoking should also be recorded.[1]

- If patients are on nonsteroidal anti-inflammatory drugs (NSAIDs) or anticoagulants long-term, these should be withheld at least one week before the procedure.
- History of any vascular insufficiency, Raynaud's phenomenon and systemic disease (like diabetes mellitus, hypertension, ischemic heart disease, etc.) should be noted.
- Results of any previous treatment undergone for the same indication and if it is a primary or a recurrent lesion is also noted.

Table 38.1: Indications for sclerotherapy.[1]

Indications	*Level of evidence*
Therapeutic indications	
Varicose veins Truncal veins, major tributaries of greater and lesser saphenous veins, lateral venous system varicosities, collateral veins, varicose veins associated with incompetent perforating veins, reticular varicose veins, residual and recurrent varicose veins (after interventions), complications like stasis dermatitis and venous ulcers	Level A
Vascular malformations Low-flow lesions (like venous or lymphatic malformations), rapidly growing or non-involuting hemangiomas	Level A
Benign vascular tumors Angiolymphoid hyperplasia with eosinophilia	Level C
Others Pyogenic granuloma, glomangioma, digital mucous cysts, venous lakes	Level C
Aesthetic indications	
Telangiectasias Spider veins Reticular veins	Level A

Examination

- Physical inspection to assess skin for stasis dermatitis, stasis ulcer, along with examination of venous system for varicosity, small and large vessels, along with the status of perforators is crucial. Examination should also include checking for evidence of any previous deep vein thrombosis.
- Arterial pulses should be identified and checked correctly.
- In case of any vascular malformations, identifying extent of malformation, any pulsation and bruit is present (to rule out an AV fistula) is also important.

Investigations

- Investigations like complete blood counts, blood sugar, blood pressure, bleeding and clotting time, and ECG should be carried out prior to the procedure.
- Venous color Doppler (duplex ultrasound) scans of patient's venous system is a must to identify the location and patency of perforators.
- Arterial Doppler studies may be done (only when considered necessary).
- In case of vascular malformations, a Doppler study indicates the direction of flow in the lesion.
- In case of vascular malformations, preferably, a magnetic resonance imaging (MRI) or a computed tomography (CT) scan to assess the depth and extent of the malformation will be useful.

Counseling

Counseling of the patient should ideally include the number of sessions, which may be needed, duration of the procedure, limitations of activity, if any after each session,

Table 38.2: Contraindications for Sclerotherapy.[1]

Absolute contraindications	*Relative contraindications*
• Acute superficial or deep vein thrombosis • Local infection in the area of sclerotherapy or severe generalized infection • Immobility, confinement to bed • Advanced peripheral arterial occlusive disease (stage 3 or 4) • Hyperthyroidism (in the case of sclerosants containing iodine) • Pregnancy in the first trimester and after the 36th week of gestation • Known allergy to the sclerosant • Severe systemic disease	• Leg edema • Sapheno-femoral junction incompetence • Thrombophilia with history of deep vein thrombosis • Long-standing diabetes • Peripheral arterial occlusive disease stage 2 • Poor general health • Myocardial decompensation • Migraine • Bronchial asthma • Marked allergic diathesis • Known hypercoagulability

Table 38.3: Comparison of various sclerosing agents.[6]

Sclerosing solution	*Advantages*	*Disadvantages*	*Vessel-treated*	*Concentration*	*Maximum volume/ dose of sclerosant*
Sodium tetradecyl sulfate	FDA approved; Painless unless injected extravascularly	May cause skin breakdown at higher concentrations	All sizes	0.1–0.2%- telangiectasias 0.2–0.5%- reticular 0.5–1.0%- varicose 1.0–3.0%- axial varicose	10 cc of 3%
Polidocanol	FDA approved; Painless	Ulcerogenic	Small to medium	0.25–0.5%-telangiectasias 0.5–1.0%- reticular 1.0–3.0%- varicose	20 cc of 3% Not to exceed 2 mg/kg
Sodium morrhuate	FDA approved	Allergic reactions (highest reported)	Small	Undiluted telangiectasias Undiluted reticular	2–5 cc of 5%, 50–250 mg depending on vein diameter
Hypertonic saline	Low risk of allergic reactions	Ulcerogenic, painful	Small	23.4–11.7%-telangiectasias 23.4%- reticular	20 cc per session Restrict volume in salt restricted diets
Hypertonic saline + dextrose	Low risk of allergic reaction, mild stinging, low ulcerogenic potential	Not FDA-approved; Relatively weak sclerosant	Small	Undiluted telangiectasias Undiluted reticular	10 cc
Chromated glycerin	Low skin ulcer potential	Not FDA-approved; Very weak sclerosant	Smallest	Undiluted telangiectasias to half strength	
Polyiodinated iodine	Highly corrosive; Allows treatment of largest veins	Not FDA-approved; Avoid use in iodine allergic patients	Largest	1–2%- for up to 5 mm veins 2-6%- for the largest veins	

followed by the need for a compression therapy and any potential adverse events and lastly the expected results.

Documentation of Case

- An informed consent should always be taken.
- Preoperative and postoperative photographs should be taken in order to document type and extent of patient's veins.
- Operative record should always include the type, concentration and volume of sclerosant used along with anatomical site treated (anatomic charts may be used). Complications, if any during the procedure, must always be noted.

PROCEDURE

Techniques

The method used to inject a sclerosant basically depends on the size of the vein to be treated.[8]

- ***Large veins***
  - *Fegan's technique*[9]: The patient is made to sit at the end of examination table with the affected leg to be treated in a dependent position and the varicosities are then marked (Figs. 38.1 and 38.2). Prominent varicosity is cannulized with a needle attached to a syringe pre-filled with desired volume and concentration of sclerosant (Fig. 38.3). The leg is next elevated and supported above the cardiac level for at least 2 minutes to allow drainage of blood from the vein to be treated. Before injecting the sclerosant, a small amount of blood is drawn into the syringe to ensure that the needle remains in the vein's lumen. After injecting 0.5–1.0 cc sclerosant, apply firm pressure by the fingers for about 1 minute, several centimeters above and below the site of injection. This helps to confine the sclerosing solution to the affected site. This is followed by immediate application of compression with a foam pad, which is secured by foam elastic tape (Fig. 38.4).

A widely used variation of Fegan's technique is the marking of varicosities with the patient standing while needle insertion is done with the patient recumbent or in slight reverse Trendelenburg position.[9]

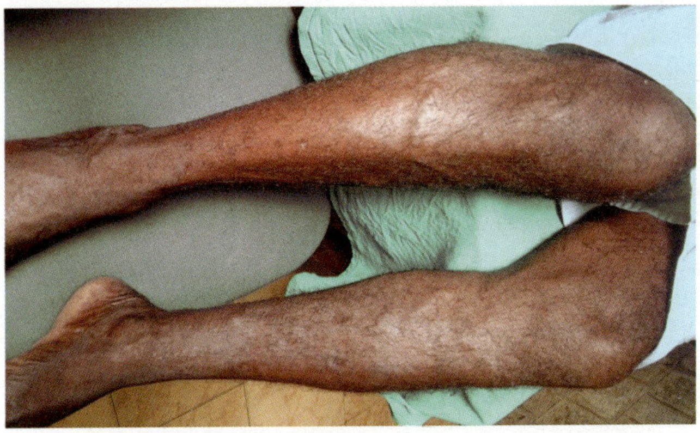

Fig. 38.1: Case of varicose veins.

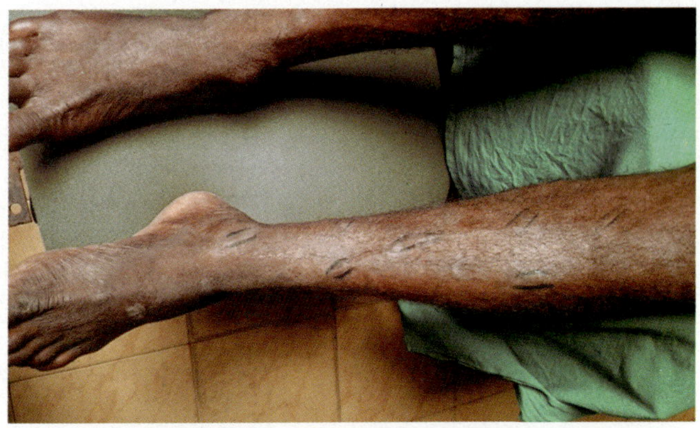

Fig. 38.2: Marking of varicosities in a dependant position.

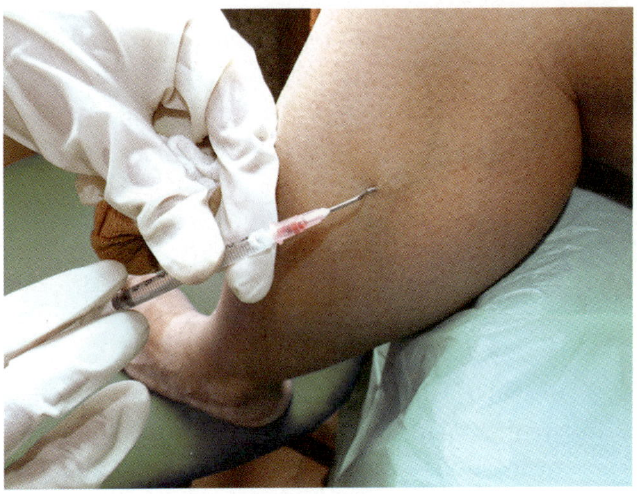

Fig. 38.3: The prominent varicosity is cannulized with a needle attached to a syringe.

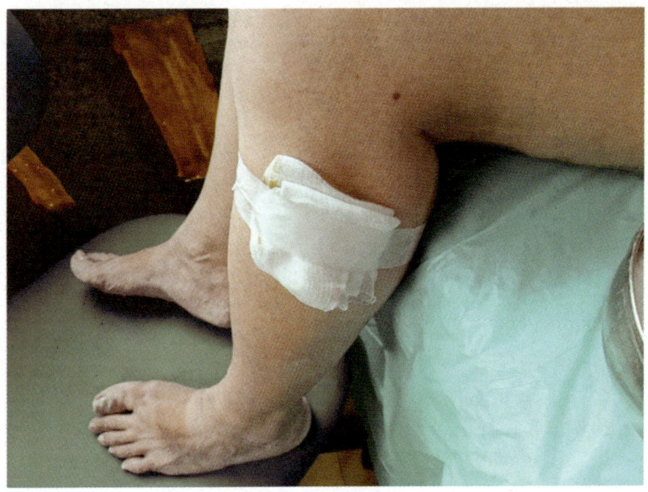

Fig. 38.4: Compression with a gauze pad is applied immediately as soon as the syringe is withdrawn. The compression is maintained for 1 minute. This is followed by immediate application of an elastic tape over the gauze to maintain the pressure.

Fegan's technique is particularly effective for incompetent perforators. The site of perforators may be marked during the venous Doppler study.

- *Sigg's technique*[9]: This method is more preferred for sclerosing the saphenous junctions. An open needle (not attached to syringe) is inserted into the skin and manipulated until blood drips from the hub, following which the sclerosant is injected.

- ***Reticular veins*:**
  The techniques are the same but the concentration, strength and volume of the sclerosant has to be reduced.[9] Subdermal reticular veins are treated only after all sources of reflux have been treated prior. Usually sodium tetradecyl sulfate in a concentration of 0.2–0.5% and volume less than 0.5 cc per injection site is used.[8]

POSTPROCEDURE CARE

- Immediately after the procedure, a continuous compression needs to be maintained. A cotton ball can be taped at the injection site with an elastocrepe compression bandage over it.[10]
- Post-treatment compression usually consists of a graduated 20–30 mm Hg support hose for larger veins and 16 mm Hg compressions for smaller veins used for 2 weeks or longer. The duration of use of compression after sclerotherapy mostly depends on the size of vessel injected, and usually varies from 1 day for spider veins to 3 weeks for larger veins.[11]
- The patient is made to walk for 30 minutes immediately postprocedure and then daily for next few days. This will reduce risk of deep vein thrombosis.

- Hot baths, intensive workouts, heavy exercise, strong UV radiation as well blood thinners (aspirin) should be avoided for couple of days.

Tips for a Good Procedure and Results

- Make the patient stand and mark all the cutaneous points on the veins to be treated.
- Then patient has to lie down in recumbent position so as to allow convenient access to all veins to be treated. A motorized table with height adjustment will better facilitate easier access to all the regions of legs.[8]
- Always inject from proximal points to distal points.
- Inject larger veins before any of the smaller veins.
- Each vein must be emptied of blood using any of the various maneuvers.
- Any reflux points should be initially determined and then treated specifically.
- Direct finger pressure needs to be exerted in compressing and spreading motion after each injection. Immediate but an adequate compression is quite important.
- Emphasize on adequate ambulation immediately post-treatment.
- Using a bent needle to inject can help in keeping the injecting hand more stable (Fig. 38.5).
- Always withdraw to look for blood in the syringe before injecting the sclerosant. Do not inject till the needle is completely inside the vein to be treated (Fig. 38.6).
- Start with lower concentrations and lower volumes of sclerosants in the initial sessions. Not more than 1 cc of the sclerosing agent should be injected at each site and only a total of 10 cc may be injected in a single session.
- The patient may be asked to mark the vessels which they feel are more troublesome.
- The resulting vessel size is the best prognostic indicator of treatment response and complications.
- Allowing 4–8 weeks between treatments helps to minimize the number of necessary sessions.

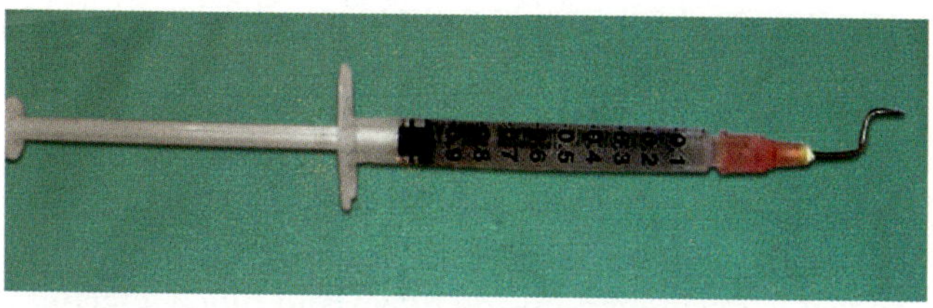

Fig. 38.5: Using a bent needle to inject will help in keeping the injecting hand more stable.

COMPLICATIONS[12]

When performed correctly with due precautions, sclerotherapy is a procedure with least complications. However, the following complications may be encountered:

- *Allergic reaction*: Anaphylaxis and systemic allergic reactions to sclerotherapy can occur rarely. Hence, it is recommended to make the patient stay in the hospital for about 30 minutes after the procedure before discharge.
- *Deep vein thrombosis and pulmonary embolism*: It probably occurs from extension of a superficial thrombus into the deep venous system. It is usually associated with injection of large quantities of sclerosant at a single site.
- *Arterial injection*: Fortunately, this dreaded complication is extremely rare. But it can lead to large areas of skin necrosis and damage to the subcutaneous tissue and muscle, which may take months to heal. Emergency treatment involves immediate application of ice, flushing the inadvertently injected artery with normal saline and heparin, injection of procaine 3% to inactivate STS and vascular surgery consultation for intravenous anticoagulation.
- *Cutaneous necrosis*: It may occur if the sclerosant spills outside the vessel into the skin. Though rare, its occurrence is serious and its treatment may be difficult. It occurs more commonly with sodium tetradecyl sulfate and very rarely with polidocanol. Normal saline in the ratio of 10:1 should be injected at the site. Application of 2% nitroglycerin paste at the extravasation site also greatly reduces the risks of necrosis.
- *Superficial thrombophlebitis*: It is characterized by a very tender, indurated and linear erythematous swelling. Transdermal glyceryl trinitrate speeds the resolution of venous inflammation.
- *Postsclerotherapy hyperpigmentation*: It is the appearance of increased visible pigmentation along the course of a treated vein. Initially, pigmentation is due to the perivascular hemosiderin deposition, but over time, the hemosiderin is replaced by melanin. Compression may help to prevent this side effect. Removal of post-sclerotherapy coagulant by a small incision using a 21 G needle and expressing it out may decrease the incidence of pigmentation. Pigmentation clears usually within 6 months and rarely persists for more than one year. Weekly subcutaneous administration of desferroxamine mesylate 500 mg reduces the time for depigmentation.

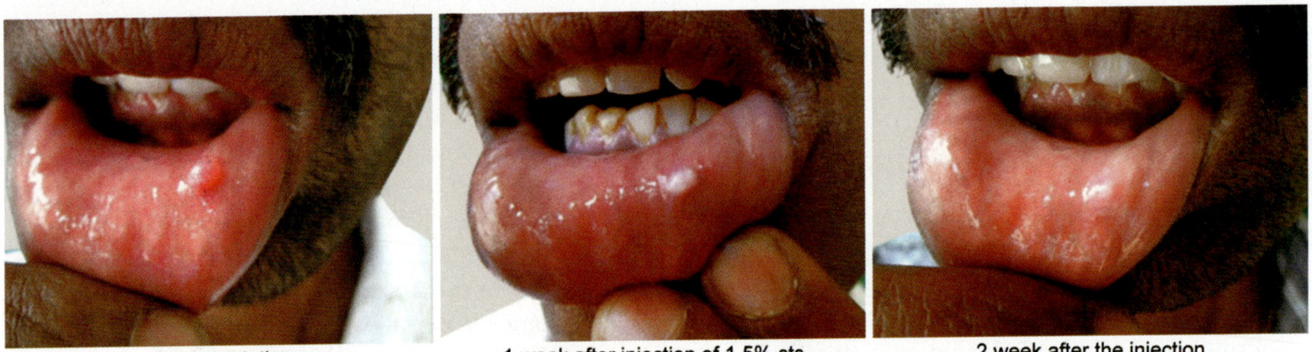

At presentation   1 week after injection of 1.5% sts   2 week after the injection

Fig. 38.6: Injecting sclerosant into mucosal cyst.

- **Matting:** It is the appearance of groups of new fine bluish telangiectasias surrounding or replacing a previously treated area. Resolution occurs spontaneously within a 3–12 month period with 70–80% spontaneous resolution within the first 6 months.
- **Others:** Rarer complications like nerve damage, small skin ulcers, urticarial reactions, scarring, visual disturbance, scintillating scotomas, orthostatic collapse, headache, and pain at the site of injection may be encountered.

SPECIAL TECHNIQUES OF SCLEROTHERAPY

Sclerotherapy Guided by Duplex Ultrasonography[13]

This technique is recommended for sclerosing the saphenous junctions, the truncal veins next to saphenous junctions, perforating veins and even low-flow vascular malformations.

The vein to be treated is visualized by duplex ultrasonography while the patient is lying down and is the vein is then punctured during visualization. The needle is visible in the ultrasound image and hence the intravascular injection can be controlled. The aim of this method is to achieve a controlled procedure that results in fewer complications and an increased effect.

Foam Sclerotherapy[14,15]

In this technique, a liquid sclerosant is mixed with air to form its foam, which is then injected into the blood vessels.

The sclerosing foam is basically a mixture of gas bubbles in a liquid solution that contains surface-active molecules. The gas used must be well-tolerated by patients, apart from being physiologic, and bubble size should be under 100 μ. Depending on the bubble diameter, foams can be classified as *froth, macrofoam, minifoam* and *microfoam*.

If the relative volume fraction of liquid is less than 5%, then that foam is *dry*, whereas if it is more than 5%, it is classified as *wet*. Wet foam (e.g. Tessari's foam) has the maximum stability. It is also known that uniform bubble diameter also provides more stability to the foam.[8]

Techniques of Foam Sclerotherapy[8]

Monfreux method: The foam is produced in a glass syringe filled with 0.3 to 0.5 cc of sclerosant. A negative pressure is produced by closing the tip of syringe with a sterile plug and maintaining this tension on piston until 2–3 cc of foam is generated. The consistency is usually low, probably due to large size of bubbles and this technique also has a relatively higher rate of side effects.

Cabrera method: Juan Cabrera used CO_2 for producing the foam.

Benigni-Sadoun method: Plastic syringes are used along with repeated and fast pulling and release of piston. But foam produced by this method is very short lasting.

Lorenzo Tessari's Tourbillon technique: Two plastic disposable syringes are connected to each other by a three-way stopcock. Foam is formed by mixing a liquid sclerosant with 4 to 5 parts of air, through 20 passes between both the syringes while rotating the hub at 30°. This rotation narrows the stopcock passage generating high turbulence, which in turn produces high quality microfoam. This is one of the more regularly used techniques.

Frullini method: The mechanism of foam generation basically uses the same turbulence effect of Tessari method. But here a connecter is inserted into a vial of STS (sclerosant) while the other end is connected to a syringe. The vial is positioned upside down and quick injection/aspiration of the solutions are performed.

Advantages and Disadvantages of Foam Sclerotherapy

Advantages of foam over liquid sclerosants are:[8]

- Foam preparations are 3–4 times more potent than equivalent concentrations and volumes of liquid sclerosants.
- There is an increase in the effective surface area while using the foam.
- There displacement of blood at the treatment site which allows undiluted intimal contact for a longer time.
- Increased vasospasm and sclerosis of veins occurs even at a distance farther away from the site of injecting the sclerosant.
- Smaller volumes and concentrations will be used.
- On duplex imaging, there is enhanced visibility due to the increased echogenicity of the foam.

Disadvantages of foam sclerotherapy

- The main disadvantage of foam is the difficulty in standardization.[16]
- The foam can lodge in the lungs and produce pulmonary fibrosis in patients of ductus arteriosus. Deep vein thrombosis and superficial thrombophlebitis are also known to occur.
- Pain and pigmentation are relatively more common.

CONCLUSION

Sclerotherapy is a simple, safe, effective, and pocket friendly procedure for treatment of varicose veins and the low-flow vascular malformations. This procedure is particularly effective for early and smaller varicosities, since it also may help in preventing the development of skin changes and is also the method preferred for residual varicosities after a varicose vein surgery. It is considered superior to any surgical and other nonsurgical treatments used to relieve symptoms and also reach optimal cosmetic results for small, localized, primary varices of the lower extremity. This procedure while being an outpatient procedure, not only reduces the cost but also the morbidity associated with a surgical treatment.

The advantages of sclerotherapy are mainly low morbidity, almost no mortality and no requirement for hospitalization; therefore, avoiding loss of work time. When the procedure is done with adequate precautions, there are relatively very few complications that may occur. Any treatment failures could be most often due to inappropriate technique rather than shortcoming of the procedure.[17] Proper training in the technique, dilution and amount of sclerosant injected is hence vital for optimal, risk-free outcomes. However, the greatest advantage of sclerotherapy is, even if it fails, it can be safely repeated any number of times.

REFERENCES

1. Khunger N, Sacchidanand S. Standard guidelines for care: Sclerotherapy in dermatology. Indian J Dermatol Venereol Leprol. 2011;77:222-31.
2. Scurr JH. Venous disorders. In: Russell RC, Williams NS, Bulstrode CJ, (Eds). Bailey and Love's Short Practice of Surgery, 24th edition. London: Arnold Publishers; 2004. p. 956.
3. Rabe E, Pannier-Fischer F, Gerlach H, et al. Guidelines for sclerotherapy of varicose veins (ICD 10: I83.0, I83.1, I83.2, and I83.9). Dermatol Surg. 2004;30:687-93; discussion 693.
4. Feied C. Sclerosing solutions. In: Bergan JJ, (Ed). The Vein Book. USA: Elsevier Academic Press; 2007:125-31.
5. Subbarao NT, Sacchidanand S, Veerabhadrappa NH. Sclerotherapy in the management of varicose veins and its dermatological complications. Indian J Dermatol Venereol Leprol. 2013;79:383-8.
6. Duffy DM. Sclerotherapy. In: Dover JS, Alam M, Nguyen TH, (Eds). Treatment of Leg Veins. USA: Elsevier Saunders; 2006:71-105.
7. Ratnavel GR. Foam sclerotherapy in various vascular and lymphatic malformations. Indian J Dermatol Venereol Leprol. 2011;77:336-8.
8. Sacchidanand S, Nagesh TS. Sclerotherapy. In: Venkataram M, (Ed). ASC(I) Textbook on Cutaneous and Aesthetic Surgery. India: Jaypee Brothers Medical Publishers; 2012:452-62.
9. Goldman MP, Weiss RA, Bergan JJ. Diagnosis and treatment of varicose veins: a review. J AM Acad Dermatol. 1994;31: 393-413.
10. Nootheti P, Cadag KM, Magpantay A, et al. Efficacy of graduated compression stockings for an additional 3 weeks after sclerotherapy treatment of reticular and telangiectatic leg veins. Dermatol Surg. 2009;35:53-8.
11. Goldman MP. How to utilize compression after sclerotherapy. Dermatol Surg. 2002;28:860-2.
12. Goldman MP. Complications and adverse sequelae of sclerotherapy. In: Bergan JJ, (Ed). The Vein Book. USA: Elsevier Academic Press; 2007;149-53.
13. Yamaki T, Nozaki M, Iwasaka S. Comparative study of duplex-guided foam sclerotherapy and duplex-guided liquid sclerotherapy for the treatment of superficial venous insufficiency. Dermatol Surg. 2004;30:718-22.
14. Breu FX, Guggenbichler S. European consensus meeting on foam sclerotherapy. Dermatol Surg. 2004;30:709-17.
15. Geroulakos G. Foam sclerotherapy for the management of varicose veins: critical reappraisal. Phlebolymphology. 2006;13:202-6.
16. Frullini A, Cavezzi A. Sclerosing foam in the treatment of varicose veins and telangiectasias: history and analysis of complications. Dermatol Surg. 2002;28:11-15.
17. Labas P, Ohradka B, Cambal M, et al. The results of compression sclerotherapy. Phlebologie. 2000;29:137-41.

CHAPTER 39

Use of Chemicals in Dermatosurgery

Niti Khunger, Shikha Bansal

INTRODUCTION

Chemosurgery is a technique of using various chemical agents to achieve therapeutic results. The chemicals act as cauterants and achieve tissue destruction to obtain the desired results. The common chemicals used are phenol, trichloroacetic acid, sodium hydroxide, potassium hydroxide, urea, salicylic acid, etc. The advantage of chemosurgery is that they are simple office procedures that do not require costly equipment or surgical expertise. Some of the commonly used chemosurgical procedures are described in this chapter.

ACNE SURGERY

Phenolization for Cystic Acne

This is a simple office procedure to drain the cysts in acne. It achieves quicker healing with minimal scarring.[1]

Principle

Early evacuation of contents of cyst reduces the risk of atrophic acne scars and application of phenol ensures complete destruction of the wall thus preventing recollection of cyst contents.

The level of evidence for this procedure is D.

Procedure

The face is first surgically cleaned with alcohol, povidone-iodine and again alcohol. The contents of cyst are drained with a no. 15 surgical blade by making a fine small nick. The cyst should then be thoroughly evacuated. The walls of the cyst are then destroyed with 88% phenol by introducing an ear bud or cotton swab on a toothpick dipped in phenol. The procedure is then repeated with fresh phenol dipped swabs, two to four times more. The phenol is then neutralized with povidone-iodine dipped cotton swabs. Intralesional and perilesional triamcinolone acetonide 5-10 mg/mL is then injected to reduce fibrosis and scarring (Figs. 39.1A to E).

The advantage of this procedure is that the cysts heal quickly, inflammation is reduced and deep scars, typical of nodulocystic acne are avoided or minimized.

The disadvantage is that improper technique can lead to complications.

Tips to reduce complications:

- It is important that the nick should be small to prevent a large scar.
- Phenol should be neutralized with povidone-iodine to prevent prolonged inflammation. This can otherwise result in postinflammatory hyperpigmentation.
- Care should be taken to prevent spillage of excess phenol on the surrounding normal skin.
- Combination of intralesional steroids is beneficial in reducing the scar.

Complications are however uncommon and it is a safe simple technique.

TCA CROSS Technique for Acne Scars

Chemical reconstruction of skin scars (CROSS) is a technique using high concentrations of trichloroacetic acid (TCA: 50–100%) focally on the atrophic acne scars to induce inflammation and collagenization.[2] The CROSS technique is an excellent treatment strategy for ice pick acne scars in all skin types including Fitzpatrick skin types IV to VI.

Principle

TCA is a caustic agent that causes precipitation of proteins and coagulative necrosis of cells in epidermis. When used in higher strengths it also causes necrosis of collagen in the papillary to upper reticular dermis. An increase in the dermal volume is also seen, which as a result of an increased collagen production, glycosaminoglycan elastin fragmentation and reorganization. It can be combined with laser skin resurfacing using fractional CO_2 laser or 1550 nm

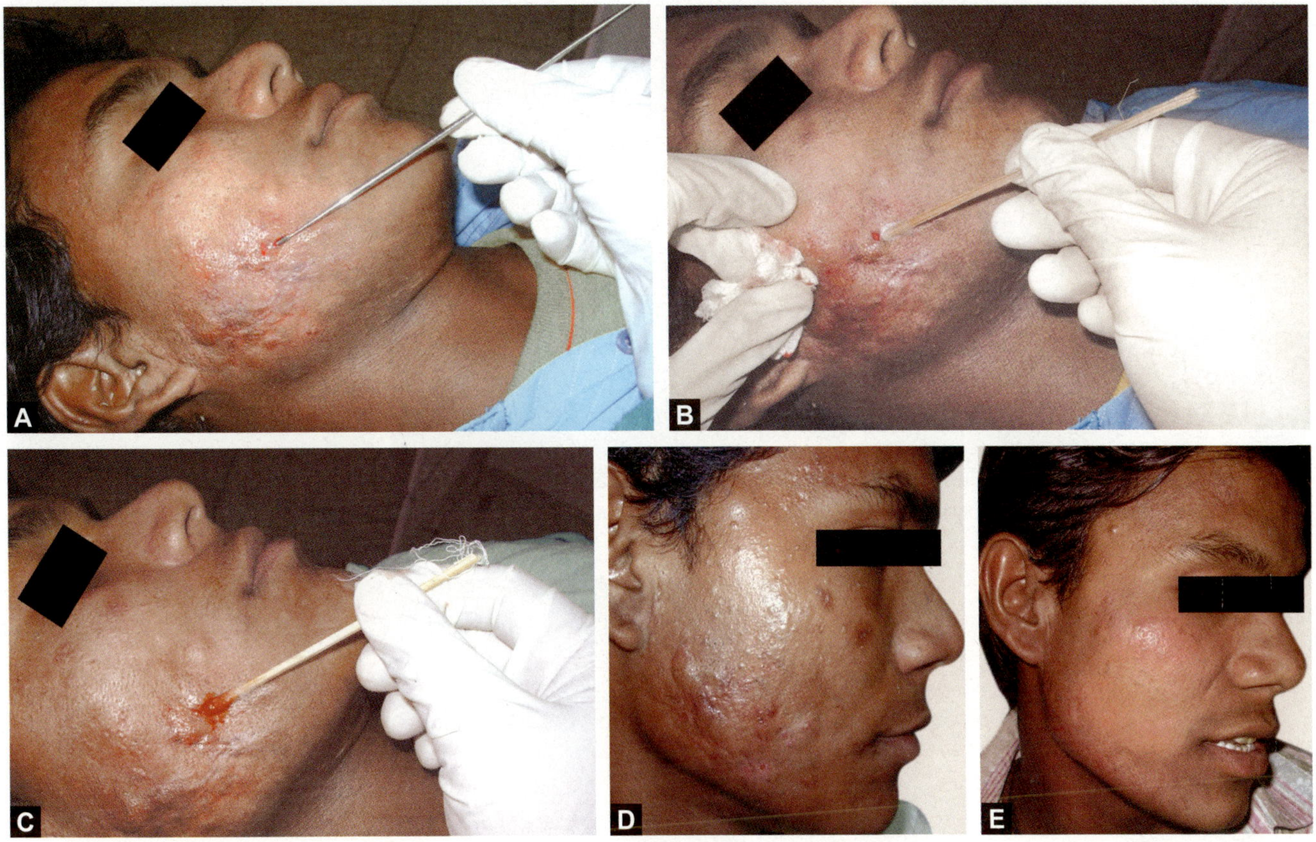

Figs. 39.1A to E: (A) Draining the cyst. (B) Phenolization. (C) Neutralizing the phenol with betadine. (D) Nodulocystic lesions before treatment. (E) Healing with no scarring after 10 days.

Erbium: Glass laser or percutaneous microneedling to further enhance the results and also improve the other type of scars.

Procedure

Priming for 2–4 weeks before the procedure is essential before doing CROSS technique as postinflammatory hyperpigmentation is common in darker skin. Tretinoin 0.025% cream at night and a sunscreen containing avobenzone, octinoxate and 2% hydroquinone in the morning is most ideal. Informed consent and pretreatment photographs are essential before treatment. It is best to do the procedure with the patient sitting or inclined at 45 degrees. A sharp pointed toothpick is dipped in the TCA solution, taking care to see that there is no dripping. The skin is stretched and TCA is focally applied to reach the bottom of the scar by pressing hard and rotating a few times, taking care to avoid spillage to the surrounding skin (Figs. 39.2A to C). The skin is kept stretched and monitored carefully until frosting occurs. The face is then washed and the patient is sent from the clinic with application of sunscreen. The procedure can be repeated every 2 to 4 weeks, till the desired results are obtained.

The advantage is that it is an efficacious cost-effective technique to treat ice pick scars.[3] Persistent erythema, postinflammatory hyperpigmentation (Fig. 39.3A) and widening of the scar (Fig. 39.3B) are complications that can occur, with improper technique.

Tips

- Preprocedure priming is must
- While dipping tooth pick care should be taken, so that only the tip is in contact with TCA
- Excess TCA to be removed to prevent spillage or dribbling
- Scar should be stretched before applying to prevent contact of TCA to surrounding skin, so that TCA is in contact only with scar base.

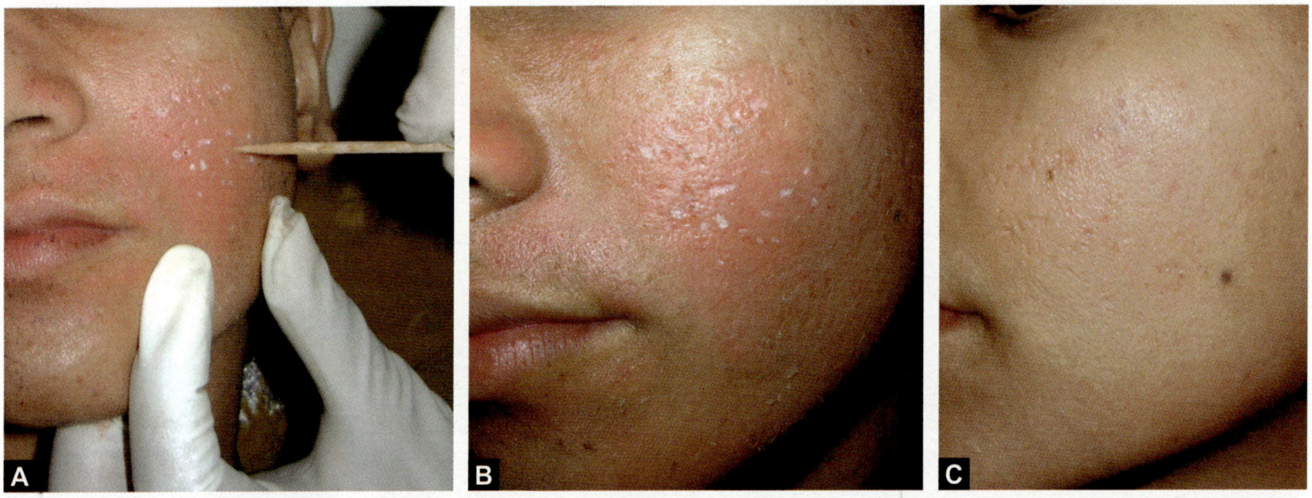

Figs. 39.2A to C: (A) Applying 100% TCA with a sharpened toothpick. (B) Pinpoint frosting. (C) Healing in 10 days.

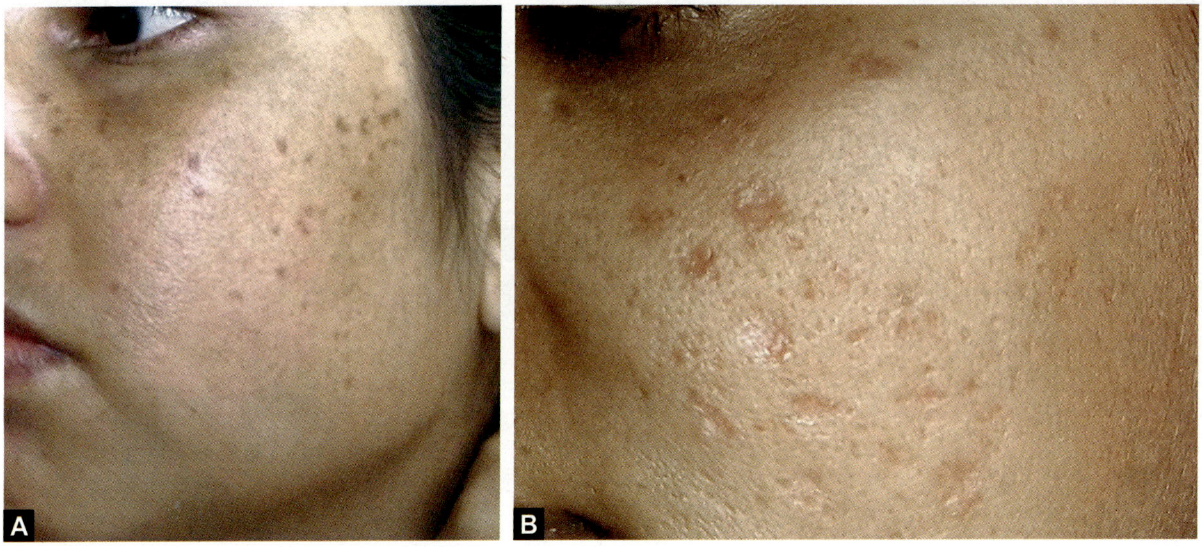

Figs. 39.3A and B: (A) Postinflammatory hyperpigmentation. (B) Widening of the scar due to spread of TCA to surrounding normal skin.

NAIL SURGERY

Chemical Matricectomy for Ingrown Toenail

Ingrown toenail is a common painful nail condition and a significant number of cases require surgical management in the form of lateral partial nail avulsion of the ingrowing edge.

Principle

A simple avulsion of the nail is associated with a high chance of recurrence. Destruction of lateral horns of matrix (lateral matricectomy) is an important component in the management of ingrown toenail. This may be managed by surgical, or more frequently by chemical destruction of the lateral matrix (chemical matricectomy). The matrix destruction should be minimalto reduce damage to surrounding normal structures, but at the same time it must be complete and valid to prevent recurrences.

Chemicals Used

Chemical matricectomy uses various chemical agents to destroy the lateral nail matrix. Among these, phenol is the most commonly used agent. It is an effective protein denaturant which has a cauterizing effect by producing a

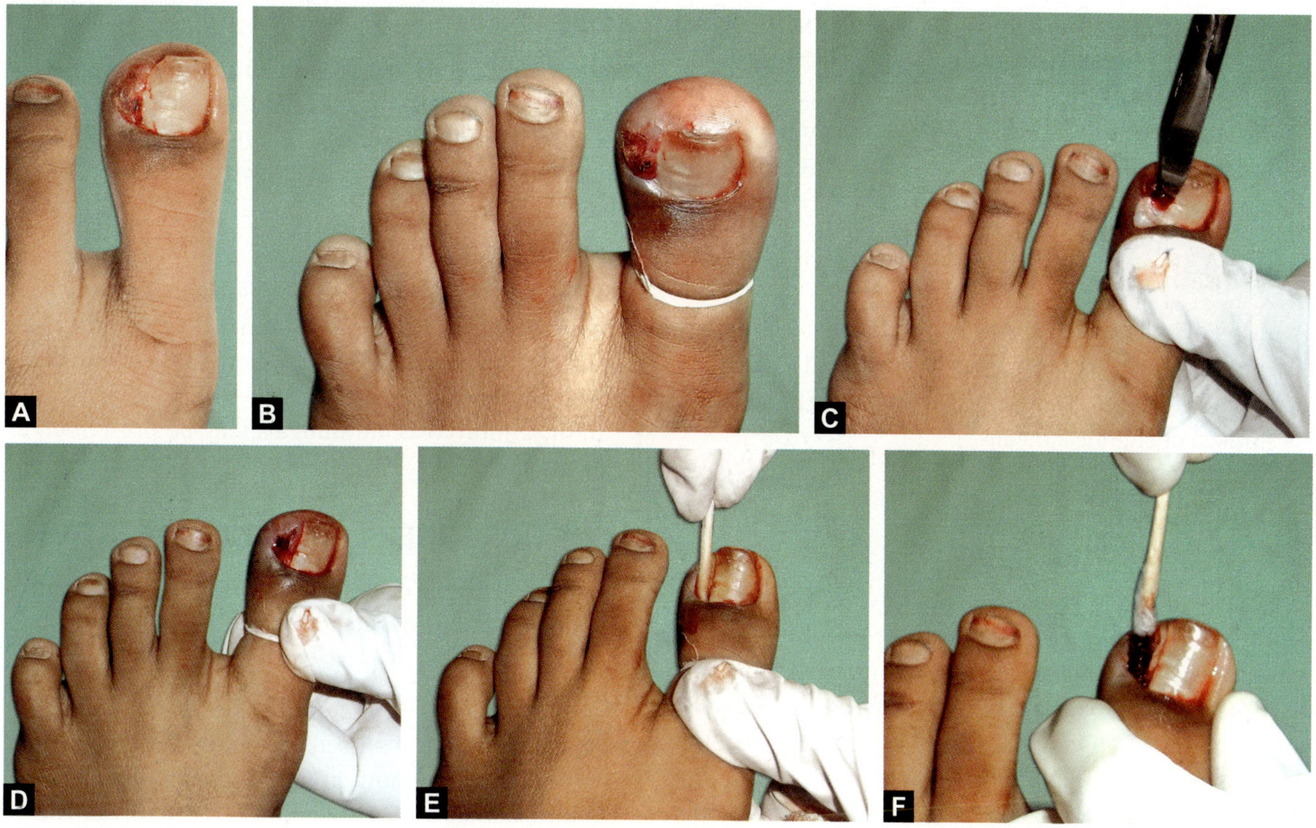

Figs. 39.4A to F: (A) Ingrown toenail. (B) Tourniquet applied. (C) Lateral nail clipped with a nail clipper. (D) Clipped nail. (E) Phenol applied. (F) Phenol neutralized with betadine.

coagulation necrosis of the area it is applied to (matrix and the surrounding soft tissue) (Figs. 39.4A to F).

Recent studies,[4] have found that 10% sodium hydroxide is as effective as 88% phenol for chemical matricectomy of ingrown toenail. Sodium hydroxide is a strong basic salt that causes basic tissue destruction and produces a liquefaction necrosis (which heals more rapidly than the coagulation necrosis produced by phenol). Thus, it has been shown to have an efficacy similar to phenol, but with a shorter recovery time. It also offers a slightly better adverse effect profile.

Procedure

After the complete or partial nail avulsion a tooth pick dipped in either phenol or sodium hydroxide is inserted into a small pocket at the lateral most end, below the proximal nail fold so that the tip is pressed gently against lateral matrix and kept for approximately one minute. And it is repeated thrice on each side to ensure complete destruction of lateral nail matrix.

Advantages

Chemical matricectomy is preferable over other methods like surgical matricectomy, ablative methods, such as carbon dioxide laser, electrocautery and radiofrequency as these techniques are more technically demanding and more expensive compared with chemical matricectomy. Phenol having antiseptic and anesthetic property reduces infection rate and postoperative pain.

Tips

- Nail avulsion should always be combined with lateral matricectomy to prevent recurrences in ingrown toe nail
- Care should be taken to avoid excess chemical on tooth pick to avoid spillage
- While applying chemical, a gentle pressure is to be applied with nondominant thumb just medial to lateral matrix to avoid contact with medial part of the matrix. This prevents excess matrix damage and nail dystrophy

- Contact time between chemical and matrix should be adequate (3 mins). Inadequate contact can result in incomplete destruction with thin nail plate regrowing.

In conclusion, chemosurgery is the most widely technique for the treatment of ingrown toenail along with partial nail avulsion.

Chemical Nail Avulsion

Avulsion of nail can be a treatment of choice in conditions like onychogryphosis, pincer nail, psoriasis and recalcitrant candidal and bacterial infections. Avulsion can be achieved by surgical or chemical means.

Principle

Though surgical avulsion is more commonly employed, chemical avulsion is more popular in the elderly population, or when the patient is not fit or unwilling for surgery or when multiple nails are involved. An urea ointment is commonly used for chemical avulsion. It is formulated to include 40% urea, 20% anhydrous lanolin, 5% white beeswax or paraffin and 35% white petrolatum.[5] Urea acts by dissolving the bond between nail bed and nail plate, and it also softens the nail plate.

Procedure

The paronychial area is first protected with an adhesive tape before applying the urea paste to prevent chemical irritation of the surrounding soft tissues. The urea ointment is then liberally applied to the nail plate, while the hypoallergenic tape is used to create a well-around the treated thickened nail in order to hold the paste in place. The patient is further instructed to keep the nail occluded and also to avoid wetting the treated area. After 1 week of continuous occlusion, the dystrophic nail is removed by using a nail elevator and a nail clipper.

Advantages

Dystrophic nails may respond better to chemical avulsion, and it is the ideal management for symptomatic dystrophic nails in patients with comobidities like diabetic neuropathy, vascular disease or immunosuppression. In addition, chemical avulsion may be used as a pain relieving, palliative therapy in cases of onychogryphosis. Minimal to absent pain, hemorrhage, a low risk of infection and lesser downtime are the advantages.

Disadvantages

Requirement of prolonged application and irritation are some disadvantages of this procedure. Further, patients with gross thickening of nail without significant nail dystrophy may respond poorly due to poor penetration of the chemical.

Tips

- Patient must be counseled that it is a temporary method of destruction of nail, as recurrence is very common.
- Cuticle and proximal nail fold should be well-protected with ample emollients.
- In onychomycosis, antifungals may be prescribed as an adjunct.

CHEMOSURGERY FOR VIRAL INFECTIONS

Chemosurgery using cauterets is useful for the treatment of warts and molluscum contagiosum.

Principle

Chemical preparations used for treatment of wart and molluscum contagiosum are salicylic acid, lactic acid, trichloro acetic acid (TCA), podophyllin, etc. TCA and other acids act by causing protein coagulation of virus infected cells thus destroying the wart tissue. Podophyllin has a cytotoxic and antimitotic action thus preventing viral multiplication.

Procedure

Wart solution containing 16.5% salicylic acid and 16.5% lactic acid is most commonly used. It is self applied by the patient as a home preparation, with proper instructions. The wart solution is carefully applied to the lesion with a pointed toothpick or cotton bud, depending on the size of the lesion. In case of plantar warts, the surrounding skin is protected with tape or Vaseline, the wart solution is allowed to dry and then the lesion is occluded with micropore tape. TCA 50–100% is an alternative. For facial verruca plana TCA 15–25% is safer. Podophyllin 25% is the agent of choice for genital warts.

Advantages

It is a preferred technique in children and in patients with multiple lesions, where ablation with radiofrequency or CO_2 laser is not feasible. It is less painful as compared to cryotherapy. In plantar warts, it is the treatment of choice as it causes least pain and scar formation as compared to ablation with electrosurgery, radiofrequency or CO_2 laser.

Disadvantages

Removal may be incomplete and recurrence rates are quite high. Irritant reactions can occur, if adequate precaution is not taken.

Tips

- Patient should be counseled about requirement about multiple sittings required and chances of recurrence
- Surrounding skin should be properly protected with Vaseline or petrolatum jelly
- Paring can be done in case of thick hyperkeratotic lesions
- Always combination techniques work well in the management of recurrent warts.

SEBORRHEIC KERATOSIS, DERMATOSES PAPULOSA NIGRA

Seborrheic keratosis is one of the most common benign epidermal tumors characterized by pigmented, flat verrucous lesions, seen commonly on the face and trunk in elderly individuals. Patients usually seek removal for cosmetic reasons. The most commonly used treatment methods are cryosurgery with liquid nitrogen and curettage, shave excision, superficial electrodessication, radiofrequency ablation or CO_2 laser vaporization.[6]

An alternative method is curettage followed by chemical cautery with 50% TCA or 100% TCA repeated at weekly intervals till the complete lesion is removed. Ammonium lactate and alpha hydroxy acids, such as 70% glycolic acid, which acts as a keratolytic have also been used to treat seborrheic keratosis.[7]

Dermatosis papulosa nigra is a variant of seborrheic keratosis seen commonly on the face and neck, that present as multiple, firm, smooth, dark brown to black, flattened papules. They are a cosmetic concern and radiofrequency ablation, electrodessication are commonly used treatment modalities. Focal 25% TCA can be used as an alternative method (Fig. 39.5).

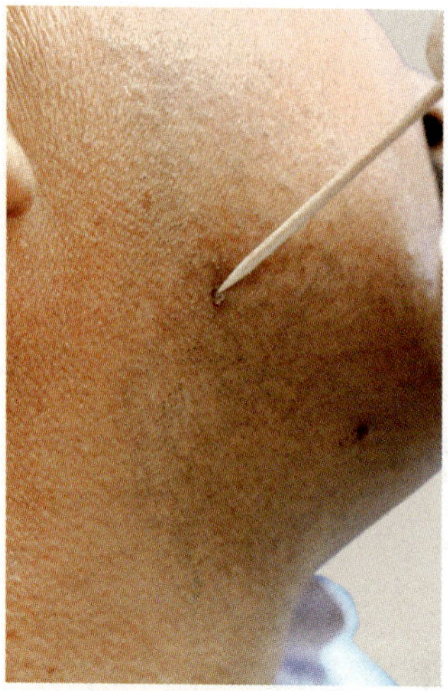

Fig. 39.5: Focal 25% TCA application in DPN.

XANTHELASMA PALPEBRARUM

Xanthelasma palpebrarum (XP) presents as yellowish cutaneous plaques, most commonly located on medial aspect of eyelids (Fig. 39.6A). Various modalities have been suggested for treatment, such as chemical cauterization with trichloroacetic acid (TCA) or liquid nitrogen, surgical excision, cryotherapy and laser ablation.

Principle

TCA is a caustic agent which acts through precipitation and coagulation of proteins and dissolution of lipids causing a nonspecific chemical injury to the skin. It offers the advantages of being simple, straightforward and nonsurgical.

Procedure

The eyelids are degreased with alcohol or acetone (Fig. 39.6B). The surrounding normal skin is protected with Vaseline® (Fig. 39.6C). The desired concentration of TCA (50–100%) is applied carefully in a spiral motion on the affected area, with the greatest amount of TCA at the margin of the lesion. An immediate after-effect of TCA application is a whitish discoloration called frosting of the lesion, which is surrounded by a zone of perilesional erythema that later subsides in a few hours (Fig. 39.6D). A dark, brownish-black crust forms, which should always be kept soft by application of petroleum jelly and must be allowed to come off by itself. This usually takes 10–14 days. If the primary lesion still persists, then TCA is reapplied.

The common side effects seen are hypo- or hyperpigmentation, which are usually transient. However scarring and ectropion formation are uncommon serious side effects especially with higher doses, 50%, 70%, or 100%. In a study by Mourad et al, 70% TCA was found to be more effective as compared to 35% or 50% TCA, with hypopigmentation seen as a side effect with 70% TCA and hyperpigmentation with 50% TCA.[8] In a comparative study by Goel et al,[9] 30% TCA was compared with the ultrapulsed

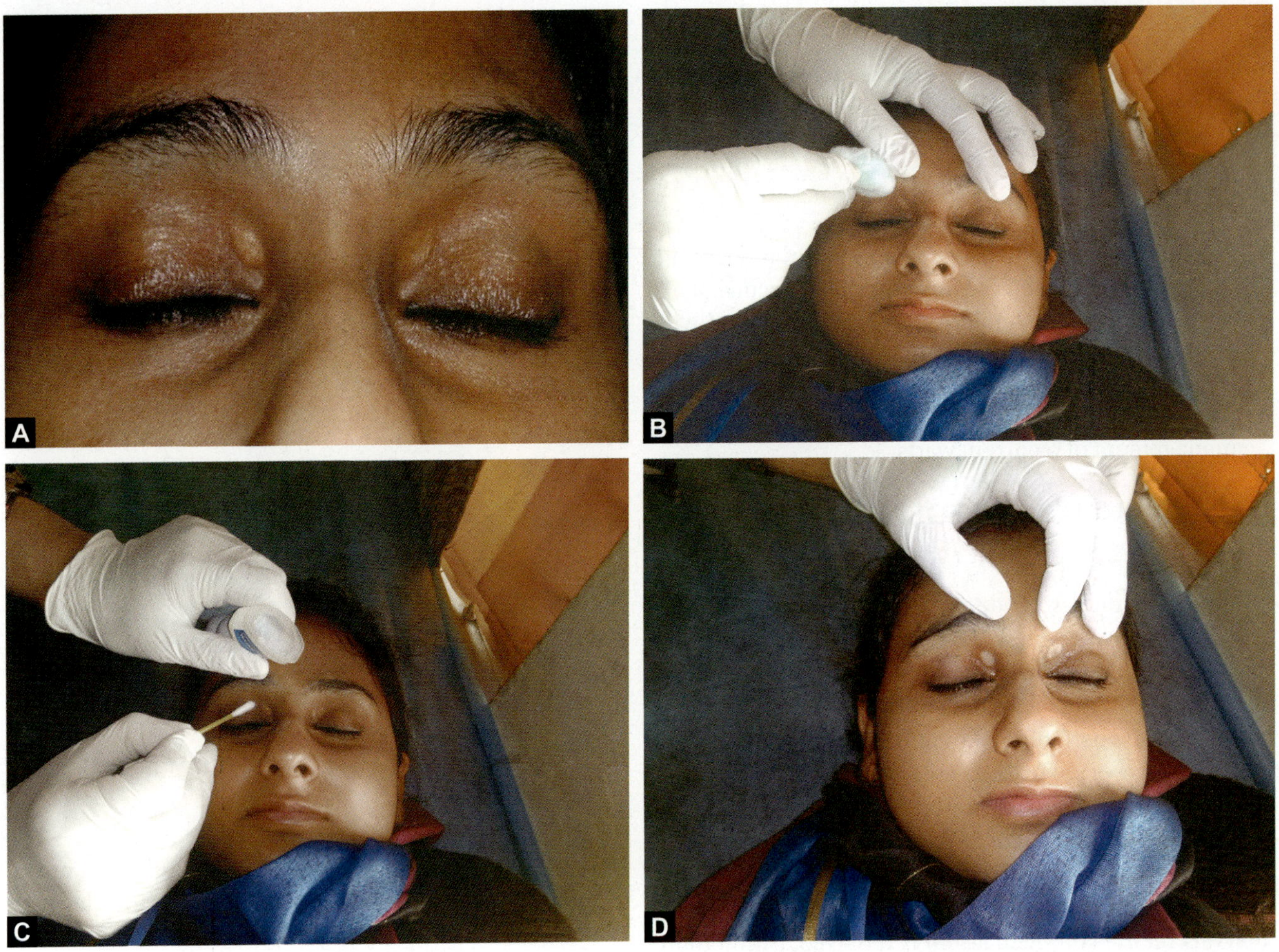

Figs. 39.6A to D: Treatment of xanthelasma palpebrarum with TCA.

CO_2 laser. It was observed that for clinically mild lesions, both TCA and laser were good options, with comparative effect, but the laser was found to be a better option for severe lesions. However, the TCA concentration used in this study was only 30%. Recurrence was seen in both groups.

Tips

- Care should be taken to avoid spillage in the eye or surrounding normal skin
- Postprocedure sun protection is must to prevent pigment mismatch.

FRECKLES AND LENTIGINES

Freckles are caused by an increase in melanin pigment in the melanocytes seen in photo exposed areas of the skin, in predisposed individuals. Lentigines are small pigmented macules, characterized histologically by hyperplasia of the epidermis and increased pigmentation of the basal layer, with a variable increase in the number of melanocytes. Treatment of freckles and lentigines carried out for cosmetic reasons.

Various treatment options include topical alpha hydroxy acids, TCA, phenol and Jessner's solution. Ablation using electrosurgery, cryotherapy or radiofrequency can also be used; Lasers, such as Q-switched Nd:YAG laser, CO_2 (both fractional and ablative) are other alternatives. All treatment options carry the risk of postinflammatory hyperpigmentation and none of them are considered completely satisfactory.

Principle

TCA is a caustic which causes coagulation of proteins and necrosis of tissue. The depth depends upon the concentration of TCA used, hence has a predictable result.[10] Necrosis of pigmented layer occurs which is reepithelialized with normal epithelium.

Procedure

The affected area is cleaned with spirit and degreased with acetone. Focal TCA application, 15–25% is done till light cloudy frosting occurs. The treatment can be repeated monthly till complete clearance. However the patient should be warned that recurrences can occur in freckles as it is an autosomal dominant condition.

Advantages

Advantages of chemosurgery with TCA are that it is a simple procedure, cost-effective and provides satisfactory results (52–86%). It is less painful with less downtime as compared to other modalities, such as cryotherapy and can be individualized on the basis of size and shape of freckles.

Disadvantages

Disadvantages include risk of accidental spillage to eyes and surrounding area and absence of an instant effect. Postinflammatory hyperpigmentation can occur which can be prevented by taking simple precautions.

Tips

- The patient should be adequately primed with sunscreens and hypopigmenting agents at least 2–4 weeks before the procedure
- Sun protection must be advised after the procedure.

EAR LOBE REPAIR (CHEMICAL ELR)

Ear lobe tear either gravitational or traumatic is usually treated with surgical correction. However when surgery is contraindicated or patient is not willing nonsurgical or chemical ELR is considered.

Procedure

Coat phenol along inner aspect of slit, to cover anterior and posterior margins till frosting. Abrade/scrape with small manual dermabraders. Reapply phenol to raw surface to induce frosting. This creates two opposing raw surfaces which are then dressed using tubular dressing for one week.

Advantages

- It is a simple procedure
- No surgical skill is required.

Disadvantages

- Does not give strength to the lobe
- Recurrences are very high.

Tips

- Care should be taken, so that the opposing surfaces are completely raw, so that better adhesion is achieved
- Avoid wearing earrings for at least 6–12 weeks
- Heavy earrings are to be avoided as this technique does not add to strength to the lobe.

CONCLUSION

Chemosurgery with various chemical agents is a simple office procedure that can be an effective tool in selected skin disorders.

REFERENCES

1. Khunger N. Standard guidelines of care for acne surgery. Indian J Dermatol Venereol Leprol. 2008;74:S28-36.
2. Lee JB, Chung WG, Kwahck H, et al. Focal treatment of acne scars with trichloroacetic acid: chemical reconstruction of skin scars method. Dermatol Surg. 2002;28(11):1017-21.
3. Khunger N, Bhardwaj D, Khunger M. Evaluation of CROSS technique with 100% TCA in the management of ice pick acne scars in darker skin types. J Cosmet Dermatol. 2011;10:51-7.
4. Grover C, Khurana A, Bhattacharya SN, et al. Controlled trial comparing the efficacy of 88% phenol versus 10% sodium hydroxide for chemical matricectomy in the management of ingrown toenail. Indian J Dermatol Venereol Leprol. 2015;81:472-7.
5. Pandhi D, Vernia P. Nail avulsion: Indications and methods (surgical nail avulsion). Indian J Dermatol Venereol Leprol. 2012;78:299-308.
6. Jackson JM, Alexis A, Berman B, et al. Current understanding of seborrheic keratosis: prevalence, etiology, clinical presentation, diagnosis, and management. J Drugs Dermatol. 2015;14(10):1119-25.
7. Van Scott EJ, Yu RJ. Alpha hydroxy acids: procedures for use in clinical practice. Cutis. 1989;43(3):222-8.
8. Mourad B, Elgarhy LH, Ellakkawy HA, et al. Assessment of efficacy and tolerability of different concentrations of trichloroacetic acid vs. carbon dioxide laser in treatment of xanthelasma palpebrarum. J Cosmet Dermatol. 2015;14(3):209-15.
9. Goel K, Sardana K, Garg VK. A prospective study comparing ultrapulse CO_2 laser and trichloroacetic acid in treatment of Xanthelasma palpebrarum. J Cosmet Dermatol. 2015;14(2):130-9.
10. Chun EY, Lee JB, Lee KH. Focal trichloroacetic acid peel method for benign pigmented lesions in dark-skinned patients. Dermatol Surg. 2004;30(4):512-6.

CHAPTER 40

Cryotherapy

Avitus John Prasad, Shruthi C

INTRODUCTION

Cryotherapy, also known as cryosurgery, is a commonly used in-office procedure for the treatment of a variety of benign and malignant lesions. The first clinical application of cryotherapy using liquid air (–190°C) was in 1889 by a New York City physician, Campbell White, who used either a swab, a spray, or a brass roller device.[1] By the 1940s, following World War II, liquid nitrogen (–196°C) became commercially available (Fig. 40.1).

In 1950 this cryogen was introduced into clinical practice by Dr. Ray Allington, who described the technique of using cotton swabs dipped in liquid nitrogen for the treatment of a variety of nonneoplastic skin diseases. Subsequently, this method became common practice for the treatment of verrucae, keratoses, and diverse other non-neoplastic lesions.[2] In 1961, Cooper and Lee,[3] introduced a closed-system apparatus to spray liquid nitrogen. In the late 1960s, metal probes became available. By 1990, 87% of dermatologists in the west used cryotherapy in their practice.[4] The general advantages of cryotherapy are its ease of use, low cost and good cosmetic results.

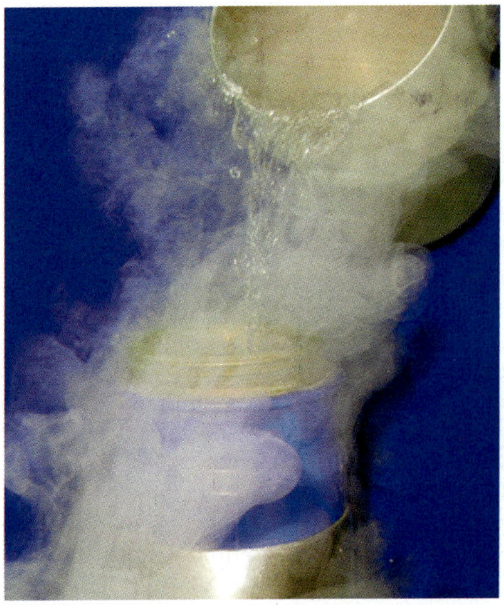

Fig. 40.1: Liquid nitrogen.

Though most skin cancers are treated with excision or other destructive procedures, such as electrodessication and curettage, superficial basal cell skin cancers,[5] and Bowen disease can be treated with cryotherapy. Recurrence rates for primary basal cell carcinoma vary with treatment modality. The 5-year recurrence rate for cryotherapy may be as low as 7.5%, if lesions are chosen judiciously.[6] Well-circumscribed lesions and tumors are most suitable for cryotherapy. The indolent local growth of these well-circumscribed tumors accounts for the high cure rates quoted in the literature.

After nearly two centuries, the technique of cryotherapy remains widely applicable. Even in the present era of lasers, cryotherapy should not be neglected and it has its place still in dermatosurgery.

INDICATIONS

- Idiopathic guttate hypomelanosis (IGH)
- Lentigo, freckles
- Dermatosis papulosa nigra, skin tags (acrocordons), pedunculated lesions
- Molluscum contagiosum
- Verrucae plana, verrucae vulgaris, plantar warts
- Seborrhoeic keratosis, actinic keratosis
- Cherry angioma, venous lake
- Fibromas
- Keloid
- Basal cell and squamous cell carcinomas.

MECHANISM OF ACTION

The mechanism of action in cryotherapy can be divided into 3 phases: (1) heat transfer (2) cell injury and (3) inflammation.

Heat Transfer

The mechanism by which cryotherapy destroys the targeted cells is the quick transfer of heat from the skin to a heat sink which in this case is liquid nitrogen which has a boiling point of –196°C. The rate of heat transfer is dependent on the temperature difference between the skin and the liquid nitrogen.

When using the spray cryotherapy technique, the liquid nitrogen is applied directly on the skin, and evaporation (boiling heat transfer) occurs in which the heat in the skin is quickly transferred to the liquid nitrogen. This process results in the liquid nitrogen evaporating (boiling) almost immediately.

Cell Injury

Cell injury occurs during the thaw, after the cell is frozen. Because of the hyperosmotic intracellular conditions, ice crystals do not form until –5°C to –10°C. The transformation of water to ice concentrates the extracellular solutes and results in an osmotic gradient across the cell membrane, causing further damage. Rapid freezing and slow thaw maximize tissue damage to epithelial cells and is most suitable for the treatment of malignancies. Fibroblasts produce less collagen after a rapid thaw.[7] Therefore, a rapid thaw may be more suitable for the treatment of keloids or benign lesions in areas prone to scarring.[8]

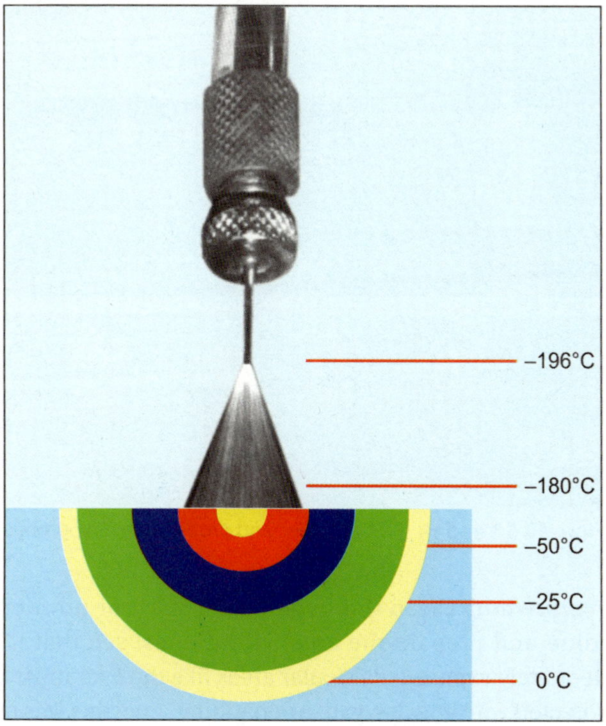

Fig. 40.2: Temperature zones in skin during cryotherapy.

Keratinocytes need to be frozen to –50°C for optimum destruction. Melanocytes are more delicate and are destroyed by temperatures as low as 5°C which often results in hypopigmentation following cryotherapy on darker-skinned individuals. Malignant skin cancers usually need a temperature of –50°C, while benign lesions only require a temperature of –20°C to –25°C.

As the liquid nitrogen is sprayed, the temperature increases from –196°C to 180°C when it touches the skin and there is drop in temperature of the skin or lesion being treated. Longer spray results in deeper freezing of tissue and more lateral spread occurs which determines the depth reached (Fig. 40.2).

Inflammation

The last response to cryotherapy is inflammation, which is usually observed as erythema and edema. Inflammation is the response to cell death and helps in local cell destruction.

A thorough cryotherapy treatment causes basement membrane separation, which may result in blister formation.

The commonly used cryogens and equipment include (Table 40.1):[9-11]

Out these, liquid nitrogen is the commonly used cryogen in dermatology practise.

CRYOSURGERY EQUIPMENT[9-11]

- *Cryogun/cryogen spray canister*: It's a specially designed portable, light weight, hand-held device to contain the liquid nitrogen. Liquid nitrogen is filled into the canister prior to treatment (Fig. 40.3)
- *Attachments*: Cryospray nozzle and sprays tips with different size opening to allow specified amount of spray of cryogen through it. A roller is used for contact cooling in treating acne vulgaris (Figs. 40.4 and 40.5)
- *Cryoprobes*: They are available in various shapes and sizes and get attached to the cryogen. As the

Table 40.1: Commonly used cryogens.

Cryogens which are used	*Boiling point*
Liquid nitrogen	–196°C
Nitrous oxide	–89°C
Solidified CO_2 (dry ice, CO_2 snow)	–78°C

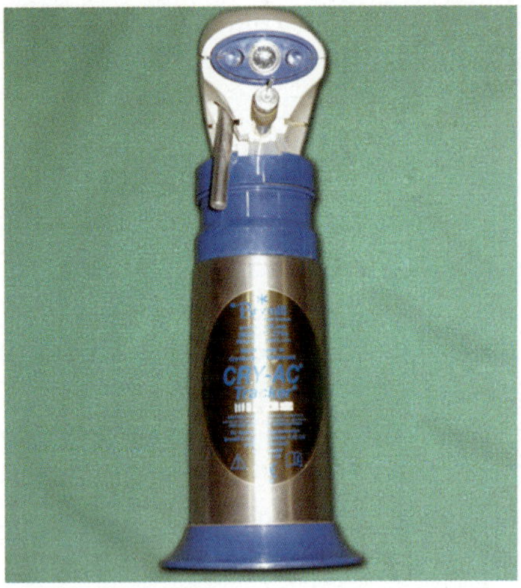

Fig. 40.3: Cryogun/cryogen spray canister.

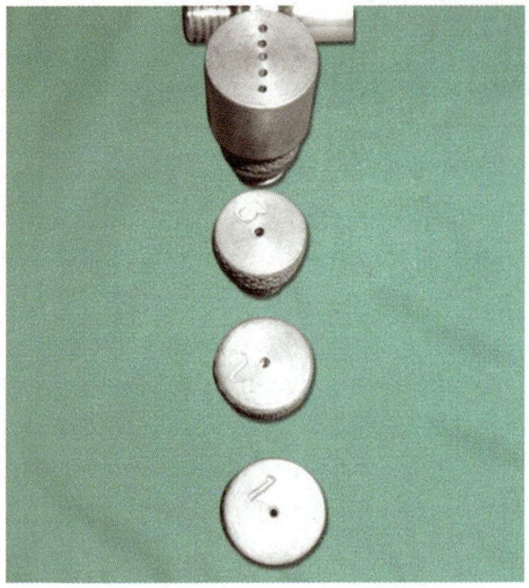

Fig. 40.4: Cryospray nozzles.

cryogen is sprayed through it, it cools and it is used in approximation to the lesion being treated. Cryoprobes are used as a conduit to transfer the temperature.

- *Cryogen storage device*: They are metal cylinders/containers that store gaseous cryogens as compressed gas and have an inbuilt internal pressure equalization mechanism, e.g. Dewar's gas container. The stored liquid nitrogen evaporates with time. The size of the tank determines how long it can contain the cryogen: usually a tank of 7 to 10 liters will hold liquid nitrogen for a week to 10 days before complete evaporation but a 35 liters tank can hold for almost 100–120 days (Fig. 40.6). The cryogen is transferred to the cryogun before the procedure by a siphon provided with the tank or by tilting the container to pour the cryogen into the gun via a funnel. Care must be taken by the operator while pouring the cryogen into the canister. Insulated gloves must be worn while transferring the cryogen.

CRYOTHERAPY PROTOCOL[12]

History taking and examination: A detailed history of the condition, its evolution, aggravating factors and previous treatment history should be taken. Patients who are sensitive to cold, history of cold urticaria, Raynaud's phenomenon or vascular insufficiency may be recorded. Physical examination taking into account the size, margin, location, depth of lesion, history of keloidal tendencies should all be recorded.

Counseling and consent: A written informed consent is obtained from the patient after explaining the procedure, the achievable results, recurrence rate and various complications of the procedure.

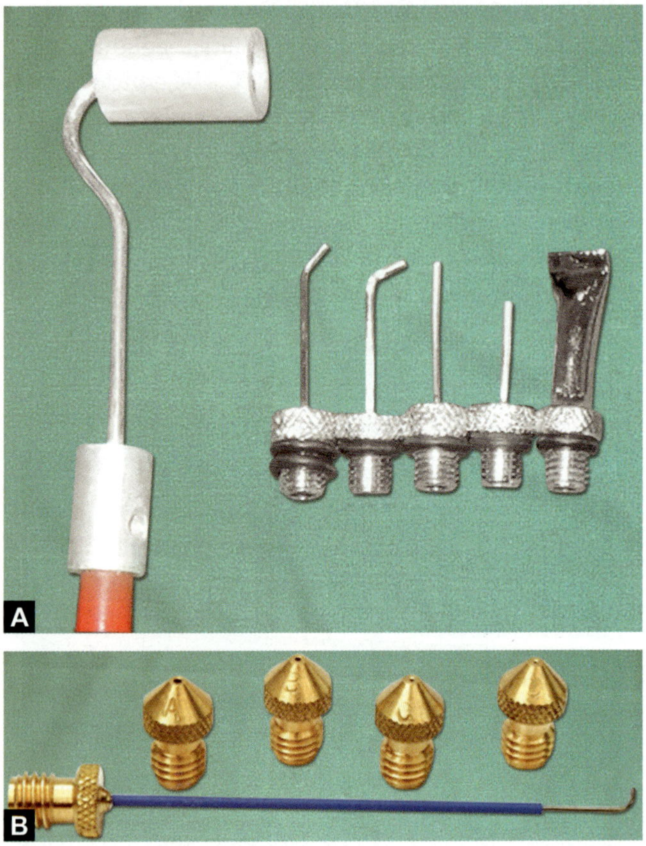

Figs. 40.5A and B: (A) Cryoroller and probes. (B) Cryoprobes.

Preprocedure: Clean thoroughly with spirit or povidone iodine and prepare the area with drapes: see that it is adequately exposed. Particular areas like the eyes must be protected with goggles, gauze or padding. Anesthesia is not required as pain is an indicator to control the amount of

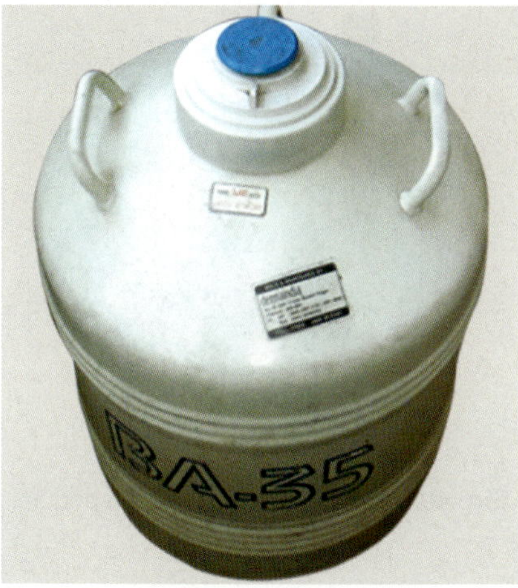

Fig. 40.6: Dewar can.

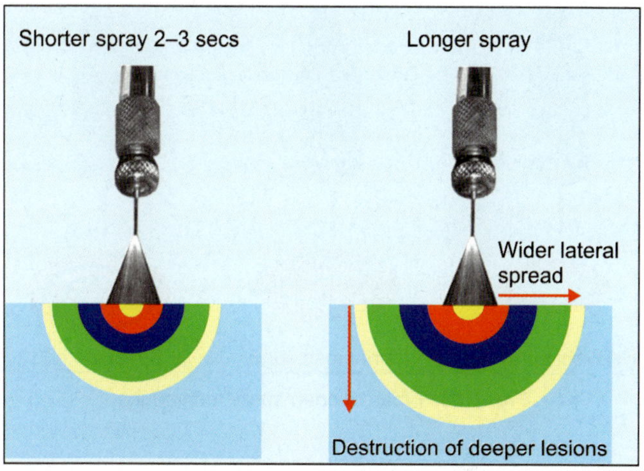

Fig. 40.7: Demonstration of lateral spread vs duration of spray.

cryospray. Intralesional anesthesia might be required when freezing larger lesions like BCC or keloid. Vocal anesthesia is enough to assure the patient and minimize the discomfort.

TREATMENT MODALITIES USING CRYOTHERAPY

Various methods have been devised in the use of cryotherapy of lesions. They include the spray freeze technique, the applicator technique, and the cryoprobe method.

Spray Freeze Technique: Timed Freeze Thaw Method

Assess the lesion: Surgical paring using 15 or 11 blade or by curettage facilitates the destruction of certain lesions like verrucae vulgaris. The cryogen is directly sprayed onto the lesion through an appropriate sized nozzle, which is chosen according to the size of the lesion. The cryogen is sprayed in the center of the lesion holding the spray tip or nozzle at least 1-2 cm away from the lesion until the desired margin is reached which encircles the whole lesion. A freeze thaw cycle is done by spraying for an adequate duration (holding time) after which the lesion is allowed to thaw to complete one freeze thaw cycle. Complete thawing is suggested by the disappearance of the frozen-white surface. For larger lesions (> 2 cm in diameter), treat separately with overlapping margins covering different parts of the lesion in the same session. In case of malignant lesions, the lateral spread of freeze should extend at least 2 mm beyond the margin in a benign lesion and 5 mm or more for adequate results (Fig. 40.7).

Freeze technique can be carried out in two ways:

- *Open spray (Fig. 40.8)*: Used when treating larger lesions like Keloids, SCC, BCC:
  - *Direct spray method*: The lesion is treated by a vertical spray technique without moving. This method is mostly used when treating well-circumscribed lesion.
  - *Paint brush method*: The lesion is treated by spraying from one side of the lesion and moving up and down across the lesion.
  - *Spiral method*: The cryogen is sprayed initially in the center of the lesion and is then moved outward in concentric circles.
- *Closed or confined spray*:[13] This technique is used in round, small, discrete lesions like verrucae, fibroma, IGH and cherry angiomas or those close to vital structures. For large, irregularly shaped lesions, sequential freezing is necessary. In this, the use of neoprene or polystyrene cones helps to confine the range of spray within the lesional area preventing damage to surrounding areas.

To concentrate the freezing and to prevent disease communication (especially in this era of conditions, such as HIV disease or hepatitis), disposable cones can be used to concentrate the liquid nitrogen. Disposable otoscope specula (Fig. 40.9) which can be bought online can be trimmed to make the aperture larger, or an angle can be cut to make a fusiform shape for oval lesions. Disposable specula come in a variety of sizes, ranging from 2.5-9 mm.[14]

The nozzle tip of the spray gun is kept on the wide opening of the cone and the narrowed opening of the cone is kept on the lesion to be treated, and liquid nitrogen is

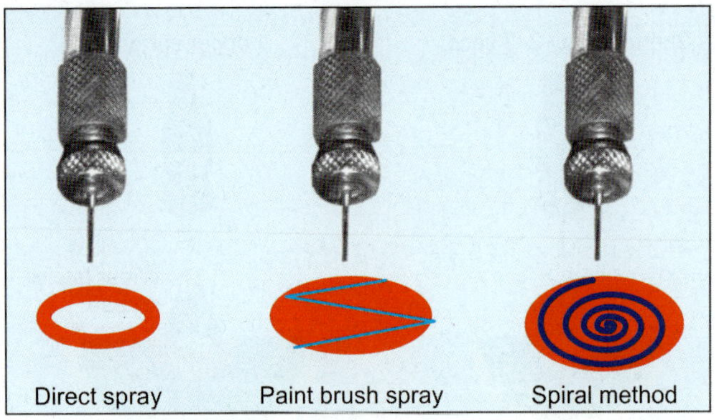

Fig. 40.8: Types of open spray techniques.

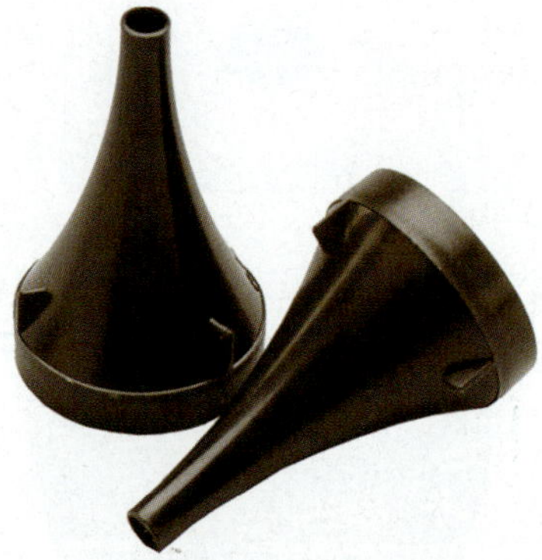

Fig. 40.9: Disposable otoscope specula.

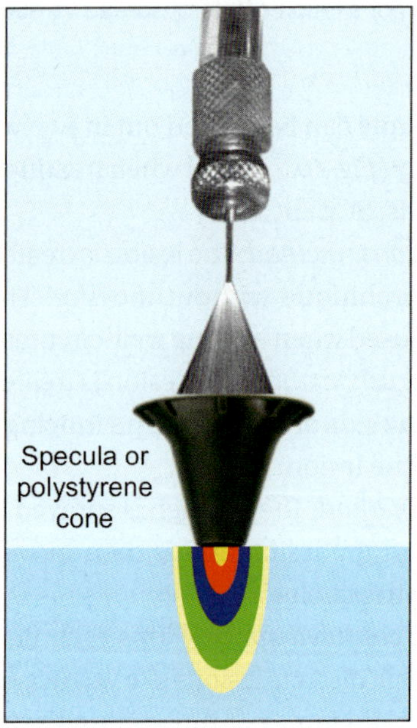

Fig. 40.10: Spray through disposable otoscope specula.

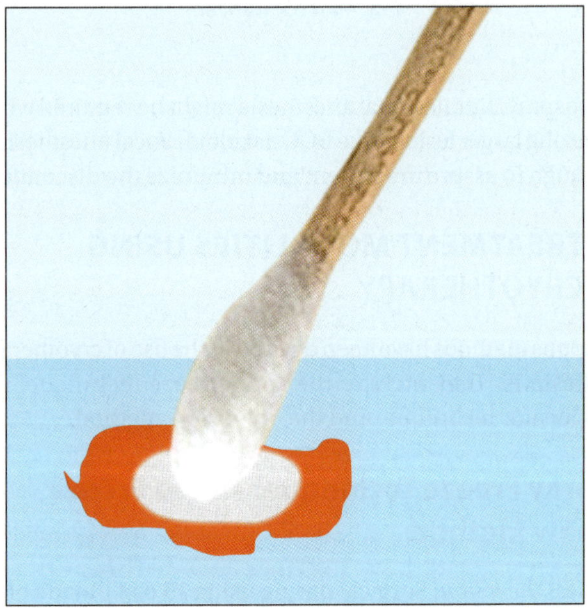

Fig. 40.11: Dipstick application method.

sprayed on the lesion through the cone. The time for which the lesion is frozen is the freeze time which is different for different lesions. This freeze-thaw cycle can be repeated, depending on the type of lesion being treated (Fig. 40.10).

TIP: The use of autoclavable cones, available with the microdermabrasion equipment can be a good substitute.

Dipstick Applicator Method[15]

The dipstick applicator method is the original method used to apply liquid nitrogen to lesions. A cotton-tipped applicator is dipped into liquid nitrogen. The dipstick applicator is then firmly pressed against the lesion delivering the cryo for the desired duration (Fig. 40.11).

The size of the bud should be smaller than the lesion. The depth of freeze can be increased by applying pressure on the lesion. Lower temperatures cannot be achieved in the dipstick applicator method as they are in the spray technique; therefore, this method is suitable only for benign and superficial lesions, e.g. freckles, verrucae plana, IGH.

Forceps Technique[16]

The use of forceps or straight artery forceps to dip into liquid nitrogen and then clamp the lesion for 15 seconds will effectively deliver the cryo to achieve the temperature needed for the destruction of the treated lesion. Brymill has special cryo tweezers for effective delivery of the cryogen (Fig. 40.12A). It can be repeated twice for larger lesions. This technique is used mostly in pedunculated lesions.

Cryoprobe Technique

Manufacturers of cryo equipments have devised various metal attachments to serve as heat-conducting probes for cryotherapy. Copper, because of its high conductivity, is typically used (Fig. 40.12B).

A thin film of white petrolatum can be applied to the treatment site, and the cryoprobe is attached to the cryogun nozzle and is firmly pressed against the lesion and the liquid nitrogen is passed.

While the cooling is occurring, the lesion gets attached to the probe, which should be raised above the surrounding normal skin by few millimeters to prevent damage to the surrounding skin.[12] Once the lesion is frozen, it is allowed to thaw. The probe should be allowed to release spontaneously from the lesion during the thawing process and must not be pulled earlier. In this technique, a longer freezing time is required as compared with the open spray technique. This technique is preferred in vascular lesions because direct application of the cryoprobe blanches the lesion and reduces the lesional temperature thus increasing the depth of the freeze. Many practitioners do not use the probe because it is cumbersome and time consuming.

Intralesional Cryotherapy

This technique is used when treating larger lesions like keloids. After obtaining adequate local anesthesia of the surgical site, the probe or large bore needle is inserted into the keloid scar by a gradual twisting motion until it penetrates the opposite end (Fig. 40.12C). A liquid nitrogen source is attached to the proximal end of the probe or needle and the gas is passed through the needle until the keloid is sufficiently frozen by visual inspection, which typically takes 10 to 60 minutes, depending on scar volume. After allowing the scar to thaw for approximately 60 seconds, the probe is gently removed and the surgical site is dressed with an antibiotic ointment and sterile gauze.

INNOVATION IN CRYOTHERAPY

Use of Microdermabrasion Tips as a Substitute for Specula

Various nozzle sizes are available in the microderm tips (Fig. 40.13). First the size of the lesion is determined. In case of plantar warts, surgical paring of the wart helps to determine the actual size of the wart. The microderm tip is kept and firmly pressed against the lesion and the liquid nitrogen is sprayed into it with the use of the canister. Depending on the lesion, the freeze time is undertaken with 2 or 3 freeze thaw cycles. The tip gets frozen and is attached to the lesion; wait till it falls off on its own. This is repeated for the other lesions (Figs. 40.14A to D). The cones are easily autoclavable making it a good alternative to disposable cones.

Modification in the Treatment of Pedunculated Lesions

Freezing the pedicle, rather than the whole lesion helps in lesser pain and faster healing (Figs. 40.15A and B). In case the whole pedunculated lesions need to be done, use a toothed forceps and pull the lesion away from the normal skin and spray. This prevents unwanted exposure of normal skin to the cryogen leading to ulceration and longer healing time (Figs. 40.16A and B).

Targeted Cryotherapy

An innovative technique devised by the author using biopsy punches ensures deeper delivery of cryo compared to the plastic cone method.

The metal cutting edge of the punch enters deeper into the lesions as the cryo is passed, sparing damage to surrounding skin.

What is unique about the use of punches is that it not only prevents lateral spread but as the cryo passes through the punch; the punch starts to sink into the lesion delivering the cryo to deeper parts of the lesion which is not possible with any other method.

Instruments

- Punches of different sizes cut to half its length (Fig. 40.17)
- Test tube holder (Fig. 40.18)
- Cryo spray can and liquid nitrogen
- Gauze
- Surgical blade 15 with blade holder for paring in case of warts.

Procedure

In case of verrucae, paring is done to reduce the thickness of the lesion and determine the size of lesion which in turns helps in deciding the size of punch which needs to be used. For all other cryo treatable conditions paring is not done. The punch is cut to half the length, the plastic part is covered

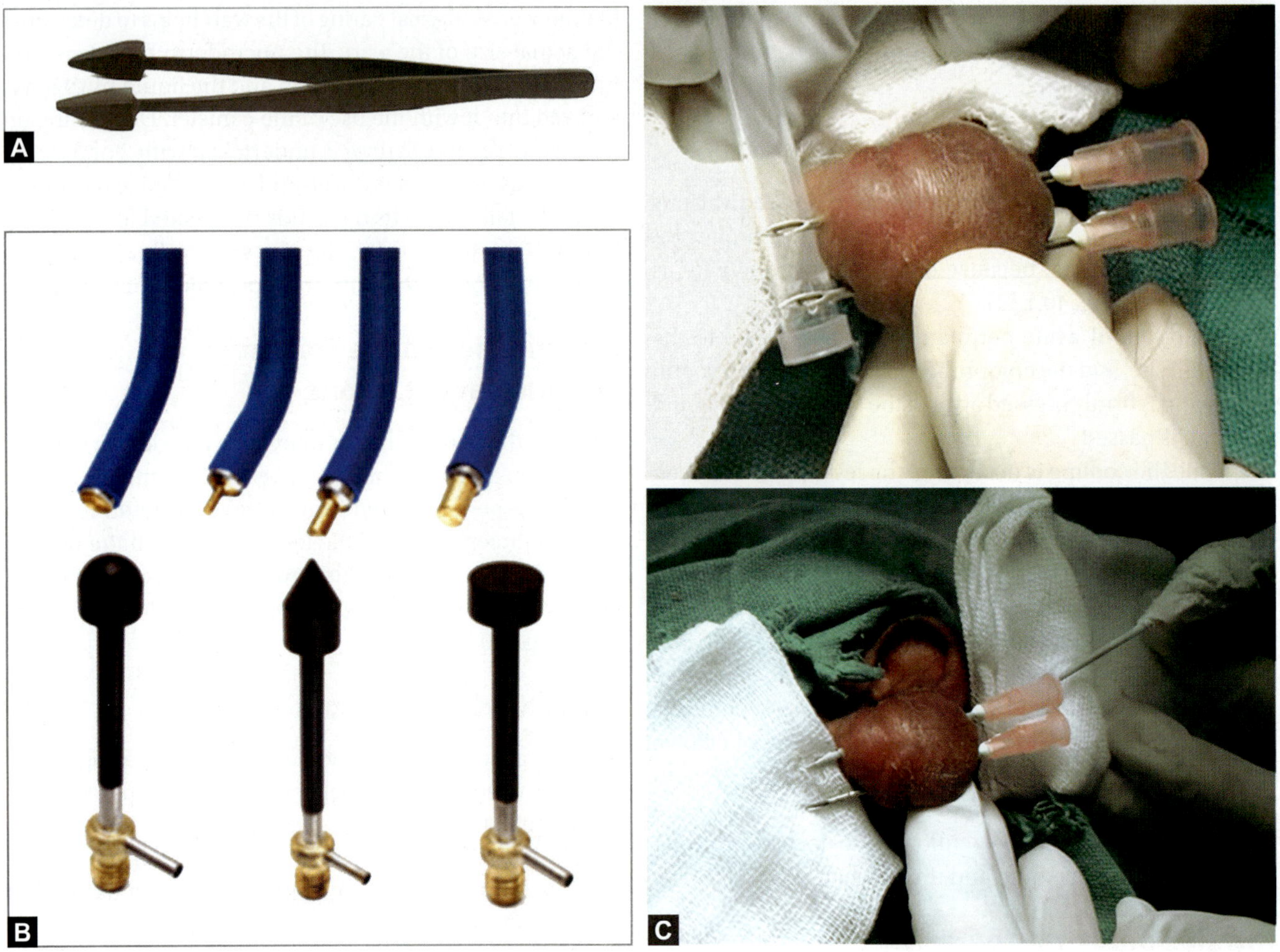

Figs. 40.12A to C: (A) Cryo forceps. (B) Metal attachments. (C) Intralesional cryotherapy.
Courtesy: Dr Kusuma MR.

with gauze and a test tube holder is used to grip it in case of smaller punches (Figs. 40.19A and B). Holding the punch with the fingers when cryo is being passed is not possible, it's very painful and can cause blisters in the fingers of the person performing the procedure.

The punch is kept on the lesion with slight pressure on the lesion, so that there is no gap between the punch metal tip and the skin. If gap is present then the cryo would seep into the normal skin which would defeat the purpose of using the punch (Fig. 40.20).

The cryo can filled with liquid nitrogen is used, the nozzle is kept on the top end of the punch. Note that when you cut the punch, make it smooth and flat, so that the nozzle sits perfectly on it. The liquid nitrogen is passed and as the cryo touches the lesion through the punch, the metal tip of the punch also get cooled which starts to enter slowly,

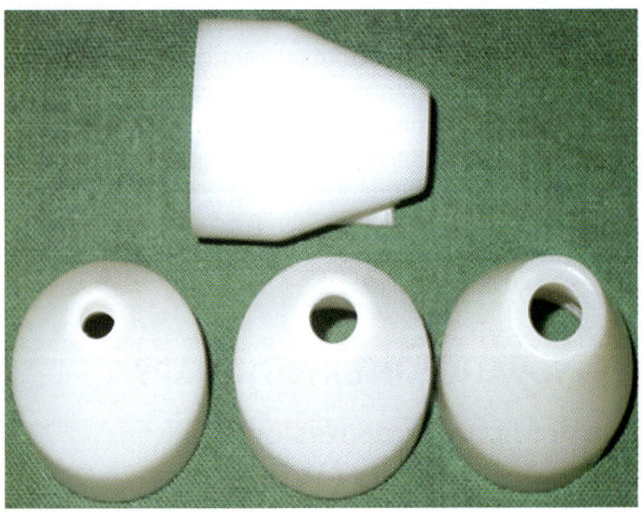

Fig. 40.13: Microdermabrasion tips.

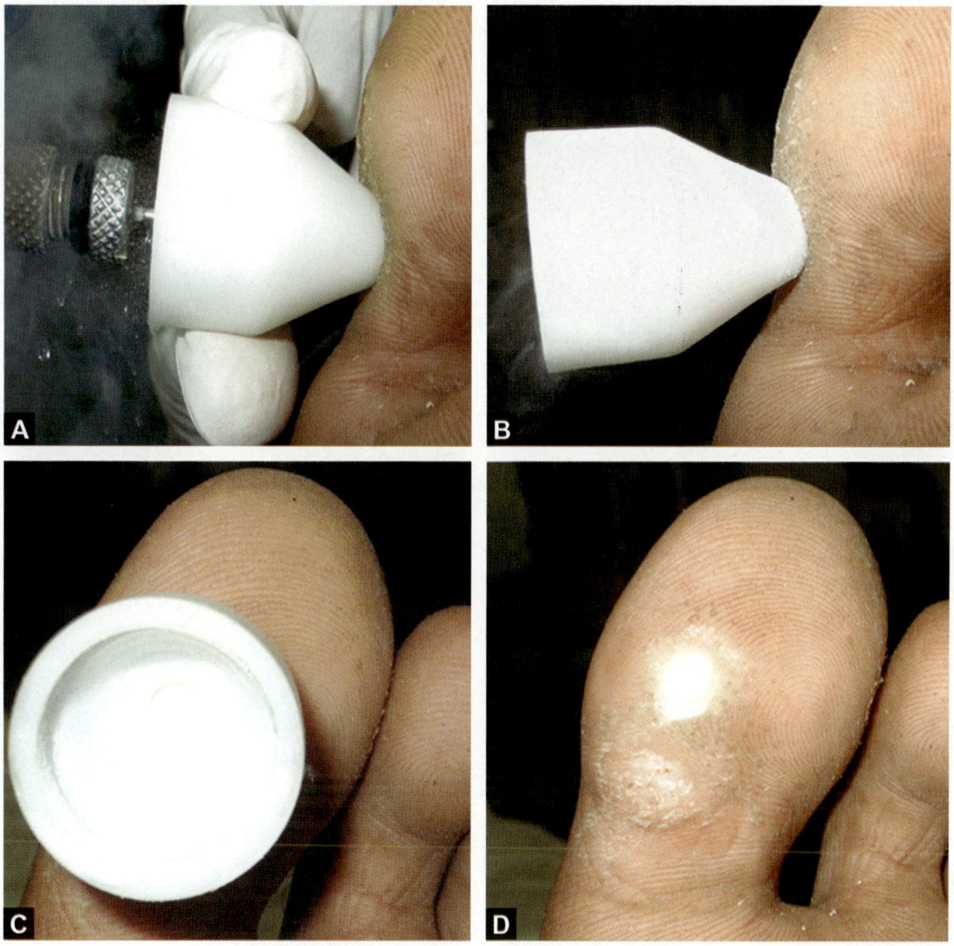

Figs. 40.14A to D: Steps of microdermabrasion.

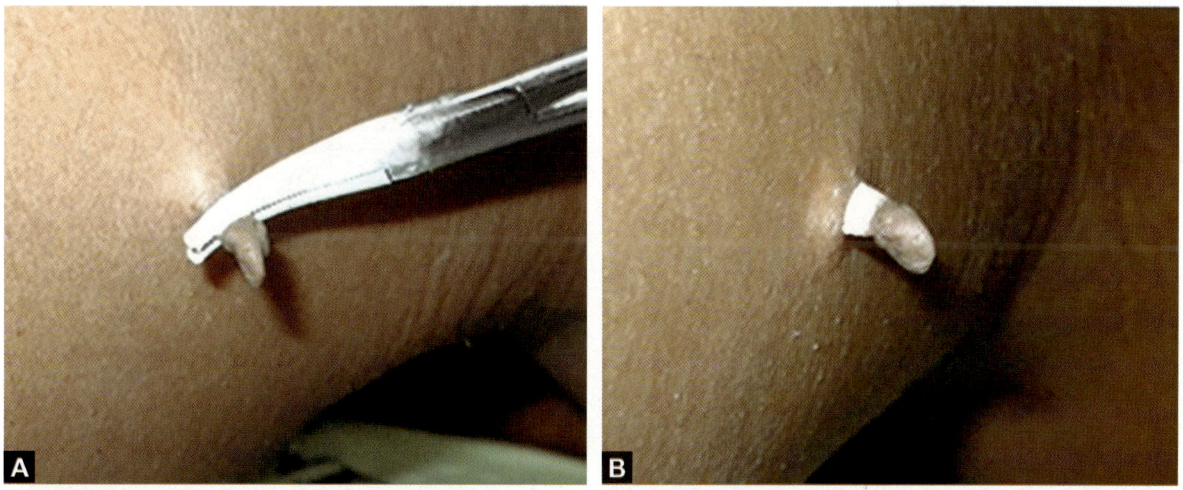

Figs. 40.15A and B: Cryotherapy for pedunculated lesion by freezing the base.

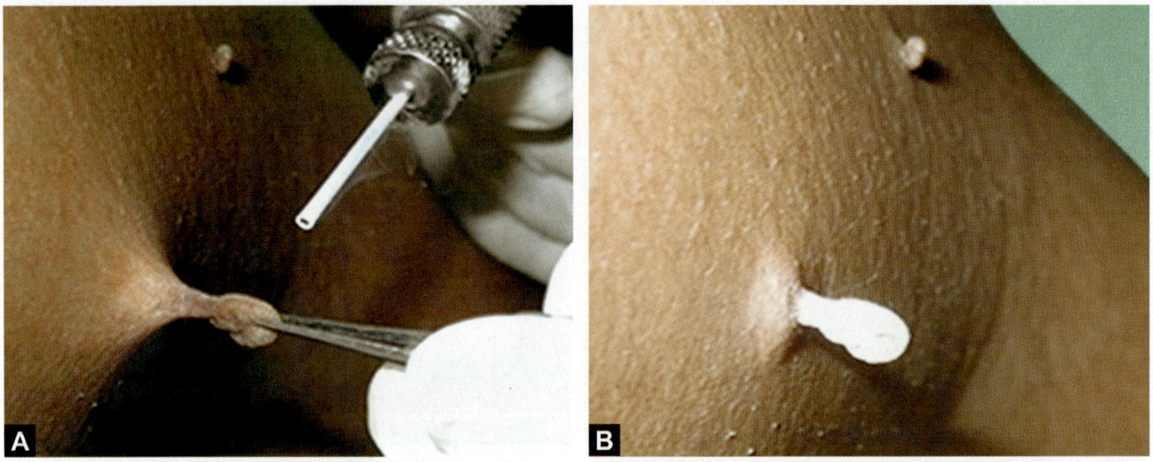

Figs. 40.16A and B: Cryotherapy for pedunculated lesion using toothed forceps.

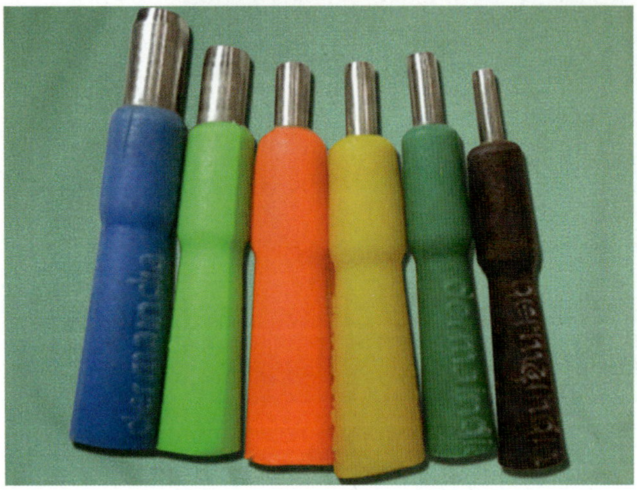

Fig. 40.17: Half cut biopsy punches.

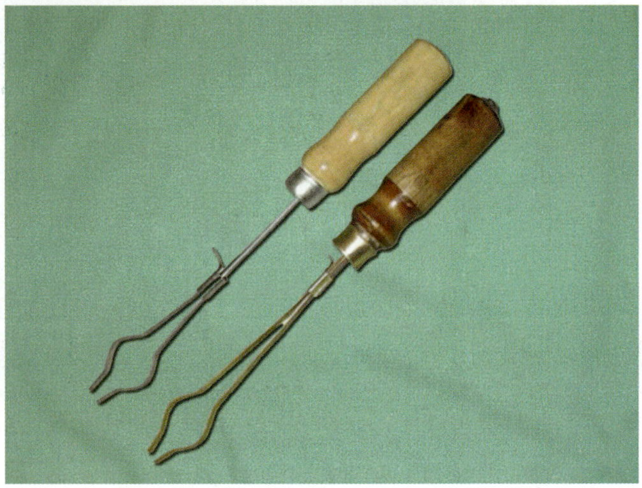

Fig. 40.18: Test tube holders.

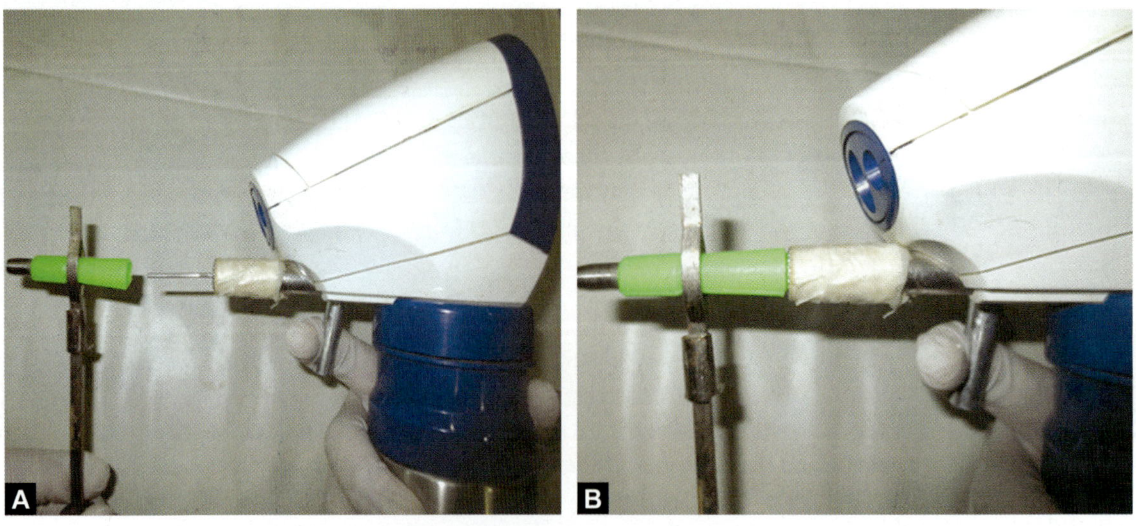

Figs. 40.19A and B: Cryospray through the punches held by test tube holder.

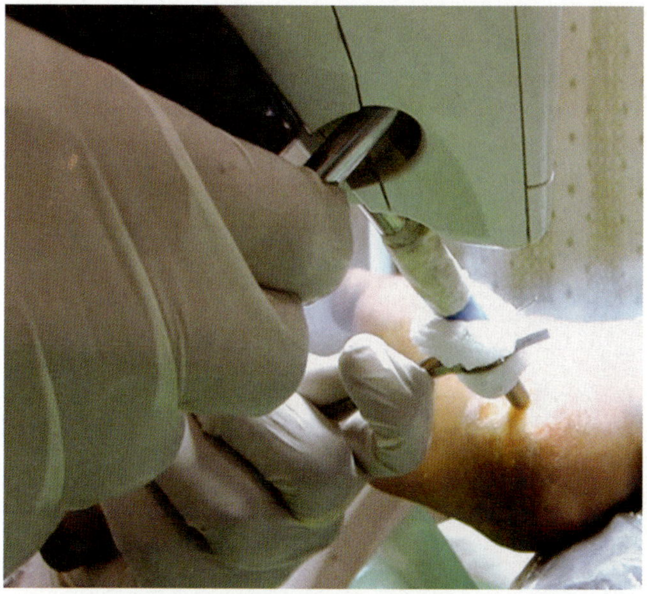

Fig. 40.20: Biopsy punch held firmly on the skin.

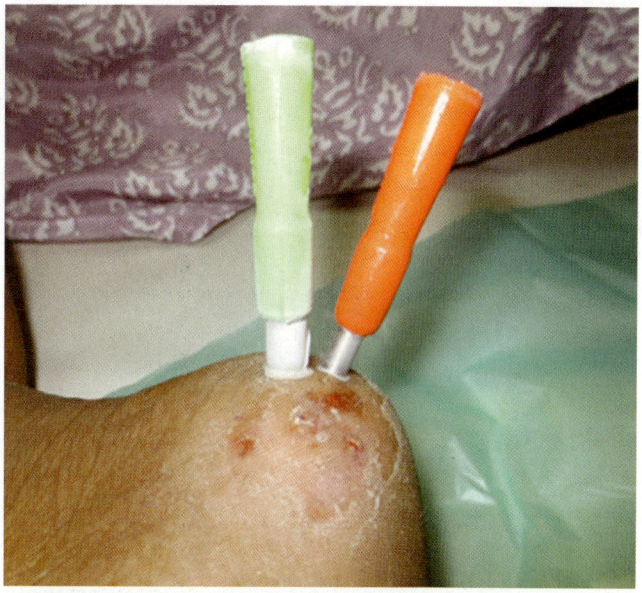

Fig. 40.21: Punches being remained over lesion after cryotherapy.

sinking into the lesion. Cryo is done till the beveled edge of the punch enters the skin in case of warts, since we need to reach up to the basal layer whereas in other conditions deeper cryo is needed. This helps in deeper delivery of the cryo and effective damage to the unwanted tissue. The punch need not be rotated to cut into the lesion, rather the effect of cooling itself makes the punch cold cut into the lesion.

The punches remain embedded after the cryo (Fig. 40.21), and they are left to fall off on their own. The punches fall off in 10 to 20 seconds depending on depth reached. The next punch can be placed adjacent to warts and the process is repeated. Depending on the lesions, the procedure can be performed two or three times on the same lesion.

The procedure is repeated after 3 weeks. Paring is done again before the next session of cryo to assess, if there is any wart tissue remaining and this time smaller punches are used to treat (Figs. 40.22A and B).

Normally, if depth has to be achieved for example in keloids,[17] the spray of cryo is done on a larger area surrounding the lesion and with longer duration of spray, But this results in severe collateral damage to normal skin resulting in large blisters and pain. But with this method the cryo can be sprayed longer, with no damage to surrounding normal tissue. This technique is useful even in larger lesions like keloid where it can be sprayed into multiple areas but lessening the pain and damage to the tissue.

Postprocedure

No dressing is required. Pain killers and anti-inflammatory drugs can be prescribed. In case, if blisters occurs (minimal chances), the fluid collected can be expressed out with a needle or syringe.

Indications in which Targeted Cryotherapy is Used

- Verrucae on plantar and palmar areas
- Dermatofibroma
- Pyogenic granuloma
- Keloid and hypertrophic scars
- Nevi.

Advantages of Targeted Cryotherapy

- Targeted damage to the unwanted tissue, sparing collateral damage to the surrounding skin.
- Reduce the blistering reaction.
- Lower incidence of hemorrhagic blisters.
- Comparatively less pain due to reduction in area traumatized.
- Deeper delivery of the cryo is possible by use of punches which slides deeper into the lesions as the cryo is being performed.
- As the cryo reaches the depth, it loses optimal temperature in normal cryotherapy method which is eliminated with this novel method.

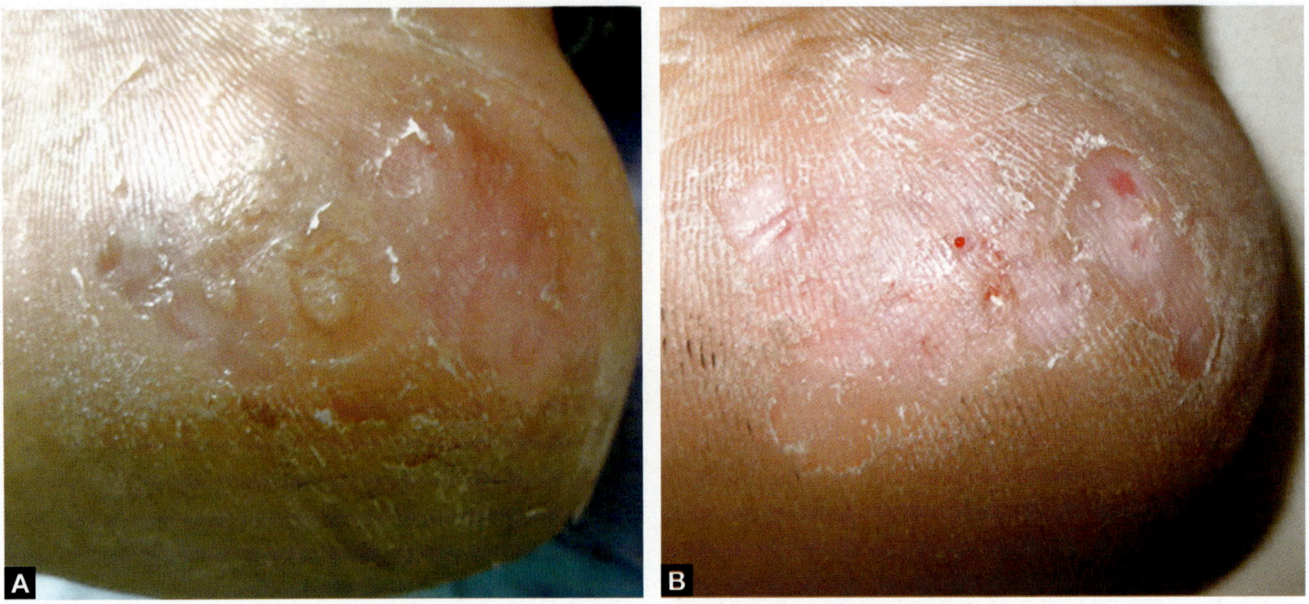

Figs. 40.22A and B: Paring prior to next session (before and after).

- The chances of recurrence are very less compared to normal cryotherapy technique because of the deeper delivery of cryotherapy to the lesion.

CASE HANDLING

Case 1 (Figs. 40.23A to D)

Patient had a visited a surgeon for a growth on the fifth toe of the left foot, the surgeon had excised the lesion which turned out to verrucae. But there was considerable damage to the periostium of the distal phalange and reoccurrence of the verrucous lesion. On examination it was diagnosed as verrucae but a biopsy was sent to rule out any malignant change. As the biopsy report confirmed the diagnosis of verrucae vulgaris, cryotherapy was done using the spiral open spray method. Patient improved after 5 sessions of cryo every 4 weeks. Once there was no evidence of verrucae, the patient was sent to an orthopedician because there was exposed damaged periostium.

Case 2 (Figs. 40.24A and B)

A 28-year-old male presented with verrucae filiformis of the glans penis since 6 months.

Cryotherapy was initiated after relevant blood tests. Dipstick method was employed in this case; 3 sessions of cryo was done once in 3 weeks. Complete clearance was seen.

It is best to treat mucosal lesions using dipstick method because the freezing is quicker and prevents unwanted damage to normal mucosa (which can happen when using spray technique which might lead to delayed healing).

COMPLICATIONS OF CRYOTHERAPY

There are common complications which are part of the treatment and there are complications associated with inappropriate patient selection, duration of freezing and number of freeze thaw cycles undertaken.[12,18 19]

Immediate Complications

- Local pain-more in the periungual area and when treating the face.
- Edema, especially on the eyelids, lips, labia and prepuce, more in infants and the elderly.
- Syncope (vasovagal shock) in anxious patients, a very common occurrence in the OT which the operator and assistant should be able to handle.
- Urticaria like wheals can occur in few patients, which is should not be confused with cold urticaria.

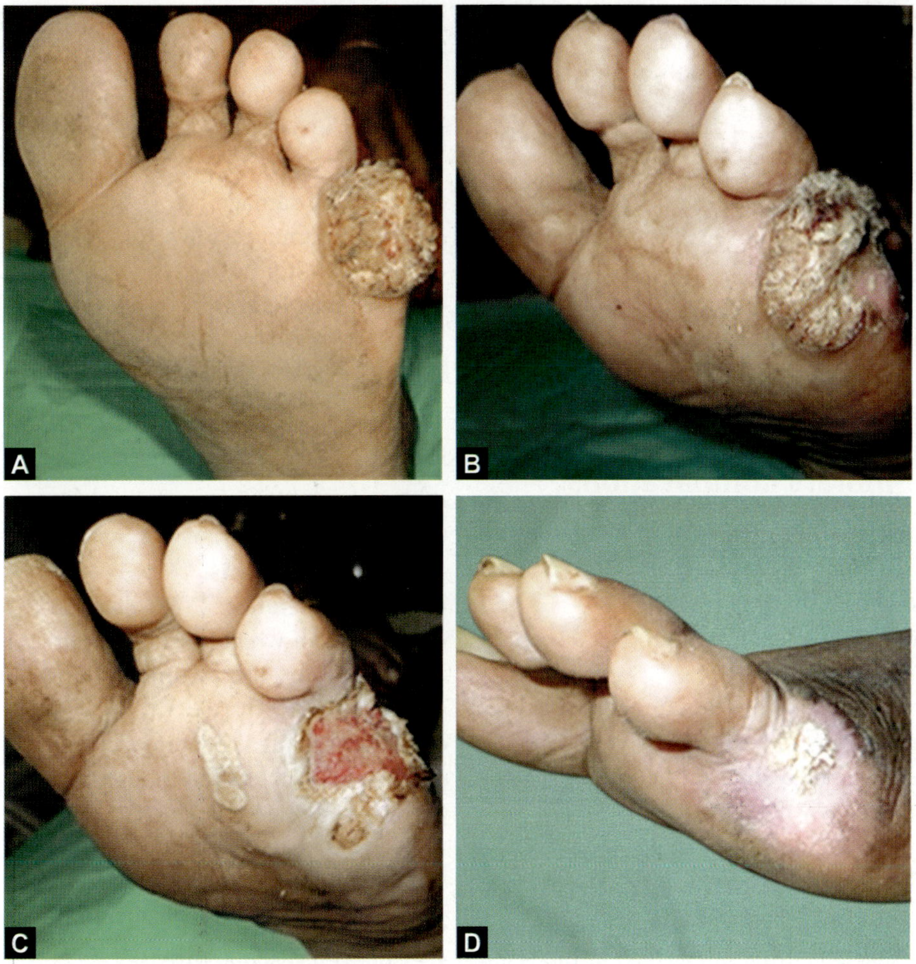

Figs. 40.23A to D: Verrucae over little toe response after 5 sessions of cryo every 4 weeks.

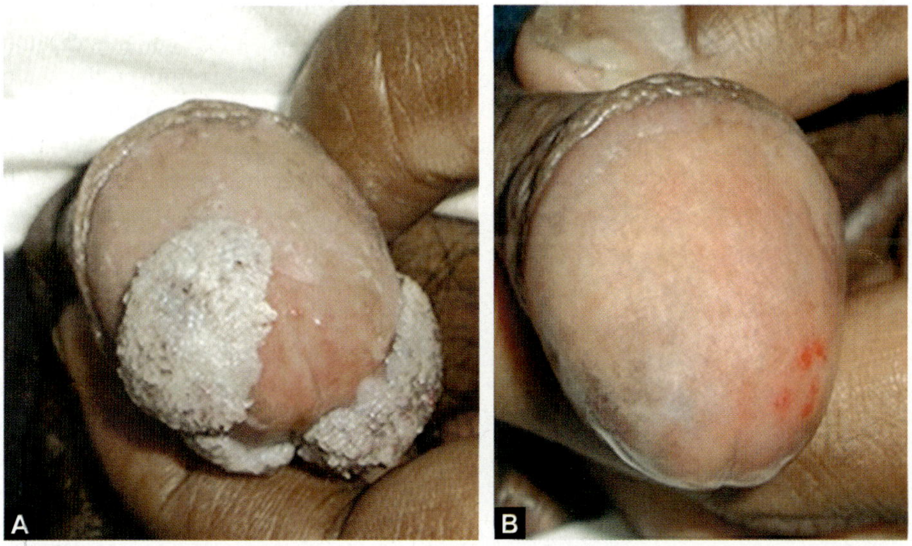

Figs. 40.24A and B: Cryotherapy for verrucae over glans penis before and after 3 sessions of cryotherapy done once in 3 weeks.

Temporary Complications

- Tingling and numbness, especially when treating verrucae on the fingers.
- Headache (migraine type) after the treatment of the head and neck area.
- Cryoblister formation (Fig. 40.25A).
- Hemorrhagic necrosis (Fig. 40.25B).
- Subcutaneous emphysema—a rare complication seen in older patients with compromised skin or in patients with broken skin. Seen when treating venous lakes in the lip. It can follow intralesional cryotherapy when needles are used into the lesions like keloids for deep cryotherapy.[20]

Prolonged-temporary Complications

- Delayed wound healing after treatment over the extremities.
- Temporary scar hypertrophy.
- Excessive granulation tissue formation.
- Milia formation.
- Local hypoesthesia due to nerve damage, especially in areas where the nerves lie superficially, such as the sides of fingers, angle of jaw, postauricular area, sides of tongue and ulnar fossa of elbow.

Permanent Complications

- Atrophic scar, which occurs when freezing time is >30 s.
- Cicatricial alopecia when treating lesions in the scalp and when longer duration of freeze time in excess of 30 seconds is employed.
- Scarring.
- Hypopigmentation, especially in dark-skinned individuals, which can be minimized by freezing for <30 s. In case it occurs, PUVA soaks helps in regaining the pigmentation.

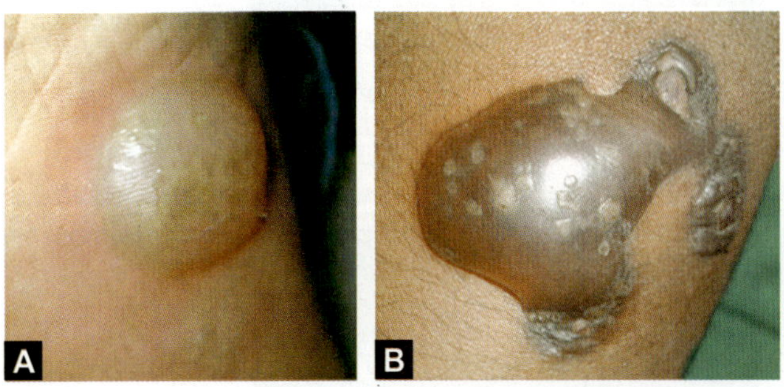

Figs. 40.25A and B: Cryoblisters and hemorrhagic necrosis respectively.

- Damage to periosteum when treating lesions on bony prominences like the distal digits, mandible with longer freeze times.

Uncommon Complications

- Cartilage damage.
- Pseudotumor recidiva.
- Fibroxanthoma.
- Traumatic neuroma.

CONTRAINDICATIONS TO CRYOTHERAPY

Absolute

- Raynaud's disease.
- Cold urticaria.
- Cryoglobulinemia.
- Cold intolerance.
- Lesions in which tissue pathology is required before cryosurgery like Actinic/seborrhoeic keratosis, BCC, SCC.
- Lesions in areas of compromised circulation.
- Skin tumors located in high-risk areas like the temple or nasolabial folds.

Relative

- Keloidal tendency.
- Collagen vascular diseases.
- Pyoderma gangrenosum.
- Dark-skinned individuals due to the high risk of developing cosmetically inacceptable protracted hypopigmentation.
- Impaired sensation: patients cannot report when they become anesthetic from cold.
- Impaired circulation: tissue damage may result from vasoconstriction.
- Lesions over the nasolabial fold, eyelid margins, ala nasi and hair-bearing areas (high risk of developing alopecia, especially cicatricial alopecia).
- Melanoma.
- Cardiac conditions: Angina pectoris, arrhythmia, myocardial infarction: for 6 months after MI, cryotherapy should be avoided. The initial shock of the ice application may cause a marked drop in blood pressure, thus causing an increase in heart attack rate.
- Common dermatological conditions where cryosurgery is useful along with parameters used for treatment is provided in Table 40.2.

Table 40.2: Common dermatological conditions in a dermatosurgery clinic where cryotherapy will be useful.

Dermatological condition	*Technique used*	*Freeze time*	*FT cycle*	*Number of sessions*
Verrucae plana and verrucae filiformis in mucosa	Dipstick	3–5 secs	1–2	1–2
Verrucae filiformis	Forceps	5–6 secs	1–2	1–2
Verrucae vulgaris	Cone assisted spray	5–10 secs depending on size	2–3	2
Verrucae in palms and soles	Targeted cryotherapy	5–10 secs depending on size	2–3	2–3
Condyloma acuminata	Open paint spray method	5–10 secs	1–2	2–3
IGH	Dipstick	3–5 secs	1	1–2
DPN	Dipstick	3–5 secs	1	1–2
Cherry angioma	Cone assisted spray	5–10 secs depending on size	1–2	1–2
Pedunculated lesions	Forceps/open spray	5–10 secs	1–2	1–2
Keloids and large lesions	Targeted cryotherapy, paint spray method, intralesional	5–15 secs depending on method employed	3–5	4–6
BCC, superficial SCC, Bowen's disease	Paint spray method 5 mm beyond margin in case of BCC	20–30 secs	2–3	2–3

(FT: Freeze thaw).

REFERENCES

1. White AC. Liquid air: its application in medicine and surgery. Med. Rec. 1899;56:109-12
2. Allington HV. Liquid nitrogen in treatment of skin diseases. Calif Med. 1950;72:153-5.
3. Cooper IS, Lee AS. Cryostatic congelation: a system for producing a limited, controlled region of cooling or freezing of biologic tissues. J Nerv Ment Dis. 1961;133:259-63.
4. Freiman A, Bouganim N. History of cryotherapy. Dermatol Online J. 2005;11(2):9.
5. Menesi W, Buchel EW, Hayakawa TJ. A reliable frozen section technique for basal cell carcinomas of the head and neck. Can J Plast Surg. 2014;22(3):179-82.
6. Kuflik EG, Gage AA. The five-year cure rate achieved by cryosurgery for skin cancer. J Am Acad Dermatol. 1991;24 (6 Pt 1):1002-4.
7. Guan H, Zhao Z, He F, et al. The effects of different thawing temperatures on morphology and collagen metabolism of -20°C dealt normal human fibroblast. Cryobiology. 2007;55(1):52-9.
8. van Leeuwen MC, Bulstra AE, van Leeuwen PA, et al. A new argon gas-based device for the treatment of keloid scars with the use of intralesional cryotherapy. J Plast Reconstr Aesthet Surg. 2014;67(12):1703-10.
9. Drake LA, Ceilley RI, Cornelison RL. Guidelines for care for cryosurgery. J Am Acad Dermatol. 1994;31:648-53.
10. Kuflik EG. Cryosurgery updated. J Am Acad Dermatol. 1994;31:925-44.
11. Graham GF. Cryosurgery. Clin Plast Surg. 1993;20:131-47.
12. Sharma VK, Khandpur S. Guidelines for cryotherapy. Indian J Dermatol Venereol Leprol. 2009;75:90-100.
13. Torre D. Cryosurgical treatment of epitheliomas using the cone-spray technique. J Dermatol Surg Oncol. 1977;3(4):432-6.
14. Kuwahara RT, Rasberry RD, Amonette RA. Use of disposable otoscope specula in cryotherapy. Dermatol Surg. 2000; 26(5):493-4.
15. Orengo I, Salasche SJ. Surgical pearl: the cotton-tipped applicator—the ever-ready, multipurpose superstar. J Am Acad Dermatol. 1994;31(4):658-60.
16. Kuwahara RT, Huber JD, Ray SH. Surgical pearl: forceps method for freezing benign lesion. J Am Acad Dermatol. 2000;43(2 Pt 1):306-7.
17. Zouboulis CC, Blume U, Buttner P, et al. Outcomes of cryosurgery in keloids and hypertrophic scars. A prospective consecutive trial of case series. Arch Dermatol. 1993;129:1146-51.
18. Elton RF. Complications of cutaneous cryosurgery. J Am Acad Dermatol. 1983;8:513-9.
19. Dawber RP. Cryosurgery: complications and contraindications. Clin Dermatol. 1991;8:96-100.
20. Martínez-Coronado J, Torres-Álvarez B, Castanedo-Cázares JP. Subcutaneous emphysema induced by cryotherapy: a complication due to previous punctures. Case Rep Dermatol Medi 2015;2015:374817.

CHAPTER 41

Radiofrequency and Electrocautery

Bipin Deshpande

INTRODUCTION

"Dermatosurgery today needs to be not just therapeutic, but 'aesthetically pleasing', whichever may be the area of body; because skin represents the surface where looks matter more than life".

Radiofrequency technique has now become an established treatment modality for surgical and nonsurgical applications in dermatologic surgery as well as in aesthetic dermatology for office and hospital-based practice.

Radiofrequency surgical modality is a 'modern electrosurgery', where all the basic needs of 'skin surgery' like 'fine cut', 'minimal tissue destruction', 'minimal intraoperative bleeding', 'faster postoperative healing' are fulfilled satisfactorily. Moreover, radiofrequency scores over older modalities of 'electrocautery' and contemporary 'ablative lasers' due to its versatility and aesthetically pleasing scars.

Electrocautery, invented in 1875, though obsolete now, is still a familiar name in dermatosurgery and hence needs mention. This will be dealt with in the later part of this chapter.

Dermatosurgery has commonly been an 'office surgery'. Majority of the skin lesions can be adequately treated in office which meets the basic requirements of a minor surgical procedure. Office cutaneous surgery is more convenient, economical and efficient as well, as it saves on the cost and time of hospital-based cutaneous surgery.

Radiofrequency and electrocautery, both are performed with portable equipment most suitable for 'Office Dermatosurgery', but can be carried outside for performing surgeries in hospitals as well. The establishment of office surgery is a matter of personal choice and thus the choice of equipment should reflect the desires and tastes of the dermatologist himself or herself.

Electrocautery as mentioned above has been a common tool with dermatologists for decades for the ease of treating most of the skin lesions and its low cost, hence still remains quite popular. Electrosurgery, though versatile with more functions, still lacks behind in the fineness, cutting-coagulation ability and hemostasis efficiency compared to radiofrequency. The surgical lasers like CO_2 and Er-Yag have the disadvantages of cost and space occupancy. Radiofrequency, being color blind scores over these lasers in applications.

When we consider the above features of each modality, it becomes obvious that radiofrequency equipment should be the basic requirement of any dermatosurgery.

FUNDAMENTALS[1,2]

The basic physical difference between Radiofrequency and Electrocautery is in three parameters:

- Type of electric current:
  - Electrocautery uses direct current
  - Radiofrequency uses alternating current
- Electric circuit:
  - In electrocautery, patient is not part of electric circuit
  - In radiofrequency, patient is part of electric circuit
- Temperature of treating electrode:
  - In electrocautery, electrode is always very hot throughout procedure
  - In radiofrequency, electrode is always cold throughout procedure.

Furthermore, kindly refer to the Table 41.1 detailing the basic differences between the two modalities.

RADIOFREQUENCY

Equipment

The Radiofrequency equipment,[2] consists of the following :

- RF generator or unit
- Handpiece which may or may not have the activating switch
- Electrodes of various shapes and sizes
- Antenna plate (nonmetal)
- Foot pedal to activate unit

Table 41.1: Parameters of radiofrequency and electrocautery compared.

Parameter	*Electrocautery*	*Radiofrequency*
Electric current	DC	AC
Treating electrode	Always hot	Always cold
Fine cutting	Inferior	Superior
Hemostasis	Very good	Good
Lateral tissue damage	Quite significant	Minimal
Postoperative healing	Slow	Fast
Cosmetic result	Inferior	Superior
Biopsy	Not possible	Possible
Applications	Limited	Many
Cost of equipment	Inexpensive	Affordable Much cheaper than lasers

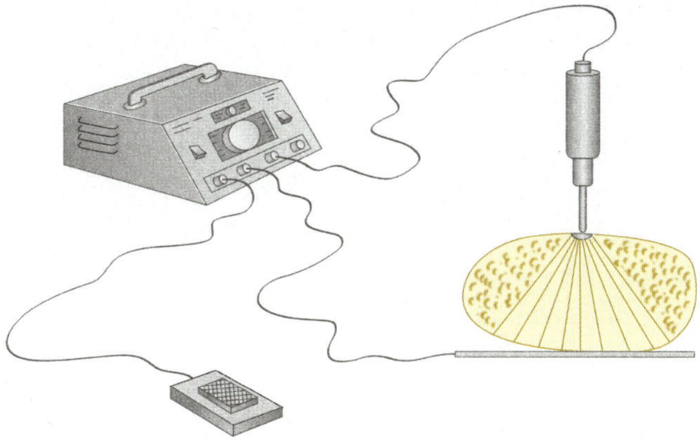

Fig. 41.1: Complete electrical circuit.

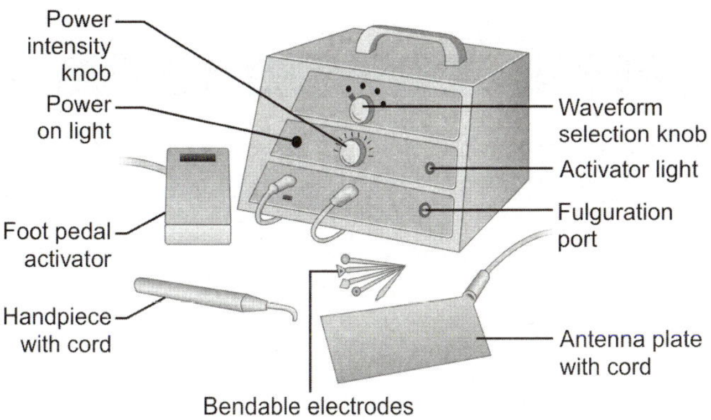

Fig. 41.2: Ellman Surgitron EMC equipment, amongst the primary and best modern radiosurgical device.

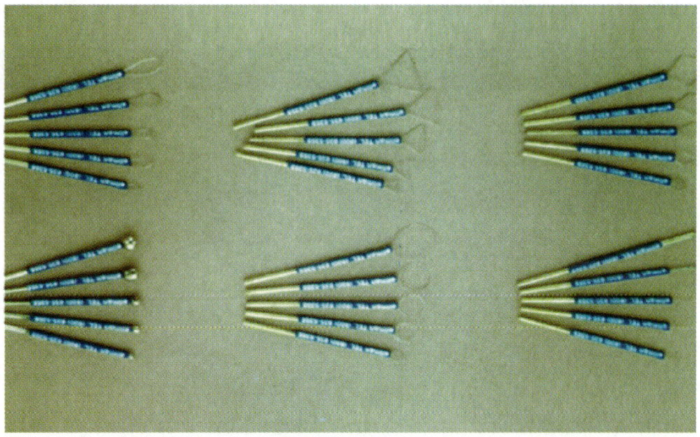

Fig. 41.3: Various probes of radiofrequency.

Figure 41.1 gives idea of the electrical circuit of the equipment for good understanding of the functionality of this technology. Figure 41.2 shows electrode touching the skin of patient during treatment. When the radio waves come in contact with skin tissue, the resistance offered helps to generate heat. These waves finally travel through patient's body to antenna plate which eventually completes the circuit. The machine is activated by the foot pedal switch or hand switch.

Figures 41.3 to 41.5 gives idea about the set of basic electrodes in various shapes and sizes which are used in dermatosurgery. These electrodes are bendable, which is advantageous.[4]

Functioning

Table 41.2[4] below will give clear idea about the ***functional features of radiofrequency*** for anybody who wishes to start it in his/ her clinical practice.

Figures 41.6 to 41.8 give clear idea of the three common functional applications of radiofrequency equipment:[5]

Figures 41.9 and 41.10 will give good idea about ***'lateral heat dispersion to adjoining tissues'.***

TIPS AND TRICKS TO MASTER RADIOFREQUENCY TECHNIQUE

- Pressureless incision
- Mechanical pressure must be avoided while operating
- Fine and light strokes (feather-like or paint brush like)
- Fine and delicate strokes give the best cosmesis
- Appropriate electrode size
- Electrode size must be customized to the lesion concerned
- Appropriate waveform selection
- Waveform selection is critical to performing operation

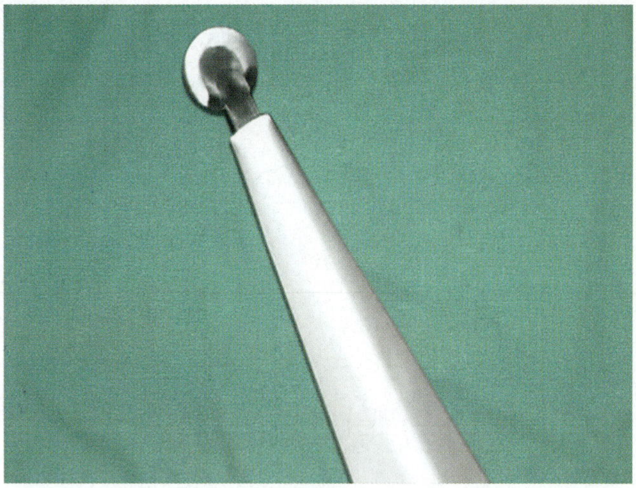

Fig. 41.4: This electrode is specially designed for scar sculpting and resurfacing.

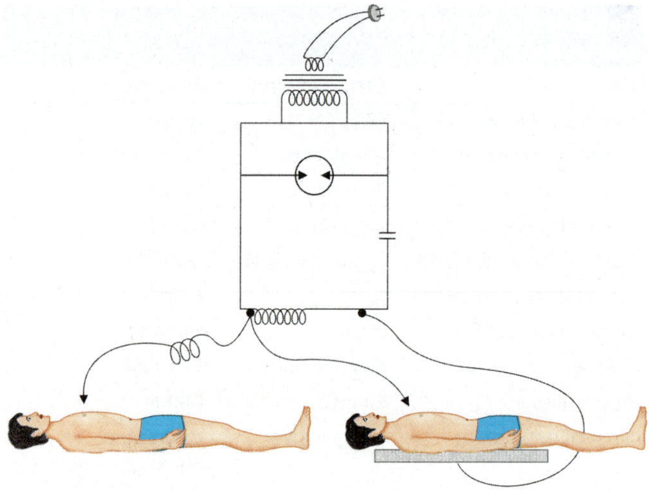

Fig. 41.5: It gives idea of the 'monopolar' and 'bipolar (with antenna plate)' features.

Table 41.2: Different waveforms of radiofrequency and their uses.

Waveform	*Function and polarity of electrodes*	*Lateral heat spread*	*Oscilloscope configuration*	*Uses*
Fully filtered and fully rectified	Electrosection Cutting (90% cut and 10% coag.) 'bipolar'	Least	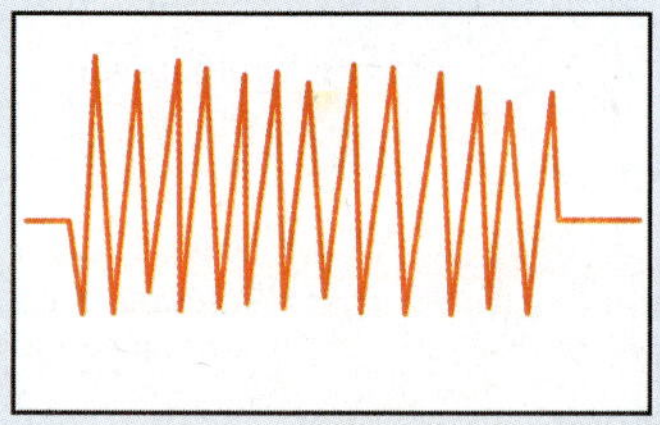	Skin Incisions excision of lesions cosmetic repairs
Fully rectified	Electrosection with coagulation (50% cut and 50% coag) 'bipolar'	More	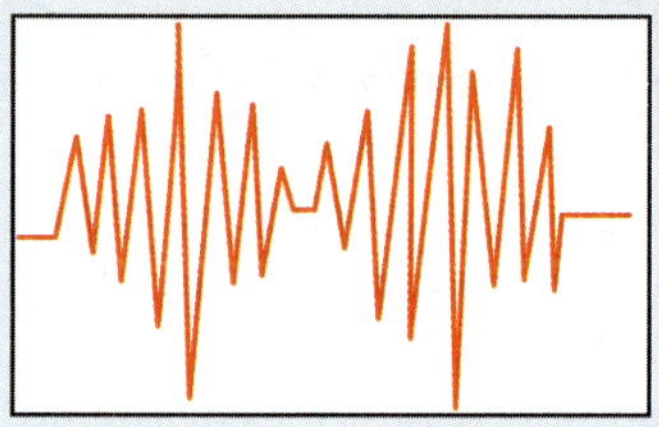	Keratoses, verrucae, neavi, Acrochordons corns, keloids, etc.
Partially rectified	Electrocoagulation (90% coag. 10% cut) 'bipolar'	Most	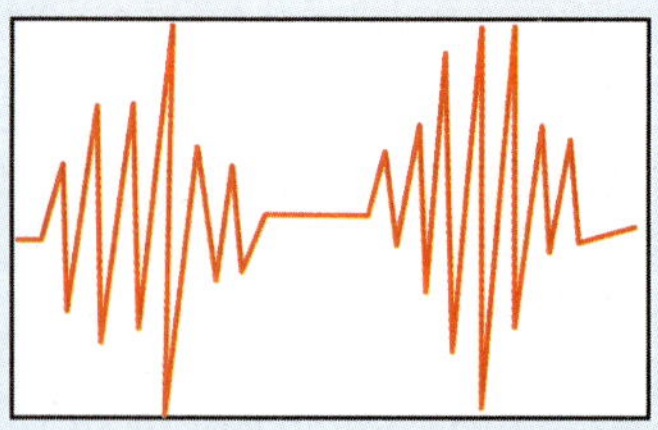	Surgical hemostasis, Benign lesions, basal cell Ca, telangiectasia epilation
Markedly damped, spark gap	Electrodessication and unipolar	More	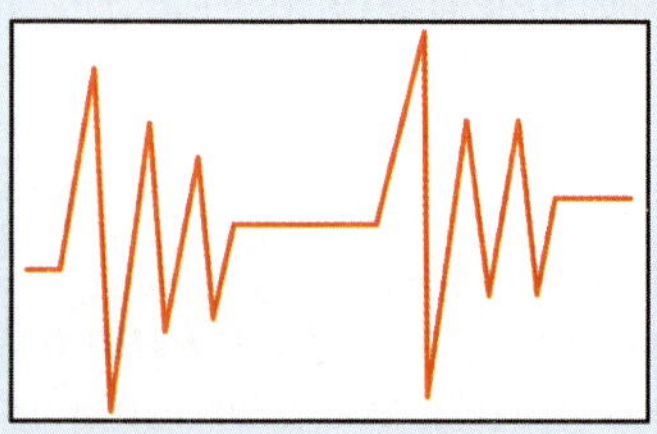	Keratoses, milia, verruca plana, xanthelasma, mol-lusscum contagiosum, etc.
Bipolar coagulation	Precise hemostasis using bipolar forceps	More		Excellent coagulation of individual vessels

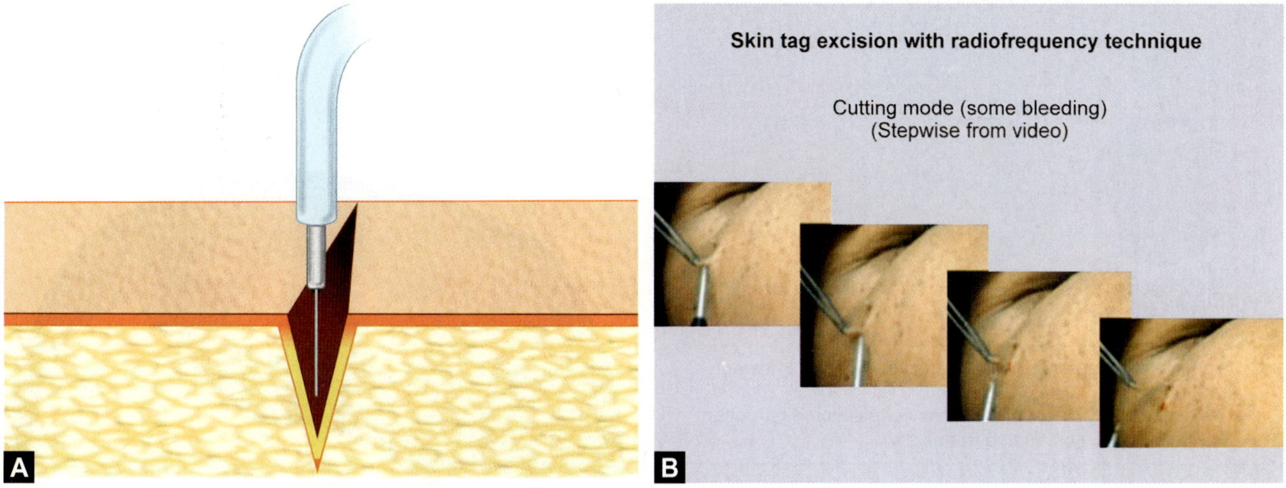

Figs. 41.6A and B: Electrosection (fully filtered waveform/CUT mode—90% cut, 10% coag).

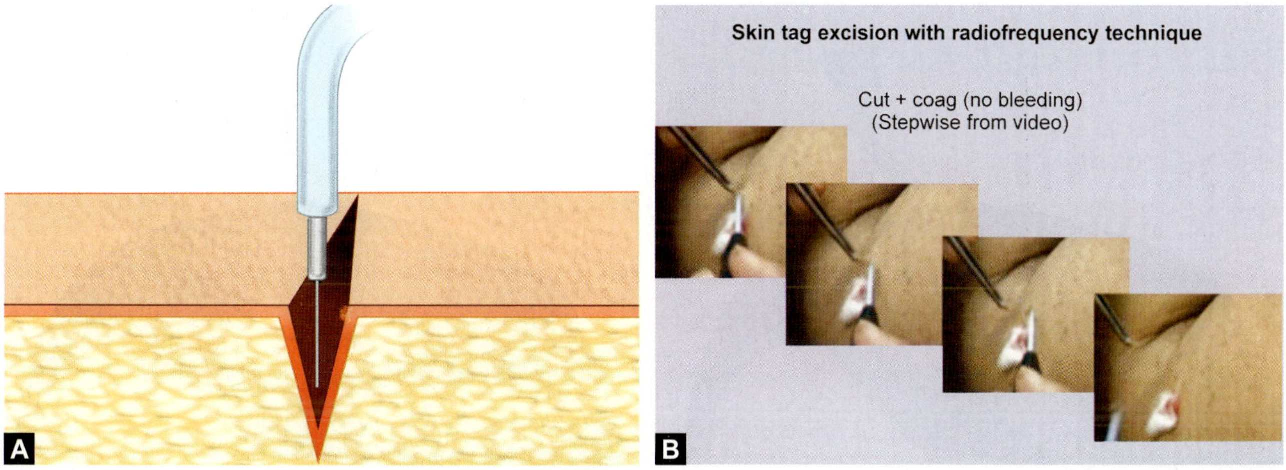

Figs. 41.7A and B: CUT + COAG (50–50) or Blended current (fully rectified waveform).

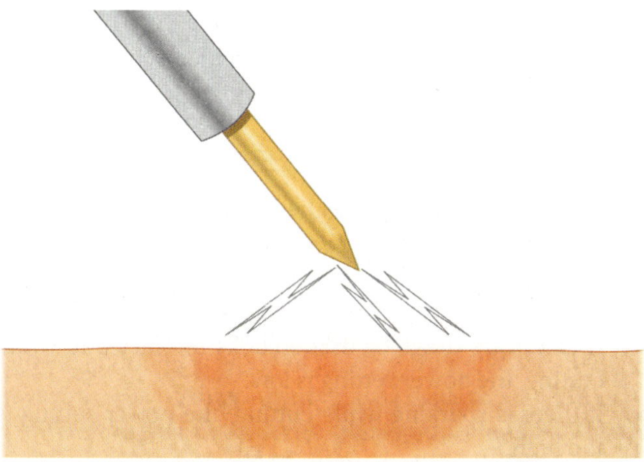

Fig. 41.8: Electrofulguration (partially rectified waveform, monopolar function).

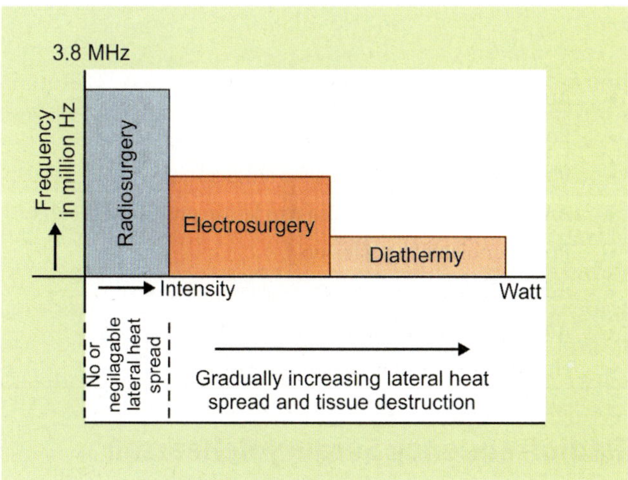

Fig. 41.9: Lateral dissipation principle.

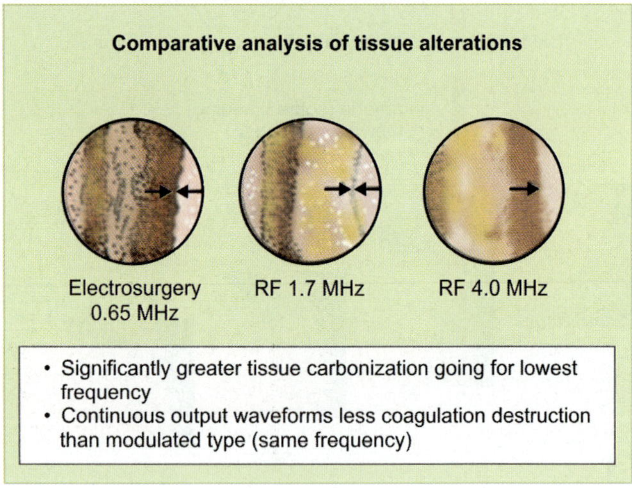

Fig. 41.10: Confirms that higher the frequency lesser the tissue alteration.

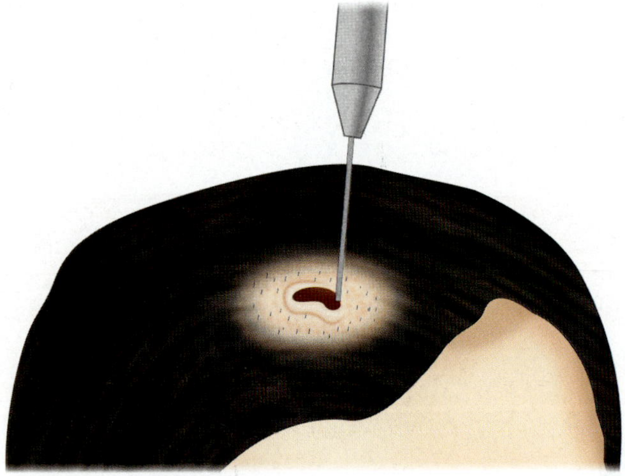

Fig. 41.11: Cutting with vari-tip electrode.

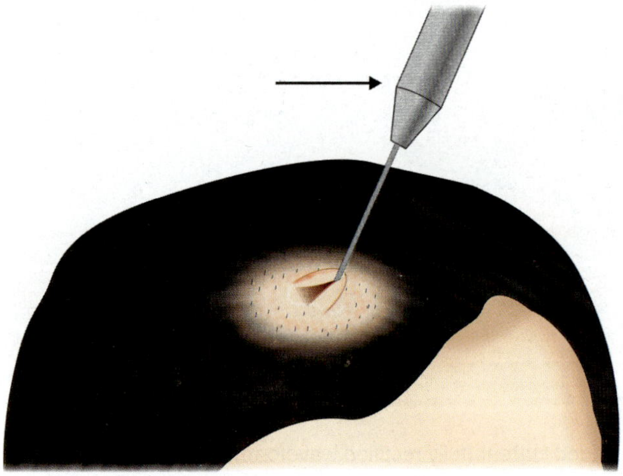

Fig. 41.12: Electrode is stuck in tissue due to low power.

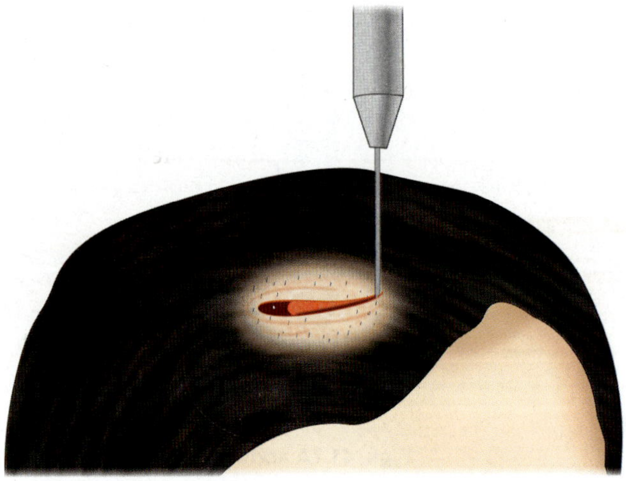

Fig. 41.13: Electrode slides smoothly when power is optimum.

- Appropriate power setting
- Power setting is critical to best operability
- Placing antenna plate close to surgical site
- Antenna plate placed closest to lesion gives best results
- Proper moistening of lesion
- Adequate hydration facilitates easy excision
- Adequate interval between two strokes
- Hurried strokes may cause charring

Radiofrequency Surgery Rehearsal:[7]

One should practice certain laboratory exercises over a meat piece before using this technique on patients. The Figures 41.11 to 41.13 will give perfect idea of using various waveforms, electrodes, power setting.

Points to Learn in Laboratory Exercises

- Antenna plate may not touch the skin of the patient
- Unit should be activated with foot switch before making electrode contact
- Never cut with 'partially rectified current' (coagulation)
- If electrode drags or tissue sticks to electrode while cutting, the power setting is low
- If there is sparking while cutting, the power setting is too high
- If the tissue does not cut in spite of increasing power, moisten the tissue

- Never stop at one point while cutting, it will deepen cut
- Cut without applying pressure.

Universal Precautions before any Radiofrequency Procedure

- *Cardiac pacemaker*[8]: Patients having cardiac pacemaker should take prior permission of his/her cardiologist before procedure
- *Alcohol-based and other inflammable antiseptics*: These should be avoided or sufficient time must be allowed for RF surgery to start after their use
- *Bowel gases*: Possibility of bowel gases leading to explosion while operating near anal area must be kept in mind
- *Electrical shock*: Avoid patient contact with any metal and let operator use latex gloves for its prevention.

Radiofrequency Application

Radiofrequency surgical method being versatile, has many applications in office dermatosurgery. Almost all superficial epidermal lesions can be very effectively cleared. Many of the deeper lesions involving the dermis and subcutaneous tissue can be very effectively tackled using this method as well.

Reader is referred to the Table 41.3 which is a ready reckoner for most of the common office nonablative applications. For the convenience of the reader and for gaining confidence in the start-up to Radiofrequency surgery, the following pages will give detailed procedures with adjoining simple sketches for a stepwise learning of important applications. This publication is accompanied by 'video demonstration' for better understanding.

Table 41.3: Parameters of RF.

Lesion	*Electrode*	*Method*	*Power*
Verruca plana	S/V	FTD	1
Molluscum contagiosum	S/D	FTD	1–2
Milia, DPN	S/V	FTD	1
Syringoma	S/D	FTD	1
Xanthelasma	S	FTD	1
Verruca vulgaris	S/D	FTD	1–2
Keratosis actinic/seborrheic	S/D	FTD	1–2
Senile comedones	S/D	FTD	1–2
Acrochordons, skin tags	S/D	FTD	1–2
Telangiectasia	V	FTD/EC	1
Cherry angioma	S/V	FTD/EC	1

(FTD: Fine touch desiccation; EC: Electrocoagulation; S: Straight needle; D: Desiccation; V: Van-tip)

Prerequisites of Office Radiofrequency Surgery

- Office minimum requirements
  - 10 × 10 feet clean room
  - Not exposed to external environment and contaminants
  - Minimum ventilation and exhaust fan (air conditioning not must)
  - Minimum sterilization requirements fully met
  - Minimum emergency injections like Inj. Adrenaline, Steroid
- Patient assessment
  - Minimum required investigations like hemogram, blood sugar levels, bleeding time, clotting time, urine examination, etc. are done as per relevance.
  - Inj. Lignocaine skin testing is done prior to surgery
- Patient counseling and informed consent
  - Patient is informed in details the operative procedure, its postoperative care, its stage-wise recovery, its final outcome, possible side effects, shortcomings, complications verbally as well as in printed format
  - Informed consent to procedure and photo-documentation is taken prior to surgery
  - Patient is informed that part or whole of the lesion will be sent for histopathology

Ready reckoner for common dermatosurgical applications using radiofrequency

Abbreviations (electrodes): S-Straight needle; V-Vari-tip (thin bendable wire); D-Desiccation (bent); L-Round loop; T- Triangular; B-Ball tip

Abbreviations (method): FTD-Fine touch desiccation; SE-Shave excision; EC-Electrocoagulation

A. ***Nonablative applications*** (monopolar, partially rectified waveform):[1,2,4,9]

Kindly refer the accompanying video for fine touch desiccation (FTD)

Fine Touch desiccation method:

- Lesions are anesthetized using topical anesthetic cream containing Lidocaine + Prilocaine after routine sterilization
- Monopolar method, hence no antenna plate
- Waveform is set as given above
- Straight needle/Vari-tip/Desiccation electrode used as per guidelines given above individualized to particular lesion
- Power setting is done according to above mentioned figures

- Single lesion is selected at a time and very finely touched multiple times to desiccate it fully (lesion turns white)
- Care should be taken not to exceed power setting even if the lesion is thick
- Care should be taken not to prolong single touch as it causes complications of dyschromia and scarring

Post-FTD skin care:

- All desiccated lesions are left untouched, no attempt should be made to remove them with pressure or scrape them
- The skin around the lesions is inflamed and there is a mild burning or stinging sensation, hence apply Aloe Vera gel for soothing effect
- Soap should be avoided for cleansing, only non-soapy like cleansing solutions containing cetyl and steryl alcohol are used
- Always pat-dry after cleansing, do not rub or wipe harshly
- Allow all lesions to form natural scabs and fall off automatically in next 4–7 days
- Topical antibiotic application is advised for one week
- Topical medium potency steroid like Mometasone may be mixed with topical antibiotic for multiple facial lesions to control inflammation faster, which can lessen or avoid postoperative dyschromia
- Oral antibiotic is given, if there are multiple lesions
- Topical sunscreen with SPF more than 30 is advised after all lesions have fallen off for minimum 4 weeks
- In spite of all precautions, there is always a possibility of postprocedure dyschromia in most of our patients.

Post-FTD Complications [4,10,11]

- Postoperative dyschromia on Fitzpatrick skin type 3 to 5
- Postoperative erythema on Fitzpatrick skin type 1 or 2
- Postoperative scarring (tiny hyperpigmented scars)

Post-FTD complications generally resolve fully without any residual problems, provided patient follows up as advised. In more than 95% patients there is no permanent problem.

B. ***Ablative Applications*** (monopolar, biterminal, fully filtered or fully rectified waveform):

All lesions which need excision under local anesthesia are treated using this technique.

These lesions are excised using the 'Cut' (fully filtered/C) or 'Cut + Coag' (fully rectified/CC) waveforms

Shave Excision Method

- Lesion is anesthetized using Inj. Lignocaine with adrenaline on all areas except nose-tip and finger-tip to avoid complication of necrosis due to vasoconstriction of end-arteries.
- Normally, 'Fully Filtered' or 'cut' waveform is selected for all lesions, which is 90% cut and 10% coag.
- For vascular lesions or for those which are likely to bleed profusely while shaving, 'fully rectified' or 'cut + coag' is selected.
- Commonly, round loop electrode of appropriate size is selected for facial and nonfacial lesions.
- Sometimes, for lesions like warts, corns, callosities, 'triangular or diamond shaped electrodes' are used

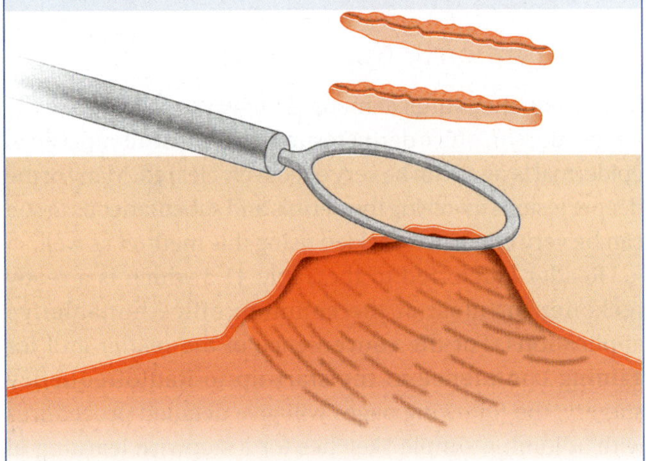

- Power of 3–5 is selected for routine shave excisions for 'cut' mode
- Power of 4–6 is selected for thicker lesions on 'cut' mode
- Power of 4–10 is selected for all lesions when 'cut + coag' mode is used
- Electrode is held at angle of 30 to 60 degrees to surface plane before shaving
- If the electrode drags (*see* Fig. 41.12) while shaving or sticks in tissue, the power is lower than optimum, hence should be increased
- If the electrode sparkles, the power is more which may char tissue, hence reduce to optimum
- Lesion is removed in stepwise manner as shown in above figure till needed using repeated delicate strokes

Table 41.4: Parameters of RF in various indications.

Lesion	Waveform	Electrode	Method	Power
Verruca vulgaris	C/CC	S/L	SE	2–3
Skin tags	C/CC	S/L	Excision of pedunculated lesion	2–3
Melanocytic nevus	C and EC, if required	L	SE	3–4
Keratoses (actinic/seborrheic)	C	L	SE	3–4
Keloids Hypertrophic scars	C and CC EC, if required	S and L and B	SE and EC, if required	3–5
Corn/Callosity	C/CC EC, if required	S and L B, if required	SE and EC, if required	4–8
Trichoepithelioma	C	L	SE	3–4
Rhinophyma	C/CC EC, if required	L and B	SE and EC, if required	3–5
Basal cell carcinoma	C and EC, if required	L and B, if required	SE and EC	3–5
Freckles	C	S	Fine superficial ablation	1
Sebaceous cyst	C	V/S	Incision followed by enucleation	3–4
Submucous cyst	C	V/S	SE and EC or Incision followed by enucleation	3–4
Pyogenica granuloma	CC and EC, if required	L and B	SE and EC, if required	3–6
Capillary hemangioma	CC	L and B	SE and EC, if required	3–4
Depressed facial scar/Boxcar/ Chicken pox scar	C	Round blade surgipen	3 step resurfacing procedure	1–3

- Hemostasis is achieved with pressure or 'electro-coagulation'
- Edges of shaved lesion is always blended with adjoining normal skin as shown in Fig. 41.38 and 'Mole Excision Video' for best cosmesis

Kindly refer to 'Mole Excision video' for live demonstration of Shave excision.

Postshave excision care (This applies to all ablative Radiofrequency procedures):

- All lesions excised by shave method are usually dressed after procedure unless these are very superficial like in freckles, depressed scars, keratoses
- Lesions of freckles, depressed scars, keratoses, pedunculated Skin tags, sebaceous cyst are covered with topical antibiotic
- Oral antibiotics are advised for one week after procedure
- Wound care dressing is done daily or alternate days till complete wound healing
- Non-soapy cleansing lotions containing cetyl and steryl alcohol are used for cleaning skin around wounds
- Once the wounds heal fully, the lesions on sun exposed area are covered with appropriate sunscreen for 1-2 months
- All patients are followed up every 2 weeks for minimum 2 months
- Follow-up visits are more and prolonged for hypertrophic scars, keloids, corns, callosities

Postshaving excision complications (apply to all ablative radiofrequency procedures): [4,10,11]

- Postoperative Dyschromia is very common in all Fitzpatrick skin type 3 to 5 patients
- Postoperative Erythema is common in fairer Indian skin patients having skin type 1 or 2
- Postoperative scarring can be a major problem which will require quite some efforts to improve appreciably
- Recurrence of moles, warts, corns, keloids

Radiofrequency applications commonly done are pictorially described below for quick and clear understanding and to facilitate as well as improvise office practice.

- *Pedunculated lesion removal*: For tips refer Table 41.4 and for visual tricks refer Figures 41.14 to 41.16.
  Another method is shown below
  If there is mild bleeding after the procedure, it can be electrocoagulated with same electrode (Figs. 41.17 to 41.19).

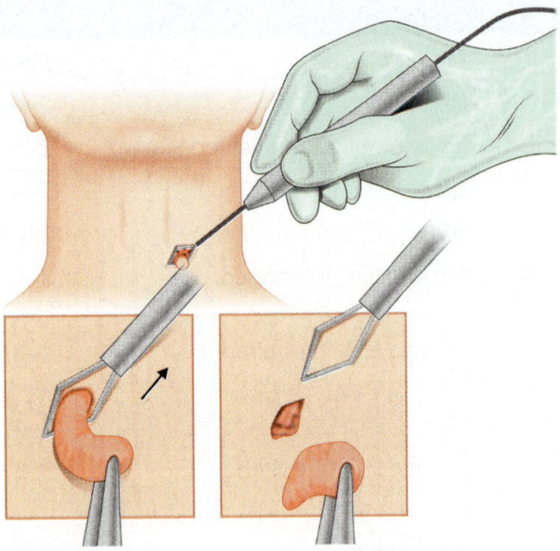

Fig. 41.14: Electrode is pushed around lesion up to its base, lesion is held by forceps and activated electrode just cuts through the lesion in one stroke.

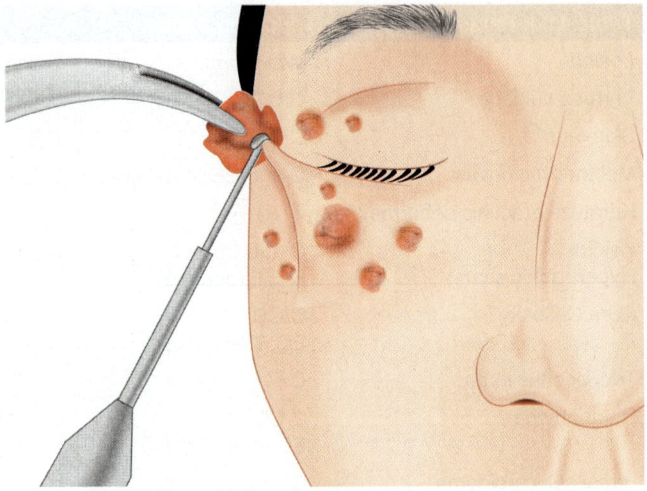

Fig. 41.15: Lesion is held with forceps and straight needle electrode is allowed to cut through the base of lesion.

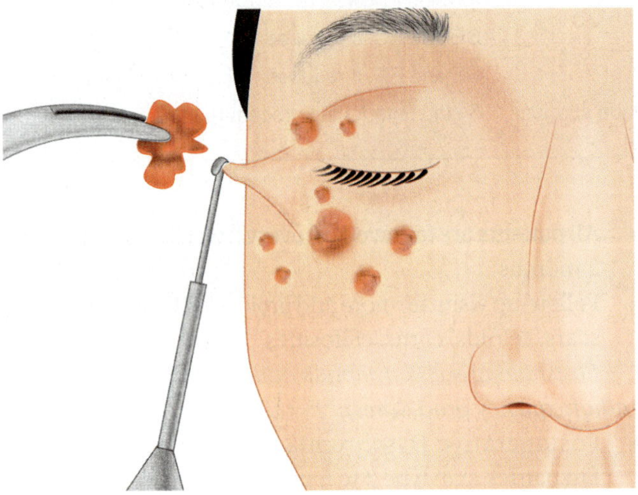

Fig. 41.16: Lesion is cut through in single stroke.

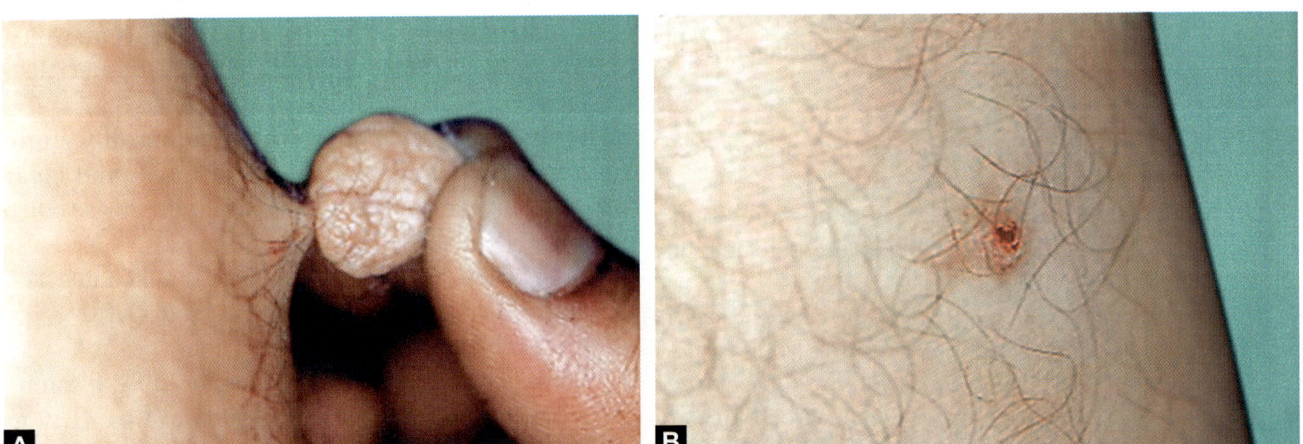

Figs. 41.17A and B: Acrochordon excised with mild bleeding.

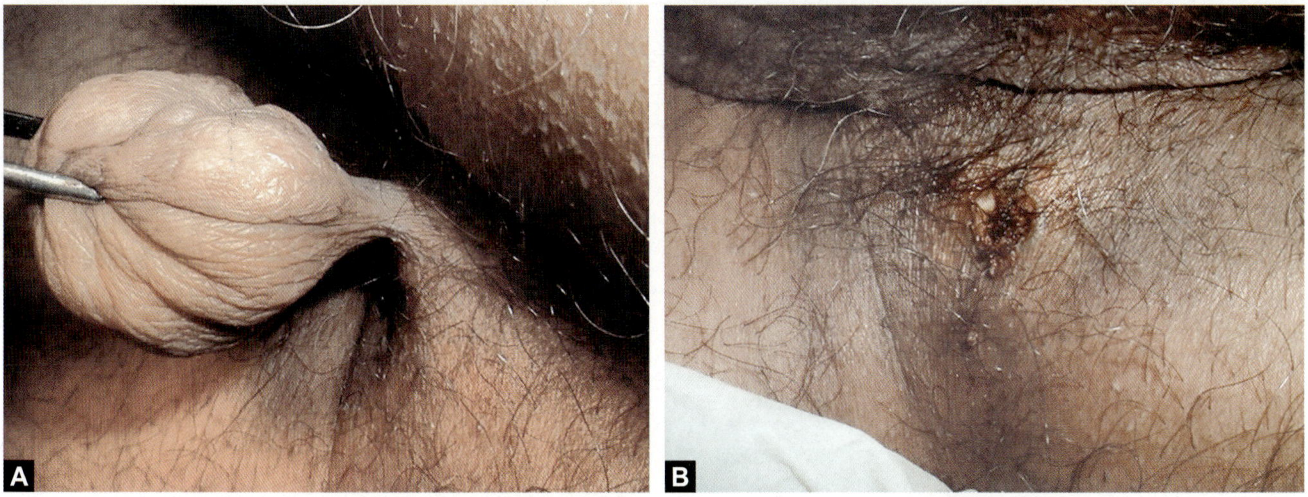

Figs. 41.18A and B: Large acrochordon excised and hemostasis achieved by electrocoagulation.

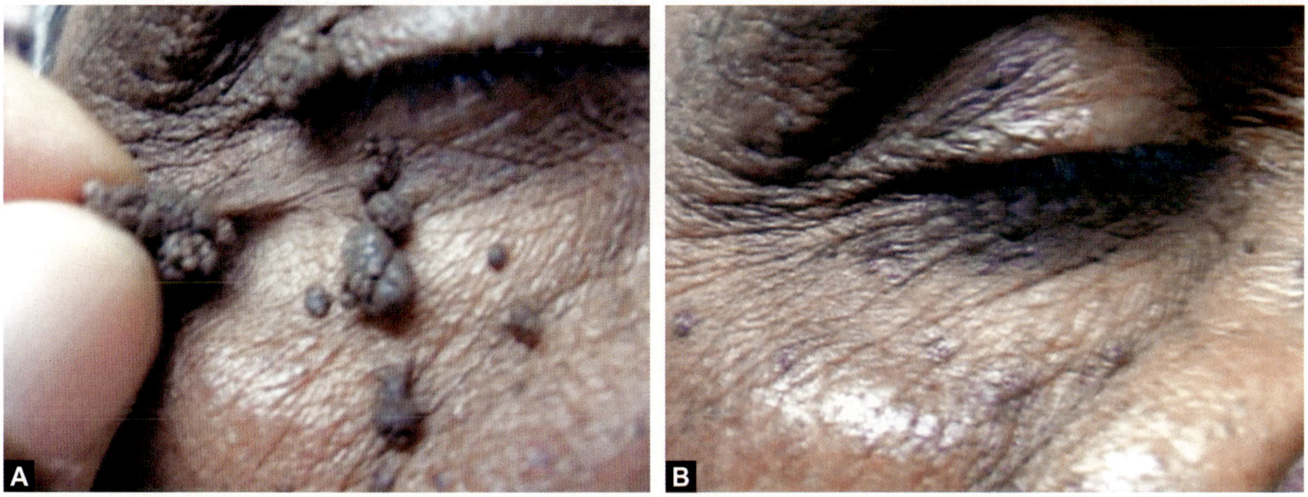

Figs. 41.19A and B: Before and after acrochordon removal (no residual dyschromia or scars).

- *Small papular lesions of dermatosis papulosa nigra, milia, syringoma, senile comedones, comedonal acne (white heads)*:
  For tips refer Table 41.3; for tricks please refer Video on Desiccation technique and Figures 41.20 and 41.21.
  Precautions for patients: Do not pull out the scabs prematurely or by scratching or wiping harshly after washing. This is very important to avoid infection and scarring. Tight clothing should also be avoided to prevent excess friction which can remove scabs prematurely and cause complications (Fig. 41.22).
- *Warts (verruca vulgaris/plana/digitate), molluscum contagiosum*:
  Please refer Table 41.3 for tips on Desiccation; refer Figure 41.23 for tricks of immediate removal following desiccation.
  Please refer the case study (Figs. 41.24 to 41.34) for better understanding. Here, electrosection or actual excision is avoided and desiccation is preferred. Desiccation will destroy the infective tissue before removal and electrocoagulation done for hemostasis will destroy any residual microscopic infective organisms in adjoining skin tissue.
- *Corn and callosity excision*: Please refer Table 41.4 for tips; please refer Figures 41.35 and 41.36 for tricks; also refer accompanying video for live demonstration.
- *Mole excision*: Please refer Table 41.4 for tips; please refer accompanying video for live demonstration and tricks; please refer the Figures 41.37 to 41.42 which show easy steps of excision.
  These give pictorial demonstration of mole (intradermal nevus) removal in brief.

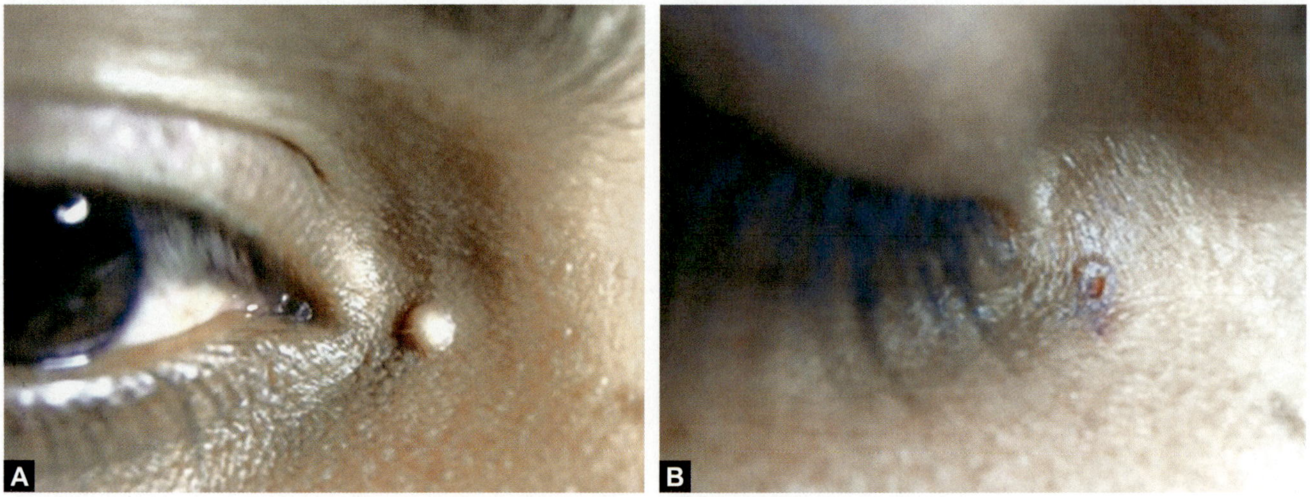

Figs. 41.20A and B: Milia immediately after desiccation.

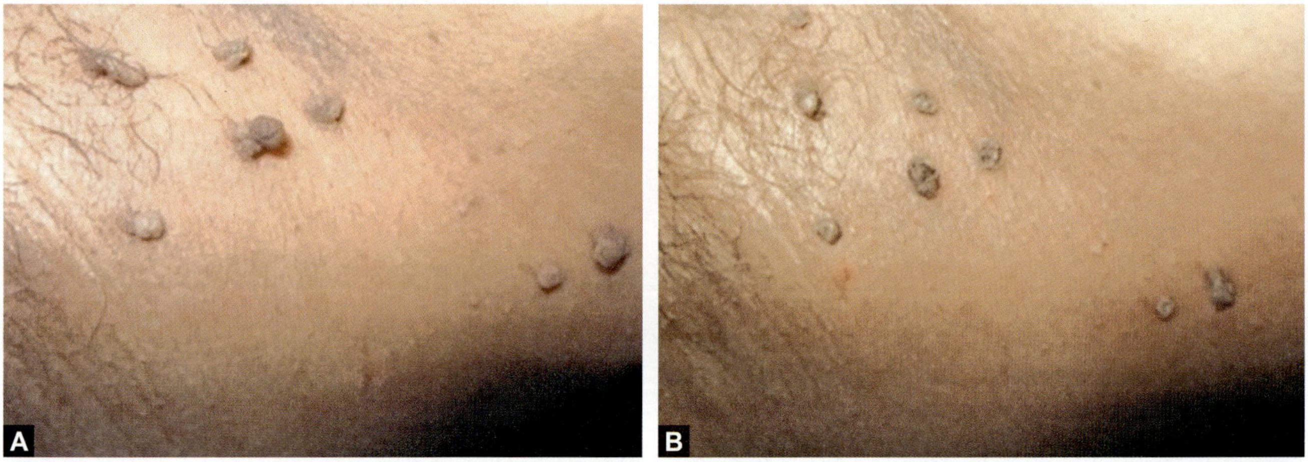

Figs. 41.21A and B: Skin tags immediately after desiccation (these lesions will form scabs and fall off automatically in a week's time).

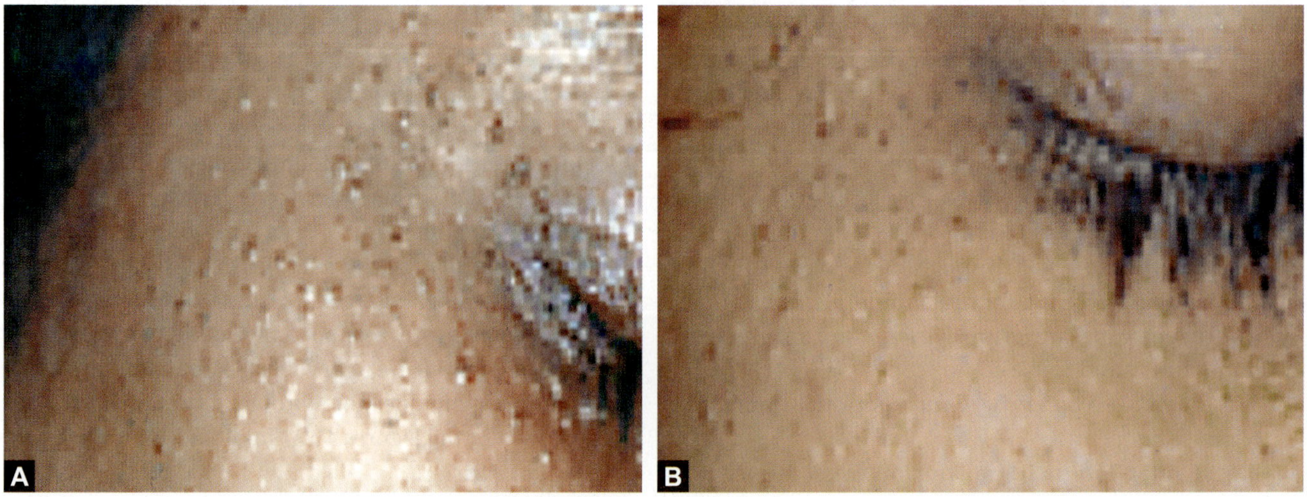

Figs. 41.22A and B: Milia cleared fully without leaving dyschromia or scars.

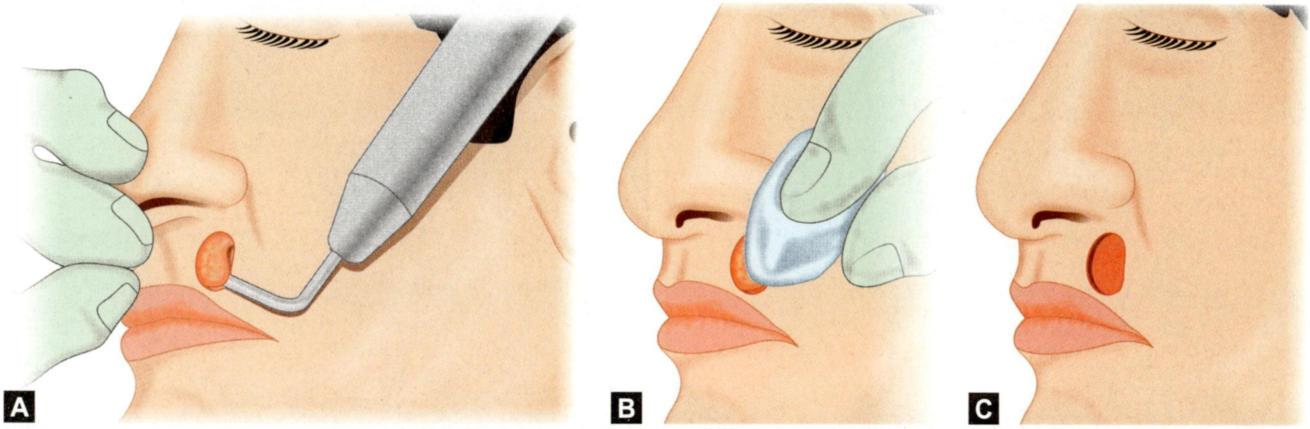

Figs. 41.23A to C: Removal of warts/molluscum. This gives step-wise desiccation followed by manual removal; this may require hemostasis with pressure or electrocoagulation.

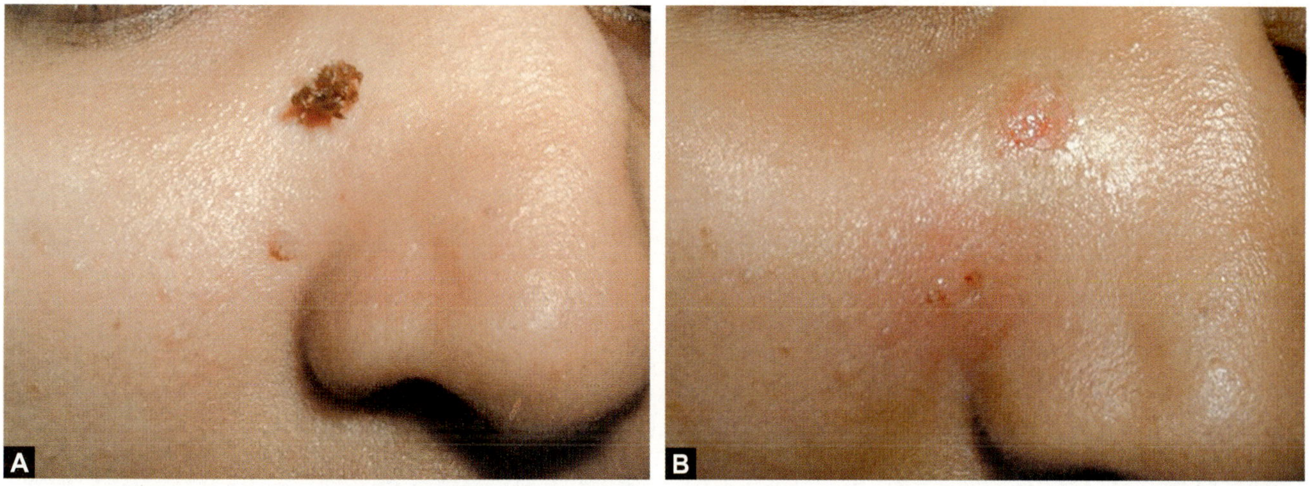

Figs. 41.24A and B: Verruca vulgaris desiccated and removed.

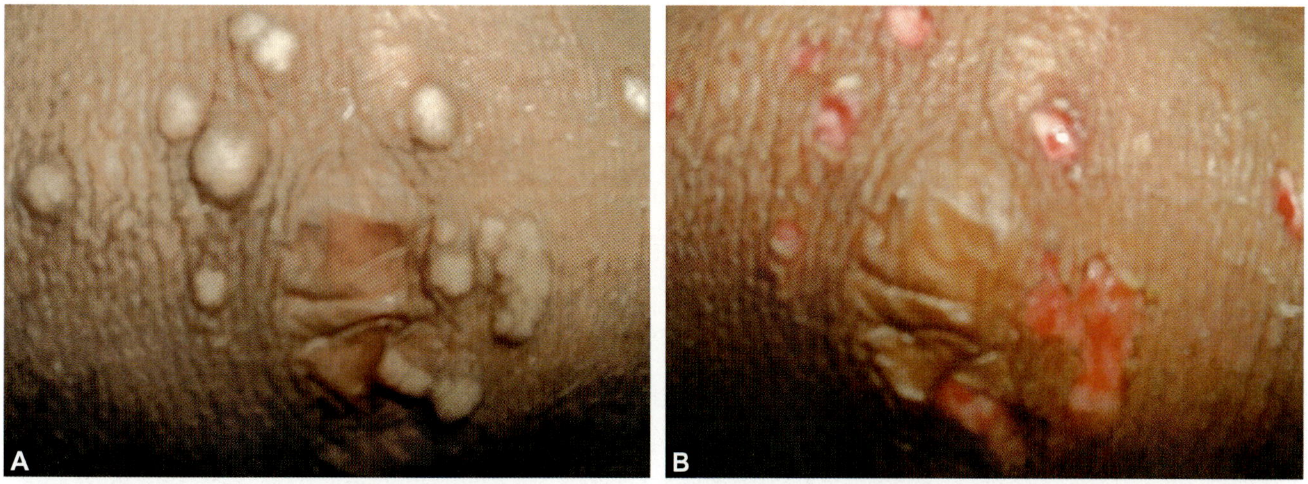

Figs. 41.25A and B: Multiple verruca vulgaris desiccated and removed and electrocoagulated; Centrally, a postelectrocautery scar after treating same problem is seen.

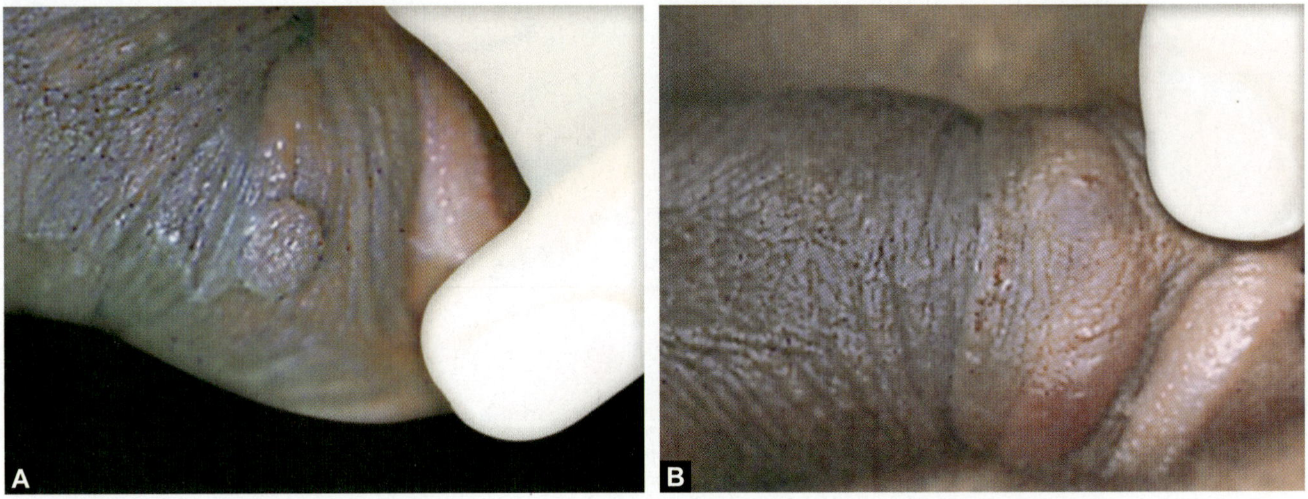

Figs. 41.26A and B: Verruca over penile shaft desiccated, removed and electrocoagulated.

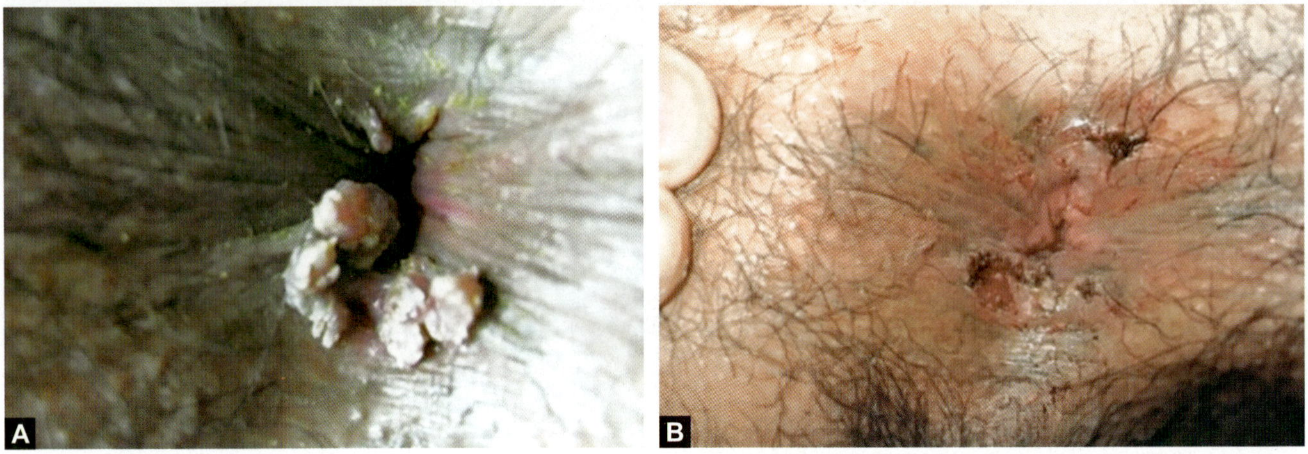

Figs. 41.27A and B: Condyloma acuminata at perianal area in a homosexual patient desiccated, removed and electrocoagulated.

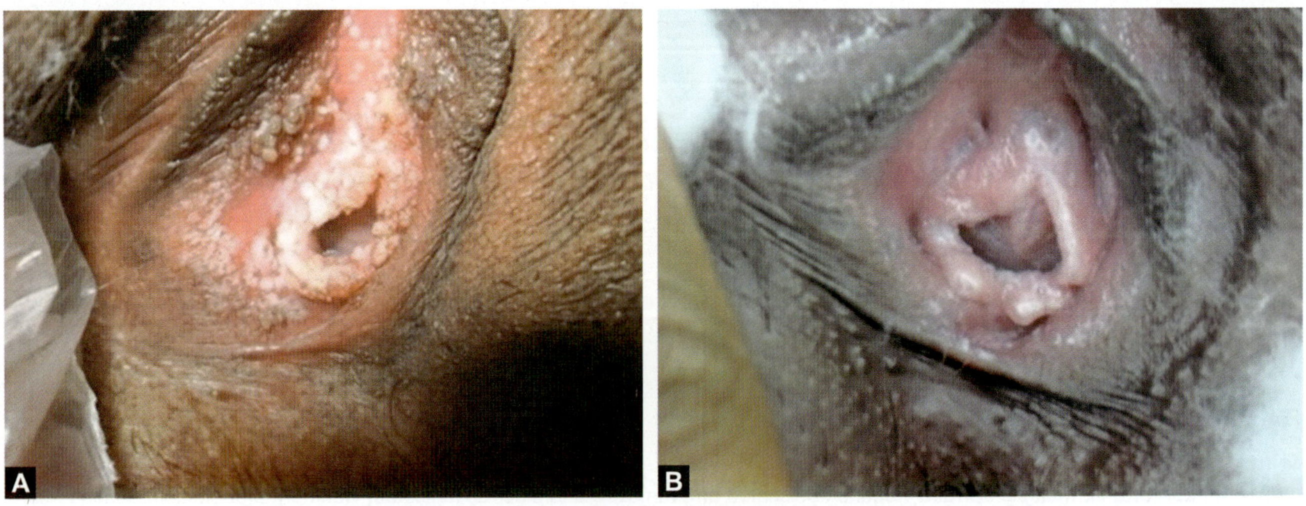

Figs. 41.28A and B: Condyloma acuminata treated as above, showing final result.

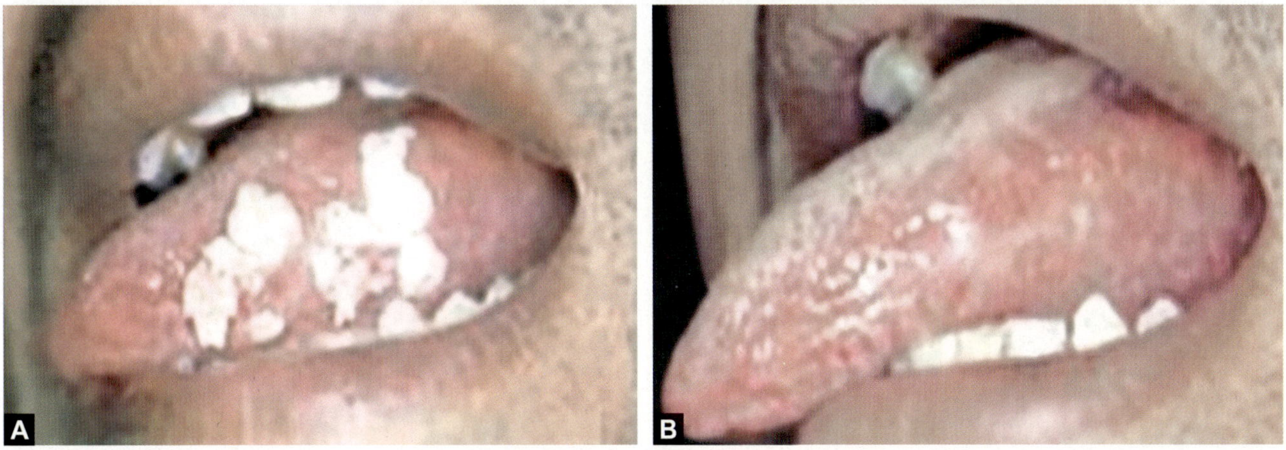

Figs. 41.29A and B: Verruca lesions over tongue desiccated in multiple sessions at weekly intervals using lignocaine viscous solution and they fully cleared without recurrence.

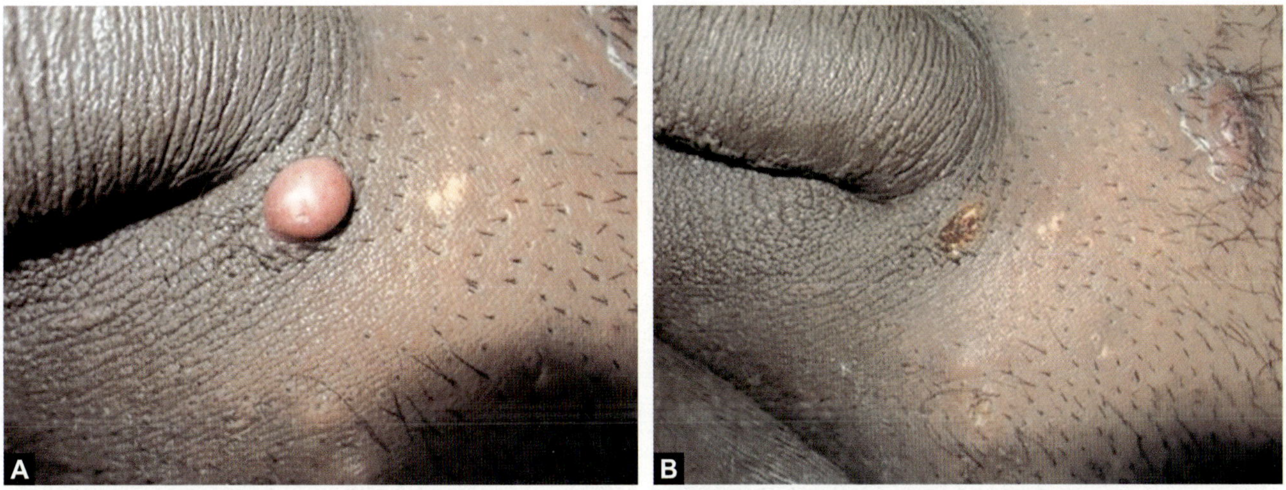

Figs. 41.30A and B: Giant molluscum contagiosum desiccated, removed and electrocoagulated.

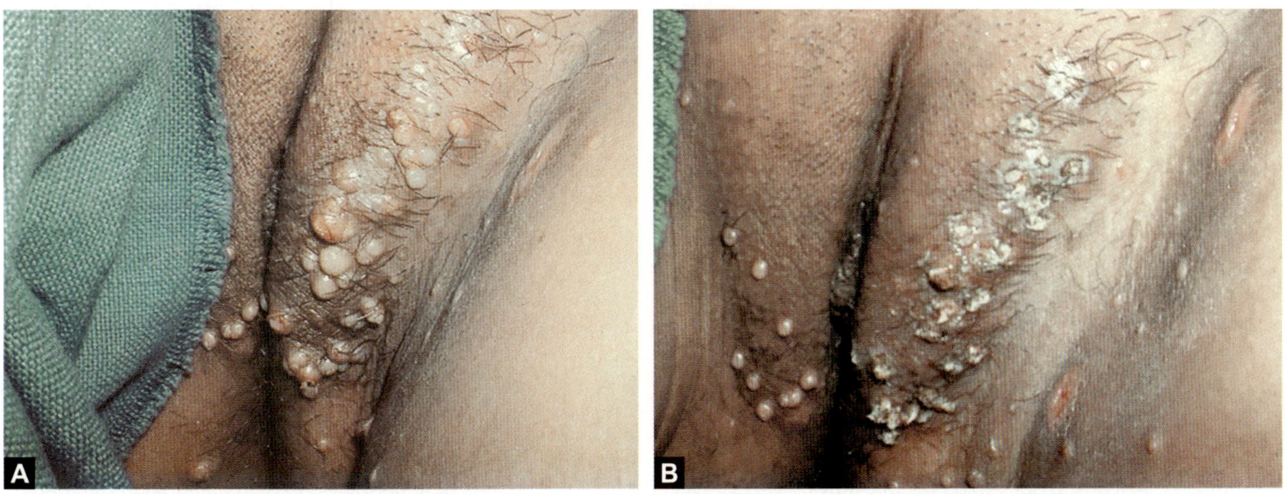

Figs. 41.31A and B: Multiple molluscum contagiosum desiccated and scabs yet to removed/scraped off.

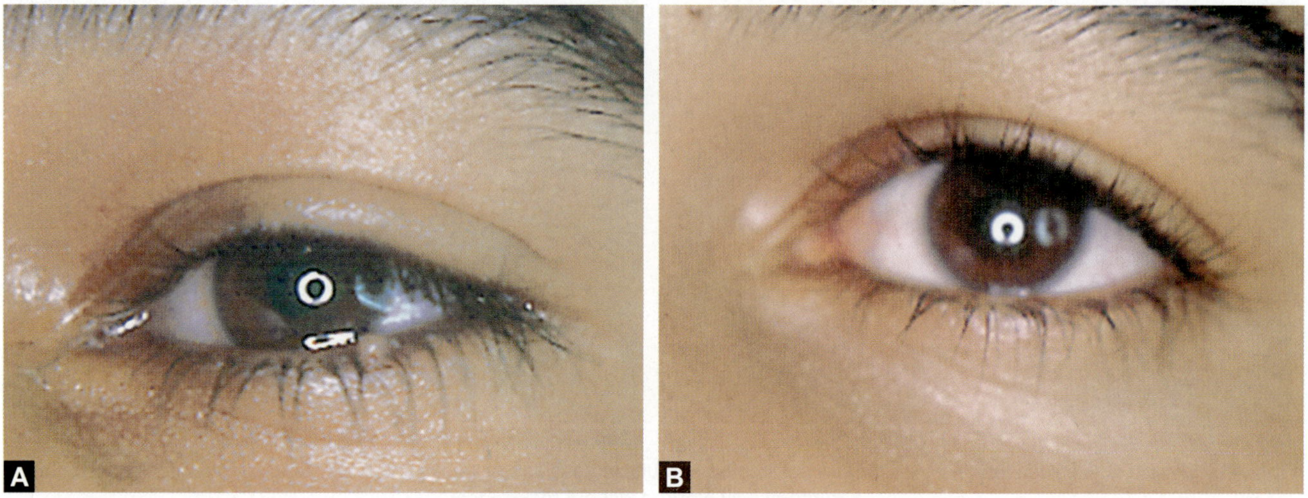

Figs. 41.32A and B: Molluscum lesion on lower eyelashes cleared fully without after desiccation.

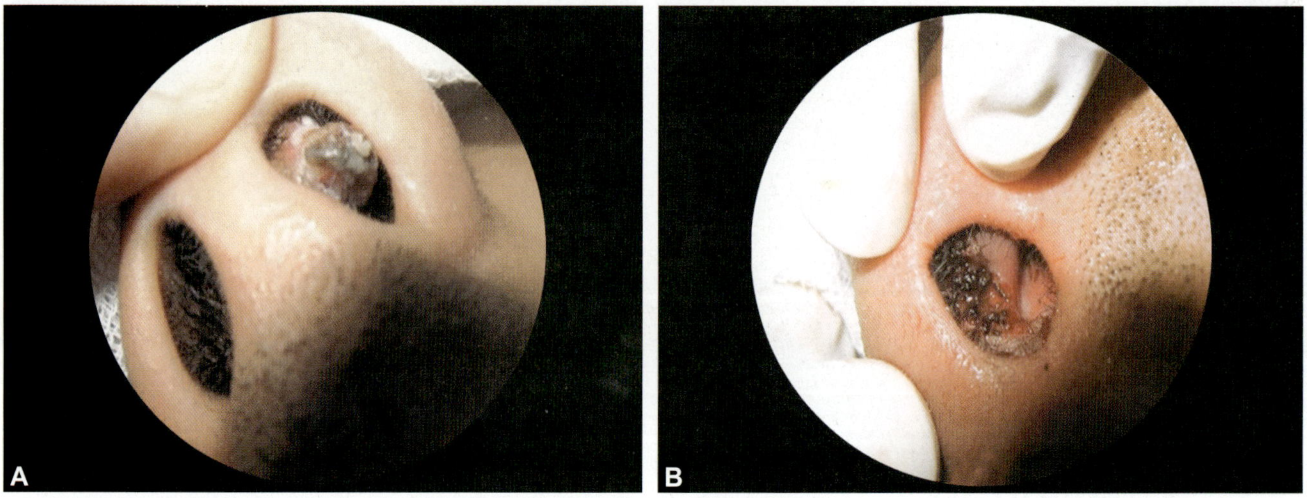

Figs. 41.33A and B: Wart in left nostril excised under lignocaine spray and Inj. Lignocaine in operation theater.

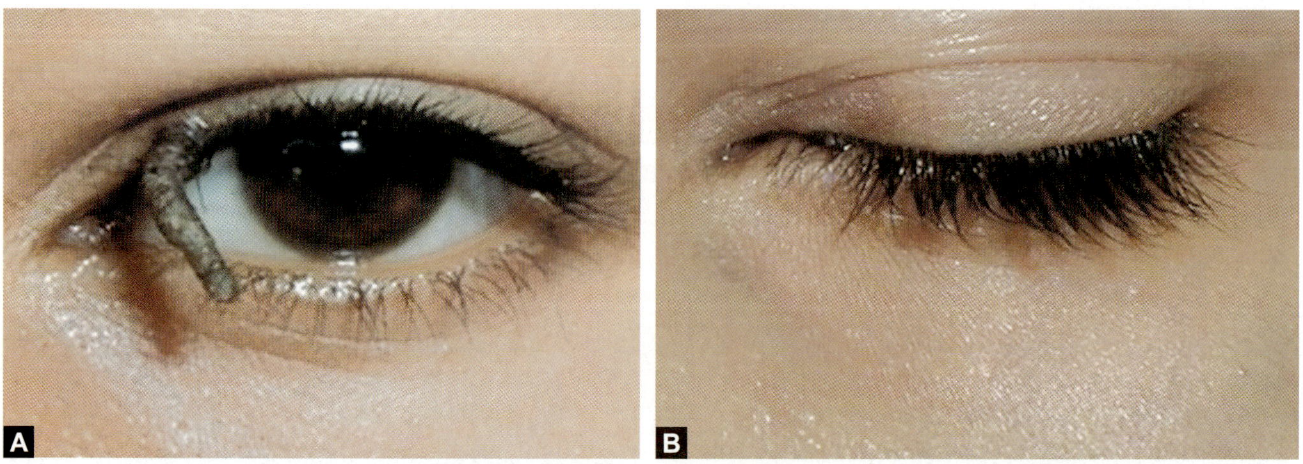

Figs. 41.34A and B: Cutaneous horn overlying verruca vulgaris in the eyelashes of upper eyelid treated under short general anesthesia; desiccated, excised on cutaneous and mucosal aspect and electrocoagulated. No recurrence.

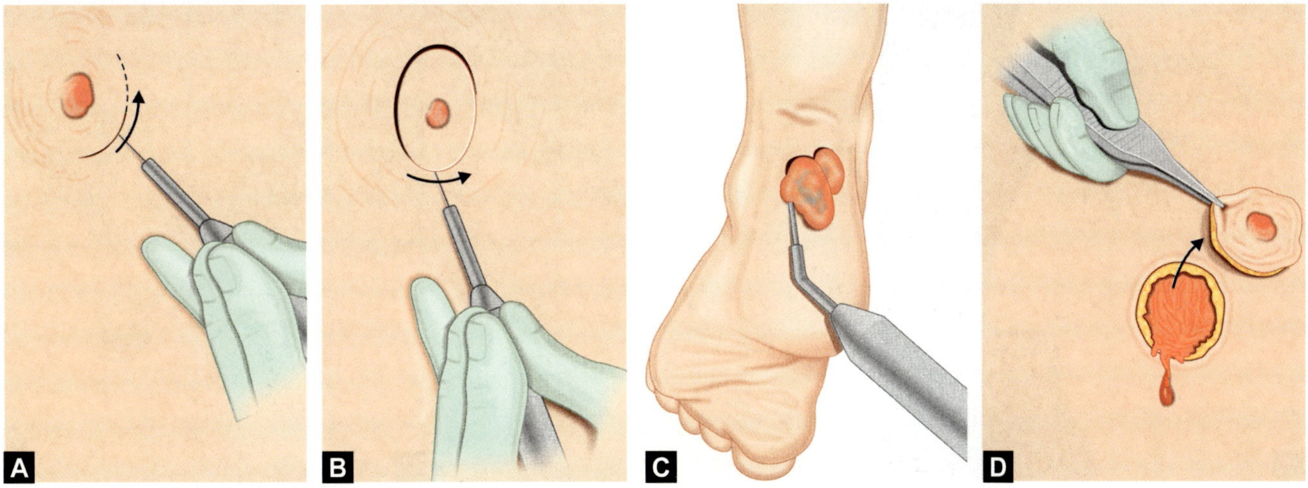

Figs. 41.35A to D: Serial steps for corn or callosity excision case study photos.

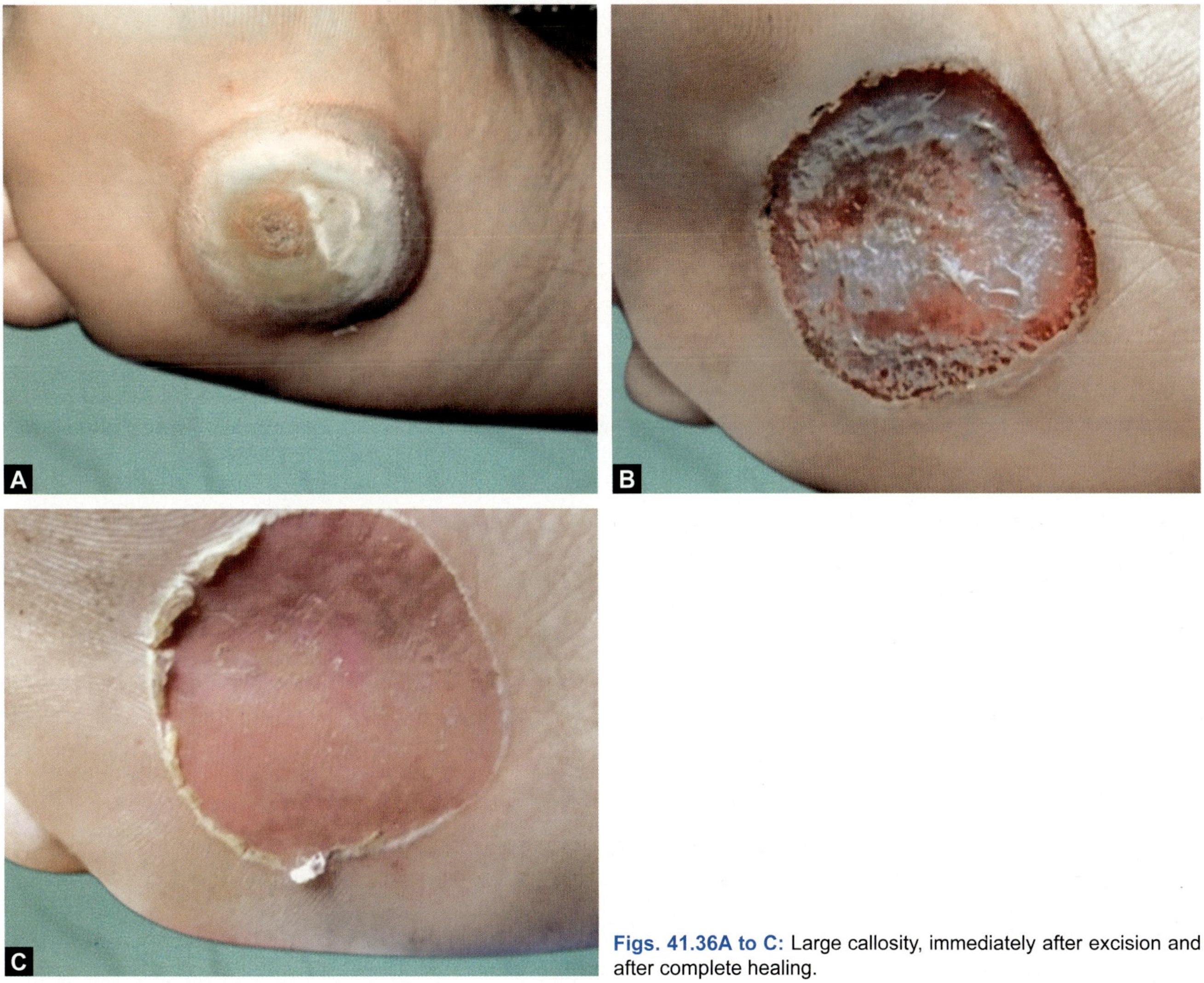

Figs. 41.36A to C: Large callosity, immediately after excision and after complete healing.

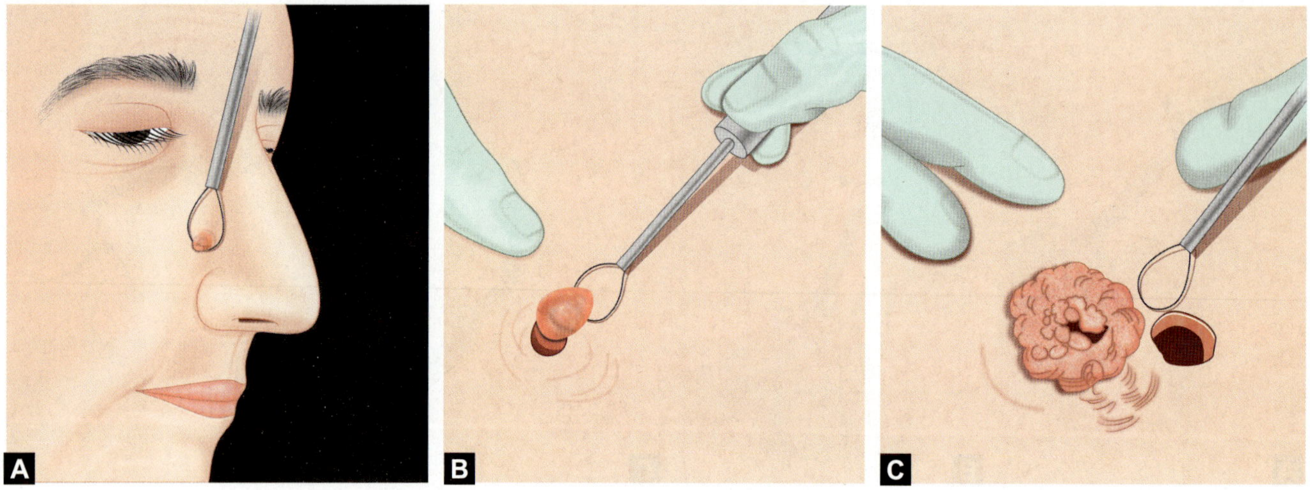

Figs. 41.37A to C: Steps of mole removal.

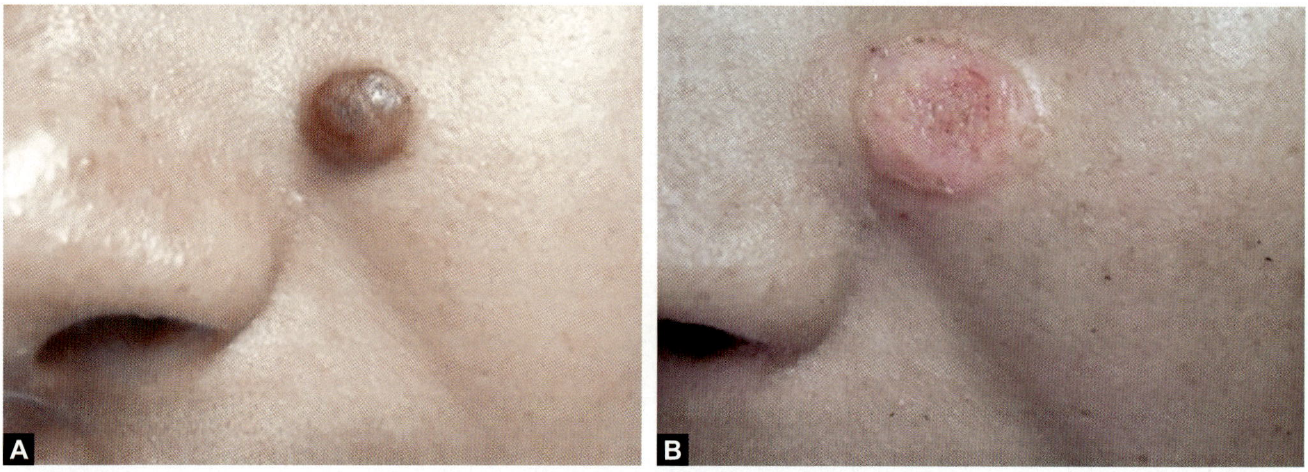

Figs. 41.38A and B: Mole removal—Immediately after picture shows very fine and clean excision, edges show blending into adjoining normal skin.

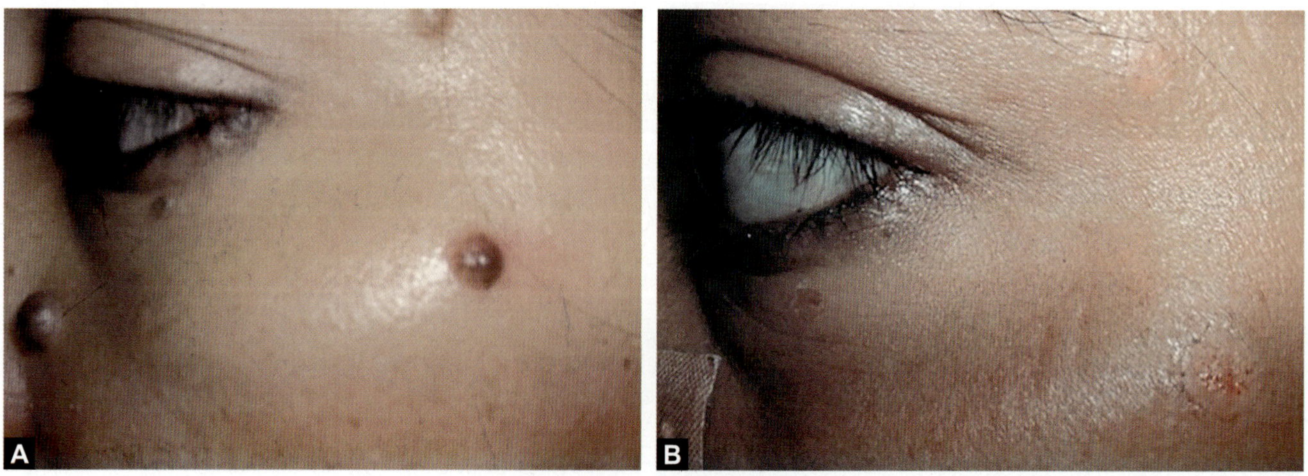

Figs. 41.39A and B: Mole removal—Immediately after picture shows excellent excision and blending.

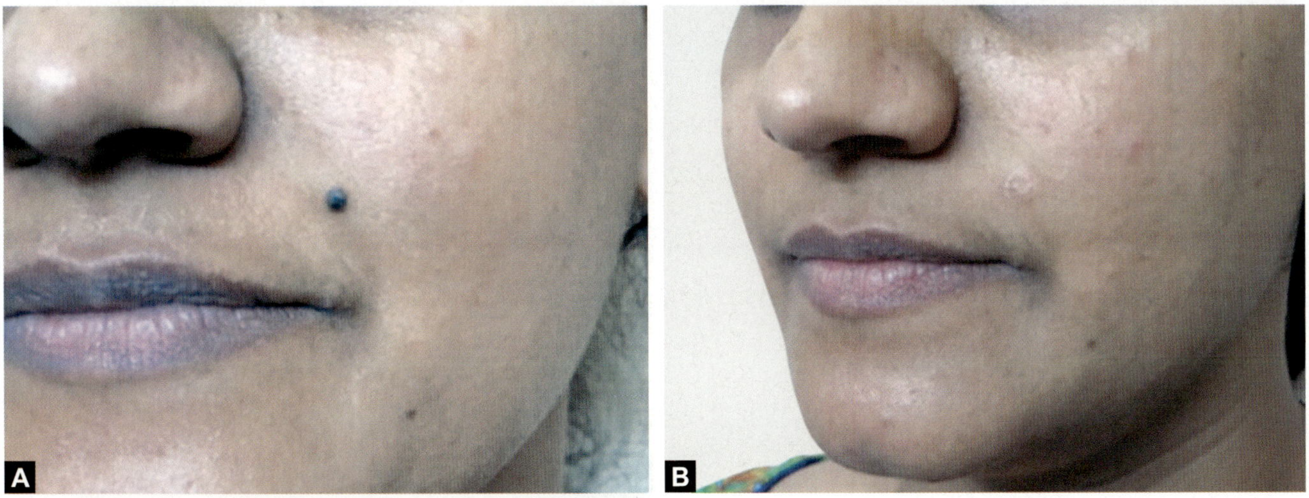

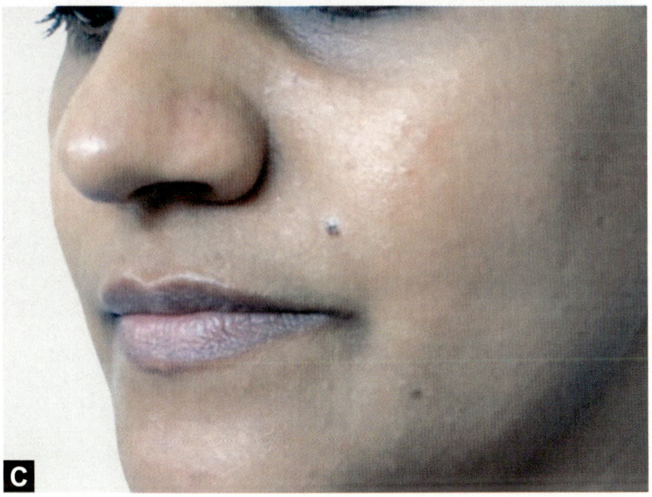

Figs. 41.40A to C: Mole removal by 'shave excision' occasionally gives recurrence as shown in. Here, the recurrent mole is excised by the same method but cutting a bit deeper than before, hence possibility of shallow scar remains.

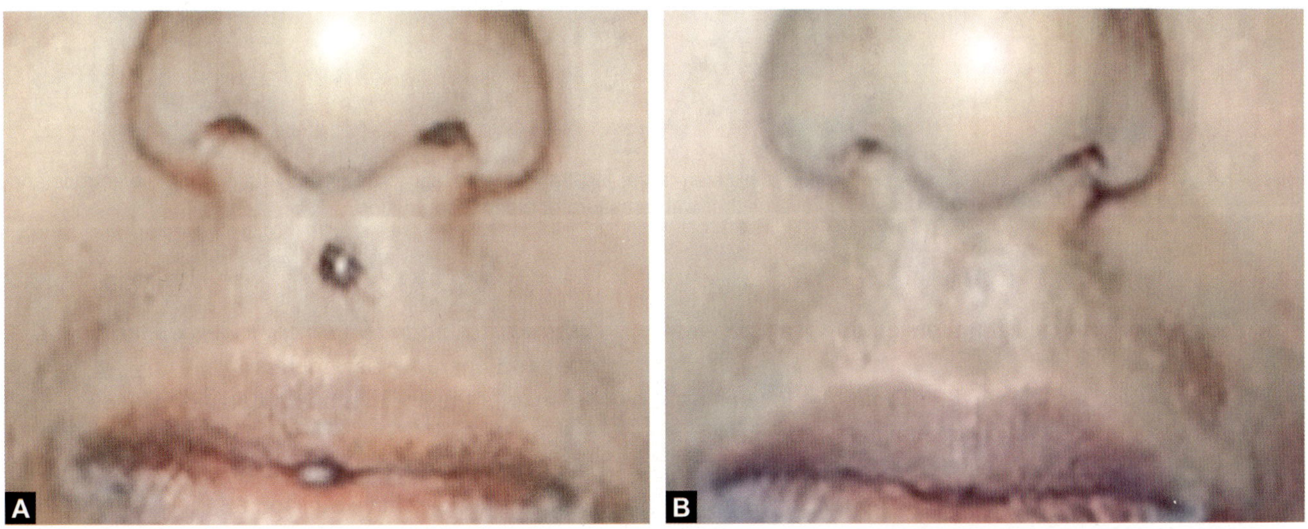

Figs. 41.41A and B: Mole before and 3 months after radiosurgery, no scar or dyschromia.

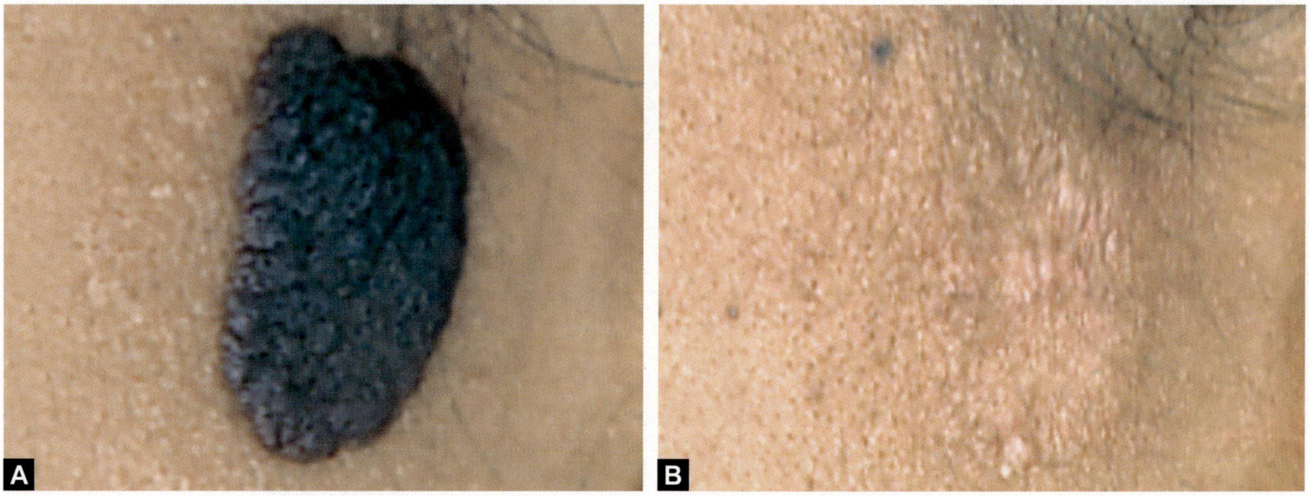

Figs. 41.42A and B: Negligible scar seen after 3 months of nevus excision.

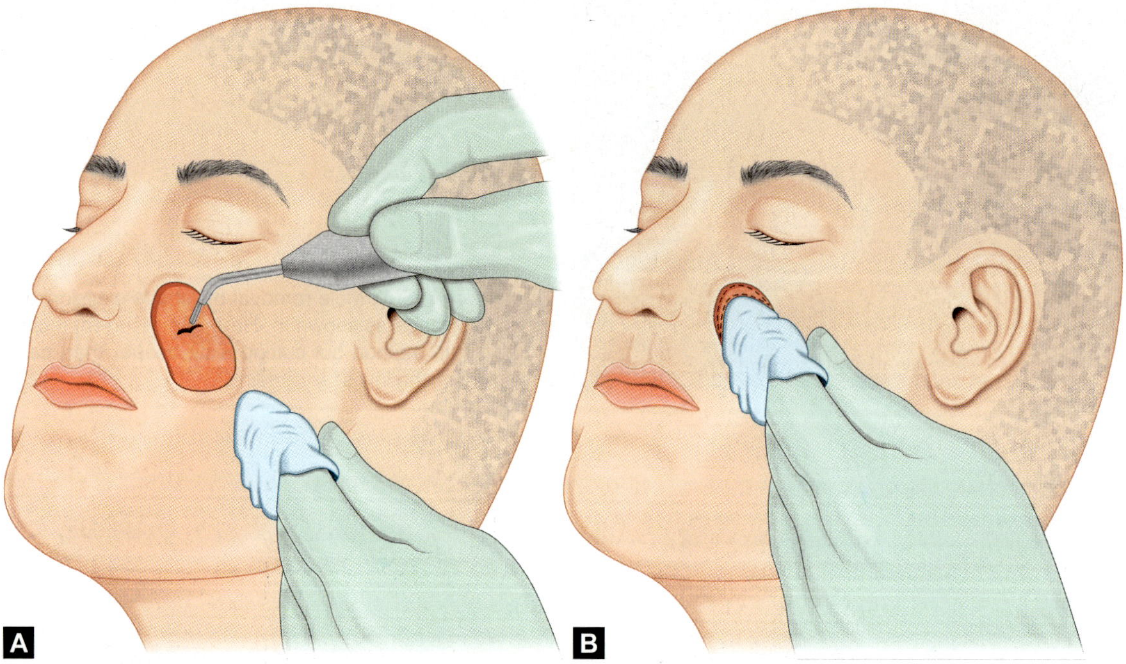

Figs. 41.43A and B: Protuberant lesions: Here, lesion is excised under local anesthesia using straight needle or vari-tip electrode and hemostasis achieved either with pressure or electrocoagulation.

Video gives easy and clear understanding of all steps of mole excision.

- *Protuberant lesions*: Please refer Table 41.4 for tips on operative parameters which are similar to mole excision.
  Please refer to the accompanying excision video for live demonstration and the case study photos given (Figs. 41.43 to 41.49):
- *Keratosis (Actinic and Seborrheic)*: Please refer Table 41.4 for tips on operative parameters.
  Please refer the live demonstration video for step-wise excision.
  Usually, all keratosis lesions can be effectively removed in one session by shave excision method with minimal scarring.

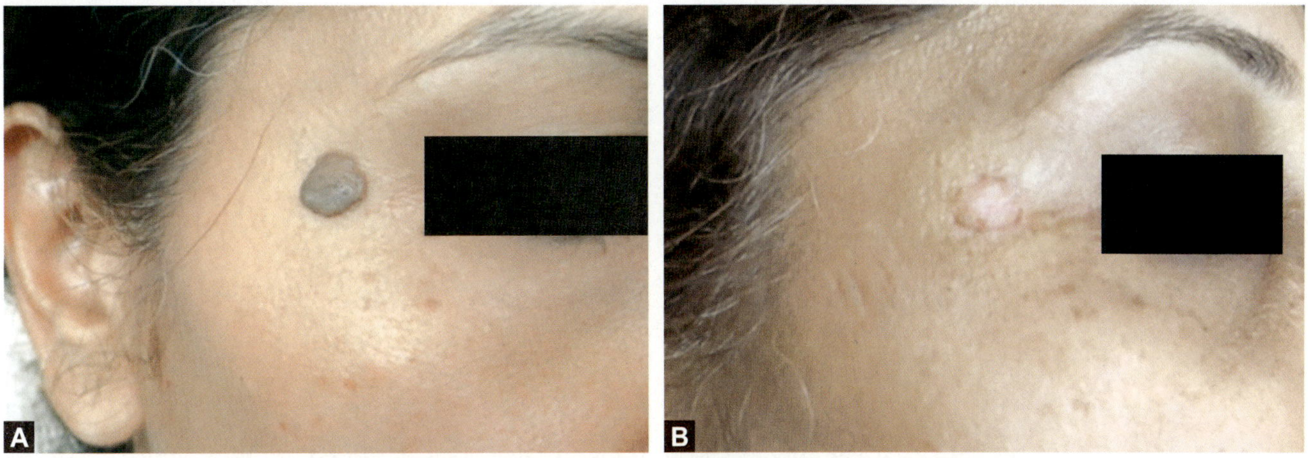

Figs. 41.44A and B: Seborrheic keratoses before and immediately after surgery picture.

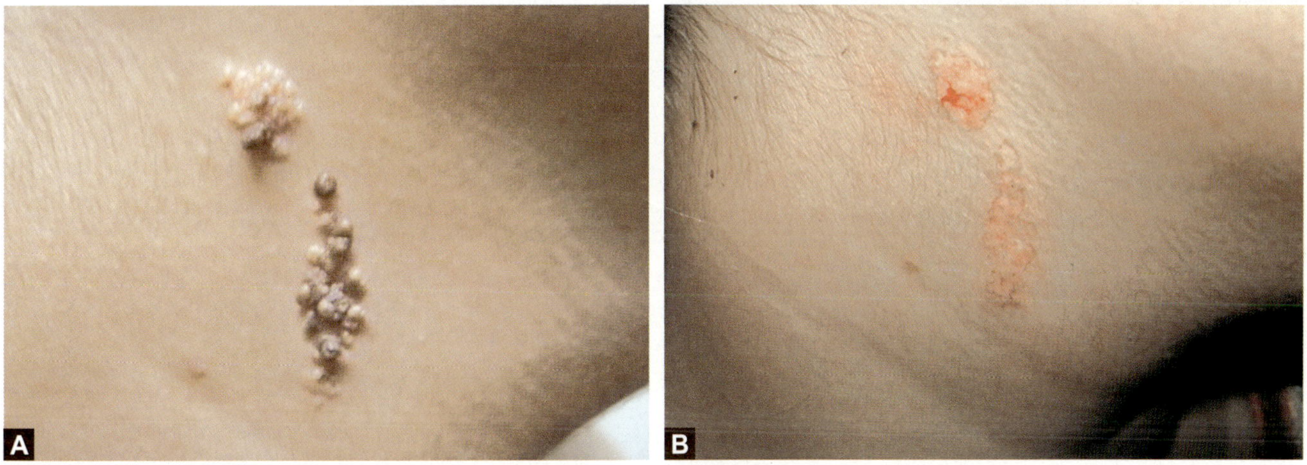

Figs. 41.45A and B: Epidermal nevus: immediately after RF excision.

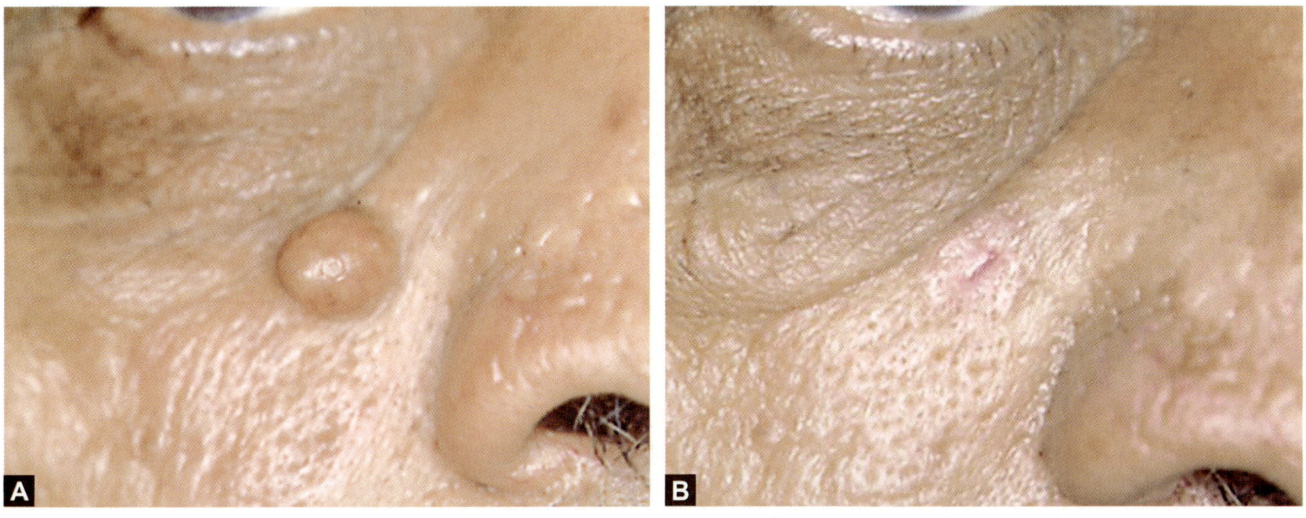

Figs. 41.46A and B: Lesion is fully removed with negligible scar.

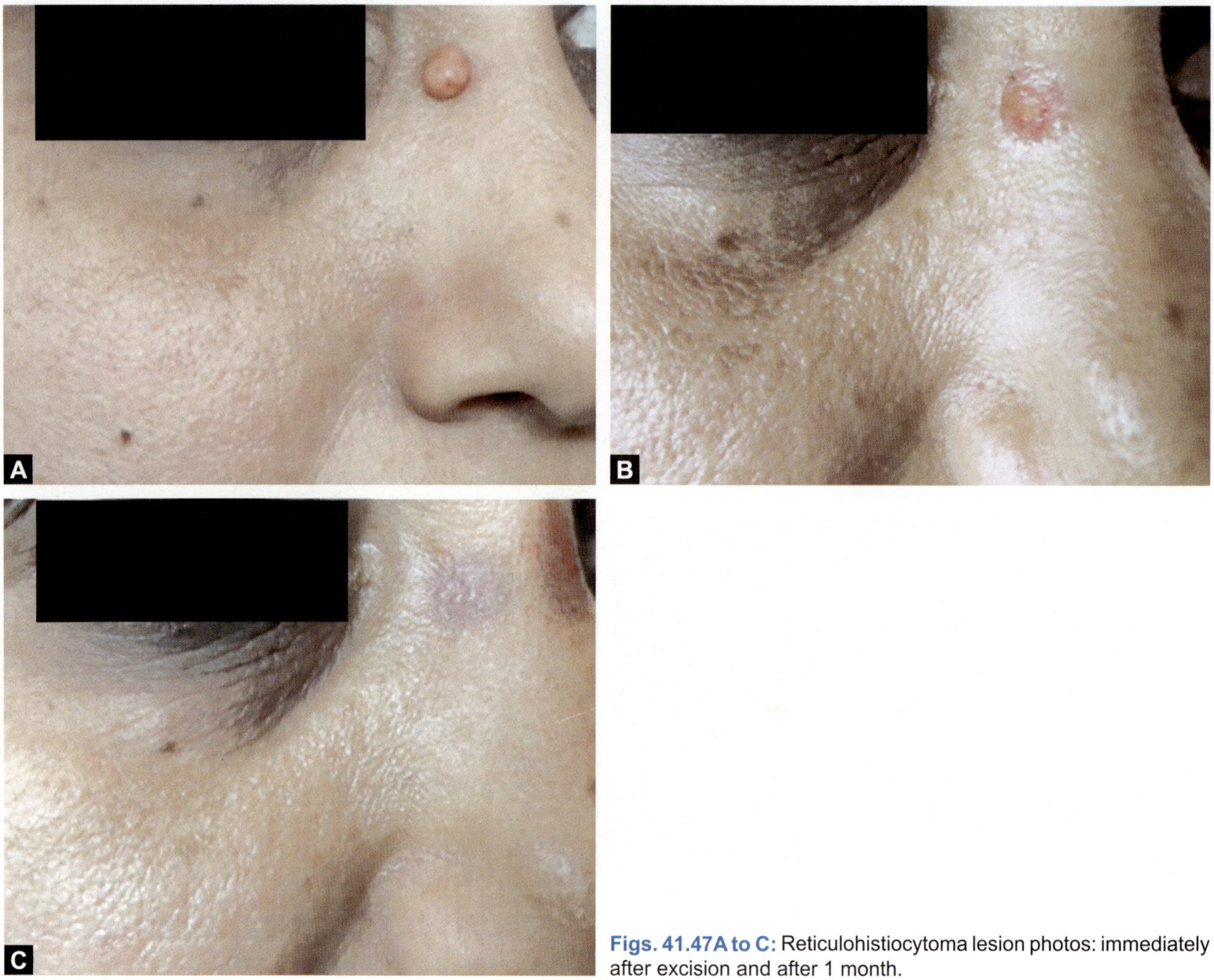

Figs. 41.47A to C: Reticulohistiocytoma lesion photos: immediately after excision and after 1 month.

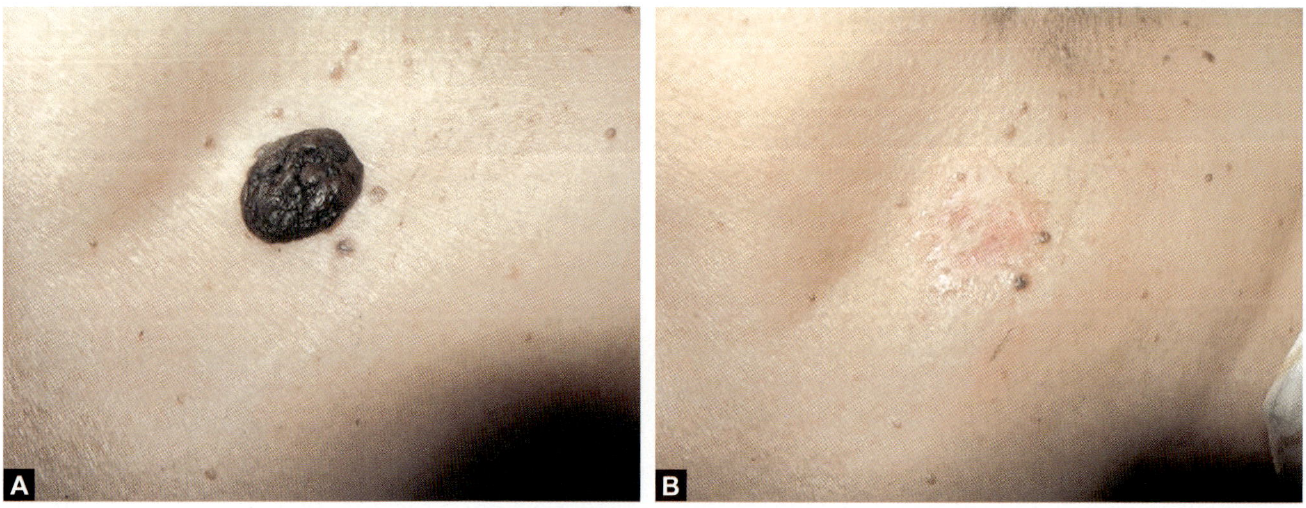

Figs. 41.48A and B: Seborrheic keratosis: immediately after excision.

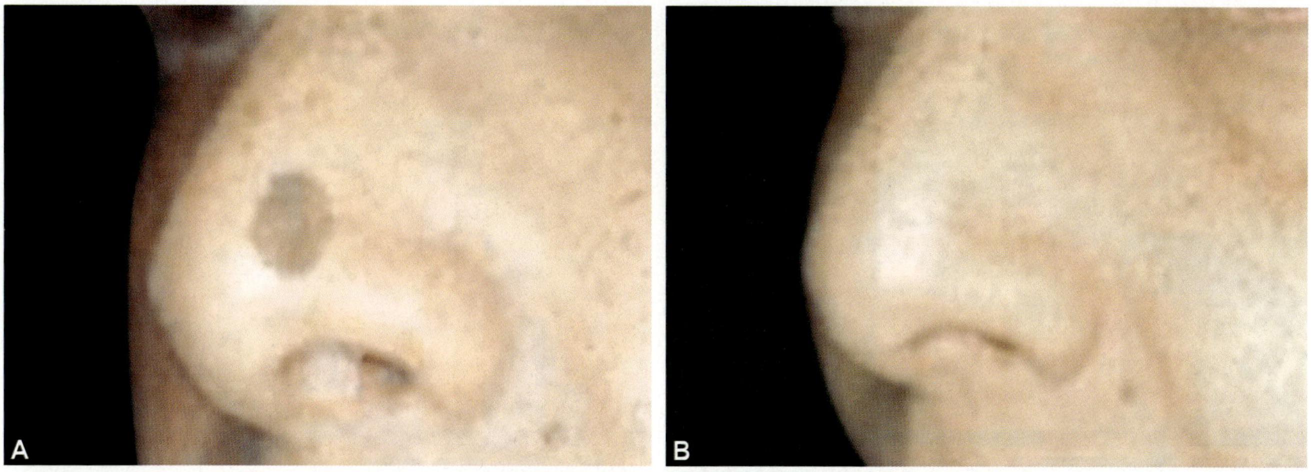

Figs. 41.49A and B: Actinic keratosis: no scar after excision.

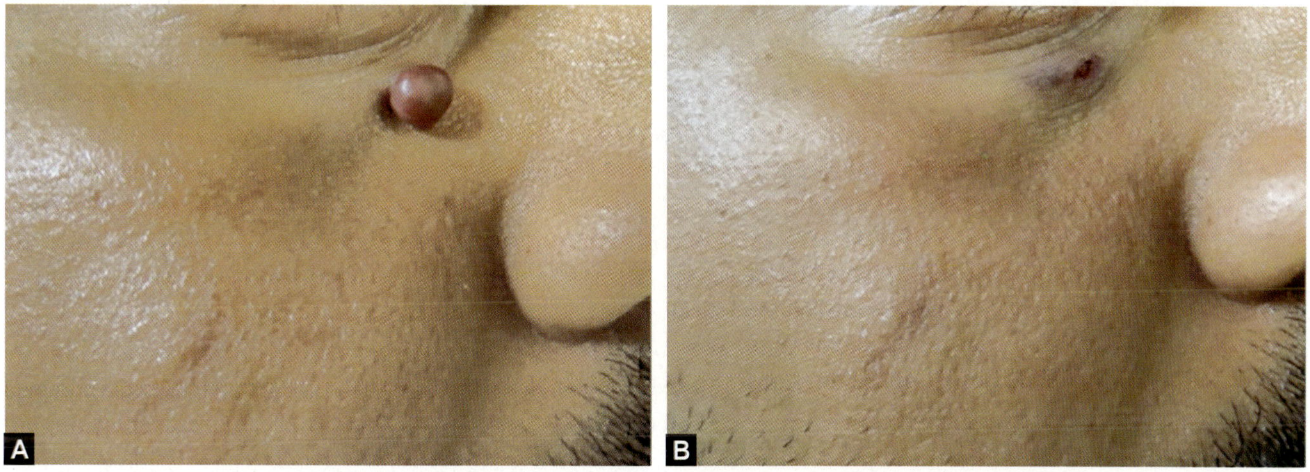

Figs. 41.50A and B: Pyogenic granuloma excised effectively and hemostasis achieved.

- *Vascular lesions*: Please refer Table 41.4 for tips on removal of vascular lesions for operative parameters. The advantage of Cut + Coag mode helps tackle, such lesions very effectively. Finally, electrocoagulation mode seals bleeding vessels very effectively (Figs. 41.50 to 41.52).

Important points to remember when tackling vascular lesions

- All small vascular lesions can be effectively tackled in office practice, but lesions in pediatric age group must preferably be tackled in operation theater under short general anesthesia
- Most of the geriatric patients and those patients on 'blood thinners' must be operated in hospital for safety purpose
- Bleeding and clotting time must be done prior to surgery
- Never work on pure Cut mode
- Periungual, nostril and scalp areas are prone for severe hemorrhage unexpectedly, hence need to be very careful when excising. Tourniquet must be used for surgery on fingers, toes, around nails
- Lesions on face are likely to leave small scar due to electrocoagulation mode which delivers more heat, hence must be explained to patients

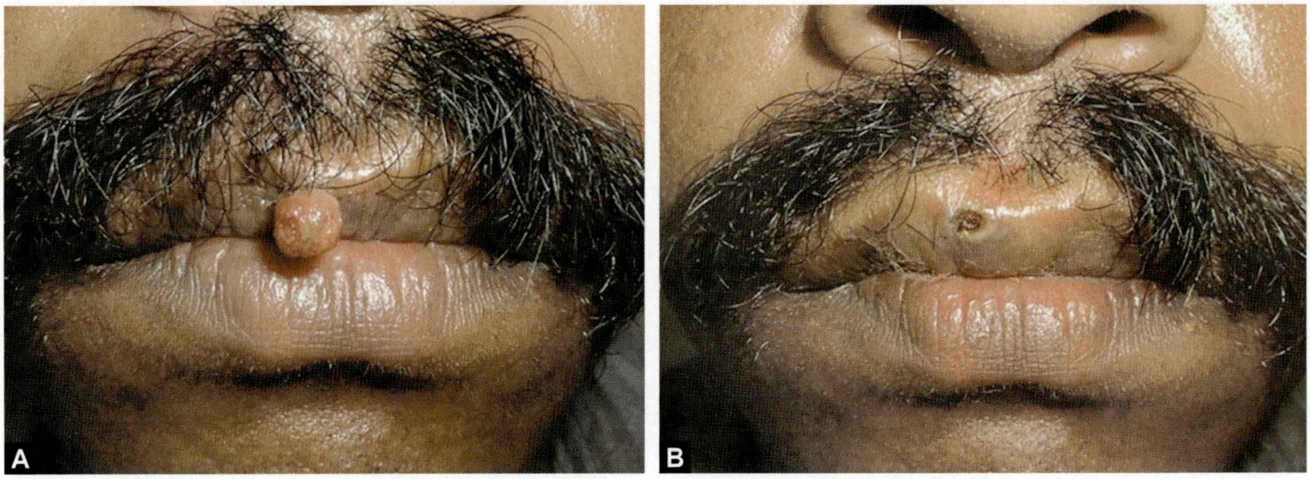

Figs. 41.51A and B: Pyogenic granuloma excised effectively and hemostasis achieved.

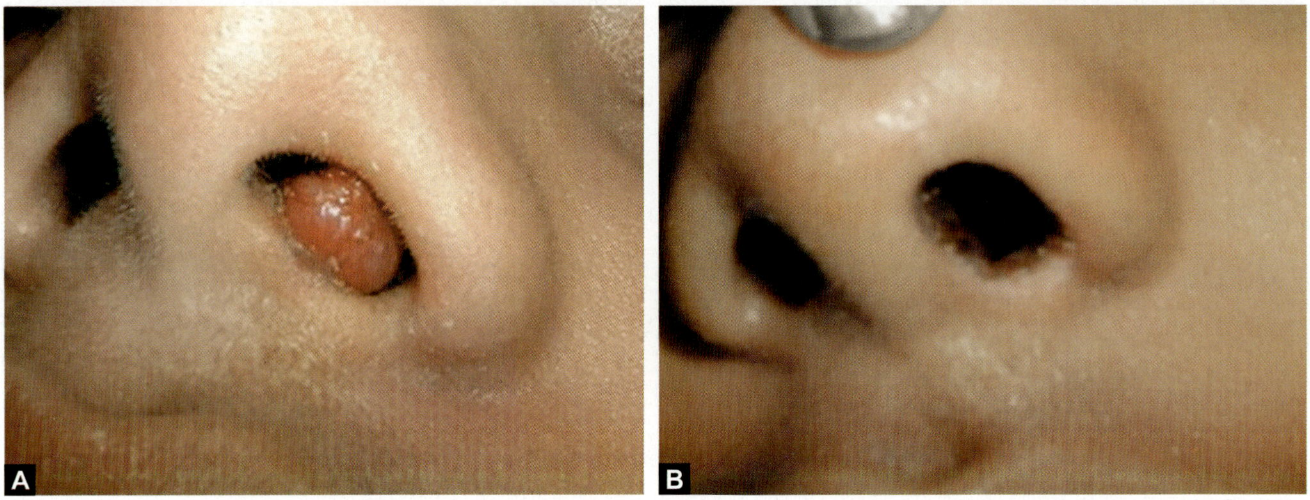

Figs. 41.52A and B: Capillary hemangioma from nostril excised under short general anesthesia in hospital. Cut + coagulation mode was used to excise followed by electrocoagulation for effective hemostasis. Finally nasal ribbon packing soaked with liquid paraffin was done.

- *Mucosal lesions*: Please refer Table 41.4 for Tips on operative parameters which remain the same as for Shave Excision. Blended mode of Cut + Coagulation is used commonly for effective bloodless excision. Tricks are same as those for shave excision (Figs. 41.53 and 41.54).

Submucous cyst or mucocele removal

- Lesion is sterilized and anesthetized as usual
- Chalazion forceps is used to hold lesion firmly
- Round loop electrode set on blended, i.e. Cut + Coagulation mode is used to shave off the lesion fully up to its base
- Hemostasis is easily achieved with ball tip electrode
- Lesion is allowed to heal with secondary intention
- Postoperatively, lignocaine viscous solution is advised for pain relief during eating and routine systemic antibiotics are prescribed.

The commonly encountered other mucosal lesions like warts are covered elsewhere in the chapter.

- *Sebaceous cyst removal*: Please refer Table 41.4 for tips on operative parameters. The Figures 41.55 to 41.62 will give fair idea of easy steps of excision.

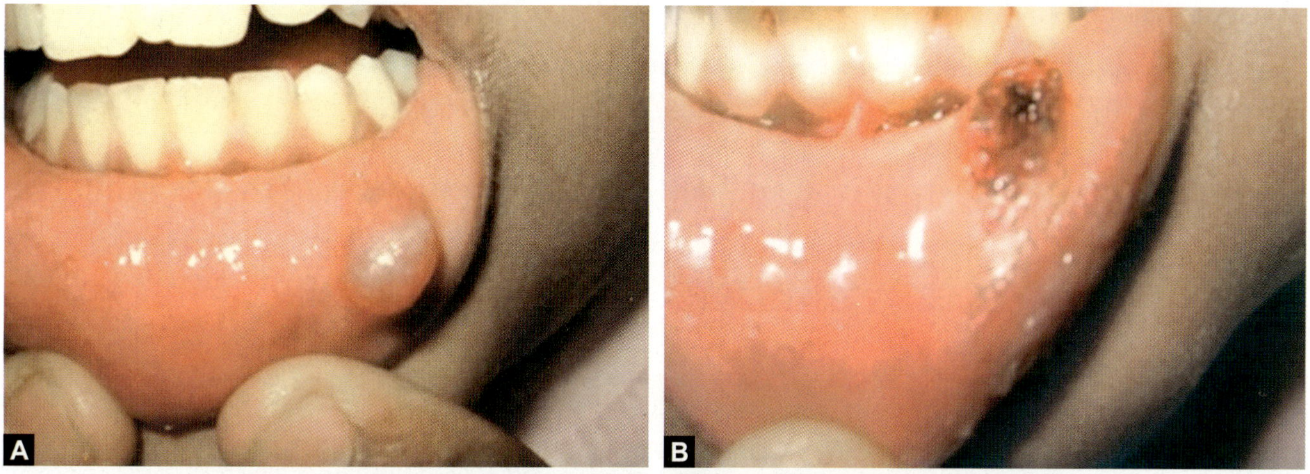

Figs. 41.53A and B: (A) Submucous cyst and, (B) a common problem after excision.

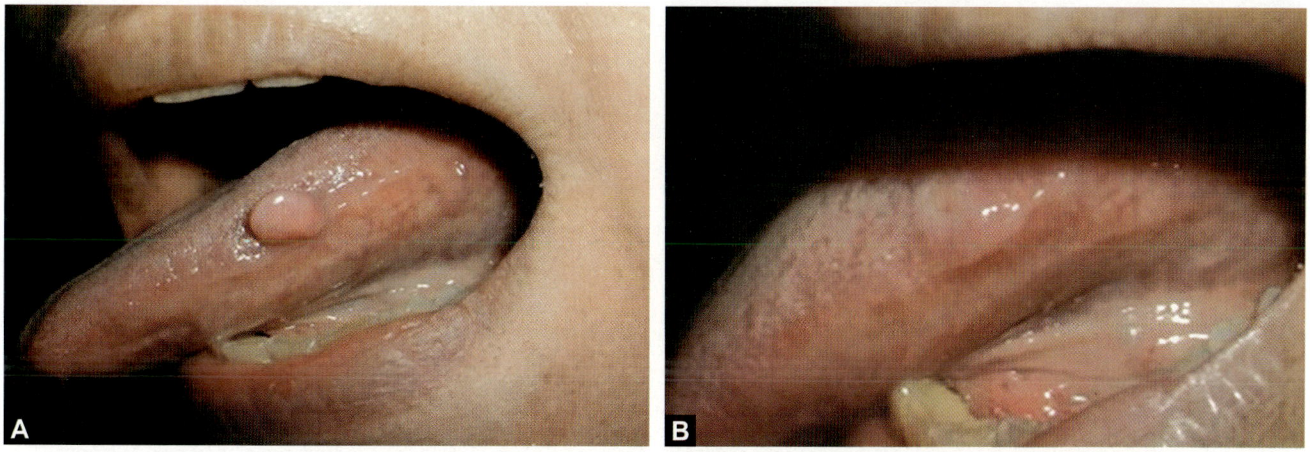

Figs. 41.54A and B: Tongue fibroma removed with shave excision healed fully without complications.

Sebaceous cyst removal

- Sebaceous cyst is sterilized and anesthetized as usual
- Very small incision is made with Vari-tip electrode just deep enough to cut open the cyst
- All sebum content is expressed out with pressure
- Cyst wall is pulled out with forceps and excised
- Small incision either is left for secondary healing or stuck with tissue glue containing cyanoacrylate
- If cyst wall is difficult to remove, insert Vari-tip electrode inside cyst and activate machine to pass on heat to wall at power of 1–2. Wall gets necrosed . Here, tissue glue is not used, wound is left open.

- *Xanthelasma treatment*: Please refer Table 41.4 for tips on parameters
- *Ear lobe repair*: Please refer Table 41.4 for operative parameters
- *Ear keloids*: Please refer Table 41.4 for operative parameters Ear keloids once excised are injected intralesionally with Inj. Triamcinolone 10 mg/mL immediately after removal and allowed to heal with secondary intention which may take 2 weeks. Once healed, topical silicone gel is applied twice daily and strictly followed up every 2 weeks for 6–8 months minimum to prevent recurrence.
- *Facial scars*[12-14]: Please refer Table 41.4 for tips on operative parameters
  - *Depressed scars:* Please refer the Figures 41.63 to 41.67 for step-wise resurfacing. Also, refer live demonstration video for details
  - *Hypertrophic scars*: These are just planed down and allowed to heal by secondary intention (Fig. 41.68).

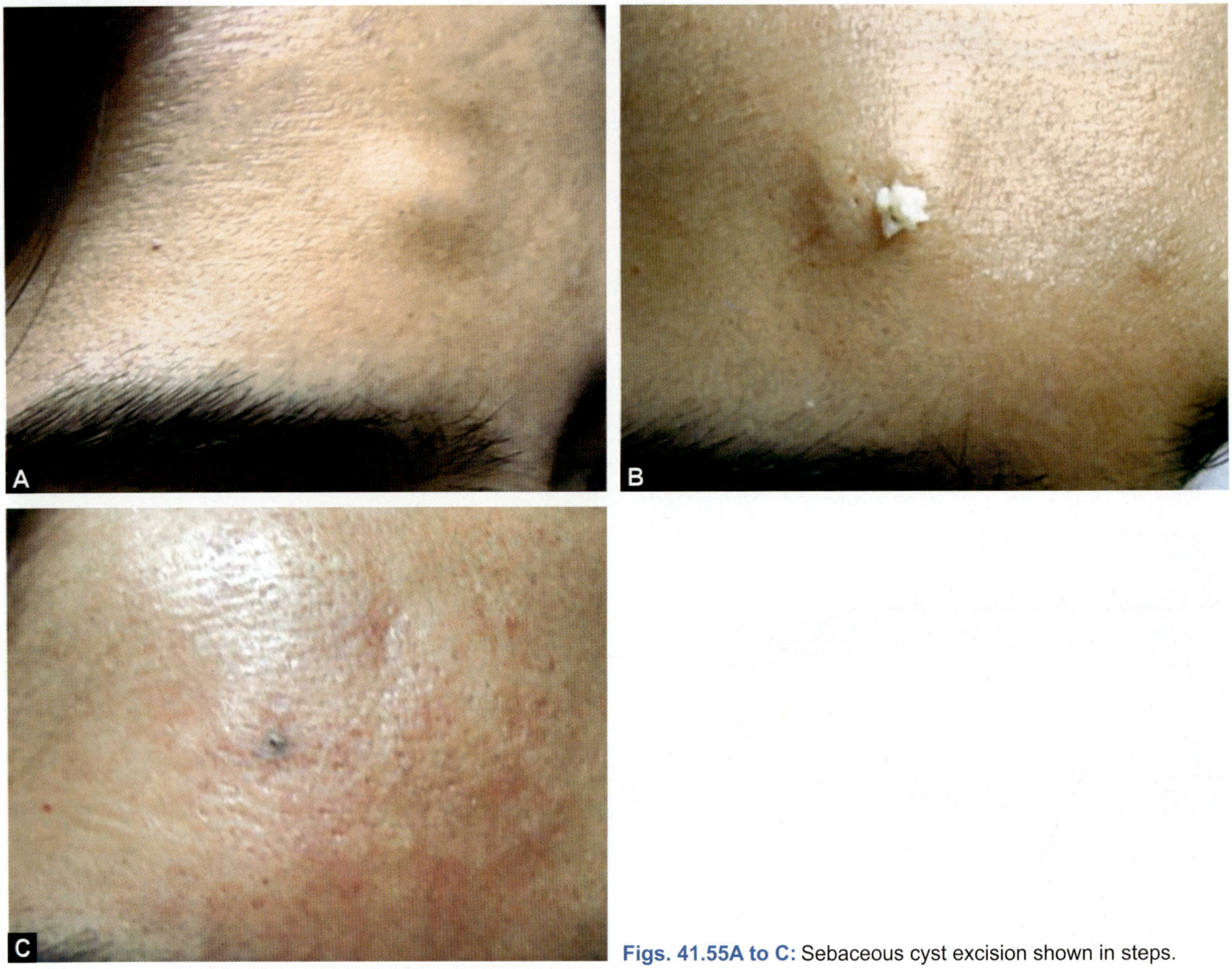

Figs. 41.55A to C: Sebaceous cyst excision shown in steps.

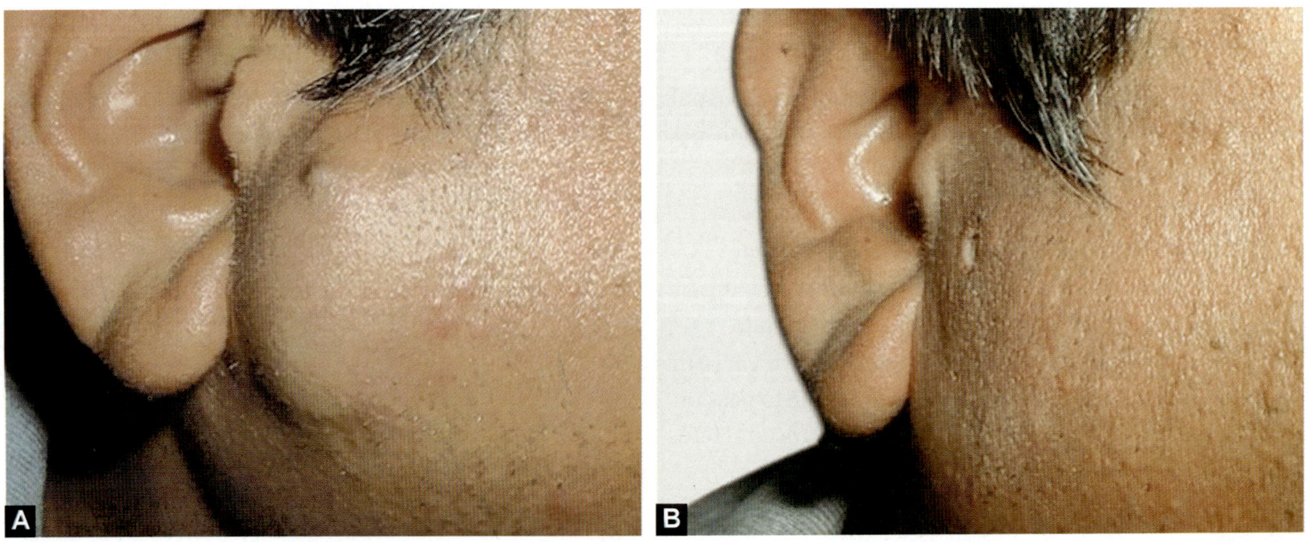

Figs. 41.56A and B: Large sebaceous cyst removed through 'small incision'.

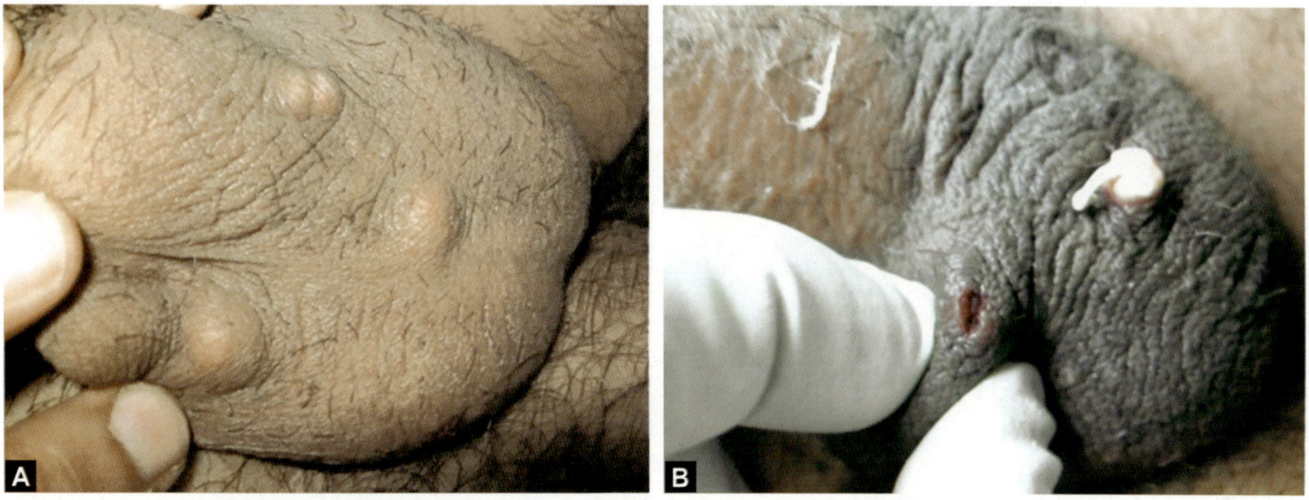

Figs. 41.57A and B: Small incision' made over cyst and sebum expressed out with pressure.

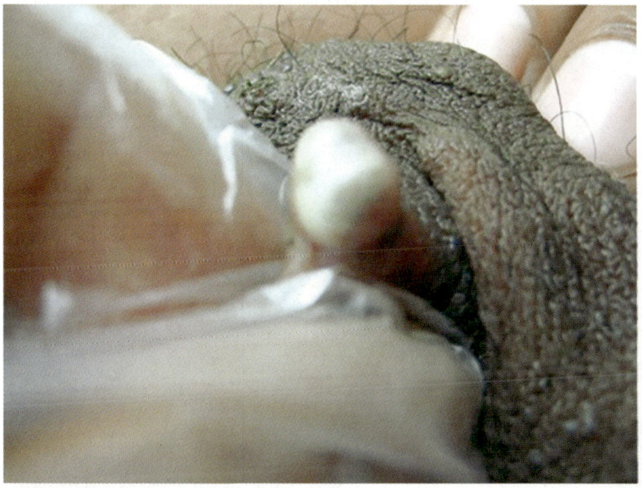

Fig. 41.58: After expressing out contents, cyst wall is pulled out and excised.

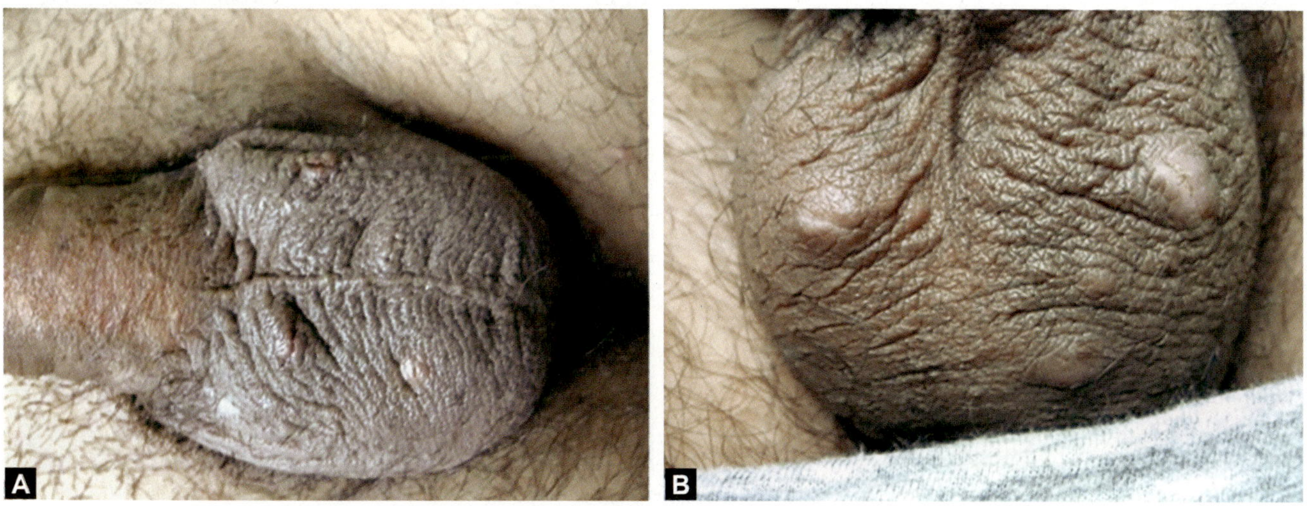

Figs. 41.59A and B: (A) Immediately post-surgery picture; (B) Complete healing with scars.

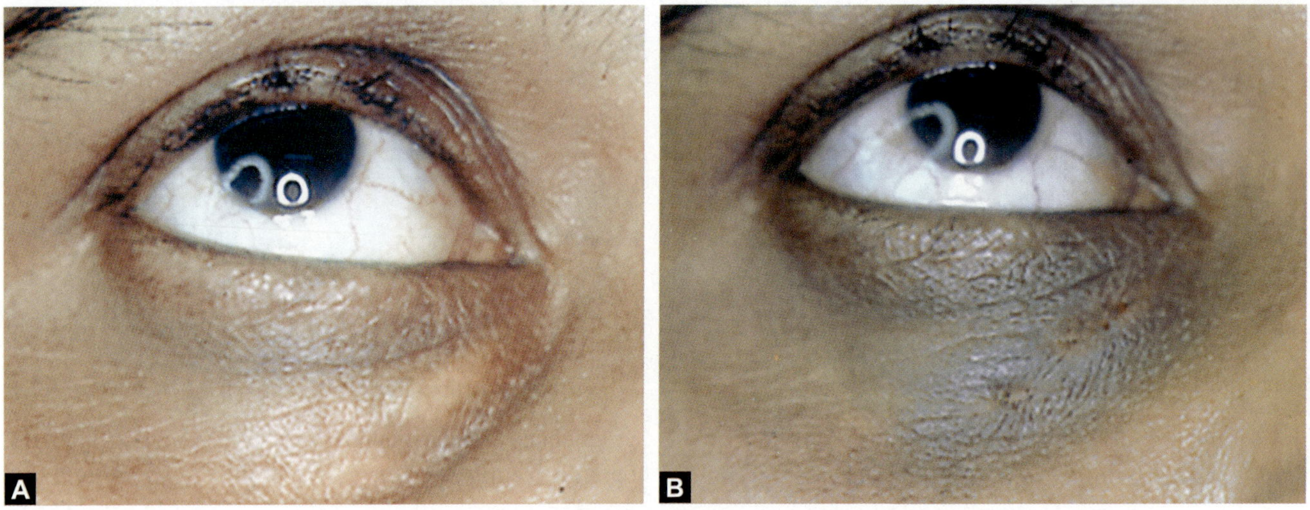

Figs. 41.60A and B: Xanthelasma desiccated superficially, it clears off.

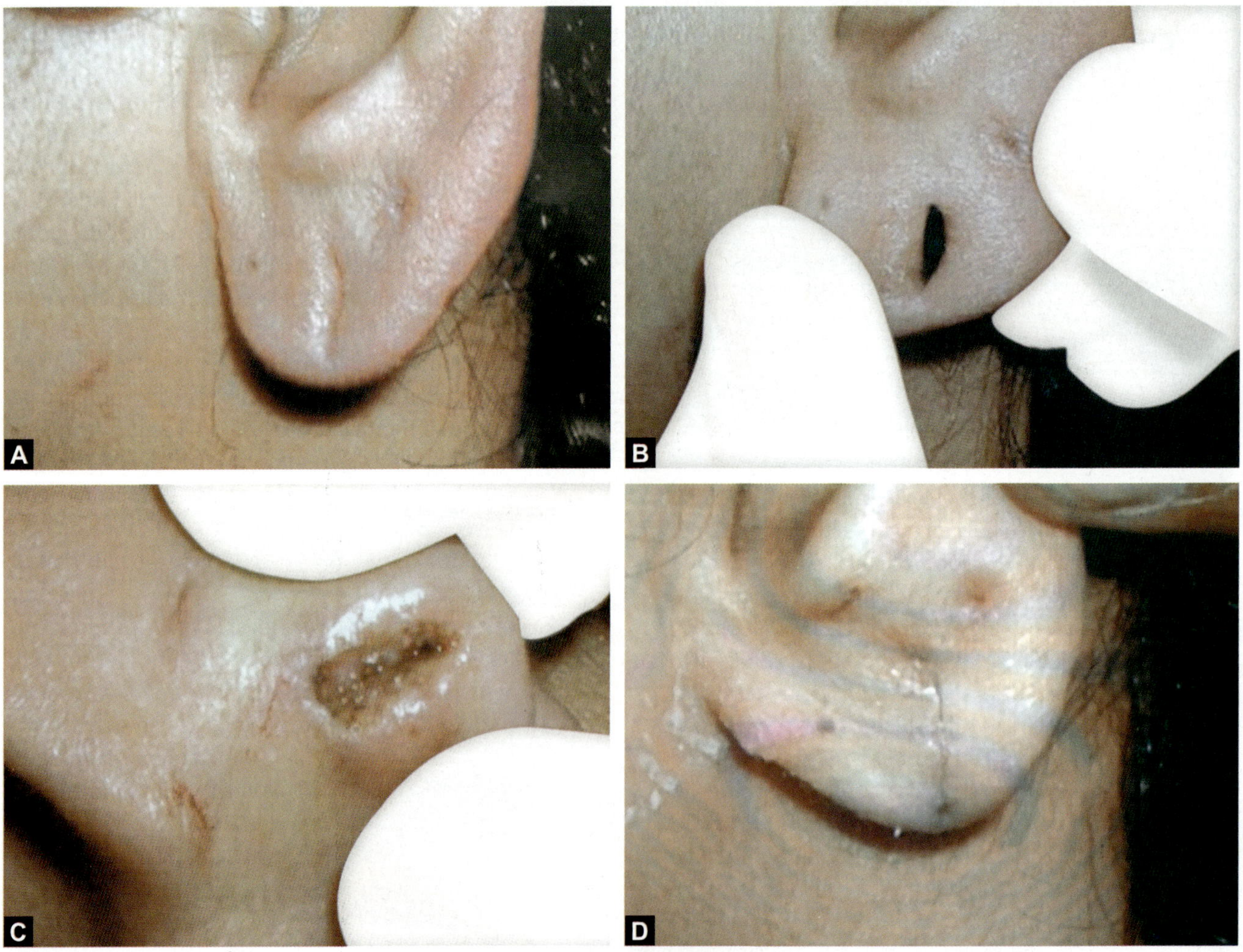

Figs. 41.61A to D

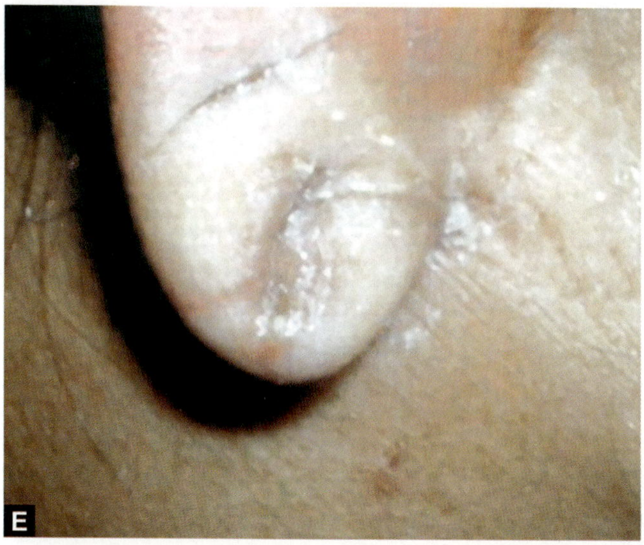

Figs. 41.61A to E: Ear lobe repair edges are refreshed with vari-tip electrode and stuck with tissue glue.

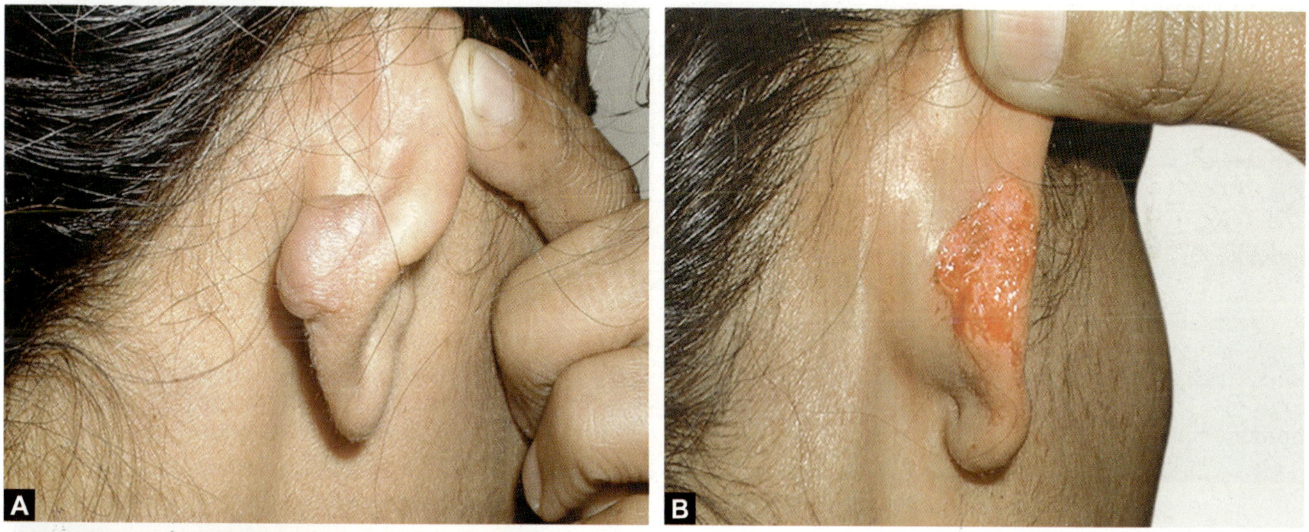

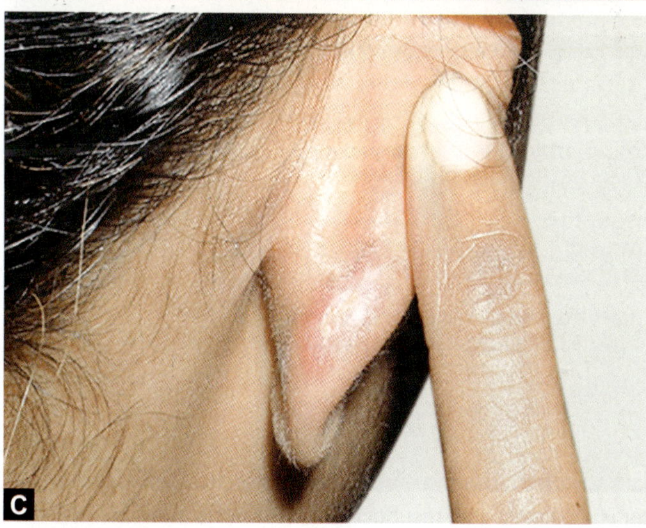

Figs. 41.62A to C: Ear keloids are easily excised.

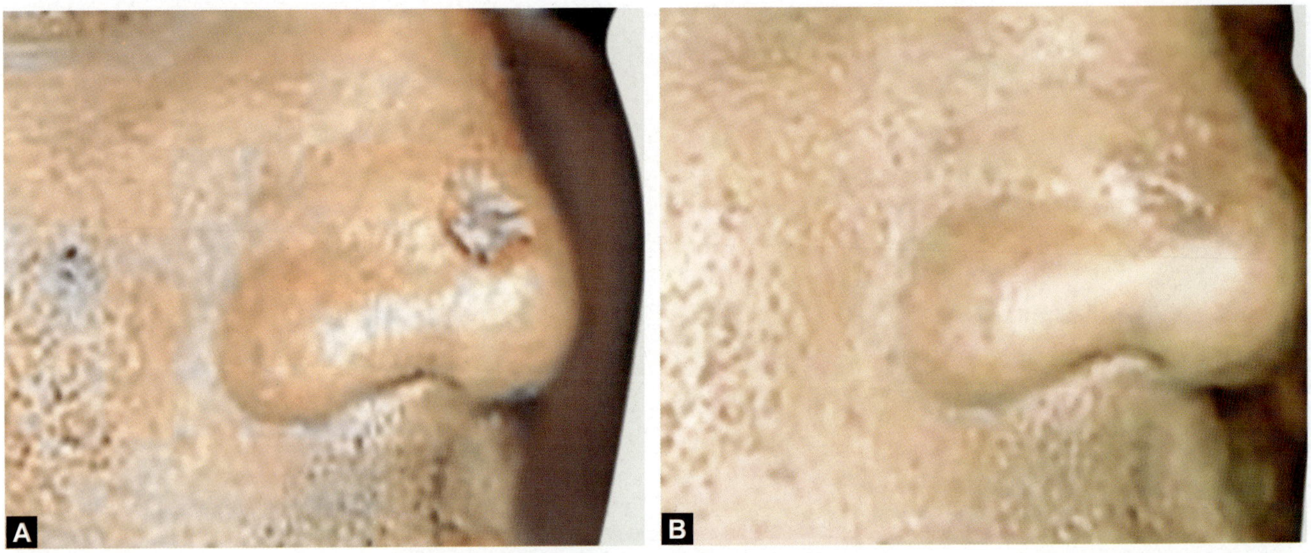

Figs. 41.63A and B: Resurfacing an atrophic scar.

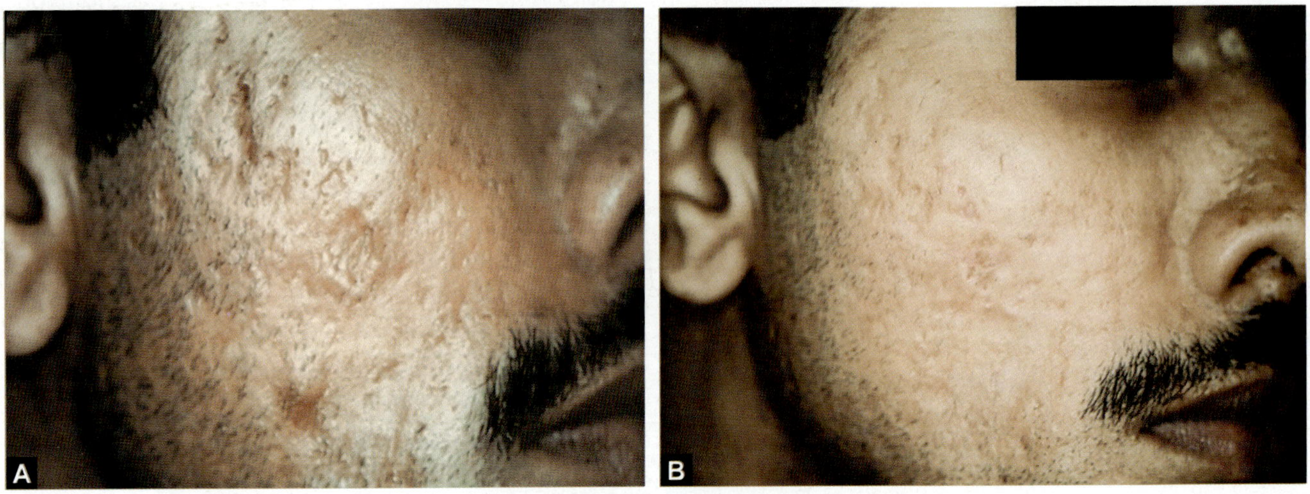

Figs. 41.64A and B: Post-trauma and postacne scar resurfaced.

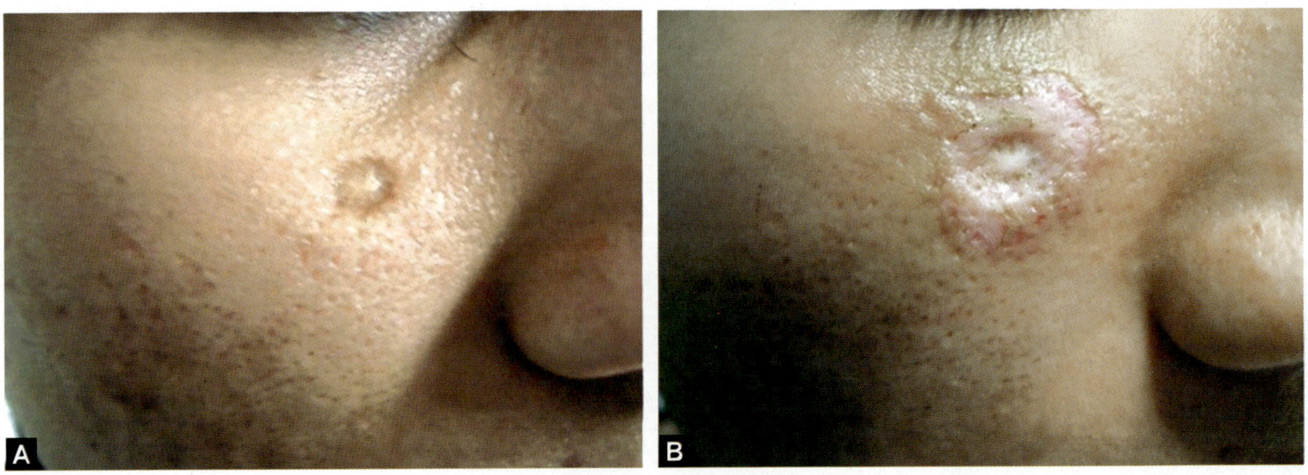

Figs. 41.65A and B: Chickenpox scar immediately after resurfacing.

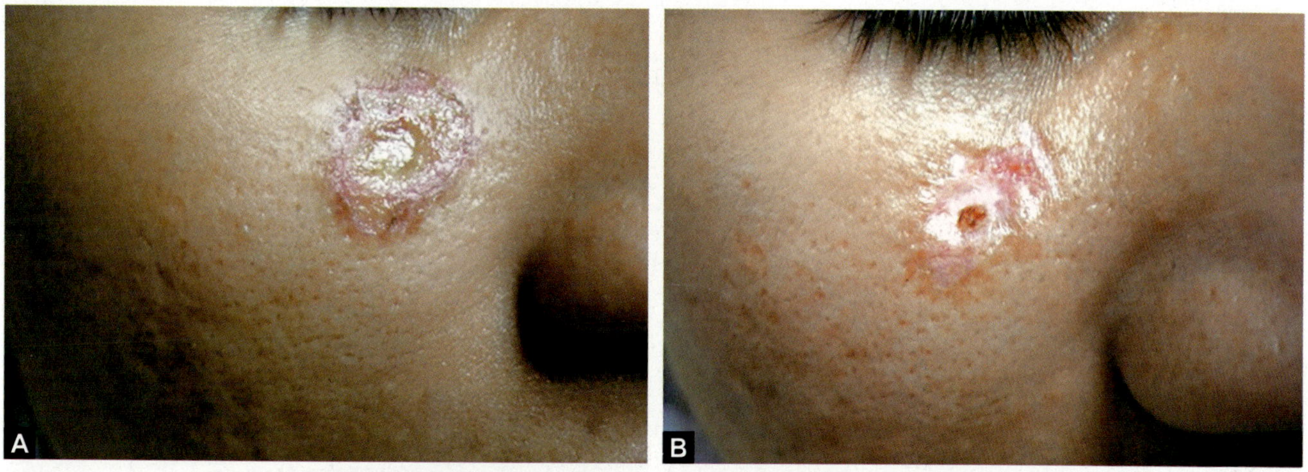

Figs. 41.66A and B: 3 days (A) and 10 days (B) after resurfacing.

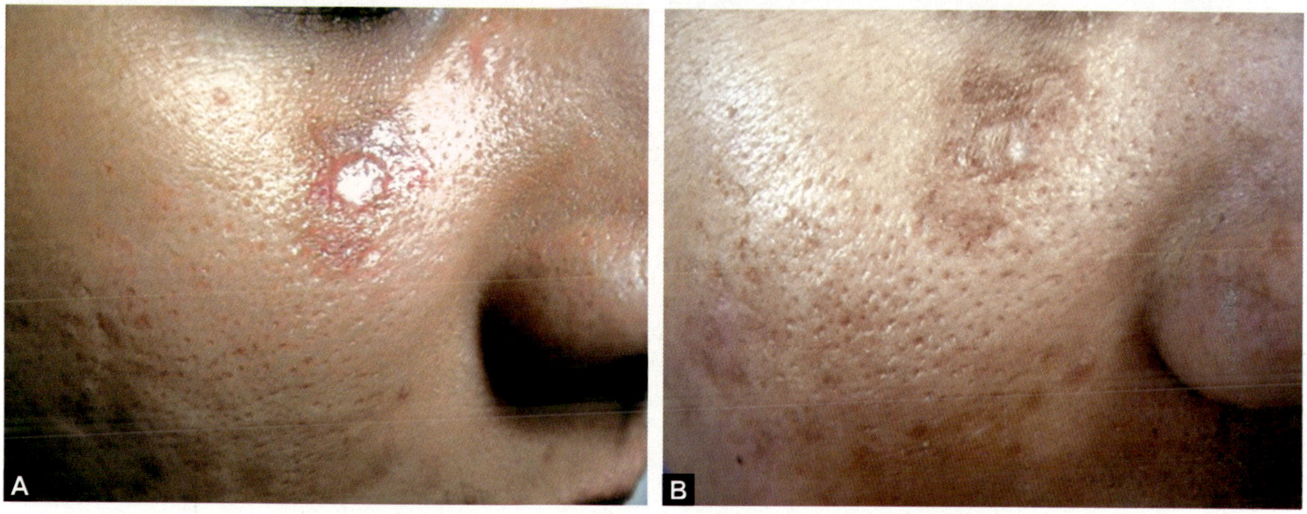

Figs. 41.67A and B: 1 month (A) and 2 months (B) after resurfacing.

Hypertrophic scars may require Inj. Triamcinolone intralesionally to prevent hypertrophy after healing.

All photos of resurfacing are at least 3 months apart (final result).

Last case study final photo is 1 year after resurfacing.

Postresurfacing dyschromia usually clears completely over 2–6 months.

- *Ingrowing toe-nails*[15]: Please refer to the Figures 41.69 to 41.73 for complete understanding of the procedure. Recurrence of this condition occurs, if the extreme horn of nail matrix is not treated effectively.
- *Rhinophyma*[16]: Please refer to the Figures 41.74 to 41.76 and method given for rhinophyma resection and resurfacing.

Rhinophyma resection and resurfacing

- Local anesthetic is given at various points around nose as shown above for good anesthesia
- Blended or 'Cut + Coagulation' current is selected
- Power is 3–5
- Round loop electrode is selected
- Shave excision is done to remove excess sebaceous tissue
- Nose is properly trimmed and reshaped removing thicker tissue
- While cutting care is taken to maintain nasal contour and symmetry

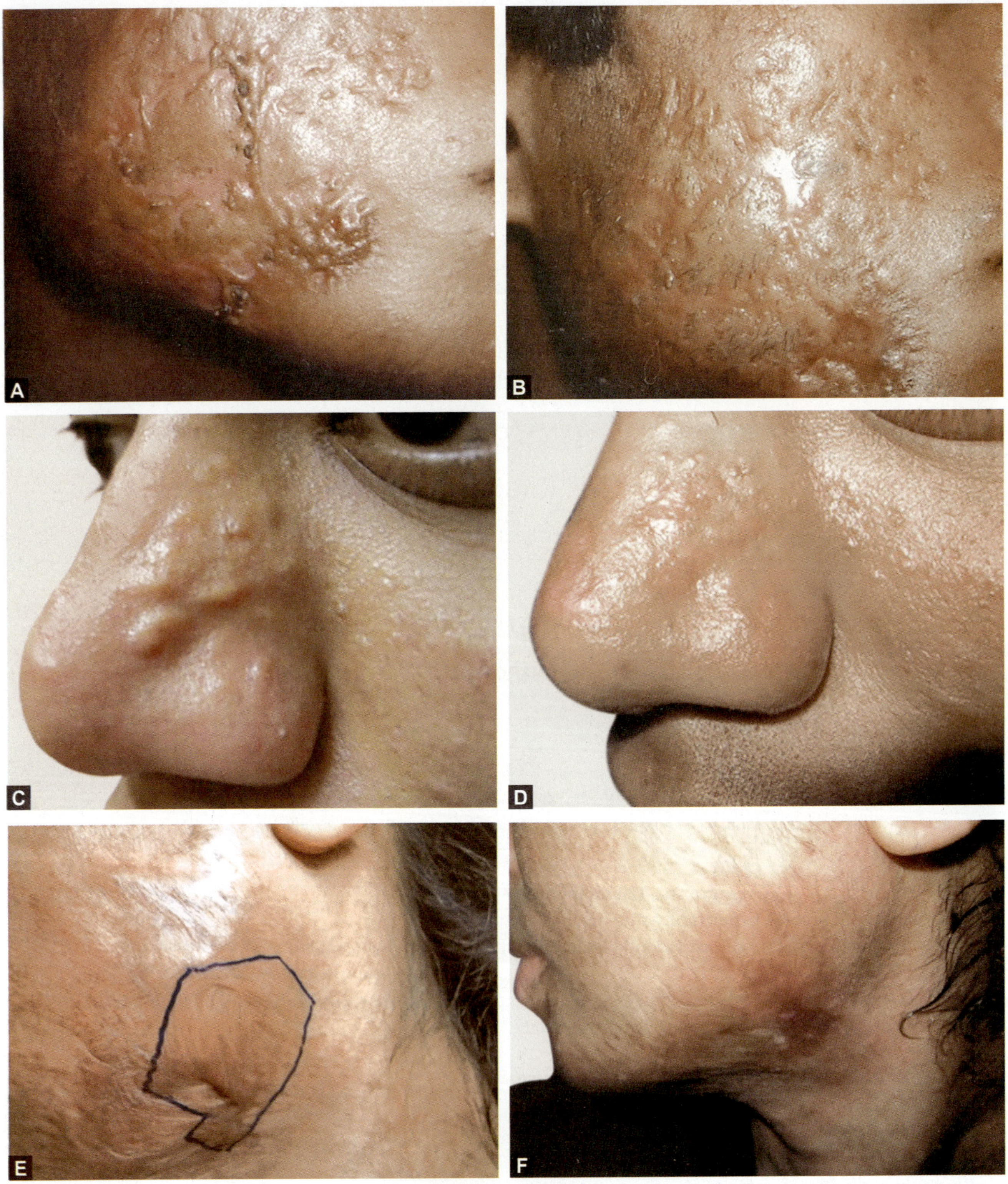

Figs. 41.68A to F: All above hypertrophic scars are resurfaced with good result.

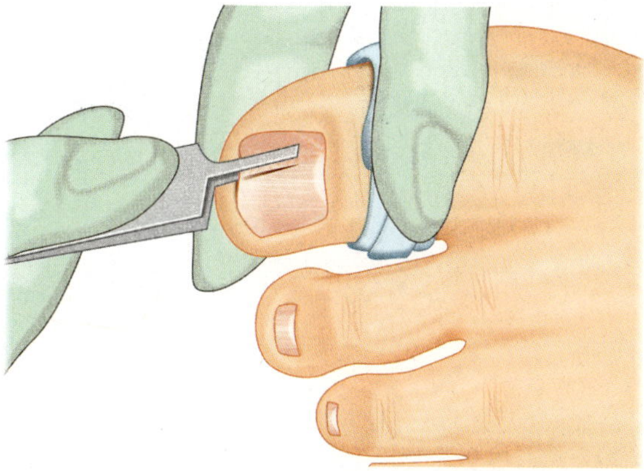

Fig. 41.69: After giving ring block with lignocaine and tying tourniquet the ingrowing toe-nail is first clipped with scissors or scalpel blade.

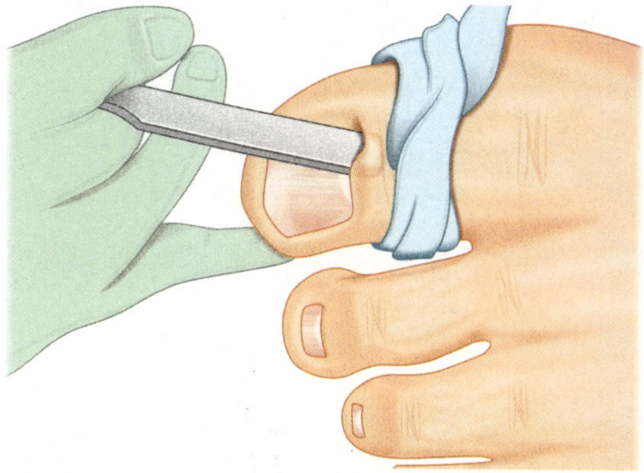

Fig. 41.70: Spatula is used to loosen proximal nail fold from underlying nail plate and nail plate from nail bed.

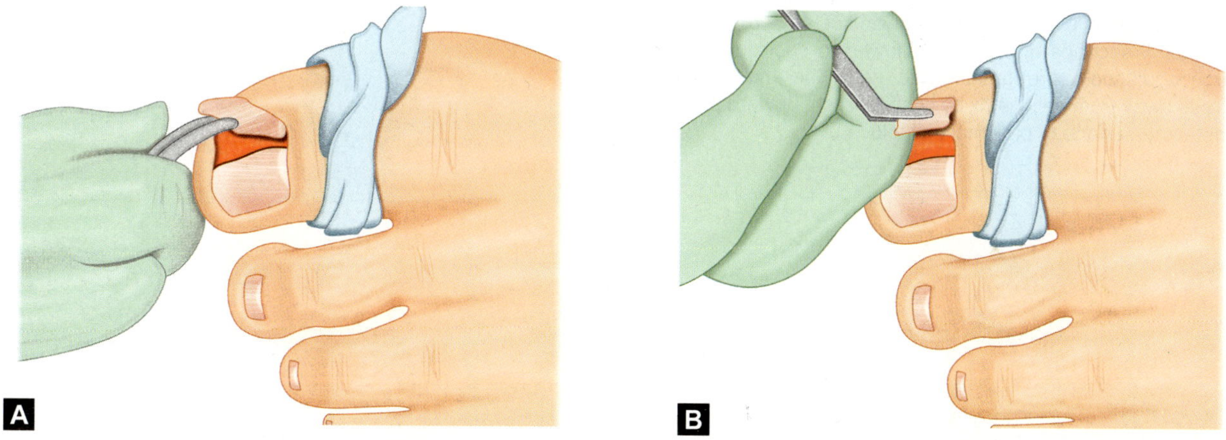

Figs. 41.71A and B: Cut nail plate is grasped with a hemostat forceps and firm pull is exerted to remove it fully taking care not to leave any portion underneath.

- Care is also taken not to have overzealous approach in order to preserve epidermal appendages which are required for healing
- Wound is allowed to heal by secondary intention
- Topical and systemic antibiotics and pain relieving medicines are advised
- Dressing is done daily
- Wound healing may require 3–4 weeks

- *Skin biopsy*[17,18]: This is a very useful application which is not only diagnostic but also therapeutic.
  Important points to remember before using this technique for skin biopsy:
  - This is always done using 'cutting current' as the lateral heating is least.
  - This is always done in one stroke whether it is incisional or excision biopsy.

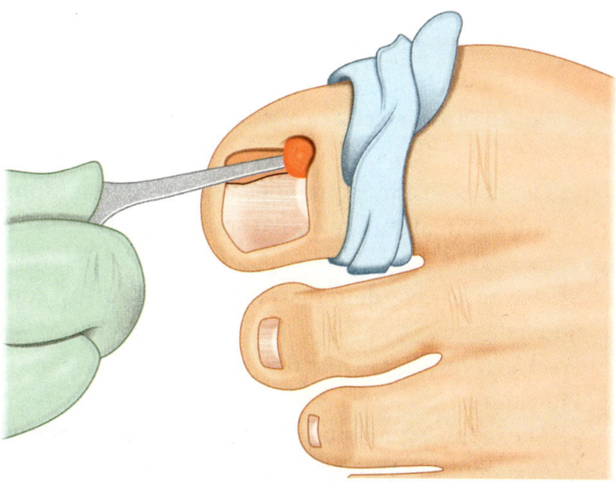

Fig. 41.72: Nail matrix to be destroyed is scraped vigorously using a curette.

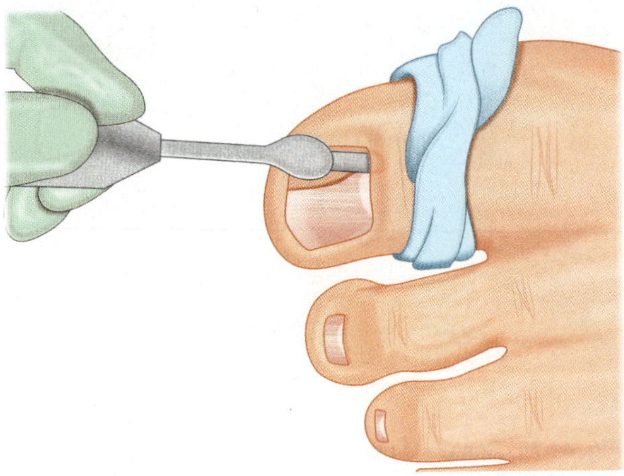

Fig. 41.73: Nail matricectomy electrode is inserted fully under proximal nail fold with its insulated side on top and metal or non-insulated side underneath close to germinal epithelium. Electrocoagulation waveform with power set at 5–6, current is applied for 5 seconds and area is allowed to cool down. While electrocoagulating, care is taken to keep the metal side of electrode away from nail matrix by keeping slight upward pressure against undersurface of proximal nail fold.

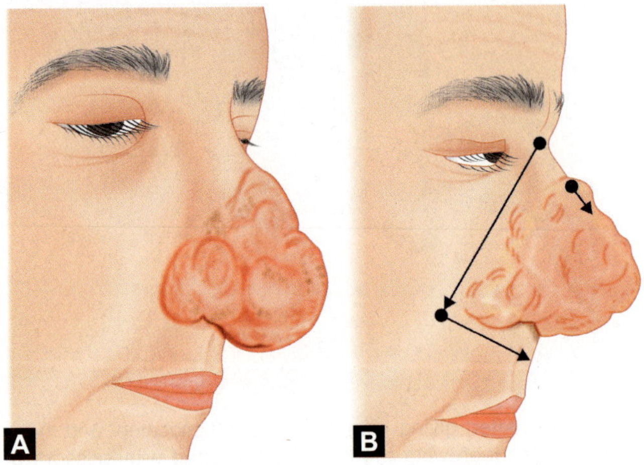

Figs. 41.74A and B: Arrows indicate plan of giving local anesthetic injection to ensure complete anesthesia during procedure.

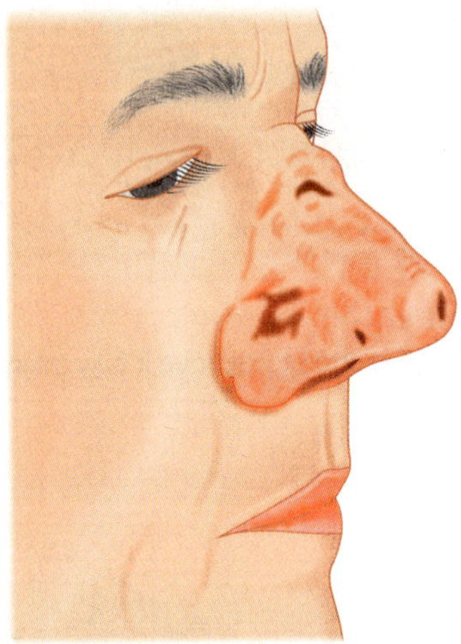

Fig. 41.75: After resection of rhinophymatous mass.

- Depth of lesion is prejudged before doing biopsy and depth of cut is planned accordingly (Figs. 41.77 to 41.82).

Please refer live demonstration of video for good understanding.

- *Freckles (Figs. 41.83A and B)*:

  Procedure:
  - After applying adequate surface anesthesia, each and every Freckle lesion is very finely ablated or scraped in single stroke
  - Straight needle electrode is used

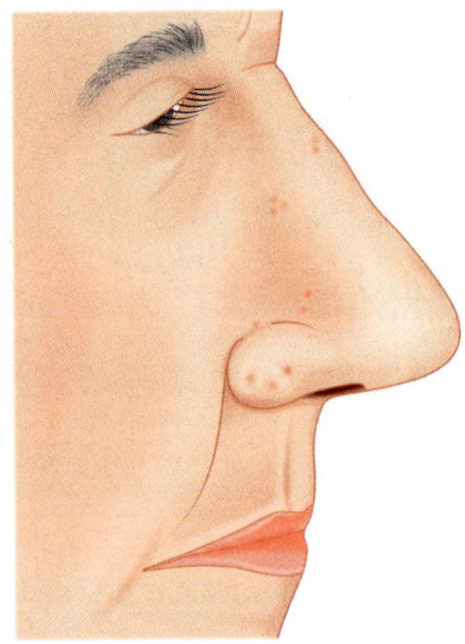

Fig. 41.76: Final result after healing of postoperative wound.

  - Angle kept is 30–60 degrees to skin surface
  - Power – 1
  - Cut or fully filtered waveform
  - Postprocedure dyschromia is common, clears off in 1–2 months.
- *Chronic lichenified eczema (Figs. 41.84A to C)*:
- *Miscellaneous important surgical applications*:
  - Prurigo nodularis
  - Dermatofibroma
  - Keratoacanthoma
  - Lipoma
  - Neurofibroma
  - Periungual and subungual lesions.

Radiofrequency is one of the most favored and popular surgical techniques in cosmetic dermatology and surgery because of its many advantages enumerated above.

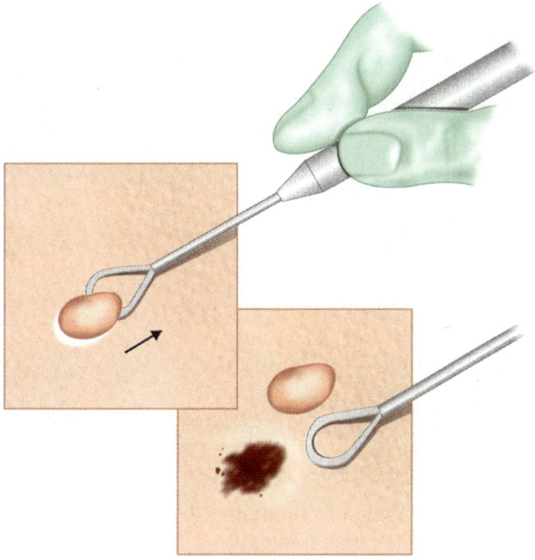

Fig. 41.77: One stroke excision biopsy.

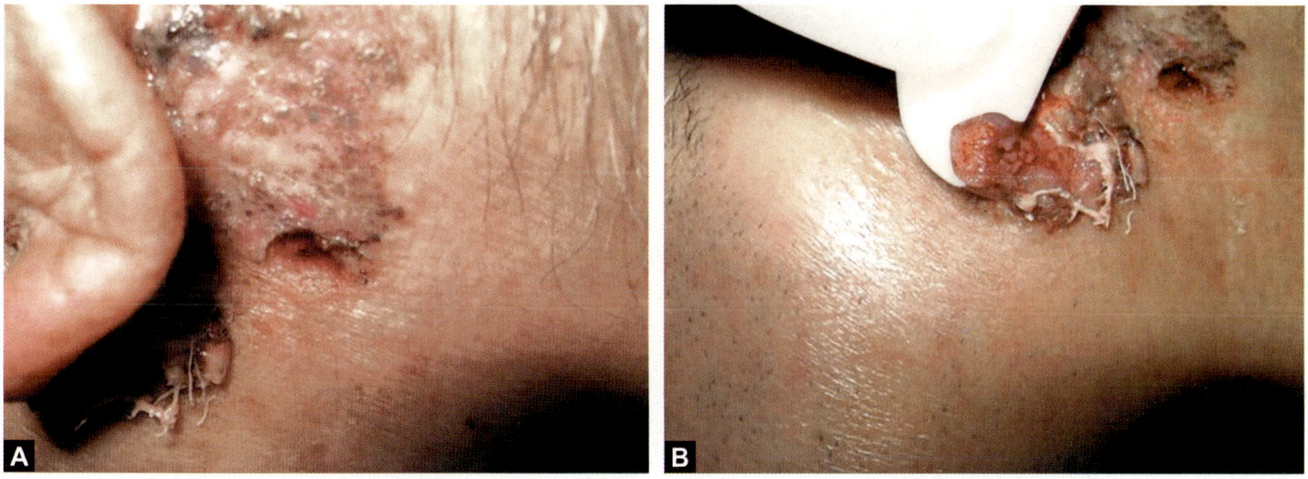

Figs. 41.78A and B: Biopsy taken from 2 areas in single stroke cut of basal cell carcinoma.

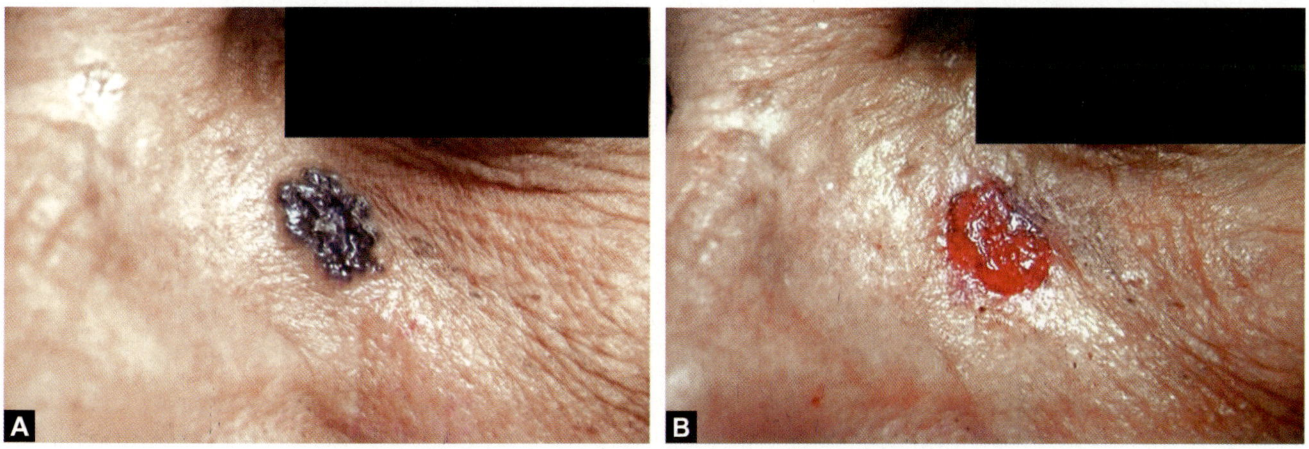

Figs. 41.79A and B: Excision biopsy of basal cell carcinoma.

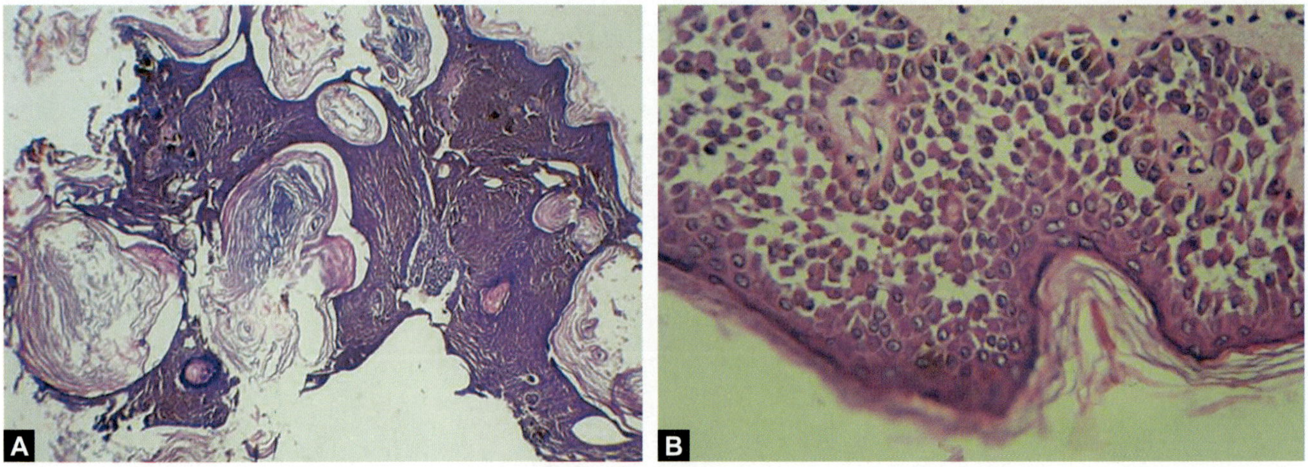

Figs. 41.80A and B: Histopathology report confirms basal cell carcinoma (tissue architecture was well-preserved, thermal damage was minimal).

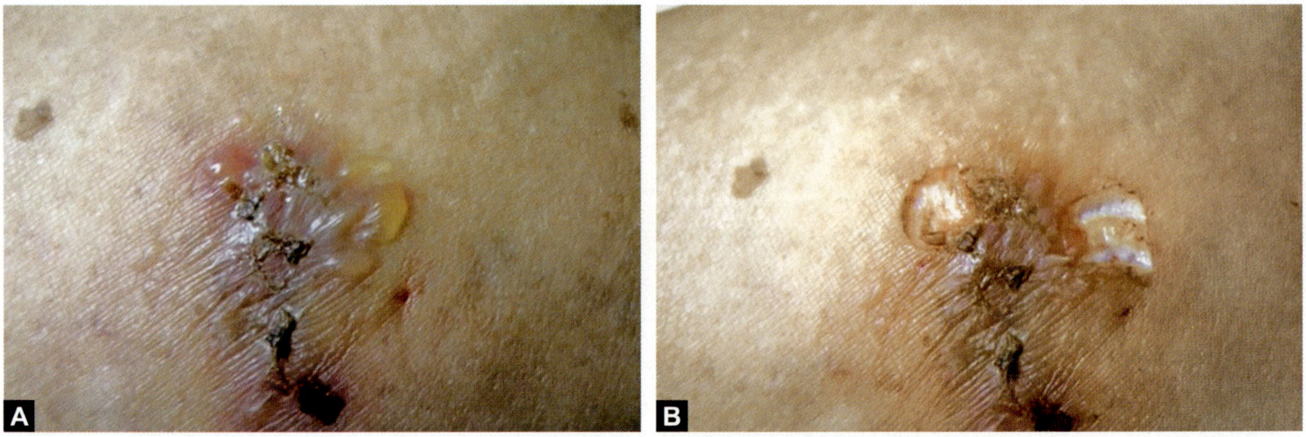

Figs. 41.81A and B: Small vesicle was selectively cut from clinically diagnosed familial benign pemphigus.

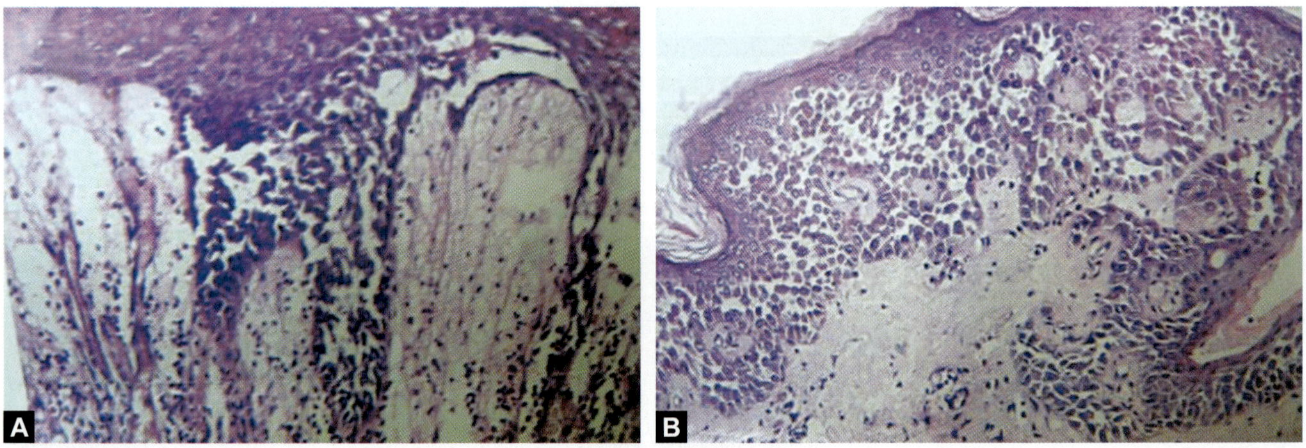

Figs. 41.82A and B: Histopathology report confirms familial benign pemphigus (Hailey Hailey disease) well-preserved tissue architecture, minimal thermal damage.

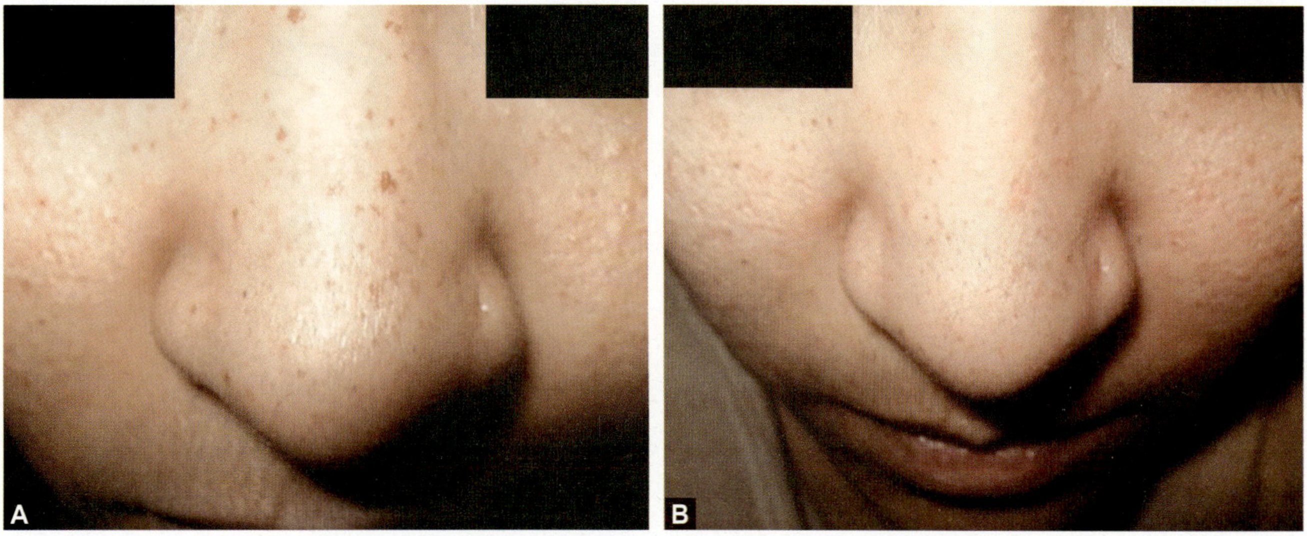

Figs. 41.83A and B: Freckles completely cleared after single session.

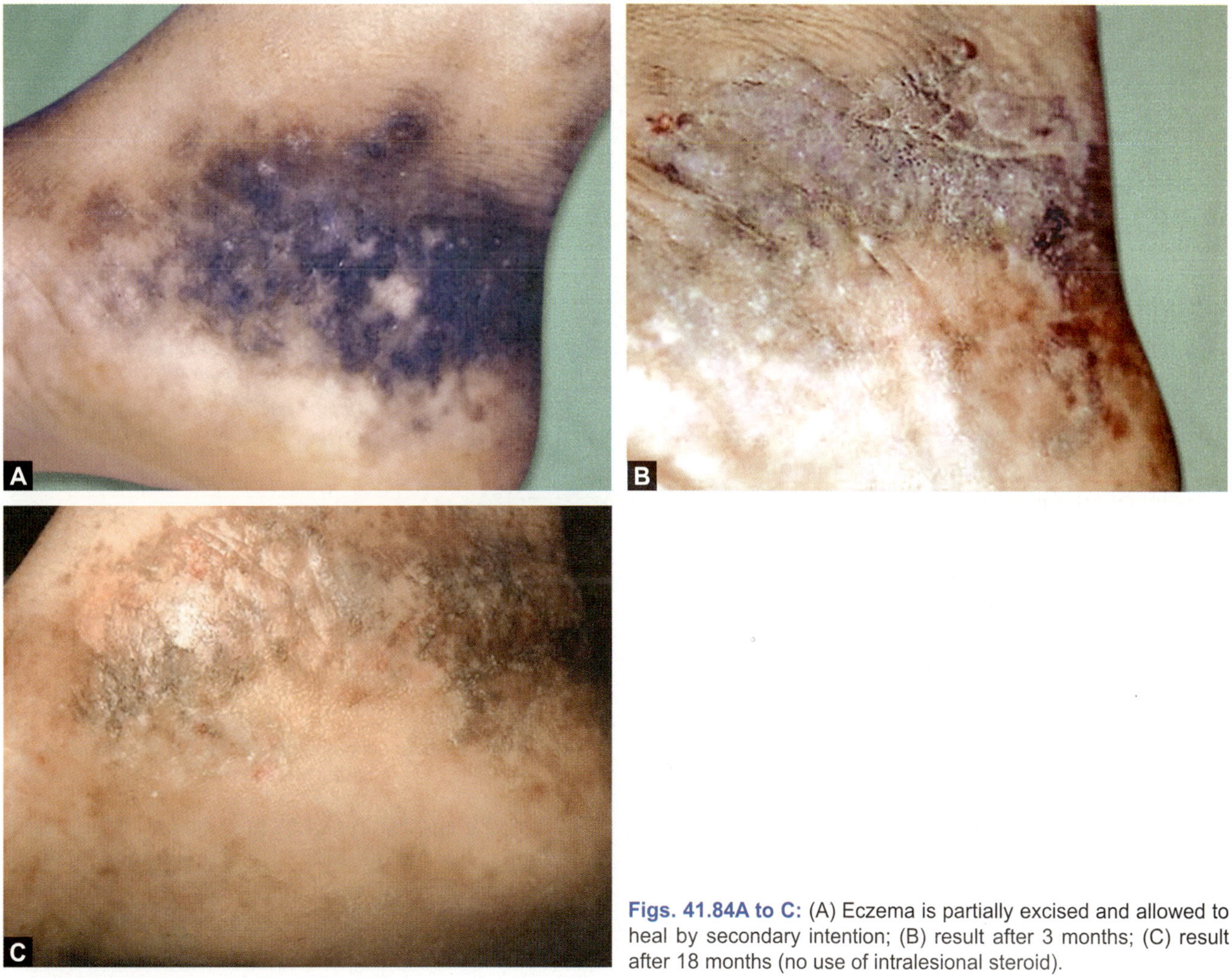

Figs. 41.84A to C: (A) Eczema is partially excised and allowed to heal by secondary intention; (B) result after 3 months; (C) result after 18 months (no use of intralesional steroid).

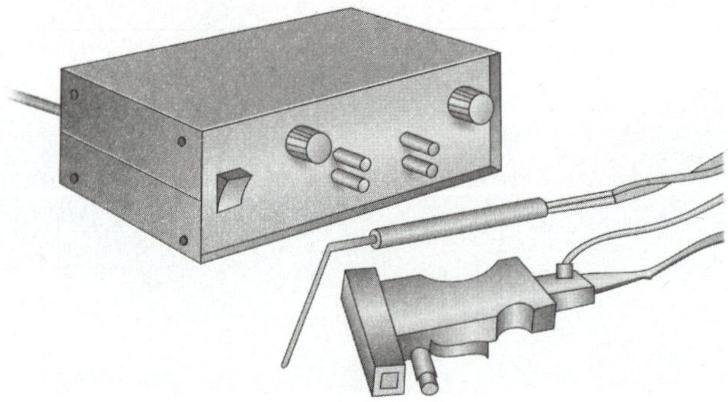

Fig. 41.85: Electrocautery machine (on mains supply).

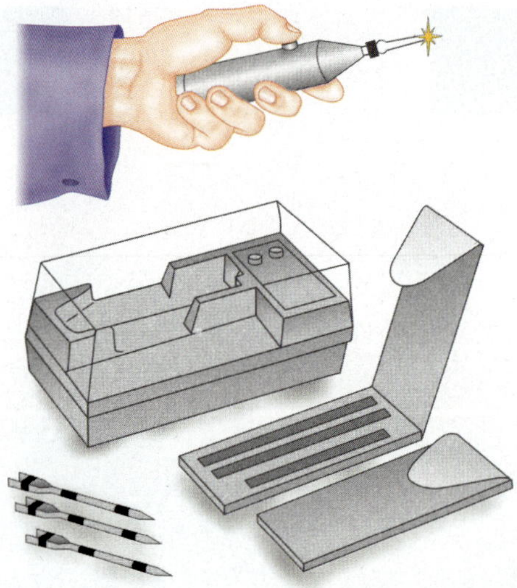

Fig. 41.86: Rechargeable electrocautery machine with electrodes.

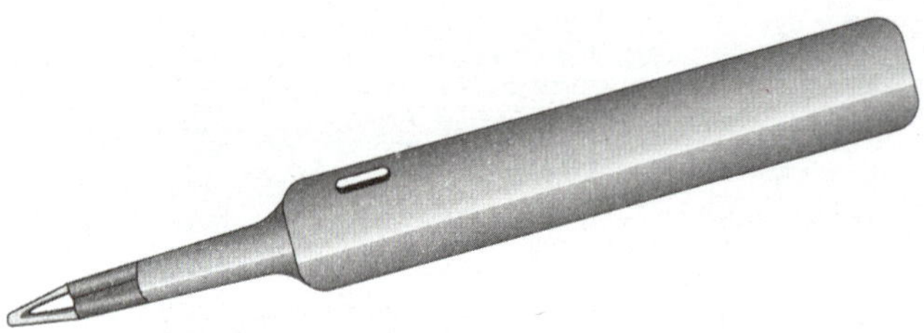

Fig. 41.87: Disposable electrocautery equipment.

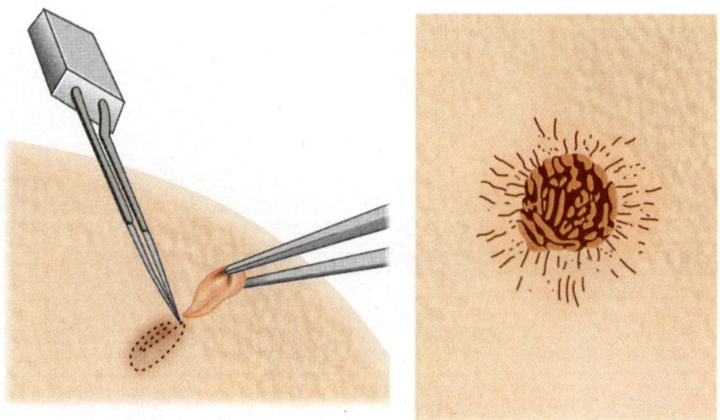

Fig. 41.88: Skin tag held with forceps and cut with electrocautery (no bleeding, but chances of scar remain).

One known and effective application of this technique is *epilation of gray hair* since radiofrequency is color blind and so is *Telangiectasia*. Radiofrequency treatment in the form of *'fractional radiofrequency'* is nowadays used commonly to treat *acne scars, stretch marks, facial ageing*. Radiofrequency is also used very commonly and effectively in cosmetic dermatology and aesthetic field by medical practitioners from different faculties for its *nonsurgical skin tightening effects either singly or in combination with ultrasound, Laser, IPL*. These effects are very useful in *facial ageing (lax and sagging skin, wrinkles and lines), doublechin, body contouring*. All above applications in the cosmetic dermatology and surgery are beyond the scope of this chapter.

- *Electrocautery*:[19] Electrocautery is perhaps the earliest electrical equipment for surgical purpose. Kindly refer Table 41.1 and Figures 41.85 to 41.89 for all the salient features. It is still quite popular as the primary mode of treatment in many dermatology clinics and almost all hospitals. In rural areas, it becomes the choice due to its advantage of cost.

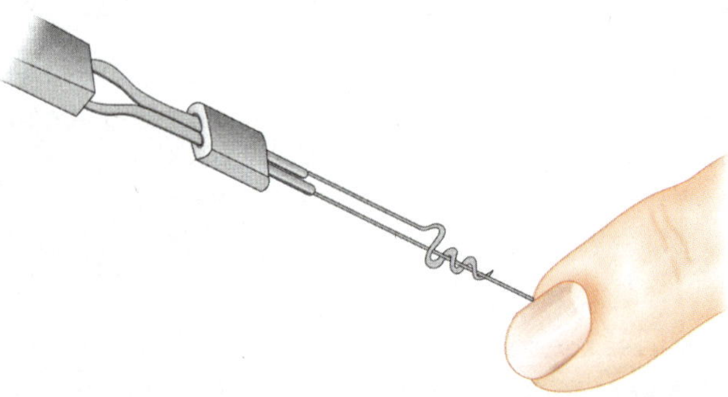

Fig. 41.89: Subungual hematoma treated with 'cold-point' cautery burner.

Cold-point burner has a central needle electrode around which is wound a heating wire. This wire heats the electrode and the heat is thus transferred to its tip. This is good for releasing subungual hematoma.

Electrocautery applications

- Skin tags, papillomas
- Warts, verrucae
- Condylomata
- Molluscum contagiosum
- Subungual hematoma
- Vascular lesions like capillary hemangioma, pyogenic granuloma

Points to remember about electrocautery

- It is the best tool for destroying a skin lesion than cutting or excising it
- It is the easiest to use tool because of its excellent property of hemostasis
- It can be used without much training as the hot electrode quickly destroys any lesion
- It should not be used for excising any lesion especially if histopathology is desired or good cosmetic result is expected
- Being portable, it can be carried anywhere for treatment
- Electrocautery is available now in three varieties: (1) Mains operated; (2) Rechargeable; (3) Disposable
- Mains operated cautery is easily and commonly available in India and is the best
- Rechargeable cautery is very portable, battery powered pocket unit (can be used in patient's home) but has limits for applications as larger lesions cannot be tackled and battery capacity may exhaust while treating
- Disposable cautery is easy on pocket for buying but too costly to maintain and also has disadvantage of battery capacity and limits for applications.

CONCLUSION

Radiofrequency or electrocautery are the basic and the most wanted dermatosurgical tools for any dermatologist whether initiating or updating practice. These techniques, especially the radiofrequency occupies the central position for the successful running of any dermatosurgical practice. Radiofrequency can be a very good addition for any other specialty practitioners who wish to diversify into dermatosurgery.

REFERENCES

1. Brown JS. Radiosurgery, In: Minor Surgery: a text and atlas, 4th edition, London; Arnold Publishers; 2000, 311-37.
2. Pollack SV. How electrosurgical devices work. In: Electrosurgery of the Skin, 1st edition. New York: Churchill Livingstone; 1991, 8:7-13.
3. Pfenninger JS, Fowler GC. Radiofrequency Surgery (Modern Electrosurgery), In: Procedures for Primary Care Physicians 2nd edition, 2003, 213-24.
4. Deshpande B. Radiofrequency treatment ablative and Nonablative. In: Practical Manual of Cosmetic Dermatology and Surgery, 1st edition, New Delhi, Mehta Publishers; 2010, 377-88.
5. Pollack SV. Electrodesiccation, electrofulguration, electroepilation. In: Electrosurgery of the Skin, 1st edition, New York: Churchill Livingstone; 1991; 31-68.
6. Niamtu J. 4.0 MHz Radiowave surgery in cosmetic facial surgery. In: Australasian Journal of Cosmetic Surgery, 2005;8:52-9.
7. Pollack SV. Laboratory Exercises, In: Electrosurgery of the Skin, 1st edition, New York: Churchill Livingstone; 1991;73-85.
8. Sebben JE. Electrosurgery and Cardiac Pacemakers. J Am Acad Dermatol 1983; 9:457-63.
9. Sawant SS, Gore D. Electrosurgery. In: Sawant SS, Gore D, Shah RA, editors, Textbook and atlas of Dermatosurgery and Cosmetology, 1st edition, Mumbai: ASCAD; 1998, 76-84
10. Pollack SV. Potential hazards of electrosurgery. In: Electrosurgery of the Skin, 1st edition, New York: Churchill Livingstone. 1991; 71-2.
11. Sebben JE. The hazards of electrosurgery. J Am Acad Dermatol 1987; 16:869.
12. Deshpande B. Single step maneuver of radiofrequency resurfacing for selected deep and punched out scars on face. in: F056: Late-breaking Research: Surgical and Cosmetic; 73rd American Academy of Dermatology, 2015.
13. Grekin RC, Tope WD, Yarborough JM, et al. Electrosurgical Facial Resurfacing. Arch Dermatol 2000; 136:1309-16.
14. Chiarello SE. Radiovaporization: Radiofrequency cutting current to vaporize and sculp skin lesions. Dermatol Surg. 2003; 2003; 29: 755-8.
15. Brown JS. Radiosurgery, In: Minor Surgery: A Text and Atlas, 4th edition, London; Arnold Publishers; 2000, 332-3.
16. Clarke DP, Hanke CW. Electrosurgical treatment of rhinophyma. J Am Acad Dermatol 1990; 22:831-7.
17. Turner RJ, Cohen RA, Voet RL et al. Analysis of margins of cone biopsy specimens obtained with Cold Knife, CO_2 and Nd:Yag Lasers and a Radiofrequency Surgical Unit. J Reproductive Med. 1992; 607-10.
18. Maness WL, Roeber FW, Clarke RE, et al. Histological evaluation of electrosurgery with varying frequency ND WAVEFORM. J Prosthetic Dent. 1978; 40; 304-8.
19. Brown JS, Electrocautery, In: Minor Surgery: a text and atlas. 4th edition, London; Arnold Publishers; 2000, 111-20.

CHAPTER 42

Lasers in Dermatosurgery: Treatment of Hyperpigmentary Disorders

BS Chandrashekar, Pavan Raj R, Madura C

INTRODUCTION

Pigmented lesions and tattoos are due to excessive or abnormally deposited melanin or other exogenous pigments. According to the depth of the pigment in the skin, the lesions are classified for the purposes of laser therapy, as epidermal, dermal and mixed lesions.

Freckles, solar lentigines, lentiginous nevus, café au lait macules and seborrheic keratosis are the epidermal pigmented lesions that may be amenable to laser therapy.Melanocytic nevi, blue nevi, drug induced hyperpigmentation and nevus of Ota and Ito are the dermal lesions which can be tackled by lasers. Mixed lesions include Becker's nevus, postinflammatory hyperpigmentation (PIH), melasma and nevus spilus, which exhibit both epidermal and dermal component[1] (Fig. 42.1).

In early 1980's treatment with pigment nonspecific lasers existed. Presently there are various lasers and light sources that treat pigmented lesions and tattoos effectively with good clinical outcome and minimal down time. This chapter summarizes various lasers for the treatment of pigmentary conditions in step wise manner for optimal results, with tips and tricks.

Here we are classifying the indications based on the clinical response to the lasers (Table 42.1).

LASER PRINCIPLES

The theory of selective photothermolysis enables site specific thermal mediated damage of pigmented lesions. The principle states that laser wavelength must be very well absorbed by target chromophore (i.e melanin/pigment) for a pulse duration shorter than thermal relaxation time (TRT) of target, with an optimal fluence conveyed to target tissue without damaging surrounding structures.

Target

While considering pigmented lesions, the foremost target to be considered is melanin. Melanin is found inside

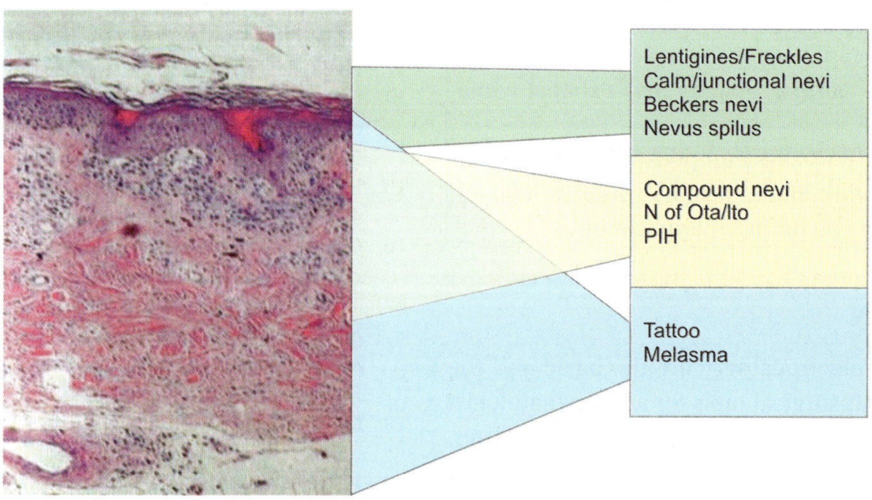

Fig. 42.1: Pigmented lesions according to the depth of the pigment.

Table 42.1: Indications for lasers in hyperpigmented disorders.

Conditions with good clinical response	*Conditions with varied response*
Freckles and lentigines	Melasma
Nevus of Ota	Cafe au lait macules (CALM)
Acquired bilateral nevus of Ota-like macules (ABNOM)	Becker's nevus
Tattoos	Melanocytic nevi
	Nevus spilus
	Drug induced hyperpigmentation/fixed drug eruption

melanosomes in the epidermis and also in a horizontal distribution along the DE junction. Melanin is also found in high concentrations in the hair follicles. Also, it is highly concentrated in hair follicles.[2] The melanin containing melanosomes are 0.5–1 μm in diameter with a TRT of 250–1000 nanoseconds. It has a broad spectrum of absorption (600–1100 nm). There is a selective disruption of melanosomes in melanocytes and keratinocytes following ultrashort, nanosecond domain pulse. The melanin is heated to 10 million degree/second and they explode. Pigment laden cells are damaged by mechanical damages from acoustic shock waves leading to cellular vacuolization and subepidermal blistering at the level of lamina lucida. Clinically it presents as ash white discoloration that decreases in 20 minutes.

Wavelength

Laser light with an appropriate absorption characteristics of melanin should be selected to attain selective photothermolysis of melanin and pigmented lesions. Melanin has a very wide absorption spectrum of 500–1100 nm. Hence many laser systems can be effectively used to tackle pigmented lesions. The various pigment removal lasers which can be used are: pulsed dye laser at 510 nm, Q-switched Alexandrite laser at 755 nm, Q-switched ruby laser at 694 nm and the Q-switched Nd:YAG laser at 1064 nm. The 532 nm frequency doubled Q-witched Nd:YAG is more suitable for epidermal lesions. QS lasers target small melanosomes by generating extremely short pulse width in nanosecond range. The lasers with shorter wavelength, such as QS 532,694 and 755 nm, are very effective in the management of epidermal lesions. 1064 nm QS Nd:YAG is used to target dermal lesions, because of its deeper penetration. Lasers which have shorter wavelengths and which emit green color have very little penetrative capability though they require much less energy to cause melanosomal thermal damage. Hence they are better suited to target pigmented lesions in the epidermis. Red light emitting lasers with much longer wavelengths penetrate more and therefore are better suited to tackle dermal lesions.[3]

Pulse Duration

The destruction of specific pigmented lesions depends both on wavelength emitted and pulse duration. The TRT of melanosomes is in the range of 250–1000 nanoseconds and therefore submicrosecond pulsed lasers are required to selectively destroy them. The shorter pulse duration lasers (40–750 ns are therefore used to target the melanosomes while the millisecond pulsed lasers are not useful here. The Laser interacts with the tissue and produces photothermal with combined photomechanical effect.[4]

Fluence

Optimal fluence required to damage the target depends on wavelength and pulse duration. The optimal fluence is one which causes immediate whitening without blistering or bleeding. Shorter wavelengths (<600 nm) require relatively less energy fluences, while at longer wavelengths higher fluences are required to produce an efficient photothermal reaction.[5] Lower fluences are used to target lesions with high density pigment. Higher fluences are required when lesions are faintly colored with less dense pigment.

Spot Size

Larger the spot size, deeper the penetration and hence, it is safe on epidermal lesions and darker skin types. Spot size can be chosen based on the size of lesion; Example: in freckles, select the spot size based on the size of the freckles. In laser toning, larger spots can decrease the duration of treatment by covering treatment area faster (Table 42.2).

Table 42.2: Lasers used for the treatment of pigmentary lesions.

Pigment specific lasers/light	*Pigment nonspecific lasers*
• IPL (500 to 1200 nm) • 532 nm KTP • 755 nm long pulsed Alexandrite • QS-Nd: YAG (1064 nm), KTP (532 nm), Ruby (694 nm) and Alexandrite (755 nm)	• 2940 nm erbium YAG • 10600 nm CO_2 • Erbium glass (1540 nm, 1550 nm, 1565 nm) • 810 nm diode

Description of Current Laser Devices

QS Nd:YAG Laser

It emits 1064 nm light, but it can also be frequency-doubled using a potassium diphosphate crystal to produce visible green light with a wavelength of 532 nm. The affinity of melanin is strong for 532 nm green light, however the longer 1064 nm red wavelength has a lower melanin absorption coefficient and penetrates deeper in the dermis. Usually there is tissue splatter leading to crusting after the use of smaller spot sizes, and may take several weeks to completely resolve.[6,7]

QS Ruby Laser (QSRL)

The Q-switched ruby laser produces wavelength of 694 nm (visible and red light) with 25–40 ns being the pulse duration. This specific range of wavelength is very strongly absorbed by melanin in the superficial layers. This can cause pigmentary reduction causing hypopigmentation to even depigmentation, which may be permanent, especially in darker individuals. Hemoglobin does not absorb this wavelength significantly.[8,9]

QS Alexandrite Laser

The Q-switched Alexandrite laser emits wavelength of 755 nm with 50–100 ns range pulse duration. The longer wavelength allows penetration to more depth leading to lesser hypopigmentation in comparison to QSRL. Postoperative healing is faster than the other Q-switch pigment specific lasers.[10]

IPL Devices

For pigment lesions, these devices employ wavelength range of 550–1200 nm. It has emission peaks at 500–670 nm and 870–1200 nm. Both oxyhemoglobin and melanin are targeted. Newer IPL devices have single and multiple pulse mode with double cut off filters. Multiple pulsed mode with long delays are safer for epidermis and in darker skin; single pulsed mode is used in lighter skin. Advantages of IPL are—it can target more superficial than deeper lesions, has larger spot size and hence has relatively shorter treatment duration and lastly it can be used when there is concomitant photodamaged skin/telangiectasia.

Other Long Pulsed (LP) Lasers

The LP lasers are 694 nm LP ruby, 755 nm Alexandrite and 810 nm diode laser. Ruby is indicated in light skin types (I-III). It has high incidence of hypopigmentation and is used rarely. 755 nm Alexandrite laser is also used in type I-III skin. 810 nm diode is safer than Alexandrite in darker skin types.

Resurfacing Lasers

CO_2 and erbium YAG lasers are pigment nonspecific lasers either used in ablative or fractional resurfacing mode. There is always a risk of pigmentary change, scarring and increased downtime (refer chapter on ablative lasers).

Pigment Specific Pulsed Dye Laser

This laser emits wavelength of 510 nm with pulse duration of 300 nanoseconds. This helps in targeting the melanosomes present superficially. The laser is very effective in treating lentigines and also various other pigmented lesions of the epidermis. Since oxyhemoglobin absorbs a lot of this energy, 50% patients may develop purpura.[11,12]

EPIDERMAL PIGMENTED LESIONS

Thus, both green light (short wavelength) and red light (long wavelength) emitting lasers can be used effectively in the treatment of epidermal pigmented lesions.

Freckles and Lentigines (Figs. 42.2 to 42.4)

Freckles are very difficult to treat because they recur frequently after any therapy. QS laser tackles them effectively; recurrences are reduced by following prevention

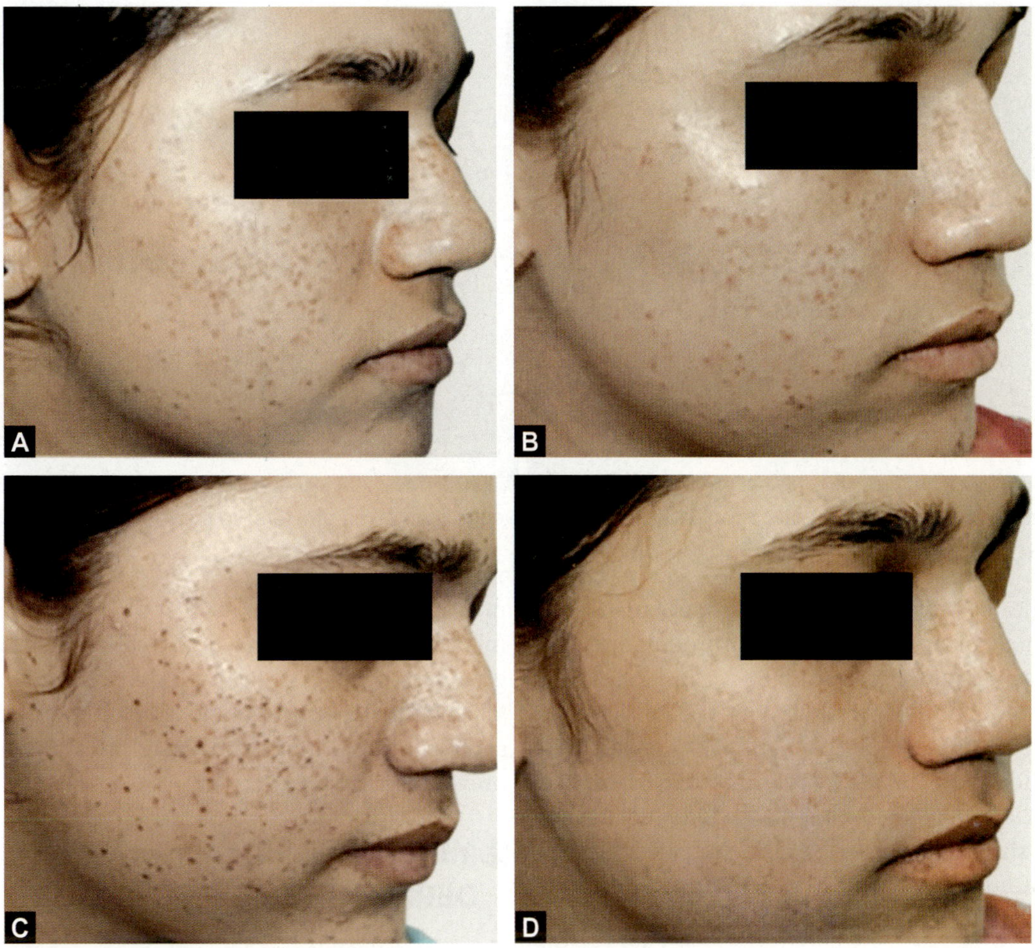

Figs. 42.2A to D: Treatment of freckles with QS Nd:YAG (660 nm); (A) Before the laser; (B) Erythema and mild frosting immediately after the procedure; (C) Scab formation at day 5; (D) 3 weeks after one session (parameters: spot size—2 mm, fluence—1.2 J/cm^2).

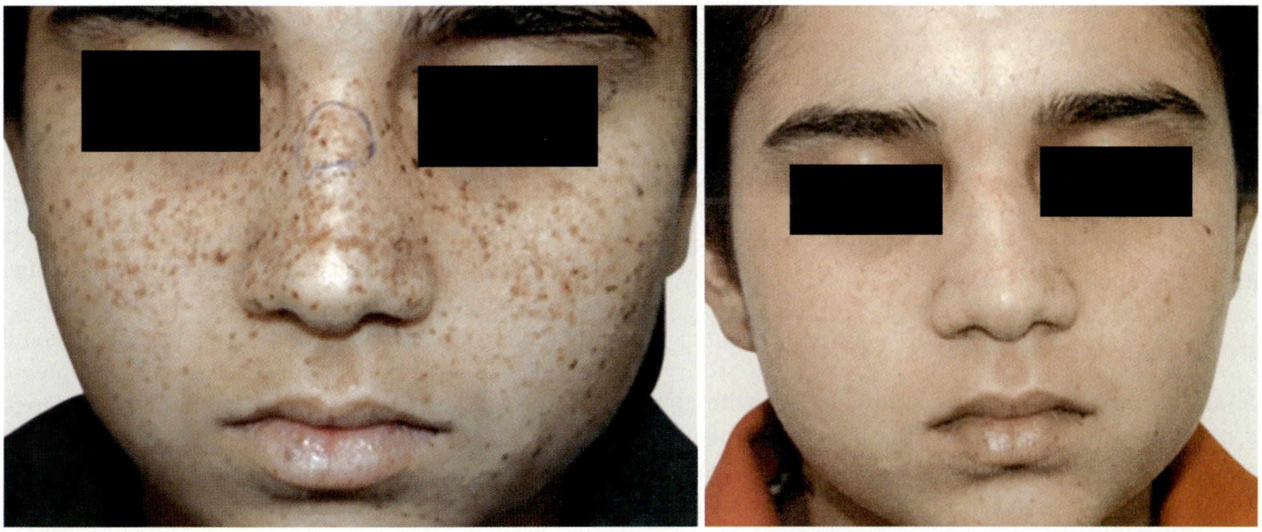

Fig. 42.3: Freckles after 4 sessions of QS Nd:YAG (660 nm) at 4 weeks interval (parameters: spot size—2 to 3 mm, fluence—0.9 to 1.6 J/cm^2).

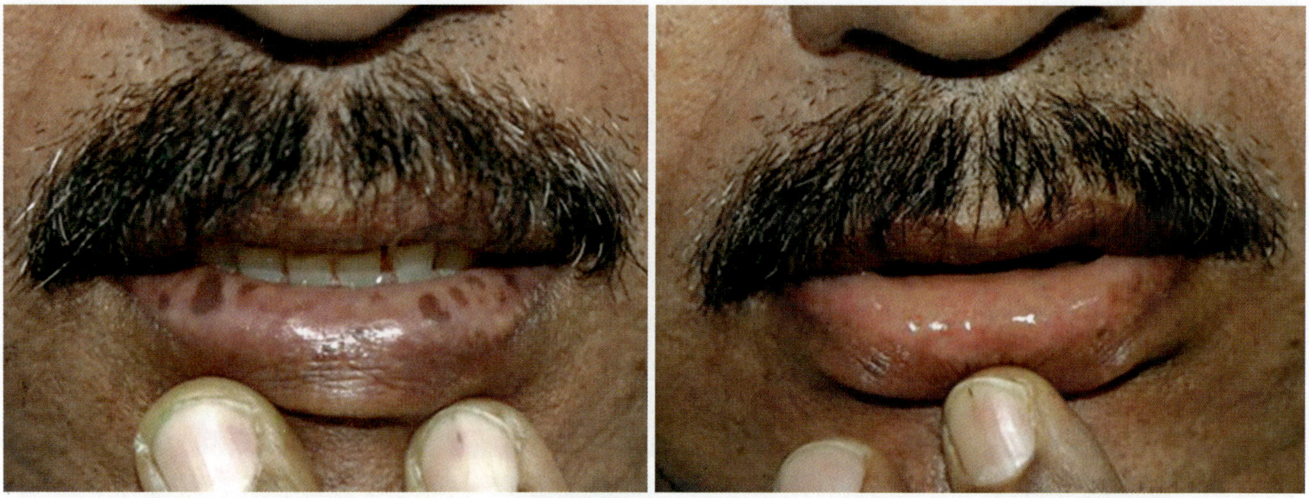

Fig. 42.4: Lentigines after 2 sessions of QS Nd:YAG (660 nm) at 4 weeks interval (parameters: spot size—3 mm, fluence—1.2 J/cm²).

regimens like sun avoidance and sunscreen usage. Beforetreatment, bleaching agents like hydroquinone may be used.[1,13] Lasings for freckles is done once in 4 to 6 weeks and usually reduction occurs by 3 to 4 sessions. Lasers of choice are 532 nm QS Nd:YAG and 660 nm Nd:YAG; alternative choices are 755 nm QS Alexandrite, QS ruby and IPL. The clinical end point is immediate whitening. Always select a spot size smaller than the lesion to avoid damage to the surrounding skin and PIH. 532 nm QS Nd:YAG produces more purpura. IPL is indicated in patients with coexisting photodamage and telangiectasia along with freckles. It is a better choice in light skinned patients with dark freckles/lentigines and large area of involvement because of larger spot size of IPL. The down time with IPL is less, but the number of sessions required to treat is more. IPL is not a choice in dark skin patients with freckles because of lesser contrast available. LP pigment lasers are also a good choice for treating pigmentation in the dark skin (LP Alexandrite, LP 532 nm Nd:YAG and 595 nm PDL).

Among all pigmented lesions, lentigines show probably the best response to laser therapy.[13,14] PIH can occur among peoplewith darker skin types, and risk is higher among lentigines compared to freckles.

Cafe-au-Lait Macules (CALM)

Cafe-au-lait macules respond variably to laser therapy and recur in as many as 50% of the patients. Repeated treatments over a long period (several months or even years) are needed to achieve maximum clearing of the lesions. At each session the complete lesion must be treated as repigmentation can occur from the adjacent untreated melanocytes.[1,13] QS lasers fail to remove the follicular melanocytic component of the café-au-lait macules and give varied results.. Both epidermal melanocytes and follicular melanocytes can be targeted by LP pigment laser, such as normal mode ruby laser or LP Alexandrite laser prevent recurrences.

MIXED EPIDERMAL/ DERMAL PIGMENTED LESIONS

The long pulsed lasers actually are the most effective ones in dealing with treatment of both epidermal as well as follicular melanocytes.[13,15] Pigmentary laser treatment is not very effective in treating postinflammatory hyperpigmentation. Improvements can only be assessed after multitude of sessions.

Melasma

It is often a therapeutic challenge to treat melasma. Pigment can be located in epidermis, or in dermis, or in both of them. Similar to other traditional methods (sunscreen, retinoic acid, hydroquinone and chemical peels), laser treatment produces variable results. Sometimes even worsening of the condition is observed.[16] Lasers and light sources should only be considered in resistant cases as there is potential risk of increase in pigmentation. The main pathogenesis is hyperactive melanocytes that results from increased activity of melanogenic enzymes.[17]

The resurfacing lasers like fractional erbium/CO_2 can remove the abnormal melanocytes in the diseased skin and alter the epidermal barrier function and enhance the

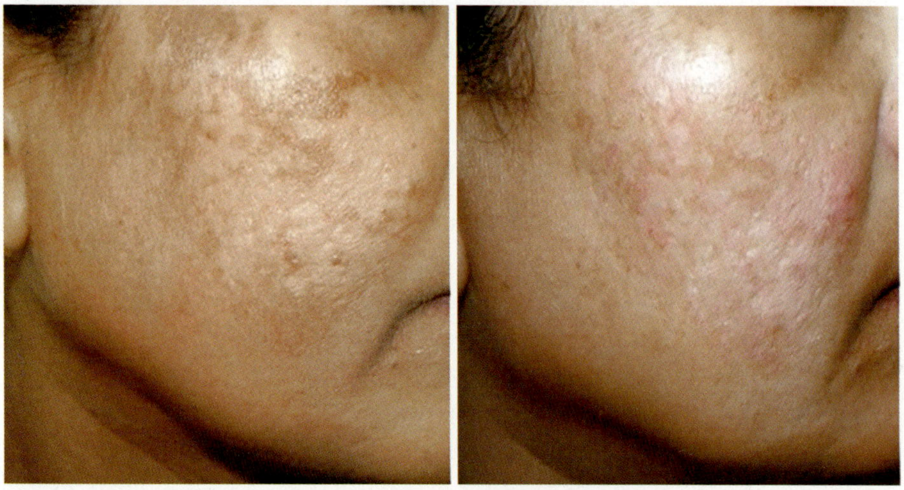

Fig. 42.5: Melasma after 6 sessions of QS Nd:YAG (1064 nm) at 1 to 2 weeks interval between 2 sessions (parameters: spot size—8 to 10 mm, fluence—1.2 J/cm^2).

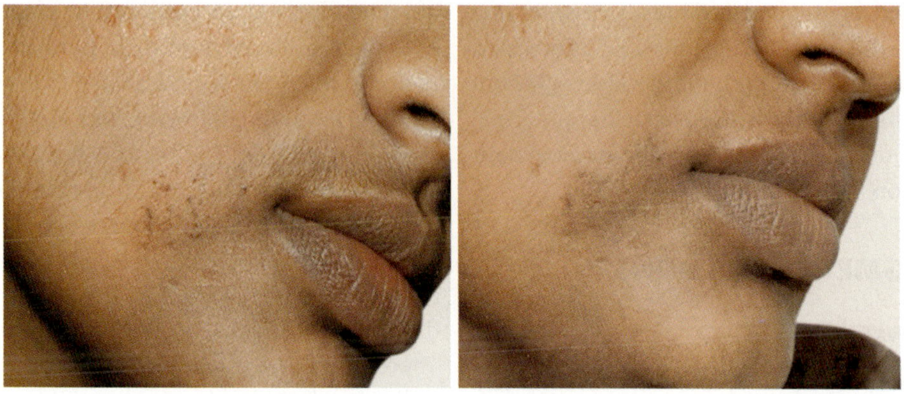

Fig. 42.6: Nevus spilus after 4 sessions of QS Nd:YAG (532 nm) (parameters: spot size—1.3 to 1.5 mm, fluence—1 to 1.4 J/cm^2) with toning of surrounding background pigment with QS Nd:YAG (1064 nm) (parameters: spot size—10 mm, fluence—0.85 J/cm^2) at an interval of 4 to 6 weeks.

absorption of topical bleaching agents postoperatively. This can lead to long-term remission, but because of risk of PIH, infection and scarring, they are unpopular.[18]

Use of LP pigment lasers (532 nm Nd:YAG, LP Alexandrite) for these cases have also been reported in literature. Author uses QS 1,064 nm Nd:YAG laser, large spot size of 8–10 mm and low fluence of 1.1 to 1.6 J/cm^2 performed at 1 or 2 weekly intervals, called the Laser toning (Fig. 42.5).[19] Appearance of mild erythema must be the clinical endpoint. Though it lightens up melasma, there is always a risk of depigmentary mottled spots.

When melasma has vascular component liketelangiectasia, vascular lasers like PDL 585 nm and IPL can be an option.[20] Lasers must be chosen weighing the risks and benefits.

Nevus Spilus (Fig. 42.6)

It is a typical cafe au lait macule with multiple darkly pigmented speckles within it. These often represent either compound or junctional nevi. There are several reports of dysplastic nevi developing within nevus spilus and of melanoma arising within these lesions. These facts make efficient laser treatment doubtful for this indication. However, in case of any atypical appearing pigment lesion with in the nevus it is recommended to take a biopsy. To

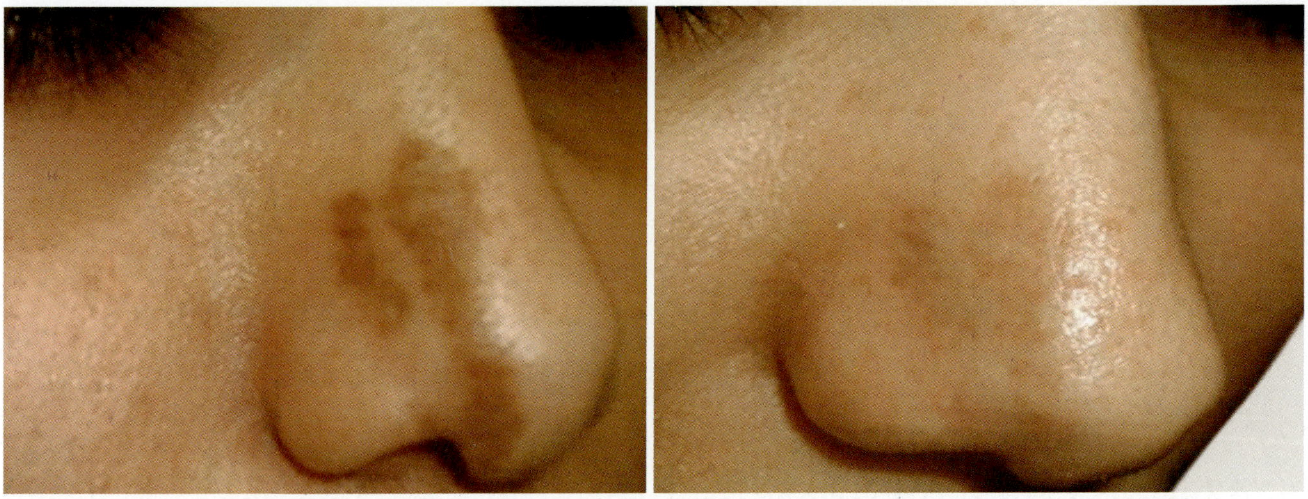

Fig. 42.7: Melanocytic nevus after 8 sessions of QS Nd:YAG (1064 nm) (parameters: spot size—4 mm, fluence—4.5 to 7.0 J/cm²) and Erb YAG laser (scan size—9 × 9, fluence—800 mJ) at 6 to 8 weeks interval.

treat the unwanted pigment several laser sessions are required to remove the unwanted pigment.[21,22] There is no specific laser of choice for this condition; QS lasers (532 nm KTP/ 755 nm Alexandrite) can be used to tackle epidermal pigmentation and long pulsed lasers can be employed for deeper pigmentation.

DERMAL PIGMENTED LESIONS

Melanocytic Nevus

Treatment of melanocytic nevi is controversial. The acquired melanocytic nevi are more concerning. They must be evaluated clinically in a detailed manner before venturing into treatment by lasers. Treatment response to short wavelength lasers is good in cases of melanocytic nevi which are both benign and junctional, while for deeper/ dermal and compound ones, longer wavelengths with longer pulse width and higher fluences are better. The latter ones recur even after this treatment.[23,24]

Congenital nevi which increase in size should always be evaluated for risk of melanoma. Therefore in such cases lasers should only be considered as distant second option only in cases where hair removal is desired or pigment reduction alone is desired. Complications of lasers when used in such situations include hypopigmentation which can be permanent, scarring, variable and incomplete responses.[25,26] Pseudomelanomas may form in these partially removed lesions and melanomas can even go undetected. Larger congenital nevi can be tackled by ablative lasers at an early age in place of dermabrasion especially when nevi occur in periorbital and perigenital regions which are critical areas.[27-29] 8–10 sessions may be required for the complete removal. Author has experience in combining CO_2 with 532 nm QS Nd:YAG; 6 sessions to give good results (Fig. 42.7). But for small moles, other treatment modalities still gives excellent results.

The longer wavelength red-light lasers can successfully-remove blue nevi. However, it must be kept in mind that differential diagnosis of blue nevi includes melanoma. Therefore, surgical excision is the safest method in this indication.[30]

Nevus of Ota (Fig. 42.8)

Nevus of Ota is dermal melanocytic hamartoma which clinically presenting as mottled, dusky blue and brown pigmentation.[31] Lasers give very good therapeutic results. Laser of choice is 1,064 nm QS Nd:YAG; while alternate choices are QS ruby and QS Alexandrite. Immediate whitening with punctate bleeding is the endpoint for 1,064 nm QS Nd:YAG laser. The treatment sessions are scheduled initially at every 6–8 weeks; pigment dilution begins after third session. When the lesion is significantly reduced, the treatment sessions are spaced at every 3 to 4 months and require higher fluence to attain the endpoint clinically. QS ruby lasers have a greater risk of hypopigmentation but clinically achieve the end point in the lowest number of treatment sessions. Earlier the onset of laser sessions, faster is the resolution and also fewer the number of sessions.[32] Periorbital involvement signifies more treatment

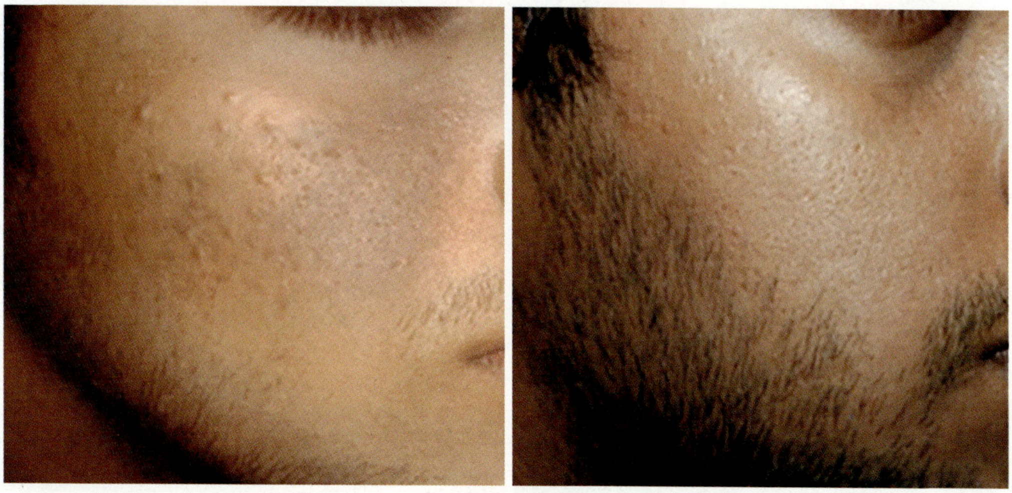

Fig. 42.8: Nevus of Ota after 8 sessions of QS Nd:YAG (1064 nm) at 8 weeks interval (parameters: spot size—4 to 8 mm, fluence—2 to 6 J/cm^2).

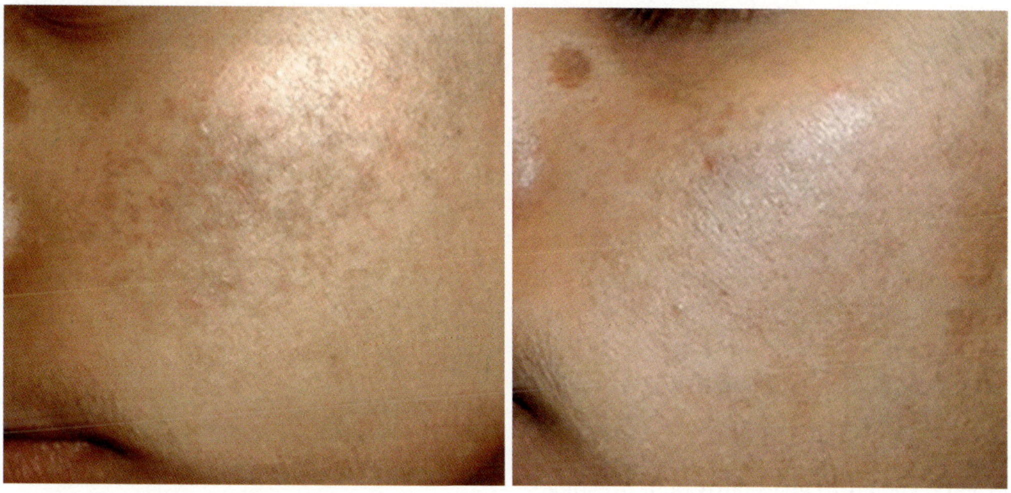

Fig. 42.9: ABNOM after 8 sessions of QS Nd:YAG (1064 nm) at 8 weeks interval (parameters: spot size—4 to 6 mm, fluence—2 to 6 J/cm^2).

sessions. Fractional resurfacing lasers can be effective, and an add on in patients who fail to respond to 1,064 nm QS Nd:YAG laser.[33]

Starting the laser treatment early in pediatric age group can have a risk of scarring also, because of thin skin and brownish pigmentation.

Acquired Bilateral Nevus of Ota-like Macules (ABNOM or Hori's Macules) (Fig. 42.9)

Hori's macules are late onset dermal hyperpigmentation seen in adulthood, and does not affect the mucosa. Treatment is similar to nevus of Ota; a combination treatment with 1064 and 532 nm QS Nd:YAG gives good results. It requires more number of sessions compared to nevus of Ota because of different depth of pigmentation. Ablative lasers can enhance penetration of QS lasers and give superior results.

Drug induced hyperpigmentation also responds very well to laser therapy. They are most commonly induced by minocycline and amiodarone.[1,13,18] Successful treatment has also been reported with the QS Alexandrite, QS ruby, 1,064 and 532 nm QS Nd:YAG laser.[34]

Becker's Nevus (Fig. 42.10)

Lasers commonly used are Er:YAG and 1,064 nm QS Nd:YAG. LP pigment lasers have also been employed

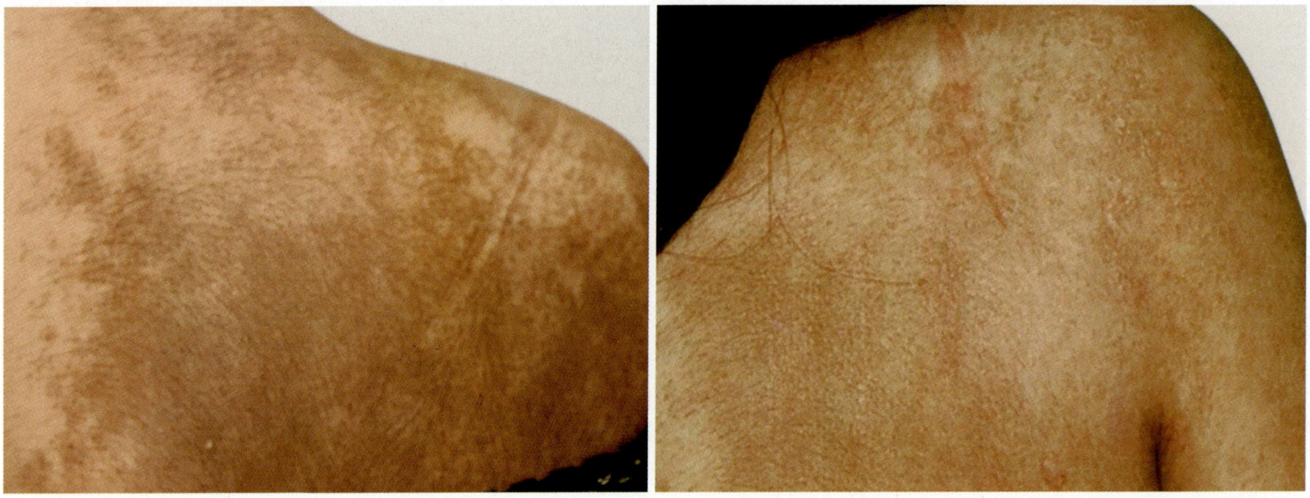

Fig. 42.10: Becker's nevus after 6 sessions of fractional CO_2 laser (10600 nm) and QS Nd:YAG (1064 nm) at 6 weeks interval.

Box 42.1: Tattoo types.

- Decorative tattoo
- Cosmetic tattoo
- Traumatic tattoo
- Medical tattoo
- Iatrogenic tattoo

Table 42.3: Comparison of professional and amateur tattoo.

Professional	Amateur
• Placed deeper in the dermis	• More superficially placed
• Larger quantity of ink	• Faint tattoos
• Variable composition of inks	• Single composition of ink
• Greater difficulty of tattoo removal	• Easy removal and require lesser sessions
• Incomplete eradication of some colors	• Usually it is black/ blue color

to remove hair and pigmentation in Becker's nevi, but textural change is a possible complication. Hence alternate choices include long-pulse 755 nm Alexandrite laser and IPL, used to target the pigment and surrounding hair follicle. In authors' experience a combination of LP Nd:YAG (1064 nm) (for hair reduction), fractional CO_2 laser (10600 nm) and QS Nd:YAG (1064 nm) gives fairly better results.

Tattoos

Tattoos may be classified as decorative, cosmetic, traumatic, medical, and iatrogenic. (Box 42.1) Decorative tattoos are most common and may be further subdivided into professional and amateur (Table 42.3). Amateur tattoos are faint and easy to treat compared to professional tattoos.

Decorative tattoos can include both inorganic and organic compounds. Inorganic pigments can be made up of compounds like cadmium, chromium, mercury, iron, titanium, aluminum, silica, copper, chlorine, bromine, sulfur, carbon, and magnesium.[34] The organic materials used in tattoos are classified as azo, non-azo or polycyclic compounds.[35]

Cosmetic and reconstructive tattoos are generally placed to improve or create the appearance of normal anatomical structures. These type of tattoos are usually done in conditions like thinning of eyebrows, eyelashes, and enhancement of vermilion border of the lips, recreation of areola following mastectomy, or camouflage of scars. Cosmetic tattoos or permanent make-up contain chemical compounds with multiple colors.[36]

Traumatic tattoos are caused by implantation of small pieces of asphalt and other debris from road traffic accidents, graphite from a pencil stab, as well as shrapnel, bullet, fireworks, or other explosive fragments. Amalgam tattoos are a result of trauma during dental procedures and usually follow implantation of metal particles into oral mucosa. Medical tattoos are frequently performed to mark radiation sites (micropigmentation for scalp). Implantation of pigmented particles into a wound during surgery, or other medical procedure result in iatrogenic tattoos.[37]

Pigment particles vary in size from less than 10 to 100 nm.[38] The depth of tattoo particles in the dermis varies from 1.1 to 2.9 mm from the granular layer, depending on whether the tattoo is professional or amateur.

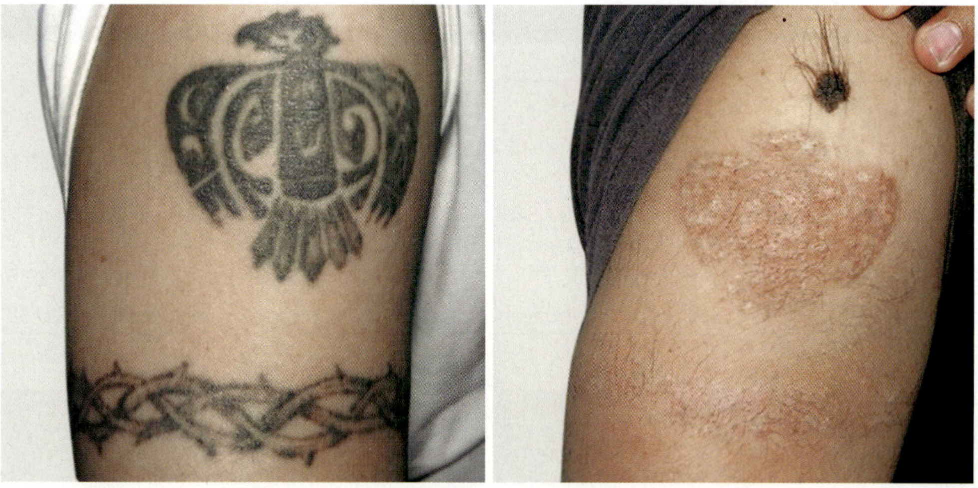

Fig. 42.11: Professional tattoo after 6 sessions of QS Nd:YAG (1064 nm) at 8 weeks interval (parameters: spot size—6 to 8 mm, fluence—2 to 4.5 J/cm^2).

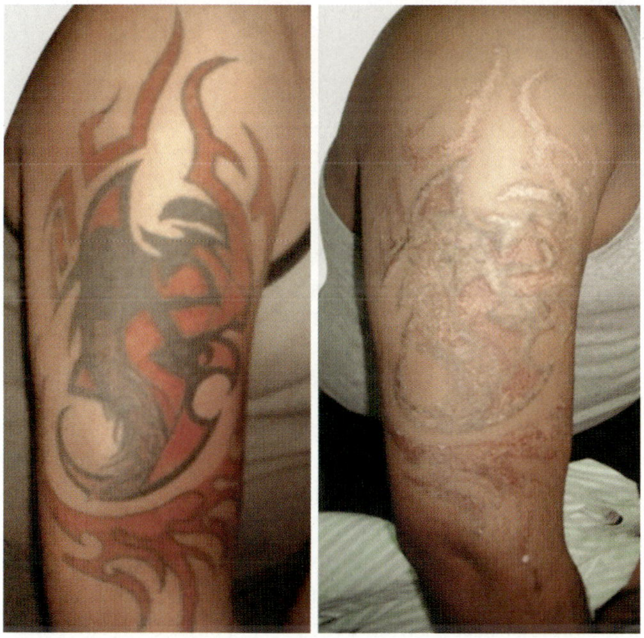

Fig. 42.12: Professional multicolor tattoo after 8 sessions QS Nd:YAG (1064 and 532 nm) at 8 weeks interval (parameters: spot size—4 to 6 mm, fluence—3 to 7 J/cm^2 for 1064 nm and spot size—2.6 mm, fluence—1.8 to 4.2 J/cm^2 for 532 nm).

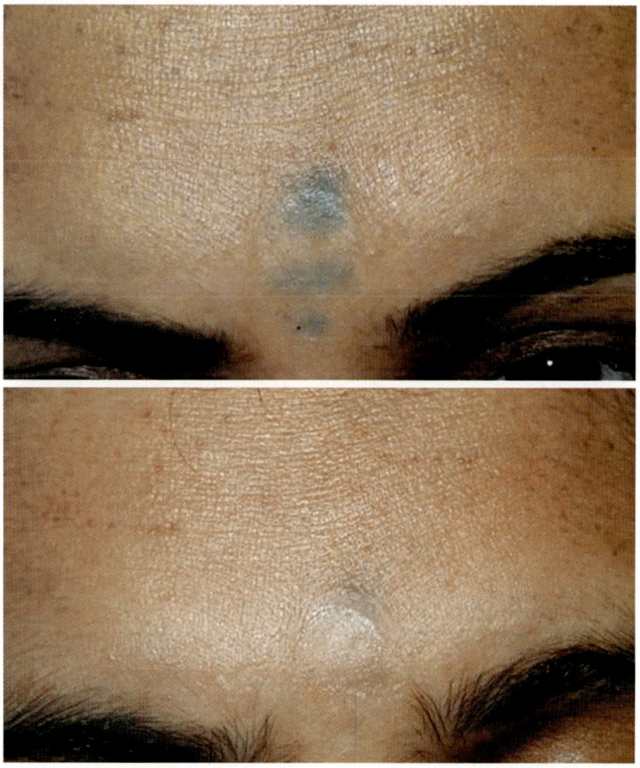

Fig. 42.13: Amateur bindi tattoo after 3 sessions of QS Nd:YAG (1064 nm) at 8 weeks interval (parameters: spot size—4 to 6 mm, fluence—2.4 to 3 J/cm^2).

Tattoo pigment is converted into small pebbles by the photoacoustic effect of Q-switched laser. These particles are then extruded via the epidermis, eliminated by vascular or lymphatic channels, or become rephagocytosed by mononuclear cells.[39,40]

The QS lasers are gold standard for tattoo removal (Figs. 42.11 to 42.13). Various wavelengths used are QS 1064, 755, 694, 532 and 585 nm. QS 1064 nm penetrates deeply and less absorbed by epidermal melanin and is the safest tattoo removal laser. Various lasers wavelength target different colors (Table 42.4) but initially tattoo can be

Table 42.4: Current wavelengths for tattoo removal.

Color of tattoo	*Pigment*	*Wavelength*
Red-Brown	Iron oxide	QS 532
Black	Carbon	QS Nd:YAG 1064 QS Alexandrite and QS Ruby
White	Titanium dioxide	QS Nd:YAG 1064
Yellow	Cadmium sulfide	QS 532
Green	Chromium salts	QS Alexandrite and QS Ruby
Blue	Cobalt, copper, ferrocyanide and ferricyanide	QS Nd:YAG 1064, QS 585

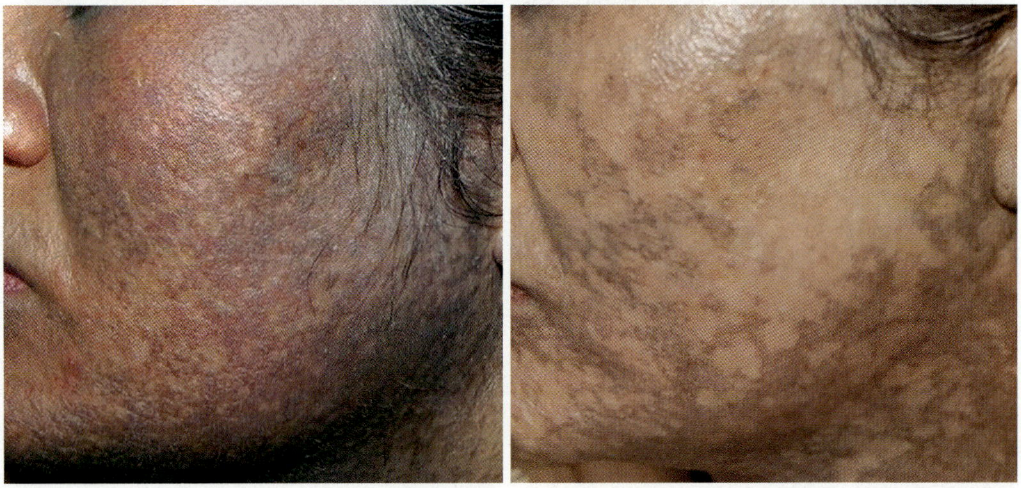

Fig. 42.14: Poikiloderma of civatte after 6 sessions of pulsed dye laser (595 nm) at 2 weeks interval, 10 sessions of QS Nd:YAG (1064 nm) at 6 weeks interval followed by 2 sessions of fractional CO_2 laser (10600 nm) spaced 3 months apart.

targeted with 1064 nm, and lateron as pigment dilutes specific laser wavelength can be chosen to treat left over color, as tattoo artist mix several colors to get the desired shade.

Picosecond Lasers

Picosecond lasers are the latest lasers, with a shortened pulse duration of 10^{12} seconds, which are used for fast and efficacious tattoo removal. Ross et al, first compared the use of nanosecond and picosecond lasers and noticed tattoo removal to be more effective with picoseconds lasers for the treatment of black tattoos in human patients, withall other parameters being equal. The shorter picoseconds pulse duration targets the tattoo pigment more effective As the diameter of common tattoo pigment is around 40 nm, with thermal relaxation time of around 1 nanosecond; also causes increased photomechanical breakup of the pigment.[38]

Controversial Indications

Authors' share their experience in treatment of lichen planus pigmentosus, poikiloderma of civatte and toxic melanosis. These are considered to be difficult to treat pigmentation. Poikiloderma of civatte (Fig. 42.14) has 3 components to tackle namely the hyperpigmentation, vascular component and textural changes which can be treated by using combination of lasers-QS Nd:YAG (1064 nm), pulsed dye laser (595 nm) and CO_2 laser (10600 nm). Similarly lichen planus pigmentosus and toxic melanosis can also be treated with a combination of QS Nd:YAG (1064 nm) and CO_2 laser (10600 nm) with good outcome (Figs. 42.15 and 42.16).

PATIENT SELECTION AND PREPROCEDURE EVALUATION

The lighter skin types are the best candidates as the treatment is highly effective with lesser number of

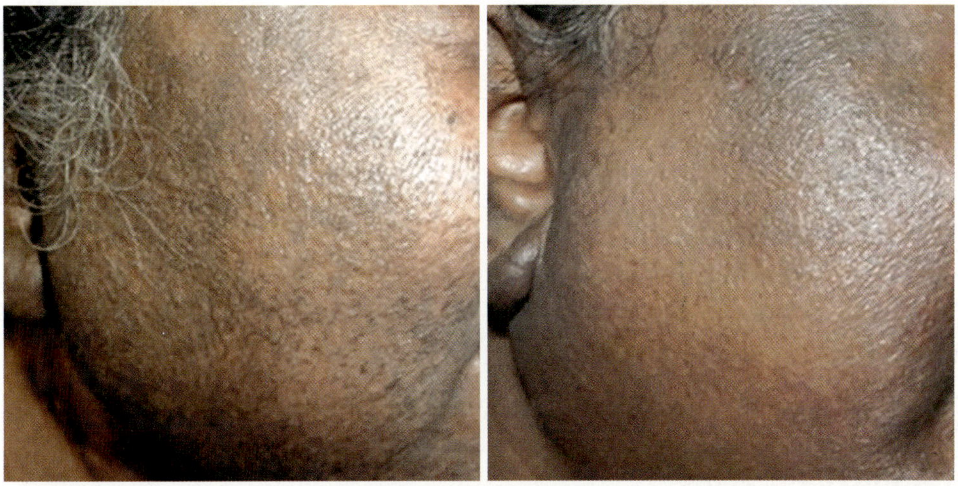

Fig. 42.15: Lichen planus pigmentosus after 4 sessions of CO_2 laser (10600 nm) done every 6 weeks followed by 6 sessions of QS Nd:YAG (1064 nm) done at 6 weeks interval (spot size—4 mm spot, fluence—4.5 to 7.0 J/cm^2).

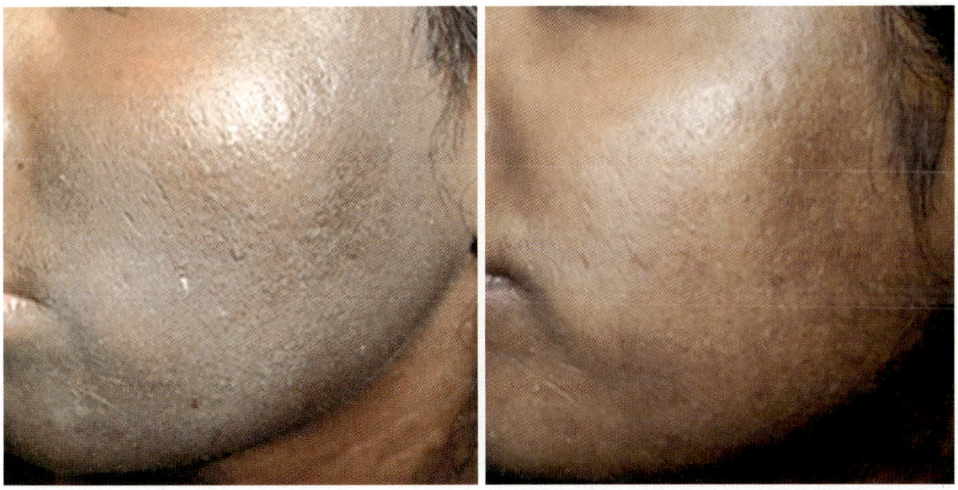

Fig. 42.16: Toxic melanosis after 6 sessions of CO_2 laser (10600 nm) followed by 6 sessions of QS Nd:YAG (1064 nm) done at 6 weeks interval.

sessions and fewer complications. The darker skin types are challenging because of the increased risk of complications. They are always managed conservatively and are counseled about the risks and benefits and more number of sessions. Also in darker skin patients, it is safe to choose a long wavelength laser like 1064 nm Nd: YAG and use lower fluences to produce less epidermal injury with same dermal effect:

- Avoid procedure in patients with recent history of tanning/sun exposure.
- In all patients it is good to prime the skin with hydroquinone and skin lightening preparations, before scheduling the treatment sessions.
- Skin biopsy to confirm the diagnosis and to determine the depth of pigmentation.
- Assess the type, color, age and site of tattoo. Any cover up tattoos done. Any allergic reaction during tattooing and past-treatment history must be elicited.
- *Counseling* of the patient regarding the laser to be used, procedure, number of sessions required, expected outcome, duration between the session, cost and the precautions that has to be taken during and after laser sessions.
- Exercise caution in patients with keloidal tendency, bleeding disorder and in patients prone for postinflammatory pigmentation and poor healing (Box 42.2).

Box 42.2: Contraindications.

- Associated photo aggravated skin diseases (e.g. SLE)
- Active infection at the site of the lesion (e.g. herpes simplex)
- Patients with unrealistic expectations
- Unstable vitiligo and psoriasis for the risk of koebnerization of treated area
- Tattoo granuloma
- Keloid and keloidal tendencies.

- A well-counseled patient with realistic expectations with the lighter skin type is the ideal candidate for laser, though dark skins are more challenging and are to be managed accordingly.

Treatment Steps in General for all Pigmentary Lesions

- *Informed consent.*
- *Digital photographs* of the lesion/tattoo should be taken prior to every session of laser with adequate lighting and proper patient position.
- *Assess skin type* and do *lesional examination* again.
- *Anesthesia*: All epidermal lesions are to be lased under topical anesthesia (EMLA) applied for about 40 min under occlusion. For fewer lesions procedure can be done without anesthesia and depends on patient's pain threshold. For nevus of Ota, larger tattoo and Becker's nevus, where resurfacing lasers are needed, infiltrative local anesthesia or nerve blocks are preferred.
- *Patient preparation*: Remove make up and jewellery. Position the patient comfortably. Shave, if hairs are more in the area. The treatment area should be cleansed with normal saline/betadine. Cover the mole or tattoo in the treatment area (not intended for treatment), if any. Mark the treatment area into grids while treating large lesions.
- Laser safety measures to be followed. Treating physician/technician to be in comfortable positions to carry out procedure.
- *Parameter settings* are determined based on the patient's Fitzpatrick skin type, degree of lesional pigmentation and clinical response to a test spot. In general, dermal lesions require higher fluences than epidermal lesions. Larger spot sizes have a greater depth of penetration, and are preferred to smaller ones. To achieve the same effect in the dermis, a larger spot size will require lower energy and therefore be gentler on the epidermis and dermoepidermal junction (Boxes 42.3 and 42.4) (Table 42.5).

Box 42.3: Guidelines for setting the parameters.

- Follow the manufacturer's guidelines about the device for first few sessions
- In dark skin types, target pigmentation is more, so more risk of epidermal injury; select safe parameters—long PW and lower fluence
- In lighter skin and in targets with sparse pigmentation—select shorter PW with higher fluence
- The frequency can be adjusted based on the expertise and how fast the hand piece can be moved. If the treating area is large, the frequency can be more to complete procedure in shorter time.

Box 42.4: Guidelines for setting parameters for tattoos.

- Select wavelength based on the ink color
- Dark skin—select large spot with low fluence
- Light skin—select small spot with higher fluence
- Dense/professional/cover up tattoos—large spot and low fluence
- Faint tattoos—small spot and high fluence
- Repetition rate must be kept less for small and fine tattoos, so that treatment is more precise. Higher repetition is kept for larger sized tattoos to complete treatment faster.

- *Test patch*: It is to be done in patients with darker skin, patients having lot of anxiety about the results, all cases of nevus spilus, melasma and poikiloderma; a small (2 × 2 cm) area of the lesion (preferably margins) should be subjected to laser, using a range of fluence, before lasing the complete lesion to determine the treatment parameters for a particular patient, as different skin type and color respond differently to lasers. The test spots have to be evaluated for 5 minutes in lighter skin and 10 min in darker skin for the desired clinical end point of pigmented lesion (whitening and signs of erythema, edema and petechiae) or any adverse clinical end points (Box 42.5). The test patch is seen after 5 days and should be followed up after 4 to 6 weeks, to decide on complete procedure.
- The test spot fluence resulting in pigmented lesion whitening, with minute to no petechiae of the surrounding skin must be selected as the treatment fluence.
- The distance guide should be in direct contact with the skin and perpendicular at all times and each spot should have an overlap of 10% to 20% with the previously treated spot. In IPL thin coat of cold gel is applied and probe is always perpendicular to surface and pressed firmly. Depending on the thickness of the lesion and clinical endpoint, number of passes is to be determined. If clinical end points are not reached, second pass must be done with same or lesser fluence and same PW is given. If any adverse reaction signs (Box 42.6) are noticed, then

Table 42.5: Laser parameters for different indications.

Indication	*Laser*	*Spot size (mm)*	*Fluence (J/cm²)*	*Hz*	*Passes*	*Interval (weeks)*	*Session*
Freckles/ lentigines	QS Nd:YAG (660 nm)	2 to 3	0.9 to 1.6	1	1	4 to 6	3 to 4
Nevus of Ota	QS Nd:YAG (1064 nm)	4 to 7	1.6 to 6	5 to 10	2 to 3	8 to 12	6 to 8; but can be up to 16 to 20
Nevus spilus	QS Nd:YAG (532 nm)	1.3 to 1.8	1 to 1.4	1	1	4 to 6	6 to 8
Postinflammatory hyper-pigmentation	QS Nd:YAG (1064 nm)	10	0.85	5 to 10	2 to 4	1 to 2	8 to 10
Cafe-au-lait macule	QS Nd:YAG (532 nm)	1.3 to 1.8	0.8 to 1.2	1	1 to 2	4 to 6	2 to 3
Melasma (laser toning)	QS Nd:YAG (1064 nm)	10	0.85	5 to 10	2 to 4	1 to 2	8 to 10
ABNOM	QS Nd:YAG (1064 nm)	4 to 7	1.6 to 6	5 to 10	2 to 3	8 to 12	8 to 10
Tattoo (blue/black/brown)	QS Nd:YAG (1064 nm)	7	2.4 to 3	1 to 2	1 to 2	4 to 6	3 to 5
Tattoo (red)	QS Nd:YAG (532 nm)	2.4	2.4	1 to 2	1 to 2	4 to 6	3 to 5

Box 42.5: Clinical end points.

- Immediate whitening with snapping sound is due to photo-acoustic vibration and formation of steam due to rapid heating of tissue, it fades in 15 min
- Perilesional erythema and edema
- Petechiae and purpura are due to tiny bleeding points in skin, appear in few minutes after treatment—indicate aggressive but optimal parameters
- In dark skin changes can be subtle
- Darkening of lesions with IPL.

Box 42.6: Adverse clinical reaction.

- Grey discoloration
- Severe whitening and frank bleeding
- Blistering.

stop the procedure and reset the parameters (Lower fluence/ increased pulse width).

- In some lesions like Nevus of Ota, cafe-au-lait macules and in tattoos, additional pass is required which is given after 20 minutes of first pass, called as the R20 technique.
- *End point*: Mild whitening (frosting) and erythema in case of freckles, nevus spilus and cafe au lait macules; frosting and mild pinpoint bleeding in case of tattoos, nevus of Ota and postinflammatory hyperpigmentation with lasers; darkening of the lesion with IPL.

Postprocedure Care

- Immediately after the laser cold compresses are given for 15 to 20 minutes to decrease inflammation and a thin layer of antibiotic/re-epithelization cream is applied.
- Thrice daily application of moderate potent steroid and antibiotic combination cream for 3 to 5 days.
- Twice daily intake of anti-inflammatory drug for 3 to 5 days.
- Strict Sun protection with repeated application of sunscreen and physical protection.
- Not to pick the lesion or scab and allow the scab to fall on its own in 1–2 weeks, encourage using hydrating creams.
- Wash with water or mild cleanser. Not to scrub the treated area for 5 to 7 days.
- Avoid using cosmetics containing retinol/AHA/alcohol for at least 5 to 7 days.

Complications

- Postinflammatory hyperpigmentation
- Postinflammatory hypopigmentation/depigmentation
- Scarring
- Thermal injury and burns
- Darkening of tattoo pigment
- Allergic tattoo reaction

TIPS AND TRICKS

- The hair over the treatment area has to be trimmed or masked before treatment.
- In nonfacial areas, use safe parameters as healing is slower.
- Purpura can be minimized by treating through a microscope slide held firmly against the skin to compress blood vessel.
- Delayed exfoliation of microcrust can be seen in few patients, it can be exfoliated gently with scrub or microdermabrasion.
- While treating large areas, mark the treatment grids to avoid skip areas and always treat the entire area in each visit.

- While changing parameters, increase the fluence or pulse width, depending on the previous experience; do not alter both together.
- If clinical end points are not reached, increase fluence in small increments as tolerated by patient.
- Keep in mind, the acne and milia postprocedure can be due to hydrating creams and steroid creams.
- Though treatment sessions are to be spaced 3 to 6 weeks, defer, if any microcrusts are still present.
- In contrast skin type, i.e. light skin with dark lesion- lesser treatment sessions are required as optimal parameters like short PW and high fluence are used.
- If tattoo is dark, thick, professional tattoo and cover up tattoos- select low fluence.
- For tattoos select larger spot size to deliver optimal fluence to proper depth. Smaller spot size has a risk of epidermal injury because more scattering.
- Professional and cover up tattoos require more sessions.
- Multicolored tattoo need to be targeted by different wavelengths.

CONCLUSION

Treating the pigmentary lesion with laser itself is a challenge in dark skin and treating the sequelae resulting from the treatment is equally tough. Freckles and lentigines respond very well to QS lasers in light-skinned patients, and in dark skinned individuals, LP pigment lasers can be a good option. Nevus of Ota and Hori's macules are best treated by QS lasers. In the treatment of melanocytic nevi, combination of LP lasers followed immediately by the use of QS lasers can be the second line treatment. Café au lait macules and Becker's nevus can be effectively treated by LP pigment lasers which target both epidermal and the follicular melanocytes. Picolasers are newer hope for tattoos and needs further studies to know their efficacy in other pigmentary lesions.

REFERENCES

1. Stratigos AJ, Dover JS, Arndt KA. Laser treatment of pigmented lesions-2000. How far have we gone? Arch Dermatol. 2000;136:915-21.
2. Polla LL, Margolis RJ, Dover JS, et al. Melanosomes are a primary target of Q-switchedru by laser irradiation in guinea pig skin. J Invest Dermatol. 1987;89:281-6.
3. Anderson RR, Parish JA. Selective photothermolysis: precise microsurgery by selective absorption of pulsed irradiation. Science.1983;22:524-7.
4. Watanabe S, Flotte T, Margolis R. The effects of pulse duration on selective pigmented cell injury by dye lasers. J Invest Dermatol. 1987;88:523.
5. Margolis RJ, Dover JS, Polla LL, et al. Visible action spectrum for melanin-specific selective photothermolysis. Lasers Surg Med. 1989;9:389-97.
6. Kilmer SL, Wheeland RG, Goldberg DJ, et al. Treatment of epidermal pigmented lesions with the frequency-doubled Q switched Nd:YAG laser: a controlled, single impact, dose-response, multicenter trial. Arch Dermatol. 1994;130:1515.
7. Li YT, Yang KC. Comparison of the frequency doubled Q-switched Nd:YAG laser and 35% trichloroacetic acid for the treatment of face lentigines. Dermatol Surg.1999;25:202-4.
8. Goldberg DJ. Benign pigmented lesions of the skin. Treatment with the Q-switched ruby laser. J Dermatol Surg Oncol. 1993;19:376-9.
9. Taylor CR, Anderson RR. Treatment of benign pigmented epidermal lesions by Q-switched ruby laser. Int J Dermatol. 1993;32:908-12.
10. Trafeli JP, Kwan JM, Meehan KJ, et al. Use of long-pulse alexandrite laser in the treatment of superficial pigmented lesions. Dermatol Surg. 2007;33(12):1477-82.
11. Tan OT, Morelli JG, Kurban AK. Pulsed dye laser treatment of benign cutaneous pigmented lesions. Lasers Surg Med. 1992;12:538-41.
12. Tanzi EL, Lupton JR, Alster TS. Lasers in dermatology: four decades of progress. J Am Acad Dermatol. 2003;49:1-31.
13. Farris PK. Combination therapy for solar lentigines. J Drugs Dermatol. 2004;3:S23-6.
14. Stern RS, Dover JS, Levin JA, et al. Laser therapy versus cryotherapy of lentigines: a comparative trial. J Am Acad Dermatol.1994;30:985-7.
15. Nanni CA, Alster TS. Successful treatment of a Becker's nevus using 694 nm long-pulsed ruby laser energy. Dermatol Surg. 1998;24:1032-4.
16. Taylor CR, Anderson RR. In effective treatment of melasma and post inflammatory hyperpigmentation by Q-switched Ruby laser. J Dermatol Surg Oncol.1994;20:592-7.
17. Kang WH, Yoon KH, Lee ES, et al. Melasma: histopathological characteristics in 56 Korean patients. Br J Dermatol. 2002;146:228-37.
18. Rokhsar C, Fitzpatrick RE. The treatment of melasma with fractional photothermolysis: a pilot study. Dermatol Surg. 2005;31:1645-50.
19. Polnikorn N. Treatment of refractory dermal melasma with the Med Lite C6 Q-switched Nd:YAG laser: two case reports. J Cosmet Laser Ther. 2008;10:167-73.
20. Kim EH, Kim YC, Lee ES, et al. The vascular characteristics of melasma. J Dermatol Sci. 2007;46:111-6.
21. Briganti S, Camera E, Picardo M. Chemical and instrumental approaches to treat hyperpigmentation. Pigment Cell Res. 2003;16:101-10.
22. Grevelink JM, Gonzales S, Bonoan R, et al. Treatment of nevus spilus with the Q-switched ruby laser. Dermatol Surg. 1997;23:365-70.
23. Hague JS, Lanigan SW. Laser treatment of pigmented lesions in clinical practice: a retrospective case series and patient satisfaction survey. Clin Exp Dermatol. 2008;33(2):139-41.

24. Suzuki H, Anderson RR. Treatment of melanocytic nevi. Dermatol Ther 2005;18(3):217-26.
25. Böer A, Wolter M, Kaufmann R. Pseudomelanoma following laser treatment or laser treated melanoma? J Dtsch Dermatol Ges. 2003;1(1):47-50.
26. Lee HW, Ahn SJ, Lee MW, et al. Pseudomelanoma following laser therapy. JEADV. 2006;20:341-62.
27. Arneja JS, Gosain AK. Giant congenital melanocytic nevi. Plast Reconstr Surg. 2009;124 (Suppl 1):1e-13e.
28. Ferguson RE Jr, Vasconez HC. Laser treatment of congenital nevi. J Craniofac Surg. 2005;16(5):908-14.
29. Zipser MC, Mangana J, Oberholzer PA, et al. Melanoma after laser therapy of pigmented lesions: circumstances and outcome. Eur J Dermatol. 2010;20(3):334-8.
30. Milgraum SS, Cohen ME, Auletta MJ. Treatment of blue nevi with Q-switched ruby laser. J Am Acad Dermatol. 1995;32:307-10.
31. Chan HH, King WW, Chan ES, et al. In vivo trial comparing patients' tolerance of Q-switched Alexandrite (QS Alex) and Q-switched neodymium: yttrium-aluminum-garnet (QS Nd:YAG) lasers in the treatment of nevus of Ota. Lasers Surg Med. 1999;24:24-8.
32. Geronemus RG. Q-switched ruby laser therapy of nevus of Ota. Arch Dermatol. 1992;128:1618-22.
33. Kouba DJ, Fincher EF, Moy RL. Nevus of Ota successfully treated by fractional photothermolysis using a fractionated 1440 nm Nd:YAG laser. Arch Dermatol. 2008;144:156-8.
34. Timko AL, Miller CH, Johnson FB, et al. In vitro quantitative chemical analysis of tattoo pigments. Arch Dermatol. 2001;137:143-7.
35. Baumler W, Eibler ET, Hohenleutner U, et al. Q-switch laser and tattoo pigments: first results of the chemical and photophysical analysis of 41 compounds. Laser Surg Med. 2000;26:13-21.
36. Suchin KR, Greenbaum SS. Successful treatment of a cosmetic tattoo using a combination of lasers. Dermatol Surg. 2004;30:105-7.
37. Amazon K, Robinson MJ, Rywlin AM. Ferrugination caused by Monsel's solution. Clinical observations and experimentations. Am J Dermatopathol. 1980;2:197-205.
38. Ross V, Naseef G, Lin G, et al. Comparison of responses of tattoos to picosecond and nanosecond Q-switched neodymium: YAG lasers. Arch Dermatol.1998;134:167-71.
39. Taylor CR, Anderson RR, Gange RW, et al. Light and electron microscopic analysis of tattoos treated by Q-switched ruby laser. J Invest Dermatol.1991;97:131-6.
40. Taylor CR, Gange RW, Dover JS, et al. Treatment of tattoos by Q-switched ruby laser. A dose response study. Arch Dermatol. 1990;126:893-9.

CHAPTER 43

Lasers in Dermatosurgery: Treatment of Hypopigmentary Disorders

BS Chandrashekar, Madura C, Shubhani Saini

INTRODUCTION

In the last decade, lasers and light devices have progressed and proved to have a key role in treating hypomelanotic disorders and vitiligo. This chapter discusses the role of laser in vitiligo, leukoderma and nevus depigmentosus. Lasers used in surgical treatment of vitiligo and also lasers used to remove the residual pigmentation in generalized vitiligo are also discussed.

EXCIMER LASER/LAMP

The 308 excimer laser and lamp are in use since 1977.[1] It was approved by FDA for vitiligo in 2001. An excimer laser typically uses a combination of a noble gas (argon, krypton, or xenon) and a reactive gas (fluorine or chlorine). Under the appropriate conditions of electrical stimulation and high pressure, an unstable pseudo-molecule called an excited dimer/excimer (or in the case of noble gas halides, exciplex) is created, which can only exist in an energized state and can give rise to laser light in the ultraviolet range. The laser light is delivered via fiber optic cable. The laser works on a theory termed "ablative decomposition", where the energy of photons from laser exceeds the energy of chemical bonds which keep organic material together. There is precise tissue ablation with minimal surrounding thermal damage. It induces apoptosis of lesional lymphocytes, with dose requirement lesser than narrow-band ultraviolet B (NBUVB).[2,3] The excimer laser produces better clinical response than NBUVB/psoralen and ultraviolet A (PUVA), as it delivers higher fluence to the targeted area.

Emission of excimer molecules is also used as a source of spontaneous ultraviolet light called excimer lamp. It is being used since 2003.[4] The excimer lamp delivers incoherent, nondirectional monochromatic light and is equally efficacious. It differs from excimer laser by being noncoherent light, being portable and less costly. The irradiation field is larger and also new devices come with hand pieces that can be adjusted to lesional size. However, it takes longer time to deliver shots compared to laser when higher doses are given and also when larger body areas need to be covered.[5]

Biological effects: The excimer light repigments, stabilizes and can be used as maintenance therapy due to its immunosuppressive and immunomodulatory properties. The monochromatic excimer light triggers apoptosis, T cell depletion, decreases antigen presentation and regulates inflammatory mediators and cytokines superior to NBUVB.[6,7] It also induces repigmentation by melanocyte migration, activation and production of melanin by upregulating endothelin-1 release from keratinocyte. It also stimulates dopa negative amelanocytic melanocytes in perifollicular region.[7,8] All these mechanisms are achieved with greater efficay in excimer light than NBUVB.[9]

Clinical response: The clinical response is termed excellent, when repigmentation is at least 75% in treated area. The response is superior to NBUVB, as it offers higher power density and also the risk of over exposure to normal skin is very less. Various studies have shown it to be effective in both pediatric and adult patients of all skin types (I–VI). The treatment response is best for face and least for bony prominence with cumulative dosage of 73.1 mJ/cm^2 for hands/feet and 3.96 mJ/cm^2 for face.[10] The frequency also affects the efficacy; most of the studies utilized thrice weekly regimen for duration of 4–36 weeks. Follow-up data in various studies have shown stability of repigmentation up to 2 years.[11-14]

Advantages of Excimer Laser Over NBUVB[15]

- Shorter treatment duration
- Lower cumulative dosage
- Fewer long-term risk
- It can be used in high-risk population group.[16]
- Increased patient compliance because of decreased treatment duration.

Box 43.1: Indications.

- Vitiligo of less than 20% body surface area
- Leukoderma
- Post-burn depigmented scars
- Hypopigmented striae (striae alba)
- Post-tattoo depigmentation[20]
- Postsurgery for vitiligo and other conditions (nevus depigmentosus, piebaldism).[21]

Indications[17-19] (Box 43.1)

Vitiligo is the primary indication. In nonvitiliginous indications, treatment stimulates residual melanocytes to produce pigment. A study showed striae and leukoderma improved with dose of 50 mJ/cm^2, however, treated area slowly depigmented on stopping the treatment.

Contraindications[22]

- Patient with photosensitivity
- Patient on photosensitizing drugs
- History of herpes simplex virus (HSV) infection.

Selection of Patient[23]

- Select limited body surface area involvement, preferably less than 20%.
- Anatomic area of treatment predicts the response of treatment—the face, scalp and neck respond well, compared to least responsive bony prominences.[24]
- Skin types III-VI respond best.
- Small lesions respond quickly.
- Counseling: Discuss risks and benefits of treatment, the cost and need for multiple sessions and long duration of treatment.

Procedural Technique (Fig. 43.1)

- Select the potential candidate.
- Informed consent and photo-documentation is obtained.
- Skin to be free of topical agents.
- Eye protection for both patient and operator.
- The patient should be protected from natural light between the treatments.
- Set the parameters: 100–150 mJ/cm^2 is starting dose on head and neck, 200 mJ/cm^2 for arms and trunk, 300–400 mJ/cm^2 bony prominence, 600 mJ/cm^2 for palms and soles and it is increased by 50–100 mJ/cm^2 per treatment until erythema develops. Determination of MED is not needed for vitiligo patients.[25]

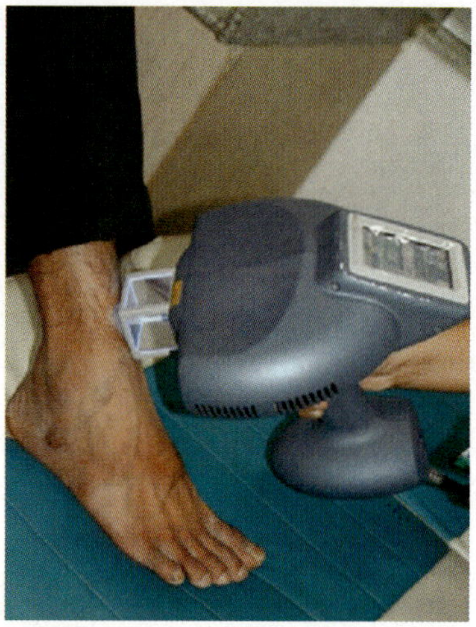

Fig. 43.1: Delivering shots from 308 nm excimer lamp.

- If patient develops severe burns, decrease the dose by 50 mJ/cm^2 or skip the session. If erythema is more, decrease dose by 100 mJ/cm^2. If this continues, avoid treatment on consecutive days. If blistering occurs, stop the treatment. Topical moderate potent corticosteroid alleviates the symptoms and treatment is resumed once the reaction subsides.
- Recommendation: 2–3 times a week for 20 weeks. Response to treatment is noted in 4 weeks; if no change in 20 weeks then it is termed as treatment failure to excimer laser.[26]

Complications

Slight tingling pain during procedure is normal. Erythema, bulla and pain occur, if started with higher doses. Sunburn reaction, freckling, variegate pigmentation and increased risk of cancer are few rare complications.

Results (Figs. 43.2 to 43.4)

- *Lasers used for depigmenting the residual pigmentation*: Lasers are an alternative option in generalized vitiligo with islands of normal pigmentation: they can be targeted with lasers. It must be reserved for small areas. Q switched Ruby laser is as effective as monobenzyl ether of hydroquinone (MBEH), but patient must be explained about risk of repigmentation in treated areas.[27] Other lasers that can be used are Q switched Alexandrite laser; an isolated case report has shown repigmentation in 1 year follow-up.[28]
- *Lasers for preparation of recipient bed in vitiligo surgeries*: There are various options for de-epidermization; they

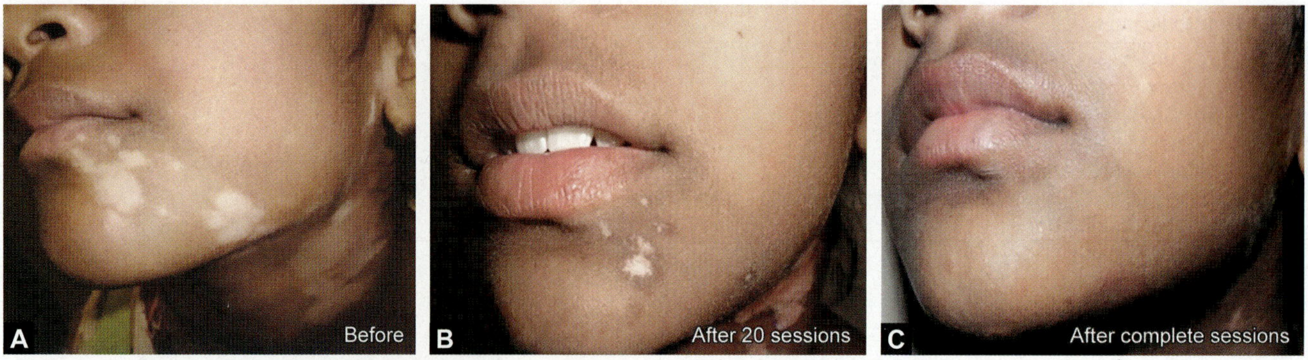

Figs. 43.2A to C: Complete repigmentation in vitiligo patch with excimer lamp.

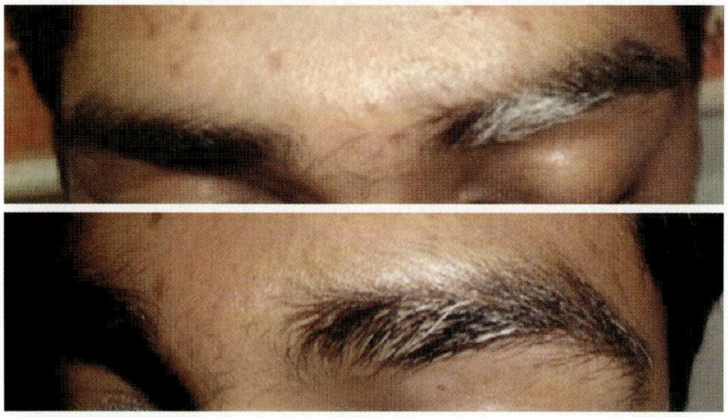

Fig. 43.3: Repigmentation of vitiligo patch after treating with excimer lamp.

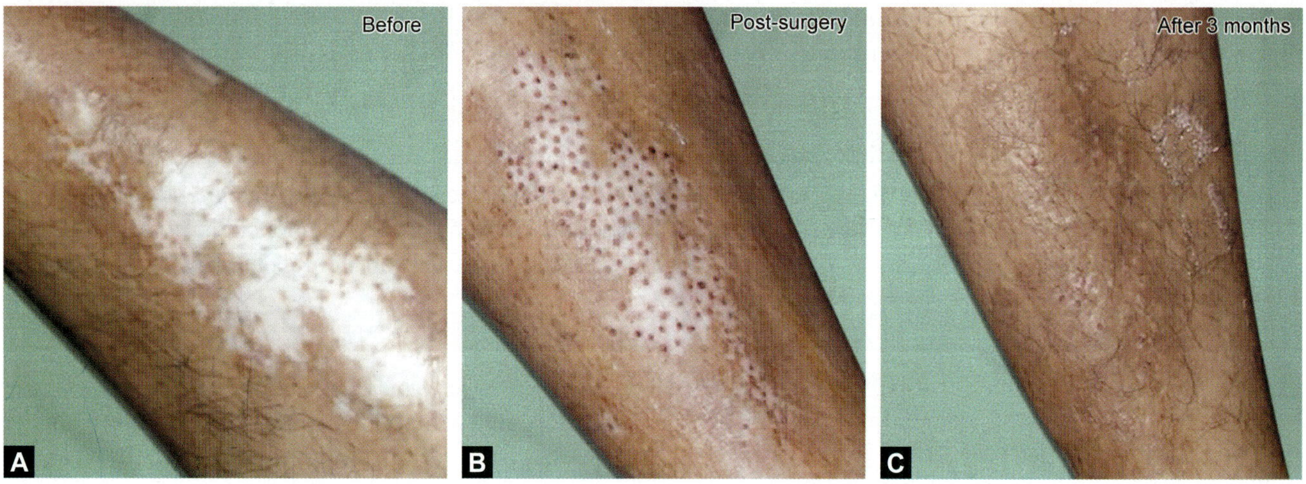

Figs. 43.4A to C: Complete repigmentation after MPG followed by excimer lamp therapy.

are manual/motor dermabrasion and radiofrequency ablation. Laser is fastest and achieves more precise and even abrasion of recipient area. Choice of lasers being either Erbium Yag,[29,30] or CO_2 laser.[31,32] Erbium Yag has 250 to 350 micro second pulse which is less than 1 millisecond (TRT of epidermis). It is 12 to 18 times more efficiently absorbed by water, leading to superficial and more precise ablation without residual damage.

Indications: Laser ablation for preparation of recipient bed is employed not only for vitiligo but also for treatment of nevus depigmentosus. A study showed successful treatment of piebaldism with permanent regimentation. Another study

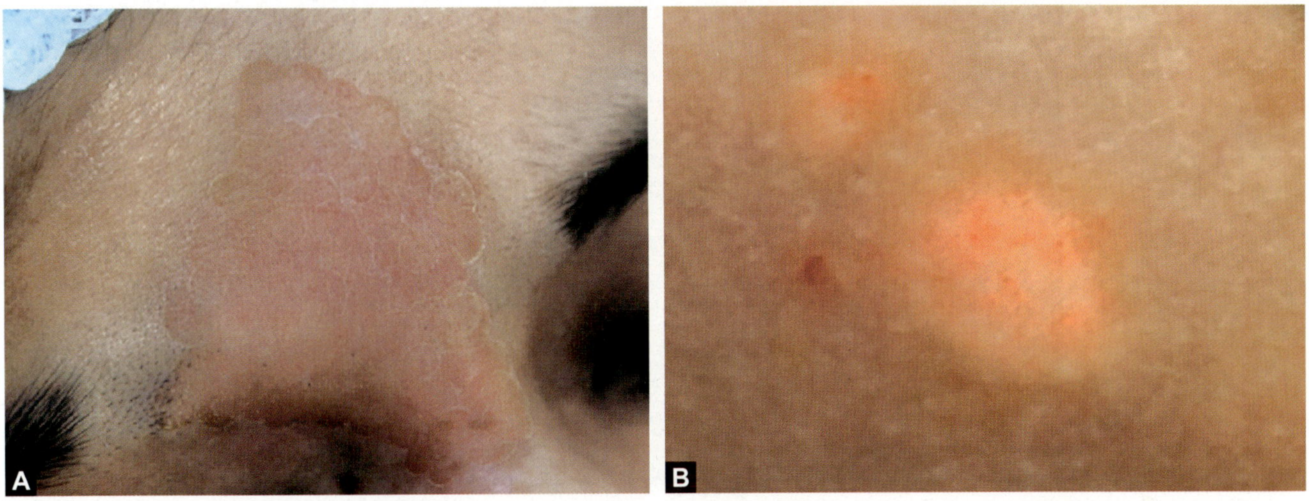

Figs. 43.5A and B: Dermabrasion with laser at recipient site (Er:YAG laser spot size—5 nm; E—7 J/cm²). Pinpoint bleeding is the surgical endpoint.

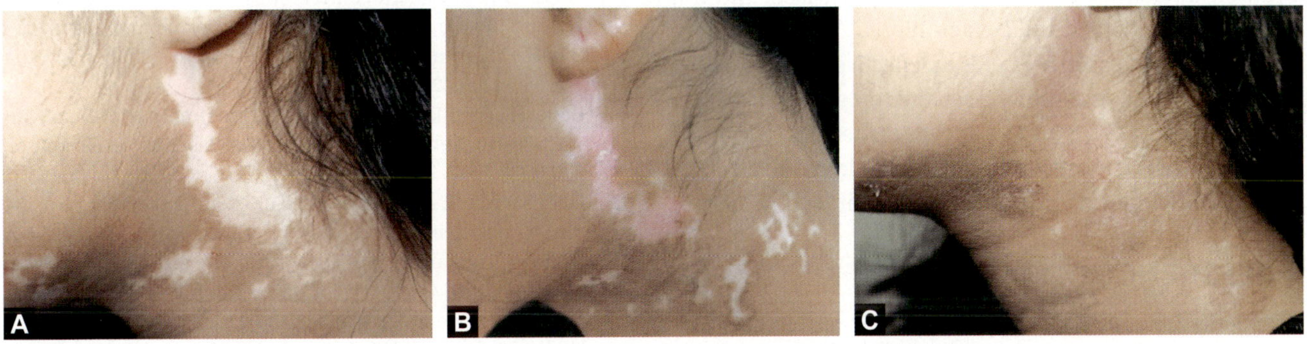

Figs. 43.6A to C: Complete repigmentation in segmental vitiligo patch after epidermal cell suspension (Er:YAG ablation done for recipient bed) followed by excimer lamp therapy.

with 50 patients of vitiligo reported good clinical outcome with Er Yag ablation with application of 5FU followed by NBUVB.[33,34]

Technical Steps

- De-epithelization is performed under anesthesia with topical EMLA under occlusion for 2 hours.
- Mark the area slightly larger than the vitiligo patch.
- Clean the area with betadine and later with normal saline; then dry the area thoroughly.
- Set the parameters: Select the spot size, frequency and fluence according to size of the patch to be ablated (5 mm, 7-8 J/cm² with 20% overlap). Do test shot with two consecutive energies and select the right parameters. Two passes are recommended in thick skin like on hands and foot.
- After the laser shots, rub the area with wet gauze. Pin- point bleeding is the end point and infers right depth of surgical ablation in creating recipient bed (Figs. 43.5A and B). This is followed by spreading the graft or cell suspension.
- Author recommends excimer laser/lamp 10 days to 2 weeks after surgery to aid faster regimentation. The pigmentation is seen as early as 2 weeks and nearly completed in 12 weeks.

Results (Figs. 43.6 and 43.7)

Combination therapy: The topical calcineurin inhibitors (tacrolimus) has shown good outcome when combined with excimer laser than when used alone.[35] A study compared excimer laser alone with excimer laser and twice daily application of tacrolimus 0.1% in vitiligo patients and found greater efficacy in combination treatment.[36,37] However,

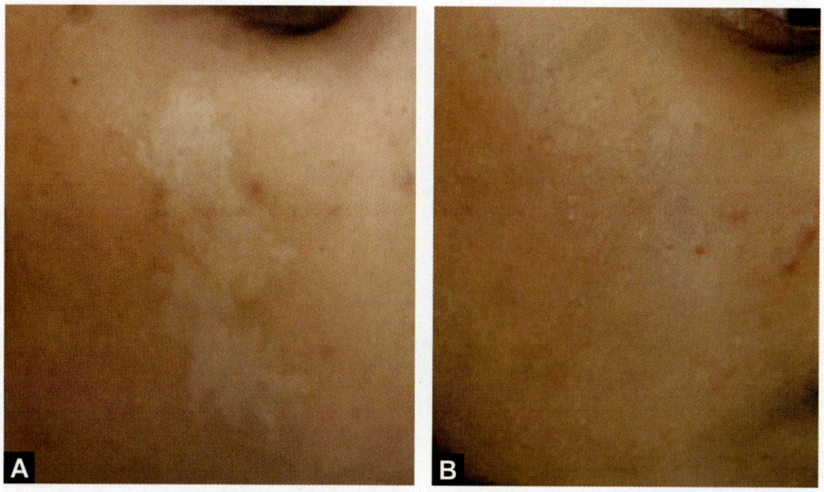

Figs. 43.7A and B: Before and after treatment of nevus depigmentosus on cheek, after erbium ablation and suction blister grafting followed by excimer lamp therapy.

addition of vitamin D_3 analog with excimer laser did not increased the efficacy, unlike tacrolimus.[37]

To conclude, excimer laser is an effective tool in treating focal vitiligo and also it increases the repigmentation rate after vitiligo surgery. It is more effective when it is combined with topical calcineurin inhibitors. The ablative lasers offer a rapid tool for dermabrasion with good clinical outcome.

REFERENCES

1. Bonis B, Kemeny L, Dobozy A, et al. 308 nm UVB excimer laser for psoriasis. Lancet. 1997;350:1522.
2. Chilbert MA, Peak MJ, Peak JG, et al. Effects of intensity and fluence upon DNA single-strand breaks induced by excimer laser radiation. Photochem Photobiol. 1988;47:523-5.
3. de With A, Greulich KO. Wavelength dependence of laser induced DNA damage in lymphocytes observed by single-cell gel electrophoresis. J Photochem Photobiol B. 1995;30:71-6.
4. Leone G, Iacovelli P, Paro Vidolin A, et al. Monochromatic excimer light 308 nm in the treatment of vitiligo: a pilot study. J Eur Acad Dermatol Venereol. 2003;17:531-7.
5. Park KK, Liao W, Murase JE. A review of monochromatic excimer light in vitiligo. Br J Dermatol. 2012;163(3):468-78.
6. Cui J, Shen LY, Wang GC. Role of hair follicles in the repigmentation of vitiligo. J Invest Dermatol. 1991;97:410-16.
7. Norris DA, Horikawa T, Morelli JG. Melanocyte destruction and repopulation in vitiligo. Pigment Cell Res. 1994; 7: 193-203.
8. Taneja A, Trehan M, Taylor CR. 308-nm excimer laser for the treatment of localized vitiligo. Int J Dermatol. 2003;42: 658-62.
9. Ostovari N, Passeron T, Zakaria W, et al. Treatment of vitiligo by 308-nm excimer laser: an evaluation of variables affecting treatment response. Lasers Surg Med. 2004;35:152-6.
10. Hong SB, Park HH, Lee MH. Short-term effects of 308-nm xenonchloride excimer laser and narrow-band ultraviolet B in the treatment of vitiligo: a comparative study. J Korean Med Sci. 2005;20:273-8.
11. Balta SE, Csoma Z, Ignacz F, et al. Treatment of vitiligo with the 308-nm xenon chloride excimer laser. Arch Dermatol. 2002;138:1619-20.
12. Hadi S, Tinio P, Al-Ghaithi K, et al. Treatment of vitiligo using the 308-nm excimer laser. Photomed Laser Surg. 2006;24:354-7.
13. Hofer A, Hassan AS, Legat FJ, et al. The efficacy of excimer laser (308 nm) for vitiligo at different body sites. J Eur Acad Dermatol Venereol. 2006;20:558-64.
14. Hadi SM, Spencer JM, Lebwohl M. The use of the 308-nm excimer laser for the treatment of vitiligo. Dermatol Surg. 2004;30:983-6.
15. Hong SB, Park HH, Lee MH. Short-term effects of 308–nm xenon-chloride excimer laser and narrow-band ultraviolet bin the treatment of vitiligo: a Comparative Study. J Korean Med Sci. 2005;20:273-8.
16. Friedman PM, Geronemus RG. Use of the 308-nm excimer laser for post resurfacing leukoderma. Arch Dermatol. 2001;137:824-5.
17. Alexiades-Armenakas MR, Bernstein LJ, Friedman PM, et al. The safety and efficacy of the 308-nm excimer laser for pigment correction of hypopigmented scars and striae alba. Arch Dermatol. 2004;140:955-60.
18. Goldberg DJ, Sarradet D, Hussain M. 308-nm excimer laser treatment of mature hypopigmented striae. Dermatol Surg. 2003;29:596-9.
19. Gundogan C, Greve B, Hausser I, et al. Repigmentation of persistent laser-induced hypopigmentation with an excimer laser following tattoo removal. Hautarzt. 2004;55:549-52.
20. Guerra L, Primavera G, Raskovic D, et al. Permanent repigmentation of piebaldism by erbium:YAG laser and autologous cultured epidermis. Br J Dermatol. 2004;150:715-21.

21. Bruce AM, Spencer J M. In: Nouri K (Ed). Lasers in Dermatology and Medicine. Springer-Verlag London Limited; 2011; 193-198.
22. Bruce AM, Spencer J M. In: Nouri K (Ed). Lasers in Dermatology and Medicine. Springer-Verlag London Limited; 2011; 198-201.
23. Hofer A, Hassan AS, Legat FJ, et al. The efficacy of excimer laser (308 nm) for vitiligo at different body sites. J Eur Acad Dermatol Venereol. 2006;20:558-64.
24. Bruce AM, Spencer J M. In: Nouri K (Ed). Lasers in Dermatology and Medicine. Springer-Verlag London Limited; 2011; 202-209.
25. Hofer A, Hassan AS, Legat FJ, et al. Optimal weekly frequency of 308-nm excimer laser treatment in vitiligo patients. Br J Dermatol. 2005;152:981-5.
26. Njoo MD, Vodegel RM, Westerhof W. Depigmentation therapy in vitiligo universalis with topical 4-methoxyphenol and the Q-switched ruby laser. J Am Acad Dermatol. 2000;42:760-9.
27. Rao J, Fitzpatrick RE. Use of the Q-switched 755-nm alexandrite laser to treat recalcitrant pigment after depigmentation therapy for vitiligo. Dermatol Surg. 2004;30:1043-5.
28. Guerra L, Primavera G, Raskovic D, et al. Erbium:YAG laser and cultured epidermis in the surgical therapy of stable vitiligo. Arch Dermatol. 2003;139:1303-10.
29. Pai GS, Vinod V, Joshi A. Efficacy of erbium YAG laser assisted autologous epidermal grafting in vitiligo. J Eur Acad Dermatol Venereol. 2002;16:604-6.
30. Oh CK, Cha JH, Lim JY, et al. Treatment of vitiligo with suction epidermal grafting by the use of an ultrapulse CO_2 laser with a computerized pattern generator. Dermatol Surg. 2001;27:565-8.
31. Kahn AM, Ostad A, Moy RL. Grafting following short-pulse carbon dioxide laser de-epithelialization. Dermatol Surg. 1996;22:965-7; discussion 967-8
32. Passeron T, OrtonneC JP. Pigmentation and hypopigmentation: vitiligo and other disorders. In Raulin C, Karrai S (Eds.), Laser and IPL Technology in Dermatology and Aesthetic Medicine. Springer; 2011.157-164.
33. Ablation plus topical 5Fluorouracil on the outcome of short-term NB-UVB phototherapy in the treatment of non-segmental vitiligo: a left-right comparative study. Photodermatol Photoimmunol Photomed. 2008;24:322-9.
34. Bae J M, Hong B Y, Lee J H, Lee J H, et al. The efficacy of 308-nm excimer laser/light (EL) and topical agent combination therapy versus EL monotherapy for vitiligo: A systematic review and meta-analysis of randomized controlled trials (RCTs). Korea J Am Acad Dermatol. 2016;74:907-15.
35. Lacour JP, et al. Topical tacrolimus and the 308-nm excimer laser: a synergistic combination for the treatment of vitiligo. Arch Dermatol. 2004;140:1065-9.
36. Kawalek AZ, Spencer JM, Phelps RG. Combined excimer laser and topical tacrolimus for the treatment of vitiligo: apilot study. Dermatol Surg. 2004;30:130-5.
37. Goldinger SM, Dummer R, Schmid P, et al. Combination of 308-nm xenon chloride excimer laser and topical calcipotriol in vitiligo. J Eur Acad Dermatol Venereol. 2007;21:504-8.

CHAPTER 44

Lasers in Dermatosurgery: Treatment of Vascular Lesions

BS Chandrashekar, Madura C

BACKGROUND

The treatment of cutaneous vascular lesions is challenging and gratifying to the dermatologist. The lesions can range from superficial cherry angiomas to deeper hemangiomas and malformations to some abnormal leg veins. When choosing the ideal device to treat a specific lesion, the depth of the intended target matters greatly. An ideal laser with optimal parameters is chosen to expect beneficial results. The technology keeps rapidly evolving and hence guidelines are reviewed periodically. This chapter covers the the current guidelines and share author's experience in using vascular lasers.

The initial treatment of vascular lesions with ruby and carbon dioxide lasers in 1960s was associated with a whole lot of side effects. The new era in laser medicine began in 1983 with the concept of selective photothermolysis (SPT) introduced by Anderson and Parish.[1] The principle states that laser or light energy produce selective heating and destruction of a targeted skin lesion which is chromophore specific, such as a blood vessel, without damaging nearby structures. Selective photothermolysis was first applied to Port wine stain (PWS), and vascular lesions were the first test cases for SPT.[1] Pulse dye laser (PDL) was the first laser to show that the concept of selectivity for chromophore was practical.

A large number of lasers (wavelength range from 532 to 1064 nm) and intense non-coherent pulsed light devices are now available for the treatment of vascular lesions. Pulsed-dye laser, potassium titanyl phosphate (KTP), alexandrite laser, diode laser, and neodymium-doped yttrium aluminum garnet (Nd:YAG) lasers, as well as Intense pulsed light (IPL) are being applied in the treatment of cutaneous vascular lesions. The laser surgeon should have complete understanding of the basics of lasers, intended target and of the device being employed for the procedure (Boxes 44.4 and 44.5).

Laser Variables

- *Target*: Oxyhemoglobin (HbO_2) is the chromophore for vascular lasers. In order to target vascular lesions, the wavelength of light chosen must be preferentially absorbed by blood vessels. Vascular lasers exploit selective absorption peak of oxyhemoglobin by 70% and rest by deoxyheomoglobin and methemoglobin. Oxyhemoglobin has three major absorption peaks at 418, 542, and 577 nm. Optimal absorption is within 577–600 nm range.[2,3]
- *Wavelength*: Wavelength is the first important factor. Choosing the appropriate wavelength involves selecting a wavelength with enough penetration depth. Shorter wavelengths of 532, 585, and 595 nm target superficial lesions. Longer wavelength like 755, 810, and 1064 nm can target both superficial and deeper pathology. The competing chromophore in the epidermis and appendages is always melanin. Sufficient fluence is required to achieve irreversible damage of the target vessel. Increase in fluence can increase the risk of damage to epidermis. Cooling is must to prevent epidermal damage. The lasers 755, 800, and 1064 nm will have less interaction with melanin because of deeper penetration.
- *Spot size*: is the second important factor for both degree of coverage and depth of effective treatment. Bigger spots go deeper and also results in faster treatment. The ratio of dermal to epidermal damage increases as the spot size increases. Treatment fluences are therefore decreased with larger spots compared to smaller spot sizes. The rule being larger the spot size, deeper the penetration and lower the fluence: vice versa is true for smaller spot size. When in doubt, smaller spot sizes are recommended, with manipulation of the fluence to achieve the desired energy at the target level (Box 44.1).[4,5]
- *Pulse width*: The third factor influencing laser outcome is pulse duration; it depends on size of the intended

Box 44.1: Spot diameter should be 10 times the size of lesion, to have no geometrical loss.

Lesion size	*Spot size*
Epidermal lesions (0.1 mm)	1 mm
PWS (1 mm)	10 mm
Tattoos (2 mm)	20 mm
Hair (3 mm)	30 mm

Box 44.2: Approximate thermal relaxation time for vessels of different diameters.

Diameter (μm)	*TRT (ms)*
10	0.048
20	0.19
50	1.2
100	4.8
200	19.0
300	42.6

Box 44.3: Factors influencing the treatment outcome.

- Vessel size
- Depth of the lesion
- Area of the body involved
- Laser spot size
- Skin type
- Fluence

Box 44.4: Vascular laser classification.[9,10]

Hemoglobin (Hb)-selective laser	
• Green yellow light sources	PDL (585/590/595/600 nm) KTP (532 nm)
• Long wavelength lasers	Diode 800 nm, Alexandrite 755 nm
• Near infrared radiation lasers (NIR)	Diode 940 nm, Nd:YAG 1064 nm
Hemoglobin (Hb)-nonselective lasers	Carbon dioxide laser (10600 nm) Erbium YAG (2940 nm)

target. High enough fluences with pulse durations equal to TRT (thermal relaxation time) will limit diffusion of heat from the target vessels and cause photocoagulation. Excessive long pulse durations, longer than the thermal relaxation time, can lead to diffusion of thermal damage to surrounding tissue. In contrast, excessively short durations can cause excessive purpura without necessarily causing elimination of the vessel (Box 44.2). As a rule shorter pulse durations are better for smaller vessels, whereas longer pulse durations are better for larger vessels.[6]

- *Cooling*: Another important factor is cooling and it is a must to prevent epidermal damage. It should form an integral part of laser treatment to minimize collateral damage and to reduce postoperative complications like swelling, scarring and pigmentation.[7] Thus, selective cooling of the epidermis before, during and after treatment allows higher temperatures in the target structures without causing damage to the epidermis. Direct contact cooling, forced cold air, and cryogen spray are methods adapted for cooling.[7,8]

Factors Influencing the Treatment Outcome

Factors influencing treatment outcome can be device or patient specific (Box 44.3). The main device specific factors are spot size and fluence.

- *Diameter of vessels*: Vessels with a diameter of 10–100 μm have TRT of 1–10 ms, whereas blood vessels with diameter >100 μm have a higher TRT, and therefore, require longer pulse duration.
- *Depth of lesions*: Superficially located lesions (papillary dermis) are treated with standard wavelengths (577, 585 nm), but the deeper vessels need longer wavelength (up to 600 nm) for deeper penetration.
- *Site of lesions*: Lesions on face and upper trunk respond better than those in lower trunk and legs. In scar prone areas and delicate skin, reduction in 10–20% of fluence is advisable. Malformations on the first and third branches of trigeminal nerve respond better than those over the second branch.
- *Age of patient*: As the blood vessels are smaller and more superficially located, young patients respond better than elderly.
- *Skin type*: Epidermal melanin is the main competitor for laser absorption and can damage the epidermis. Hence darker skin types require longer pulse duration, higher fluence, and longer pulse intervals.

An optimal fluence is chosen based mainly on vessel color, vessel size, intravascular pressure and depth of lesion. Purple and blue vessels absorb more energy than pink and red vessels, and require less fluence. Greater intravascular pressure (nose or legs) require higher fluences to achieve effective thermocoagulation.

Tips to Remember

- If lesion is dark red compared to the surrounding tissue, a case can be made for hemoglobin selective technology.
- Ratio of absorption of the vascular target versus surrounding skin should not exceed 10:1.
- Wavelength selectivity should be based on optimal ratio of vascular to pigment destruction.
- Large spot size minimizes Polka dot effect.
- Beam profile must be flat topped.
- Surface cooling is by contact sapphire window/copper plate/cryogen spray/DCD (dynamic cooling device).

LASER DEVICES (BOX 44.5)[10,11]

There are many laser and light devices to treat a wide array of common vascular lesions. Each device is unique. Devices from different companies can have different pulse structures, hand piece specifications, and cooling abilities. Follow the manufacturer's recommendations and correlate them with personal experience.

Frequency-doubled Nd:YAG Potassium Titanyl Phosphate (KTP)

Potassium titanyl phosphate crystals are used to double the frequency, which halves the wavelength from 1,064 to 532 nm. The shorter wavelength effectively destroys the most superficial vessels. As melanin is the competing chromophore, efficient epidermal cooling is necessary when using these devices, especially in darker skin.

Pulsed Dye Lasers (PDL)

Pulsed dye lasers penetrates deeper than frequency-doubled Nd:YAG and is more selectively absorbed by hemoglobin. These lasers have become a mainstay of vascular lesion treatment. The original PDLs employed 585 nm and had short pulse widths of 0.45 ms. The next generation of PDLs have the ability to deliver high frequency pulses that could be combined into longer combined pulse widths of 1.5 ms. The longer pulse widths allow treatment of larger vessels with less extravasation of blood and therefore less purpura. The new generation of PDLs also produce wavelengths of 585, 590, 595, or 600 nm. The most recent versions of pulsed dye lasers have only the 595 nm wavelength but have adjustable pulse widths ranging from 0.45 to 40 ms to provide optimal treatment parameters for various vessel sizes.

Box 44.5: Types of lasers used for vascular lesions.[10]

Laser/Light source	*Wavelength (nm)*	*Pulse duration (ms)*
Pulsed KTP	532	1–200
Pulsed dye (PDL)	585	0.45
Long-pulsed dye	585, 590, 595, 600	1.5–40
Long-pulsed Alexandrite	755	3–20
Diodes	800,810,940	1–250
Long-pulsed Nd:YAG	1064	1–100
Intense pulsed light source (IPL)	515–1200	0.5-30

Alexandrite Lasers

Alexandrite lasers produce 755 nm wavelengths light that can better target deoxygenated hemoglobin. The long pulsed Alexandrite laser is found to be effective against violaceous deeper vascular lesions. The long pulsed Alexandrite lasers with longer wavelength allow deeper penetration to further target larger vessels.

Neodymium-doped Yttrium Aluminum Garnet (Nd:YAG) Laser

Neodymium-doped yttrium aluminum garnet lasers are less vascular specific lasers. The longer wavelength penetrates deeper and oxyhemoglobin no longer absorbs the energy better than the surrounding dermis and needs higher fluence to be effective and hence higher risk of causing dermal damage and scarring. To avoid complications, fluences and pulse width are adjusted according to vessel size, location, and the oxygenation of hemoglobin. Vessels with larger diameters needs longer pulse widths and small vessels need shorter pulse widths, but require higher fluences, as there is less chromophore (Hb) present. Combination of PDL and Nd:YAG laser can selectively target vessels that have both superficial and deep components.

Intense Pulsed Light (IPL)

Intense pulsed light devices produce high-energy broad spectrum noncoherent light that can be selectively filtered to target vascular lesions. Cut-off filters are used to limit the spectrum to 580–590 nm. Newer devices filter out the longer infra-red wavelengths, reducing many of the adverse effects of earlier devices. The larger application tips have advantage to cover larger treatment areas. It is important to remember when using IPL devices that the pulsing, filters, and cooling are different from one device to another.

PATIENT SELECTION AND PREOPERATIVE EVALUATION

The best candidates for treatment of vascular lesions are fair skin and with high degree of contrast between background and target. In dark skin patient, melanin is also a competing chromophore and hence risk of complications is more.

A thorough medical history is to be taken, to rule out photosensitive disorders, keloidal tendencies, medications that worsen redness, and any past treatments.

In the examination, assess the type of skin. Detailed examination includes recording size, thickness, color, site of lesion and presence of type of vessels (telangiectasias and feeding vessels).

The patients must be counseled about results and number of sessions required, expected outcome and should have realistic expectations.

Consent and photography is must in all patients.

Contraindications

- Active infection over areas to be treated.
- Sun exposure within the preceding 4 weeks with red or tanned face.
- Photosensitizing medication/photosensitive disorders.
- Unrealistic expectation.

Preoperative Instructions

- Avoid sun exposure
- Priming of background skin in dark skinned (IV–VI skin type) patients.
- Antiviral medications to be started 48 hours prior to lasers and continued for 5 days in suspected cases of herpes.
- Hair in the treatment area to be trimmed.

Test spots are done in patients with darker skin type and also in patients with lot of anxiety about the outcome. Based on lesional characteristics, skin type and manufacturer guide lines, parameters are chosen: a small area is treated initially and observed for erythema, crusting, blistering and any adverse side effects. Full sessions can be taken up after 3 to 6 weeks.

Anesthesia

Topical anesthesia can cause vasoconstriction, reduced vascular targets and reduced treatment efficacy. For treatment of large lesions and in children, general anesthesia is preferred; especially for hemangiomas and large port wine stain. It can also be done under nerve blocks/ring block.

Selecting Parameters

Follow manufacturer's guidelines in the beginning:

- *Fitzpatrick darker skin type*: Use safe parameters, low fluence and long pulse width and vice versa for lighter skin.
- *Lesional characteristics*: If lesions are more red, target chromophore is more; so use low fluence and long pulse width. If faint red lesions: use high fluence and short pulse width.
- *If telangiectasia are large and deeper*: Use longer wavelength lasers, long pulse width and high fluence to increase the penetration and efficacy. Small telangiectasia are superficial: use green yellow light, short pulse width and high fluence.
- *If treatment area has pigmented lesions*: More number of competing chromophores, then use safe parameters. For example, Telangiectasia with pigmentary blemishes in background.
- *Presence of dark hair in treatment area*: Use safe parameters. Protect the hair with mask and treat only telengiectasia, to avoid permanent hair reduction.
- If treatment area is large: keep faster repetition rate
- *Nonfacial areas*: Keep safe parameters, as healing is impaired in extremities.

TECHNIQUES

- Patient preparation (remove makeup, jewelry and clean the area).
- Proper position of patient and safety precautions.
- The treatment site to be marked into grids, and while treating face: mark the aesthetic units of face with white marker.
- The laser probe must be perpendicular to the surface. Laser shots must be spaced with 10% to 20% overlap. In case of IPL, thin gel is applied. Always place tip firmly on marking, do not press too much.
- Initial laser shots must begin always at the lateral margin of the lesion and pre auricular area in case of face and look for clinical end point.
- Exceeding >20% overlap in treatment area leads to adverse reactions. In such cases, cool the area, wait for 5min, and change the parameters for next pass.

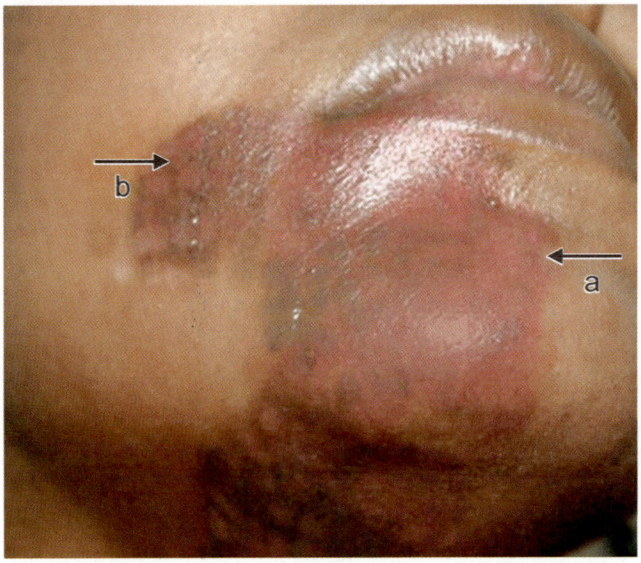

Fig. 44.1: (a) Ideal end point; (b) Ash gray color indicating over treatment.

- Inspect the treatment area, if adequate clinical end point is lacking, then give 2nd pass.
- *Immediate post-procedure care*: Ice compressions, topical antibiotic and steroid application followed by sun screen.
- Follow-up after 5 days.

Clinical End Point

Expected end point
- Intense erythema and swelling (long pulsed lasers)
- Blanching
- Darkening of the lesion with greyish discoloration (Fig. 44.1, arrow a)
- Purpura (green yellow light)

Adverse reaction
- Blistering

Ash gray color indicates over treatment (Fig. 44.1, arrow b).

Post-procedure Sequelae and Care

- The intense redness and edema decreases in 48 hours—Patients are advised ice compression till it reduces. Moderate potent corticosteroid application thrice a day is advised for 5 days. If erythema persists after 5 days, it indicates impending complication.
- Telangiectasia and purpura fade gradually in 2–3 weeks.
- Soothing hydrating creams are advised till crust gets dislodged.
- Broad spectrum sunscreen and physical sun protection are advised.

Tips

- If erythema decreases with treatment sessions- increase the fluence and decrease the pulse width.
- Change one parameter at a time, like increase the fluence by 2–4 J/cm^2 and decrease PW by 5 ms.
- If there is prolonged edema then increase fluence in small increments and pretreatment with antihistamines can be a remedy.
- Delay treatment by 2 weeks, if crusts are visible.

Complications

- Temporary sequelae of pain, erythema and edema are well known, and decrease promptly.
- Persisting erythema and edema lasting for 5 to 15 days.
- Reactivation of HSV.
- Petechia and purpura is relieved in 2 weeks.
- Visible egg crater or strip appearance: represents the laser tip shape surrounded by untreated skin. Space laser shots with 10–20% over lap to avoid this.
- Hyperpigmentation and hypopigmentation are seen more in dark skinned patients.
- Scarring results due to aggressive parameters and persistent intense erythema indicates future scarring.
- There can be decreased density of hair in treated area.

TREATMENT OF SPECIFIC CONDITIONS

There are various indications for vascular lasers that includes both congenital and acquired conditions (Box 44.6).

Facial Telangiectasia[11,12]

Facial telangiectasia is common presentation, either occurring as an isolated entity or associated with acne rosacea or photodamage. Both lasers and IPLs have proven to be effective. The improvement of telangiectasia is achieved by direct heating of hemoglobin (Hb). The choice of lasers for smaller telangiectasia (0.1 to 0.6 mm) are PDL/KTP and IPL. For larger telangiectasia of >1 mm, the choices are Long pulse Nd:YAG and Alexandrite laser. Diode 940 nm is an alternative choice.

As vessels are superficial on face, high-powered 532-nm lasers with large spot treatments and cooling are clinically useful and very effective without producing

Box 44.6: Indications for vascular lasers.[9,10]

- Capillary malformations
  - Infantile PWS
  - Macular PWS in adults
  - Hypertrophic PWS in adults
- Hemangioma
  - Superficial hemangioma
  - Mixed type hemangioma
  - Evolving hemangioma
- Venous malformations
- Telangiectasias
  - Spider angiomata
  - Actinic telangiectasia
  - CREST syndrome
  - Essential telangiectasia
  - Hereditary hemorrhagic telangiectasia
  - Radiation dermatitis
- Rosacea
- Facial erythema
  - Associated with rosacea
  - Flushing and blushing
- Cherry angiomas
- Venous lakes
- Poikiloderma of Civatte
- Miscellaneous
  - Angiokeratomas
  - Glomus tumors
  - Pyogenic granuloma
  - Blue rubber bleb nevi
  - Warts
  - Erythematous and hypertrophic scars

purpura. PDLs at 585 and 595 nm have been reliable tools in the treatment of facial telangiectasia and diffuse erythema. The short pulsed PDLs results in purpura due to the rupture of smaller blood vessels due to high peak powers achieved during procedure. The new generation long pulsed PDLs address this problem.[13,14] It delivers multiple individual pulselets of durations of 150–200 μs, over an interval of 2–40 ms. But due to the low peak power of these subpulses, multiple stack pulses and multiple passes are necessary for purpura free treatments (Figs. 44.2A and B).

A combination of PDL and LP-Nd:YAG gives good results. The smaller vessels of 150 to 400 mm are best treated in the 10-ms pulse range of PDL and the Nd:YAG laser. The larger vessels, measuring 400–1,000 mm, are ideally treated with the 40-ms pulse duration. There is approximately 75% clearance rate in most patients with one to two treatments. The LP-Nd:YAG with spot size smaller than vessel size and high energy can eradicate telangiectatic vessels.[15] The only concern is the narrow margin of safety noted between the therapeutic and toxic doses.

Intense pulsed light devices are unique and as they come from different manufacturers, cutoff filters and the optic spectrum are often very different. The power of some of these devices makes it difficult to treat smaller vessels at pulse durations as short as 5 ms. Like lasers, IPLs are often best used with multiple passes to treat facial telangiectasia.

Parameters of Laser Used for Facial Telangiectasia

- *IPL (Filter -550/560/570 nm)*: Fluence of 12–45 J/cm^2; Double pulse width - 2.4 ms/6.0 ms; pulse delay - 10–30 ms.

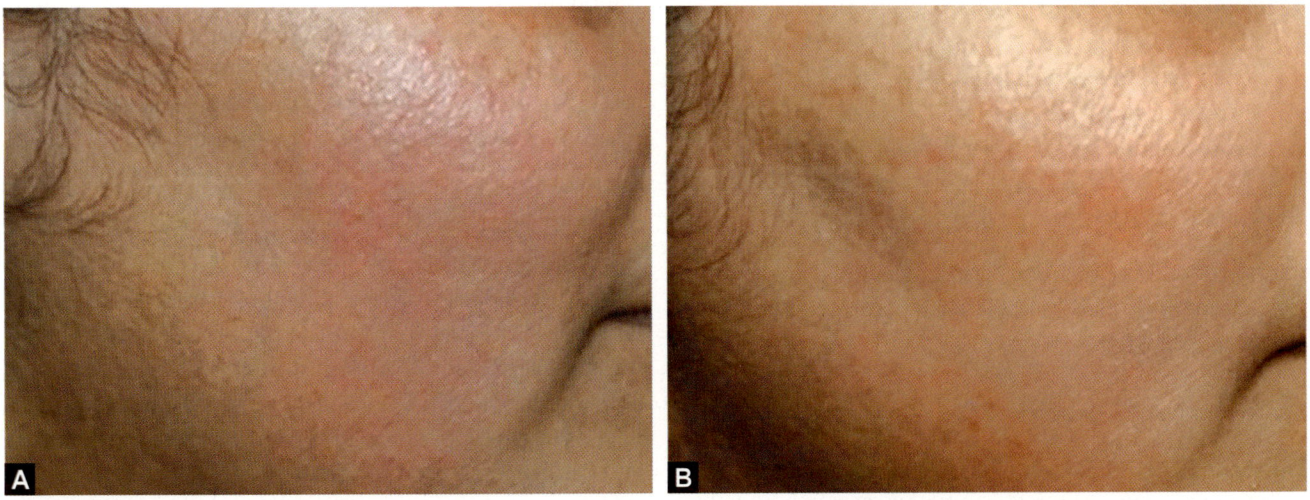

Figs. 44.2A and B: (A) Facial telangiectasia. (B) After 6 sessions of PDL (E - 6 J/cm^2, pulse width - 0.45 ms, spot size - 5 mm; device set parameters).

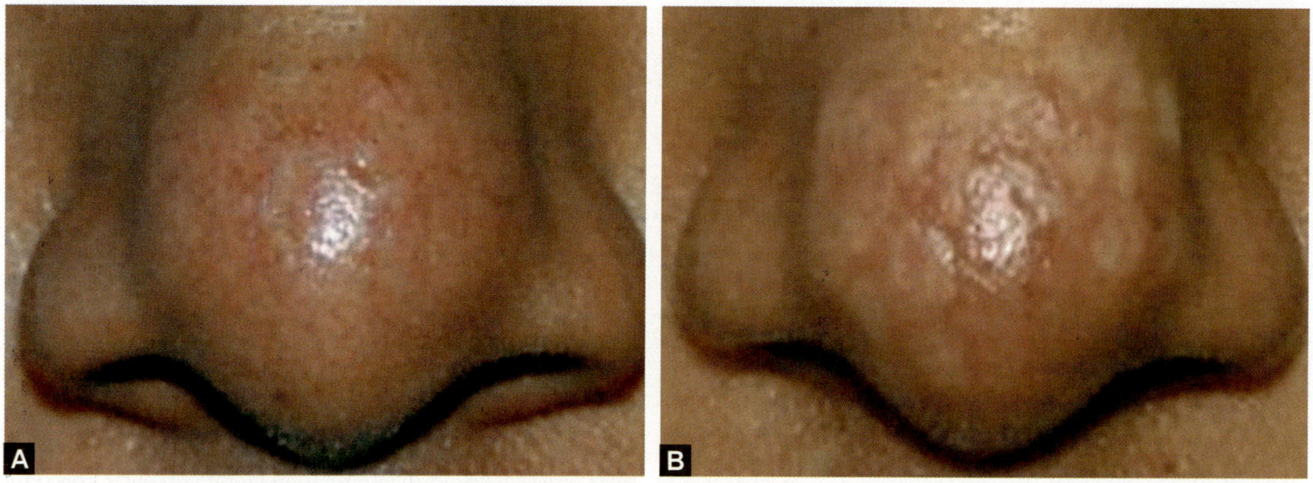

Figs. 44.3A and B: (A) Generalized essential telangiectasia. (B) After 2 sessions of PDL (E - 6 J/cm^2, pulse width - 0.45 ms, spot size - 5 mm).

- *LP Nd:YAG-1064 nm*: Fluence of 120 to 170 J/cm^2; Pulse width - 5 to 40 ms; spot size - 3 to 6 mm.
- *PDL-585 nm*: Fluence of 6 J/cm^2; pulse width - 0.45 ms; spot size - 3–5 mm
- *Diode 940 nm*: Fluence of 140 J/cm^2; Pulse width - 20 ms; spot size - 3 mm.

One should expect epidermal desquamation; if it is to be avoided, then use longer wavelength or increase delay time between double/triple pulses. Advantages of IPL are lack of purpura and adverse sequelae.

Pearl

- Always use smallest spot size and smallest of fluence
- The efficacy of millisecond laser can be improved by using plastic mask to protect the surrounding skin.
- HbO_2 absorption of 1064 is 10 times lesser than 532/595, hence need to use high fluence.
- More the spot size, greater is the scarring; hence recommended spot size is less than 2 mm.

Spider Angiomas/Telangiectasia

Laser of choice is PDL. Alternate choices are IPL with small tip adaptor and small spot KTP with parameters similar to that of facial telangiectasia.

Generalized Essential Telangiectasia

Large spot KTP is the laser of choice with Fluence of 6–8 J/cm^2; Spot size 10 mm; Pulse width 18–22 ms and contact cooling. PDL is the alternate choice with fluence of 6–7 J/cm^2 (Figs. 44.3A and B).[16]

Rosacea

Intense pulsed light (Filter 550/560) is the device of choice. The main advantage of IPL in rosacea is thermal destruction of demodex mites that contributes to the therapeutic effects of IPL. Erythema usually recurs within 6 months of laser treatment, most likely due to resurgence of demodex population and associated inflammation and hence control of disease requires maintenance treatment twice a year.[19,20] Parameters are: Double pulse - 2.4 and 4 ms; Pulse delay - 10 ms; Fluence 18 to 26 J/cm^2. The treatment interval is every 4 weeks for 6 to 8 sessions followed by maintenance of twice a year.[21]

Alternate device used is PDL 595 nm (Figs. 44.4 and 44.5). The parameters are Fluence 7 to 9 J/cm^2; Pulse width - 6 ms and cryogen spray cooling.[22] Resistant Rosacea responds best to aminolevulinic acid-photodynamic therapy (ALA PDT).[23]

Poikiloderma of Civatte[24,25]

In Poikiloderma of Civatte, the degree of hyperpigmentation and erythema varies in each patient. The epidermal melanin is the first chromophore in the path of any light device; the fluence should be appropriate and not to exceed the ability of a particular device to cool both the epidermis and dermis. If the pigment load is more, over heating occurs and can significantly damage the dermis and appendages, resulting in a scar.

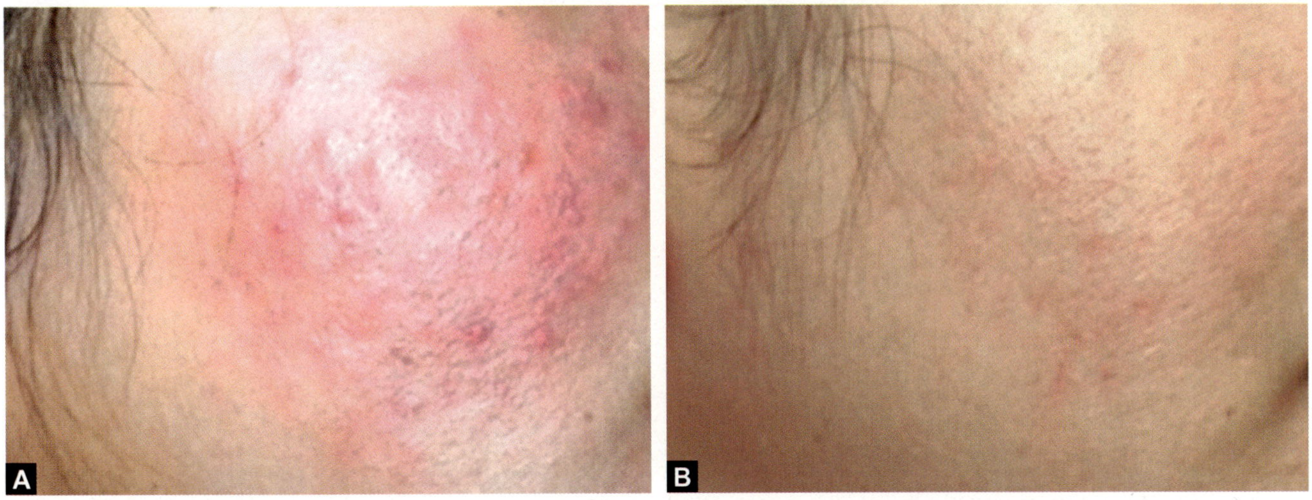

Figs. 44.4A and B: (A) Rosacea; (B) After 6 sessions of PDL (E - 5 J/cm^2, pulse width - 0.45 ms, spot size - 5 mm).

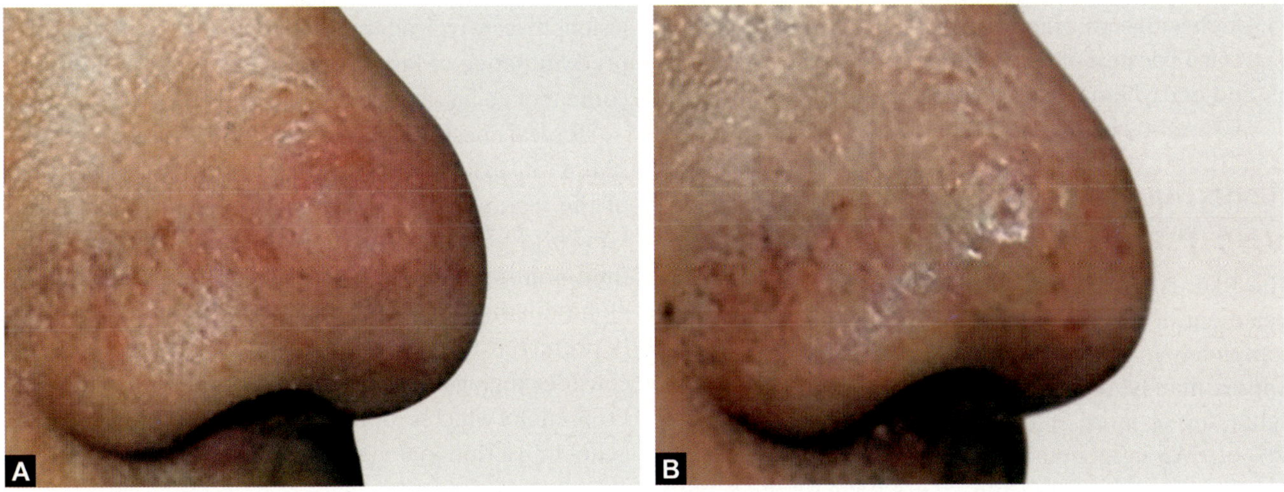

Figs. 44.5A and B: (A) Rosacea; (B) After 2 sessions of PDL (E - 5 J/cm^2, pulse width - 0.45 ms, spot size - 5 mm).

Device of choice is IPL, due to the spectrum of action against melanin as well as Hb. Alternate choices are Large spot KTP, extended pulse PDL and 1550 – Erbium glass.

The PDL parameters are: Fluence of 5 to 6 J/cm^2; pulse width of 1.5 ms and spot size of 10 mm with cryo spray cooling. Fluence of 7 to 9 J/cm^2; pulse width of 10 to 20 ms are adapted in non-purpuric approach. The test spot is highly recommended, with an evaluation after 24–48 hours to know the tolerance of treatment plan (Figs. 44.6A and B).

Pearls

- Demelanizing agents and hydroquinone application to detan for a month increases ratio of vascular to melanin heating leading to better efficacy and safety.
- Choosing IPL has an advantage of clearing both pigment and vessels. Settings are device specific. Purpura is intravascular and resolves in 3 to 5 days. Foot print of contact crystal may be present for first two sessions; patients need to be informed.

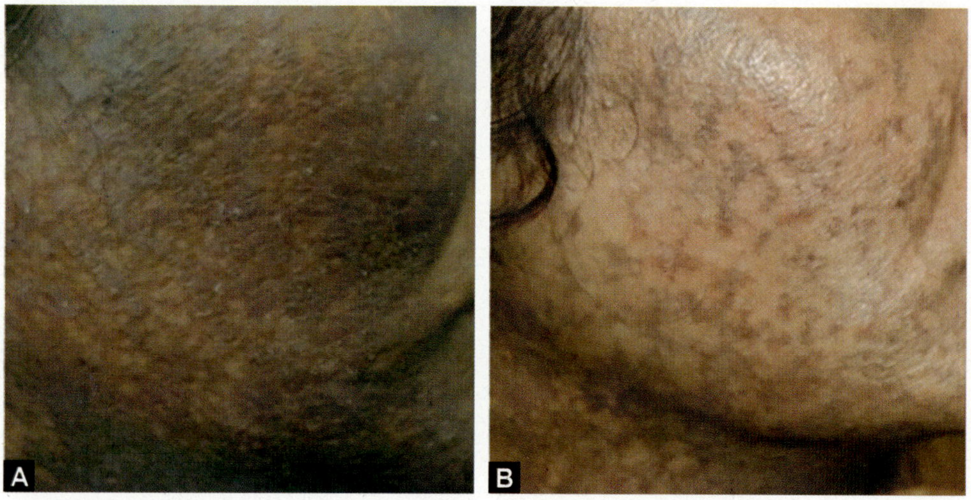

Figs. 44.6A and B: (A) Poikiloderma of Civatte. (B) After 4 sessions of QSNd:YAG (E - 4.6 J/cm², spot size - 5 mm) + fractional CO_2 (E - 30 mJ/cm², Power - 20 W, 100 spots/cm²) with 11 sessions of PDL (E - 5 J/cm², pulse width 0.45 ms, spot size - 5 mm) and 2 sessions of fractional Er:YAG (E - 16 J/cm², 2 passes, frequency 1 Hz, spot size - 12 x 12 mm).

- One has to keep in mind that pigmentation in poikiloderma is also because of deoxyhemoglobin, because melanin and deoxyhemoglobin shares common reflectances at 560 nm which is the deoxyhemoglobin peak.

Nevus Simplex or Salmon Patch/Port Wine Stain (PWS)

The PDL is considered the best laser for the overall treatment of a mixed population. Port wine stains clears completely in only minority of patients after treatment. Approximately 40% of patients with PWS achieved 75% lightening or more after laser treatment and more than 80% of PWS lightened by at least 50%.[26] To improve the results, second-generation lasers have evolved with several modifications like longer pulse widths, longer wavelengths, higher fluences, and the use of dynamic cooling devices. Many of these lasers have proved to be useful in the treatment of PWS.[27]

The gold standard treatment of PWS is PDL[9] (Figs. 44.7A to D). The alternate options include new generation IPL and KTP laser. The KTP laser can further lighten the PDL-resistant lesions. It causes less discomfort and purpura. The shorter wavelength, long pulses and better response to higher fluence can cause significant epidermal injury and higher scar rate compared to new generation PDLs. **Not to be used lasers are Nd:YAG, and Copper vapor** but there are few indications where they can be employed.[35] Longer-wavelength lasers such as the Alexandrite (755 nm) and Nd:YAG (1,064 nm) may have a role in treating bulky malformations and mature PWSs; lesions that are typically more resistant to PDL because of the predominance of larger and deeper vessels and higher content of deoxygenated hemoglobin.[36]

Topical anesthesia in treating PWS is better avoided as EMLA causes local vasoconstriction impeding visualization of the lesion. Prilocaine constituent of EMLA is also known to induce methemoglobinemia in children less than 6 months of age, particularly if they have hemoglobinopathies or G6PD deficiency. General anesthesia is preferred in infants and small children.[21] One can consider angiogenesis inhibitors like topical Rapamycin or Propranolol which suppresses VEGF and hypoxia sensitive gene- transcriptional regulators.[37,38]

Parameters of Laser used for PWS

- *PDL (Pink/Red PWS - 585 nm and for Blue/Dark red is PWS 595 nm)*:
  - Fluence - 12 J/cm² for first pass and - 10 J/cm² for second pass
  - Pulse width - 1.5 ms for first pass 0.45 ms second pass
  - Pulse duration - for dense PWS is 1.5 ms and for lighter PWS - 0.45 ms.
  - Spot size 7 mm with [10% overlap with cryospray/dynamic cooling device (DCD)].
  - Treatment interval - 3 to 6 weeks for up to 8–10 sessions.[39]
- *IPL:*[9]
  - Fluence - 25 to 40 J/cm² for first pass, 40 to 60 J/cm² for second pass

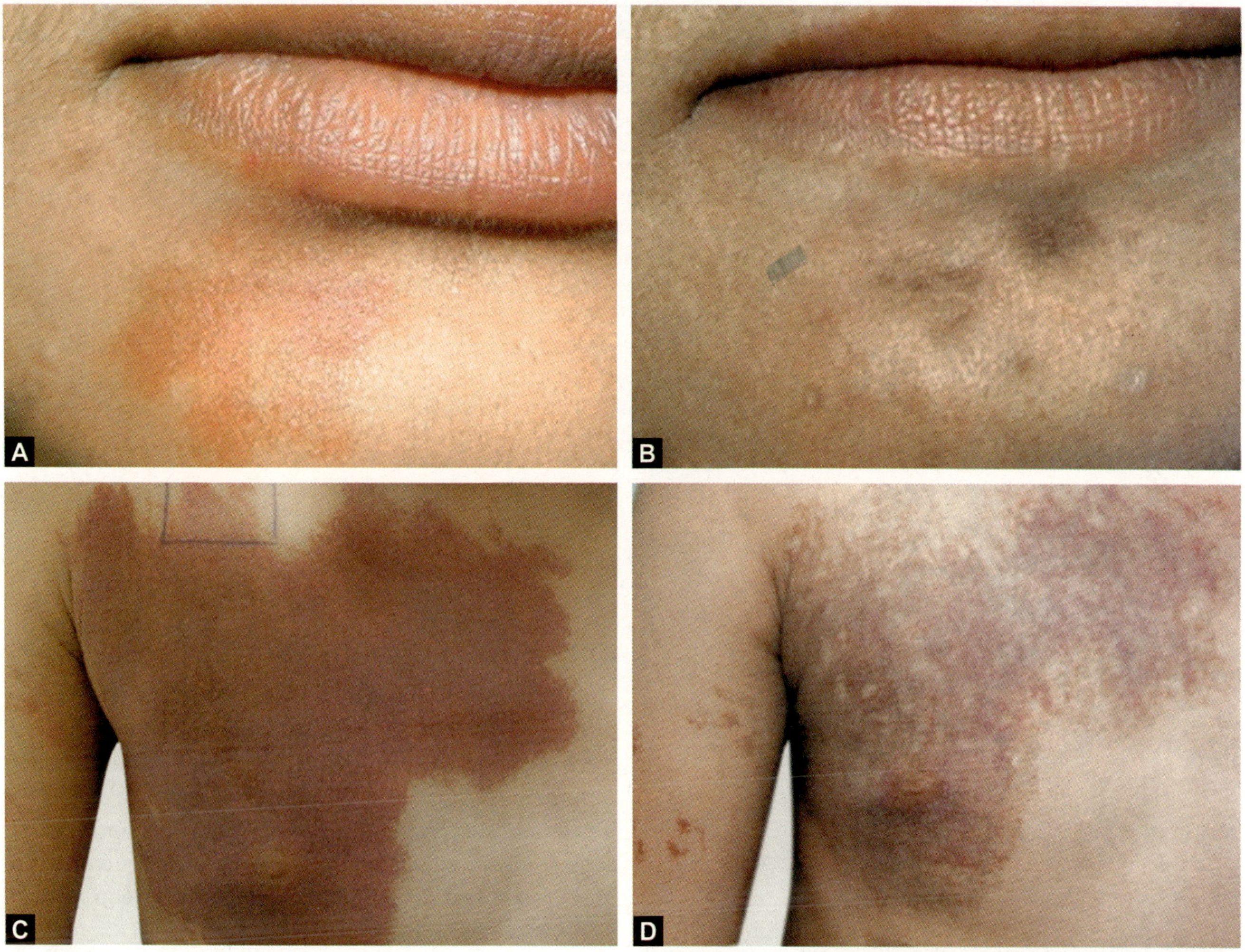

Figs. 44.7A to D: (A) Port wine stain; (B) After 8 sessions of PDL (E - 6 J/cm^2, pulse width - 0.45 ms, spot size - 5 mm) along with 3 sessions of long pulsed Nd:YAG (E - 140 J/cm^2, pulse width 20 ms, spot size - 3 mm). (C) Port wine stain; (D) After 4 sessions of PDL (E - 6 J/cm^2, pulse width - 0.45 ms, spot size - 5 mm).

  - Pulse width - 10 ms for first pass and 100 ms for second pass
  - Pulse delay - 60 ms for first and second pass.
- *Aminolevulinic acid–photodynamic therapy (ALA-PDT)*: Laser used is copper vapor/CO_2 in Gaussian mode with a Power of 800 to 1000 W/cm^2, Spot size of 9 cm and DLI (Drug and Light administration interval) - 40 to 55 minutes.[40,41]
- *Other lasers for Resistant or Dark PWS*: Alexandrite: Fluence - 25 to 80 J/cm^2, Pulse width - 3 to 20 ms, Spot size 12 to 15 mm. Diode: 810 nm– 3.5 to 60 J/cm^2: spot 1 cm^2.[42,43] Nd:YAG 1064 is best reserved for exophytic lesions with Spot size same as nodule size and fluence of 60 to 120 J/cm^2.
- *The end point is slight blueing of the lesion*: Deep greying signifies over treatment and pandermal necrosis.[43,44]

CO_2 can also be used for nodules with an advantage of coagulation of ectatic vessels.[35]

Tips in Treating PWS

- Treatment responses are variable due to differing anatomic sites, gross and microscopic anatomy of lesions and hence treatment response curve is more for lateral facial lesions > midface lesions > nonfacial lesions.
- Initial breakup of lesions allows better penetration of light in subsequent sessions.
- Reasons for requirement of multiple treatment sessions are: variable depth, variable locational anatomy and angiogenesis in between treatment sessions (Table 44.1).

Table 44.1: Factors affecting the treatment outcome of PWS.

Color of port wine stain	Few studies show best results with pink lesions and few show better results with red lesions. In a study of 261 patients, color of PWS was not found to be of prognostic value.[26]
Age of patient	It is considered that younger children require less treatment sessions because of smaller size of the lesion, smaller diameter of vessels which are superficial, and also reduced permanent adverse sequelae.[28,29] Van der Horst et al.,[32] found treating PWS in early childhood was not more effective than treatment at a later stage. Alster and Wilson,[27] reported that younger children may require more treatments because of the rapid growth of residual blood vessels between treatments.
Site of the PWS	PWS on the face and neck respond better than those on the leg and hand.[32] Lesions on forehead, i.e. area of second branch of the trigeminal nerve[33] respond better than middle face. The chest, upper arm, and shoulder generally respond well.
Size of the nevus	PWSs less than 20 cm² at the initial examination cleared more than those greater than 20 cm² irrespective of age.[34]
Number of sessions	The patients shows satisfactory lightening, in their first four to ten treatments, later on improvements may have small benefits that should be balanced against the morbidity from treatment.[27]

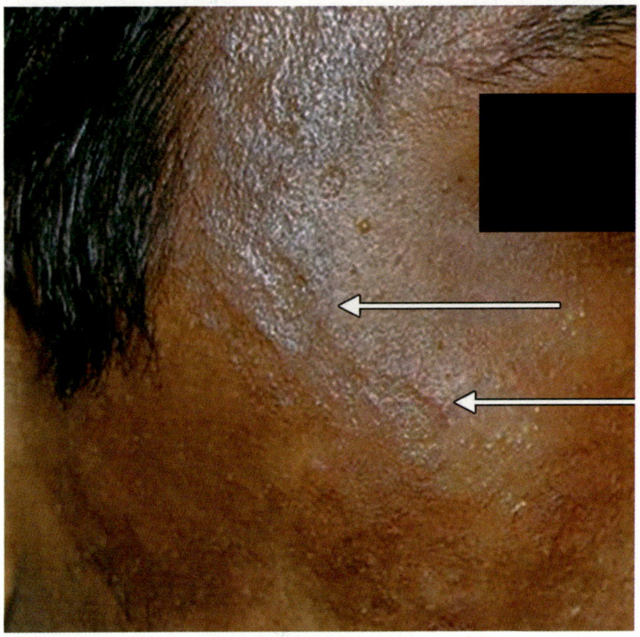

Fig. 44.8: Laser imprint.

- Multiple passes of longer pulses, progressing to shorter pulses in subsequent passes within 30 minutes interval could be the key to early clearance of lesion.
- Expect atrophic scars at laser impact sites (Laser imprint - Fig. 44.8) in some cases indicating excessive delivery of energy, absence of cooling, spot overlap and post treatment trauma.
- Side effects: blistering, crusting, scarring hypertrophic/ atrophic and pigmentary changes.
- Perform test spot of about 4 to 8 laser pulses.
- To make patient comfortable, analgesics are given half an hour before procedure.
- Average number of treatment in children up to 14 years is 4 to 8, and in adults it is minimum 6 to 20 treatments.

Hemangiomas (Figs. 44.9A and B)

The only indication with predicable results till today is ulcerative lesion with active ulcer. PDL with 5 to 7 J/cm² with cryogen cooling minimizes further ulceration. Mean number of treatment sessions are two. The use of PDL for uncomplicated proliferative hemangiomas is controversial. The limitations are focal scaring, diffuse ulceration, pain, cost and questionable impact on deep lesions (Figs. 44.10A and B).[9,45,46]

Leg Veins (Box 44.7)

Sclerotherapy is the "gold standard," treatment. Lasers still have a role in patients who desire for laser or are not tolerant to sclerotherapy. The 1,064-nm long-pulsed laser has been used with good success to treat leg veins (Figs. 44.11A and B).[17,18] Some practitioners use a large spot (6–7 mm) device with appropriate fluences, whereas others use a smaller 3 mm spot with higher fluences. Unwanted thermal damage is the concern because of narrower therapeutic window of a 1,064-nm device.

Miscellaneous Conditions (Box 44.8)

A large number of miscellaneous vascular disorders can be treated by lasers. Both PDL and Nd:YAG lasers are used to treat Pyogenic granuloma especially in children. Hypertrophic scar, vascular keloid and venous lakes respond to PDL treatment (Figs. 44.12 and 44.13). Angiokeratomas

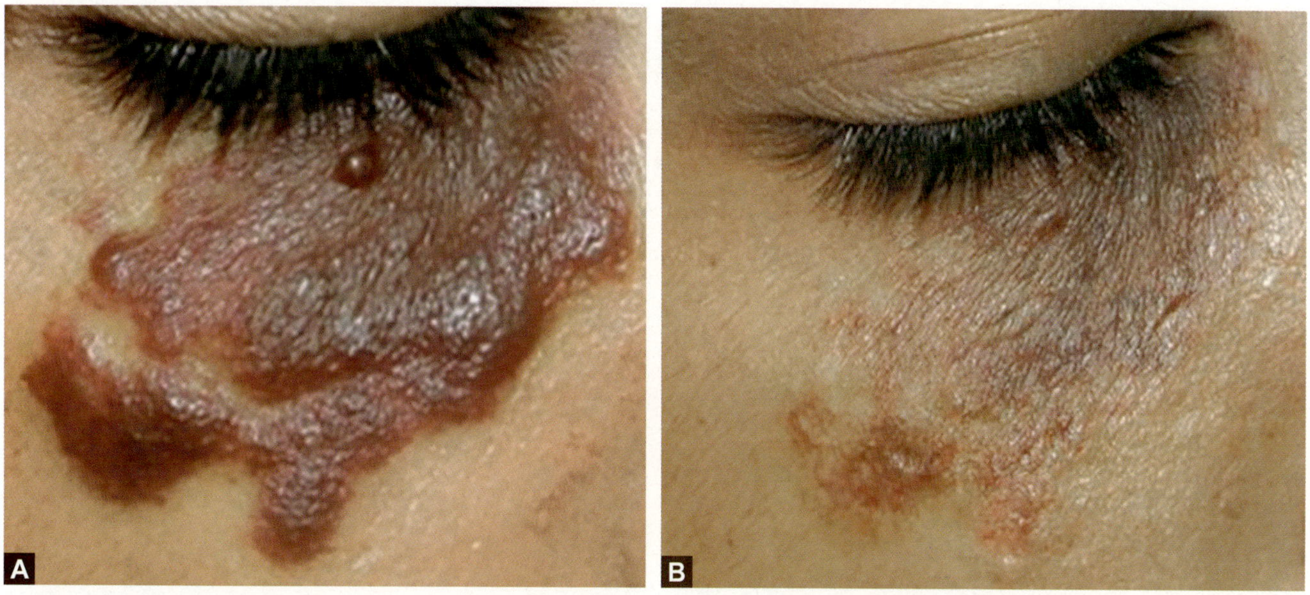

Figs. 44.9A and B: (A) Hemangioma; (B) After 15 sessions of PDL (E - 5 J/cm², pulse width - 0.45 ms, spot size - 5 mm) with 2 sessions of long pulsed Nd:YAG (E - 120 J/cm², pulse width - 20 ms, spot size - 3 mm).

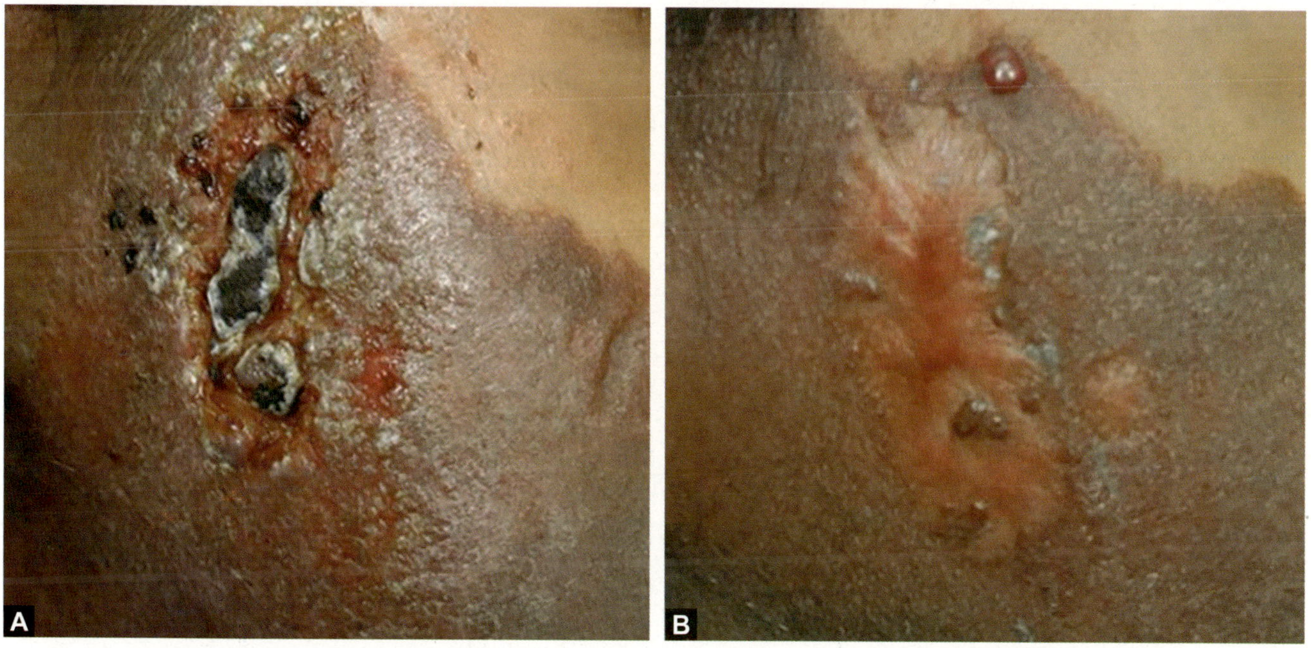

Figs. 44.10A and B: (A) Pandermal necrosis following LP Nd:YAG. (B) Healing with atrophic scarring.

Box 44.7: Summary of leg veins treatment.

Vessels	*Lasers*	*Remarks*
Smaller red vessels measuring 300 mm	532 nm lasers and 595 nm PDLs	
Larger and deeper vessels of 0.3 mm and larger	755 nm Alexandrite lasers LP 1,064 nm lasers Combination of 595 nm/1,064 nm devices	For LP 1,064 nm lasers • 0.2 and 0.5 mm, PW of 5–20 ms • 0.6–1 mm, PW of 30–60 ms

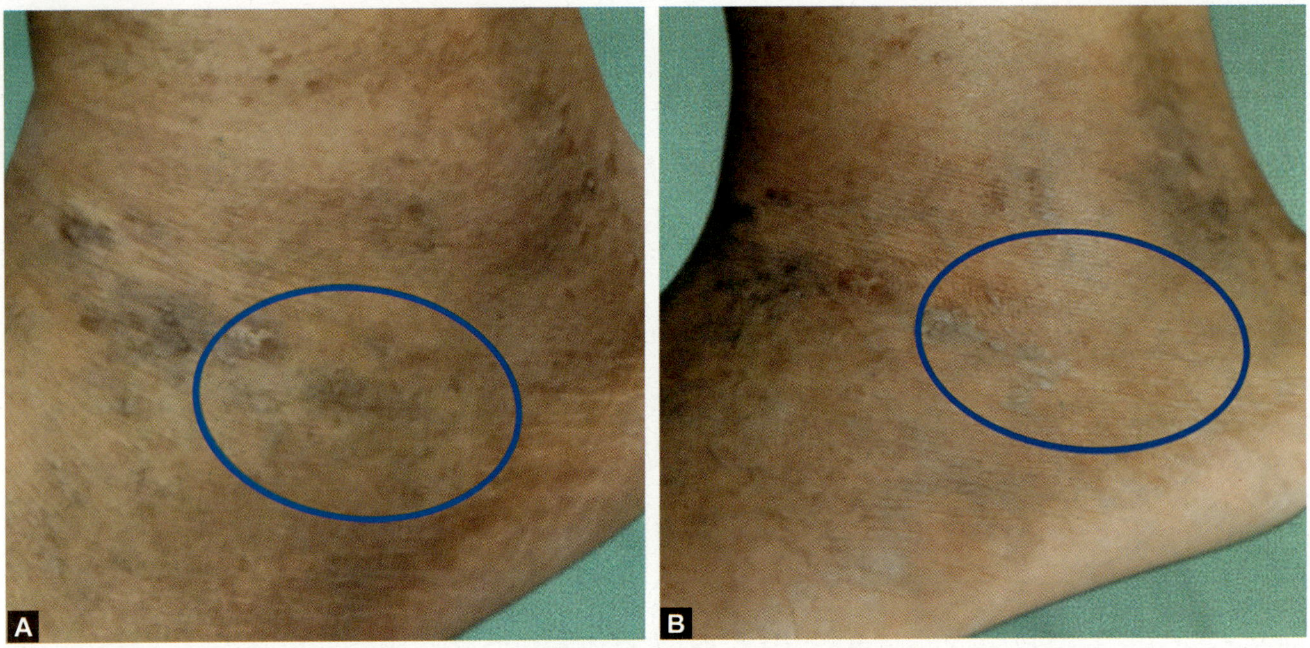

Figs. 44.11 A and B: (A) Spider telangiectasia. (B) After 1 session of long pulsed Nd:YAG (E - 240 J/cm^2, pulse width - 40 ms, spot size - 3 mm).

(Figs. 44.14A and B) of Fordyce presenting as blue-to-red papules often located on the scrotum are easily treated with both the pulsed dye laser and long-pulsed Nd:YAG lasers. Hereditary multiple glomus tumors are characterized by pain; PDL can relive pain though it is not curative.

Superficial lymphatic malformations of lymphangioma circumscriptum containing blood can be targeted with the pulsed dye laser though there are other better options like CO_2 ablation. Hereditary hemorrhagic telangiectasia can cause recurrent bleeding and cosmetic problems and can be treated with long pulsed Nd:YAG laser and PDL. Venous malformations can be mucosal or cutaneous; early Nd:YAG laser therapy can cause shrinkage of the tissue and induce dermal fibrosis.

General Tips

- To avoid full thickness burns over moles/tattoos or permanent hair reduction on beard region, cover or mask the lesion.
- To avoid laser imprints, avoid skip areas by keeping shots closer.
- Apply thin film of gel, do not put excessive pressure on hand piece as it can blanch vessels and diminish treatment efficacy.
- Anesthesia can blanch the lesion and also patient's feedback.
- On treating telangiectasia, observe for vessel blanching on pressure and refill after release. Absence of blanching indicates good treatment. If blanching is present it indicates inadequate treatment. Slow refilling indicates partial treatment. Telangiectasia may need multiple passes.

SUMMARY

Undoubtedly vascular lasers are the treatment of choice for congenital and acquired cutaneous vascular lesions. Appropriate treatment begins with the correct diagnosis. The choice of device type and treatment parameters must be set according to the type of lesion being treated. Vessel ssize and depth, blood flow, skin type, melanin content, recent suntan must be assessed prior to treatment. Available vascular lasers are more suitable for western skin types and the parameters used in western skin may not always suit all colored skin. The technology keeps rapidly evolving and hence guidelines are reviewed periodically. We present the current guidelines and parameters for various disorders and devices while sharing our experience in using vascular lasers on Indian skin.

Box 44.8: Miscellaneous conditions.[34-41]

Indication	*Laser*	*Spot size (mm)*	*Fluence (J/cm²)*	*Pulse width (ms)*	*Comments*
Venous lakes[9]	KTP/PDL				Slight pressure on hand piece for better absorption and penetration of laser.
Smaller lesion	Alexandrite	6	60–80	3	
Bigger lesion	Nd:YAG	3–5	50–100	35–60	
Glomus tumor[46]	Nd:YAG	3	120–200	50	Larger the lesion smaller is the fluence and smaller the lesion larger the fluence.
Blue rubber bleb nevus[9]	Nd:YAG	2–4	80–130	50	
Angiofibromas/fibrous papules:[47]	Carbon dioxide	Continuous mode	2–5 watts (Power)		
Striae rubra[9]	PDL	7–10	5–6	1.5	
Sebaceous hyperplasia[54]	PDL	3	15	1.5	Stacked pulses at 1.5 Hz. End point is yellow to gray color.
Ecchymosis[48]	PDL	6–10	5–6	10	
Molluscum contagiosum[49]	PDL	7	6–7	6.45	
Warts[50,51]	PDL	5–7	12–15		Give 2 to 4 passes without cooling to achieve the end point of grayish discoloration. Flat lesions require lower fluence and 1 to 2 passes only.
	IPL		30–45	10	Use bole punch index card for better clearance and surrounding skin protection.
Lymphangioma circumscriptum[52]	PDL				Blue/red lesions are amenable for PDL.
Pyogenic granuloma[53]	PDL	3	6–9		The lesion is compressed with glass slide and treated.
	Nd-YAG	3–7	100–250	20–50	CO_2 vaporisation works best for Pyogenic granuloma.
Post fillers bruises/scars/vascular keloids[54]	PDL	6–10	4–6	6–10	Clears within 1 to 3 days with IPL treatment. Parameters of minimum purpuric settings are to be employed.

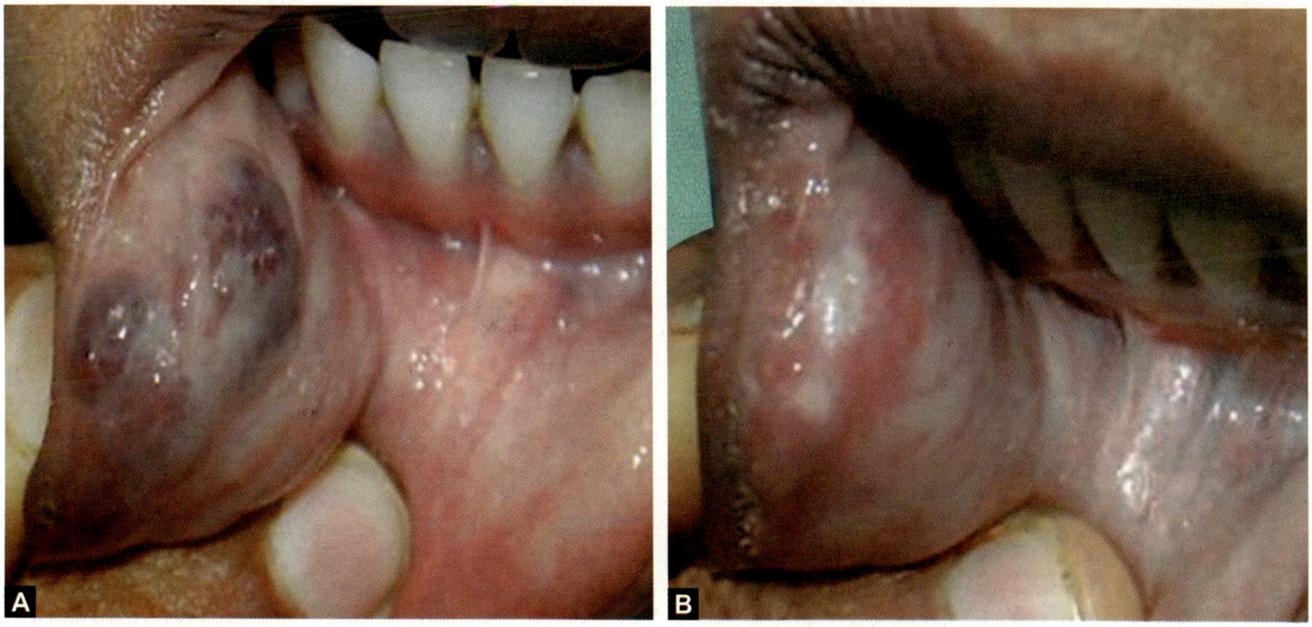

Figs. 44.12A and B: (A) Venous lakes. (B) After 1 session of long pulsed Nd:YAG (E - 220 J/cm², pulse width - 40 ms, spot size - 3 mm).

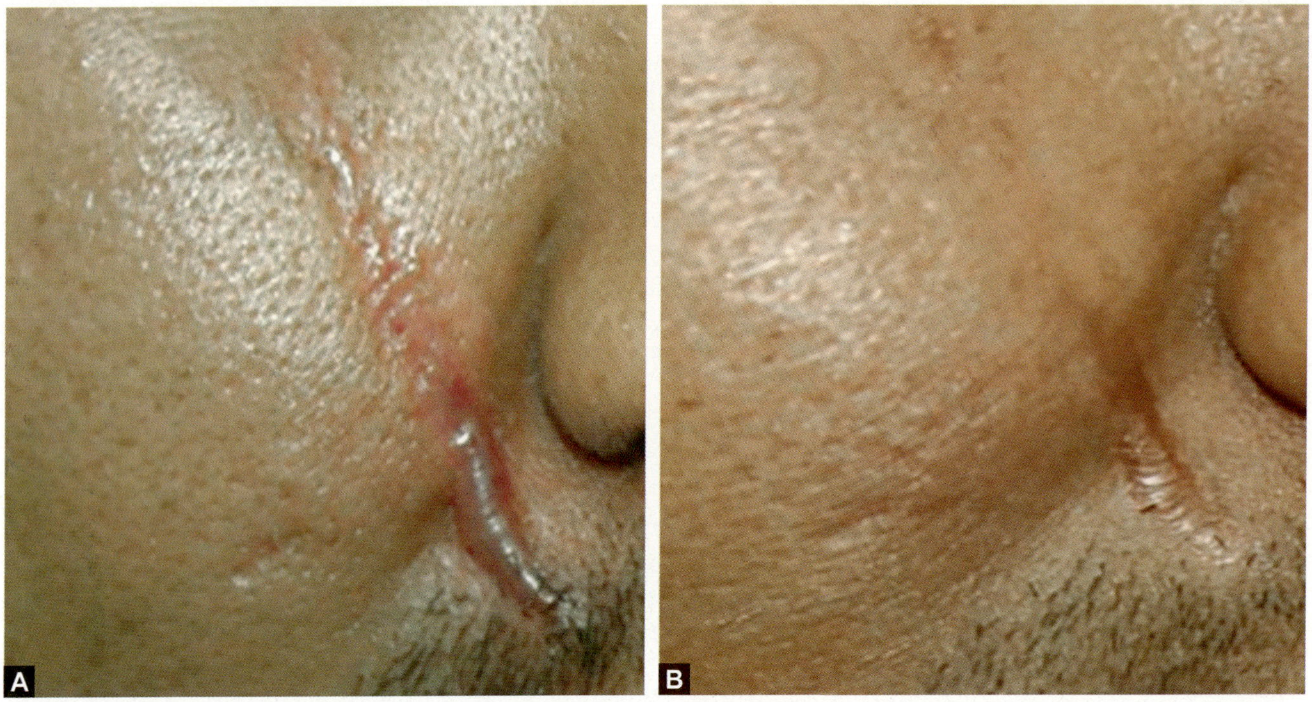

Figs. 44.13A and B: (A) Hypertrophic scar. (B) After 4 sessions of PDL (E - 5 J/cm², pulse width - 0.45 ms, spot size - 5 mm).

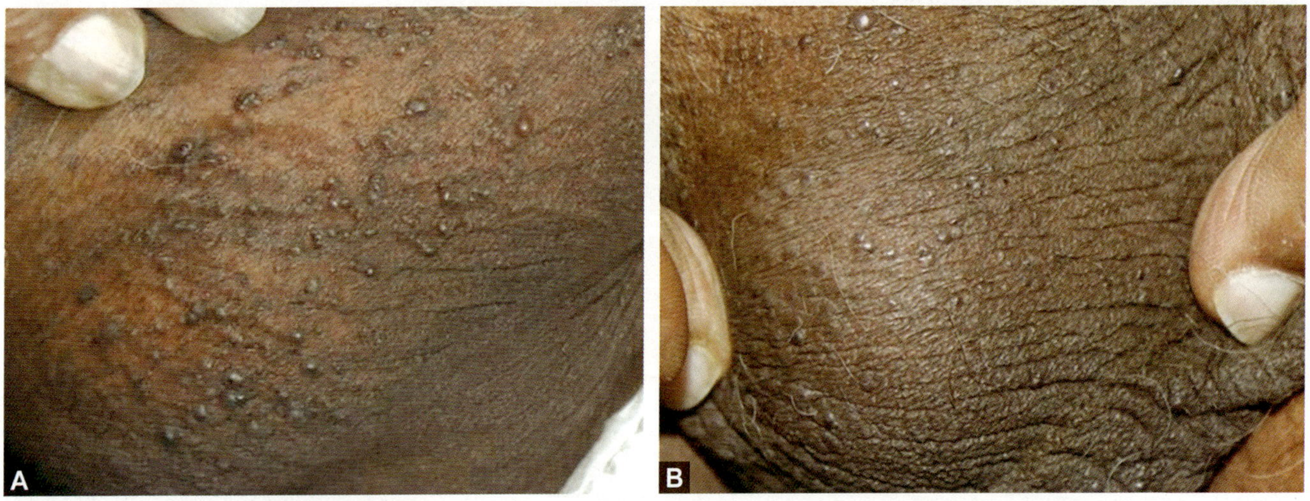

Figs. 44.14A and B: (A) Before; (B) after treatment of angiokeratoma on scrotum with LP Nd:YAG.

REFERENCES

1. Anderson RR, Parrish JA. Microvasculature can be selectively damaged using dye lasers: a basic theory and experimental evidence in human skin. Lasers Surg Med. 1981;1:263-76.
2. Dai T, Pikkula BM, Wang LV, et al. Comparison of human skin opto-thermal response to near-infrared and visible laser irradiations: a theoretical investigation. Phys Med Biol. 2004;49(21):4861-77.
3. Basschaart N, Faber DJ, van Leeuwen TG, et al. In vivo low coherence spectroscopic measurements of local hemoglobin in absorption spectra in human skin. J Biomed Opt. 2011:16:100504.
4. Keijzer M, Pickering JW, van Gemert MJ. Laser beam diameter for port wines stain treatment. Laser Surg Med. 1991:11:601-5.
5. Lucassen GW, Verkruysse W, Keijzer M, et al. Light distributions in port-wine stain model containing multiple cylindrical and curved blood vessels. Lasers Surg Med. 1996;18:345-57.

6. Kimel S, Svaasand LO, Cao D, et al. Vascular response to laser photothermolysis as a function of pulse duration, vessel type, and diameter: Implications for port wine stain laser therapy. Lasers Surg Med. 2002;30(2):160-9.
7. Nelson JS, Milner TE, Anvari B, et al. Dynamic epidermal cooling in conjunction with laser induced photothermolysis of port wine stain blood vessels. Lasers Surg Med. 1996;19:224.
8. Anvari B, Milner TE, Tanenbaum BS, et al. Selective cooling of biological tissues: application for thermally medicated therapeutic procedures. Phys Med Biol. 1995;40:241.
9. Ross EV, Krakowski AC. Laser treatment for vascular laser. In: Goldman MP, Fitzpatrick RE, Ross EV (Eds). Lasers and Energy Devices for the Skin, 2nd edition, Goldman MP: CRP Press; 2013.
10. Laser and Light Treatment of Acquired and Congenital Vascular Lesions, Text book of Surgery of skin, 2nd edition,
11. Michael D, Kilmer S. Lasers for treatment of vascular lesions. In: Nouri K. (Ed). Lasers in Dermatology and Medicine. London: Springer-Verlag; 2011. pp. 33-43.
12. Goldberg DJ, Marcus J. The use of the frequency-doubled Qswitched Nd:YAG laser in the treatment of small cutaneous vascular lesions. Dermatol Surg. 1996;22:841-4.
13. Kauvar AN, Rosen N, Khrom T. A newly modified 595 nm pulsed dye laser with compression hand piece for the treatment of photo damaged skin. Laser Surg Med. 2006;38: 808-13.
14. Dierickx CC, Casparian JM, Venugopalan V, et al. Thermal relaxation of port-wine stain vessels probed in vivo: the need for 1-10-millisecond laser pulse treatment. J Invest Dermatol. 1995;105:709-14.
15. Sarradet DM, Hussain M, Goldberg DJ. Millisecond 1064-nm neodymium:YAG laser treatment of facial telangiectases. Dermatol Surg. 2003;29:56-8.
16. Goldman MP, Bennett RG. Treatment of telangiectasia: a review. J Am Acad Dermatol. 1987;17(2 Pt 1):167-82.
17. Ozturk S, Hoopman J, Brown SA, et al. A useful algorithm for determining fluence and pulse width for vascular targets using 1,064 nm Nd:YAG laser in and animal model. Lasers Surg Med. 2004;34:420-5.
18. Parlette EC, Groff WF, Kinshella MJ, et al. Optimal pulse durations for the treatment of leg telangiectasias with a neodymium YAG laser. Lasers Surg Med. 2006;38: 98-105.
19. Schmidt N, Gans E. Demodex and rosacea I: the prevalence and numbers of Demodex mites in rosacea. Cosmetic Dermatol. 2004;17:497-502.
20. Schroeter CA, Haaf-von Below S, Neumann HA. Effective treatment of rosacea using intense pulsed light systems. Dermatol Surg. 2005;31:1285-9.
21. Menezes N, Moreira A, Mota G, et al. Quality of life and rosacea: pulse dye laser impact. J Cosmet Laser Ther. 2009;11:139-41.
22. Jasim ZF, Woo WK, Handley JM. Long-pulsed (6-ms) pulsed dye laser treatment of rosacea-associated telangiectasia using subpurpuric clinical threshold. Dermatol Surg. 2004;30:37-40.
23. Baglieri F, Scuderi G. Treatment of recalcitrant granulomatous rosacea with ALA-PDT: report of case. Indian J Dermatol Venereol Leprol. 2011;77:356.
24. Weiss RA, Goldman MP, Weiss MA. Treatment of poikiloderma of Civatte with an intense pulsed light source. Dermatol Surg. 2000;26:823-7; Discussion 828.
25. Goldman MP, Weiss RA. Treatment of poikiloderma of Civatteon the neck with an intense pulsed light source. Plast Reconstr Surgery. 2001;107:1376-81.
26. Katugampola GA, Lanigan SW. Five years' experience of treating port wine stains with the flashlamp-pumped pulsed dye laser. Br J Dermatol. 1997;137:750-4.
27. Alster TS, Wilson F. Treatment of port-wine stains with the flashlamp-pumped pulsed dye laser: extended clinical experience in children and adults. Ann Plast Surg. 1994;32(5):478-84.
28. Stier MF, Click SA, Hirsch RJ. Laser treatment of pediatric vascular lesions: port wine stains and hemangiomas. J Am Acad Dermatol. 2008;58:261-85.
29. Chapas AM, Eickhorst K, Geronemus RG. Effective of early treatment of facial port wine stains in newborns: a review of 49 cases. Laser Surg Med. 2007;39:563-5.
30. Lanigan SW. Port wine stains on the lower limb: response to pulsed dye laser therapy. Clin Exp Dermatol. 1996;21(2): 88-92.
31. Kauvar AN, Geronemus RG. Repetitive pulsed dye laser treatments improve persistent port-wine stains. Dermatol Surg. 1995;21(6):515-21.
32. van der Horst CM, Koster PH, de Borgie CA, et al. Effect of the timing of treatment of port-wine stains with the flash-lamp-pumped pulsed-dye laser. N Engl J Med. 1998;338(15):1028-33.
33. Renfro L, Geronemus RG. Anatomical differences of port-wine stains in response to treatment with the pulsed dye laser. Arch Dermatol. 1993;129(2):182-8.
34. Morelli JG, Weston WL, Huff JC, et al. Initial lesion size as a predictive factor in determining the response of port-wine stains in children treated with the pulsed dye laser. Arch Pediatr Adolesc Med. 1995;149(10):1142-4.
35. Buecker JW, Ratz JL, Richfield DF. Histology of port-wine stains treated with carbon dioxide laser. J Am Acad Dermatol. 1984;10:1014-9.
36. Lanigan S. Vascular lesions: port wine stains. In: Raulin and S. Karsai. Laser and IPL Technology in Dermatology and Aesthetic Medicine. Springer-Verlag Berlin Heidelberg; 2011. pp. 241-4.
37. Jia W, Sun V, Tran N. et al. Long term blood vessel removal with combined laser and topical rapamycin antiangiogenic therapy: implication for effective port wine stain treatment. Laser Surg Med. 2010;42:105-12.
38. Moehrle M, Leaute-Labreze C, Schmidt V, et al. Topical timolol for small hemangiomas of infancy. Pediatr Dermatol. 2012;30:245-9.
39. Goldman MP, Fitzpatrick RE, Ruiz-Esparza J. Treatment of port-wine stains (capillary malformation) with the flashlamp-pumped pulsed dye laser. J Pediatr. 1993;122: 71-7.

40. Lu YG, Wu JJ, Yang YD, et al. Photodynamic therapy of port wine stains. J Dermatolog Treat. 2010;21:240-4.
41. Huang N, Cheng G, Li X, et al. Influence of drug-light interval on photodynamic therapy of port wine stains simulation and validation of mathematic models. Photodiagnosis Photodynther. 2008;5;120-6.
42. Jasim ZF, Handley JM. Treatment of pulsed dye laser-resistant port wine stain birthmarks. J Am Acad Dermatol. 2007;57:677-82.
43. Izikson L, Nelson JS, Anderson RR. Treatment of hypertrophic and resistant port wine stain with a 755 nm laser: a case series of 20 patients. Laser Surg Med. 2009;41: 427-32.
44. Geronemus RG. Long pulsed Neodymium:Yttrium-Aluminum-Garnet laser treatment for port wine stains. J Am Acad Dermatol. 2006;54:923.
45. Morelli JG, Tan OT, Weston WL. Treatment of uncreated hemangiomas with the pulsed tunable dye lasers. Am J Dis Child. 1991;145:1062-4.
46. Hughes R, Lacour JP, Chiaverini C, et al. Nd-YAG Laser treatment for multiple cutaneous glomangiomas: report of 3 cases Arch Dermatol. 2011;147:255-6.
47. Weiss ET, Geronemus RG. New technique using combined pulsed dye laser and fractional resurfacing for treating facial angiofibromas in tuberous sclerosis. Laser Surg Med. 2010;42;357-60.
48. Karen JK, Hale EK, Geronemus RG. A simple solution to the common problem of ecchymosis. Arch Dermatol. 2010;146:94-5.
49. Binder B, Weger W, Kemericki P, et al. Treatment of molluscum contagiosum with pulsed dye laser: pilot study with 19 children. Dermatol Surg. 2008;6:121-5.
50. Sethuraman G, Richards KA, Herimagalore RN, et al. Effectiveness of pulsed dye laser in treatment of recalcitrant warts in children. Dermatol Surg. 2010;36:58-65.
51. Tan OT, Hurwitz RM, Stafford TJ. Pulsed dye laser treatment of recalcitrant verrucae: a preliminary report. Lasers Surg Med. 1993;13:127-37.
52. Lai CH, Hanson SG, Mallory SB. Lymphangioma circumscriptum treated with pulsed dye laser. Pediatr Dermatol. 2001;18:509-10.
53. Gonzalez S, Vibhagool C, Falo LD Jr, et al. Treatment of pyogenic granulomas with the 585-nm pulsed dye laser. J Am Acad Dermatol. 1996;35:428-31.
54. Goldman MP (Ed). Lasers and Energy Devices for the Skin, 2nd edition; 2013. pp. 31-53.

CHAPTER 45

Lasers in Dermatosurgery: Treating Exophytic Lesions

BS Chandrashekar, Madura C, Varsha DV

INTRODUCTION

Patients with epidermal and dermal lesions often seek treatment for cosmetic improvement. As the laser technology is advancing, the list of heterogeneous lesions that can be well tackled with lasers are also increasing. The ablative laser can treat array of lesions from epidermal to dermal exophytic miscellaneous conditions with precise results. Ablative lasers (CO_2 and Er:YAG) are the main stay for the therapy, though vascular specific laser like long pulsed Nd:YAG has a role in few conditions, but cannot destroy the tissue to the extent of ablative lasers. They vaporize the tissue removing the epidermal layer and part of dermal tissue which forms the bulk of the lesion. CO_2 laser, the "workhorse" for dermatologists was invented by an Indian scientist, Kumar Patel in 1964. The older conventional CO_2 laser has undergone tremendous modifications to short pulsed scanned CO_2 lasers with minimal thermal damage and good clinical outcome. This chapter encapsulates the various indications of ablative lasers, choosing right technique with practical tips for optimal outcome.[1,2]

LASER PRINCIPLES: LASER DEVICES AND LASER TISSUE INTERACTION

Water is the main target chromophore for epidermal or dermal lesions, others being hemoglobin and melanin. For CO_2 laser and Er:YAG laser, water is the only target chromophore. Ablative lasers vaporize the tissue removing the epidermal layer and part of dermal tissue, followed by wound healing giving rise to neocollagenesis and collagen remodeling.[1,2]

CO_2 Laser

The CO_2 laser has changed the path of treating various exophytic skin conditions. It is an infrared laser emitting the beam at 10,600 nm wavelength, with carbon dioxide gas as its medium. It has an aiming beam which helps the operator to focus laser beam at the point on target tissue. It works under the principle of selective photothermolysis, where water in tissue is the chromophore which absorbs laser resulting in thermal damage.[1,2]

The CO_2 laser can ablate 20-30 μm of skin in one single pass. Though the tissue ablated is 20–30 μm (zone of ablation), the zone of necrosis extends up to 1 mm in continuous wave (CW) mode and 40–120 μm in pulsed mode. The damage can vary and depends on water content of tissue, spot size and duration of laser exposure on tissue (Table 45.1).

Expected laser tissue interactions, are different in focused and defocused mode. Laser vaporization is a mode between focused (laser incision) and defocused mode (coagulation mode), producing good outcome (Figs. 45.1 and 45.2).

Table 45.1: Modes of ablation of CO_2 or erbium YAG or pulsed CO_2.

	Continuous mode CO_2	*Pulsed mode CO_2*	*Erbium YAG*
Laser ablation	20–30 μm	100 μm	10–20 μm
Zone of thermal damage	0.2–1 mm	50 to 150 μm	>10 μm
Uses	It is reserved for thick lesions, such as verrucae, condyloma acuminata and rhinophyma or when significant dermal damage with resulting dermal fibrosis is desired.	It is indicated for precise tissue ablation with less residual damage	Indicated for superficial lesional ablation

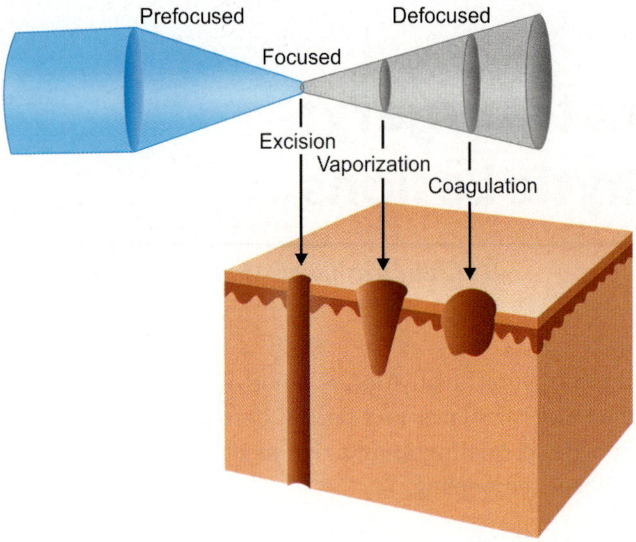

Fig. 45.1: Parameters on which laser efficacy depends.

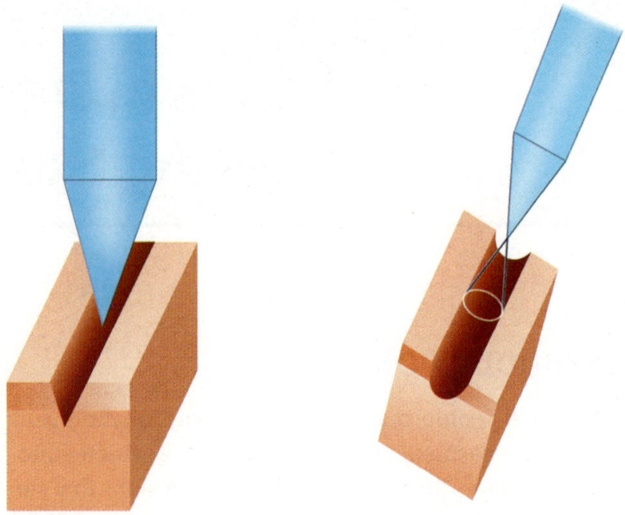

Fig. 45.2: Focused and defocused modes of laser tissue interaction.

The Relationship between Beam Size, Power of Laser and Duration of Exposure

The power density is indirectly proportional to beam size (Fig. 45.3). Most of the machines have a spot size of < 1mm. The spot size can be altered by moving hand piece closer or farther from target surface. The power density (power per unit area) or irradiance is higher with small beam size at same laser power and laser penetrates deeper (focus mode). The power density drops with larger spot size with same laser power (defocused mode). A beam size must be appropriately selected to have desirable power density; the beam of lower power density will result in shallow ablation of tissue.[1,2]

The duration of exposure can be controlled by manual movement or by using mechanical shutters. The zone of thermal damage is directly proportional to the duration of exposure and power density. The long irradiance time and low power density produces larger thermal necrosis because as explained above: beam of low power density, will ablate only thin layer of tissue, and it requires more number of passes to remove the complete lesion. The heat is conducted to underlying unablated tissue causing residual damage called thermal necrosis. A beam with high power will ablate tissue in few passes with less residual damage, good clinical out come and minimal scar (Figs. 45.4A and B).[1,2]

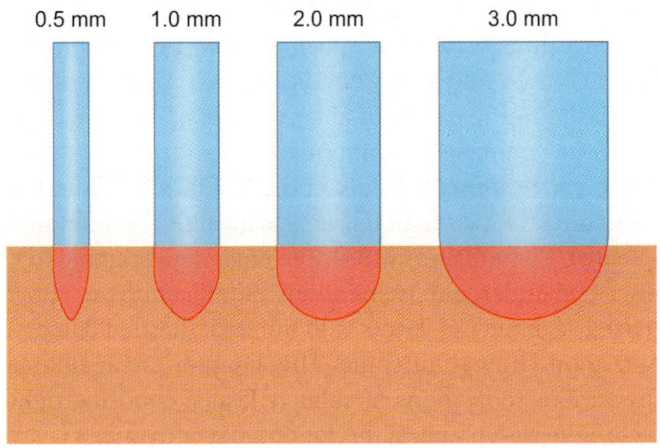

Fig. 45.3: The relationship between beam size and power density with respect to ablation.

Thermal Relaxation Time and Thermal Necrosis

If the exposure time of laser energy is less than TRT of tissue, there is lesser damage to adjacent tissue. The thermal relaxation time (TRT) for skin tissue is approximately 1ms. Hence short exposure time with high power density will ablate same volume of tissue as a longer exposure time at low power density, but with lesser damage to adjacent tissue and it is more precise with less healing time and good aesthetic results. This formed the base for emergence of pulsed CO_2 laser. The pulsed CO_2 lasers cause minimal thermal damage (50 to 150 micrometer) with more precise ablation as pulse duration of laser is less than the thermal relaxation time of target tissue. This application is greatly utilized in ablation of various cutaneous lesions. As penetration depth of CO_2 laser is more, proper energy assessment and good control on probe while targeting the lesion can avoid the side effects most of the time (Figs. 45.5A to C).[1,2]

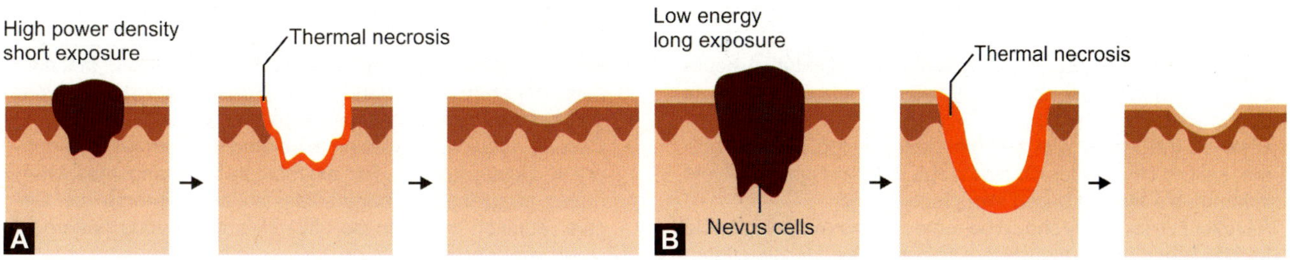

Figs. 45.4A and B: (A) Thermal damage and scar caused by a laser beam with a low power density and a short exposure time (supplement from Lutronic corp) (B) Thermal damage and scar caused by a laser beam with a low power density and a long exposure time (supplement from Lutronic corp).

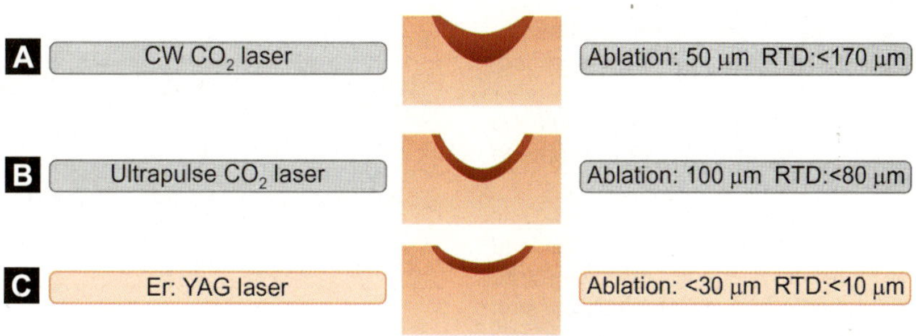

Figs. 45.5A to C: (A) Penetration depth and residual thermal damage (RTD) of CW CO_2 laser. (B) Much narrower zone of residual thermal damage with precise tissue ablation (C) Narrow zone of residual thermal damage with shallow and precise tissue ablation.

Er:YAG Laser

Er: YAG laser emitted at 2,940 nm wavelength has absorption coefficient of water 16 times more than CO_2 laser. This is the reason why its penetration depth is limited to epidermis with thermal damage zone of less than 10 microns (*see* Table 45.1). Thermal damage zone does not increase with additional passes with the Er:YAG laser;[3-6] This serves as an advantage of being more precise in targeting the lesion with less chances of pigmentary alterations and less downtime. However, there is almost no hemostasis, and ablation beyond the papillary dermis is not practical. To overcome this limitation, Er: YAG lasers with variable pulse durations have been developed. With these variable-pulse Er:YAG lasers, ablation is relatively hemostatic; the effectiveness of hemostasis and the thickness of the thermal damage zone are between those of a resurfacing CO_2 laser and a short-pulse Er:YAG laser.[7] Indications for ablative lasers are given in Table 45.2.

Table 45.2: Indications for ablative laser. The ablative laser can treat wide range of cutaneous lesions.

Common indications	*Uncommon indications*
• Dermatosis papulosa nigra, skin tag and Stucco keratoses • Warts and condyloma acuminatum • Syringoma[1,2,8] and Neurofibroma[9-11] • Nevi[12,13] melanocytic nevi, epidermal nevus and nevus sebaceous • Xanthelasma[14] • Keratoses[15,16] • Angiofibroma, pyogenic granuloma, angiokeratoma • Papular scars	• Cutaneous cysts-milia, steatocystoma multiplex, epidermoid cysts and myxoid cyst • Appendageal lesions-sebaceous adenoma, sebaceous hyperplasia and small pilomatricomas • Hidradenitis suppurativa • Acanthosis nigricans • Scars and keloids[17,18] • To prepare recipient area in vitiligo • Rhinophyma, lymphangioma circumscriptum • Nail surgery

Parameters (*see* Figs. 45.1 and 45.2)

- The parameters vary with the device. Selecting the parameters depends on choice of laser and lesion to be treated.
- *Focused or cutting mode*: It is used for excising lesions and most of the dermal lesions like papular scars, nodules of rhynophyma, neurofibroma, etc.
- *Vaporization mode*: Employed for most of the epidermal lesions.
- *Defocused mode*: To coagulate the bleeding points.

Technique of laser resurfacing: General principles and safety measures are provided in Box 45.1. Select higher power density and lesser pulse duration to achieve precise ablation. The laser hand piece must be held steadily

Box: 45.1 General principles and safety.

- Laser procedure must be carried out under all safety precautions. Protective laser specific eyewear should be worn both by the doctor and patient.
- Cleanse the lesion with betadine solution followed by normal saline. Dry the lesion thoroughly with wet gauze. Avoid inflammable alcohol based skin preparations.
- All reflective jewellery should be removed. Instruments should be blackened or roughened to eliminate specular reflections.
- Laser room door should be closed, and laser warning signs should be posted on door.
- The surgical field should be surrounded with wet towels, and dry gauze and oxygen must be kept away from the treatment field to avoid fire hazards.
- Patients under general anesthesia must have a nonflammable endotracheal tube or one that is wrapped in a nonreflective, nonflammable material.
- When working in the perianal area, wet gauze should be inserted into the anal canal to eliminate the risk of methane gas explosion.[19]
- Prophylactic antivirals to be considered when indicated.
- The laser plume contains carbonized particles of cell and tissue fragments. It is more carcinogenic than cigarette smoke and also poses a potential risk of viral transmission from patient to operator.[20-22] High-efficiency smoke evacuator must be held immediately around less than 1 cm away the hand piece once procedure is started.

perpendicular to the skin surface. The hand piece is moved across and the focused beam will vaporize the tissue. The spot size can be altered by moving hand piece closer or farther from target surface. Based on movement of hand piece, we can have point ablation, circular ablation and paint brush type of ablation (Box 45.2). Once the lesion is vaporized, the charred tissue debris is wiped with wet gauze after drying; ablate the lesion sequentially till desired depth is reached. The depth to be achieved varies with the type of lesion. A dermal curette can also be used to separate thick epidermal lesions from the underlying dermis. The white glistening layer seen after removing debris is the papillary dermis. At the end of the procedure, if bleeding is seen at the base of the lesion, coagulation is done by moving hand piece away to get defocused beam.

PATIENT SELECTION

Patients must have realistic expectations. History of keloid tendency and past history of HSV infection mandates precautions. Give prophylactic antivirals 48 hours prior to procedure and continue till complete epithelialization. In patients with keloidal tendency, do not ablate deeper than papillary dermis. Be cautious while working around eyes. Patient should be counseled in his own language regarding the procedure, number of sittings required, cost, frequency of the procedure (once in 6 weeks), side effects and strict use

Box 45.2: Types of ablations.

- *Point beam ablation*: The laser beam ablates tissue at single point without moving hand piece. For example, DPN, syringoma, small trichoepithelioma, small moles, etc.
- *Circular ablation*: The lesion is ablated from center to periphery in circular fashion. For example in big syringomas, wart, moles, papular scars, nodular lesions, neurofibroma, etc. Circular ablation can also be utilized in continuous pattern to cover larger areas.
- *Paint brush type of ablation*: It is movement of hand piece slowly to ablate large areas like rhinophymas, polyps, condylomas, xanthelasma, etc.

Box 45.3: Contraindications.

There are no absolute contraindications. The relative contraindications are as follows:
- Bleeding disorders
- Uncontrolled diabetes mellitus
- Infection at the site of lesion
- Keloidal tendency (avoid on keloid prone areas like chest, arms and upper back).

of sunscreen. Based on type of lesion and skin type, laser is chosen. In skin type IV and V, either CO_2 laser or Er:YAG laser is indicated, whereas in skin type VI and superficial and epidermal lesions, Er:YAG laser is preferred. Associated comorbidities which affect healing like diabetes mellitus and bleeding disorders should be ruled out (Box 45.3).

PREPROCEDURE PREPARATION

Routine investigations like clotting time, bleeding time, random blood sugar, HIV and HBsAg are done when ablating large lesions. Priming with topical retinoids is considered for facial lesions like acne scars, extensive syringomas and trichoepitheliomas.

ANESTHESIA

Ablative lasers like CO_2 require complete anesthesia of treatment site. Anesthesia is achieved by infiltrative anesthesia (1 to 2% lignocaine), ring block or nerve block. Superficial lesions can be managed under topical EMLA for 45 to 60 minutes especially while using erbium YAG laser. For small lesions, local infiltration of 2% lignocaine is effective and field block for bigger lesions.

SPECIFIC INDICATIONS

Dermatosis Papulosa Nigra (DPN)

The DPN are benign growths, easily treated with radiofrequency. CO_2 laser vaporizes the DPN superficially with a single pulse leaving behind scabs. Scabs actually act like a biological dressing with subsequent re-epithelialization beneath it, thus preventing development of pigmentary changes. It requires expertise for pin point precise ablation when compared to radiofrequency.

Seborrheic Keratoses

Seborrheic keratoses are common benign tumors. The treatment of choice is still RF and curettage. Lasers are indicated in cases with extensive lesions and also for giant seborrheic keratosis near nose or eye. Laser of choice is Er:YAG laser based on thickness and size of lesion, spot size and fluence are chosen. Lesion is sequentially ablated in 2 to 3 passes, care is taken to remove the charred tissue after each ablation till the entire lesion is removed. The minute bleeding points determine that the laser has reached the dermis and treatment is adequate. Author suggests stopping treatment before bleeding points occur. Alternate choice is CO_2 laser. The thick lesions are ablated in vaporization mode to remove most of the lesion, followed by single pass in coagulation mode. Do not rub, after using coagulation mode. For thin lesion, the parameters are set closer to coagulation mode for shallow ablation.

Acrochordon (Skin Tag)

CO_2 laser can be advantageous in removing large skin tags. The lesion is clamped with artery forceps under infiltrative anesthesia. In focused mode, cut the skin tag along the upper margin of the clamped tissue and coagulate the base for hemostasis. CO_2 laser parameters: E—6 J/cm^2, Power—30 W, 30–60 Hz.

Verrucae

Carbon dioxide laser (continuous-wave or super pulsed) is used to treat verrucae. As human papilloma virus (HPV) can be found even more than 1 cm away from the clinically visible wart,[23] it is recommended to vaporize 3 to 5 mm area of normal-appearing epidermis around the clinically apparent wart. The disadvantages of CO_2 over other treatment modalities are more cost, discomfort, and prolonged healing. Hence it is indicated in resistant warts, periungual and palmoplantar warts with response rate of 56% to 81%.[24-27] The thick stratum corneum and the additional callus that often develops over warts on the feet can be efficiently vaporized with the CO_2 laser with excellent control over the depth of destruction. Flat warts can be ablated with a short-pulsed Er:YAG laser. The CO_2 laser should not be used in such cases because of the risk of hypopigmentation and scarring. CO_2 laser is effective in debulking all visible anogenital warts (condyloma acuminatum) with 5 mm surrounding skin, to achieve long term remission rates of approximately 50% to 70% .[28-30] Follow universal precautions as the plume generated during CO_2 laser vaporization of warts has been found to contain viable HPV particles.[31,32]

Fordyce Spots

These are benign spots on the lips, best ablated by Erb:YAG: with 1 to 2 mm spot size, 20 mJ of fluence and heals well without scaring. CO_2 can be an alternate choice (Figs. 45.6A to C).

Benign Dermal Growths

The CO_2 laser has been shown to ablate various small superficial dermal growths precisely, including adenoma

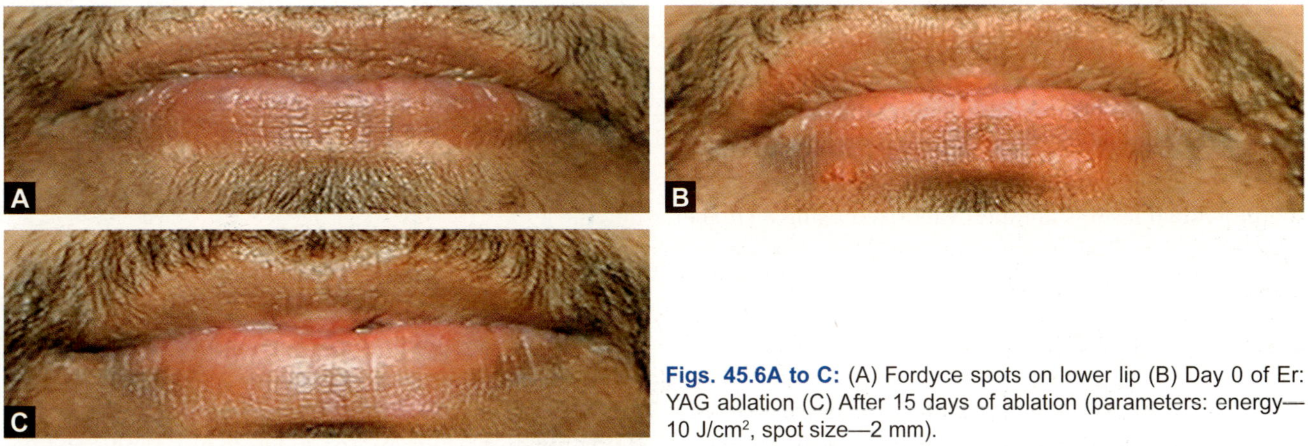

Figs. 45.6A to C: (A) Fordyce spots on lower lip (B) Day 0 of Er: YAG ablation (C) After 15 days of ablation (parameters: energy—10 J/cm^2, spot size—2 mm).

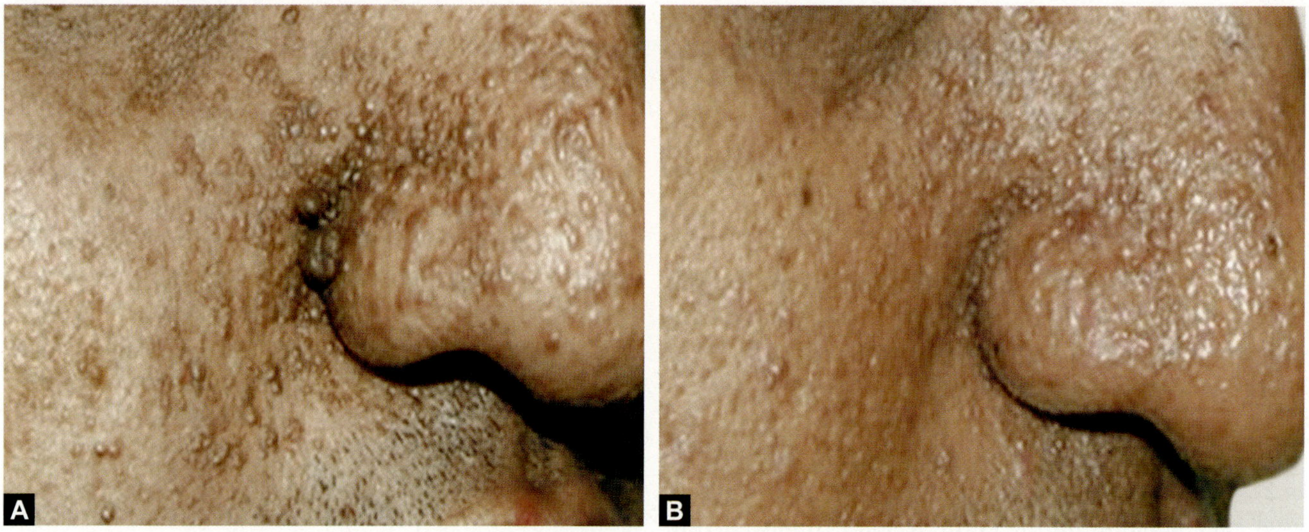

Figs. 45.7A and B: (A) Angiofibromas (B) After 3 sessions of ablative CO_2 laser (E—5–6 J/cm^2, power—30 W, pulse rate—40 Hz) along with 2 sessions of microablative Er-YAG (E—10–15 J/cm^2, spot size—2 mm).

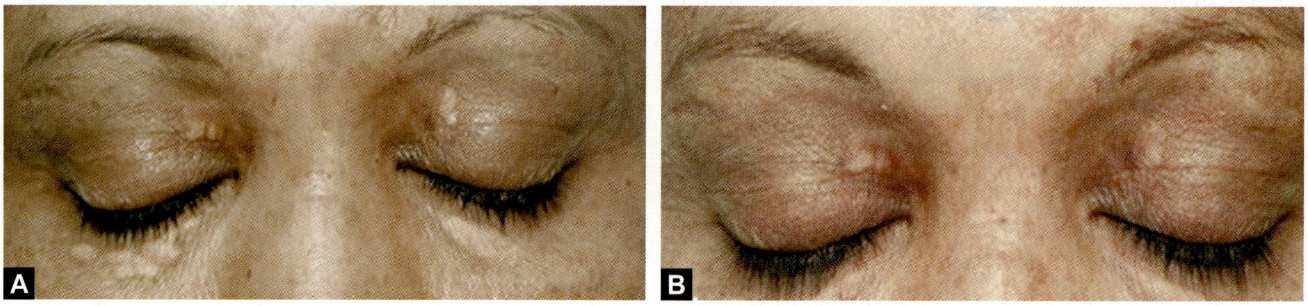

Figs. 45.8A and B: (A) Xanthelasma around eyes (B) After 1 session of Er: YAG laser ablation (parameters: energy—14–20 J/cm^2, spot size—3 mm).

sebaceum (Figs. 45.7A and B),[33] syringoma,[34] trichoepithelioma,[35,36] apocrine hidrocystoma,[37] and xanthelasma.[38,39] For individual lesions, the growth is vaporized by using relatively low-power settings in the 3 to 5 W range with a spot size that matches the size of the lesion. The removal is continued into the dermis, but the entire lesion is not completely removed, because the residual thermal damage will extend the depth of the defect by 0.5 to 1 mm. When a large number of lesions are treated, the entire cosmetic unit is de-epithelialized with a large spot size, and the individual lesions are then vaporized using a smaller spot size. Re-epithelialization following this procedure is usually complete within 2 weeks.

Xanthelasma

The best treatment option for xanthelasma is excision, but CO_2/erbium laser can be one of the choices of treatment. Flat lesion can be treated with a single session of CO_2. Thick lesions require multiple sessions (Figs. 45.8A and B).

Syringoma

Syringoma is a common condition but difficult to treat and can result in pigmentary alterations and require multiple sessions to clear. The laser of choice is CO_2. Er:YAG is the alternate choice. Hasson et al., in his study of 5 patients, showed that using low-energy parameters on the CO_2 laser in combination with low energy on the radiofrequency, could maximize the destruction of the tumors and minimize the adverse effects, and results could be achieved in only two sessions.[40] The CO_2 laser is a dependable, safe, and nonscarring method (if used appropriately) for the treatment of periorbital syringomas.[41,42] Other treatment modalities are known to produce nonsatisfactory results unlike ablative lasers. Author prefers to use combination of

CO_2 and Er:YAG laser. The center core of the lesion is treated with CO_2 laser while the erbium, targets the entire lesion with spot size equal to size of target lesion with optimal fluence. This method gives cosmetically better results (Box 45.4, Figs. 45.9 and 45.10).

Lymphangioma Circumscriptum

The CO_2 laser can be used to coagulate the superficial lesions of lymphangioma circumscriptum. If the lesion is only superficial, CO_2 laser treatment may eliminate the problem permanently, but most cases have an associated deeper component that requires resection.

Box 45.4: Syringoma.

Laser of choice CO_2/erbium procedure:
- The lesions are small and commonly seen around eyes, they are targeted precisely with small spot size and focused beam, pulsed mode with 2–3 J/cm^2 to produce good results.
- Eye protection is mandatory.
- The nondominant hand stretches the skin and the lesion is lased either in circular pattern or in loop pattern from center to outside, more precisely without much collateral damage.
- The upper charred tissue is removed with wet gauze and the same is repeated till the white glistening dermal tissue is seen.
- It heals with slight hypopigmentation and mild scarring that becomes inconspicuous in few weeks. In patients with periorbital melanosis, these can be more prominent.
- Recommended sessions: 2 to 4 and retouch procedure when required can be spaced at 4 to 6 week intervals.

Nevi

Epidermal nevus is a hamartoma with varying size and, can either present as soft papillomas or verrucous lesions. The laser of choice is CO_2 laser. The alternative options include Erb:YAG laser. Carbon dioxide laser vaporization of epidermal nevi provides good clinical result and offers unique advantage of effective intraoperative hemostasis with excellent lesional visualization.[12-14]

The verrucous lesion may need high fluence, focus mode with evenly spaced ablation. Soft nevus can be vaporized with lesser fluence. Erbium is alternative choice, but CO_2 is advantageous for large nevus as bleeding hampers visibility and ablative result of CO_2 scores over Er:Yag. If the treatment is too superficial, with only the epidermis removed, the nevus regrows. If the treatment goes too deep into the reticular dermis, a hypertrophic scar can develop. Therefore, vaporization or coagulation should be carried out up to the papillary dermis.

Melanocytic Nevus

Dermal nevi are amenable to the treatment with superior results, but one should be cautious in removal of the nevi,

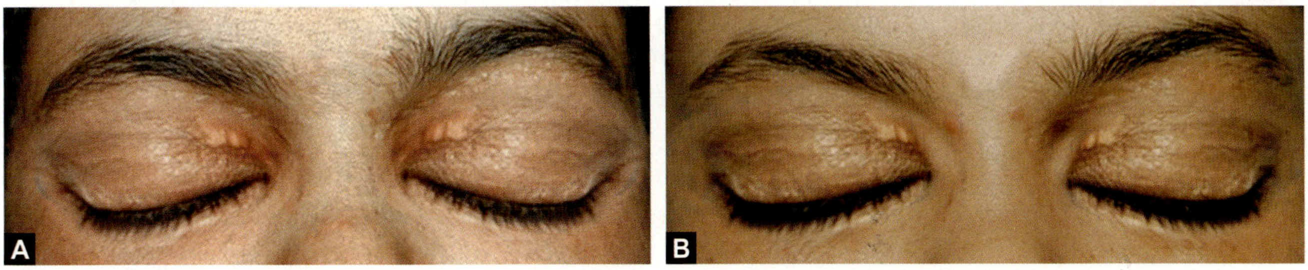

Figs. 45.9A and B: (A) Periorbital syringomas. (B) After 4 sessions of CO_2 laser ablation (parameters: energy—2–3 J/cm^2, power—30 W, 10 to 20 Hz).

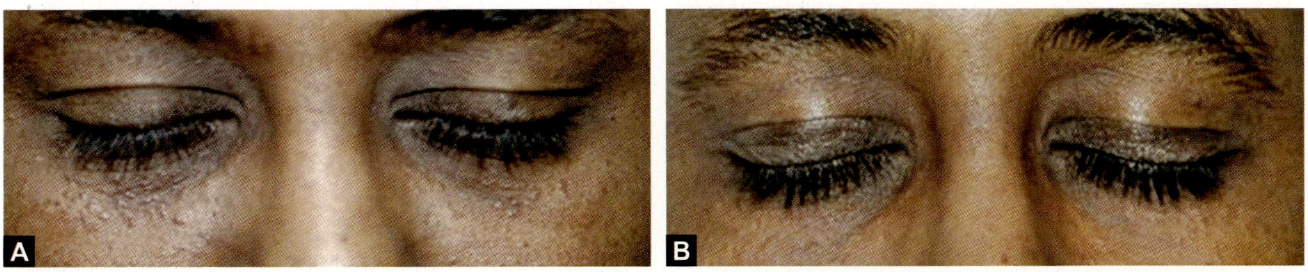

Figs. 45.10A and B: Periorbital syringomas (A) Before (B) After two sessions of CO_2 laser ablation (parameters: energy—2–3 J/cm^2, power—30 W, 10 to 20 Hz).

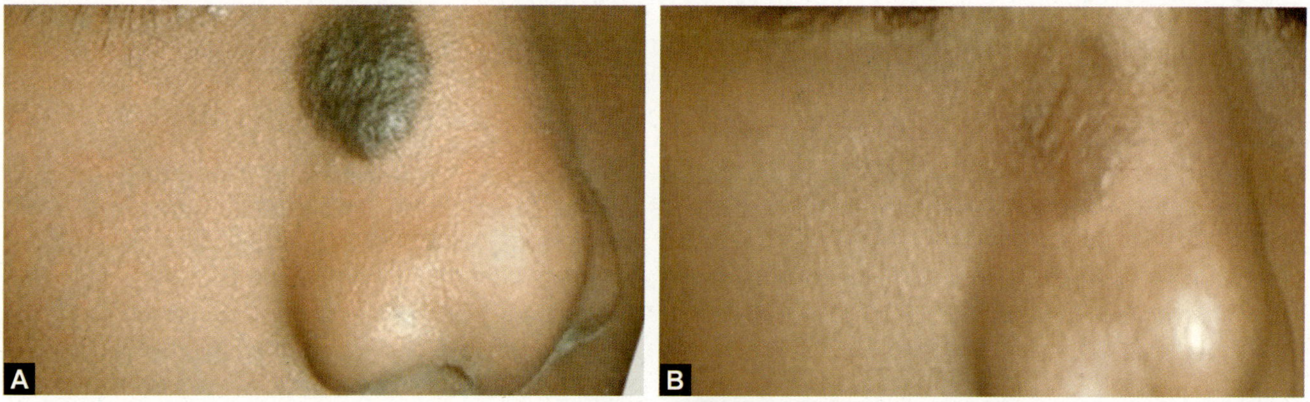

Figs. 45.11A and B: (A) Melanocytic nevus on face (B) After 4 months of CO_2 laser ablation (parameters: energy—3 to 5 J/cm^2, power —20 to 30 W, 20 Hz).

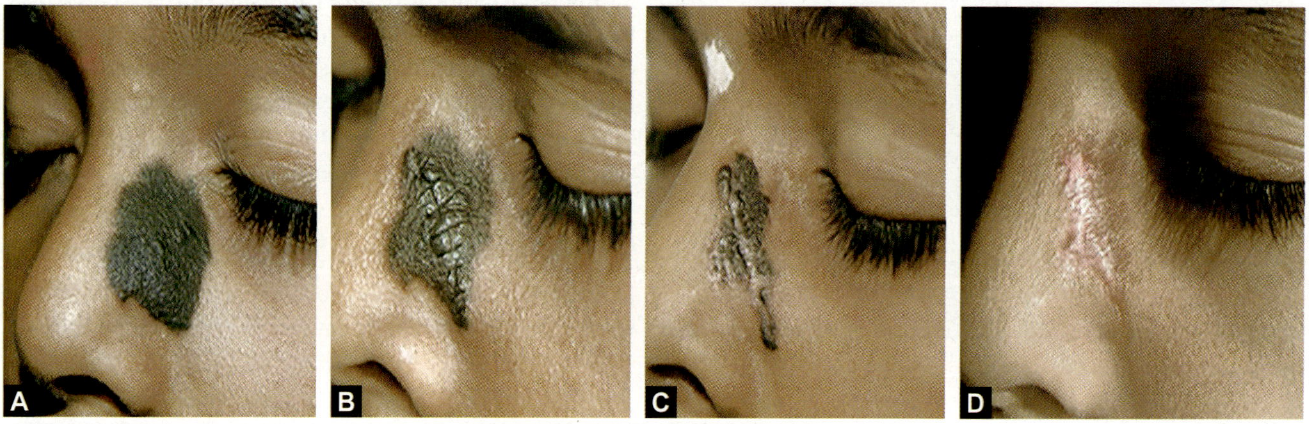

Figs. 45.12A to D: (A) Congenital nevus (B) After one session of serial excision (C) After one session of CO_2 laser (D) After serial alternate excision and CO_2 laser.

as incomplete removal can lead to pseudomelanomas. Dermal nevus can be vaporized with CO_2. Small nevi can be vaporized with erbium sequentially, till complete removal (Figs. 45.11 and 45.12).

Nevus Sebaceous

Nevus sebaceous is a commonly seen hamartoma on scalp and the treatment of choice is surgical excision. For broader lesion not amenable for excision in one session, laser gives equally good results. Since nevus sebaceous is deeper, complete removal needs deeper ablation and hence more downtime. Superficial ablation is associated with recurrences. Sebaceous nevi have been partially ablated with a CO_2 laser for cosmetic improvement (Figs. 45.13A to C).[43]

Neurofibroma

Neurofibromas can be easily and rapidly treated using the CO_2 laser with results equal to or better than excision. Patients with large numbers of small- or medium-sized cutaneous neurofibromas are most benefitted (Figs. 45.14A to F).[9-11] The neurofibromas are removed only for cosmetic reasons especially on face in patients who wants to get rid of them, though they understand it is a noncurable disease. The objective of treatment is only remission and new lesions occur in all cases. Laser of choice CO_2 (CW mode) (Box 45.5).

Rhinophyma

The ablation of rhinophyma is time consuming as compared to other conventional treatment like scalpel excision and

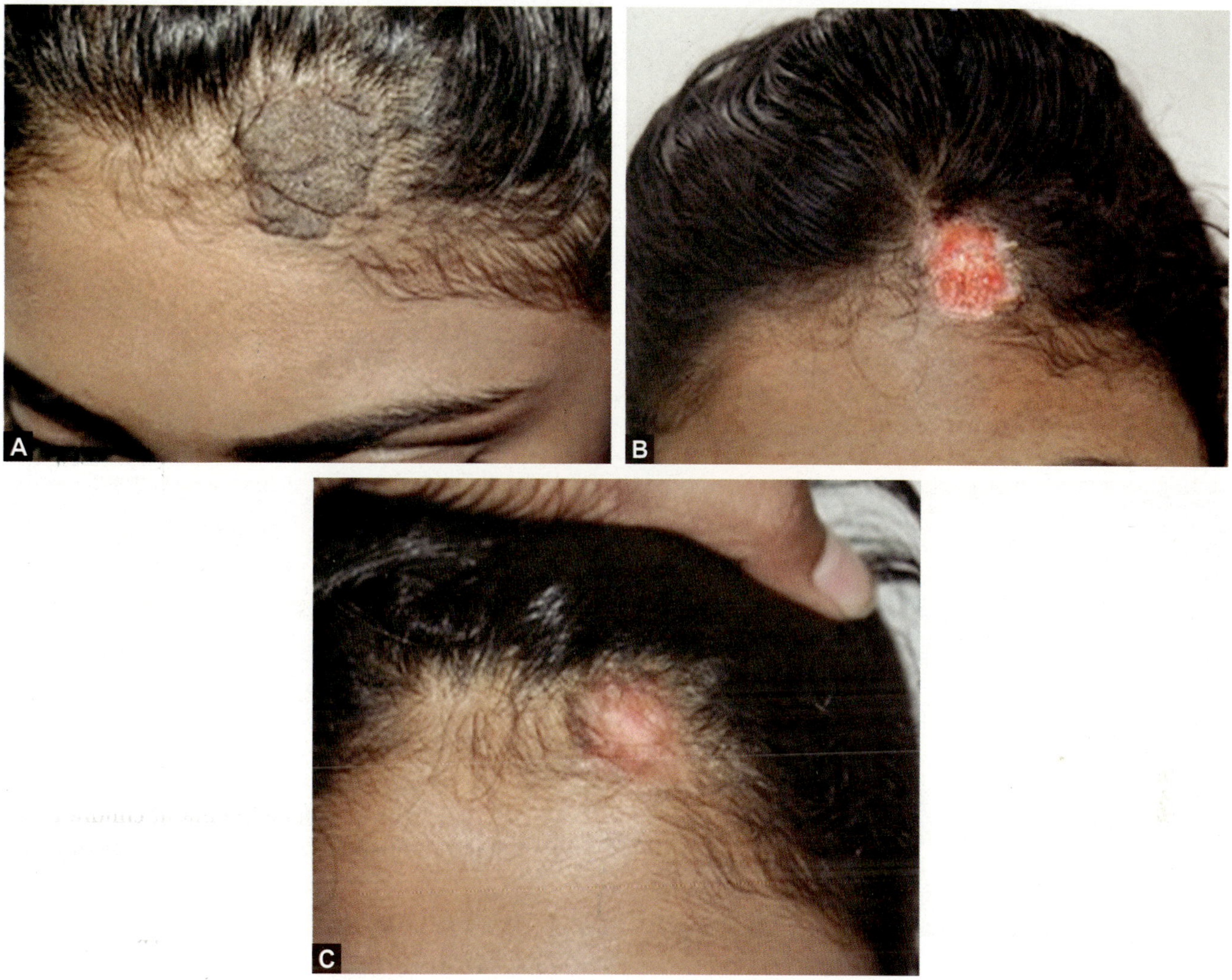

Figs. 45.13A to C: (A) Nevus sebaceous along hairline (B) After 15 days of CO_2 laser ablation (C) After one month of secondary healing (parameters: energy—9 J/cm^2, power—30 W, 10 to 20 Hz).

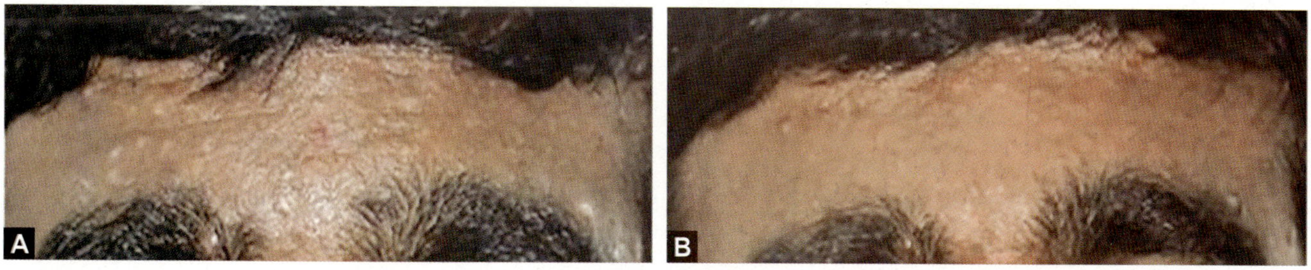

Figs. 45.14A and B

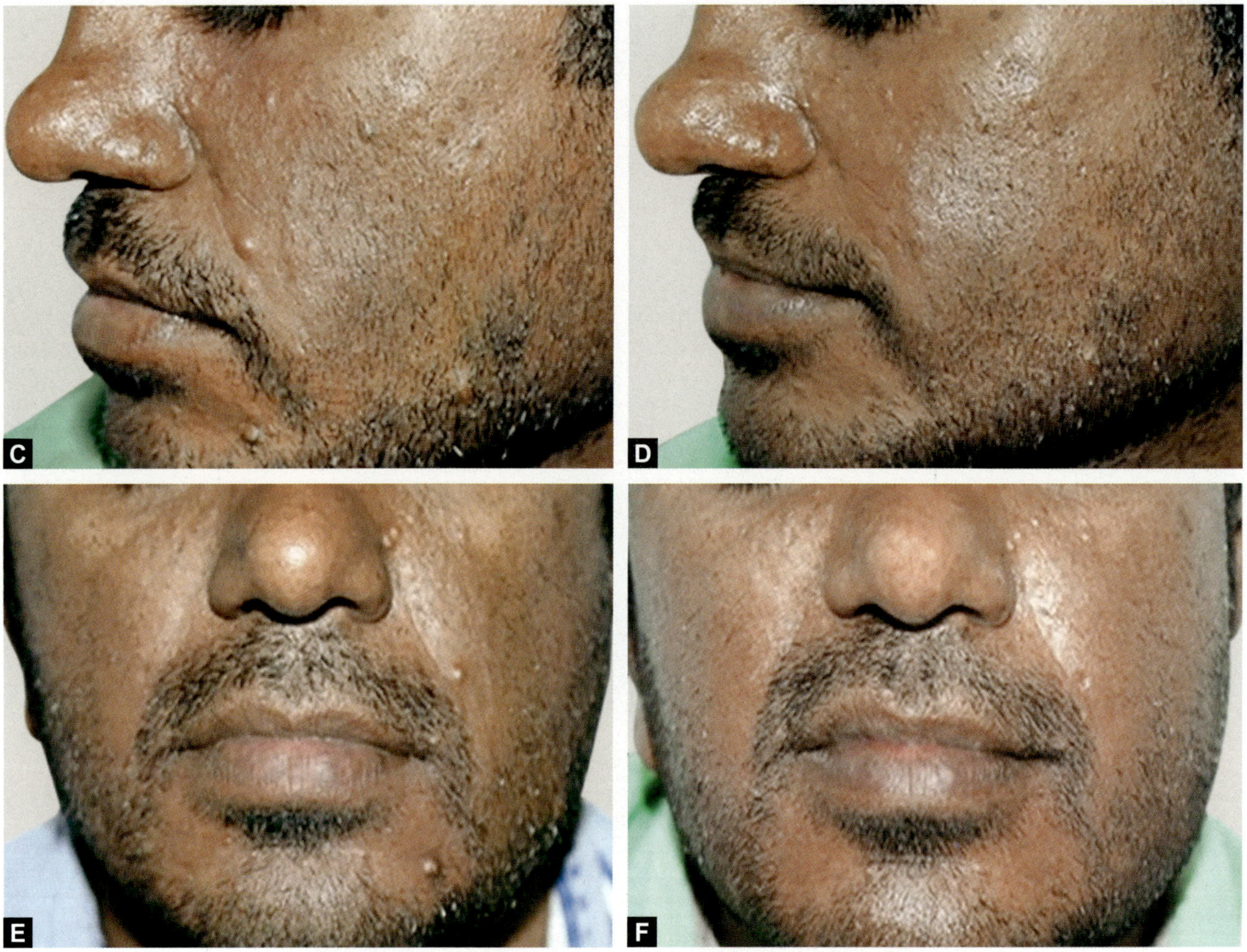

Figs. 45.14A to F: (A, C and E) Baseline multiple neurofibromas on face. (B, D and F) After 3 months of CO_2 laser ablation (parameters: energy—5 to 8 J/cm^2, power—20 to 30 W, 20 Hz).

Box 45.5: Author suggests two techniques for removal of neurofibroma (NF).

Small NF (drill hole technique)

Stabilize the lesion with index and thumb finger. The center of lesion is lased using high fluence 6–9 J/cm^2, 30 W and 40 Hz, to create a drill hole, through which entire dermal component is lased by maneuvering the lesion with nondominant hand. Removal must be complete up to base to prevent early recurrence.

Medium sized NF (cut and coagulate)

At fluence of 9 to 10 J/cm^2, 30 W, 60 Hz, CO_2 laser is used like skin knife to incise the neurofibroma circumferentially. After incising, hold the central circular tissue with forceps and separate it from surrounding tissue. Lastly, the base is coagulated and left to heal by secondary intention.

radiofrequency (RF), the only advantage being hemostasis. The continuous (Cw) mode is recommended to debulk the tissue. Pulsed mode is used to precisely shape the target site.

Cysts

The cysts encountered in dermatosurgery include epidermal cyst, trichilemmal cyst, steatocystoma, mucosal cyst, eccrine hydrocystoma and eruptive vellus cyst. Choice of laser is CO_2 in pulsed mode/continuous mode (Box 45.6).

Actinic Keratoses

CO_2 laser is an alternative to surgical treatment of premalignant lesions (actinic keratosis) on face and can be used effectively without significant complications.[17] But the resulting thermal damage leaves the patient with hypopigmentation and an increased risk of scarring. The most valuable use of these lasers is for the treatment of diffuse actinic keratoses. The entire face, scalp, or dorsal hand can be treated in one session. Moist wound

Box 45.6: Laser in cysts.

	CO_2 laser parameters	Remarks
Epidermal cyst	E—8–9 J/cm^2, power—30 W	The CO_2 laser in focus mode can be used to make an incision over the cyst followed by blunt dissection with an artery to reach the plane and rest of the steps will be same as cyst enucleation. Advantage is that bleeding and procedural time is lessened.
Steatocystoma and other cysts	E—4–5 J/cm^2, power—30 W	Regular vaporization and coagulation.

healing with bio-occlusive dressings helps speed re-epithelialization.

Skin Tumors

CO_2 laser is least opted method for removal of skin cancer as other proven and less expensive methods are available.[1,44] Superficial basal cell carcinomas,[45] Bowen's disease,[46-48] Lentigo maligna and erythroplasia of queyrat,[49] can be treated with CO_2. The advantage of CO_2 vaporization is efficient concurrent hemostasis. Using a resurfacing CO_2 or variable-pulsed Er:YAG laser reduces the amount of residual thermal damage and speeds healing.

Tattoos

Ablative lasers are indicated in patients who have developed an allergic reaction to the tattoo; patients who want to have the tattoo removed in one treatment and ready to accept scar and patients who seek tattoo removal early, i.e. less than 3 weeks of tattooing, might benefit from CO_2 laser vaporization. Only 30% to 50% of the ink is vaporized to minimize scaring. The rest of the ink is leached out from the skin with 40% to 50% urea paste applications for 10 to 14 days after laser treatment[50,51] To avoid ghost tattoo, the entire region of the tattoo must be vaporized to have a patch of scar that resembles a superficial burn scar. The ghost tattoo following Q-switched laser treatment can be efficiently ablated with a resurfacing laser in fractional mode.

Excisional Surgeries

Any lesion that can be excised with a scalpel is amenable to CO_2 laser excision. The CO_2 laser acts like a light scalpel. The focus beam of spot size 0.1 to 0.2 mm has high irradiances of 50,000 W/cm^2 or more, that makes it ideal for laser excision. Laser excision is significantly slower than cold-steel surgery, and initially wound healing is also delayed.[52,53] The main advantage of this method is that the laser excision is relatively hemostatic.[53] Excision by CO_2 laser may be useful in patients with bleeding disorders, in patients taking warfarin, or when excising vascular lesions. The CO_2 laser has been useful for the debridement of burn wounds [54,55] Smart laser systems are being developed that will ablate devitalized tissue and stop ablating once viable tissue has been reached. The endpoint is found through a feedback system using indocyanine green that is taken up only by viable tissue and has characteristic green fluorescence.[56]

Nail Surgery

The CO_2 laser can be helpful in selected cases of nail surgery.[57-59] In the defocused mode, the laser can be used to vaporize the nail matrix to treat ingrown toenails or other conditions requiring permanent destruction of the nail matrix. Koenen tumors can be efficiently vaporized by CO_2 laser with less operating time, minimal bleeding, good functional and cosmetic outcome.

Miscellaneous Indications

CO_2 laser is used in various other indications like acne keloidalis nuchae, papular scars (Figs. 45.15A to D) and fibroepithelial polyp (Figs. 45.16A and B) because of efficient hemostasis. Fibrous papule of nose is a regressed fibrosed nevus or fibroma, a cosmetically disturbing entity. CO_2 or Er:YAG laser can ablate the fibrous papule and may require 2 to 3 sessions for sequential scar free removal. Mucosal lesions like mucosal fibroma, papillomas, Bowenoid papulosis, sublingual keratosis can be treated with CO_2 laser and sebaceous hyperplasia with either CO_2 or Er:YAG laser.[1]

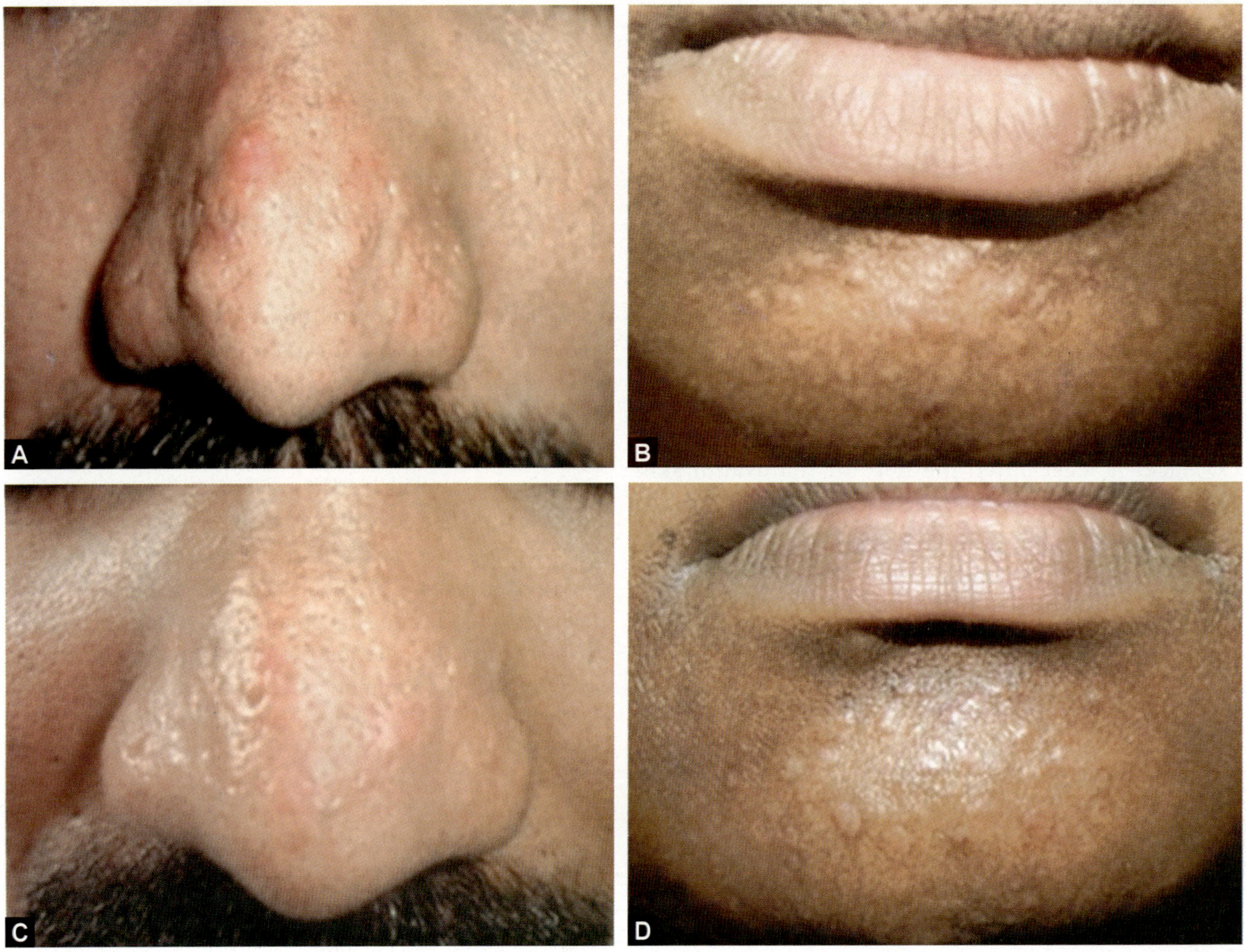

Figs. 45.15A to D: (A and B) Papular scars on nose and chin (C and D) After CO_2 ablation (parameters: energy—2 to 3 J/cm^2, power—20 W, 10 to 20 Hz).

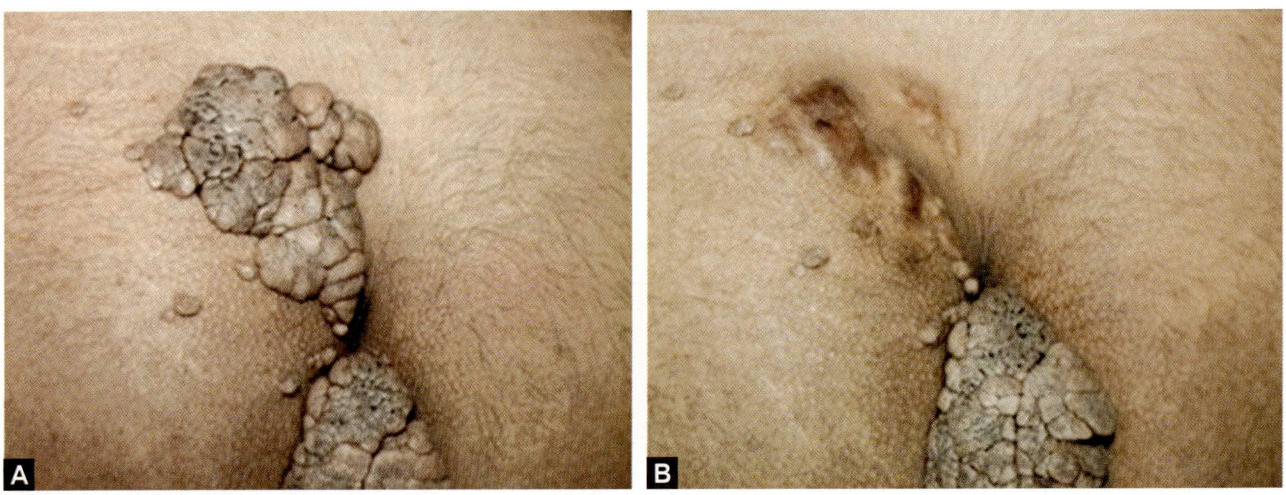

Figs. 45.16A and B: (A) Fibroepithelial polyp on back (B) After 1 session CO_2 ablation (parameters: energy—10–12 J/cm^2, power—30 W).

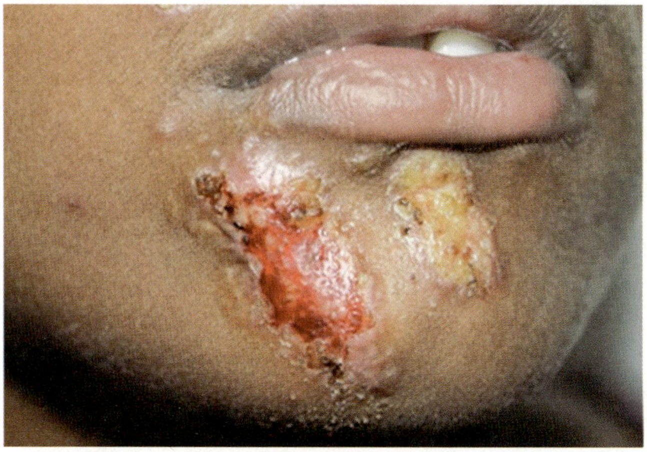

Fig. 45.17: Herpes simplex infection after CO_2 laser.

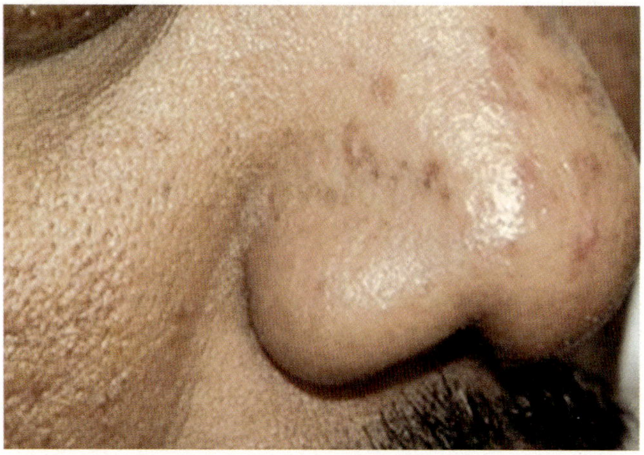

Fig. 45.18: Postinflammatory hyperpigmentation, after CO_2 laser ablation for papular scars on nose.

POSTLASER INSTRUCTIONS

- Antibiotic ointment for one week
- Systemic antibiotics and analgesics for 5 days in case of large lesions
- Strict sun screen application to avoid PIH
- In case of superficial lesions, scab falls off in 5 to 7 days and hence no dressing is required
- Whereas in deeper lesions like sebaceous nevus, regular occlusive dressings are carried out every 3 days till it heals completely
- Follow-up after 6 weeks to decide on repeating the next session of laser.

SEQUELAE

Pain, erythema, oozing, edema and crusting, which are well taken care of by anti-inflammatory drugs.

SIDE EFFECTS

- *Persistent scab or crust*: It will be susceptible to infection which heals with bad scar.
- *Infections*: Viral (Fig. 45.17) and bacterial infections.
- *Persistent erythema*: More risk of PIH, after crust falls off. With sun exposure, it may worsen giving rise to postinflammatory hyperpigmentation.
- Postinflammatory hyperpigmentation (Fig. 45.18) can be transient or permanent.
- *Hypopigmentation*: The amount of hypopigmentation (Figs. 45.19 and 45.20) is related to the amount of injury caused by the laser.[60]
- *Scarring*: Hypertrophic scarring,[61] or keloid
- Milia formation.

Parameters of the various Lasers for different indications are summarized in Table 45.3.

TIPS AND TRICKS

- Dry the lesion completely after cleansing, since water is the chromophore.
- Always remove the debris and then vaporize. The sequence should be dry - lase - wipe - lase - coagulate.
- Do not rub after using coagulation mode. Do not lase on bleeding surface as it boils and do not coagulate bleeding vessel.
- After initial ablation, wiping off with wet gauze or curetting the charred tissue avoids residual damage and speeds healing process.
- The laser hand piece must always be perpendicular in order to deliver intended energy more precisely and nondominant hand must stabilize the target area.
- Always assess the depth properly and target precisely. Do not overdo. Avoid collateral injury.
- Do not wipe off the scab after vaporizing DPN. Let it act as biological dressing.
- Closed dressing is indicated after deeper ablation. Once epithelization begins, follow open dressing, if needed. Saline compresses can be advocated to remove crust.
- Apply thin layer of topical antibiotic to facilitate epithelization.
- Clamping the skin tag and targeting upper border leaves behind a part of tissue which helps in healing without depigmented spots.
- Defer the procedure in case of prolonged sun exposure and sunburn, or else it results in PIH.
- During infiltrative anesthesia, always inject into subcutaneous tissue.
- Always take biopsy whenever question of benign nature is doubtful.
- Do a test patch when treating multiple lesions especially in over conscious and anxious patients.

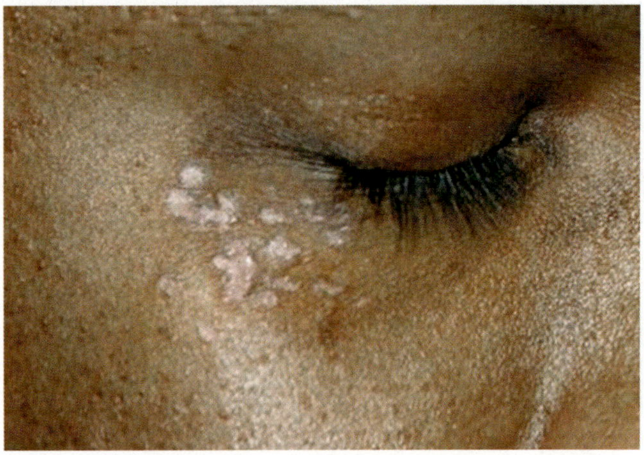

Fig. 45.19: Postinflammatory depigmentation after CO_2 ablation of periorbital syringomas.

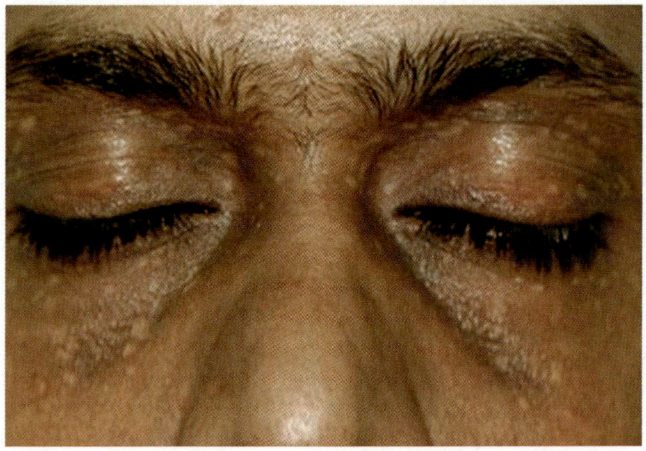

Fig. 45.20: Postinflammatory hypopigmentation after CO_2 laser ablation for periorbital syringomas.

Table 45.3: Parameters for various lesions (setting of parameters varies with type of device. The energy mentioned below is specific to the Lutronic corporation ECO_2 laser and Erbium YAG action II laser machines).

Type of lesion	*CO_2 laser*	*Er:YAG laser*	*Sessions*	*Remarks*
DPN	E: 1 J/cm^2, P: 20 W	E: 10–20 J/cm^2, spot size: 1 mm	1	Do not remove scab
Lentigo	E: 0.5–1 J/cm^2, P: 20 W	E: 10 J/cm^2, spot size: 2–3 mm	1	For thick lesions ablate it first with CO_2
Freckle		E: 5 J/cm^2, spot size: 1–2 mm	1–2	
Skin tag	E: 4–6 J/cm^2, P: 30 W		1	
Cysts	E: 8 J/cm^2, P: 30 W		1	
Fordyce spots	E: 0.5 J/cm^2, P: 15 W	E: 10 J/cm^2, spot size: 1 mm	1–2	
Syringomas	E: 2–3 J/cm^2, P: 30 W	E: 10 J/cm^2, spot size: varies on size of the lesion	2–6	
Neurofibroma	E: 8–10 J/cm^2, P: 30 W		1	
Papular scars	E: 1–2 J/cm^2, P: 20 W	E: 10–20 J/cm^2, spot size: 3 mm		
Xanthelasma	E: 1–2 J/cm^2, P: 20 W	E: 20 J/cm^2, spot size: 3–4 mm		Ablate till reddish fibers of muscle are seen
Seborrheic keratoses	E: 1–3 J/cm^2, P: 20 W	E: 30–50 J/cm^2, vary with spot size	1	Keep higher repetition rate, stop before you see bleeding points
Epidermal nevus	E: 3–5 J/cm^2, P: 20 W	E: 30–50 J/cm^2	1	CO_2 is preferred for verru cous, and erbium can be used for soft lesions
Nevus sebaceous	E: 6–9 J/cm^2, P: 30 W		1	If ablate deeper risk of scarring, if superficial it recurs
Rhinophyma	E: 6–10 J/cm^2, P: 30 W		1–2	
Warts	E: 3–5 J/cm^2, P: 20 W	E: 20–30 J/cm^2, varies with spot size (plane warts)	1	
Incision surgery	E: 9–10 J/cm^2, P: 30 W		1	
Moles	E: 1–3 J/cm^2, P: 20 W	E: 10–40 J/cm^2, varies with spot size	1	Ablate it sequentially with higher repetition rates for erbium YAG laser

CONCLUSION

The ablative lasers (CO_2/erbium) can treat many epidermal and dermal lesions. CO_2 laser is a versatile, efficient and popular tool for such lesions, where there is no easily targeted chromophore other than water. The knowledge of laser basics and safety, assessing the clinical end point of treatment, using the optimal parameters and good post-procedure care will give best outcome.

REFERENCES

1. Hruza GJ. Laser treatment of warts and other epidermal and dermal lesions. Dermatol Clin. 2002;20(1).
2. Rosenbach A, Alster TS. Multiple trichoepithelioma streated with a high-energy, pulsed carbon dioxide laser. Dermatol Surg. 1997;23:708-10.
3. Kaufmann R, Hartmann A, Hibst R. Cutting and skin-ablative properties of pulsed mid-infrared laser surgery. J Dermatol Surg Oncolo. 1994;20:112-8.
4. Kaufmann R, Hibst R. Pulsed 2.94 microns erbium-YAG laser skin ablation: experimental results and first clinical application. Clin Exp Dermatol. 1990;15:389-93.
5. Kaufmann R, Hibst R. Pulsed Er:YAG and 308 nm UV-excimer laser: An in vitro and in vivo study of skin-ablative effects. Lasers Surg Med. 1989;9:132-40.
6. Walsh JJ, Deutsch TF. Er:YAG laser ablation of tissue: measurement of ablation rates. Lasers Surg Med. 1989;9:327-37.
7. Alster TS. Clinical and histologic evaluation of six erbium: YAG lasers for cutaneous resurfacing. Lasers Surg Med. 1999;24:87-92.
8. Nerad JA, Anderson RL. CO2 laser treatment of eyelid syringomas. Ophthal Plast Reconstr Surg. 1988;4:91-4.
9. Lapid-Gortzak R, Lapid O, Monos T, et al. CO2 laser in the removal of a plexiform neurofibroma from the eyelid. Ophthalmic Surg Lasers. 2000;31:432-4.
10. Becker DW. Use of the carbon dioxide laser in treating multiple cutaneous neurofibromas. Ann Plast Surg. 1991;26:582-6.
11. Roenigk RK, Ratz JL. CO2 laser treatment of cutaneous neurofibromas. J Dermatol Surg Oncol. 1987;13:187-90.
12. Verma KK, Ovung EM. Epidermal and sebaceous nevi treatment with CO2 laser. Indian J Dermatol Venereol Leprol. 2002;68:23-4.
13. Ratz JL, Bailin PL, Wheeland RG. Carbon dioxide laser treatment of epidermal nevi. J Dermatol Surg Oncol. 1986;12: 567-70.
14. Gladstone GJ, Beckman H, Elson LM. CO2 laser excision of xanthelasma lesion. Arch Ophthalmol. 1985;103:440-2.
15. Trimas SJ, Ellis DA, Metz RD. The carbon dioxide laser: An alternative for the treatment of actinically damaged skin. Dermatol Surg. 1997;23:885-9.
16. Ward PD, Baker SR. Long-term results of carbon dioxide laser resurfacing of the face. Arch Facial Plast Surg. 2008;10(4):238-43, discussion 244-5.
17. Cheng ET, Pollard JD, Koch RJ. Effect of blended CO_2 and erbium: YAG laser irradiation on normal and keloid fibroblasts: A serum-free study. J Clin Laser Med Surg. 2003;21:337-43.
18. Nowak KC, McCormack M, Koch RJ. The effect of superpulsed carbon dioxide laser energy on keloid and normal dermal fibroblast secretion of growth factors: A serum-free study. Plast Reconstr Surg. 2000;105:2039-48.
19. Macdonald AG. A brief historical review of nonanaesthetic causes of fires and explosions in the operating room. Br J Anaesth. 1994;73:847-56.
20. Baggish MS, Elbakry M. The effects of laser smoke on the lungs of rats. Am J Obstet Gynecol. 1987;156:1260.
21. Nezhat C, Winer WK, Nezhat F, et al. Smoke from laser surgery: Is there a health hazard? Lasers Surg Med. 1987;7: 376-82.
22. Tomita Y, Mihashi S, Nagata K, et al. Mutagenicity of smoke condensates induced by CO2 laser irradiation and electrocauterization. Mutat Res. 1981;89:145-9.
23. Ferenczy A, Mitao M, Nagai N, et al. Latent papilloma virus and recurring genital warts. N Engl J Med. 1985;313: 784-8.
24. Lim JT, Goh CL. Carbon dioxide laser treatment of periungual and subungual viral warts. Australas J Dermatol. 1992;33: 87-91.
25. Logan RA, Zachary CB. Outcome of carbon dioxide laser therapy for persistent cutaneous viral warts. Br J Dermatol. 1989;121:99-105.
26. McBurney EI, Rosen DA. Carbon dioxide laser treatment of verrucae vulgaris. J Dermatol Surg Oncolo. 1984;10:45-8.
27. Kaufmann R, Hibst R. Pulsed 2.94 microns erbium-YAG laser skin ablation: experimental results and first clinical application. Clin Exp Dermatol. 1990;15:389-93.
28. Baggish MS. Carbon dioxide laser treatment for condylomata acuminata venereal infections. Obstet Gynecol. 1980;55: 711-5.
29. Bellina JH. The use of the carbon dioxide laser in the management of condylomata acuminatum with eight-year follow-up. Am J Obstet Gynecol. 1983;147:375-8.
30. Calkins JW, Masterson BJ, Magrina JF, et al. Management of condylomata acuminata with the carbon dioxide laser. Obstet Gynecol. 1982;59:105-8.
31. Bergbrant IM, Samuelsson L, Olofsson S, et al. Polymerase chain reaction for monitoring human papilloma virus contamination of medical personnel during treatment of genital warts with CO2 laser and electrocoagulation. Acta Derm Venereol. 1994;74:393-5.
32. Garden JM, O'Banion K, Shelnitz LS, et al. Papilloma virus in the vapor of carbon dioxide laser-treated verrucae. JAMA. 1988;259:1199-202.
33. Wheeland RG, Bailin PL, Kantor GR, et al. Treatment of adenoma sebaceum with carbon dioxide laser vaporization. J Dermatol Surg Oncolo. 1985;11:861-4.
34. Apfelberg DB, Maser MR, Lash H, et al. Superpulse CO2 laser treatment of facial syringomata. Lasers Surg Med. 1987;7: 533-7.

35. Rosenbach A, Alster TS. Multiple trichoepithelioma streated with a high-energy, pulsed carbon dioxide laser. Dermatol Surg. 1997;23:708-10.
36. Wheeland RG, Bailin PL, Kronberg E. Carbon dioxide (CO_2) laser vaporization for the treatment of multiple trichoepithelioma. J Dermatol Surg Oncolo.1984;10:470-5.
37. Bickley LK, Goldberg DJ, Imaeda S, et al. Treatment of multiple apocrine hidrocystomas with the carbon dioxide (CO_2) laser. J Dermatol Surg Oncolo. 1989;15:599-602.
38. Alster TS, West TB. Ultrapulse CO2 laser ablation of xanthelasma. J Am Acad Dermatol. 1996;34:848-9.
39. Apfelberg DB, Maser MR, Lash H, et al. Treatment of xanthelasma palpebrum with the carbon dioxide laser. J Dermatol Surg Oncolo. 1987;13:149-51.
40. Wang JI, Roenigk HH Jr. Treatment of multiple facial syringomas with the carbon dioxide laser. Dermatol Surg. 1999;25:136-9.
41. Wheeland RG, Bailin PL, Reynolds OD, et al. Carbon dioxide laser vaporization of multiple facial syringomas. J Dermatol Surg Oncol. 1986;12:225-8.
42. Nerad JA, Anderson RL. CO2 laser treatment of eyelid syringomas. Ophthal Plast Reconstr Surg. 1988;4:91-4.
43. Ashinoff R. Linear nevus sebaceous of Jadassohn treated with the carbon dioxide laser. Pediatr Dermatol. 1993;10:189-91.
44. Goldman L, Rockwell RJ, Meyer R, et al. Investigative studies with the laser in the treatment of basal cell epitheliomas. South Med J. 1968;61:735-42.
45. Landthaler M, Szeimies RM, Hohenleutner U. Laser therapy of skin tumors. Recent Results Cancer Res. 1995;139:417-21.
46. Gordon KB, Garden JM, Robinson JK. Bowen's disease of the distal digit. Outcome of treatment with carbon dioxide laser vaporization. Dermatol Surg. 1996;22:723-8.
47. Gordon KB, Robinson J. Carbon dioxide laser vaporization for Bowen's disease of the finger. Arch Dermatol. 1994;130:1250-2.
48. Landthaler M, Haina D, Brunner R, et al. Laser therapy of bowenoid papulosis and Bowen's disease. J Dermatol Surg Oncolo. 1986;12:1253-7.
49. Baggish MS, Poiesz BJ, Joret D, et al. Presence of human immunodeficiency virus DNA in laser smoke. Lasers Surg Med.1991;11:197-203.
50. Chernoff G, Slatkine M, Zair E, et al. Silk touch: a new technology for skin resurfacing in aesthetic surgery. J Clin Laser Med Surg. 1995;13:97-100.
51. Robson KJ, Cunningham NM, Kruzan KL, et al. Pulsed-dye laser versus conventional therapy in the treatment of warts: A prospective randomized trial. J Am Acad Dermatol.2000;43:275-80.
52. Calkins JW, Masterson BJ, Magrina JF, et al. Management of condylomaacuminata with the carbon dioxide laser. Obstet Gynecol.1982;59:105-8.
53. Montgomery TC, Sharp JB, Bellina JH, et al. Comparative gross and histological study of the effects of scalpel, electric knife, and carbon dioxide laser on skin and uterine incisions in dogs. Lasers Surg Med.1983;3:9-22.
54. Stellar S, Levine N, Ger R, et al. Laser excision of acute third-degree burns followed by immediate autograft replacement: An experimental study in the pig. J Trauma. 1973;13:45-53.
55. Green HA, Domankevitz Y, Nishioka NS. Pulsed carbon dioxide laser ablation of burned skin: in vitro and in vivo analysis. Lasers Surg Med.1990;10:476-84.
56. Green HA, Bua D, Anderson RR, et al. Burn depth estimation using indocyanine green fluorescence. Arch Dermatol.1992;128:43-9.
57. Geronemus RG. Laser surgery of the nail unit. J Dermatol Surg Oncolo. 1992;18:735-43.
58. Leshin B, Whitaker DC. Carbon dioxide laser matricectomy. J Dermatol Surg Oncolo. 1988;14:608-11.
59. Rothermel E, Apfelberg DB. Carbon dioxide laser use for certain diseases of the toenails. Clin Podiatr Med Surg.1987;4:809-21.
60. Ward PD, Baker SR. Long-term results of carbon dioxide laser resurfacing of the face. Arch Facial Plast Surg. 2008;104:238-43.
61. Ostertag JU, Theunissen CC, Neumann HA. Hypertrophic scars after therapy with CO2 laser for treatment of multiple cutaneous neurofibromas. Dermatol Surg. 2002;28:296-8.

CHAPTER 46

Lasers in Dermatosurgery: Treating Scars

BS Chandrashekar, Madura C, Sushmitha Jayaprasad

INTRODUCTION

A scar is the fibrous mass that results from healing of tissue which is destroyed by injury or disease. Scars can be secondary to surgery, burns, trauma, chronic wounds, disease conditions like acne, chicken pox scar, etc and also includes striae. Acne scars form the majority of these scars.[1] The indications for scar improvement can be functional, esthetic or psychological. It is important to classify the scars, which helps in choosing the most appropriate treatment (Box 46.1). This chapter will not only address the use of lasers and light sources for acne scars, other atrophic scars, hypertrophic and miscellaneous scars but also discuss the strategies to minimize the scar formation. The expected outcome of laser treatment is reduction of erythema and height with improved pliability and cosmetic appearance of scar.[2]

PRELASER EVALUATION

It is important to have good patient evaluation before laser treatment.

History

- Etiology of scar
- *Duration*: Lesions of less than a year are ideal for laser therapy

Box 46.1: The international advisory panel on scar management has classified scars into 6 types.

- *Mature scar:* It is light colored, flat scar.
- *Immature scar:* It is red, itchy or painful and slightly elevated scar, still in process of remodeling.
- *Linear hypertrophic scar:* It is red, raised, sometimes itchy confined to the border of original scar, e.g. surgical or traumatic scar.
- *Widespread hypertrophic scar:* It is widespread, red, raised sometimes itchy scar confined to the border of burn injury, e.g. burn injury.
- *Minor keloid*: A focally raised, itchy scar extending beyond normal tissue.
- *Major keloid*: A large raised > 0.5 cm scar, possibly painful and extending beyond normal tissue.

- *Previous treatment modalities and outcome*: These help us in choosing appropriate laser, and also modify parameters accordingly, e.g. After cryotherapy, lot of fibrosis is expected
- *Active disease process*: Treat active acne before scar revision. Treat infection in case of keloid or hypertrophic scar
- *Associated comorbidities*: Be cautious while using ablative lasers in diabetic patients
- History of HSV infection is important.

Examination

- *Skin type*: The response is good with Fitzpatrick skin types I to III with fewer side effects, whereas Fitzpatrick skin types IV to VI have an increased risk of postoperative hypo- or hyperpigmentation.
- *Lesion type*: Lesional scar assessment include, assessment of size, color, height and pliability after removal of the makeup and creams, if any. This helps choosing the right laser for therapy. The early scars are red and raised and lasers targeting vascular component would be the better choice in such cases.
- *Location of scar*: Facial scars respond better to treatment than in other locations.

Investigations: Extensive investigations are not needed. In clinically suspected cases do routine investigations to rule out comorbidities especially while treating larger areas and while using ablative lasers.

Patient Selection and Preoperative Measures

- The patient must be well-counseled for realistic expectations and must be explained about the laser to be used, procedural details, number of sessions required, expected outcome, duration between the session, cost and the precautions that has to be taken during and after laser sessions.

- In all patients of acne scars, it is good to prime their skin with hydroquinone and skin lightening preparations, before scheduling the treatment sessions.
- Exercise caution in patients with keloidal tendency, bleeding disorders, history of HSV infection in past and in patient sprone for postinflammatory pigmentation and poor healing. In patients with keloidal tendency, do not ablate deeper than papillary dermis. Give prophylactic antivirals 48 hours prior to procedure and continue till complete epithelialization.
- Priming with depigmenting agents and sun screens and initiation of treatment at lower fluences are advised in patients prone to hyperpigmentation.
- Associated bacterial infections of the facial skin may require prescription of oral antibiotics
- Patients are advised to protect against sun exposure for 2 weeks prior to procedure and use a broad-spectrum sunscreen.
- Avoid procedure (resurfacing) in patients with recent history of tanning/sun exposure.
- Contraindications for Laser scar revision are provided in Box 46.2.

Anesthesia

Ablative lasers like CO_2 require complete anesthesia of treatment site. Anesthesia is achieved by infiltrative anesthesia (1 to 2% lignocaine) or ring block in case of keloid. Fractional resurfacing can be managed under topical EMLA for 45 to 60 minutes. PDL lasers and nonablative lasers can be done without topical anesthesia, if patient is comfortable.

POSTPROCEDURE CARE

- Immediately after the laser, cold compresses are given for 15 to 20 minutes to decrease inflammation and a thin layer of antibiotic/re-epithelializing cream is applied.
- Thrice daily application of moisturizing antibiotic cream for 3 to 5 days after fractional ablative lasers.
- Twice daily intake of anti-inflammatory drug for 3 to 5 days (when large areas are treated)

Box 46.2: Contraindications.

- Active infection at the site of the lesion (e.g. herpes simplex).
- Patients with unrealistic expectations.
- Unstable vitiligo and psoriasis in treated area due to risk of koebnerization.
- Keloidal tendencies.
- Associated photo aggravated skin diseases (e.g. SLE) and uncontrolled diabetes.

- Strict sun protection with repeated application of sunscreen and physical protection.
- Not to pick the lesion and to allow the scab to fall on its own in 1–2 weeks. Encourage using hydrating creams.
- Wash with water or mild cleanser. Not to scrub the treated area for 5 to 7 days.
- Avoid using cosmetics containing retinol/AHA/alcohol for at least 5 to 7 days.

ACNE SCARS

Acne scars are polymorphous and require a multimodal approach for successful outcome. Icepick scars, Box scars and Rolling scars are 3 basic types of scars (Box 46.3). These form the atrophic scars. Other scar types include hypertrophic scars, keloidal scars, and sinus tracts.

Goodman et al. has proposed a qualitative grading system, in four grades according to scar severity as Grade I corresponding to macular involvement (including erythematous, hyperpigmented, or hypopigmented scars), whereas Grades II, III, and IV correspond to mild, moderate, and severe atrophic and hypertrophic lesions, respectively (Table 46.1). The selection of treatment modality depends on type and grade of acne scars.

Choice of Laser

Lasers: The choice of laser and light energy device is dependent on the type and depth of the scarring as well as the patient's skin type and risk tolerance (Table 46.2).

Ablative Lasers[1]

CO_2 laser (10600 nm): The treatment is more aggressive and deeper: it targets extracellular and intracellular water. It is usually bloodless but can achieve total ablation of the epidermis and a portion of the dermis. In addition to the destructive nature, there may also be stimulation of collagen by

Box 46.3: Classification of acne scars for an appropriate treatment modality.[4]

- *Ice-pick scars:* < 2 mm in diameter, sharply defined edges and penetrate deep into the skin. Treatment of choice includes TCA cross, punch excision and closure followed by resurfacing treatments.
- *Boxcar scars:* 1.5–4 mm in diameter, shallow or deep, sharply defined vertical walls. Treatment of choice includes subcision, punch excision and closure followed by resurfacing treatments.
- *Rolling scars:* >4 mm in diameter, soft edges and may be circular or linear. Full face resurfacing procedures, that will peel the skin and stimulate new collagen.

Table 46.1: Goodman and Baron qualitative global acne scarring grading system.[3]

Grade	Level of disease	Clinical features	Examples of Scars
1	Macular disease	Erythematous, hyper- or hypopigmented flat marks visible to patient or observer irrespective of distance	Erythematous, hyper- or hypopigmented flat marks
2	Mild disease	Mild atrophy or hypertrophy that may not be obvious at social distances of 50 cm or greater and may be covered adequately by makeup or the normal shadow of shaved beard hair in males or normal body hair, if extrafacial	Mild rolling, small soft papular
3	Moderate disease	Moderate atrophic or hypertrophic scarring that is obvious at social distances of 50 cm or greater and is not covered easily by makeup or the normal shadow of shaved beard hair in males or body hair, if extrafacial, but is still able to be flattened by manual stretching of the skin	More significant rolling, shallow "box car," mild to moderate hypertrophic or papular scars
4	Severe disease	Severe atrophic or hypertrophic scarring that is obvious at social distances of 50 cm or greater and is not covered easily by makeup or the normal shadow of shaved beard hair in males or body hair (if extrafacial) and is not able to be flattened by manual stretching of the skin	Punched out atrophic (deep "box car"), "ice pick", bridges and tunnels, gross atrophy, dystrophic scars, significant hypertrophy or keloid

Table 46.2: Types of lasers and light devises.

Ablative nonfractional	Ablative fractional	Nonablative nonfractional	Nonablative fractional	Light sources
Carbon dioxide (CO_2)—10,600 nm	Nd:YAG—10,600 nm	Nd:YAG—1320 nm	Nd:YAG—1440 nm	IPL
Erbium doped yttrium aluminum garnet (Er:YAG)—2940 nm	Er:YAG—2940 nm	Diode—1450 nm	Erbium glass—1550 nm	
	Er:YSSG—2790 nm	PDL—585 nm	Thulium fiber—1927 nm	

the procedure. CO_2 laser resurfacing is an effective treatment for mild acne scarring but often produces limited improvement in severe scarring when used as monotherapy.[5]

Er:YAG laser (2940 nm): It is a more superficial ablative therapy than the carbon-dioxide laser. The target chromophore being water, but there is 16 times more energy absorption as compared to carbon-dioxide laser. There is more superficial penetration, in turn, leading to less collateral damage and more rapid healing but lesser efficacy in terms of dermal remodeling and collagen stimulation.[1]

Fractional Lasers[6]

Fractional photothermolysis was introduced in 2004. It ablates tissue in columnar fashion leaving intermingling rings that helps in stimulating collagen remodeling and neo-collagenesis and better healing and remodeling of acne scars.

Nonablative Lasers

The nonablative lasers cause a controlled tissue injury in the dermis and stimulate dermal remodeling and collagen production. The complications associated with nonablative lasers are significantly less compared to ablative lasers (downtime of redness and peeling).[7] The most important benefit of these lasers is their significant reduction in downtime after treatment compared with ablative lasers. The nonablative lasers are best suited for darker skin tones as there is lesser risk of abnormal pigmentation, which often arises with ablative laser in darker skin types.[8]

Nd: YAG (1320 nm): The long-pulsed 1320 nm Nd:YAG laser functions by not damaging the epidermis. It targets dermis and stimulates new collagen growth. The water being the chromophore creates an even distribution of energy without damaging melanin or hemoglobin. This laser is effective in managing acne scars and it also decreases size and activity of sebaceous gland and prevent recurrence.[9]

Diode laser (1450 nm): The target chromophore is water. It partially damages sebaceous glands in upper dermis sparing the epidermis. Hence it is efficient in treating inflammatory acne and acne scars with less down time.

PDL (585 nm): This laser is used in inflammatory acne and erythematous scars as the target chromophore is oxyhemoglobin and porphyrin produced by Propionibacterium acnes. One of the studies demonstrated an increase in TGF-beta1 messenger RNA levels after PDL treatment and it was thought to be significant in promoting collagen synthesis.[10]

Nd:YAG (1440 nm): It targets the water chromophore. There is heating of dermal microcolumns leading to microrejuvenation and improvement of rhytides and acne scars.

Erbium glass (1550 nm) and thulium fiber (1927 nm): These lasers treat both epidermal and dermal scarring. It treats epidermal pigmentation, photoaging, melasma,

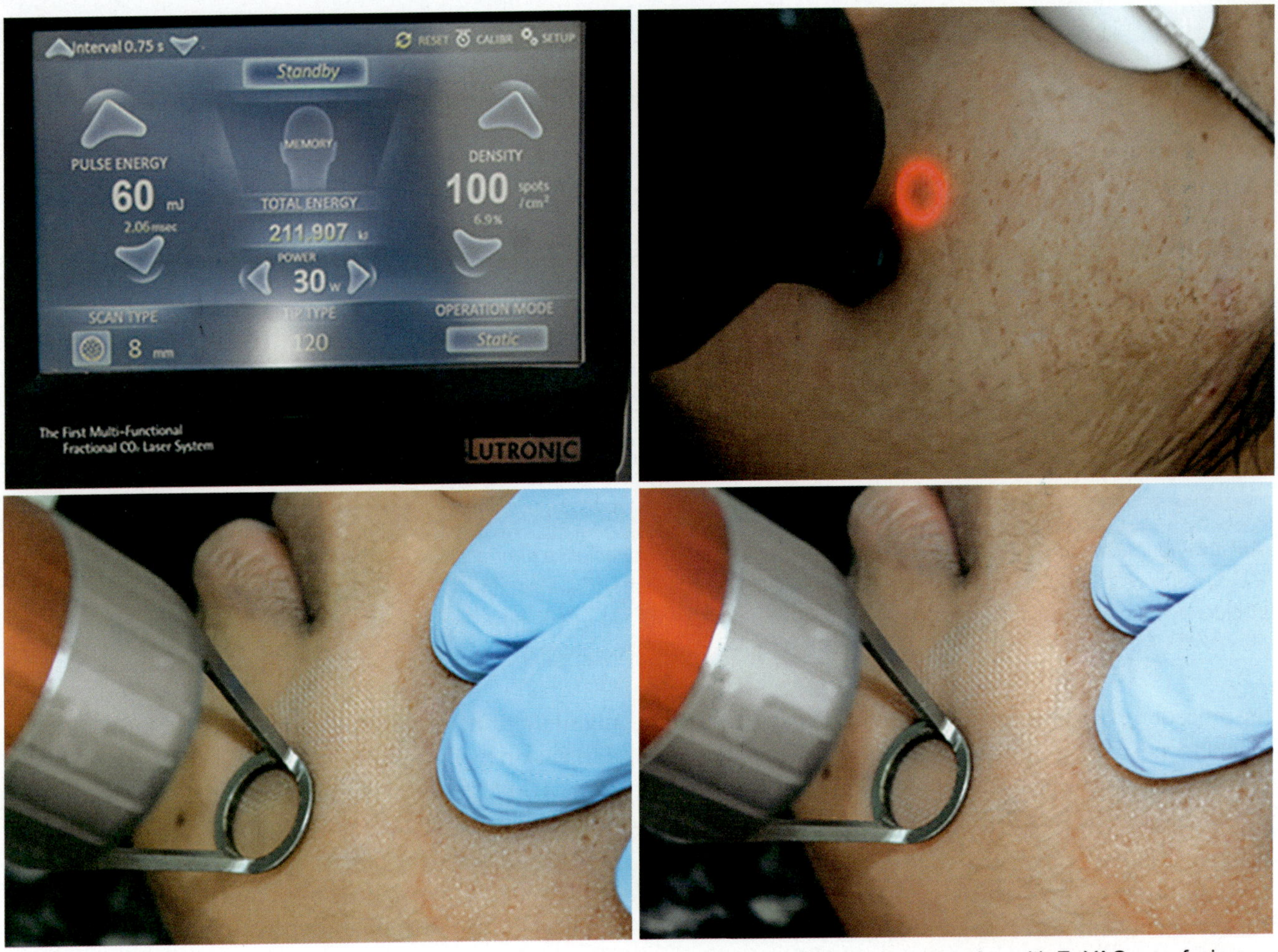

Fig. 46.1: Fractional CO_2 parameters and the scan type, showing 20% overlap during the laser session with Er:YAG resurfacing.

atrophic scars, postsurgical scars and postacne scarring and additional textural abnormalities.

Intense pulse light: Light based treatment of acne and erythematous acne scars has aimed at producing a photochemical effect. The target chromophore in acne and erythematous acne scars is porphyrin produced by the Propionibacterium acnes and hemoglobin in the capillaries supplying the sebaceous glands.

Steps of Laser Procedure (Figs. 46.1 and 46.2)

- Informed consent and preprocedure photography is mandatory for all patients.
- Patients with previous history of herpes labialis, should receive prophylactic oral antivirals, such as acyclovir, famciclovir or valacyclovir (starting 48 hrs before fractional resurfacing and continuing for 5 days postoperatively).
- Assess skin type and scars again.
- Anesthesia: Depends on laser used.
- Patient preparation: Remove make up and jewellery. Position the patient comfortably. The area to be treated must be cleaned with a mild acetone-based cleanser to facilitate adequate degreasing of the skin.
- While treating facial scars, mark the treatment area and also type of scars to be targeted (e.g. Ice pick scars for laser pinpoint ablation technique or shouldering box scars). Treatment grids have to be drawn appropriately.
- Laser safety measures to be followed. Treating physician/ technician to be in comfortable position.
- Parameter settings are determined based on the patient's Fitzpatrick skin type and type of scar and laser used.
- The distance guide should be in direct contact with the skin and perpendicular at all times and each spot should have an overlap of 10% to 20% with the previously treated spot.
- Scars require 2–3 passes of the laser beam.
- Feathering over the normal skin surface is essential.

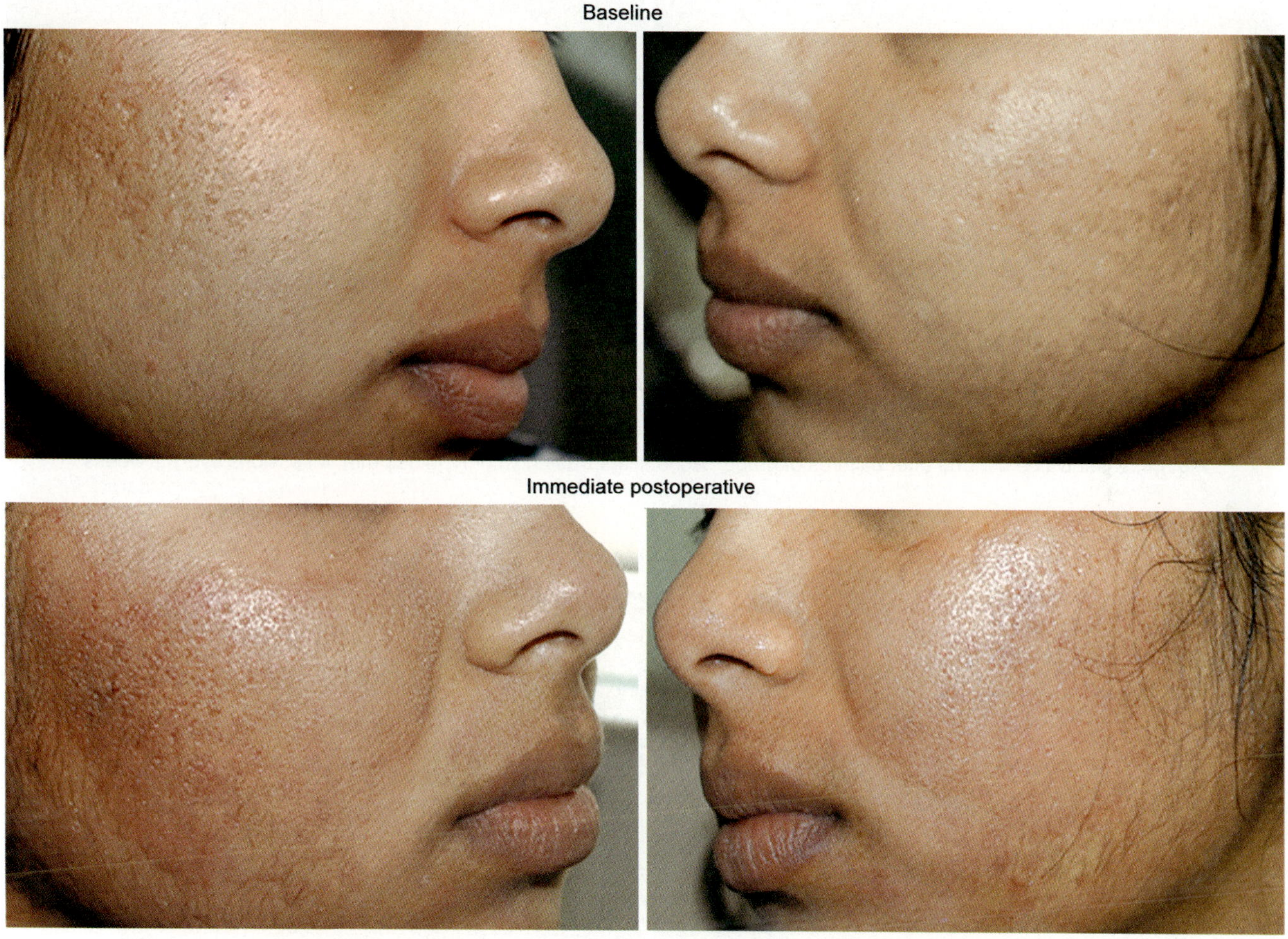

Fig. 46.2: Pretreatment and immediate post-treatment with fractional CO_2.

Postoperative Measures

- Broad spectrum sunscreens and avoidance of direct sun exposure is mandatory.
- Moisturizers to be used every 3 hours for 5 days.
- Mild topical steroid may be prescribed, if erythema and edema persists.
- In author's experience, patient must be warned to report in case of any unusual or mauve erythema, which implies risk of hyperpigmentation in Indian skin.

Complications of Laser scar revision are provided in Box 46.4

Results for all grades of acne scars (Figs. 46.3 to 46.7).

Box 46.4: Complications of acne scar laser resurfacing.

Ablative:
- *Short-term side effects*: Erythema, edema, crusting, milia and acneiform eruptions.
- *Delayed side effects*: The incidence of post-CO_2 hyperpigmentation varies with skin type but ranges from 26% to 36%.[11] Hypopigmentation is a delayed complication occurring in 8% to 19% of patients.[10] Peripheral feathering at the borders of the treatment site or treating with a gradient of passes that attenuates at the periphery, can minimize the color and texture contrast between sun-damaged and resurfaced skin. Hypertrophic scars and keloids can be seen rarely.

Nonablative:
- Temporary erythema, edema and hyperpigmentation.

HYPERTROPHIC SCAR AND KELOID (FIGS. 46.8 TO 46.10 AND TABLE 46.3)

Hypertrophic scar is linear, red, raised firm scar, confined to the original injury site; sometimes pruritic, occurs on sites under constant pressure and stretching and usually arise within 1 month of injury. It is known to improve spontaneously during first 6 months. Keloids are dome shaped claw like outgrowths, which are often out of proportion to the severity of wound and so, not limited

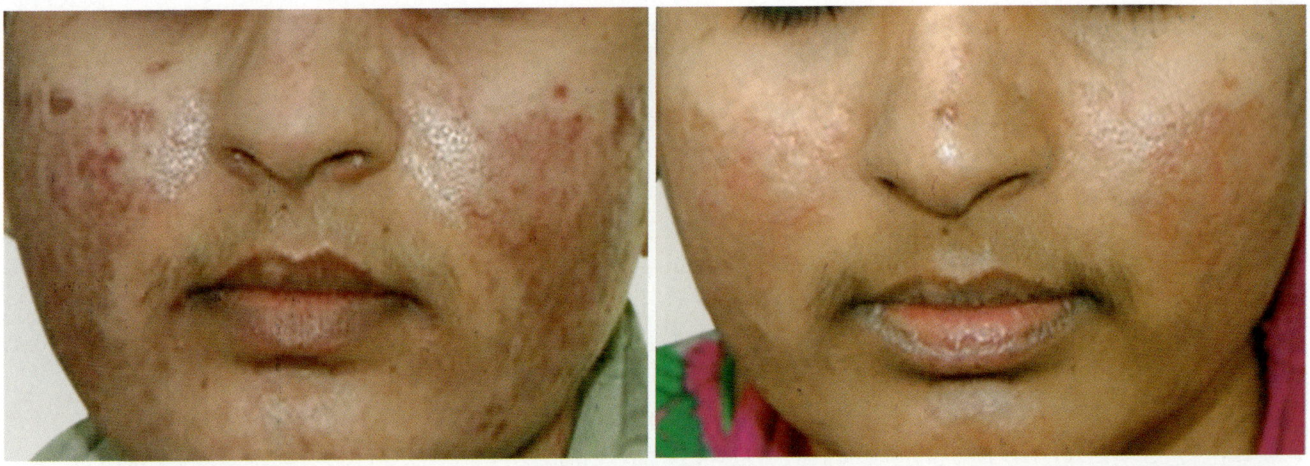

Fig. 46.3: Shows before and after pictures of grade I Acne scars treated with PDL 585 mm, 4 sessions every 2 weeks (E—4–5 J/cm^2, 7 mm).

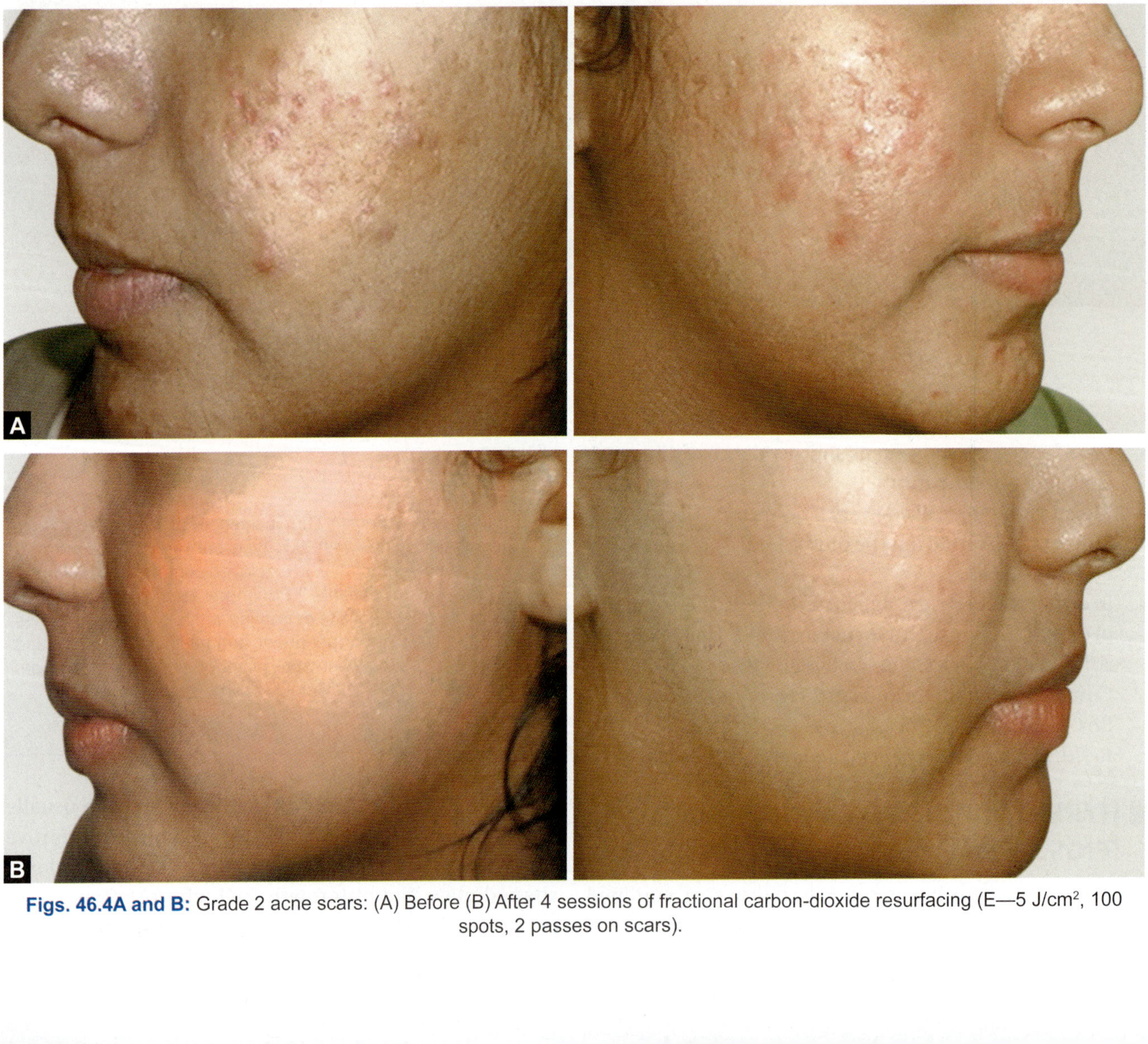

Figs. 46.4A and B: Grade 2 acne scars: (A) Before (B) After 4 sessions of fractional carbon-dioxide resurfacing (E—5 J/cm^2, 100 spots, 2 passes on scars).

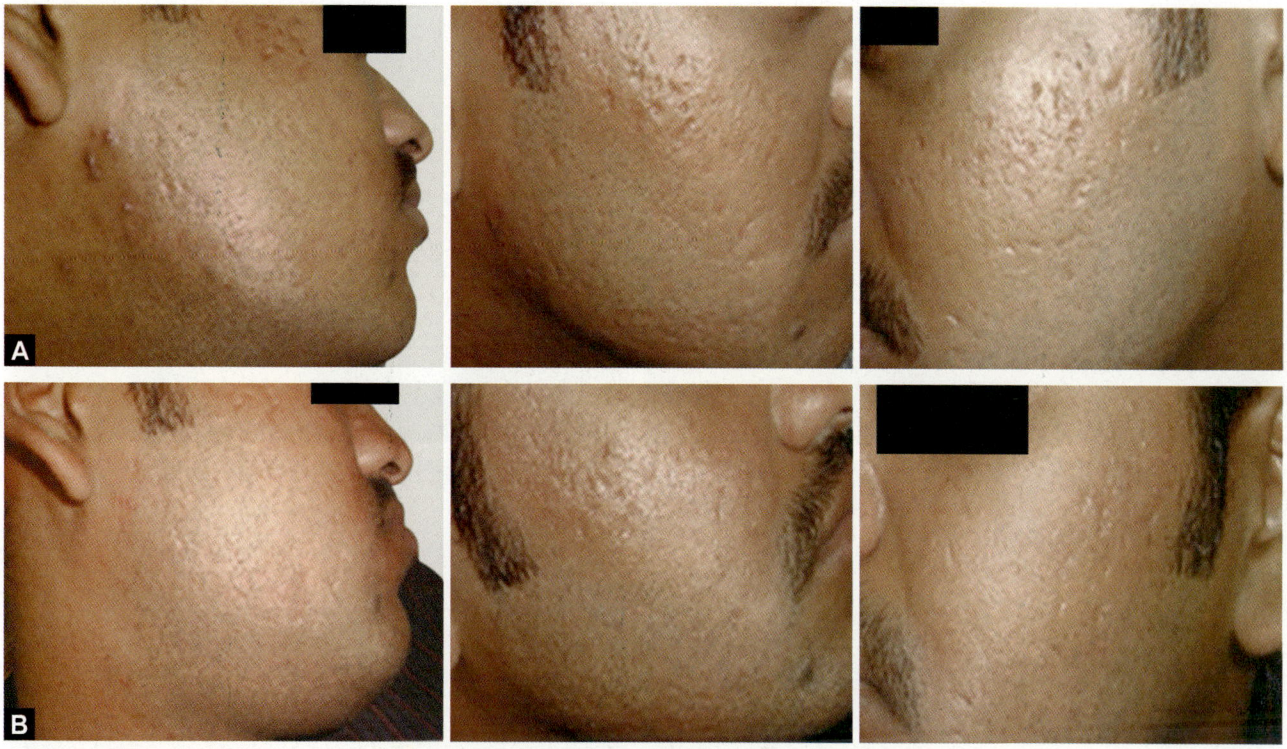

Figs. 46.5A and B: Grade 3 acne scars: (A) Before (B) After 4 sessions of fractional carbon-dioxide resurfacing (E—6 J/cm^2, 100 spots, 2 passes on scars). Shouldering of box scars with point beam ablation (E—2 J/cm^2).

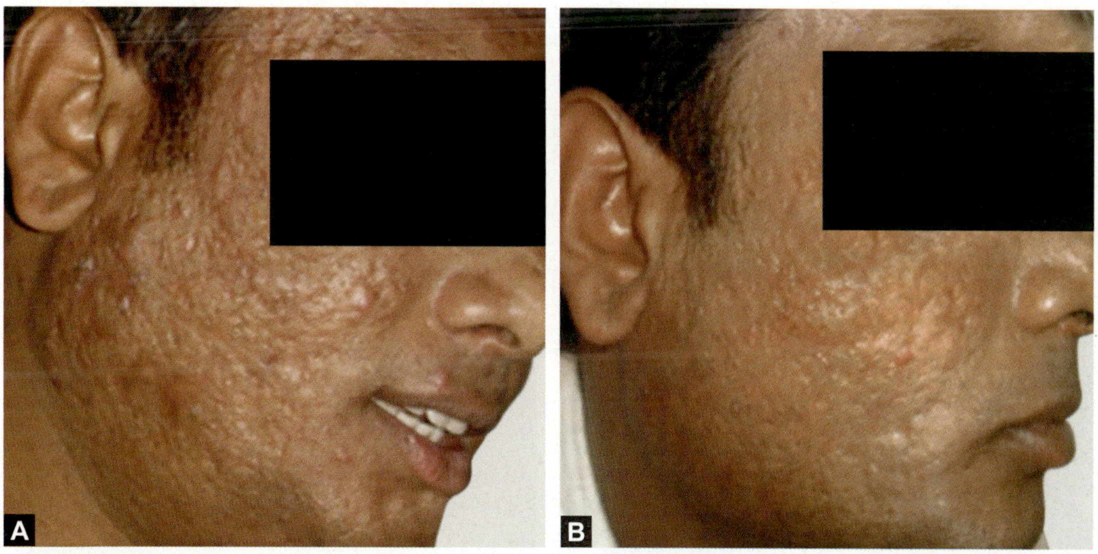

Figs. 46.6A and B: Grade 4 acne scars: (A) Before (B) After 6 sessions of fractional carbon-dioxide resurfacing (E—7–8 J/cm^2, full face laser resurfacing).

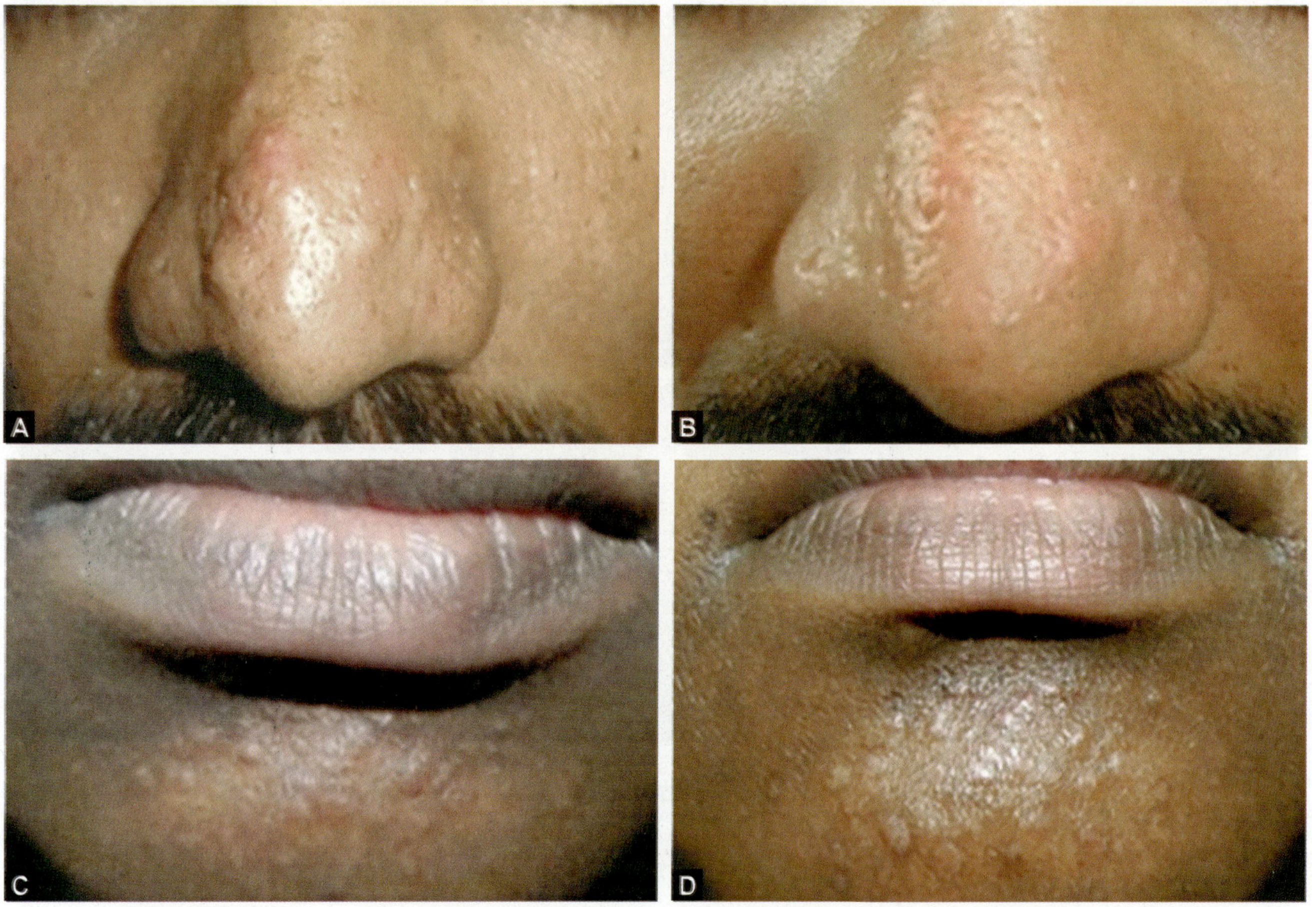

Figs. 46.7A to D: (A and B) Papular scars on nose and chin (C and D) After CO_2 ablation (parameters: energy—2 to 3 J/cm^2, power—20 W, 10 to 20 Hz). The lesions are ablated sequentially.

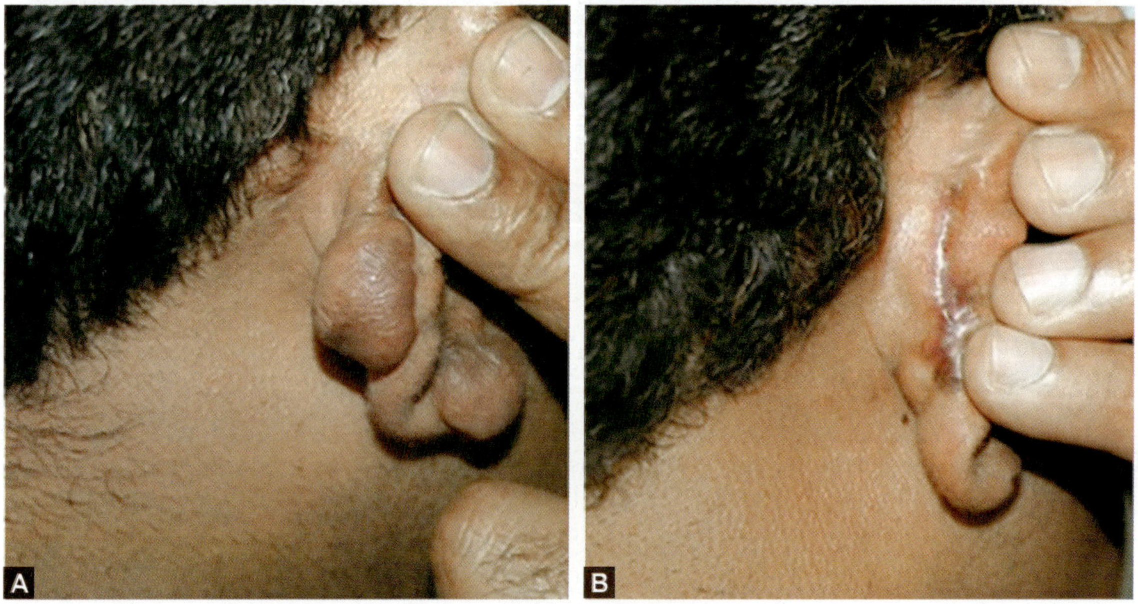

Figs. 46.8A and B: (A) Keloid on ear (B) After one session CO_2 ablation (parameters: energy—9 J/cm^2, power—30 W).

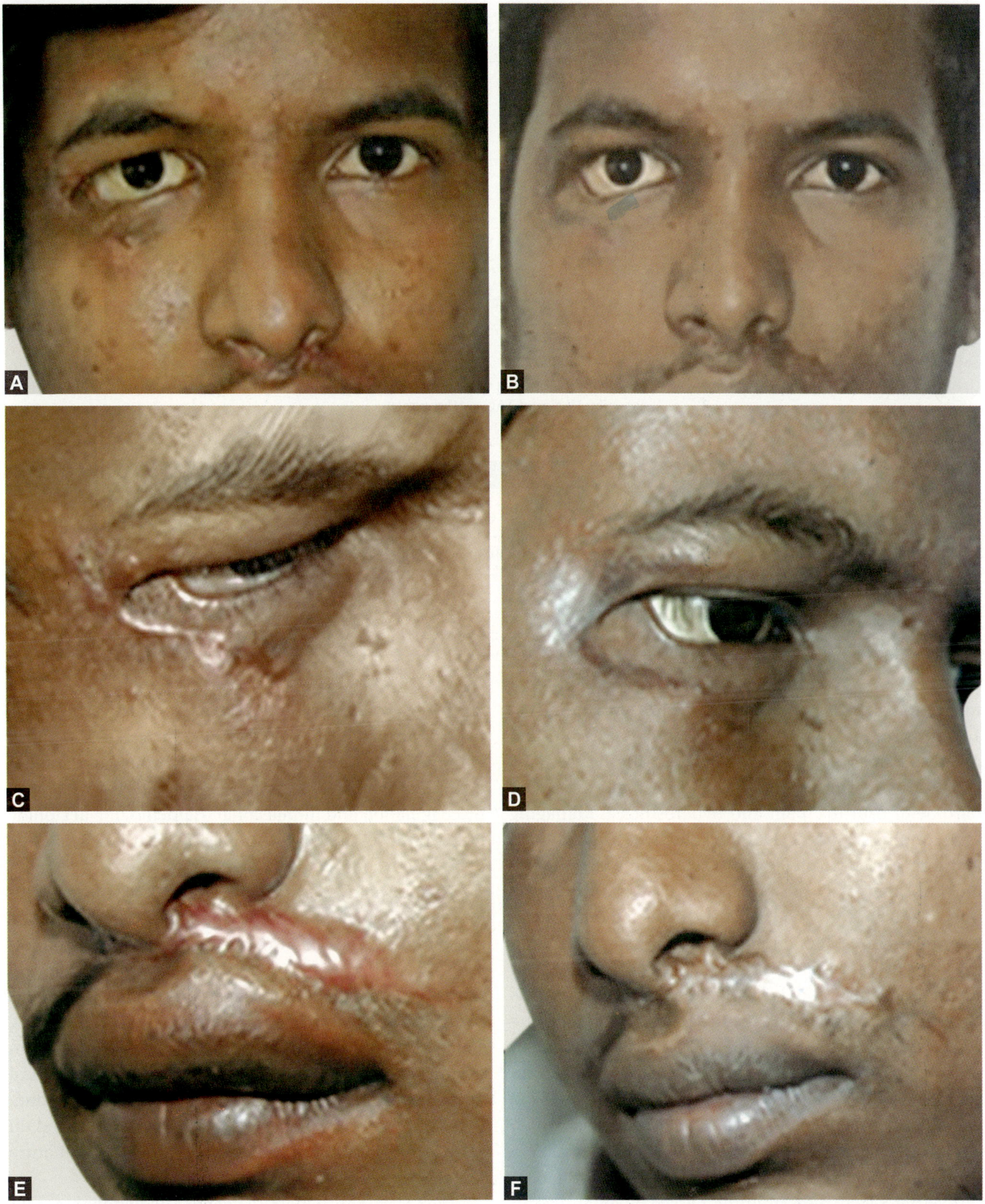

Figs. 46.9A to F: (A to C) Post-traumatic scar with ectropion (D to F) After 3 sessions of CO_2 laser with significant improvement in ectropion (parameters: E—80 mJ, P—30 W).

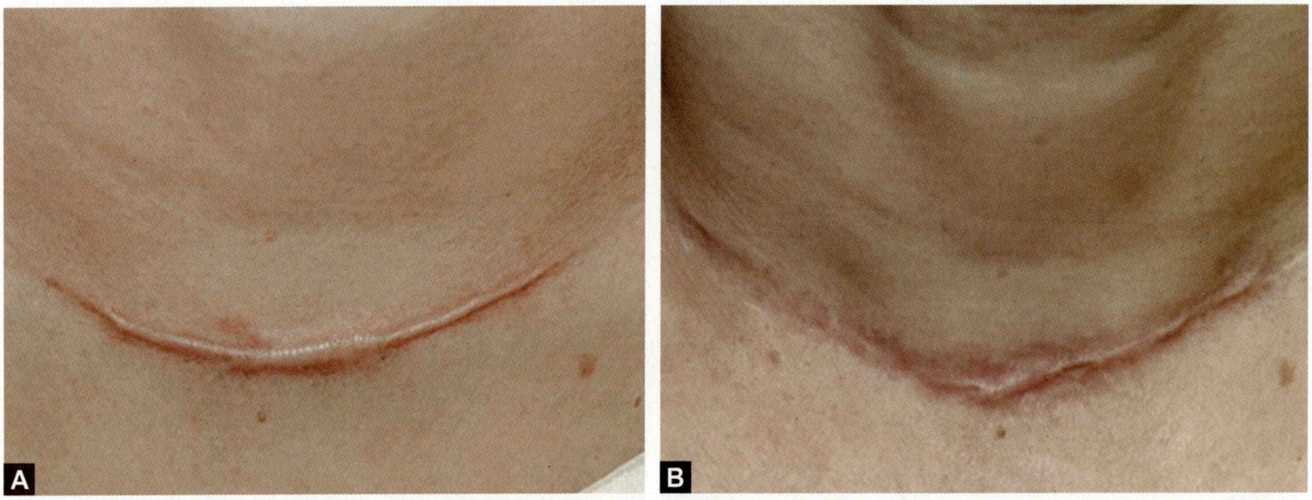

Figs. 46.10A and B: Improvement in hypertrophic scar following 6 sessions of PDL (4 J/cm², 5 mm, every 3–4 weeks followed by intralesional TAC—10 mg/mL).

Table 46.3: Laser for keloids and hypertrophic scars.

Type of scar and parameters	*CO_2 laser*	*QS Nd: YAG 1064*	*PDL 585*	*LP-Nd: YAG 1064 nm*
Hypertrophic scar	E: 20 to 30 mJ, Power: 20 W	1.8–2.2 J/cm², 7 mm spot size and 5–6 passes with 5–15% overlap	5.0 J/cm², every 2 weeks for 6 sessions	E: 65–75 J/cm², spot size 5 mm, an exposure time per pulse of 250 μs and 2 Hz.
Keloid	E: 60 to 90 mJ, Power: 40 W	Same	–	Same

to site and size of trauma. It can occur from 1 month to 1 year of trauma, with no spontaneous regression and mainly on areas of high anatomical risk. The early lesions are erythematous and tender. Old lesions are brown, hard, with pruritus, pain and hyperesthesia. Managing hypertrophic scars is easier than keloids, as prevention of recurrence itself is a challenge in keloids. The lasers in use include Ablative CO_2, Erbium:YAG, Pulsed dye laser, Long pulsed and QS Nd: YAG lasers. The expected outcome of laser treatment is reduction of symptoms, erythema and thickness of scar with improved pliability and cosmesis.[12-14]

The CO_2 ablation of keloids and hypertrophic scars is documented, however, the recurrence rates are high. The advantage of CO_2 laser is creating a dry surgical environment with minimal tissue trauma.[15] The author uses CO_2 ablation in ear lobe keloids (*see* Figs. 46.8A and B) and also for breaking the bridge between painful butterfly keloids on chest which is followed by preventive regimen for keloids.[16,17]

Procedure: The hypertrophic scar can be flattened to skin surface level with multiple passes by ablating and removing the charred tissue layer by layer. Since the wound is left for secondary healing, regular wound dressings have to be done till it heals. Keloids with narrow stalk are pulled with the forceps and cut through and through under focus beam. Ear lobe keloid can be excised with laser followed by coagulation and intralesional triamcinolone acetonide injection into and under the lesion. Flat keloid can be debulked in continuous mode.

The pulsed dye laser (PDL) is the choice of treatment for hypertrophic scars. The erythematous and early scars respond best. The 585 nm wavelength specifically targets blood vessels causing microvascular destruction and ischemia, alters the local collagen production, stimulates production of matrix metalloproteinase, including collagenase and causes flattening of scar.[18,19] Combination of intralesional corticosteroids and PDL gives better clinical outcomes (Figs. 46.9 and 46.10).[20-22] However, the data suggests recurrence are less, if treatment is continued till complete resolution of redness and induration (mature scars).

The LP Nd:YAG penetrate deeper and flattens resistant thick scars, by decreasing collagen production by

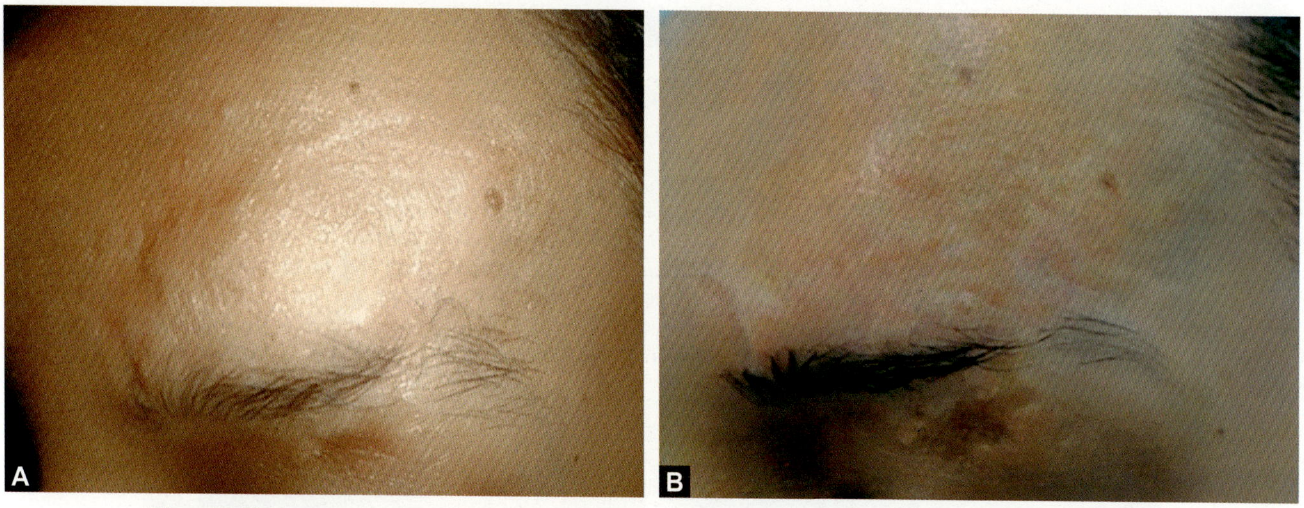

Figs. 46.11A and B: Improvement in post-traumatic atrophic scar following 6 sessions of fractional CO_2.

stimulating matrix metalloproteinases.[23] The 1064 nm Nd:YAG laser reduce the vascularity of pathological scar, this in turn may decrease cytokine or growth factor levels in the tissue, which, in turn promotes collagen deposition.[24-27.]

QS Nd:YAG 1064 nm with low fluence can be used in the treatment of keloids and hypertrophic scars.[28] The laser causes coagulation necrosis of vessels, breakdown of collagen, synthesis and realignment of new collagen.[21] QS Nd:YAG-induced neocollagen (nonkeloidal collagen) production and collagen remodeling by thermal damage might also have a role in the clinical improvement of keloids and hypertrophic scars.[29,30]

532 nm, frequency-doubled, Nd:YAG laser targets both oxyhemoglobin and melanin and can be a promising treatment for pigmented keloid and hypertrophic.[31] The decrease of pigmentation in scars, will obscure the distinctive border between the scar and surrounding skin. There can be a risk of post-therapy dyschromia.

Nonablative fractional photothermolysis with near infrared 1,540 and 1,550 nm erbium-doped fiber lasers is a new modality to tackle hypertrophic scars. Ablative fractional resurfacing lasers are employed for scar drug delivery to improve outcomes in future. A single case report recently demonstrated marked improvement in a meshed split grafted burn scar after a single treatment with ablative fractional CO_2 laser.[32,33] Author uses fractional resurfacing followed by triamcinolone acetonide 10 mg/mL to be spread on resurfaced area, to increase the pliability of scar. It improves scar in 2 to 4 sessions depending on thickness.

ATROPHIC SCARS

Atrophic scars are depressed scars resulting due to inflammatory process, such as trauma, acne or varicella and surgical incisions (Figs. 46.11A and B). Atrophy is due to inflammatory destruction of collagen with resultant dermal atrophy. Early lesions are erythematous and with time, become increasingly fibrotic and hypopigmented. In recent era, lasers are the mainstay of treatment.

Laser Treatment of Atrophic Scars

Include use of ablative lasers (CO_2, Erbium), nonablative lasers, ablative and nonablative fractional modalities, and PDLs that target vascular components of atrophic scars (Table 46.4). Ablative Er:YAG lasers is the best option for mild atrophic scars like varicella scars. Both Fractional CO_2 and erbium lasers are preferable for more extensive atrophic scars as in acne scaring.

LASERS FOR SCAR PREVENTION

Lasers for scar prevention are becoming increasingly popular. The treatment must target both the mechanism of abnormal scar formation and scar morphology itself.Author prefers to use laser that targets the vascular component of scar (PDL 585 nm/595 nm Nd:YAG toning) in severe grade acne, fresh scars and postscar revision surgeries to decrease inflammation and resulting in better remodeled scars (Figs. 46.12 and 46.13).

PDL selectively targets local microcirculation and decreases the TGF-β1expression. It also reduces fibroblast proliferation and collagen deposition.[39]

Table 46.4: Laser parameters for atrophic scaring.

Laser	*Parameters*	*Comments*
PDL[20,34,35]	4.5–5.5 J/cm^2 (average of 5.0 J/cm^2), once in 2 weeks for 4–6 sessions	It is the choice in all early or red /pink scars. 585 nm PDL use alone led to substantial clinical and histological improvement
Long-pulsed frequency doubled Nd:YAG laser[28]	Energy density is 17 J/cm^2 for pigmentation and 22 J/cm^2 for vascularity, with the laser automatically selecting pulse duration.	Choice in mature scars. An endpoint of vessel disappearance for vascular scars or darkening or graying of pigmented scars must be noted.
Er:YAG laser [36]	500–1200 mJ/pulse at 3.5–9 W was used. Two to five passes performed, every 6 weeks for 4 sessions	Scars from scratching, knife injury, laceration, simple excision and focal burn scars
1550 nm NAFL (nonablative fractional laser)[37,38]	40 mJ and treatment level 4 and subsequently increased in each visit according to the patients' tolerance level	Post surgical scars shows improvement in pigmentation, thickness, and pliability

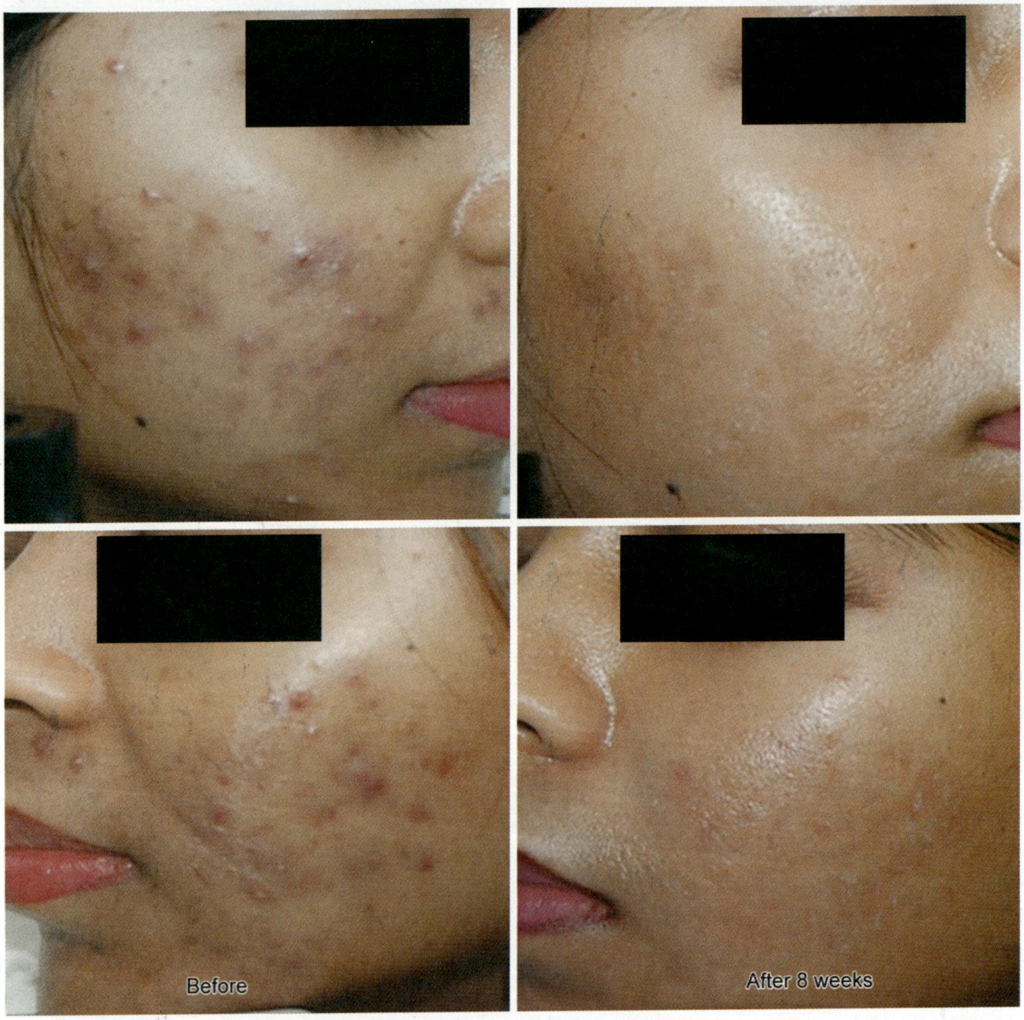

Fig. 46.12: Shows remodeling of acne scars after 595 QS Nd:YAG toning, 6 sessions, every 10 days.

McCraw et al showed in a study, that 585 nm PDL laser at initially low energy followed by standard-fluence starting 2 weeks after surgery or 1–2 weeks after suture removal for 3–6 sessions every 3–4 week sprevented scar hypertrophy.

In a study conducted by Nouri et al, the half of the scar treated with 3-monthly 585 nm PDL treatments scored over the other half that was not treated. The ideal PDL parameters for scar prevention is 585 nm wavelength;

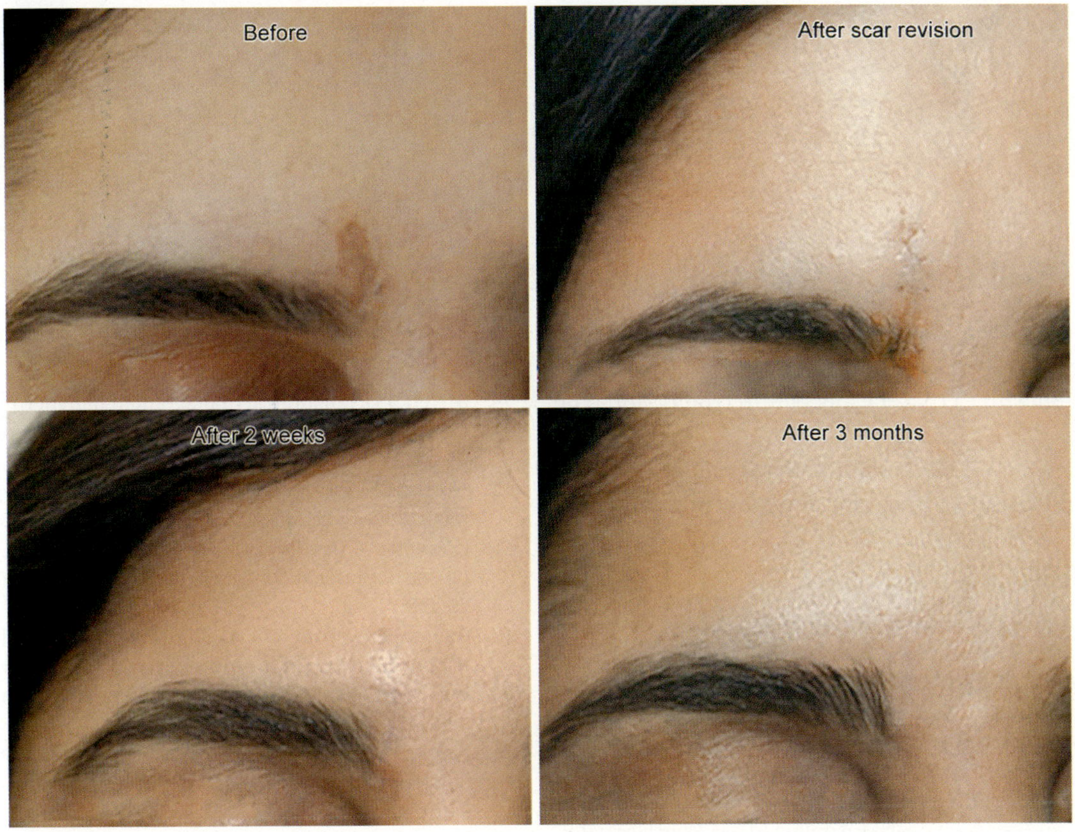

Fig. 46.13: Shows improvement in revised scar on forehead after 4 sessions PDL 585 nm, 4 J/cm^2, 2 to 3 passes, every week.

10 mm spot size; 3.5–5.5 J/cm^2 fluence; 450 ns–1.5 ms pulse duration; and two to three treatment sessions.[40-42]

Nonablative fractional Er: glass-Choe showed good scar improvement with 4-monthly treatments with the 1550 nm fractional Er: glass laser. 810 nm diode laser demonstrated that dermal heating in the postoperative period induces elevation of heat shock protein 70 that results in reduction in the synthesis of other proteins, causing a temporary cessation of cell proliferation.[43] Capon conducted study on surgical scar with patients receiving either a high dose (80–130 J/cm^2) or low dose (<80 J/cm^2) treatment with the 810 nm diode laser to half the scar; the other half of the scar was left untreated, the high-energy-treated group showed greater improvement.[44-47]

STRETCH MARKS

Stretch marks are benign, but can have great psychological implications especially in female.[48] They results due to changes in extracellular matrix, elastin and collagen.[49] Elastin is the primary target and later affects other components. In early stage they are red/violaceous and later stage, they are white and atrophic. Though various treatment modalities exist (tretinoin 0.1%, glycolic acid 20% or combination of glycolic acid and tretinoin), there is no effective remedy. Various lasers and lights are used widely, that include 585 nm pulsed dye laser, 308 nm excimer laser, 1064 nm long pulsed Nd:YAG laser, fractional laser and IPL.

The 585 PDL is employed in early red striae. PDL: 7 mm, fluence of 2–4 J/cm^2, single pass with 20% overlap can significantly remodel the stretch marks and bring desired response in stria rubra. Author suggests 6 sessions every 2 weeks (Fig. 46.14).[50,51]

The excimer 308 nm laser, improves the stretch marks by improving the pigmentation.[21]

Long pulsed Nd-Yag 1064 nm has shown satisfactory results in early striae.[52,53]

The fractional CO_2 and erbium Yag laser significantly improves the mature stretch marks, by stimulating new collagen and elastin synthesis. A study evaluated efficacy of IPL (monthly twice) and fractional CO_2(monthly once) and found fractional CO_2 to be more effective.

IPL works through fibroblast stimulation and collagen deposition, with minimal side effects. There is a risk of hyper

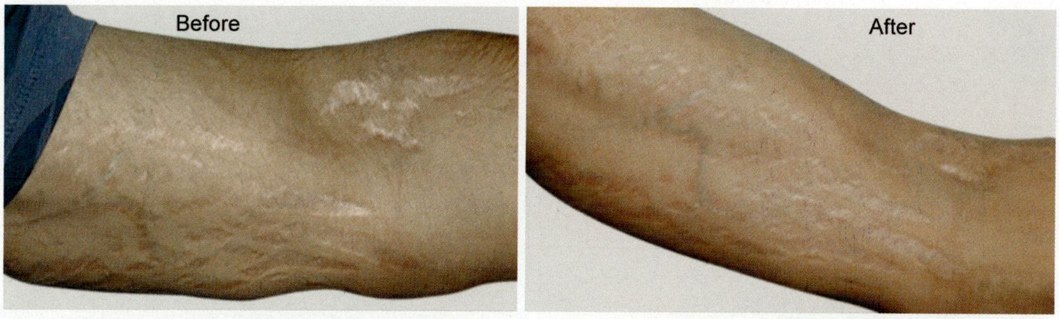

Fig. 46.14: Improvement in striae following 6 sessions of PDL 585 nm, 5 J/cm², every 2 weeks.

pigmentation with CO_2 laser especially in type IV and type V skin types.[54-56]

Nonablative 1550 nm, erbium doped fiber laser improved the color and texture of striae alba and rubra in Asian skin.[57]

REFERENCES

1. Rivera AE. Acne scarring: a review and current treatment modalities. J Am Acad Dermatol. 2008;59:659-76.
2. Gladstone HB, Berg D, McDonald M. Scar revision. Dermatol Res Pract. 2010;2010: 545796.
3. Goodman GJ, Baron JA. Postacne scarring: a qualitative global scarring grading system. Dermatol Surg. 2006;32:1458-66.
4. Jacob CI, Dover JS, Kaminer MS. Acne scarring: a classification system and review of treatment options. J AM Acad Dermatol. 2001;45:109-17.
5. Apfelberg DB. A critical appraisal of high-energy pulsed carbon dioxide laser facial resurfacing for acne scars. Ann Plast Surg. 1997;38:95-100.
6. Manstein D, Herron GS, Sink RK, et al. Fractional photothermolysis: a new concept for cutaneous remodeling using microscopic patterns of thermal injury. Lasers Surg Med. 2004;34:426-38.
7. Ciocon DH, Doshi D, Goldberg DJ. Nonablative lasers. Curr Probl Dermatol. 2011;42:48-55.
8. DeHoratius DM, Dover JS. Nonablative tissue remodeling and photorejuvenation. Clin Dermatol. 2007;25(5):474-9.
9. Yaghmai D, Garden JM, Bakus AD, et al. Comparison of a 1,064 nm laser and a 1,320 nm laser for the nonablative treatment of acne scars. Dermatol Surg. 2005;31(8 Pt 1):903-9.
10. Seaton ED, Mouser PE, Charakida A, et al. Investigation of the mechanism of action of nonablative pulsed-dye laser therapy in photorejuvination and inflammatory acne vulgaris. Br J Dermatol. 2006;155:748-55.
11. Manuskiatti W, Fitzpatrick RE, Goldman MP. Long-term effectiveness and side effects of carbon dioxide laser resurfacing for photoaged facial skin. J Am Acad Dermatol. 1999;40:401-11.
12. Bouzari N, Davis SC, Nouri K. Laser treatment of keloids and hypertrophic scars. Int J Dermatol. 2007;46:80-8.
13. Ketchum LD, Cohen IK, Masters FW. Hypertrophic scars and keloids: a collective review. Plast Reconstr Surg. 1974;53: 140-54.
14. Atiyeh BS. Nonsurgical management of hypertrophic scars: evidence-based therapies, standard practices, and emerging methods. Aesthetic Plast Surg. 2007;31:468-92.
15. Norris JCE. The effect of carbon dioxide laser surgery on the recurrence of keloids. Plast Reconstr Surg. 1991;87:44-53.
16. Connell PG, Harland CC. Treatment of keloid scars with pulsed dye laser and intralesional steroid. J Cutan Laser Ther. 2000;2:147-50.
17. Asilian A, Darougheh A, Shariati F. New combination of triamcinolone, 5-Fluorouracil, and pulsed-dye laser for treatment of keloid and hypertrophic scars. Dermatol Surg. 2006;32:907-15.
18. Paquet P, Hermanns JF, Piérard GE. Effect of the 585 nm flash lamp-pumped pulsed dye laser for the treatment of keloids. Dermatol Surg. 2001;27:171-4.
19. Dierickx C, Goldman MP, Fitzpatrick RE. Laser treatment of erythematous/hypertrophic and pigmented scars in 26 patients. Plast Reconstr Surg. 1995;95:84-90; discussion 91-2.
20. Alster T. Laser scar revision: comparison study of 585 nm pulsed-dye laser with and without intralesional corticosteroids. Dermatol Surg. 2003;29:25-9.
21. Bowes LE, Nouri K, Berman B, et al. Treatment of pigmented hypertrophic scars with the 585 nm pulsed dye laser and the 532 nm frequency-doubled Nd:YAG laser in the Q-switched and variable pulse modes: a comparative study. Dermatol Surg. 2002;28: 714-9.
22. Manuskiatti W, Wanitphakdeedecha R, Fitzpatrick RE. Effect of pulsed width of a 595 nm flash lamp-pumped pulsed dye laser on the treatment response of keloidal and hypertrophic sternotomy scars. Dermatol Surg. 2007;33:152-61.
23. Koike et al. Nd:YAG Laser treatment for keloids and hypertrophic scars. Plast Reconstr Surg. Glob Open. 2014;2:e272.
24. Akaishi S, Koike S, Dohi T, et al. Nd:YAG laser treatment of keloids and hypertrophic scars. E plasty. 2012;12:e1.
25. Akaishi S, Akimoto M, Ogawa R, et al. The relationship between keloid growth pattern and stretching tension: visual analysis using the finite element method. Ann Plast Surg. 2008;60:445-51.
26. Rossi A, Lu R, Frey MK, et al. The use of the 300 microsecond1064 nm Nd:YAG laser in the treatment of keloids. J Drugs Dermatol. 2013;12:1256-62.
27. Landthaler M, Haina D, Brunner R, et al. Neodymium-YAG laser therapy for vascular lesions. J Am Acad Dermatol.1986;14:107-17.

28. Cho SB, Lee JH, Lee SH, et al. Efficacy and safety of 1064 nm Q-switched Nd:YAG laser with low fluence for keloids and hypertrophic scars. JEADV. 2010;24;1070-4.
29. Lee MC, Hu S, Chen MC, et al. Skin rejuvenation with 1,064 nm Q-switched Nd:YAG laser in Asian patients. Dermatol Surg. 2009;35:929-32.
30. Godberg DJ, Silapunt S. Histological evaluation of a Q-switched Nd:YAG laser in the nonablative treatment of wrinkles. Dermatol Surg. 2001;27:744-6.
31. Bouzari N, Davis SC, Nouri K. Laser treatment of keloids and hypertrophic scars. Int J Dermatol. 2007;46:80-8.
32. Haedersdal M. Fractional ablative CO_2 laser resurfacing improves a thermal burn scar. J Eur Acad Dermatol Venereol. 2009;23(11):1340-1.
33. Haedersdal M, Moreau KE, et al. Fractional nonablative 1540 nm laser resurfacing for thermal burn scars: a randomized controlled trial. Lasers Surg Med. 2009;41(3):189-95.
34. Alster T, Zaulyanov L. Laser scar revision: a review. Dermatol Surg. 2007;33:131-40.
35. Kerwin LY, El Tal AK, Stiff MA, et al. Scar prevention and remodeling: a review of the medical, surgical, topical and light treatment approaches. Int J Dermatol. 2014; 53:922-36.
36. Kwon SD, Kye YC. Treatment of scars with a pulsed Er:YAG laser. J Cutan Laser Ther. 2000;2:27-31.
37. Pham AM, Greene RM, Woolery-Lloyd H, et al. 1550 nm nonablative laser resurfacing for facial surgical scars. Arch Facial Plast Surg. 2011;13:203-10.
38. Tierney E, Mahmoud BH, Srivastava D, et al. Treatment of surgical scars with nonablative fractional laser versus pulsed dye laser: a randomized controlled trial. Dermatol Surg. 2009;35:1172-80.
39. Kuo YR, Jeng SF, Wang FS, et al. Flash lamp pulsed dye laser (PDL) suppression of keloid proliferation through down-regulation of TGF-beta1 expression and extracellular matrix expression. Lasers Surg Med. 2004;34:104-8.
40. Nouri K, Rivas MP, Stevens M, et al. Comparison of thee effectiveness of the pulsed dye laser 585 nm versus 595 nm in the treatment of new surgical scars. Lasers Med Sci. 2009;24:801-10.
41. Alam M, Pon K, van Laborde S, et al. Clinical effect of a single pulsed dye laser treatment of fresh surgical scars: randomized controlled trial. Dermatol Surg. 2006; 32:21-5.
42. Conologue TD, Norwood C. Treatment of surgical scars with the cryogen-cooled 595 nm pulsed dye laser starting on the day of suture removal. Dermatol Surg. 2006;32:13-20.
43. Souil E, Capon A, Mordon S, et al. Treatment with 815 nm diode laser induces long-lasting expression of 72-kDa heat shock protein in normal rat skin. Br J Dermatol. 2001;144:260-6.
44. McCraw JB, McCraw JA, McMellin A, et al. Prevention of unfavorable scars using early pulse dye laser treatments: a preliminary report. Ann Plast Surg. 1999;42:7-14.
45. Nouri K, Jimenez GP, Harrison-Balestra C, et al. 585 nm pulsed dye laser in the treatment of surgical scars starting on the suture removal day. Dermatol Surg. 2003;29:65-73.
46. Choe JH, Park YL, Kim BJ, et al. Prevention of thyroidectomy scar using a new 1,550 nm fractional erbium-glass laser. Dermatol Surg. 2009;35:1199-205.
47. Capon A, Iarmarcoval G, Gonnelli D, et al. Scar prevention using laser-assisted skin healing (LASH) in plastic surgery. Aesthet Plast Surg. 2010;34:438-46.
48. El Taieb MA, Ibrahim AK. Fractional CO_2 laser versus intense pulsed light in treating striae distensae. Indian J Dermatol. 2016;61:174-80.
49. Elsaie ML, Baumann LS, Elsaaiee LT. Striae distensae (stretch marks) and different modalities of therapy: An update. Dermatol Surg. 2009;35:563-73.
50. McDaniel DH, Ash K, Zukowski M. Treatment of stretch marks with the 585 nm flash lamp-pumped pulsed dye laser. Dermatol Surg. 1996;22:332-7.
51. Jimenez GP, Flores F, Berman B, et al. Treatment of striae rubra and striae alba with the 585 nm pulsed-dye laser. Dermatol Surg. 2003;29:362-5.
52. Goldberg DJ, Marmur ES, Hussain M. 308 nm excimer laser treatment of mature hypopigmented striae. Dermatol Surg. 2003;29:596-9.
53. Goldman A, Rossato F, Prati C. Stretch marks: Treatment using the 1,064 nm Nd:YAG laser. Dermatol Surg. 2008;34;686-91.
54. Savas JA, Ledon JA, Franca K, et al. Lasers and lights for the treatment of striae distensae. Lasers Med Sci. 2014;29:1735-43.
55. Lee SE, Kim JH, Lee SJ, et al. Treatment of striae distensae using an ablative 10,600 nm carbon dioxide fractional laser: A retrospective review of 27 participants. Dermatol Surg. 2010;36:1683-90.
56. Cho SB, Lee SJ, Lee JE, et al. Treatment of striae alba using the 10,600 nm carbon dioxide fractional laser. J Cosmet Laser Ther. 2010;12:118-9.
57. Wanner M, Tanzi EL, Alster TS. Fractional photothermolysis: Treatment of facial and nonfacial cutaneous photodamage with a 1,550 nm erbium-doped fiber laser. Dermatol Surg. 2007;33:23-8.

CHAPTER 47

Lasers in Dermatosurgery: Treating Excessive Hair

BS Chandrashekar, Teena Ramesh, Madura C

INTRODUCTION

Laser hair removal (LHR) is a well-established treatment for hirsutism or unwanted body hair. Photoepilation by laser or light-based devices is one of the most common procedures in aesthetic practice. But, it was not until Anderson and Parrish proposed the, "Theory of selective photothermolysis", that the concept of selectively targeting a particular chromophore on the basis of its absorption spectra and size was realized.[1] Laser hair removal was first done in 1996 when the long-pulse ruby laser was introduced. Alternative methods for hair removal include plucking, bleaching, shaving, waxing and chemical depilation but none of these provide a long lasting solution.[2] Electrolysis causes permanent hair removal of terminal, nonterminal as well as non-pigmented; however, this technique is impractical while treating large areas.[3]

Increased hair growth congenital or otherwise at aberrant body sites leads to functional impairment and psychological morbidity affects the psyche of the individual. This chapter deals with the application of laser hair removal for treating noncosmetic indications, such as acne keloidalis nuchae, hidradenitis suppurativa, trichostasis spinulosa and also for aesthetic correction of hairline post hair transplant.

MECHANISM OF LASER HAIR REMOVAL

The wavelength range of hair removal lasers is between 600 nm and 1100 nm, and the melanin present in the hair shaft and the hair follicle can absorb the laser energy within this wavelength. There are classically three ways by which lasers can destroy the hair follicles: (a) by producing local heating, (b) mechanically by shock waves and cavitation and (c) photochemically by generating singlet oxygen and free radicals which act as toxic mediators. Removal of hair has been attempted by all three means (Table 47.1)

The theory of selective photothermolysis aids one to selectively target the melanin in the hair shaft and bulb of the pigmented hair follicle as chromophore. To achieve optimum results, this theory of selective photothermolysis must be modified for laser hair removal. The theory states that, by using the appropriate wavelength, adequate pulse duration and correct fluence, thermal injury can be limited to the chromophore, thereby protecting the surrounding tissue.[1]

The pulse duration should be shorter than or equal to the thermal relaxation time of the hair shaft which is estimated to be in the range of 10–100 milliseconds. Thermal relaxation time (TRT) is defined as the time required for the targeted heated tissue to lose half its heat.

The heat into the surrounding tissues of the hair follicle and not only the bulb and hair shaft, is required for more permanent hair reduction. Taking this into account, longer pulse durations are necessary to achieve targeted thermal destruction of the entire hair follicle.[4]

Melanocytic outer root sheath, the shaft and matrix are the major targets for laser within the follicular unit. Stem cells play a crucial role in the hair development and growth. Lasers must destroy not only the hair follicle, but also the progenitor cells for permanent inhibition of hair growth. The "split fuse" hypothesis mentions two main

Table 47.1: Mechanisms for hair removal.

Photothermal destruction
• Long-pulsed ruby laser
• Long-pulsed alexandrite laser
• Long-pulsed diode laser
• Long-pulsed Nd:YAG laser
• Pulsed, noncoherent broadband light source
Photomechanical destruction
• Q-switched Nd:YAG laser
• Carbon suspension Q-switched Nd:YAG laser
Photochemical destruction
• Photodynamic therapy

stem cells reservoirs in the anagen hair follicle. A group of amelanotic cells located at proximal outer root sheath, which may also be the melanocytic reservoir. The second group is hypothesized to be located in the distal outer root sheath.[5]

In the human hair follicle, the location of the bulge is thought to reside in the lower third of the follicle of the outer root sheath. Therefore, to achieve permanent hair reduction with lasers, an extended theory of selective photothermolysis was proposed which requires diffusion of heat from the chromophore to the desired target for destruction.[6] In order to accomplish this goal, longer pulse durations are necessary to propagate heat to the entire hair follicle.[7]

DIVERSE APPLICATIONS OF LASER HAIR REMOVAL[8]

- Hypertrichosis and hirsutism
- Pseudofolliculitis barbae
- Acne keloidalis nuchae
- Hidradenitis suppurativa
- Pilonidal sinus
- Pseudofolliculitis
- Hair-bearing skin flaps/grafts
- Hairy Becker's nevus
- Trichostasis spinulosa
- Keratosis pilaris
- Miscellaneous conditions like recurrent folliculitis of the bikini area, aesthetic correction of hairline after hair transplant, fawn tail nevus, etc.

HYPERTRICHOSIS AND HIRSUTISM

Hypertrichosis refers to the growth of hair on any part of the body in excess of the amount usually present in persons of the same age, race, and sex, excluding androgen-induced hair growth whereas, hirsutism is defined as excessive growth of androgen dependent sexual hair. Irrespective of the cause, the cosmetic embarrassment caused, results in a significant emotional burden. LHR has proved to be beneficial in the management of both. Choice of laser depends on the thickness of hair and the skin type (Figs. 47.1 to 47.3).

Pseudofolliculitis barbae (PFB) is an inflammatory condition affecting the hair in the beard area. The growing

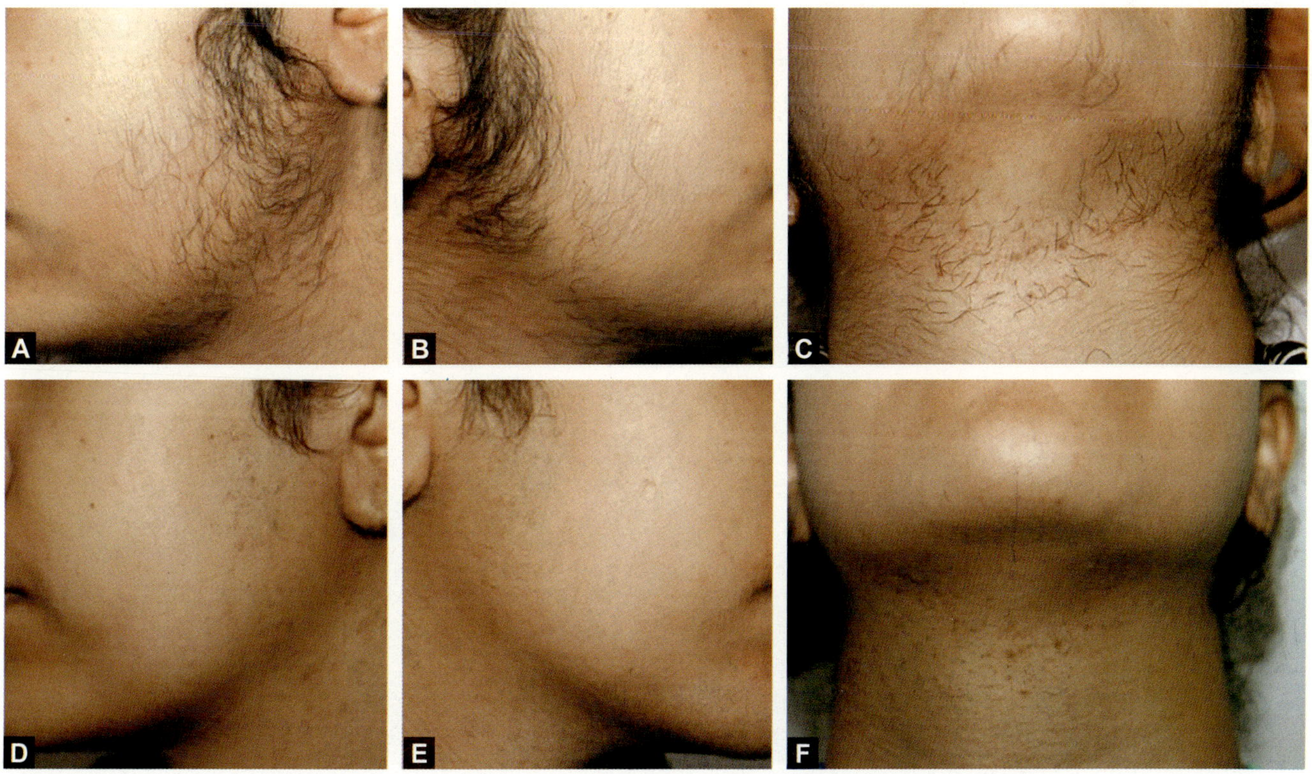

Figs. 47.1A to F: (A to C) Hirsutism; (D to F). After 8 sessions of diode laser, 808 nm, fluence 28–30 J/cm^2; spot 50 mm x 15 mm, PW 30–40 ms; interval of 4–6 weeks.

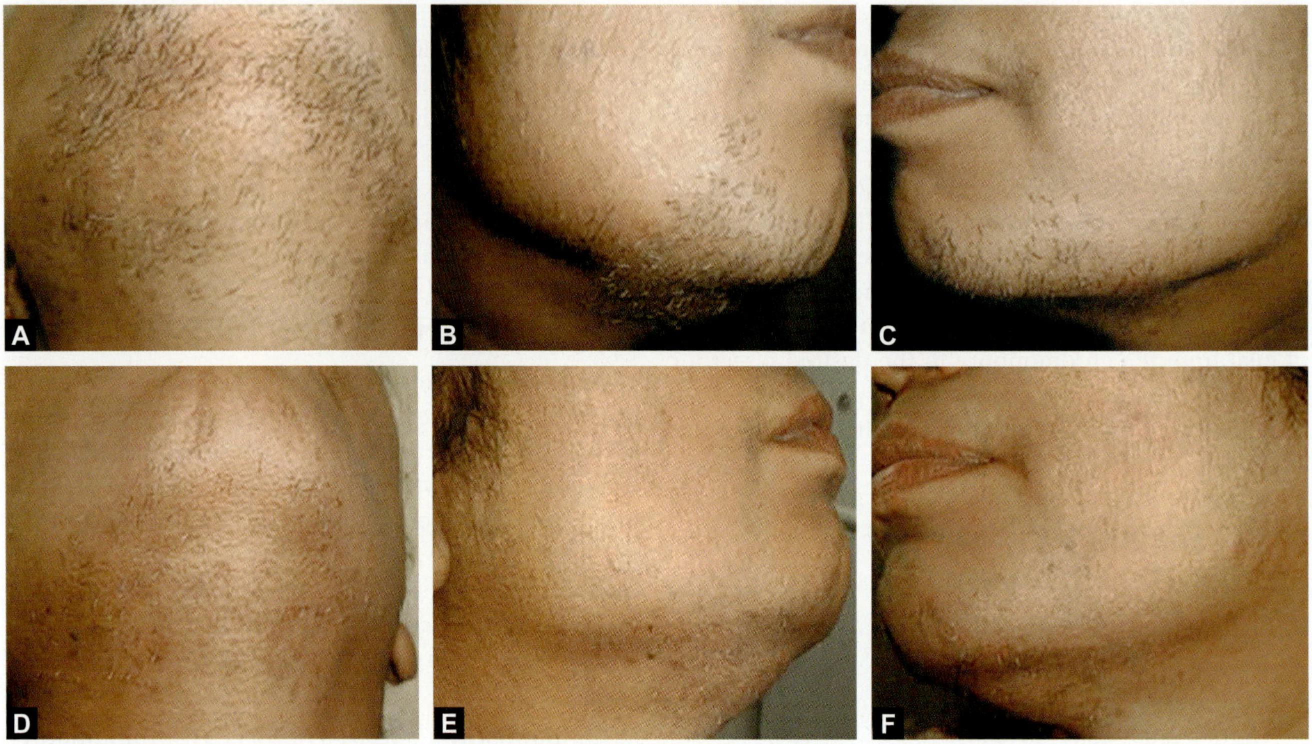

Figs. 47.2A to F: (A to C) Hirsutism; (D to F). After 8 sessions of LP Nd: YAG, 1064 nm, fluence 28–32 J/cm^2; spot 15 mm, PW 30–40 ms; interval of 4–6 weeks.

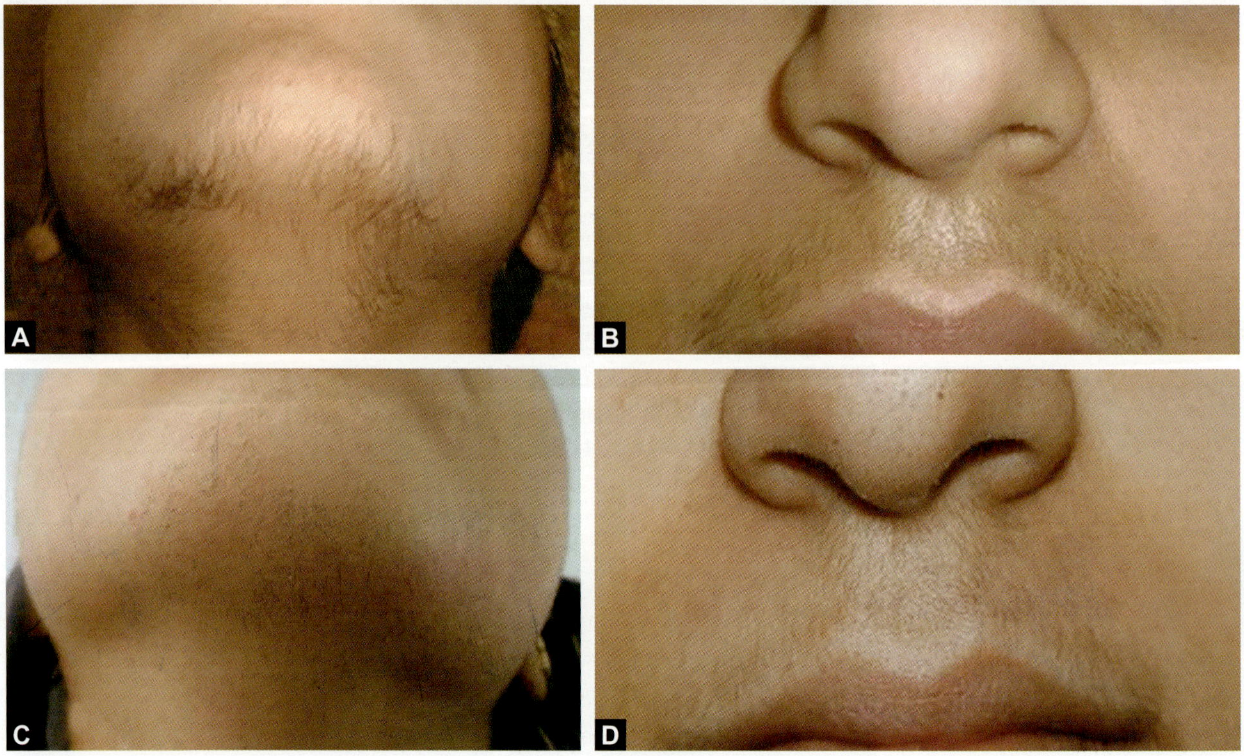

Figs. 47.3A to D: (A and B) Hirsutism; (C and D). After 6 sessions of IPL laser, 645 nm, fluence 9–15 J/cm^2; spot 10 mm × 48 mm, PW 20–40 ms; interval of 4 weeks.

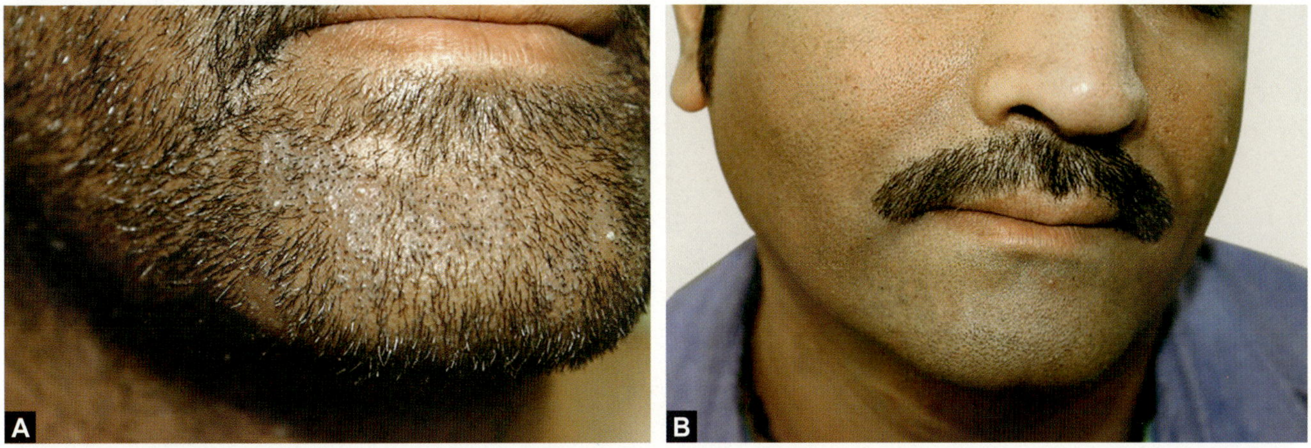

Figs. 47.4A and B: (A) Pseudofolliculitis barbae; (B) After 4 sessions of LP Nd: YAG, 1064 nm, fluence 28–32 J/cm^2; spot 12 mm, PW 30 ms; Interval of 8 weeks.

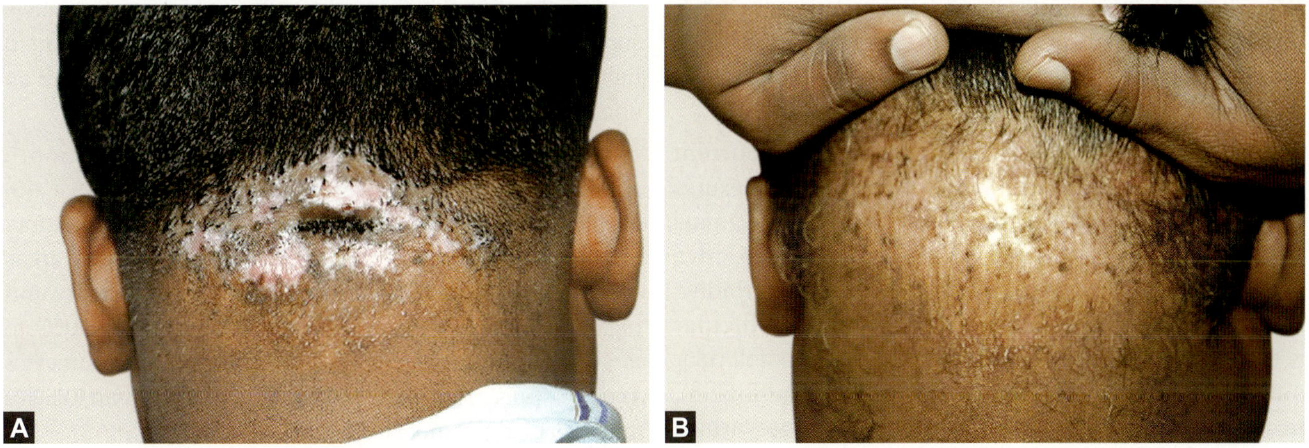

Figs. 47.5A and B: (A) Acne keloidalis nuchae; (B) After 10 sessions of Nd:YAG (fluence 36 J/cm^2, pulse width 40 ms, spot size 15 mm).

follicles, which are placed at an acute angle to the surface of the skin re-enters the skin at or next to the follicular opening. These misdirected follicles lead to formation of inflammatory papules and pustules causing discomfort, secondary infection, and occasionally hypertrophic or keloidal scars (Figs. 47.4A and B). Six sessions of LHR done 6 to 8 weeks apart represents an effective option for reducing thickness of hair and subsequent papule formation in these patients.

Acne keloidalis nuchae (AKN) is a chronic inflammatory disorder of the posterior aspect of the neck and occipital region of the scalp. Despite numerous medical and surgical treatment modalities available only few offer cure or a superior cosmetic result for patients with extensive disease. Laser hair reduction can significantly improve this disfiguring early imitation of the treatment achieves better results and can limit the progression of the disease (Figs. 47.5A and B). Starting treatment as early as possible achieves the best results and can stop the disease process, if followed by maintenance sessions. Author follows a comprehensive regimen of surgical excision of large lesions, punch excision of small lesions, surface/intralesional cryotherapy for tumor stage of AKN in combination with intralesional triamcinolone acetonide to target the active and chronic stage of the disease. This is followed by LHR to achieve long-term remission (Figs. 47.6A and B). There must be no active infection during LHR. The long pulse Nd:YAG laser (1064 nm) and diode laser is the laser of choice and targets thick terminal hair. In AKN, the follicles are deeper and always follow tortuous course, especially in the tumor

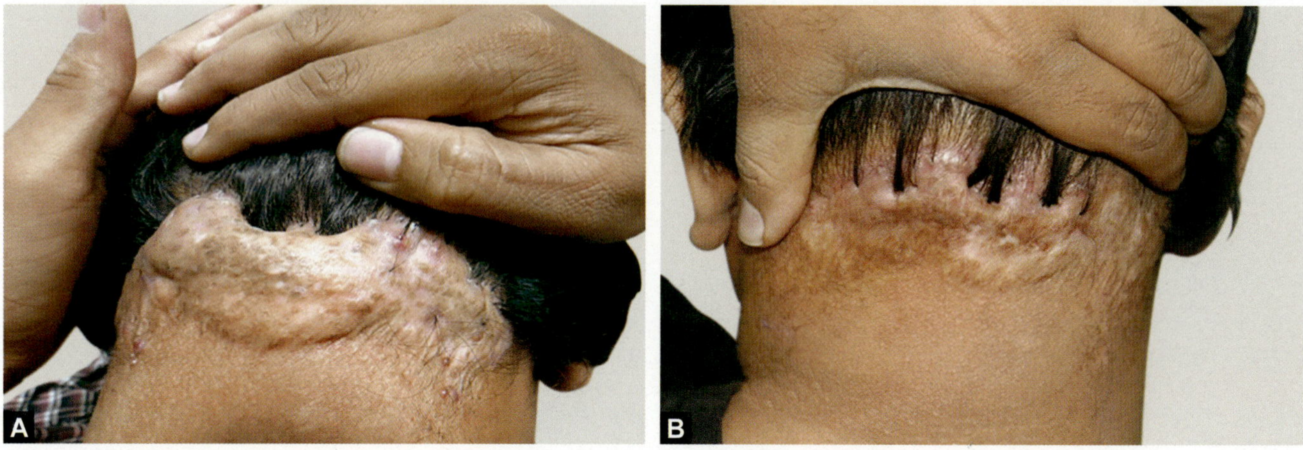

Figs. 47.6A and B: (A) Acne keloidalis nuchae; (B) After 10 sessions of LP Nd:YAG (1064 nm) (fluence 36 J/cm^2, pulse width 40 ms, spot size 15 mm) along with intralesional cryotherapy and intralesional triamcinolone acetonide.

stage. It is difficult to target; such hairs may require many sessions, as lasers cannot reach the target through such tunnels. It can be facilitated by using plastic cones to reach the target.

Hidradenitis suppurativa (HS) is a chronic, recurrent inflammatory disease primarily affecting the skin in flexures of the body, such as the axilla, inframammary and inguinal areas. It has been shown to have a significant negative impact on quality of life along with increased morbidity. Histopathologic studies have demonstrated follicular occlusion as the inciting event, this is followed by perifollicular inflammation and rupture of the follicular infundibulum, manifesting clinically as painful nodules and abscesses, which leads to the end result—sinus tract formation and scarring. LHR has dual action in the lesions of HS. First is, it helps in resolution of the active lesions and it also induces remission by photoepilation of the follicular unit and destruction of organized inflammatory lesions in the superficial to mid dermis.[9] It takes 4–6 sessions for complete reduction of hairs. The sessions are spaced once in 6–8 weeks, later increased to 8–10 weeks. The author has experience in using LP Nd:YAG 1064 nm for HS (Figs. 47.7A to D). The sessions are started in the inactive phase of the disease.

Pilonidal sinus disease is a persistent focus of sepsis initiated by a down-growth into the skin of unwanted hair. The hair serves as a breach in the dermis through which bacteria enter. They commonly occur in the natal cleft (Figs. 47.8A and B), but can also occur in the umbilicus, the axilla, and the interdigital web spaces. LHR represents an alternative and effective method of treatment, with a low complication rate, giving the sinus an opportunity to heal by prolonging the hair-free interval.[10]

Hair-bearing skin flaps and grafts used for reconstructive surgeries in the head and neck area might contain unwanted hair, leading to unacceptable cosmesis.[11] LHR provides an effective management of this condition.

Becker's nevus is an uncommon pigmented smooth muscle hamartoma that develops during adolescence and is characterized by hypertrichosis and hyperpigmentation. Shoulder, upper arm, and scapula are the common areas of involvement. LHR can decrease both hair density and pigmentation.[12] Authors use a combination of fractional CO_2 to target the keratinocytes, QS-Nd:YAG to target the melanocytes and long-pulsed Nd:YAG (1064 nm) to target the hair follicles and follicular melanocyte (Figs. 47.9A and B).

Trichostasis spinulosa is a common follicular disorder that results from the retention of multiple vellus hairs within pilosebaceous follicles (Figs. 47.10A and B). A variety of treatment modalities have been used with variable but largely transient success. LHR provides a safe and long-term effective treatment.[13] The laser of choice is LP Nd:YAG (1064 nm) because of variable spot size and adequate energy.

Laser hair removal is also utilized for miscellaneous conditions like keratosis pilaris, recurrent folliculitis of the bikini area, for aesthetic correction of hairline after hair transplantation (Figs. 47.11A and B), synophrys (Figs. 47.12A and B), etc.

DIFFERENT HAIR REMOVAL DEVICES

Long-pulsed Ruby Laser

The long-pulsed ruby laser (694 nm): The first device to be used for selective hair reduction was long-pulsed Ruby

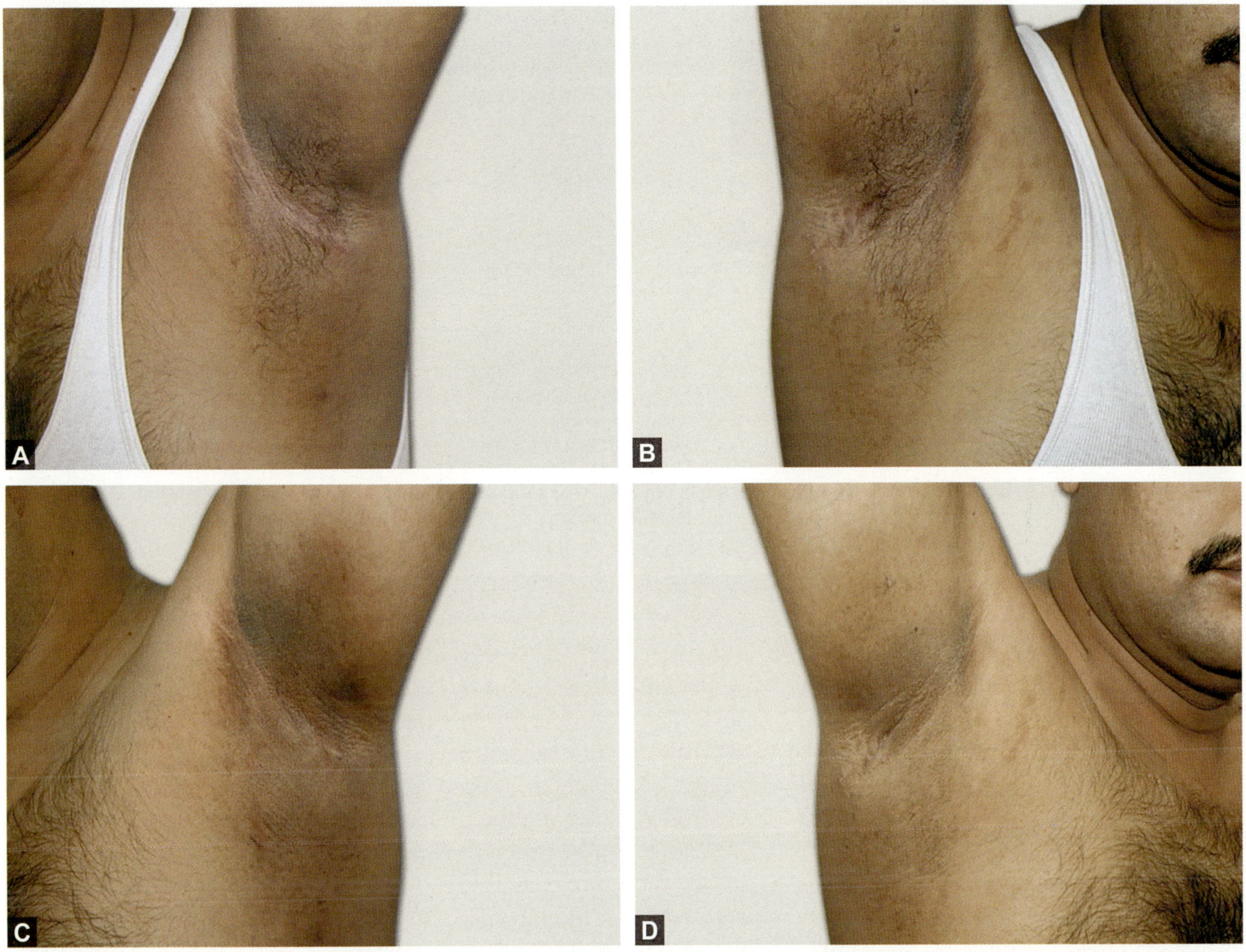

Figs. 47.7A to D: (A and B) Hidradenitis suppurativa; (C and D) after 6 sessions of LP Nd: YAG, 1064 nm, fluence 28–32 J/cm^2; spot size 15 mm, PW 30 ms; interval of 6 weeks.

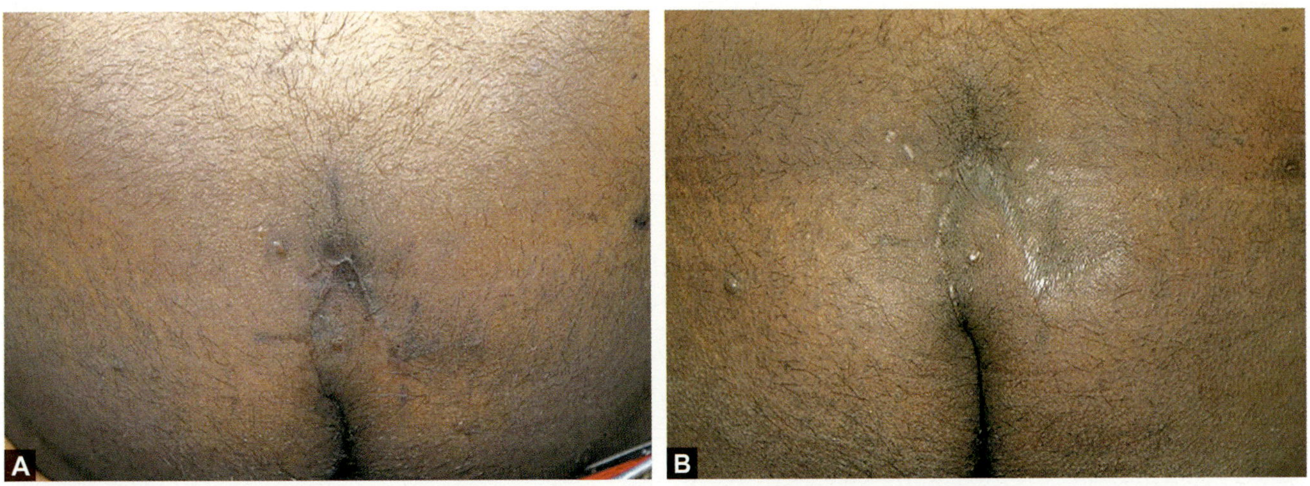

Figs. 47.8A and B: (A) Pilonidal sinus disease, post surgery; (B) After 5 sessions of LP Nd:YAG (1064 nm) fluence 26–34 J/cm^2, pulse width 20 ms, spot size 15 mm).

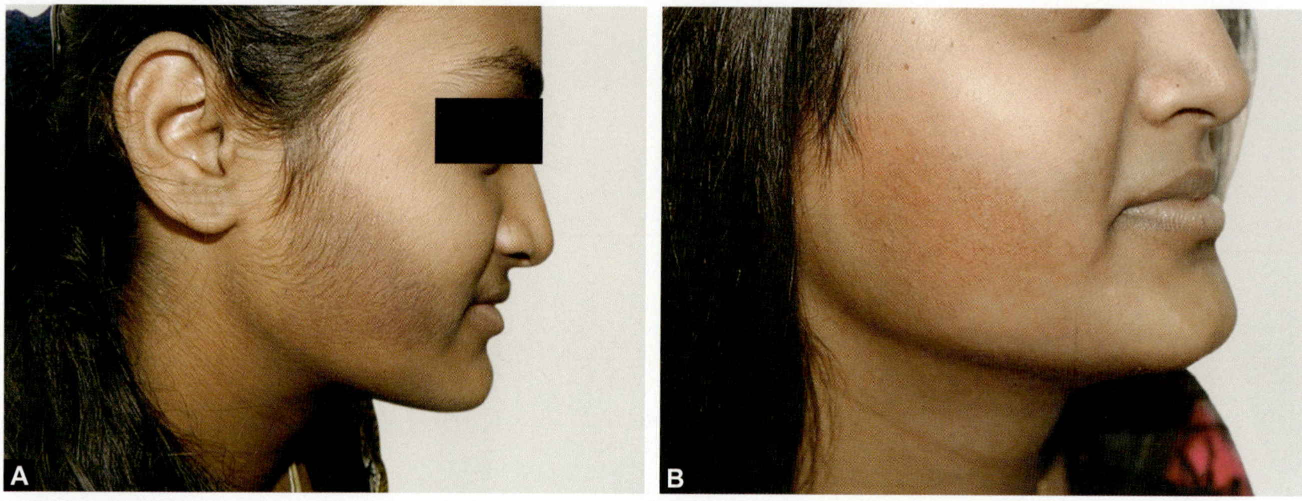

Figs. 47.9A and B: (A) Becker's nevus. (B) After 7 sessions of LPNd:YAG (1064 nm) (fluence 24–32 J/cm^2, pulse width 20 ms, spot size 15 mm).

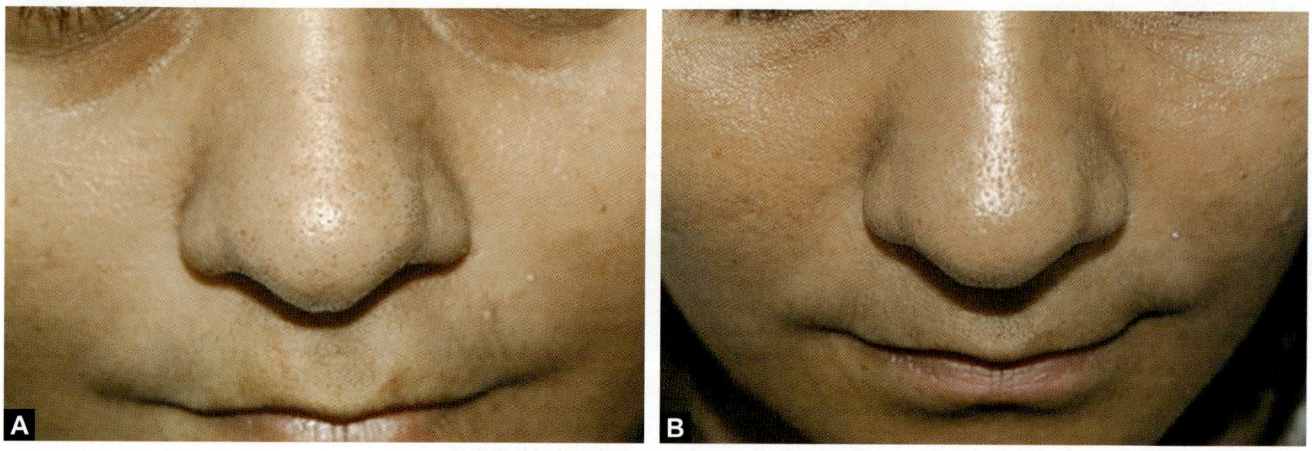

Figs. 47.10A and B: (A) Trichostasis spinulosa; (B) After 6 sessions of LP Nd:YAG (1064 nm) (fluence 24–32 J/cm^2, pulse width 5–12 ms, spot size 15 mm).

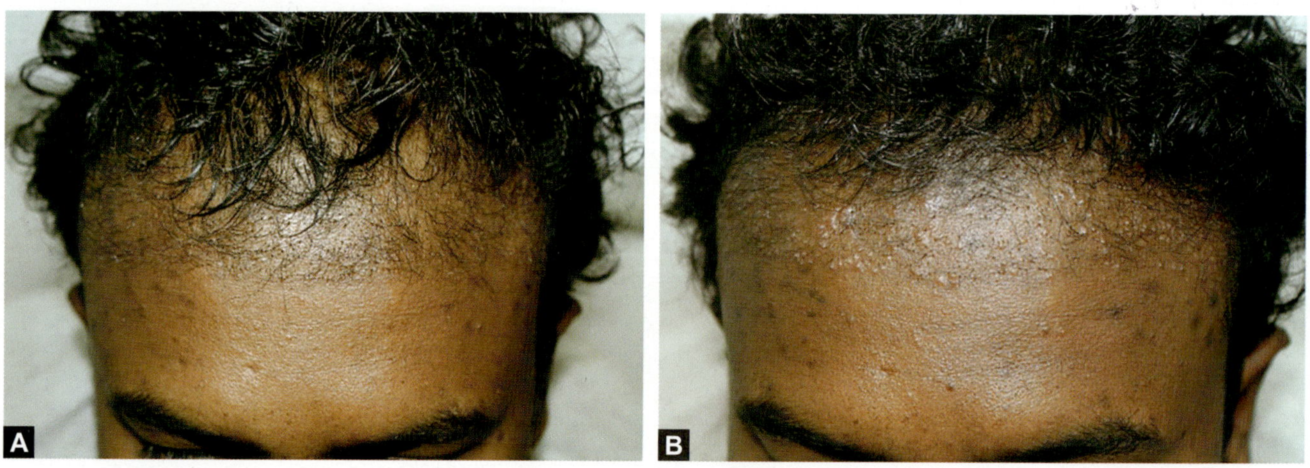

Figs. 47.11A and B: (A) Post hair transplant, unsatisfactory hairline: (B) After 2 sessions of LP Nd:YAG (1064 nm) (fluence 28–34 J/cm^2, pulse width 40 ms, spot size 15 mm).

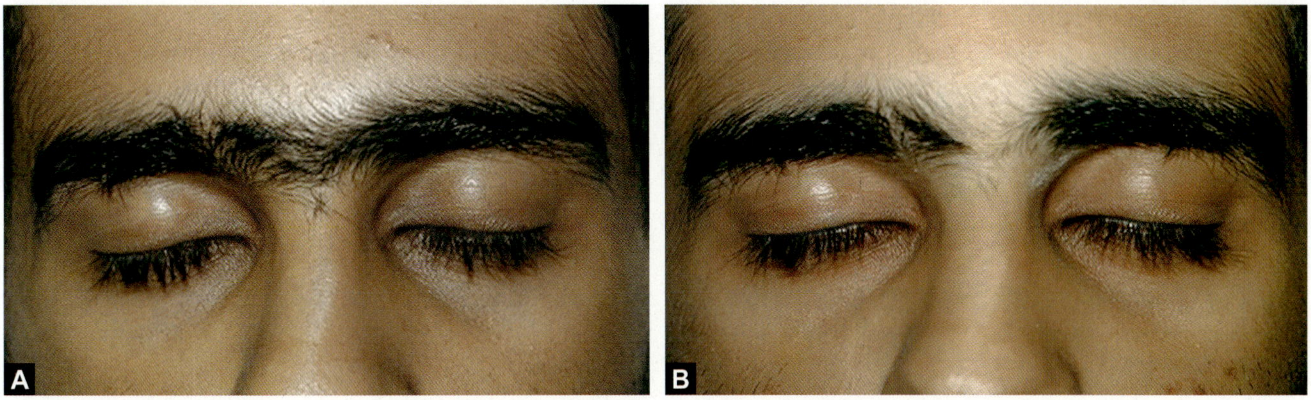

Figs. 47.12A and B: (A) Synophrys: (B) After 4 sessions of LP Nd:YAG 1064 nm (fluence 28–34 J/cm^2, pulse width 30–40 ms, spot size 12 mm).

laser (694 nm), with a long-term hair reduction even at a follow-up of 2 years).[14] The long-pulsed ruby laser is indicated in light-skinned (phototypes I–III) individuals with dark hair.[15] With 20% to 60% reduction after a single session of laser and 50% to 78% after multiple laser sessions, the efficacy of this laser has been established.[16]

But, as this is the shortest wavelength of the laser hair removal systems, the long-pulsed ruby laser is not suitable for skin of color as the risk of adverse effects such scarring and pigment alterations are higher as compared with the longer wavelength devices. RubyStar™ (Aesclepion-Meditec), Sinon™ (Wavelight), EpitouchRuby™ (Sharplan), E2000™ (Palomar), and Chromos™ (MehlBiophile) are the commercially available long-pulsed ruby devices.

Alexandrite Laser 755 nm

The long-pulsed alexandrite laser can be used in patients with skin type III to V as the longer wavelength allows for greater depth of penetration, provided adequate precautions and cooling measures are in place. [17,18] Commercial systems in use include the Apogee™ (Cyanosure), EpitouchAlex™ (Lumenis), Epicare™ (LightAge) GentleLase™ (Candela), Ultrawave II–III™ (Adept Medical), and Clarity™ (Lutronic).

Diode Laser 800–1000 nm

The diode laser, because of its longer wavelength, longer pulse widths and active contact cooling allows its use in darker skin types.[15] For safe use in dark skin types, it utilizes pulse durations of 100 milliseconds or more, but to treat phototype VI, very long pulse durations (400 milliseconds and longer) as well as adequate contact cooling is recommended.[7] Commercial systems include the LightSheer™ (Lumenis), Apex- 800™ (Iridex), SLP1000™ (Palomar), MedioStar™ (Aesclepion-Meditec), F1 Diode Laser™ (Opusmed), EpiStar™ (Nidek) and LinScan808™ (Geosmatic).

Long-pulsed 1064 nm Nd:YAG Lasers

The Nd:YAG lasers (1064 nm) is considered to be the safest hair removal device in patients with dark skin.[18,] Epidermal melanin absorption is minimized by the longer wavelength and this also maximizes wavelength penetration to the dermal hair follicular unit leading to a lower side effect profile and better tolerance.This in turn also means, the poorer absorption by melanin at 1064 nm, necessitating higher fluences and more treatment sessions for effect hair removal. However, due to close approximation of its pulse duration to thermal relaxation time of hair, it is possible that the long-pulsed Nd:YAG laser, can provide permanent hair loss.[16]

Commercial systems using this long-pulsed wavelength include the CoolGlide™ (Cutera), Lyra/Gemini™ (Laserscope), Ultrawave™ (Adept Medical), Athos™ (Quantel), GentleYAG™ (Candela), Profile™ (Sciton), VascuLight™ (Lumenis), SmartEpill™ and Acclaim™ (Cyanosure), Dualis™ (Fotona), Varia™ (CoolTouch), Mydon™ (Wavelight) and Clarity™ (Lutronic).

Intense-pulsed Light (IPL) Systems

Intense-pulsed light are xenon flash lamps, which emit strongly in the near-infrared spectrum. It is composed of noncoherent, polychromatic light ranging from 400 to 1200 nm. Various filters can be used to target particular chromophores, including melanin.[14] Shorter wavelengths are excluded by the cut off filters that limit the range of wavelengths that are used with these devices. As a result, patients with darker skin can be treated safely with the help of suitable filters.[16]

Commercially available systems include the Epilight™ (Lumenis), Quantum HR™ (Lumenis), Ellipse™ (DDD), Photolight™ (Cyanosure), Estelux™ (Palomar), ProLite™ (Alderm), Spatouch™ (Radiancy), Quadra Q4™ (Derma Med USA) and SpectraPulse™ (Primary Technology).

DEVICE VARIABLES

Wavelength: Melanin is the target chromophore for laser hair removal. It is principally located within the hair shaft, although the outer root sheath and matrix area also contain melanin. Melanin absorbs wavelengths in the red and near-infrared portion of the electromagnetic spectrum, and therefore can be targeted by ruby, alexandrite, diode, and Nd:YAG lasers, as well as IPL devices.[19]

Fluence: Fluence is defined as the amount of energy delivered per unit area and is expressed as J/cm^2. Higher fluences have been associated with greater permanency in hair removal; but frequency of untoward side effects also increase. However, giving a test spot of laser is a more appropriate method of determining the optimal treatment fluence for a given patient to evaluate for the desired clinical endpoint of perifollicular erythema and edema. The highest possible tolerated fluence, without any adverse effects can be used for the session.[14]

Pulse duration:Pulse duration is defined as the duration in seconds of laser exposure per shot. Thermal relaxation time (TRT) can be the guiding factor enabling the laser surgeon to select an optimal pulse duration.[1] (TRT of a 200 μm hair follicle is 40 ms).

Spot size: The spot size is the diameter in millimeters of the laser beam. Larger spot sizes are preferable to smaller spot sizes. As photons within a laser beam penetrate the dermis, collagen fibers cause the scattering, and those that are scattered outside the area of the laser beam are essentially wasted. The likelihood of scattering of photons is larger for a smaller spot sizes, whereas in a larger spot size, the photons are likely to remain within the beam area following scatter. Using the largest possible spot size also translates into faster treatment session.[14] Moreover, a larger spot has deeper penetration; thus, reducing the risk of stimulating the surrounding melanocytes and chances of hyperpigmentation.

Skin cooling: Epidermal melanin, particularly in skin of color, presents a competing chromophore to melanin in the hair follicle. Cooling of the skin surface minimizes the epidermal damage, allowing the laser physician to use higher fluence with greater safety.[20] Techniques employed to cool tissue vary between different laser manufacturers. Principles of convection and conduction are the basis for all cooling methods used. They can be broadly classified into contact and noncontact cooling devices. A few of them are mentioned in brief below: surface of the skin through one or more of the following processes:[17]

Cold air convection: A closed loop cooling circuit reduces the air in the treatment area to –30°C. It also has added advantage of minimizing pain during treatment session.

Contact cooling: Sapphire is a better conductor of heat when in comparison to glass. Its thermal conductivity is almost as good as that of metals. Chilled moving solids, such as copper have been used as means for heat extraction in certain devices. Cold gel extract heat via passive contact cooling.

Dynamic cryogen cooling: Cryogen liquid is sprayed on to target areas to precool the skin just before the laser pulse. Another burst of cryogen lasting a few milliseconds may also be delivered just after the laser pulse for post cooling.[14] Cooling of the tissue up to a depth and temperature of 1 mm and –20°C, respectively may be achieved by this method.[20] Certain technologies allow the tissue cooling to be sustained during the entire laser pulse.

TREATMENT GUIDELINES

Patient Selection

Although LHR seems like a simple cosmetic procedure, preoperative evaluation should always include a complete medical history, physical examination and informed consent. Potential risks should be informed to the patient prior to any laser treatment, including setting realistic patient expectations.

Preoperative Considerations (Box 47.1)

History:

- Presence of conditions that may cause hypertrichosis:
  - Hormonal
  - Familial
  - Medications
  - Tumor
- *History of herpes simplex*: Particularly important for treating face and the inguinal region.

- History of keloids/hypertrophic scarring.
- *History of previous treatment modalities*: Shaving, waxing, tweezing, depilatory creams, electrolysis, lasers; frequency and last treatment session; and response.
- Present medications and isotretinoin use within 1 year. Although this was previously thought to be contraindicated, the authors have published a report confirming its safety.

Examination:

- Site
- Hair thickness, density color
- Skin type
- Pigmentary or scarring changes
- Presence of nevi or tattoo within treatment site
- Any signs of other medical problems.

TREATMENT TECHNIQUE (BOXES 47.2 TO 47.4)

The procedure for hair removal using all of the above devices can be summarized as follows:

- *Skin preparation*: Completely remove makeup, or other skin creams/powders. Hair should be trimmed in case of tunneling in AKN. Any discharging sinuses should have healed before undergoing LHR.
- *Visibility*: A treatment grid can be applied in order to provide the operator with an outline of the area to be treated. Careful attention must be paid to prevent double-pulsing and to avoid skipped areas in the absence of a grid.
- *Treatment parameters*: The ideal treatment parameters must be individualized for each patient: test sites can be placed at inconspicuous locations in the sites to be treated. The fluence is carefully increased while

Box 47.1: Pretreatment care.

Six weeks before laser treatment:
- Sunscreen: A broad-spectrum sunscreen is recommended and sun avoidance must be practiced, if hair removal is planned in exposed sites
- Priming agents like demelanizing creams, advised three weeks prior to starting the procedure
- No plucking, waxing, or electrolysis. Research has shown greater hair loss at shaved versus epilated sites, suggesting that light absorption by the pigmented hair shaft itself plays an important role
- Shaving and depilatory creams may be used

Day before laser treatment:
- The patient is instructed not to depilate or shave the area as it is necessary to assess the hair growth to set optimal parameters for laser hair removal
- Start a prophylactic antiviral when indicated
- Start an oral antibiotic when indicated (e.g. nasal and perianal skin)

Day of treatment:
- Area to be treated should be clean and free of makeup
- Although EMLA cream can be applied prior to treatment, the authors do not recommend the use of a topical anesthetic

Box 47.2: Selecting parameters.

Skin type	Darker skin type has higher risk of epidermal injury, hence use long pulse width and low fluence (safe parameters). Longer wavelength lasers are preferred Light skin type—short pulse width, high fluence
Skin color	Areas like the axilla and perineum are darker than other areas. Select safe parameters based on patient skin type
Hair	If the hair is thick, dark and dense—use safe parameters If the hair is thick, light and sparse- use high fluence and short pulse width
Pigmentation	If there is an underlying pigmentary blemish (hyperpigmentation) use safe parameters
Large areas	If the treatment area is large, the laser frequency can be increased to reduce the treatment time
Skin contour	Frequency can be reduced while treating areas like the axilla and perineum as there is a change in the skin contour
Bony prominences	Reduced fluence while treating over bony prominences.
Tunneling and sinuses	Double passes are recommended over tunnels and sinuses like HS and AKN

Box 47.3: Clinical endpoints.

Favorable endpoints	*Unfavorable/adverse endpoints*
• Perifollicular erythema	• Graying
• Singed hair	• Severe whitening
• Hair cast	• Blistering

Box 47.4: Post-treatment care and advice.

- Application of cold packs in the immediate post procedure period reduces pain and minimizes swelling
- Analgesics are not usually required unless extensive areas are treated
- Prophylactic courses of antivirals may be given, if previous history of herpes simplex present in the treatment area
- Topical antibiotic ointment should be applied twice daily, if epidermal injury occurs
- Mild topical steroid creams can be prescribed to reduce swelling and erythema
- Avoid any trauma such as picking or scratching of the area.
- Avoid sun exposure. Use sunblock with SPF-30
- Makeup may be applied on the next day unless blistering or crusting develops
- Shedding of hair casts: seen particularly on the face. The damaged hair shafts are often shed during the first week after treatment. Patients should be reassured that this is not a sign of hair regrowth

observing the skin for signs of acute epidermal injury, such as whitening, blistering, or mauve erythema. Test sites should be observed for 10 minutes in light skinned patients and 20 minutes in patients with dark skin (Box 47.2 and Table 47.2).

- *Technique*: Nonoverlapping laser pulses are delivered with a predetermined spot size. It is recommended that the largest spot size and the highest tolerable fluence be used to obtain the best results.
- *Adequate cooling of the epidermis* should be done before the treatment.
- *Postoperative changes*: The ideal immediate response is vaporization of the hair shaft with no other apparent tissue effect. After a few minutes, perifollicular edema and erythema appears. The intensity and duration depends on the hair color and hair density. If there is a sign of epidermal damage, the fluence should be reduced.

Treatment Interval

The interval between treatments depends on the growth cycle of the hairs in the treatment area. The longer the telogen (resting) phase, the longer the interval between treatments should be (Table 47.3). It is most efficient to plan the second treatment as soon as a large number of hairs are in the anagen or growing phase (Table 47.4).

Table 47.2: Laser hair removal parameters for specific indications.*

Indications	*IPL*	*Nd:YAG*	*Alexandrite*	*Diode*
Pseudofolliculitis barbae	F: 12–15 J/cm^2 PW: 30–55 ms SS: 10 mm x 48 mm	F: 40–60 J/cm^2 SS: 15 mm PW: 30–40 ms	F: 12–15 J/cm^2 SS: 12 mm PW: 5 ms	F:18–30 J/cm^2 PW: 30–60 ms SS: 50 mm × 15 mm
Acne keloidalis nuchae	F:12–15 J/cm^2 PW: 30–55 ms SS: 10 mm × 48 mm	F: 40–50 J/cm^2 SS: 15 mm PW: 12–40 ms	F: 12–18 J/cm^2 SS: 18 mm PW: 5 ms	F: 18–24 J/cm^2 PW: 30–80 ms SS: 50 mm × 15 mm
Hidradenitis suppurativa	F: 7–16 J/cm^2 PW: 20–40 ms SS: 10 mm × 48 mm	F: 30–40 J/cm^2 SS: 15 mm PW: 20–40 ms	F: 12–18 J/cm^2 SS: 18 mm PW: 5 ms	F: 14–24 J/cm^2 PW: 30–50 ms SS: 50 mm × 15 mm
Pilonodal sinus	F: 10–16 J/cm^2 PW: 20–40 ms SS: 10 mm × 48 mm	F: 40 J/cm^2 SS:15 mm PW: 40 ms	F: 8–12 J/cm^2 SS: 15 mm PW: 5 ms	F: 30–60 J/cm^2 PW: 30–40 ms SS: 50 mm × 15 mm
Pseudofolliculitis	F:10–15 J/cm^2 PW:20–55 ms SS: 10 mm × 48 mm	F: 40–60 J/cm^2 SS:15 mm PW: 20–40 ms	F: 12–16 J/cm^2 SS: 18/20 mm PW: 5 ms	F: 18–30 J/cm^2 PW: 15–24 ms SS: 50 mm × 15 mm
Hair bearing skin flaps	F:12–15 J/cm^2 PW: 30–55 ms SS: 10 mm × 48 mm	F: 26–40 J/cm^2 SS:15 mm PW:30–40 ms	F: 12–16 J/cm^2 SS: 18/20 mm PW: 5 ms	F:18–30 J/cm^2 PW: 30–60 ms SS: 50 mm x 15 mm
Hairy Becker's nevus	F:9–15 J/cm^2 PW: 30–55 ms SS: 10 mm × 48 mm	F: 24–40 J/cm^2 SS: 15 mm PW: 20–40 ms	F: 12–18 J/cm^2 SS: 12–18 mm PW: 5 ms	F: 14–24 J/cm^2 PW: 30–60 ms SS: 50 mm × 15 mm

(F: Fluence; PW: Pulse width; SS: Spot size)

*The parameters mentioned above should be modified according to the skin type, the thickness of hair and the site. Every laser machine comes with its own settings, which have to be modified accordingly with subsequent sessions, but it is advisable to use the preset factory settings for the initial sessions.

Table 47.3: Growth cycle of hair in different treatment areas.

Body site	*Telogen (%)*	*Telogen duration*	*Anagen (%)*	*Anagen duration*	*Depth of follicle*
Scalp	13	3–4 months	85	2–6 years	3–5
Cheeks	30–50		50–70		2–4
Beard/Chin	20	10 months	70	1 year	3–5
Moustache	35	6 weeks	65	16 weeks	2–4
Axillae	70	3 months	30	4 months	3.5–4.5
Trunk					2–4.5
Arms	80	18 weeks	20	13 weeks	2–4.5
Legs-thighs	80	24 weeks	20	16 weeks	2.5–4

Table 47.4: Treatment interval.

Area	*Interval after first treatment*	*Interval after subsequent treatments*
Upper lip	6 weeks	6–8 weeks
Chin and cheeks Ears and eyebrows	6 weeks	8 weeks
Underarms, bikini areas	8 weeks	10 weeks
Arms	10 weeks	12 weeks
Legs	12 weeks	12–14 weeks
Male back	12 weeks	12–16 weeks

COMPLICATIONS OF LASER HAIR REMOVAL

The complications and various side effects are listed in Table 47.5.

The advantage of choosing melanin as the chromophore is that, it is present in both the hair follicle and shaft. Unfortunately, in terms of complications, melanin is found in the epidermis as well. Since light must initially pass through the epidermis in order to get to the deeper hair follicle, it is therefore potentially absorbed first in the epidermis. This results in adverse effects such as vesiculation, crusting, burns, and dyspigmentation.

Patients with darker colored skin, especially skin types V and VI, are more likely to experience cutaneous adverse effects due to the abundance of melanin in theirepidermis. This is both patient and wavelength dependent.[22] It should be noted that such complications are not just limited to genetically determined dark skin but also to patients with sun tanning and lentiginous photoaging.

The wavelength used, pulse duration fluence, utilized handpiece spot size and the use of appropriate cooling are the factors determining the occurrence of adverse effects. Epidermal melanin absorbs less energy when treated with laser of longer wavelength and with longer pulse duration. While it is true that wavelengths with lower absorption coefficients will decrease the amount of light absorbed by epidermal melanin, these longer wavelengths also decrease the amount of light absorbed by hair, and longerpulse duration will decrease the rate of heat generation in hair and hair shaft containing melanin. Thus, in the end, the laser parameters need to be chosen to limit thermal diffusion to the size of the hair follicles and limit its diffusion into surrounding tissue.[23]

Pigmentary Changes

Hypopigmentation: What causes hypopigmentation after laser hair removal is not really clear? It may be due to the melanocyte destruction, melanogenesis suppression or melanin redistribution in keratinocytes. The tyrosine activity may be reduced due to the sustained subdisruptive damage to the melanocytes and this explains the reversible hypopigmentation which results. [24,25]

Hyperpigmentation: Comparatively the transient hyperpigmentation which occurs after laser hair treatment happens in about 14–25% patients. This can be attributed to melanocyte stimulation. Delayed tanning and injury to the epidermis can cause immediate transient pigment darkening phenomenon due to photo-oxidation of the pre-existing melanin. This may be transient, lasting 3–4 weeks and usually resolves spontaneously without any sequelae. However, the hyperpigmentation which occurs due to epidermolysis or blistering occurs at a higher energy threshold and can be permanent and more grave. This has the potential for permanent dyschromia, both in very dark-skinned individuals and darkly tanned individuals. Post-inflammatory hyperpigmentation due to cold air convection techniques have also been reported.[26]

Table 47.5: Principal adverse effects of laser/IPL hair removal.[21]

Acute short-term effects (lasting hours to days)

- Pain*
- Perifollicular erythema*
- Edema*
- Blistering+
- Crusting+
- Folliculitis
- Purpura
- Thrombophlebitis
- Cold urticaria

Postinflammatory transient effects (lasting weeks to months)

- Hyperpigmentation
- Hypopigmentation
- Leukotrichia
- Reticulate erythema

Permanent adverse effects (rare)

- Hyperpigmentation
- Hypopigmentation
- Atrophy
- Scarring
- Leukotrichia
- Treatment failure

*Expected, favorable side effects suggestive of using optimum parameters;
+Side effects suggestive of using aggressive parameters.

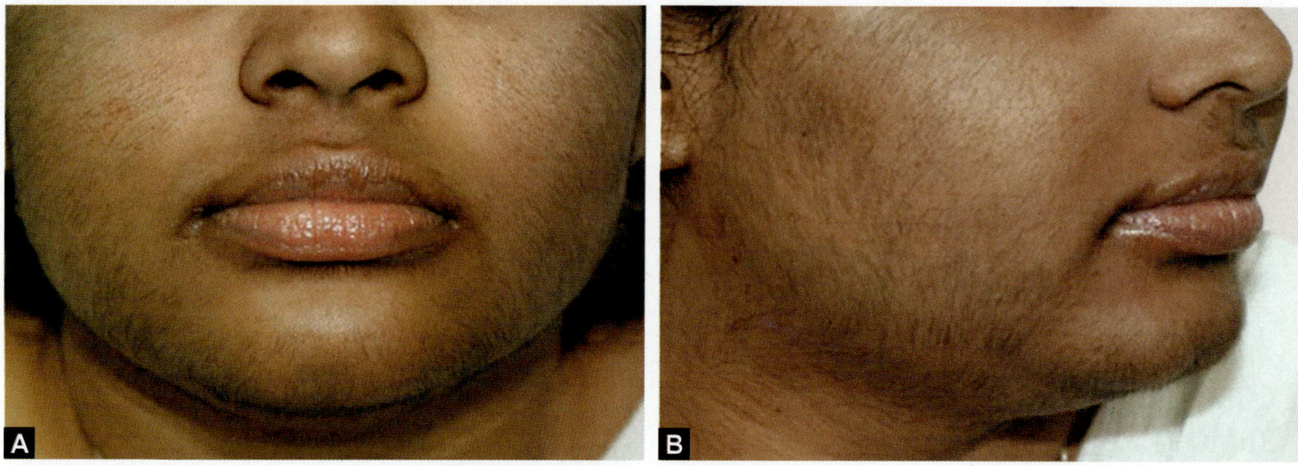

Figs. 47.13A and B: Paradoxical hair growth.

Blistering

Direct thermal injury may occur in 10–15% of patients especially when post and preprocedure instructions are not followed by the patient.[27]

Scarring and Textural Changes

The normal appearance and distribution of both collagen and elastin in laser-treated skin suggest that textural changes in skin are unlikely after laser-assisted hair removal except in cases of over-aggressive treatment, inadequate cooling, or postoperative infection.[23]

Infections

Herpes simplex: Herpes simplex outbreaks are uncommon after laser and light source-treatment of hair removal, but may occur in patients with a strong history of outbreaks. This is most commonly seen on, or around, the lip.

Bacterial infection: The risk of bacterial infection is extremely low; it may occur following epidermal damage induced by any form of trauma, including aggressive laser hair removal.

Paradoxical Hair Growth (Paradoxical Hypertrichosis)

Treatment of vellus hairs, especially of the lateral cheeks and chin area, may result in the induction of terminal hairs, a phenomenon known as paradoxical hypertrichosis (Figs. 47.13A and B). This has been reported to occur more commonly in females of Mediterranean, Middle Eastern, Asian, and South Asian descent.[28]

The reason for this can be attributed to the possibility of using an incorrect pulse duration or energy. If hairs are treated with too low an energy or too long a pulse duration, the target cells may not be heated sufficiently and can stimulate hair growth. If paradoxical hair growth is noted, the recommended course of action is to cease treatment for a period of 6 months and later recommence the treatments.

Reticulate Erythema

Reticulate erythema, a rarely reported complication after laser hair removal, appears to be the result of cumulative laser fluencies associated with multiple episodes of laser hair removal. The complication is generally subtle andoften missed.[29]

SAFETY

- Patients should be placed in a room with a treatment chair that makes the desired treatment area easily accessible.
- The room should be adequately cooled to keep the laser device from overheating and be free of any hanging mirrors or uncovered windows.
- A fire extinguisher should be readily available.
- Having a vacuum device on hand during treatment can minimize the plume and unpleasant odor created by each laser pulse.
- As the retina contains melanin that can be damaged by all LHR devices, proper eye protection is absolutely critical for both the patient and laser surgeon. Each device requires the use of protective goggles that are unique to the device's particular wavelengths and they cannot be interchanged.

Box 47.5: Contraindications.

- Active infections at the site of treatment
- Keloidal tendency
- Patients with unrealistic expectations

- Because of the risk of retinal damage, one should never treat a patient for LHR within the bony orbit.
- There is a small but real risk of infection with contact cooling devices. The handpiece should be adequately disinfected.

DURING PREGNANCY

Treatment of a pregnant woman for non-urgent conditions is discouraged, although there is no evidence suggesting a potential risk to pregnant women undergoing LHR (Box 47.5).[14]

FUTURE DIRECTIONS

Pain Control

Laser hair removal is not a painless procedure, most patients experience some discomfort during and immediately after treatment. According to the Gate theory of pain transmission, the stimulation of pressure receptors on the skin, blocks the activation of pain fibers. Utilizing this theory, is a novel technique to reduce LHR-associated pain with the pneumatic skin flattening (PSF). It works by coupling a vacuum chamber that generates a negative pressure and flattens the skin against the treatment window of the handpiece.[30] PSF is just beginning to be incorporated into commercially available lasers.

Home Use Devices

A number of devices that can achieve hair removal at home have been developed. They are based on IPL, laser and thermal technologies. However, the lack of proper training and the risk of eye injuries with improper use of these devices preclude its popularity.

Alternative Technologies for Hair Removal

Electro-Optical Synergy (ELOS): This technology combines the electrical [radiofrequency (RF)] and optical (laser/light) energies. The optical component heats up the hair shaft and then concentrates the bipolar RF energy to the surrounding hair follicle.[31]Based on this combination, lower fluences are needed, thus suggesting that it be well tolerated in all skin phototypes and also potentially effective in removal of white and poorly pigmented hair.[32]

Low Fluence High Repetition Rate Lasers

The approach of using low fluences with repetitive millisecond pulses to achieve heat stacking in the hair bulb and bulge represents a paradigm shift in laser hair removal methodology. Multiple passes of diode laser at low fluences but with high average power results in permanent hair removal with less discomfort and fewer adverse effects, especially on darker skin.[33]

The tips and tricks for the outcome with laser hair removal is summarized in Box 47.6.

Box 47.6: Tips and tricks for optimum outcome with laser hair removal.

- Proper patient evaluation prior to treatment is the key to successful LHR
- To achieve maximum benefit, an appropriate wavelength, pulse duration, and fluence must be tailored to each individual. Choose minimum fluence producing desired tissue effect
- Light/blond hair require more sittings, higher fluence and low PW
- Dark hair- low fluence and long PW. Keep low and safe parameters if there is a lower contrast between the skin color and hair, and higher parameters can be attempted if the contrast is high
- Lower fluence required in highly dense areas, e.g. pseudofolliculitis barbae

In darker skin, there is increased risk of side effects. Type VI skin absorbs 40% more energy when compared to type I

- Some dark skin patients may have lighter skin but their ethnic background and genetic darker skin descent must be kept in mind
- Darker skin may require more number of sessions. Discuss potential risk of scarring/hypo/hyperpigmentation
- Cooling allows higher fluences to be used for more permanent hair removal
- Cooling is important but avoid cold injuries
- A laser test spot should be considered for any patient in whom there is a concern about the potential for side effects like dark skin.Wait for 48 hrs to decide about optimum parameters as there may be delayed reaction to exposure

Avoid jawline vellus hairs as chances of paradoxical hair stimulation risk is more

- Wait for 6 weeks after waxing/plucking. Avoid direct sun exposure for at least 2 weeks
- Delay the treatment interval, if there is no growth

REFERENCES

1. Anderson RR, Parrish JA. Selective photothermolysis: precise microsurgery by selective absorption of pulsed radiation. Science. 1983:220(4596):524-7.
2. Shapiro J, Lui H. Treatments for unwanted facial hair. Skin Ther Lett. 2005;10 (10):1-4.
3. Richards RN, Meharg GE. Electrolysis: observations from 13 years and 140,000 hours of experience. J Am Acad Dermatol. 1995; 33(4):662–6.
4. Van Gemert MJC, Welch AJ. Time constants in thermal laser medicine. Lasers Surg Med. 1989;9:405-21.
5. Commo S, Gaillardo O, Bernard BA. The human hair follicle contains two distinct K19 positive compartments in the outer root sheath: A unifying hypothesis for stem cell reservoir? Differentiation. 2000;66:157-64.
6. Altshuler GB, Anderson RR, Manstein D, et al. Extended theory of selective photothermolysis. Lasers Surg Med. 2001;29(5):416-32.
7. Battle EF Jr, Hobbs LM. Laser-assisted hair removal for darker skin types. Dermatol Ther. 2004;17:177-83.
8. Koch D, Pratsou P, Szczecinska W, et al. The diverse application of laser hair removal therapy: A tertiary laser unit's experience with less common indications and a literature overview. Lasers Med Sci. 2015;30:453-67.
9. Xu LY, Wright D, Mahmoud BH, et al. Histopathologic study of hidradenitis suppurativa following long-pulsed 1064-nm Nd:YAG Laser treatment. Arch Dermatol. 2011;147(1):21-8.
10. Odili J, Gault D. Laser depilation of the natal cleft—an aid to healing the pilonidal sinus. Annals of The Royal College of Surgeons of England. 2002;84(1):29-32.
11. Shim TN, Abdullah A, Lanigan S, et al. Hairy intraoral flap–an unusual indication for laser epilation: A series of 5 cases and review of the literature. Br J Oral Maxillofac Surg. 2011;49:50-2.
12. Nanni CA, Alster TS. Treatment of a becker's nevus using a 694-nm long-pulsed ruby laser. Dermatologis. 1998;24.
13. Manuskiatti W, Tantikun N. Treatment of trichostasis spinulosa in skin phototypes III, IV, and V with an 800-nm pulsed diode laser. Dermatologic Surgery. 2003;29:85-8.
14. Ibrahimi OA, Avram MM, Hanke CW, et al. Laser hair removal. Dermatol Ther. 2011;24(1):94-107.
15. Dierickx CC. Laser-assisted hair removal: state of the art. Dermatol Ther. 2000;13:80-89.
16. Wanner M. Laser hair removal. Dermatol Ther. 2005;18: 209-16.
17. Garcia C, Alamoudi H, Nakib M, et al. Alexandrite laser hair removal is safe for Fitzpatrick skin types IV–VI. Dermatol Surg. 2000;26(2):130-4.
18. Galadari I. Comparative evaluation of different hair removal lasers in skin types IV, V, and VI. Int J Dermatol. 2003;42(1): 68-70.
19. Anderson RR, Parrish JA. The optics of human skin. J Invest Dermatol. 1981;77(1):13-9.
20. Zenzie HH, Altshuler GB, Smirnov MZ, et al. Evaluation of cooling methods for laser dermatology. Lasers Surg Med 2000;26(2):130-44.
21. Su-Ping Lim R. Laser hair removal in the Asian skin. In: Textbook of Laser and Light Dermatology in the Asian Skin. USA: EBSCO Publishing; 2011;p 69-81.
22. Liew SH. Laser hair removal: Guidelines for management. Am J Clin Dermatol. 2002;3:107-15.
23. Goldberg D. Laser complicatons: Hair removal. J of Cosmetic and Laser Therapy. 2006;8:197-202.
24. Liew SH, Grobbelaar AO, Gault DT, et al. Ruby laser hair removal: Clinical efficacy in Fitzpatrick skin type I–V and histological changes in epidermal melanocytes. Br J Dermatol. 1999;140:1105-9.
25. Liew SH, Grobbelaar AO, Gault DT, et al. Ruby laser- assisted hair removal: Repeated treatments and clinical efficacy. Eur J Plast Surg. 2000;23:121-6
26. Manuskiatti W, Eimpunth S, Wanitphakdeedecha R. Effect of cold air cooling on the incidence of postinflammatory hyperpigmentation after Q-switched Nd:YAG laser treatment of acquired bilateral nevus of Ota like macules. Arch Dermatol 2007;143:1139-43.
27. Nanni CA, Alster TS. Laser-assisted hair removal: side effects of Q-switched Nd:YAG, long-pulsed ruby, and alexandrite lasers. J Am Acad Dermatol. 1999:41:165-71.
28. Desai S, Mahmoud BH, Bhatia AC, et al. Paradoxical hypertrichosis after laser therapy: a review. Dermatol Surg. 2010;36(3): 291-8.
29. Lapidoth M, Shafirstein G, Ben Amitai D, et al. Reticulate erythema after diode laser- assisted hair removal. J Am Acad Dermatol. 2004;51:774-7.
30. Lask G, Friedman D, Elman M, et al. Pneumatic Skin Flattening (PSF): A novel technology for marked pain reduction with high energy density lasers and IPLs. J Cosmet Laser Ther. 2006;8:76-81.
31. Waldman A, Kriendle M. New technology in aesthetic medicine: ELOS electro optical synergy. J Cosmet Laser Ther. 2003; 5: 204-6.
32. Ibrahimi OA, Suzanne KL. Hair removal. In: Goldman MP, Fitzpatrick RE, Ross EV, et al. (Eds). Lasers and Energy Devices for the Skin. 2nd edition. CRC Press, India. 2013;94.
33. Braun M. Permanent laser hair removal with low fluence high repetition rate versus high fluence low repetition rate 810 nm diode laser-a split leg comparison study. J Drugs Dermatol. 2009;8:14-7.

CHAPTER 48

Lasers in Dermatosurgery: Safety and Complications

BS Chandrashekar, Chaithra Shenoy

INTRODUCTION

With newer applications of laser and light devices, arise newer complications. Lasers being an ever evolving field, changes are relentlessly pursued to make them safer and more efficacious. The principle of selective photo thermolysis (SPT) by Anderson and Parrish has revolutionized the concept of laser application and helped confine the tissue injury to specifically targeted chromophores, making it possible to treat infinite conditions with least complications.[1] Laser complication has been defined as "any undesirable effect, even if expected, that occurs with the laser treatment".[2] It is mandatory that the laser physician be equipped with the knowledge of basic principles of laser, the device in hand and laser-tissue interaction to understand how the laser acts. This is helpful in maximum utilization of the laser with minimal complications.

GENERAL SAFETY MEASURES

Laser safety measures and stringent post-laser care can prevent many of the complications.

- Laser operations should be supervised directly by an individual knowledgeable in laser safety.
- Diffusely reflecting materials should be used near the beam, where appropriate.
- Personnel within the laser controlled area should use appropriate laser protective eyewear at all times.
- There must be a sign on the door indicating that the laser is in use.
- The laser machines have to be kept dust free and serviced regularly to maintain the efficacy of the device.
- Patient must be made to wear appropriate eye shields and if the laser is being done within the orbital margin, then corneal shield is mandatory.
- Written instructions regarding the dos and don'ts have to be given to the patients after the procedure. This reinforces the post procedural care instructions given orally.
- The laser physician should insist on frequent follow-ups in the immediate post-laser period to look out for any early signs of complications.
- The patients should be educated as to what is to be expected after the procedure and has to report back immediately, if any untoward reactions are suspected.

The cause of complications occurring due to laser and light-based devices can be classified into two broad categories: operator dependent and patient dependent. The operator dependent variables are faulty parameters causing damage to the epidermis or faulty technique in handling the lasers, such as not placing the hand piece probe perpendicular to the skin, inadequate cooling, placing the probe too close or too far to the skin while operating the laser and not using adequate protective gears: both by the operating personnel and the patient. The causal factors dependent on the patients are skin type, type of lesion, hormonal status in the female patient for laser hair reduction, inadequate and improper sunscreen application and recent tanning.

LASER HAIR REDUCTION

Laser hair reduction (LHR) is one of the most common laser procedure in a laser set-up. Although the procedure is relatively safe, side effects are known to occur. The devices used for LHR are long-pulsed Nd:YAG, Diode, Alexandrite, Ruby and Intense Pulse Light (IPL).

Complications[3-5]

Immediate	Transient	Persistent
Burning sensation Edema Crusting (Fig. 48. 1) Superficial thrombophlebitis Cold urticaria Palpable purpura	Acneform eruptions Folliculitis Postinflammatory hyperpigmentation (PIH) (Fig. 48.2) Postinflammatory hypopigmentation (Fig. 48.3) Skip areas (Fig. 48.4) Reticulate erythema	Scarring Paradoxical hypertrichosis (Fig. 48.5) Undesired styling of the hair line

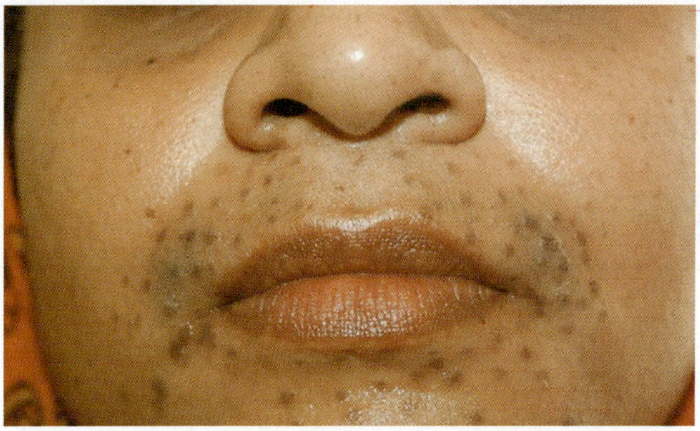

Fig. 48.1: Atrophic scarring following long-pulsed Nd:YAG laser for port wine stain.

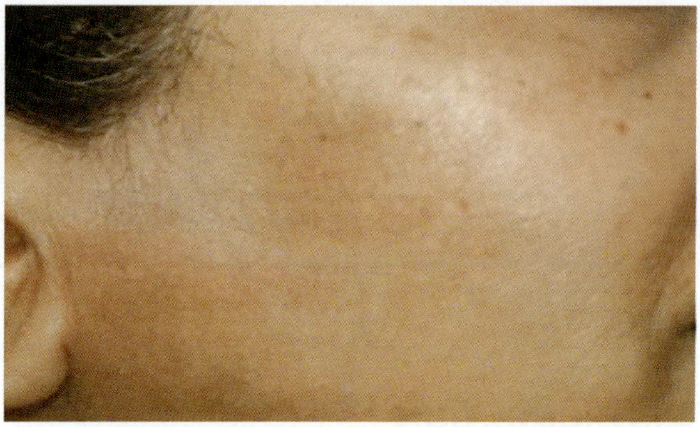

Fig. 48.2: PIH following IPL for LHR. (PIH: Postinflammatory hyperpigmentation; LHR: Laser hair reduction).

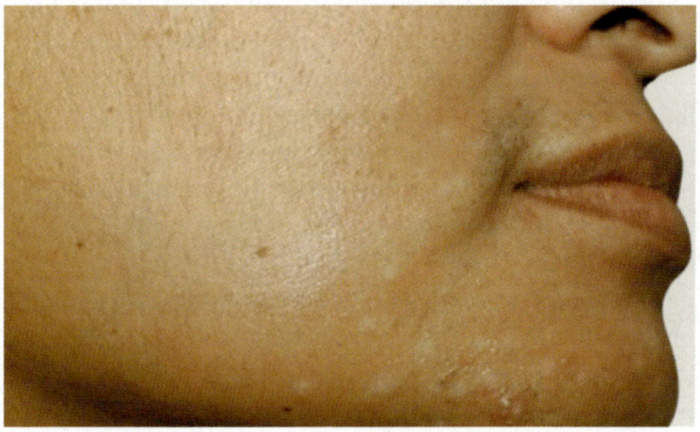

Fig. 48.3: Postinflammatory hypopigmentation following laser hair removal by long-pulsed Nd:YAG 1064 nm.

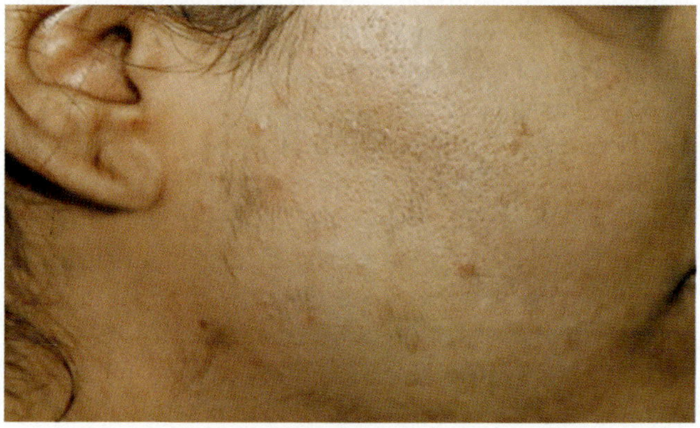

Fig. 48.4: Skip areas following laser hair reduction.

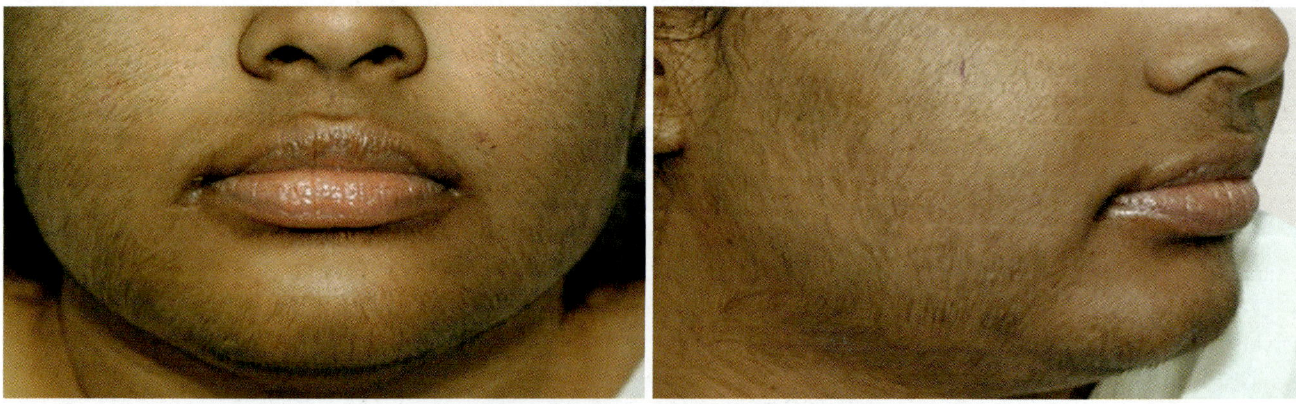

Fig. 48.5: Paradoxical hypertrichosis following laser hair removal by long-pulsed Nd:YAG.

Proper skin cooling is essential to minimize epidermal damage while permitting treatment with higher fluence. The immediate side complications, such as burning sensation, pain, edema and crusting can be reduced with a good precooling and postcooling protocol. Laser burns require early recognition and immediate treatment. Moderate potency topical steroids, such as Mometasone or Fluticasone can be used for a short period of time to reduce the inflammation due to inhibition of release of arachidonate derived inflammatory mediators such as prostaglandins and leukotrienes.[6] Cold urticaria, superficial thrombophlebitis and palpable purpura are few of the self-limiting uncommon side effects seen with laser hair reduction.[4,5,7]

Acneform eruptions occur in around 6% of the patients undergoing laser hair reduction. The incidence of acneform eruption is not dependent on the Polycystic Ovarian syndrome, neither on the sex of the patient nor on the number of sessions of laser previously undergone by them. Folliculitis and acneform eruptions should be treated with oral Doxycycline or Minocycline for a duration of 10–20 days alongside topical antibiotics.[8]

Reticulate erythema is a transient complication reported after hair removal treatment with Diode laser in lighter skin. Six out of the ten patients has prior history of chill blain. Hence it is prudent to avoid patients with collagen vascular disease for laser hair removal.[9]

The line of treatment for postinflammatory hyperpigmentation repeated includes meticulous usage of broad spectrum sunscreen and topical depigmenting creams like Hydroquinone, Kojic acid and Glycolic acid. Postinflammatory hypopigmentation is treated with topical tacrolimus as it stimulates tyrosinase activity and also enhances melanocyte migration.[10] A good amount of counseling is necessary to convince the patient about repigmentation. Post-laser depigmentation can be treated with TCA CROSS technique by using 65–100% Trichloroacetic acid (TCA) on the depigmented spot.[11]

Paradoxical hypertrichosis can occur in 0.6% to 10% of the patients undergoing laser hair reduction. The definitive cause has not been determined even though various hypotheses have been proposed. All the devices have the potential to produce paradoxical hypertrichosis but more commonly seen with IPL. Subtherapeutic thermal injury to the surrounding vellus hair which stimulates them to convert into terminal follicle has been the most accepted mechanism. Also effects of inflammatory mediators and upregulatory cytokines have been described. LHR in the head and neck areas—more so in the chin, mandibular and zygomatic areas, in patients with darker skin types and thick dark hair and in patients with underlying hormonal imbalance are predisposing factors for paradoxical hypertrichosis.[12,13] This can be avoided by protecting the surrounding non lased areas with cold packs during the procedure.

Undesired styling of hair line is a common complaint when shaping the eyebrows and side locks in women and beard line in men. Hence it is worthwhile that the desired hairline margin is marked with a white marking pencil, photographed and stored for future reference.

Ocular complications have been reported with laser hair reduction, especially when attempting epilation within the bony margin of the orbit. When the eyelid closes, the iris and other pigmented parts of the eyeball roll up owing to the Bell's phenomena. This makes them vulnerable to laser damage. Hence any attempt to epilate the hair on the lower part of the eyebrow with laser has to be done only after the metallic corneal eye shield is in place.[14]

Leukotrichia may develop following IPL and laser hair removal therapy may be temporary or permanent. It has been explained based on the difference in the thermal relaxation times of melanocytes and germinative cells, as light absorbed and the heat produced by melanin may be sufficient enough to destroy or impair the function of melanocytes but insufficient to damage the hair follicle cells.[15] Epilation or to a certain extent Electro-optical synergy (ELOS) technology of hair removal can be employed for removal of grey hairs.[16]

ABLATIVE AND FRACTIONAL RESURFACING LASER

Ablative and fractional lasers have significantly evolved over time to improve the efficacy and more importantly the safety profile of the devices. This technology has garnered interest from doctors across specialty due to its versatile nature and varied applications. Ablative full face resurfacing technique has a higher risk of hyperpigmentation and scarring especially in Types IV, V and VI Fitzpatrick skin types. Fractional resurfacing on the other hand has gained popularity especially in Asia for the treatment of acne scars and photoageing.

Complete history and counseling sessions prior to the procedure should include enquiry into occupational details to determine the number of hours the patient is exposed to direct or indirect sunlight, and tendency toward keloids, hypertrophic scars or postinflammatory hyperpigmentation (it can be checked by examining an old scar). History of prior herpes simplex infections have to be determined. Patient has to be counseled regarding downtime required after each laser session and enquiry has to be made into any significant life events in the near future, to avoid unpleasant surprises. Aggressive parameters, such as increased energy or density and faulty technique are common causes of complications with fractional and ablative lasers.

Complications[17-19]

Immediate	Transient	Persistent
Pain Erythema and edema Burning sensation Crusting Acneform eruptions Reactivation of herpes simplex virus (HSV) (Fig. 48.6)	Prolonged redness (Fig. 48.7) Postinflammatory hyperpigmentation Postinflammatory hypopigmentation Demarcation lines	Scarring—more common in nonfacial skin Keloids and hypertrophic scars Ocular complications

Reactivation of herpes simplex virus (HSV) following the laser is more common after resurfacing lasers. The HSV infection can lead to delay in re-epithelialization, wide spread facial lesions and post-laser scarring. It is advisable to start therapy with oral antiviral such as Valacyclovir or Famciclovir at a minimum of two hours before the procedure and continue it ten days thereafter in all patients undergoing lasers for resurfacing.[20]

Prolonged redness is known to occur with ablative and sometimes even with non-ablative resurfacing of skin. Temporary fragility of skin and peeling can occur up to a month. Strict photoprotection and moisturizers are helpful in treatment. Postinflammatory hyperpigmentation can occur in 26–36% of the patients undergoing resurfacing lasers depending on their skin type.[21] Demarcation lines are areas of contrast in between the lased and non-lased skin. This can be avoided by peripheral feathering of the laser beam into the borders of the treated areas.

PIGMENT LASER

The commonly used lasers to treat pigment are Quality (Q) switched Nd:YAG at 1064 nm, potassium titanyl phosphate (KTP) crystal frequency doubled Q-switched Nd:YAG at 532 nm, IPL, Q-switched Alexandrite laser at 755 nm and Q-switched Ruby at 694 nm. These laser devices are used to target a variety of conditions such as Nevus of Ota, freckles, lentigines, tattoos, melasma, postinflammatory hyperpigmentation and acquired bilateral Nevus of Ota-like macules (ABNOM).

Complications[2,22]

Immediate	Transient	Persistent
Pain Erythema Edema Blistering Petechiae Crusting	Postinflammatory hyperpigmentation Postinflammatory hypopigmentation Reactivation of herpes simplex virus infection	Depigmentation (Fig. 48.8) Scarring (Fig. 48.9) Hypertrophic scars Darkening of flesh color tattoos

Immediate complications, such as pain, erythema, edema and blistering are directly proportionate to the energy used during the procedure. When using higher energy, as in the treatment of dermal lesions, such as Nevi or a tattoo, the patient can be put at ease by using a topical anesthetic cream 45 minutes prior to the starting of the procedure. Cold compresses following the session helps in mitigating the pain and burning sensation. Blistering or crusting usually resolves over a period of seven to ten days. A topical antibiotic cream alongside a moisturizer is advised to prevent secondary infection. Depigmentary macules are a known complication while treating Nevus of Ota. It can be treated with TCA CROSS technique by using 65–100% TCA on the depigmented spot (Figs. 48.10A to C).[11]

Adverse reactions to tattoo ink after laser removal, including eczematous reactions and generalized urticaria is well known.[23] Anaphylactic reaction has also been reported after laser removal of tattoos, presumably due to release of ink particles into the systemic circulation. Immediate cutaneous hypersensitivity and delayed anaphylaxis following laser

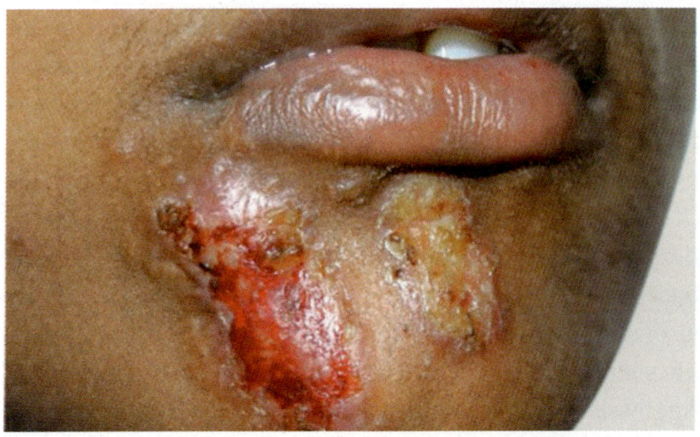

Fig. 48.6: Herpes virus reactivation after fractional CO_2 on posttraumatic scar.

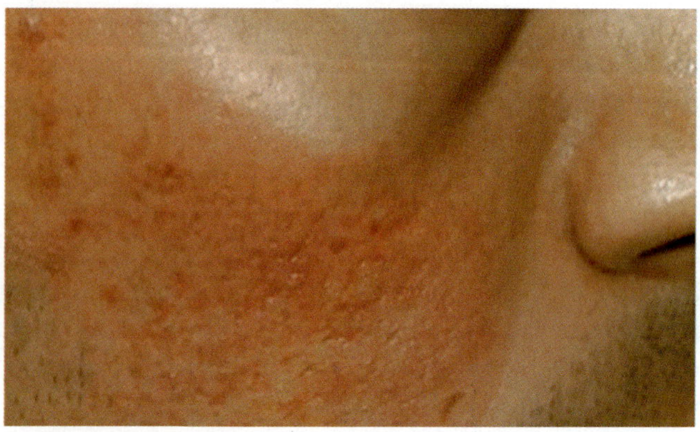

Fig. 48.7: Persistent erythema following laser resurfacing.

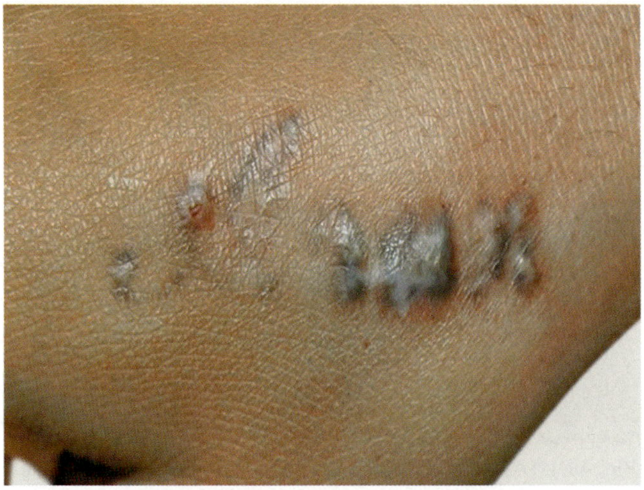

Fig. 48.8: Depigmentation and hyper trophic scar following Q-switched Nd:YAG laser for tattoo removal.

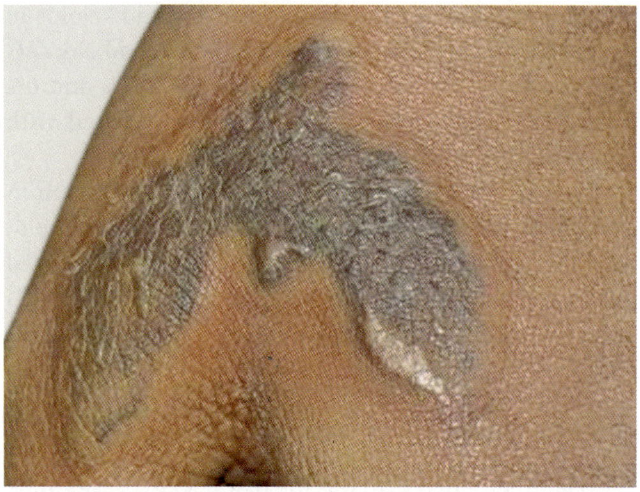

Fig. 48.9: Hypertrophic scar following Q-switched Nd:YAG laser for tattoo removal.

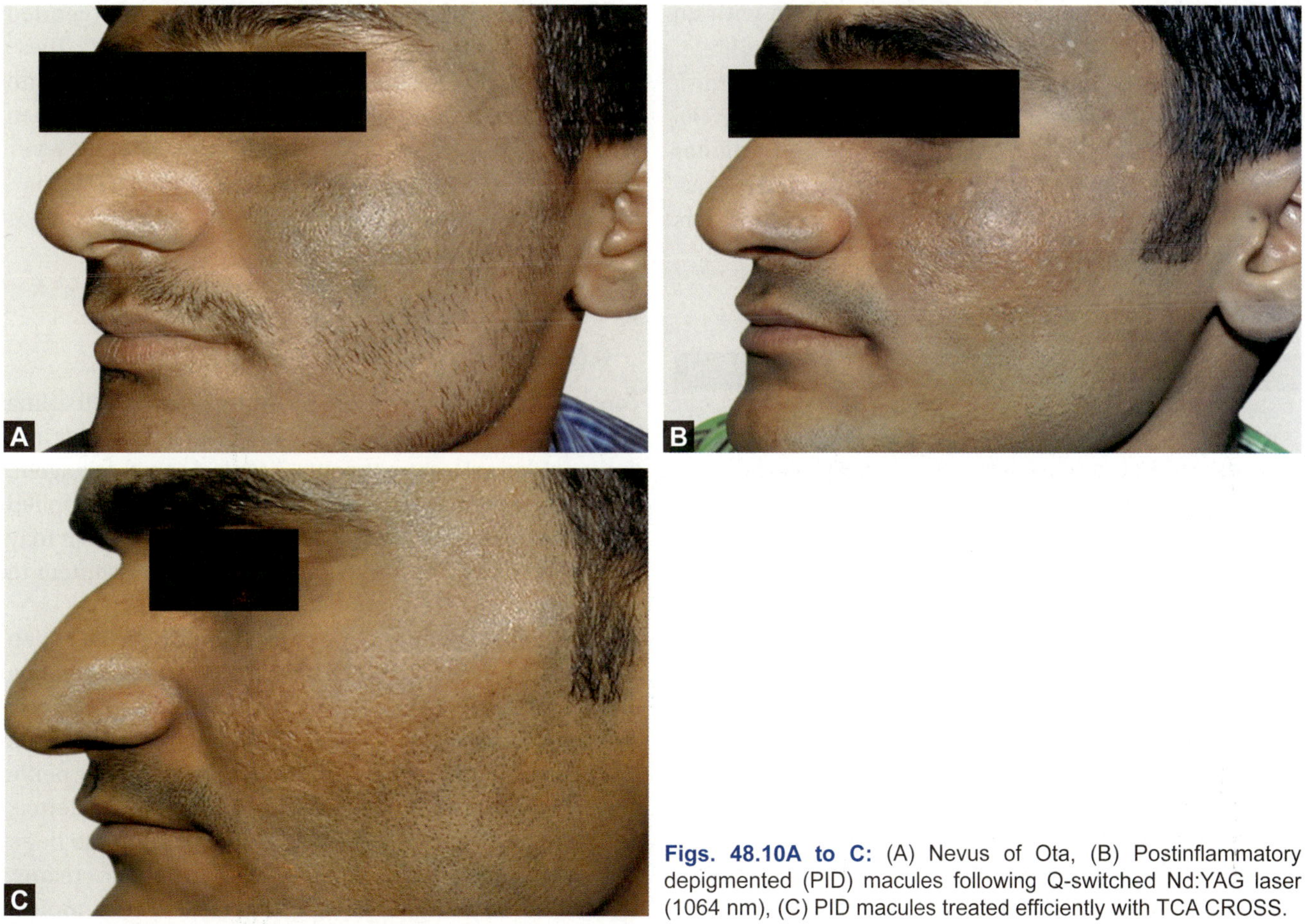

Figs. 48.10A to C: (A) Nevus of Ota, (B) Postinflammatory depigmented (PID) macules following Q-switched Nd:YAG laser (1064 nm), (C) PID macules treated efficiently with TCA CROSS.

for tattoo removal have been reported. In such cases either pretreatment with antihistamines and topical or oral corticosteroids have been successful in suppressing allergic sequelae. Other ablative modalities, such as CO_2 or Erbium:YAG laser for clearance of the tattoo can also be used.[2,24]

The incidence of hypertrophic scarring and keloids in patients following treatment with a Q-switched Nd:YAG laser for tattoo removal was found to be 0.28% and 0% respectively.[25] The hypertrophic scars are treated with intralesional triamcinolone acetonide injections.

Darkening of tattoos made-up of ferric and titanium oxide after treatment with Q-switched Nd:YAG is due to oxidation and discoloration of the tattoo pigment. Oxidized tattoos can only lighten up to a certain extent with Nd:YAG laser. CO_2 laser ablation or surgical excision may become necessary for complete removal.[2]

VASCULAR LASERS

Flash lamp pumped PDL was the first selective laser to be developed on the basis of selective photothermolysis theory for the treatment of port wine stain.[1] The chromophore for a vascular lesion is oxyhemoglobin with a absorption peak at 418, 542 and 577 nm and deoxyhemoglobin with an absorption peak at 430 and 555 nm.[26]

Pulsed potassium titanyl phosphate (KTP-532 nm), pulsed dye laser (585 nm), long-pulsed dye laser (585, 590, 595, 600 nm), long-pulsed alexandrite (755 nm), diodes (800, 810, 940), long-pulsed Nd:YAG (1064 nm) and intense pulsed light source (515–1200 nm) are the various lasers used for the treatment of vascular lesions.

Complications

Immediate	Transient	Persistent
Pain	Postinflammatory hyper-pigmentation	Atrophic scarring-laser imprint (Fig. 48.11)
Bleeding		
Purpura	Uneven resolution	Hypertrophic scars
Edema	Pyogenic granuloma	Depigmentation

The available vascular lasers are more suitable for the fairer skin rather than the type IV and V Fitzpatrick skin types. In comparison to the longer pulse width lasers, PDL is a relatively safer technology to be used for superficial vascular lasers. End point of yellow green light is purpura.

While preparing for the vascular laser sessions, the patient has to be well counseled, especially regarding the number of sessions and the prolonged duration of treatment. The reasons for multiple sessions are variable depth of the lesions, locational anatomy and angiogenesis in between sessions.[27] There is an uneven resolution of the vascular lesion at times; port wine stain for example resolves faster on the lateral aspect of the face than the medial. The nonfacial lesions respond last to treatment with PDL, due to extensive distribution of the vessels from the dermis into the subcutaneous tissue in the central face and nonfacial lesions. [28]

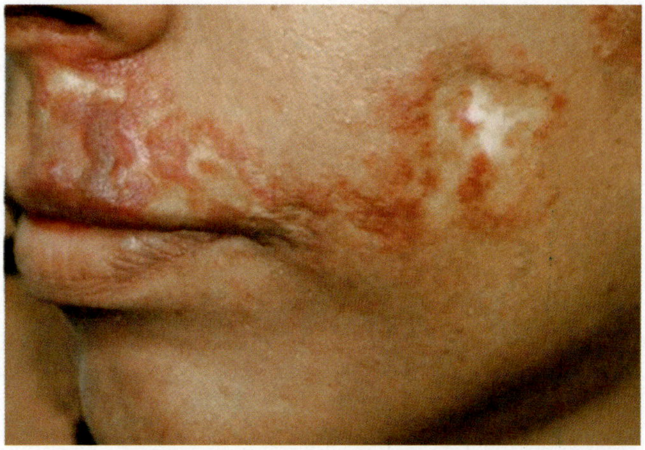

Fig. 48.11: Atrophic scarring following long-pulsed Nd:YAG laser for port wine stain.

Occurrence of pyogenic granuloma is a well-reported phenomenon in port wine stains treated with PDL. These growths can either be treated with PDL itself or excised with a radiofrequency cautery.[29] Egg crater like appearance is often seen with PDL lasers and is due to skip areas. Atrophic scars, also known as "laser imprints" can occur at laser impact sites in some treated cases indicating excessive delivery of energy, absence of cooling or spot overlap.[27]

COMPLICATIONS DUE TO TOPICAL ANESTHESIA

Topical anesthetic agents are recommended as a first-line method of anesthesia for nonablative laser treatments and limited ablative laser treatments. A topical anesthetic agent, such as lidocaine and prilocaine cream (EMLA) is applied for 1 hour before the procedure. Cold packs or cold air may be applied during or immediately after laser treatment to alleviate any further discomfort.[30]

Sensitivity reaction to the topical anesthetic has been well documented (Fig. 48.12). If the patient develops itching or erythema post the application of topical anesthetic cream, the procedure has to be postponed to a later date and other options such as infiltration anesthesia or nerve blocks have to be considered. In authors experience, seborrheic melanosis (Fig. 48.13) like picture has been known to occur as a reaction to topical anesthetic creams. This has to be recognized early and treated with topical moderate potency corticosteroid creams, depigmenting creams and broad spectrum sunscreen.

Caution must be exercised when topical anesthetics are used over large surface areas. Methemoglobinemia is belie-

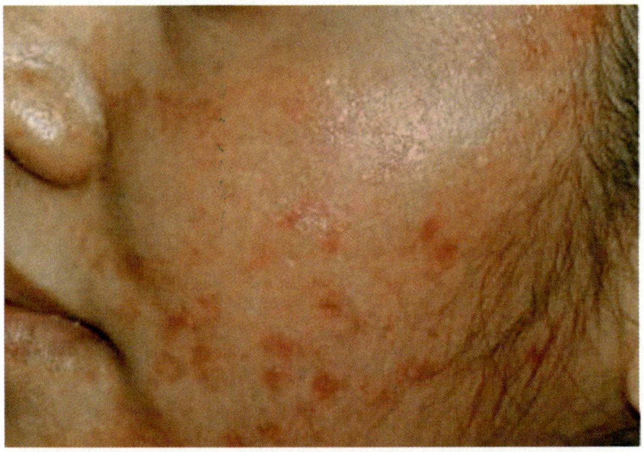

Fig. 48.12: Erythema and edema due to sensitivity reaction to topical EMLA.

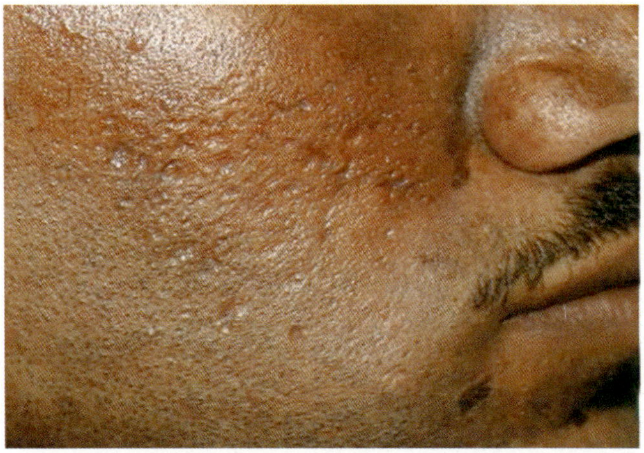

Fig. 48.13: Seborrheic melanosis like pigmentation due to reaction to topical anesthetic cream.

ved to be mechanism of action of severe toxicity when large areas are treated with topical anesthesia under occlusion. Anesthesia-related methemoglobinemia may occur even more commonly in infants.[31]

OCULAR COMPLICATIONS DUE TO LASERS[2,32,33]

Laser glasses are rated by optical density at various wavelengths. An optical density of >4 is considered safe for that particular wavelength. Adherence to strict laser protection guidelines can prevent ocular injury due to laser. The ocular injury to the eye depends on the wavelength of laser used, duration of exposure, beam size and incidence of the laser beam. The likely chromophores in the eye are water and melanin. The lasers in the range of 400–1100 nm target melanin present in the pigmented structure of the eyes such as the retina, iris, choroid and the sclera causing color flashes (after images in the color complementary to the color of the exposed beam) or immediate vision loss with no warning signs due to damage to fovea. Cornea and lens is targeted by the laser of wavelength in between 1400 and 10600 nm leading to thermal damage which manifests as immediate burning pain.

LASER SAFETY AND APPLICATION IN CHILDHOOD AND PREGNANCY

In the pediatric population, standard protective eye equipment may be too large or uncomfortable to provide adequate protection. Use of overlapping patches of white gauze to fit to the contour and size of the periorbital area and securing with paper tape increases the safety profile. Formation of a parent-child tent for procedures below the head and neck is particularly useful in younger children.[34]

Port wine stains in children are flatter and thinner, also lack large ectatic vessels or a nodular component, making them amenable to PDL therapy. In adults with hypertrophied lesions, a laser with longer wavelength such as alexandrite or Nd:YAG gives better response.

There are two schools of thought when it comes to the treatment of nevus of Ota. Early treatment of the lesion in childhood, when the lesion is still brownish can reduce the number of treatment sessions and in doing so lowers the risk of complications. The second group supports the thought that treatment is to be undertaken once the individual is above the age of 16 years as the patient is more cooperative. The pilosebaceous glands are fully developed and the dermal melanocytes are completely positioned leading to lesser complications. The author practices the latter with good results.[34,35]

Lasers for cosmetic indications are better avoided during pregnancy. There are no reports of any adverse effects to the fetus due to laser procedures conducted during the period of gestation.[36]

SUMMARY

A careful and open-minded discussion with patient about results and complications, with documentation and protection of both patient and physician are indispensable. The proper diagnosis, patient selection and optimal parameters of laser are helpful in avoiding most of the complications. The common sources of error leading to complications are choosing wrong equipment/settings and inadequate patient evaluation and care or lack of experience.

Hence success rate of laser treatment directly rests on laser physician's understanding of technology, equipment and its working physics. The aim of laser surgery should maximize patient benefit, minimize risks and avoid permanent sequelae.

REFERENCES

1. Anderson RR, Parrish JA. Selective photothermolysis: precise microsurgery by selective absorption of pulsed radiation. Science. 1983;220(4596):524-7.
2. Isenhath S, Willey A, Bouzari N, et al. Complications of laser Surgery. In: Nouri K (Ed). Complications of Dermatologic Surgery. Mosby Elsevier; 2008. pp. 159-78.
3. Lim SP, Regina. Laser hair removal in the Asian skin. In: Tay Y-K, Chan Y-C (Eds). Textbook of Laser and Light Dermatology in Asian Skin. World Scientific; 2011. pp. 69-81.
4. Lanigan SW. Incidence of side effects after laser hair removal. J Am Acad Dermatol. 2003;49(5):882-6.
5. Lim SP, Lanigan SW. A review of the adverse effects of laser hair removal. Lasers Med Sci. 2006;21(3):121-5.
6. Callender VD, St Surin-Lord S, Davis EC, et al. Post-inflammatory hyperpigmentation: etiologic and therapeutic considerations. Am J ClinDermatol. 2011;12:87-99.
7. Nasiri S, Saeedi M. Palpable purpura: an uncommon side effects of alexandrite laser hair removal. Iran J Dermatol. 2010;13:62-3.
8. Carter JJ, Lanigan SW. Incidence of Acneform reactions after laser hair removal. Laser Med Sci. 2006;21(2):82-5.
9. Lapidoth M, Shafirstein G, Ben Amitai D, et al. Reticulate erythema following diode laser assisted hair removal: a new side effect of a common procedure. J Am Acad Dermatol. 2004;51(5):774-7.
10. Kang HY, Choi YM. FK506 increases pigmentation and migration of human melanocytes. Br J Dermatol. 2006;155 (5):1037-40.
11. Chandrashekar BS, Sriram R, Madura C. Novel method of treatment of post-Q-switched Nd-YAG laser depigmentation with trichloroacetic acid: a report of two cases. J Cutan Aesthet Surg. 2014;7:56-7.
12. Kontoes P, Vlachos S, Konstantinos M, et al. Hiar induction after laser assisted hair removal and its treatment. J Am Acad Dermatol. 2004;54(1):64-7.
13. Desai S, Mahmoud BH, Bhatia AC, et al. Paradoxical hypertrichosis after laser therapy:a review. Dermatol Surg. 2010;36(3):291-8.
14. Remington. Complications of removal lasers. In: Tosti A, Beer KR, DePadova MP (Eds). Management of Complications of Cosmetic Procedures: Handling Common and More Uncommon Problems. Springer; 2012. pp. 47-56.
15. Radmanesh M, Mostaghimi M, Yousefi I, et al. Leukotrichia developed following application of intense pulsed light for hair removal. Dematol Surg. 2002;28(7):572-4.
16. Karsai S, Schmitt L, Raulin C, et al. Combination of short- and long-pulsed mode of electro-optical synergy technology for photoepilation: a retrospective study with short- and long-term follow-up. J Eur Acad Dermatol Venereol. 2009;23(1):46-51.
17. Brightman LA, Brauer JA, Anolik R, et al. Ablative and fractional ablative lasers. Dermatol Clin. 2009;27:479-89.
18. Petrov A, Pljakovska V. Fractional carbon dioxide laser in treatment of acne scars. Maced J Med Sci. 2016;4(1):38-42.
19. Hirsch R. Iatrogenic laser complications. Clin Dermatol. 2011;29:691-5.
20. Gilbert S. Improving the outcome of facial resurfacing: prevention of Herpes Simplex virus type I reactivation. J Antimicrob Chemother. 2001;47(T1):29-34.
21. Riggs K, Keller M, Humphrey TR. Ablative resurfacing: high energy pulsed carbon dioxide and Er:YAG. Clin Dermatol. 2007;25:462-73.
22. Tay YK. Treatment of pigmented lesions in the Asian skin. In: Tay YK (Ed). Textbook of Laser and Light Dermatology in Asian skin. World Scientific; 2011. pp. 37-57.
23. Ashinoff R, Levine VJ, Soccer AN. Allergic reaction to tattoo pigment after laser treatment. Dermatol Surg. 1995;21(4):291-4.
24. Hibler BP, Rossi AM. A case of delayed anaphylaxis after laser tattoo removal. JAAD Case Rep. 2015;1(2):80-1.
25. Kirby W, Alston DB, Chen AH. Incidence of hypertrophic scarring and keloid formation following laser tattoo removal with quality switched Nd:YAG laser. J Clin Aesth Dermatol. 2016;9(5):43-7.
26. Ross EV, Krakowski AC. Laser treatment for vascular laser. In: Goldmann MP, Fitzpatrick R, Ross V, Kilmer SL (Eds). Lasers and Energy Devices for the Skin. 2nd ed. CRP Press. 2013.
27. Chandrashekar BS, Madura C, Pavan RR, et al. Complications in vascular lasers. In: Pai GS (Ed). Complications of Cosmetology: Crafting Cures. 1st ed. New Delhi: Jaypee Brothers Medical Pvt Ltd. 2016.
28. Yu W, Ma G, Qiu Y, et al. Why do port-wine stains (PWS) on the lateral face respond better to pulsed dye laser (PDL) than those located on the central face? J Am Acad Dermatol. 2016;74(3):527-35.
29. Meeker J, Bruce M, Powers R. Pyogenic granuloma appearing in a port wine stain after pulsed dye laser treatment. J Am Acad Dermatol. 2016;74(5):290.
30. Kouba DJ, LoPiccolo MC, Alam M, et al. Guidelines for the use of local anesthesia in office based dermatological surgery. J Am Acad Dermatol. 2016;74(6):1201-19.
31. Minkis K, Whittinton A, Alam M. Dermatologic surgery emergency. J Am Acad Dermatol. 2016;75(2):265-84.
32. Lolis M, Dunbar SW, Goldberg DJ, et al. Patient safety in procedural dermatology: Part II—safety related to cosmetic procedure. J Am Acad Dermatol. 2015;73(1):15-23.
33. Yates B, Keena ST, D'souza L, et al. Laser treatment of periocular skin conditions. Clin Dermatol. 2015;33:197-206.
34. Shahriari M, Makkar H, Finch J. Lasers in dermatology: kids are not just little people. Clin Dermatol. 2015;33:681-6.
35. Kim J. Nevus of ota. In: Cho E. (Ed). Laser and Light Treatment in Asian Skin: Practical Approaches. 1st ed. Koonjna Publishing; 2016.
36. Goldberg D, Maloney M. Dermatologic surgery and cosmetic procedures during pregnancy and the postpartum period. Dermatologic Therapy. 2013;26:321-30.

CHAPTER 49

Lasers: Algorithms

BS Chandrashekar, Madura C, Neelima Ravipati

Flowchart 49.1: Ablation of epidermal and dermal growths.

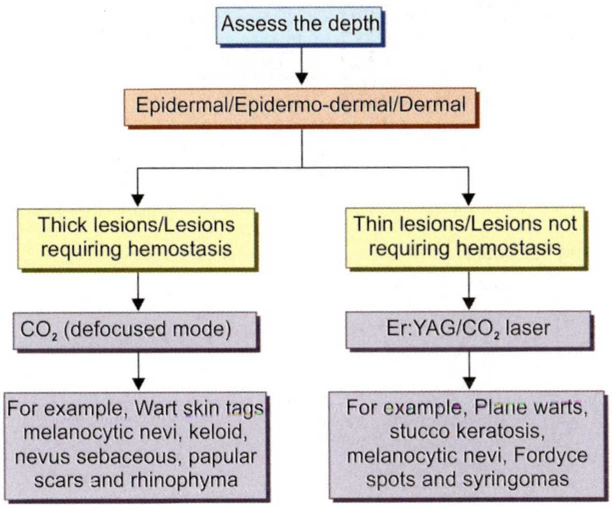

Flowchart 49.2: Treatment of nevus.

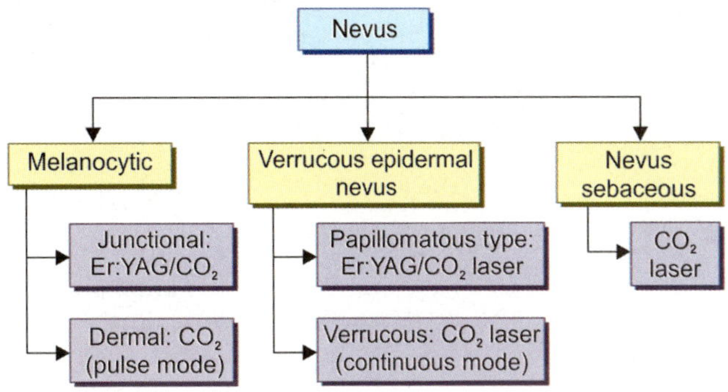

Flowchart 49.3: Managing pigmentary lesions.

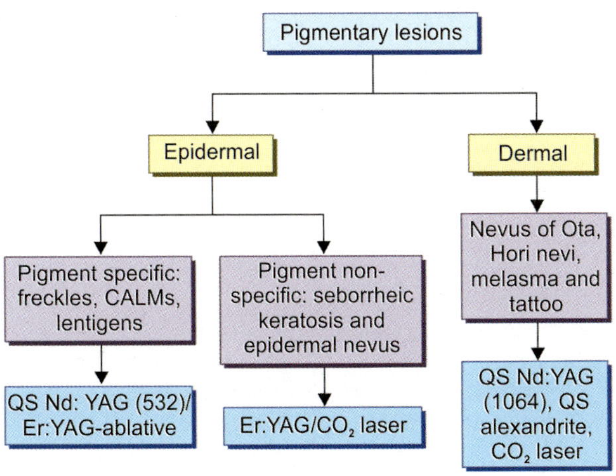

Flowchart 49.4: Tattoo removal.

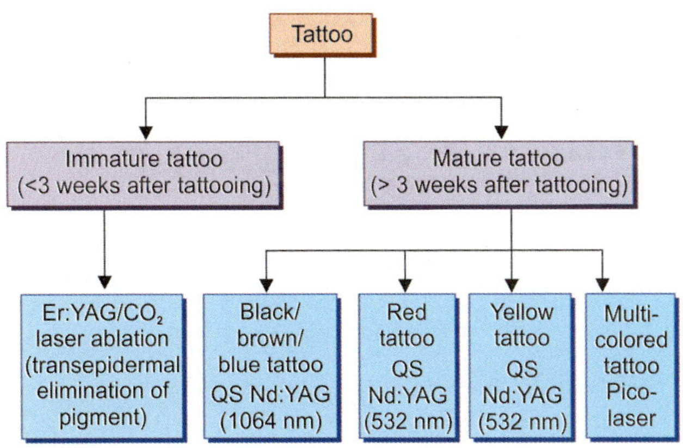

Flowchart 49.5: Keloid and hypertrophic scar.

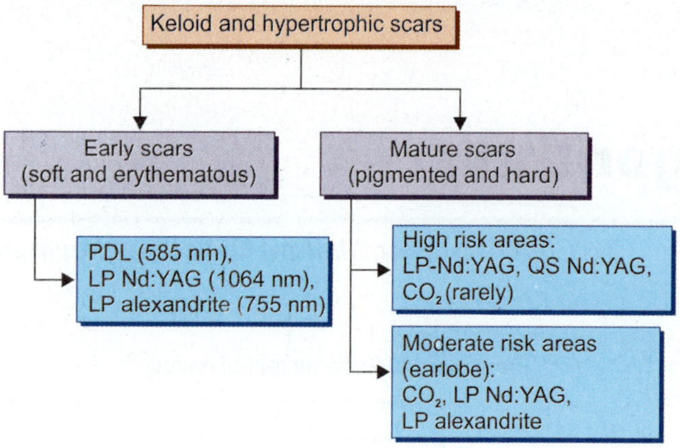

Flowchart 49.6: Managing acne scars with lasers.

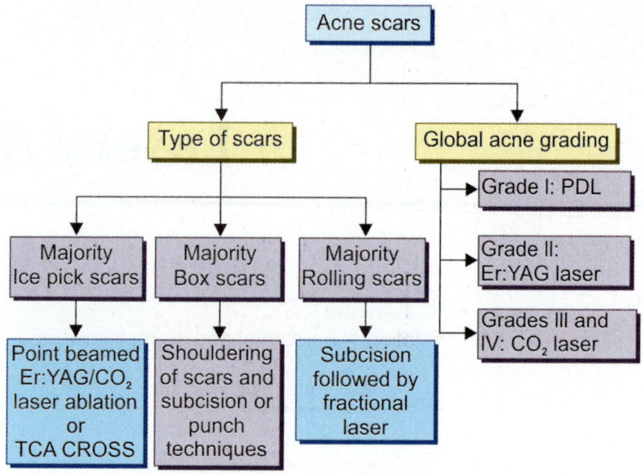

Flowchart 49.7: Managing flat scars.

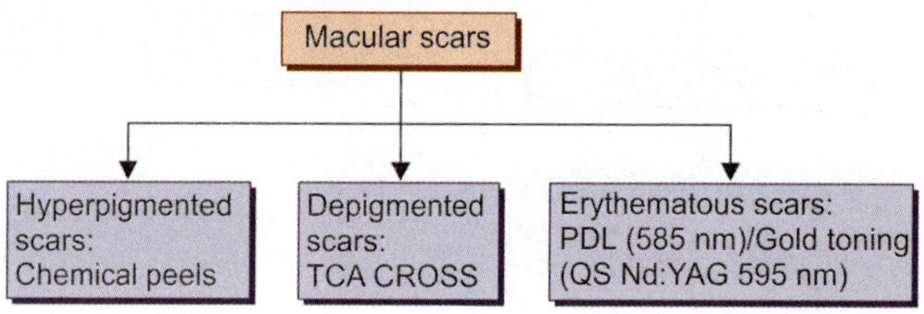

CHAPTER 50

Botulinum Toxin in Dermatosurgery

Shehnaz Arsiwala, Pradeep Kumari, Rasya Dixit, Chaithra Shenoy

INTRODUCTION

Botulinum toxin is a powerful neurotoxin produced by gram-positive anaerobic bacterium clostridium botulinum. The therapeutic efficacy of botulinum toxin (BTX) was first seen with marked improvement of 67 patients with strabismus.[1] Results of the therapy were seen in a week without any systemic side effects. Though the effects lasted for a few months this success opened up avenues for use of BTX in medicine.

There has been an exponential rise in the use of botulinum toxin in the recent years. As time has gone by the number of indications have only increased. The exotoxin has been a novel modality to treat rhytids, the outcome though temporary is unmatched in efficacy by any other method of treatment for dynamic rejuvenation.

Botulinum toxin in dermatology has been available for more than three decades for cosmetic and noncosmetic indications. Wrinkle reduction and rejuvenation are the cosmetic indications while facial spasms, other spastic conditions, calf hypertrophy, migraine, dystonias, dysphonias, hyperhidrosis are some of noncosmetic ones.

DEFINITION

Types of botulinum toxin: Translocation and endopeptidase activity basis.

Seven different antigenic variants of botulinum toxins have been described in the literature. However human nervous system, is susceptible only to 5 types of toxins (A, B, E, F, G) and unaffected by two (C, D). Currently commercially available serotypes are only botulinum toxin types A and B. A is reported to be the most potent of the seven serotypes. B can be as a second line therapy for therapeutic nonresponders to type A. Botulinum toxin does not penetrate the skin therefore there is no topical formulation.[2-4]

Mechanism of action (Figs. 50.1A to E): Botulinum toxin acts by blocking the release of Acetylcholine (Ach) from the presynaptic nerve terminals, causing a chemical denervation of the end organ (muscle or secretory gland). End organ function returns after 12 to 16 weeks when the new nerve terminals sprout and establish reconnection with the muscle endplate, ending the clinical effect of the toxin. This is why the effect of botulinum toxin is not permanent. The blockage of Ach release after BTX injection is a multistep process, including binding, internalization, translocation and cleavage. The steps of the mechanism have been illustrated below; however a detailed explanation of this is beyond the scope of this chapter.

Preparation and Interactions[5]

BTX-A is most commonly used toxin. The vial available is a 100 or 50 unit freeze dried powder which contains purified clostridium botulinum toxin type A neurotoxin complex-BTX-A.

- The vial must be stored in a freezer at or below –5°C until reconstitution.
- Sterile saline (0.9% sodium chloride) with or without preservative is used to reconstitute the BTX injection by gentle mixing.
- Sterile saline solution with preservative (0.9% benzyl alcohol) used as reconstituting diluents reduces microbial contamination and provides a weak local anesthetic effect. However, contamination is rarely a problem, and the anesthetic effect is modest.
- The standard practice is to use 2.5 mL of diluent to 100 units of toxin to prepare a solution of 4U/0.1 mL.
- Once reconstituted, botulinum toxin should be refrigerated at 2–8°C till it is used. (Table 50.1)
- It is recommended to use the reconstituted botulinum toxin within 4 hours for best results. The vial is however usable up to 4 weeks after reconstitution.
- Use a 30-gauge 1-inch needle with a tuberculin syringe to perform the injection procedure.

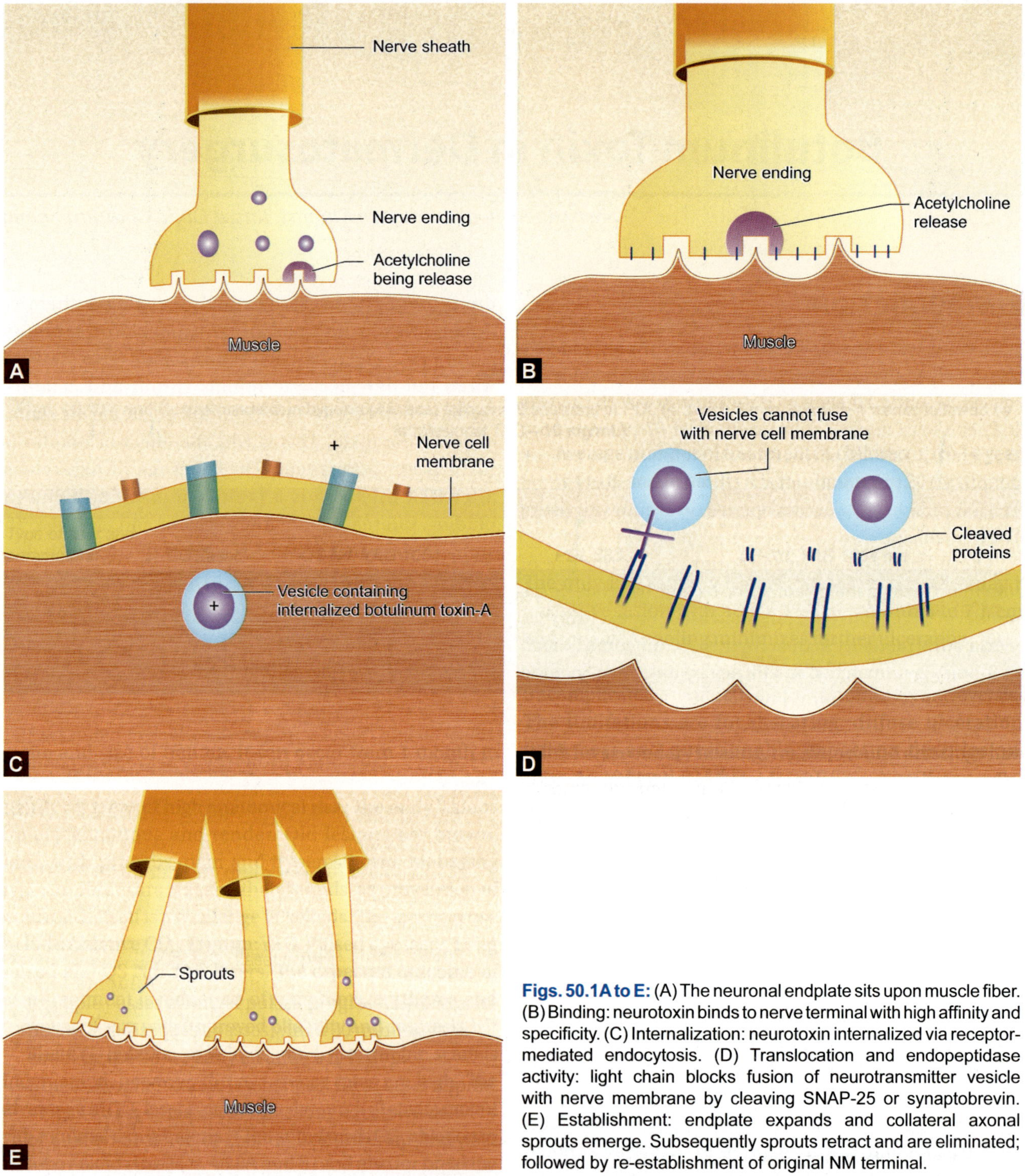

Figs. 50.1A to E: (A) The neuronal endplate sits upon muscle fiber. (B) Binding: neurotoxin binds to nerve terminal with high affinity and specificity. (C) Internalization: neurotoxin internalized via receptor-mediated endocytosis. (D) Translocation and endopeptidase activity: light chain blocks fusion of neurotransmitter vesicle with nerve membrane by cleaving SNAP-25 or synaptobrevin. (E) Establishment: endplate expands and collateral axonal sprouts emerge. Subsequently sprouts retract and are eliminated; followed by re-establishment of original NM terminal.

- More than 50 units per site and more than 400 units per session should be avoided as chance of BTX antibodies is high.[5] Action of BTX-A on skin starts within a week, peak response is seen at 2 months and action wears off in 4–6 months.[6] For a 70 kg person the lethal dose of BTX is estimated to be 3000 U.[7]

Table 50.1: Dilution and storage of BTX.

Diluent	0.9% nonpreserved sterile saline
Concentration	Ratio of 100 U/2.5 mL
Storage	
• Before reconstitution	2°C to 8°C for up to 24 months
• After reconstitution	Up to 6 weeks at 4°C
Handling	Maintain cold chain while transporting

- In a study it was found that no loss of activity at 6 hours but a 44% loss after 12 hours and a 70% loss with refreezing at 1-2 weeks. Contradictory to this other authors report no substantial loss of potency in a 10 U/1 mL reconstituted solution kept refrigerated for 1 month.

There are ever expanding applications of BTX in medicine (Table 50.2).

Table 50.2: Indications of BTX in medicine.

Noncosmetic indications of BTX in medicine
Achalasia
Anismus
Blepharospasm*
Cervical dystonia*
Detrusor hyperreflexia*
Essential tremor
Hemifacial spasm*
Axillary hyperhidrosis*
Palmoplantar hyperhidrosis and facial hyperhidrosis
Migraine and headache*
Myofascial pain syndrome
Occupational dystonia
Pain due to muscle spasm
Rectal fissure
Sialorrhea
Spasmodic dysphonia
Strabismus*
Spasticity
Thoracic outlet syndrome
Traumatic brain injury
Writer's cramp

*US FDA approved indications.

CLINICAL APPLICATION OF BTX IN DERMATOLOGY[5]

Cosmetic indications: of BTX are well-known, and are beyond the scope of this chapter.

Noncosmetic indications of BTX in dermatology include:[5]

- Hyperhidrosis
- Scars—hypertrophic scars and keloids, Acne scars, painful scars
- Lichen simplex chronicus and other neurodermatitis
- Postherpetic neuralgia
- Blepharospasm
- Multiple eccrine hidrocystomas

The advantages of using BTX for the management of these conditions, is manifold.

Demonstrated clinical efficacy
Wide margin of safety data
Low incidence and short time of side effects
Easily available therapy, simple to administer
Quick treatment, single treatment twice a year
Excellent safety and tolerability
Offers chance of treatment, where many other options may not be feasible

General considerations before injecting BTX:

- Evaluate (by animation in blepharospasm)
- Rule out contraindications
- Understand patient desire
- Explain realistic expectations, including the temporary nature of treatment, and need for repeat treatment in 6 to 8 months time
- Take informed valid written consent
- Counsel regarding all other available invasive and non-invasive modalities
- Take photographs/videos with animation
- Use surface anesthesia to make the injections more comfortable
- Mark injection points
- Change needles frequently to avoid pain due to needle blunting
- Estimate total units given and make a record of the same in the treatment chart, so the doses can be repeated and results can be duplicated at a later date.

CONTRAINDICATIONS FOR BTX TREATMENT

- During pregnancy and breastfeeding
- Neuromuscular junction diseases: Eaton Lambert syndrome, myasthenia gravis

- Disorders of muscle weakness: multiple sclerosis, amyotrophic lateral sclerosis, concomitant use of aminoglycoside antibiotics
- Patient with unrealistic expectations.

HYPERHIDROSIS

Botulinum toxin is an FDA approved minimally invasive nonsurgical therapy for axillary hyperhidrosis, however BTX has been used to treat palmoplantar, facial and scalp hyperhidrosis.

Hyperhidrosis may be focal or generalized. Focal hyperhidrosis usually affects localized areas like axillae, palms, soles of the feet, face, and rarely, other areas. It can affect quality of life when severe. It usually appears during the second or third decade of life.[6]

Other treatments for hyperhidrosis
Antiperspirants
Oral anticholinergics
Iontophoresis
Curettage
Bipolar radiofrequency
Microwave based therapies
Transthoracic sympathectomy[6]

Botulinum Treatment in Hyperhidrosis

Treatment with BTX-A reduces perspiration in the axilla, on the palms, and on the soles of the feet, in patients with hyperhidrosis.[7]

Mechanism of action: Intradermal use of BTX is found to be beneficial in patients with hyperhidrosis due to its action on Ach receptors which are important end effectors in autonomic nervous system where sweat glands are targeted. It acts by blocking the release of acetylcholine temporarily thus preventing synaptic transmission and producing an effective chemodenervation of the gland. This results in temporary cessation of sweating. BTX-A is superior to topical therapies in controlling sweating. Hornberger et al[8] reported that the mean sweat production was still below 50% of the preinjection levelat 24 weeks post-injection without any adverse effects and satisfaction rate of over 92% in injected patients and also reported its efficacy in auriculotemporal syndrome.

Injection Sites

Before injecting, the hyperhidrotic field (particularly in axillary hyperhidrosis) may be demarcated using the minor starch-iodine test.

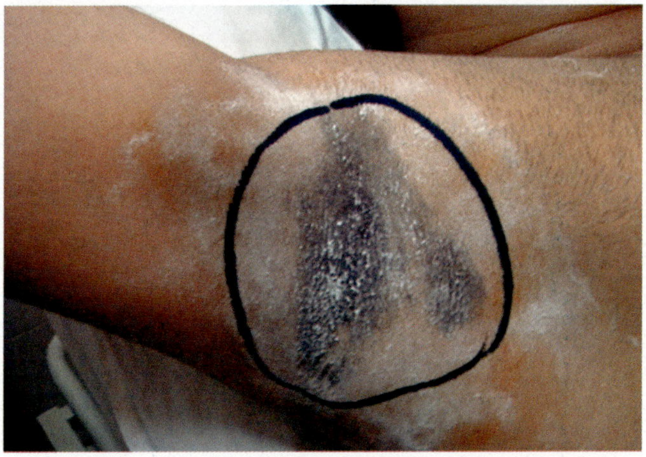

Fig. 50.2: Starch iodine test to mark demarcate sweating activity zone in axilla.
Courtesy: Dr Shehnaz Arsiwala.

Starch iodine test: Cleanse the skin and paint the axilla with povidone iodine solution. After the solution dries on the skin, dusty corn starch powder. Wait for the sweating. The areas of sweating show a bluish black discoloration. A photograph of the area of sweating helps to document the pretreatment image.

In most cases the axillary sweat glands are concentrated in a circular or ovoid area approximately 4–5 cm in diameter, although there may be some peripheral sweat glands also. The starch-iodine test will locate the exact area to be treated including any peripheral glands (Fig. 50.2).[9-11]

- 30–40 intradermal injection sites within defined area using 1.5–2 cm grid spacing of injections (Figs. 50.3 and 50.4)
- Injections are made intradermally and small wheals/blebs are raised at a level at deep dermis as the sweat glands are located in the reticular dermis or subcutis (Fig. 50.5).
- Injection at this level prevents diffusion to the deeper muscles
- The 31 G needle is introduced at angle of 45° to reach a depth of 2–3 bevels, and the toxin deposited in the dermis. An oblique introduction of the needle, prevents wastage and helps ease the needle point more comfortably into the skin
- Use of ice helps to alleviate any discomfort
- Injections need to be repeated every 6–7 months. Starch iodine test can be done to check response (Fig. 50.6)

Complications: This is a simple procedure and usually devoid of complications. However, compensatory increase in sweating over the body has been described.

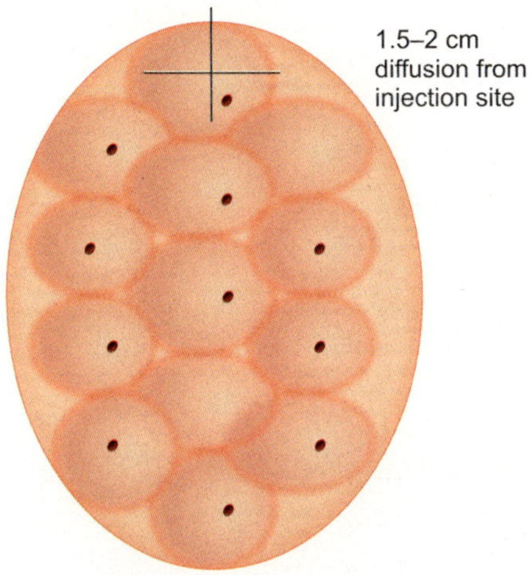

Fig. 50.3: Injection points axilla.

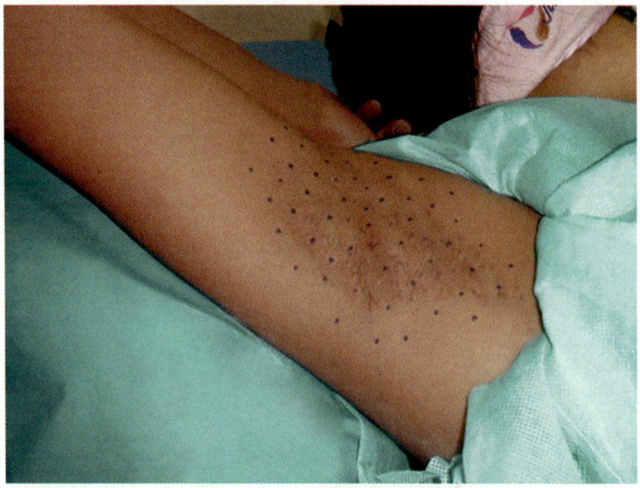

Fig. 50.4: Injection points axilla.
Courtesy: Dr Shehnaz Arsiwala.

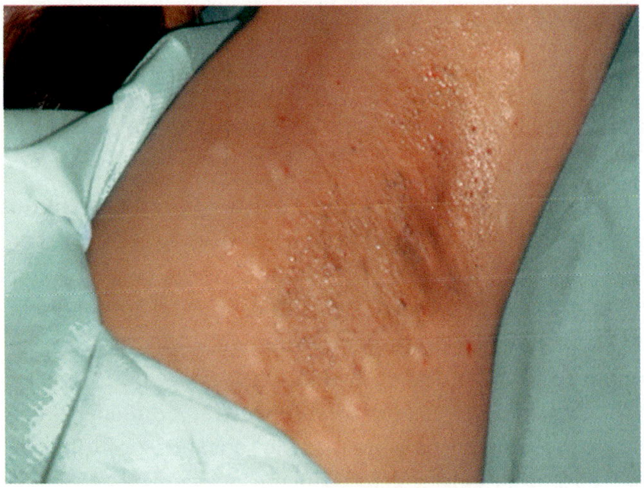

Fig. 50.5: Classical blebs formed after intradermal BTX-A injection.
Courtesy: Dr Shehnaz Arsiwala.

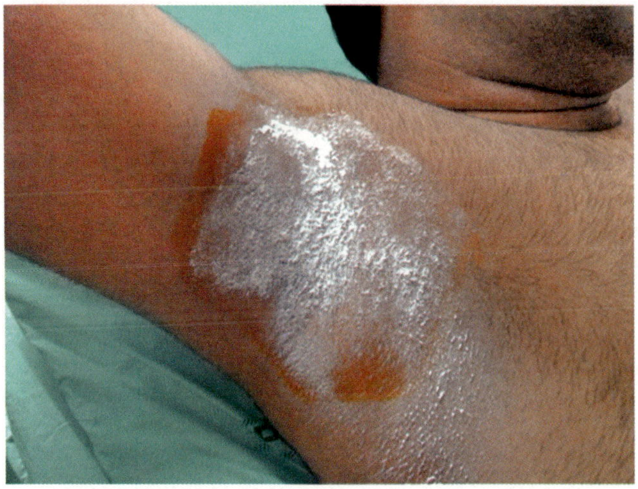

Fig. 50.6: Negative starch iodine test 2 weeks after BTX-A injection.
Courtesy: Dr Shehnaz Arsiwala.

Dilution/100 unit vial	4.0 mL
Total volume/axilla	2.0 mL
Volume/injection site	0.13–0.2 mL
Units/injection site	3–3.5 U
Total dose/axilla	50 U

BTX IN PALMAR HYPERHIDROSIS (OFF LABEL INDICATION)

BTX treatment can help in the management of primary palmoplantar hyperhidrosis, and also in palmar hyperhidrosis associated with conditions, such as EB simplex or pachyonychia congenita. In pompholyx associated dyshidrosis, the condition of pruritus as well as the associated hyperhidrosis improves.

Dilution/100 unit vial	:	4.0 mL
Total volume/palm	:	2.0 mL
Volume/injection site	:	0.13–0.2 mL
Units/injection site	:	3–3.5 U
Total dose/palm	:	100–150 U
Total dose/sole	:	50–250 U

- BTX reconstituted with saline 100 U/4 mL.
- 2-4 U of BTX-A was injected intradermally on palmar aspects of fingers and palms

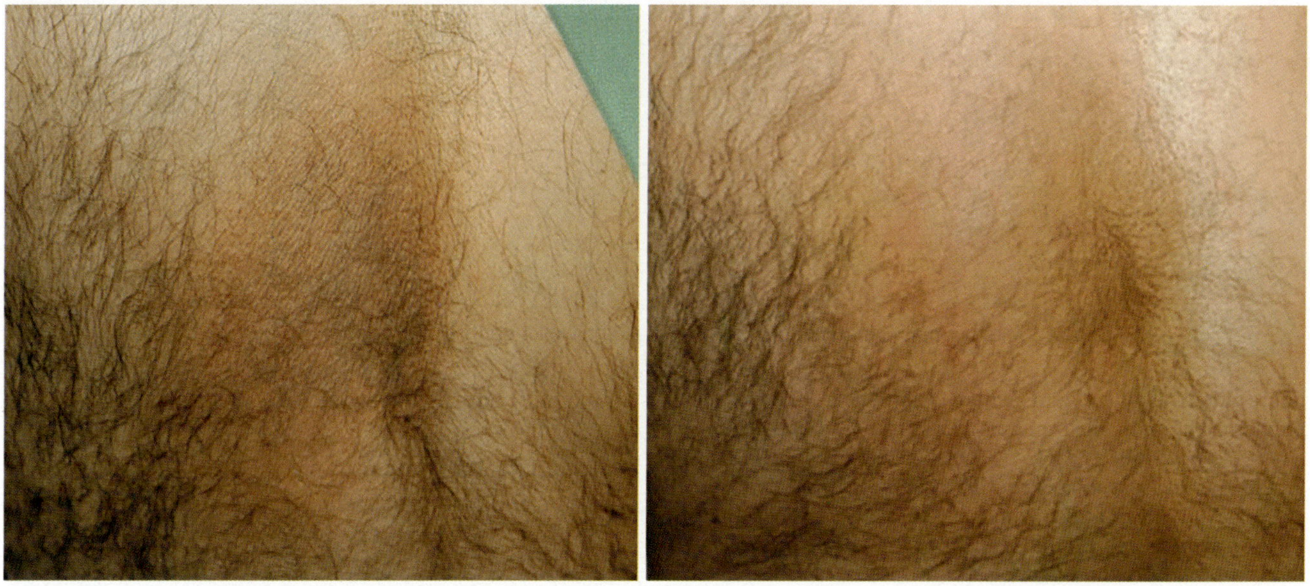

Fig. 50.7: Lichen simplex chronicus: resolution of lichenification after two sessions of BTX injection.
Courtesy: Cutis Academy of Cutaneous Science.

- Injection is introduced at a 45° angle and advanced just beyond the stratum corneum, where the resistance gives. The toxin is deposited in this plane.
- Around 100–150 units/hand can be injected as total dose.
- Significant pain is expected in this area, use multiple needles, use of nerve blocks recommended in addition to topical anesthesia.
- A keratolytic product applied for a few weeks prior to treatment can help with sole injections.
- Complications include weakness of the thenar and hypothenar muscles which may cause changes in handwriting temporarily.
- Musicians who use their fingers must be cautioned about the temporary weakness of these muscles.

Other conditions which can be treated in the same manner include:

Craniofacial hyperhidrosis
Frey's syndrome
Submammary hyperhidrosis
Perianal and groin hyperhidrosis
Compensatory hyperhidrosis
Hailey Hailey disease

BTX IN LICHEN SIMPLEX CHRONICUS

Lichen simplex chronicus is an eczematous condition characterized by intractable pruritus.[12] BTX-A has proved beneficial when injected intradermally in these lesions (Fig. 50.7).[13]

Mechanism of action: ACh-sensitive C-fibers explain pruritus in LSC patients.[14] The action of ACh on the fibers is modulated by BTX-A injections. In a broader perspective other pruritic conditions may be amenable to BTX therapy like pompholyx where dyshidrosis plays an important role and as shown in a study[15,16] where 7 out of 10 patients improved after treatment. BTX-A directly affects neurotransmitters causing pruritic sensation or indirectly decreases that sensation by reducing localized perspiration.

Technique of injection: About 4–16 units of BTX is injected intradermally in the lichenified lesions with associated pruritus.

Dilution/100 unit vial	2.5 mL
Volume/injection site	0.13–0.2 mL
Units/injection site	3–3.5 U
Total dose/area	10–15 U

BOTULINUM TOXIN IN SCARS[17,18]

Botulinum toxin acts mainly as adjunctive treatment and has been used for treatment of acne scars, atrophic/hypertrophic scars and keloids.

Acne scars: BTX in scars has mainly been used to prevent widening of newly formed scars as an adjunctive treatment. The proposed mechanism of action is that BTX may help immobilize the local muscles and thereby reduce muscle pull leading to less skin tension, and therefore, leads to reduced microtrauma and subsequent inflammation.

Hypertrophic Scars

- Inject intradermally, till slight blanching of scar is seen
- Dose of 2.5 units per cubic cm of scar, maximum dose 100 units
- Repeat injections at monthly intervals till symptomatic relief is attained.

Hypertrophic scars have been reported to show satisfactory improvement when followed up till 6 months.[19]

Mechanism of action: In hypertrophic scars, botulinum toxin is believed to temporarily denervate smooth muscle fibers and thus decrease tension in scar, in turn leading to reduced scar formation.[20]

Keloids: BTX is supposed to act in this indication by reducing tensile forces during cicatrization and by effectively regulating the balance between fibroblast proliferation and cellular apoptosis.

Dilution	2.5 mL/100 U
Dose per session	70–140 U
Intervals between treatments	3 months
Maximum treatments	4

In keloids; neoplastic fibroblasts are the target for BTX-A injection and the intended effect is on primary trophic and metabolic changes and not on muscle immobilization. Thus the timing of injection in keloid is late rather than during surgery like surgical scars.[21]

Surgical or traumatic scars: Mechanism of action—In these scars, BTX has been postulated to help by chemo denervating the muscle and thus immobilising the muscle, this helps in better healing of the scars. BTX-A in this indication has also been postulated to help by having a positive effect on cutaneous healing. BTX-A injection leads to superior apposition of wound edges and finally to smooth skin overlying soft tissues (Figs. 50.8A to D).

Ideal time of injection	Intraoperatively, so wound heals without tension
Site of injection	Just adjacent to the scar
Dilution	2.5 mL/100 U vial
Dose	15 units over each side

Gassner and colleagues could demonstrate that botulinum toxin injections into the musculature adjacent to the wound (15 U of BTA (Botox, Allergan, Irvine, CA, USA) per 2 cm intraoperative length) within 24 hours after wound closure resulted in enhanced wound healing and less noticeable scars compared with placebo.[22]

POSTHERPETIC NEURALGIA

Therapeutic benefits of BTX-A in patients have been studied by various random controlled studies. The improvement reported by the patient is quantified by using the visual analogue scale. The affected area is marked with the help of the patient and toxin is injected intradermally or subdermally in the range of 1-2 units/cm^2.

BTX-A has been shown to block release of pain-mediating substance P, CGRP and glutamate from motor and sensory neurons. The mechanism of action may be dual, first by blocking peripheral sensitization and by indirectly reducing central sensitization. Second mechanism may be due to reduction in various substances that sensitize nociceptors.[23,24]

BLEPHAROSPASM[25,26]

Botulinum toxin in blepharospasm was one of the early noncosmetic indications of BTX-A usage and has become mainstay therapy for blepharospasm. This was the first FDA approved indication of noncosmetic usage of BTX-A. Blepharospasm may occur in isolation or increase gradually to other areas.

Treatment is mainly indicated to avoid functional blindness, to prevent complications like corneal abrasions and maintain quality of life. Blepharospasm is typically more common in elderly, bilateral and involuntary.[26]

Botulinum toxin is now considered a standard treatment option in patients that are 12 years or older. Cumulative dosage in a 30 day period for blepharospasm should not exceed 200 units

The 10 most recommended injections sites are marked on the diagram (Fig. 50.9).

Dilution	1 mL/100 unit vial
Dosage	2–3 units per site
Frequency	Once in 3–6 months, effect may wear off earlier due to smaller doses used

- A patient with furrows should be injected in corrugator supercilii. Preferably injections should be close to the lid margin.
- Injections in the lower lid should be only on lateral side to avoid functional ectropion/tearing.
- Other injections sites can be lateral to orbicularis oculi, if this area is also affected by spasm. Injection of

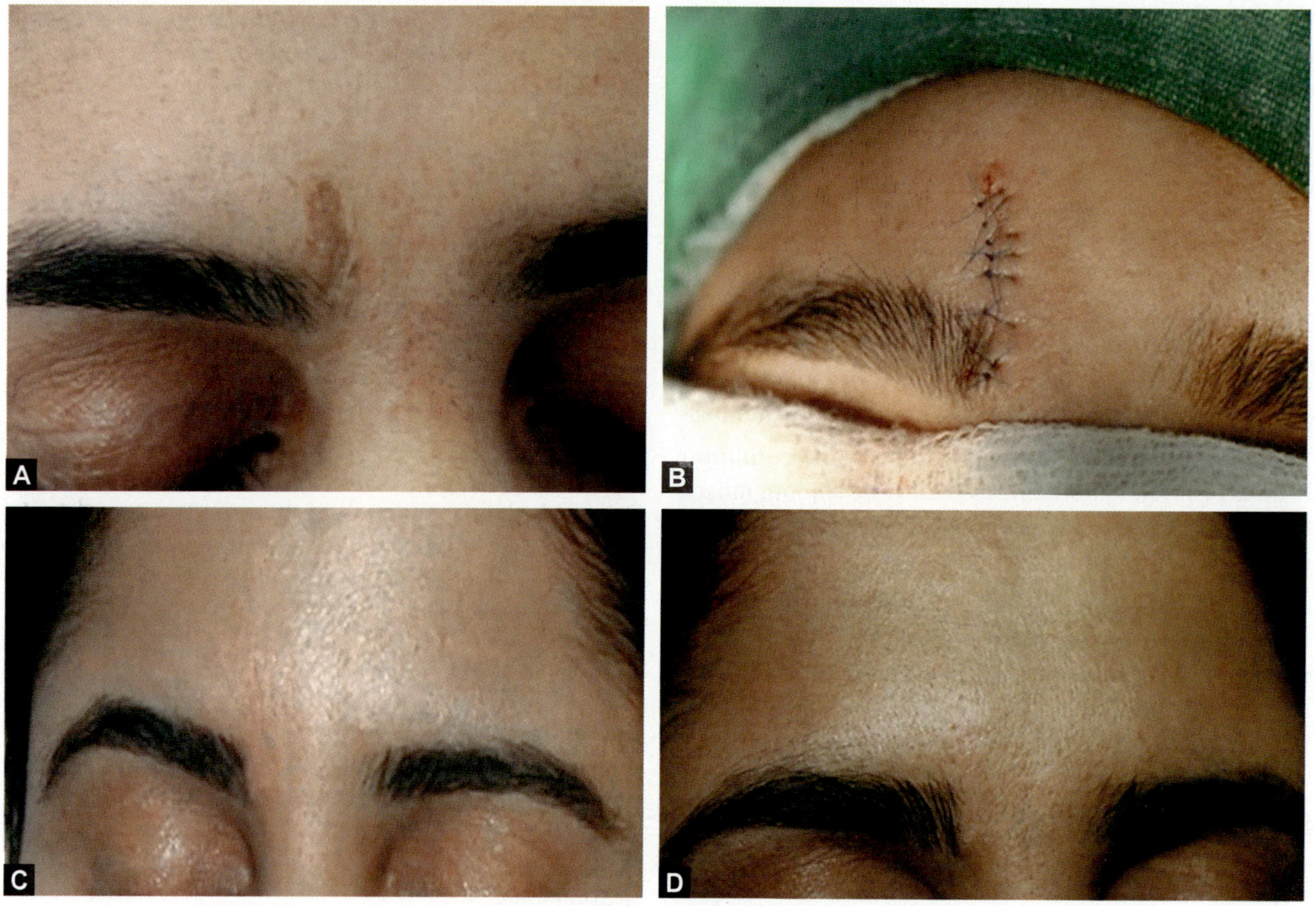

Figs. 50.8A to D: Serial pictures of scar excision followed by BTX injection in the intraoperative period. Note the elevation of right eyebrow in third image due to the injection of BTX into medial corrugators and the procerus muscle.
Courtesy: Cutis Academy of Cutaneous Science.

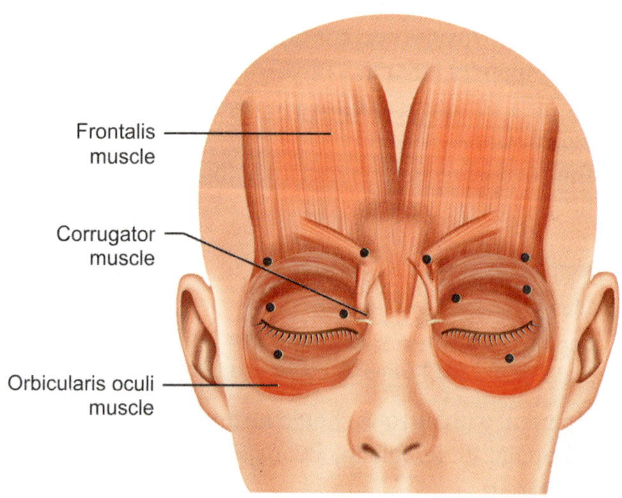

Fig. 50.9: Treatment of Blepharospasm: 10 most common injection sites.

the procerus, levator labii superioris nasi may also be helpful.

- Avoid injecting near the levator palpebrae superioris to avoid ptosis.
- Injecting into medial part of the lower lid should be avoided to prevent diplopia.
- Initial effect of the injections is generally seen within 3 days and reaches a peak 1 to 2 weeks post-treatment. The effect lasts for approximately 3 months, following which the procedure can be repeated.[1]
- At repeat treatment sessions, dose can be increased, if initial response was insufficient. However, there appears to be little benefit obtainable from injecting more than 5 units.

Inappropriate techniques, site and dosage of botulinum toxin injection can result in complications like ptosis (7–11%), corneal exposure/lagophthalmos (5–12%), symptomatic dry eye (7.5%), entropion, ectropion, epiphora, photophobia (2.5%), diplopia (<1%), ecchymosis, and lower facial weakness.[27,28]

MULTIPLE ECCRINE HIDROCYSTOMA

Eccrine hidrocystomas are benign cystic multiple shining small translucent skin-colored dome shaped papules arising from eccrine or apocrine glands, with a predilection for the central face. The condition runs a chronic course with seasonal variability, exacerbated in summer due to increased sweat production.

The recommended dosage on BTX injection is superficial injections of 1–2 units/cm^2, given annually at the beginning of summer. The lesion begin to resolve in 7 days.[29]

CONCLUSION

In the last decade a large number of indications in dermatology that are noncosmetic have emerged in the application of BTX in dermatology. An in depth knowledge helps one to apply these indications to clinical practice albeit safely and effectively. One has to keep abreast with latest developments for uses in conditions like lichen simplex chronicus and scars, as they have shown valuable results in pilot studies. More scientific studies are needed to evaluate the efficacy of BTX in these conditions and to expand the horizon.

REFERENCES

1. Scott AB. Botulinum toxin injection of eye muscles to correct strabismus. Trans Am Ophthalmol Soc. 1981;79:734-70.
2. Eleopra R, Tugnoli V, Quatrale R, et al. Different types of botulinum toxin in humans. Mov Disord. 2004;19:S53-9.
3. Dressler D. Botulinum toxin mechanisms of action. Suppl Clin Neurophysiol. 2004;57:159-66.
4. Breidenbach MA, Brunger AT. New insights into clostridial neurotoxin-SNARE interactions. Trends Mol Med. 2005;11: 377-81.
5. Klein AW. The clinical use of botulinum toxin. Dermatologic Clinics. 2004;22.
6. Zacherl J, Huber ER, Imhof M, et al. Long-term results of 630 thoracoscopic sympathectomies for primary hyperhidrosis: the Vienna experience. Eur J Surg.1998;80(suppl 5):43-6.
7. Herbst F, Plas EG, Odderson IR. Axillary hyperhidrosis treated with botulinum toxin A. Arch Phys Med Rehabil. 1998;79:350-2.
8. Hornberger J, Grimes K, Naumann M, et al. Recognition, diagnosis, and treatment of primary focal hyperhidrosis (review). J Am Acad Dermatol. 2004;51:274-86.
9. Karamfilov T, Konrad H, Karte K, et al. Lower relapse rate of botulinum toxin A therapy for axillary hyperhidrosis by dose increase. Arch Dermatol. 2000;136:487-90.
10. Wollina U, Karamfilov T, Konrad H. High-dose botulinum toxin A therapy for axillary hyperhidrosis markedly prolongs the relapse-free interval. J Am Acad Dermatol. 2002;46:536-40.
11. Naumann M. Evidence-based medicine: botulinum toxin in focal hyperhidrosis. J Neurol. 2001;248:31-3.
12. Wallengren J. Neuroanatomy and neurophysiology of itch. Dermatol Ther. 2005;18:292-303.
13. Heckmann M, Heyer G, Brunner B, et al. Botulinum toxin type A injection in the treatment of lichen simplex: An open pilot study. J Am Acad Dermatol. 2002;46:617-9.
14. Schmelz M, Schmidt R, Bickel A, et al. Specific C-receptors for itch in human skin. J Neuroscience. 1997;17:8003-8.
15. Swartling C, Naver H, Lindberg M, et al. Treatment of dyshidrotic hand dermatitis with intradermal botulinum toxin. J Am Acad Dermatol. 2002;47:667-71.
16. Wollina U, Karamfilov T. Adjuvant botulinum toxin A in dyshidrotic hand eczema: A controlled prospective pilot study with left-right comparison. J Eur Acad Dermatol Venereol. 2002;16:40-2.
17. Sherris DA, Gassner HG. Botulinum toxin to minimize facial scarring. Facial Plastic Surgery. 2002;18(1):35-40.
18. Xiao Z, Zhang M, Liu Y, et al. Botulinum toxin type a inhibits connective tissue growth factor expression in fibroblasts derived from hypertrophic scar. Aesthetic Plastic Surgery. 2011;35(5):802-7.
19. Xiao Z, Zhang F, Cui Z. Treatment of hypertrophic scars with intralesional botulinum toxin type A injection: a preliminary report. Aesth Plast Surg. 2009;33(3):409-12.
20. Scheffer AR, Erasmus C, van Hulst K, et al. Efficacy and duration of botulinum toxin treatment for drooling in 131 children. Arch Otolaryngol Head Neck Surg. 2010;136:873-7.
21. Zhibo X, Miaobo Z. Intralesional botulinum toxin type A injection as a new treatment measure for keloids. Plast Reconstr Surg. 2009;124(5):275e-7e.
22. Gassner HG, Brissett AE, Otley CC, et al. Botulinum toxin to improve facial wound healing: A prospective, blinded, placebo-controlled study. Mayo Clin Proc. 2006;81(8):1023-8.
23. Ali S, Noah A, et al. Botulinum toxin: noncosmetic and off-label dermatological uses. J Dermatology Dermatologic Sur. 2015;19:1-8.
24. Wollina U. Botulinum toxin: noncosmetic indications and possible mechanisms of action. J Cutan Aesthe Surg. 2008;1(1):3-6.
25. Costa J, Espirito-Santo C, Borges A, et al. Botulinum toxin type a therapy for blepharospasm. Cochrane Database Syst Rev. 2005;1:CD004900.
26. Hallett M, Albanese A, Dressler D, et al. Evidence-based review and assessment of botulinum neurotoxin for the treatment of movement disorders. Toxicon. 2013;67:94-114.
27. Cote TR, Mohan AK, Polder JA. Botulinum toxin type A injections: adverse events reported to the US Food and Drug Administration in therapeutic and cosmetic cases. J Am Acad Dermatol. 2005;53(3):407-15.
28. Grandas F, Elston J, Quinn N, et al. Blepharospasm: a review of 264 patients. J Neurol Neurosurg Psychiatry. 1988;51(6):767-72.
29. Correia O, et al. Multiple eccrine hidrocystomas - from diagnosis to treatment: the role of dermatoscopy and botulinum toxin. Dermatology. 219;1:77-9.

CHAPTER 51

Fillers in Dermatosurgery

Rasya Dixit, Harish Prasad, Chaithra Shenoy

INTRODUCTION

Dermal fillers are an important tool in the armamentarium of aesthetic physicians. However, they also have an equally significant role in the management of noncosmetic indications. The use of dermal fillers is gratifying because the improvement they offer is immediate and does not involve any long surgery or downtime.

DEFINITION

Dermal filler refers to enhancing or replacing the volume, by natural or synthetic substance to improve the appearance. The specific procedure that is performed depends on the material of filler used, the plane in which it is injected and the limiting factors being the physical property of the filler itself; and the characteristics of the patient's skin.

TYPES OF FILLERS

There are various types of fillers available today. A simple classification system is described in Table 51.1.

This chapter deals with only hyalorunic acid (HA) filler, though the same techniques and methods of injection can be substituted for any other filler molecule.

Table 51.1: Classification of fillers.

Filler class	*Average clinical efficacy*	*Examples*
Temporary fillers	3 months–18 months	Hyalorunic acid (HA) fillers and collagen
Semi-permanent fillers	Upto 24 months	Poly-l-lactic acid (PLLA) and calcium hydroxyapatite
Permanent fillers	Many years, if not life long	Silicon, polyacrylamide, polymethylmethacrylate (PMMA), hydroxyethyl-methacrylate

PRINCIPLE OF FILLERS

Hyalorunic acid (HA), also called hyaluronan, is chemically a glycosaminoglycan, which consists of regularly repeating nonsulfated disaccharide units of both glucuronic acid and N-acetylglucosamine.[1] HA pharmacologically is a highly hydrophilic molecule which attracts water leading to the formation of higher concentrations occupying large volumes, compared to its mass. HA can form gels even at low concentrations. When water is drawn into the HA matrix, turgor/pressure is created across the gradient which allows the HA to resist compressive forces. HA is inert, i.e. it does not exhibit tissue or species specificity and therefore immunologic reactions and rejections are not seen.

Deciding the Type of HA Filler

The various characteristics of the filler is given in Table 51.2.

The HA fillers mainly differ from each other based on concentration, cross-linking, type of agent which cross links, particulate size, monophasic/biphasic and presence or absence of anesthetic. The concentration of HA filler is probably the most important of theses. Those with higher HA concentrations have longer duration of effect because they are likely to displace more tissue. Concentrations of 20 mg/g or more are considered ideal. It is a single ether cross-link bonding which is utilized to stabilize the HA fillers. Double cross-linked, multi crossed-linked, and monophasic gels are presently available in the newer nonparticulate form. The long chains of HA are bound to 1,4-butanediol diglycidylether (BDDA) and the shorter HA chains are bound to the network, also with BDDA. This results in a homogeneous mass which is potentially less resistant to degradation, making it a longer-lasting HA filler. Although as previously discussed, HA concentration is a principal parameter in influencing product duration, it is not the total HA concentration that affects duration, but rather the amount of cross-linked HA gel that plays an important role in filler performance. Unmodified HA is completely metabolized a few days after injection.

Table 51.2: Characteristics of fillers.

Filler characteristics	*Effect*	*Depth of injection*	*Longevity*
Concentration of HA	–	–	Higher concentration of HA linked to longevity
Cross linking	Higher concentration of cross-linked product may need a larger bore of needle to inject	More cross-linked HA should be injected deeper	Higher concentration of cross-linked HA linked to longevity
Monophasic or biphasic	–	Biphasic gels come in different particulate sizes and may be customized to individual treatment area	Monophasic may last longer and be more cohesive
G Prime	Gel hardness	Higher G, deeper injections, wider bore needles may be needed for injection	–
Hydration of filler	Ability to absorb water	Inject smaller volumes as product will swell, under-correction recommended	–
Preincorporated local anesthetic	No/ minimal pain during injection	–	–

Because of above facts, the newer gels are nonparticulate requiring higher HA concentration for the same duration of effect. Cross-linking of HA is mainly required to prevent its biodegradation due to free radicals and enzymes and to increase the duration of effect. BDDA has been used with good efficacy. A newer agent named 1, 2, 7, 8-diepoxyoctane is found to have a further increased duration of action. Larger HA particles last longer and are therefore reserved for deep dermal injections and defects. Monophasic HA fillers are more like cohesive gels rather than just being HA particles. Biphasic HA fillers are however mainly particle forms. The monophasic HA fillers last longer and usually do not migrate after the injection. The biphasic HA fillers can however be customized to the indication and area being treated by altering the particle size.[2]

Whether the filler would cause a swelling depends on the filler's ability to reach an equilibrium with bound water. HA gel's capacity to swell differs from product to product and depends on various parameters like the concentration, cross-linking density, and what process has been used to hydrate the gel. The fully hydrated or equilibrium gels are the fillers which have already reached their utmost hydration capacity; so they will not swell up after injecting into dermis. Nonequilibrium gels which have not yet reached their hydration capacity are the ones which tend to swell post the injection, and therefore consideration must be given to underfilling defects when performing such corrections.[3]

Another important factor among the properties of fillers is the role of the hardness of the gel or G Prime in its performance. This in turn depends on factors like HA concentration, initial molecular weight, modification type and the presence or absence of the unmodified HA in finished product. Firm gels with higher G provide much better resistance to deformation though they may be stiffer or lumpier when injected and compared to the softer gels. Firmer gels can induce more tissue trauma than softer gels, which can lead to more pain, inflammation, edema, and erythema post the injection. Softer gels with a lower G' however do not resist deformation as much as the firmer gels, and provide a more natural feel when they are injected.[3]

Hyaluronic acid fillers offer the following advantages over the other groups of fillers.

- Low allergenic potential as the newer generations of fillers are obtained from bacterial synthesis.
- Availability of a wide range of options to address defects in various layers of the skin.
- Relatively painless due to the addition of anesthetic agents along with the product which makes injections comfortable.
- Opportunity of a rapid correction of nodules or over filling by the use of hyaluronidase injection.[4]

Assess the Deformity

The deformity should be analyzed in relation to the following aspects:

- Its anatomical location
- Its proximity to vital structures
- Direction with respect to cosmetic units

- Length, width and shape
- Contour
- Color (hypo/hyperpigmentation).

Examination of the Surrounding Tissue

- Local landmarks
- Tension in surrounding tissues
- Distortion of angle of eyes, mouth, vermilion border of lips
- Skin texture, pigmentation, laxity, and adnexal structures.

Counseling

- Foremost duty is to explain that no deformity can be made to vanish completely
- It can only be modified to make it more aesthetic and functionally viable
- Temporary nature of dermal fillers should be explained in detail
- Objective to be achieved should be explained
- Discuss all other available invasive and noninvasive modalities
- Patients with underlying psychiatric disease who blame their deformity for their psychological difficulties, who are soon to be married, who are involved in litigation related to their scar, are poor candidates for filler treatments.

GENERAL TECHNICAL CONSIDERATIONS FOR DERMAL FILLERS

- *Anesthesia*: Most hyaluronic acid fillers are now available with anesthetic preincorporated in the syringe. If not, a topical local anesthetic cream under occlusion can be used over the treatment area. However, as topical anesthetic can cause mild edema over the treatment area obscuring the defects. Clinical photographs need to be taken before local anesthetic application for the same reason. Local nerve blocks can be used if possible.
- *Assessment of deformity*: The correct assessment of the depth and relations of the deformity decides the type of HA filler to be used. So, it is important to understand the basic level at which the deformity exists. For example in En coup de sabre, there is a full thickness deformity, which may even involve bone. In such a condition, two different HAs may be used, one on top of the other. The bottom layer of the filler would be an HA with a greater G prime with higher cohesivity, to provide the support and the lift, the superficial layer would be an HA with lesser G prime and lower cohesivity to help the skin merge with the surrounding tissue. In a patient with acne scars or post-accident scars, it is also important to complete all other complementary scar revision techniques, achieve the maximum improvement with the other techniques, before attempting filler. This is because once the filler is integrated into the skin, further treatment aimed at scar revision, may introduce inflammatory cell mediators which can affect the longevity of the filler molecule.
- *Techniques of injection*: The choice of the injection technique depends on many factors like the indication, its location, the filler material and its qualities, the choice of needle vs cannula and the experience of the injector.

Linear Threading Technique

Indications

- Linear scars
- Post surgical depressed scars.

Principle or Technique

This technique is used in the management of linear atrophic scars or depressions. The full length of the needle is inserted in the middle of the line and the filler is injected while withdrawing the needle slowly backwards, so that the threads of the gel are placed linearly along the length of the scar (Fig. 51.1).

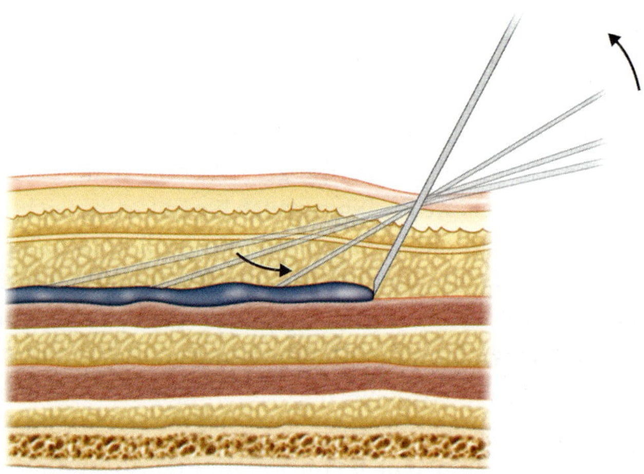

Fig. 51.1: Linear threading.

Tips

The angle of entry into the skin is around 30 to 45° from the skin. Injection can be antegrade or retrograde. In the antegrade technique, filler is injected as the needle is being pushed forward, so that the product displaces any small blood vessel in its way. In the retrograde technique, the full length of the needle is injected and the product is injected as the needle is withdrawn. Since this is a technique where the needle enters the skin tangentially, the depth of injection is intradermal or supramuscular. If a deeper plane of injection is desired, then change to the serial puncture technique.

It is important to stop injecting when withdrawing the needle or cannula from the skin. This prevents a track of filler forming which can keep the skin from re-epithelializing and allows infection to track back into the filler.

Serial Puncture Technique

Indications

This is used again for the management of linear scars especially in anatomical areas where improvement is needed along a line, however the linear threading is contraindicated due to vascular elements in the area, or if the depth of injection is necessary to be deep due to the thickness of the product being used. Here serial puncture along the avascular zone is preferred (Fig. 51.2).

Technique of Injection

Multiple injections are placed serially along the length of the deformity. It is made closely together, so that it merges into a smooth continuous line which lifts the overlying tissue.

The needle entry into the skin is perpendicular to the skin. Here the depth of injection depends on the deformity to be corrected. As the depth of injection can be varied, different depths can be chosen for different deformities. However, care has to be taken in depositing equal amounts of product in each site to avoid a bumpy appearance. If excess product is deposited in a single site, using a gentle but firm pressure, the filler product can be massaged into the surrounding dermis. If the whole procedure involves multiple serial puncture technique, change the needles frequently to avoid blunting of the needle and unnecessary pain or discomfort to the patient.

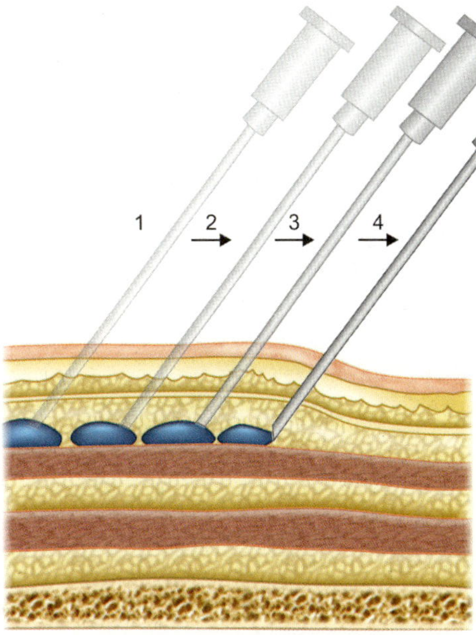

Fig. 51.2: Serial puncture technique.

Fanning Technique

Indication

Larger area of volume loss is targeted.

Technique

The needle is inserted at the periphery of the area to be treated as when using the linear threading technique. After injecting one line, the needle is withdrawn till the tip is almost exiting the skin, then, the direction of the needle is changed to the new desired direction and injected as before along a new line. This technique helps in covering a larger area with a single point of entry (Fig. 51.3).

Tips

Though it is easy to deposit product with a single point of entry, this method has most chances of bruising.[5]

Cross-hatching Technique

Indication

Used to volumize large areas of volume loss.

Methods and Techniques

The needle is inserted at the periphery of the area intended to be augmented and injected using the linear threading

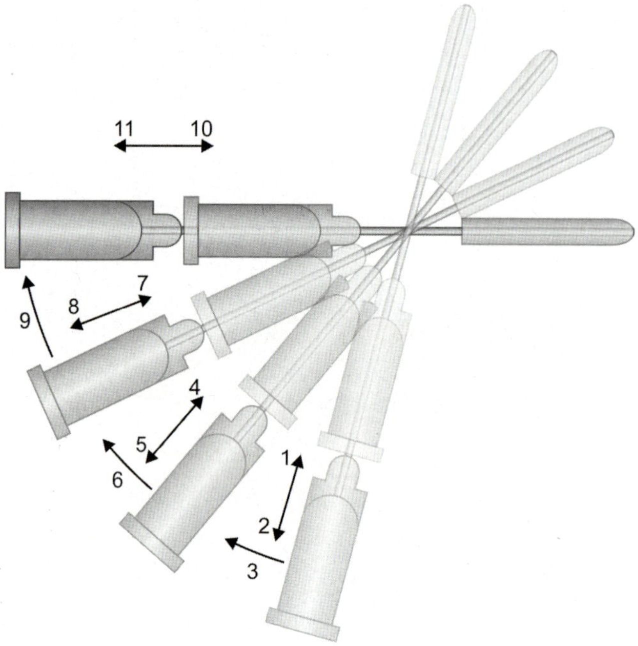

Fig. 51.3: Fanning technique.

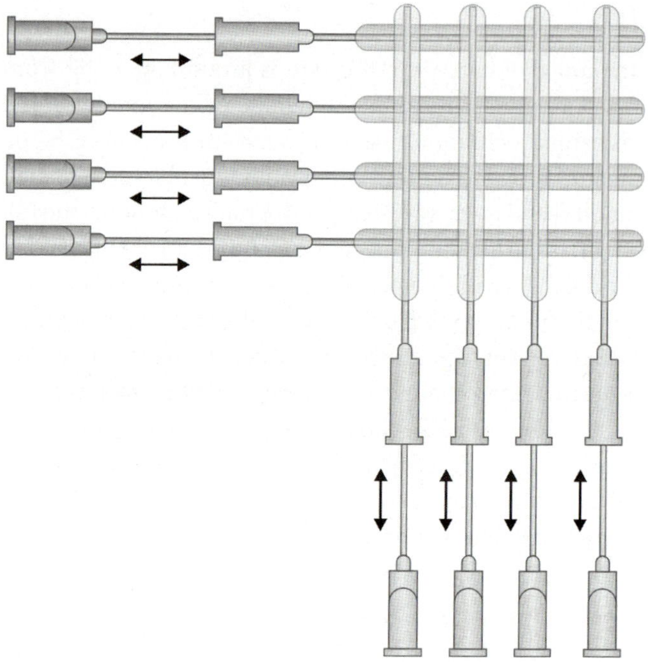

Fig. 51.4: Cross-hatching technique.

technique. The needle is withdrawn from the skin and inserted 5–10 nm away from the first injection site and injected in the same way. Same procedure can then be repeated perpendicular to the original lines (Fig. 51.4). This helps augment a broad area with an even distribution of product. This can be used to form the base or foundation of the filler platform and can reduce the volumes of product used.

Depot Technique

Indication

This technique is used when the defect is to be repaired at a single point.

Technique

The needle is inserted perpendicular to the skin and a small bolus of product is deposited. Then the needle is withdrawn (Fig. 51.5).

Cone/Tower Technique

Indication

Repair of defects at a single point, however, the tower is built from the bony support and lifts up the skin like a tent.

Technique

This is a modification of the Depot technique. The needle is inserted perpendicular to the skin till it reaches bone. Then a small bolus of product is deposited. As the needle is withdrawn, product is continually injected so a cone or pyramid shape is formed. The needle may have to be reinserted along another edge of the pyramid, so the use of a small quantity of product can lift up or support the overlying tissue like the pillars of a tent (Fig. 51.6).

Dual Plane Technique/Sandwich Technique

Indication

Large volume deficits, with smaller, localized deficits in the dermis (e.g. Acne scarring with acne induced lipoatrophy).

Technique

In this technique, the fillers are injected in two planes, a deep plane and a superficial plane. Any technique described above can be used, and even two different types of HA can be combined. For example, a product with a higher viscosity can be placed deeper, as it has greater ability to lift, and a more smoother HA product can be

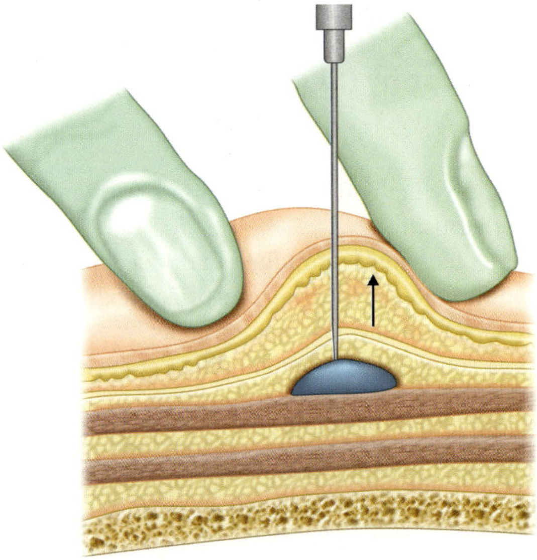

Fig. 51.5: Depot technique.

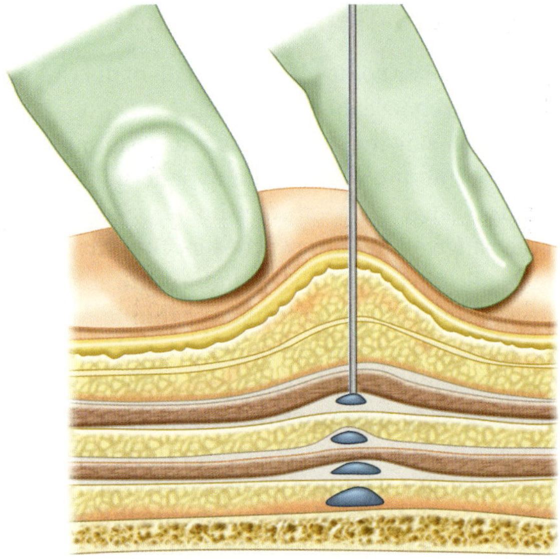

Fig. 51.6: Towering technique.

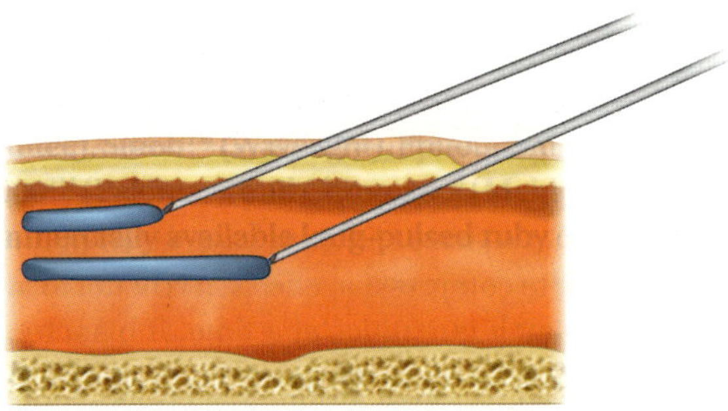

Fig. 51.7: Dual plane technique/Sandwich technique.

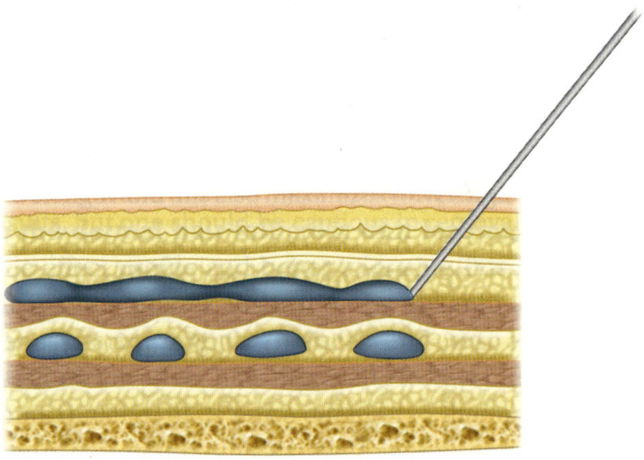

Fig. 51.8: Pillar and bridge technique.

placed on top of it. The use of two layers addresses the deficit in both the superficial and deep compartments (Fig. 51.7).

Pillar and Bridge Technique

Indication

In areas of great volume loss, it is difficult to replace all the lost volume with product. Greater volumes of product increase the cost as well as can cause compression of the surrounding vascular elements giving rise to complications. To minimize the use of product, a pillar and bridge technique is used.

Technique

The pillars are depots or cones of product which are deposited close to one another over a bony support, and then the bridge of a linear thread of filler is deposited superficially over it (Fig. 51.8).

NEEDLES VERSUS CANNULA

The most dreaded complication of any filler technique is an intravascular deposition of filler product into the blood vessel. This could cause skin necrosis or even lead to blindness when associated with retrograde blood flow in the face regions. The recent availability of blunt-tipped cannulas have minimized the damage to the neurovascular bundles.[6]

Use of a Blunt-Tipped Microcannula

Choosing the entry point—Use the length of the cannula as a reference to choose the entry point.

After cleansing the skin to ensure asepsis, puncture an entry point into the skin using a hypodermic disposable needle, the gauge of the needle should be slightly bigger than the gauge of the cannula chosen. The entry direction of the needle track is 60 to 90°. A more acute angle of entry is not advised as the blunt-tipped cannula may not be able to enter. Remove the sharp needle, and introduce the microcannula into the same entry point. The entry direction has to be the same as made by the needle.

Tips to Help Easy Entry of Cannula

Pinch the skin to create a small drop of blood so the entry point can be better visualized. Else have your assistant pull out the needle while you are ready to introduce the cannula.

Hold the cannula like a pen, and stretch the skin in the opposite direction with the noninjecting hand to increase the diameter of the entry hole.

Do not touch the length of the cannula with your glove as it increases the chances of infection.

Slide the length of the cannula into the skin. If you encounter resistance, then withdraw partially and move back and forth without forcing the cannula. The non-injecting hand can be used to palpate the tip of the cannula to assess the depth and direction of injection.

Inject the filler in a retrograde manner as you withdraw the cannula.

To change directions of injection, withdraw the cannula almost out of the skin, with just the tip remaining inside at the desired depth and reintroduce in a different direction.

COMPLICATIONS AND THEIR PREVENTION

Injection techniques that results in dissection of the subepidermal plane (e.g. fanlike needle use, rapid injection, rapid flow rates, and higher volumes) increase the risks of local adverse events. Injection techniques that increase epidermal damage or subcutaneous exposure (e.g. multiple punctures or deep subcutaneous injection) have no effect on adverse events. Furthermore, single injection correction, depth of injection, and nonanimal stabilized hyaluronic acid (NASHA) product injected have no effect on local adverse events.[5]

SPECIFIC INDICATIONS FOR FILLERS

Lipodystrophy (Figs. 51.9A to D)

Tips

- Use a product with higher G prime with a cannula to avoid bruising.
- A cross hatching technique can be used to increase the volume followed by tower and bridge technique to help under specifically low volume areas.
- Large volume loss is better addressed by fat grafting as there can be a big economic burden.[7]
- Products which enhance collagen remodeling and stimulate fibroblast action may be better suited as they reduce need for frequent reinjections.[8]

Lip Repair (Post Cleft Lip Surgery/Post-Accident)

Tips

- Use a product with low G prime as it is softer and does not make the lip stiff.
- Respect the anatomy of the lip, and inject below the white line to avoid the vessels.
- Single depot injections are preferred under the surgical line, and linear threading can be used to volumize the lip.[9]
- Excess product injected can cause vascular compromise in the lip due to compression effects. It is better to inject slowly and small quantities at a time. If blanching is noted, stop injection, use a warm compress. If no improvement is noted, hyaluronidase can be injected.

Acne Scars/Chicken Pox Scars (Figs. 51.10 to 51.12)

The goal of using dermal fillers in the treatment of atrophic acne scarring is to replace volume lost by the atrophic effects of acne. Rolling scars are most amenable to treatment by fillers. Fillers are chosen as a last option as a quick fix to the management of scars.

Technique

- The depot technique is used to treat the superficial scars.
- The needle is introduced into the middle of the scar vertically and the product is placed in the mid-dermis.
- The product chosen is of a mid level viscosity.

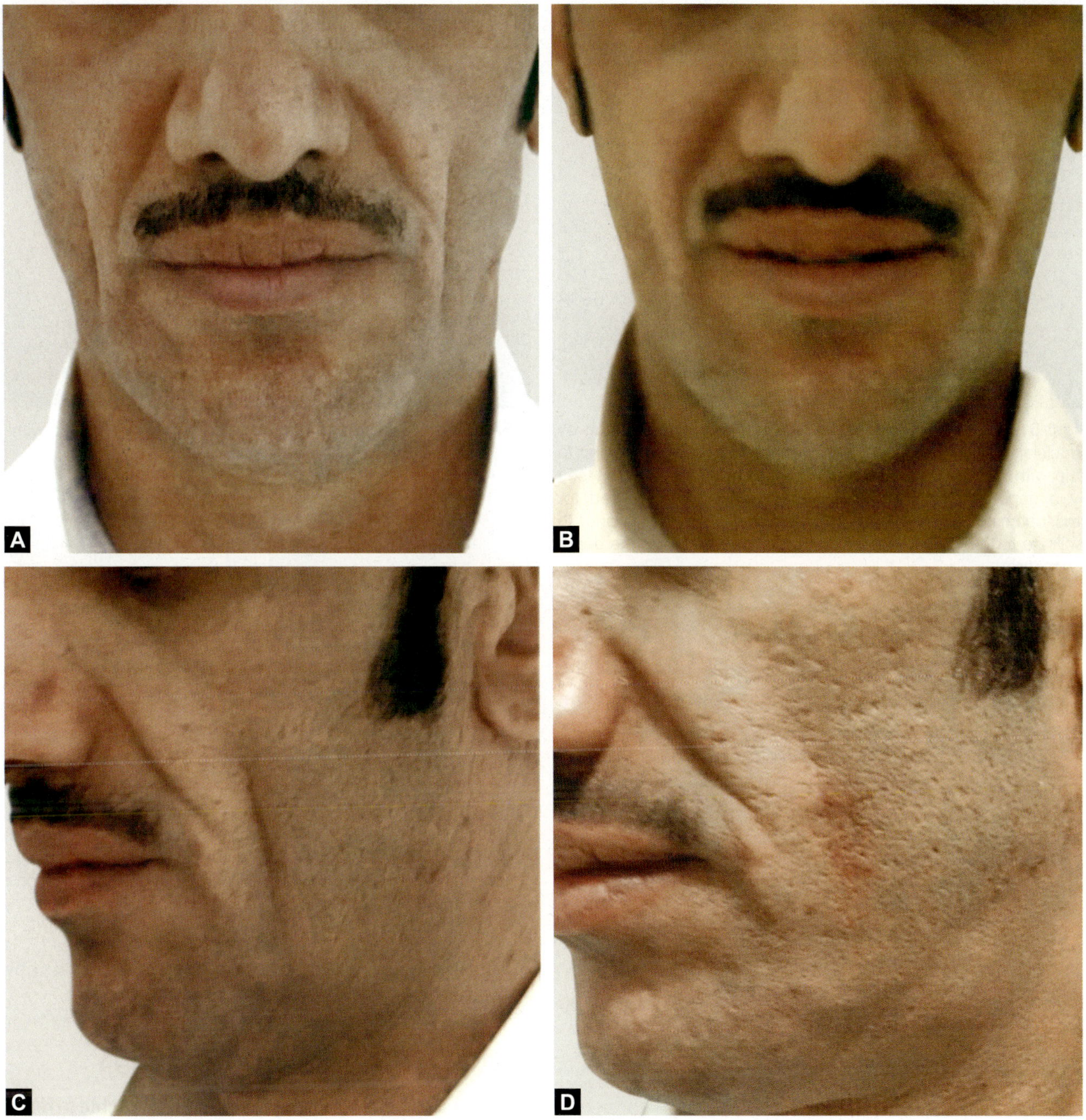

Figs. 51.9A to D: Lipodystrophy treated with a filler of high G prime. Improvement is noted in the hollows of the cheeks after 1 mL was injected into each cheek. Further improvement can be delivered by injecting more volume of product into the cheeks, however a maximum of 2 to 3 mL is injected into each cheek per session. Autologous fat as a filler is more appropriate where larger volumes are required.

- A tower technique has been recently described using a higher viscosity product for the management of acne scars.[10]

Tips

- Avoid high viscosity products as they can form lumps.
- In severe acne scarring, with associated lipoatrophy, first a higher viscosity filler is deposited in the supramuscular plane using a fanning or cross hatching technique to restore volume. Then the superficial individual scars are addressed by depot technique.
- Subcision of the acne scars a week prior to the filler injection is better than subcision on the same day as the formation of a hematoma and edema can obscure the quantity of filler needed for improvement.

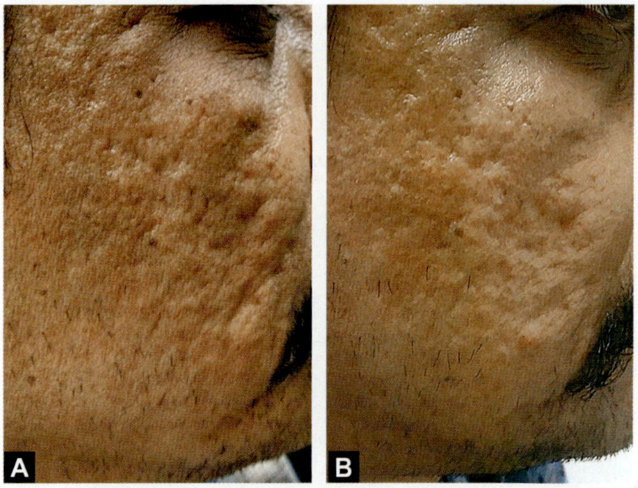

Figs. 51.10A and B: This severe acne scarring was treated by subcision. A week later, HA filler was added by cross hatching to help with the lipoatrophy. Individual large scars were addressed by a depot and/or tower technique. A cannula was used for crosshatching to avoid inadvertent vascular damage and to facilitate further subsicion. A 27 G needle was used for the depot procedure.

- However, the ideal filling agent should be the one that restores volume to the defect by stimulating the surrounding tissue to produce collagen thus giving a long-lasting effect, as opposed to those temporary agents that provide a short-term effect based on the volume of injected material and gets absorbed over a time. Semi-permanent fillers like PLLA and calcium hydroxyapatite have been used to treat acne scars.[11,12] However, in the case of a nodule formation, these materials cannot be dissolved (as HA filler can be, with hyaluronidase). That makes HA a better molecule for a novice injector.

En Coup de Sabre/Localized Scleroderma (Figs. 51.13A and B)

Tips

- Assess the deformity to know the extent of the damage to select the filler appropriately.
- In the forehead area, use a blunt-tipped microcannula to avoid inadvertent intravascular injection.[13]
- Else, serial puncture to deposit filler product on bone is preferred. In areas with deep volume deficits, a tower and bridge technique or a sandwich technique is used to reduce the volume of product being used.

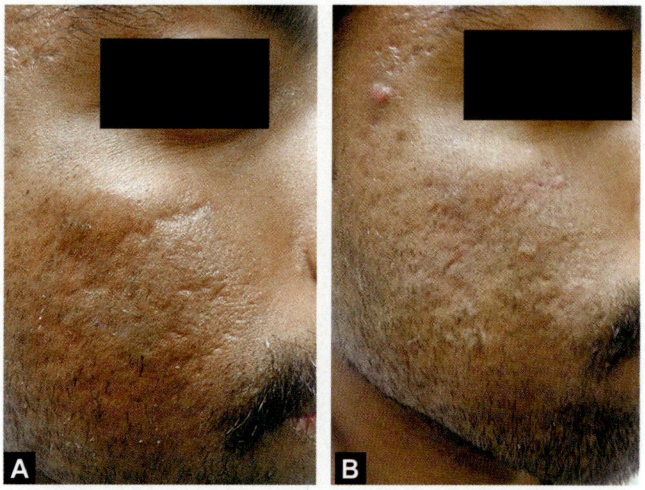

Figs. 51.11A and B: Another case of acne scars treated with filler.

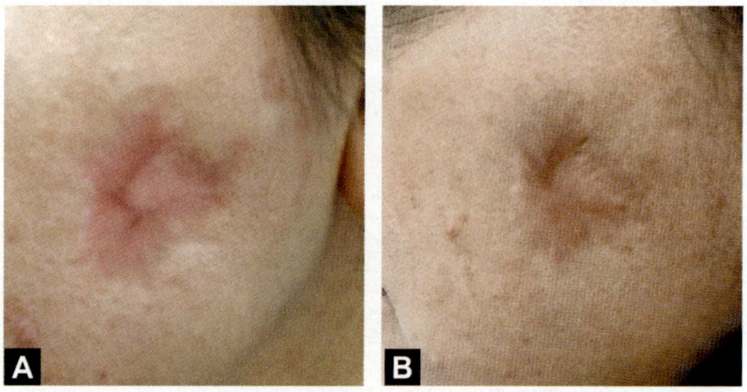

Figs. 51.12A and B: These depressed scars were treated with HA with medium thickness in order to give support. The filler was laid down in a cross hatching method to support the base of the scar. The change in depth as well as color is noted as the hydration of the skin improves.

- In large areas of volume loss, fat grafting is a more viable option.

Depressed Surgical Scar/Scar Edge

- In areas where surgical scars are not amenable to repair, the scar depth and/or edges can be restored with fillers.
- A depot technique/tower technique is used to support the scar.

Tips

- To allow the edges of the scar to merge with the surrounding skin, a filler with a low G Prime can be used to soften the edges.[14]

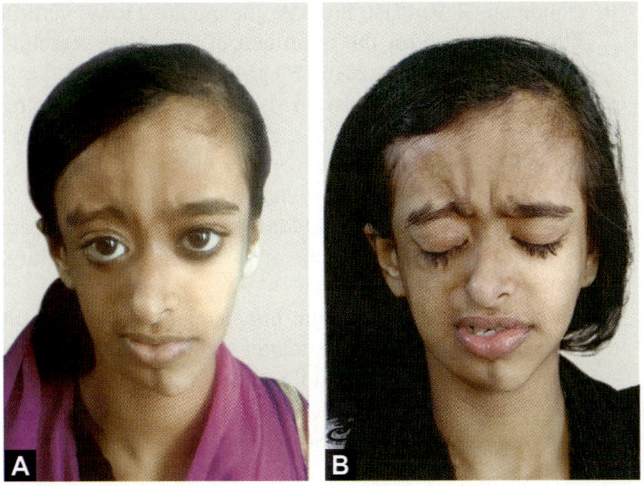

Figs. 51.13A and B: A cannula was used to deliver the filler under the lesion to avoid neurovascular bundle. Product is then massaged to prevent any appearance of bumps. A Q-Switched Nd:YAG laser can help with the hyperpigmentation. Laser can precede the filler or follow after a 2-week interval after filler. Laser is not done on the same day, as edema caused by laser can obscure the deformity.

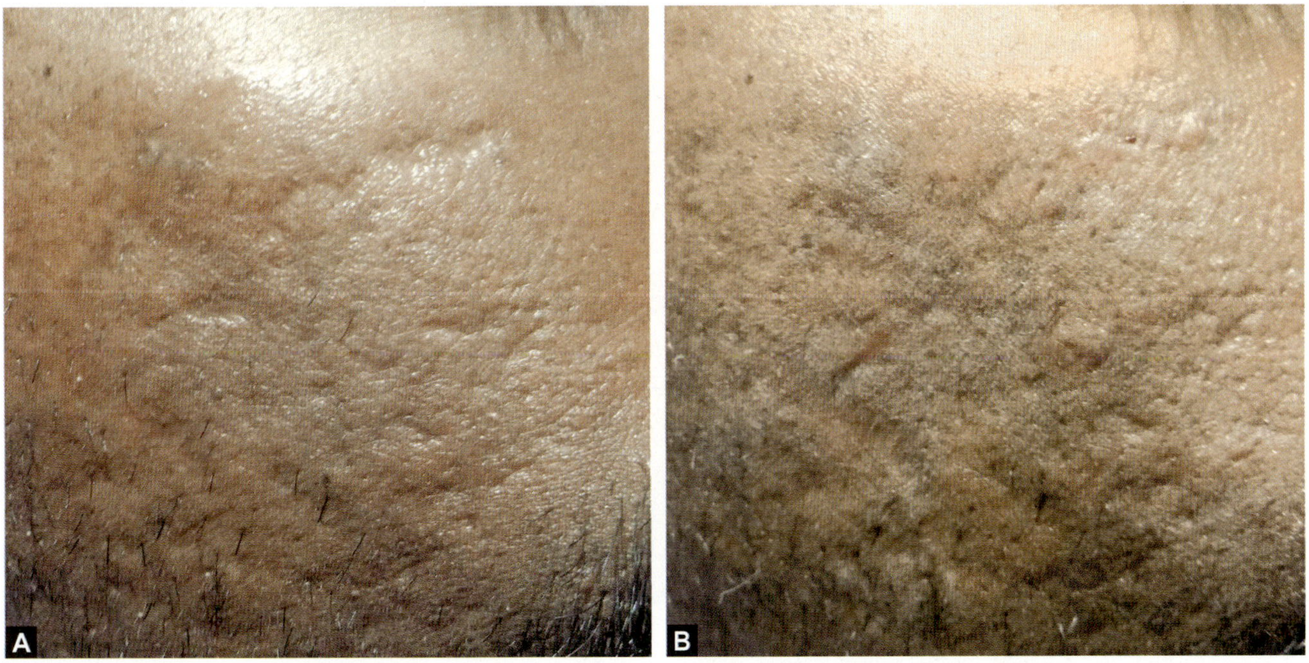

Figs. 51.14A and B: Photography tips for getting better pre- and post images.

- The angle of photography, amount of light falling and contrast are importance while presenting pre and post results for documentation and patient information (Figs. 51.14A and B).

REFERENCES

1. Alberts B, Johnson A, Lewis J, et al. (Eds). The Molecular Biology of the Cell: Cell Junctions, Cell Adhesion, and the Extracellular Matrix 1065. New York: Garland Science;2002.
2. Medical Insight, Inc 2006. Global market for dermal fillers; 2005-2011.
3. Kablik J, Monheit GD, Yu L, et al. Comparative physical properties of hyaluronic acid dermal fillers. Dermatol Surg. 2009;35:302-12.
4. Rzany B, Becker-Wegerich P, Bachmann F, et al. Hyaluronidase in the correction of hyaluronic acid-based fillers: A review and a recommendation for use. J Cosmet Dermatol. 2009;8(4):317-23.
5. Glogou RG, Kane MAC. Effect of injection techniques on the rate of local adverse events in patients implanted with

nonanimal hyaluronic acid gel dermal fillers. Dermatol Surg. 2008;34(1):S105-S9.
6. Fulton J, Caperton C, Weinkle S, et al. Filler injections with the blunt-tip microcannula. J Drugs Dermatol. 2012;11(9):1098-103.
7. Shuck J, Iorio ML, Hung R, et al. Autologous fat grafting and injectable dermal fillers for human immunodeficiency virus-associated facial lipodystrophy: a comparison of safety, efficacy, and long-term treatment outcomes. Plast Reconstr Surg. 2013;131(3):499-506.
8. Strand A, Wolters M. HIV-related lipodystrophy and facial lipoatrophy: the role of RestylaneSubQ in reversing facial wasting. Lipodystrophy Aesthet Surg. J 2006;26(1S):S35-40.
9. Schweiger ES, Riddle CC, Tonkovic-Capin V, et al. Successful treatment with injected hyaluronic acid in a patient with lip asymmetry after surgical correction ofcleft lip. Dermatol Surg. 2008;34(5):717-9.
10. Goodman GJ, Van Den Broek A. The modified tower vertical filler technique for the treatment of post-acne scarring. Australas J Dermatol. 2016;57(1):19-23.
11. Goldberg DJ, Amin S, Hussain M. Acne scar correction using calcium hydroxylapatite in a carrier-based gel. J Cosmet Laser Ther. 2006;8(3):134-6.
12. Beer K. A single-center, open-label study on the use of injectable poly-L-lactic acid for the treatment of moderate to severe scarring from acne or varicella. Dermatol Surg. 2007;33:S159-67.
13. Sivek R, Emer J. Use of a blunt-tipped microcannula for soft tissue filler injection in the treatment of linear scleroderma (en coup de sabre). Dermatol Surg. 2014;40(12):1439-41.
14. Garg S, Dahiya N, Gupta S. Surgical scar revision: An overview. J Cutan Aesthet Surg. 2014;7(1):3-13.

CHAPTER 52

Micropigmentation

Amit Kerure, Satish Udare, Madhulika Mhatre

INTRODUCTION

Tattooing is the art of inserting metabolically inert pigments in a desired pattern and at the optimum level into the skin. The process is performed using manual or electrically driven needles, whereby the pigment that is deposited beyond the epidermis is taken up by the dermal macrophages and fibroblasts where it resides permanently, resulting in the desired change in color and pattern on the skin.[1,2] The terms "micropigmentation" and "dermatography", often used interchangeably, reflect the medical application of tattooing.

History

Tattooing, first introduced by Captain Cook in 1976 literally means implantation of black pigment into the skin.[1,2] Tattooing has been practiced since over 4000 years and was performed in ancient Egypt to indicate worship to a God. In today's world, tattooing is associated with high risk activity, such as drug abuse, substance abuse, interpersonal violence, intercourse at early age, school failures and hence may act as an identity marker for those adolescents involved in high risk activity.[3]

Van der Velden reported the use of tattoos for medical purposes for the first time in 1990. The term micropigmentation denotes the esthetic use of tattooing in medical field, which is being used commonly in dermatology and plastic surgery for various skin conditions of cosmetic importance like vitiligo, burn scars, alopecia patches, etc. The Japanese used dermainjector, a modified apparatus for medical tattooing and termed it as 'Dermatography'.[4]

Definition

Micropigmentation/dermatography is the uniform implantation of minute, metabolically inert pigment granules into the dermis using manual or electrically driven needles.

Basic Principles

- The pigments used are inert, nontoxic, nonallergenic, tissue-stable with a minute particle size of about 6 μm. They are implanted intradermally between the superficial and middle dermis.
- These pigment particles are permanently fixed, both intracellularly and extracellularly within dermal mononuclear cells and collagen fibers, respectively.[2-5] After few years, a small amount of this pigment may be taken up by the regional lymph nodes which causes color fading at the treatment site.
- Immediately after the procedure, the pigment lies mostly intracellular and over a period of time, it migrates into extracellular spaces and lies among collagen bundles, blood vessels, and hair follicles without causing foreign body inflammation.

Pigments

Iron oxide is most commonly used chemical as a pigment. Various other chemicals used for attaining different shades are as follows:[2]

- White: titanium dioxide
- Red: cinnabar, mercuric sulfate (cadmium sulfide added to make red brighter)
- Black: iron oxide
- Yellow: cadmium sulfide
- Camel yellow: iron oxide
- Light brown: iron oxide
- Dark brown: iron oxide.

Instruments

Various machines can be used for micropigmentation ranging from the basic machine that is used by tattoo artists to specialized medical tattoo machines (Fig. 52.1).

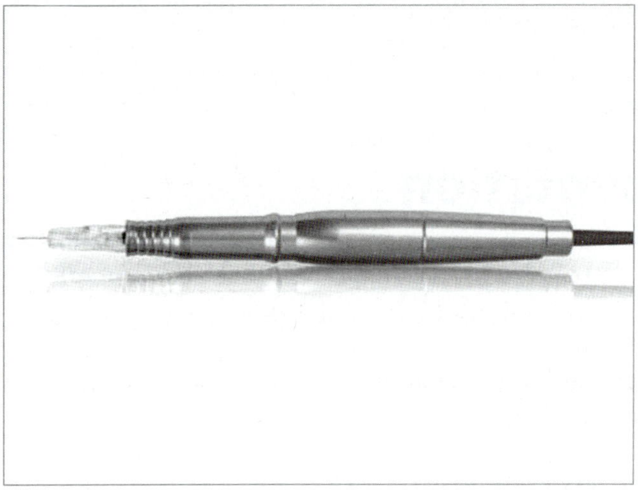

Fig. 52.1: Specialized medical tattooing machine.

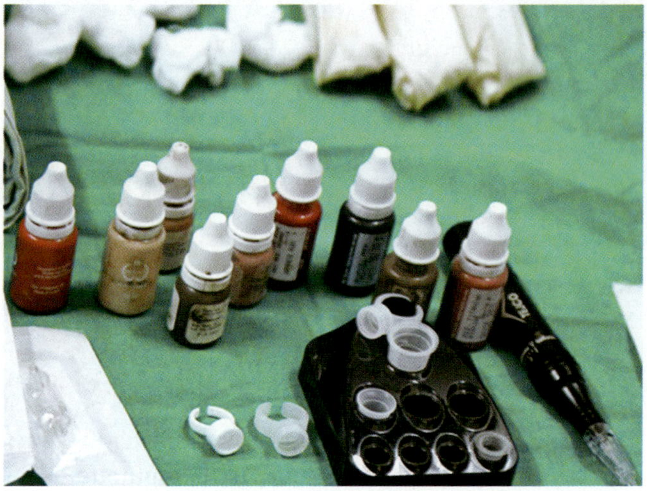

Fig. 52.2: Various inks used for micropigmentation.

The specialized medical tattooing machine has its advantages over its conventional counterpart by being light in weight and allowing precision for accurate needle depth insertion to the ideal depth of 0.8–1.0 mm and thereby also decreasing the pain and discomfort caused to the patient. In the conventional tattoo machine, the needle length has to be set manually by rough estimation by adjusting the needle chamber and locking it on the handle using a screw. Both the machines have provisions for selecting the desired rotor speed as needed.

The conventional tattoo machine has a power adapter attached to a primary unit which has a digital display and dial to adjust the speed of the rotor. The unit is connected to the handle with a wire which supplies the current for achieving the desired speed. The handle has a hollow center through which the needle (single or triple pronged) is inserted and a disposable transparent plastic chamber is placed over the needle which covers the needle. The cylindrical tube at the tip of the plastic chamber acts as reservoir to hold the dye while performing micropigmentation.

The medical tattooing machine consists of a single hand piece which is attached to a power supply. The hand piece has a button to select one of the desired presets of rotor speed. The tip of the hand piece has to be attached to a disposable cartridge which has a prefixed needle inside which can be used for micropigmentation. The cartridge has a conical tip through which the needle projects and it also acts as a reservoir for the ink during the procedure.

The tattoo inks are available in gel base as well as alcohol base. The alcohol-based dye is the one commonly used and in patients with oily scalp, the gel-based dye is preferred. There are various inks available in the markets, that have a wide range in their quality and cost (Fig. 52.2).

Micropigmentation machine is electrically driven and has a reusable detachable cartridge which can be sterilized after every use. These cartridges have a single needle or an assembly of two to seven needles held on a needle bar. The needles are usually of 25 gauge, with an approximate length of 36 mm and a thickness of 0.36 mm, and are placed about 0.3 mm away from each other. The speed ranges from 1,500 to 9,500 strokes per minute, and the depth of needle penetration is adjustable from 1 to 3 mm.

Indications and Patient Selection

Micropigmentation has been routinely done as an adjuvant in reconstructive and cancer surgeries. For dermatological indications, patient selection is very crucial and the patient has to be selected after detailed counseling as in any general considerations.

Micropigmentation as a Therapeutic Treatment in Skin Conditions

- For skin conditions like stable vitiligo, nevus depigmentosus, idiopathic guttate hypomelanosis (IGH), post inflammatory hypopigmentation, etc. Micropigmentation serves as an effective treatment modality.
- Patients who have failed to respond to medical line of therapy, e.g. recalcitrant stable vitiligo not responding to oral or topical modalities and phototherapy.

- Patients not fit for or unwilling for corrective surgery.
- Patients whose quality of life (QOL) is affected by the cosmetic defect.
- Patients needing a quick fix for disturbed QOL, inter-personal relationships, upcoming marriage, professional difficulties because of the defect.

Micropigmentation as a Permanent Make-up

Micropigmentation is an excellent tool for individuals seeking a more permanent and longer lasting cosmetic enhancement or make-up option. However, this option is ideal for:

- Patient with realistic expectations.
- Working women who need makeup regularly and do not have time to hassle with a makeup routine.
- Women with poor eye sight, unsteady hands or trouble applying makeup.
- Patients having less prominent features and would like to enhance them. For example: thin eyebrows.

Micropigmentation in Miscellaneous Conditions

Other conditions where micropigmentation can be used include:

- Scalp micropigmentation in cases of cicatricial or noncicatricial alopecias
- Correction of scars
- Correction of striae

However, such patients should be explained in detail about the expected outcome and should be primed about having realistic expectations.

Contraindications

- Patient with known allergy to pigments
- Major skin disorders or systemic illnesses, such as SLE, bleeding disorders, uncontrolled diabetes
- Seropositive for syphilis and HIV
- History of malignancies especially melanoma
- Patient with unrealistic expectations
- Adult nonconsenting patient
- Pregnancy-though the pigments are mainly iron oxide based, there is no adverse effects on pregnancy outcomes
- Unstable vitiligo
- Children below age of 18, as their disease may get modified in either directions easily
- For nevus depigmentosus, can be done after age of 18.

Preprocedural Counseling

Understanding the patient's motivation for surgery and their expectations of the outcomes are the keys to achieving satisfied patients postoperatively:

- Managing the patient's expectations requires full patient education
- Second consultations are almost always necessary preoperatively
- Be sure to discuss your policy for revision surgery during the preoperative period.
- Postoperative follow-up should include detailed written instructions and the surgeon's contact details
- Regular follow-up visits are needed during the early postoperative period to assist the patient through the recovery
- Unhappy patients or those with unsatisfactory outcomes should be seen more often to improve communication.

Micropigmentation is usually done either for correction of underlying conditions or as a permanent makeup.When it is done for correction, one has to explain the limitations of micropigmentation to the patient. Micropigmentation can achieve excellent results and the corrections might be undetectable but in reality it will never match the skin color by 100%. The desired result may need multiple sessions and this should be informed before the procedure.

Micropigmentation is a procedure for correcting small deformities and not for larger defects. It is very difficult to achieve good results on a large area. Micropigmentation for larger areas should be undertaken only when all other treatment modalities have failed to achieve the normal skin appearance.

For permanent makeup, one has to understand the patient's expectations from the procedure. Unrealistic expectations should not be entertained.

Preprocedure Work-up

- Routine blood investigations should be done including CT, BT, HIV 1, 2 and Hep B
- Drugs like aspirin should be stopped 3 days prior to the procedure.
- Patch test is advisable to rule out any pigment allergy if present
- Medical history, allergies and intolerances to medications, anesthesia or other agents (specify reaction type), surgical history
- History of trauma (major) and risk factors for development of surgical site infection (e.g., smoking,

diabetes, obesity, malnutrition, chronic skin disease) should be elicited
- Skin should be calm, free from any rashes, infections or healing scars.
- Avoid tanning and procedures like chemical peels before procedure.
- Avoid consumption of medicines like aspirin, smoking, drinking coffee, before procedure.

Preparation of Pigment

Achieving exact color matching is difficult and is a matter of experience and expertise. With practice, one can achieve an almost similar color which can give excellent results.

Steps

- Sterilized container with a fixed base should be used to prepare the pigment. A scoop shaped stirrer can be used for mixing as well as transfer of pigment to the treated site
- While preparing the pigment for micropigmentation, pigment with a lighter shade is taken as the base color first and a darker shade of the same color is added drop-by-drop and mixed simultaneously, till it matches the skin color. Stirrer can be used to mix the two pigments.
- During the color matching process, the prepared pigment is put on the border of normal skin and the area to be treated to check the color match with the normal skin. With every addition of new colored pigment or a darker shade, this step is repeated till the desired colored pigment is prepared. For example, If beige color is taken as a base and dark brown color is added drop-by-drop, simultaneously mixing with a stirrer and similarity checked by applying on the treatment site every time additional drops are added (Fig. 52.3).

TIPS AND TRICKS

- First assess the size of the area to be treated and prepare the pigment accordingly.
- Always treat the entire affected area in one session to avoid difference in the pigment color
- Shake the pigment bottle before starting in order to disperse the pigment evenly and to get a thick homogenous pigment.
- Glycerin can be added, if the pigment is too thick or too dry.
- Prepare a slightly darker shade than the surrounding skin as the color fades by 30–50% after the first sitting
- Patch test is advisable.

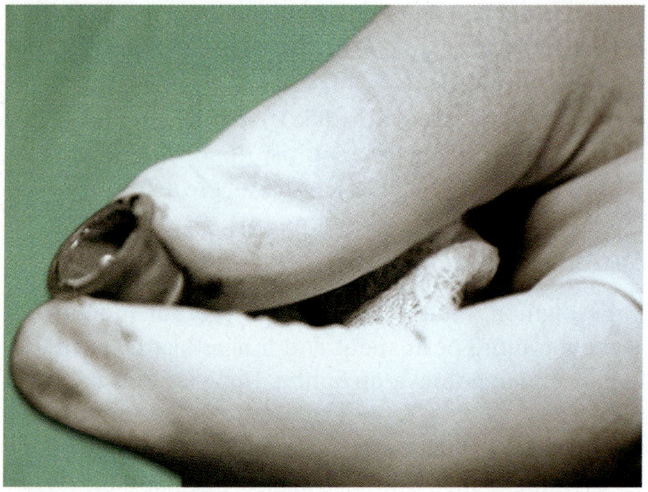

Fig. 52.3: Mixing up of colors to get desired color match in a sterile container.

Procedure Steps

- Preprocedure photos and consent are a must before the actual procedure.
- Make the patient lie down comfortably. Surgeon's position should be comfortable and site to be treated should be easily accessible
- Explain the procedure to the patient in detail before starting and answer doubts, if any

Site Preparation

- Clean the area with spirit and betadine.
- Mark the border of the lesion to be treated with a skin marker
- Use a new cartridge of appropriate number of needles for the micropigmentation machine.
  - Array of needles available
  - Selection of needles
  - Tips and tricks how to choose needle arrays.

Anesthesia

Topical EMLA cream under occlusion is used one hour prior to the procedure as in Figure 52.4. In vascular areas like face or lips, injectable anesthesia like 2% lignocaine can be used along with adrenaline.

Generally the pain is tolerable by the patient.

Steps

- Apply a thick paste of pigment over the site to be treated and spread uniformly. If the area is larger, treat the area

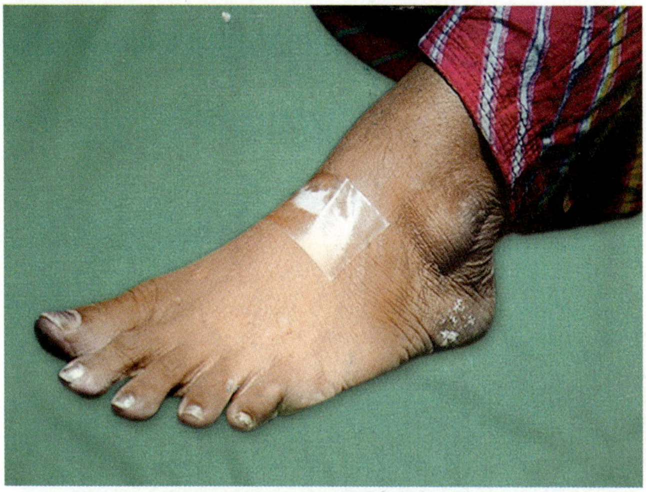

Fig. 52.4: EML application one hour before the procedure to achieve adequate anesthesia.

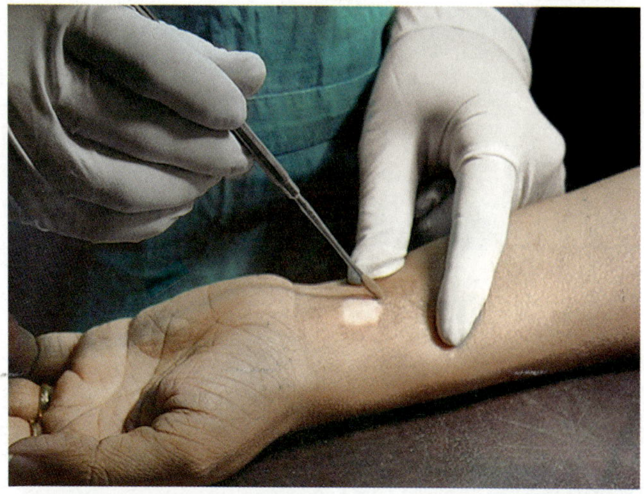

Fig. 52.5: Application of pigment paste as a thick film over the patch.

in parts (variation—pigment can be sucked at the tip of cartridge by dipping it in the pigment when the machine is on Figure 52.5).

- Make sure the area treated is in the horizontal plane.
- Start the machine at around 1500–4500 rpm and keep the length of the needle around 1.2–1.5 mm. The length can be reduced to 1 mm for lesions on face and can be increased accordingly, if used on thicker areas like theback.
- Hold the machine at a 90° angle to the skin surface and in a pen holding manner (Fig. 52.6).
- Stretch the area to be treated with the thumb and index finger of the left hand while machine is being operated by the right hand.
- Keep it on the surface of skin firmly and gently, without pressing it too forcefully. Rotate the machine slowly in a circular and overlapping manner.
- Avoid making big loops during circular motion. Speed of movement should be slow and steady.
- Pinpoint bleeding will be visible on the area where repeated movements have been done.
- After completing the tattooing over the patch where pigment was spread, wipe out the pigment with Vaseline. Look out for areas where pigment insertion is not uniform or if any skip areas are present.
- Reapply the pigment over those areas only and repeat the tattooing in the same manner only over that area.
- If the treatment area is larger, tattooing should be done in parts but the whole area should be treated in one sitting to avoid any pigment mismatch.

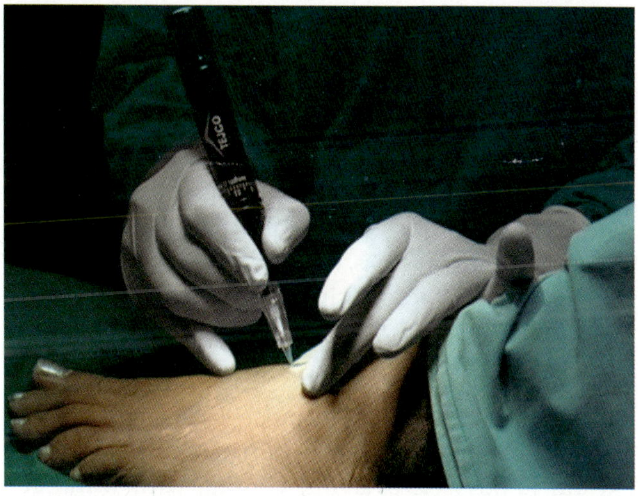

Fig. 52.6: Machine held at a 90° angle to the skin surface in a pen holding manner.

- Make sure that uniform pigmentation is achieved by the end of the procedure.

TIPS AND TRICKS

Excessive bleeding while tattooing can cause pigment dilution. If more bleeding occurs, wipe out with Vaseline petroleum jelly and press it with a gauze piece for few seconds and resume the tattooing.

For Permanent Makeup

- Lips (Fig. 52.7A)
- Eyebrows (Fig. 52.7B)
- Scalp micropigmentation
- Artificial mole.

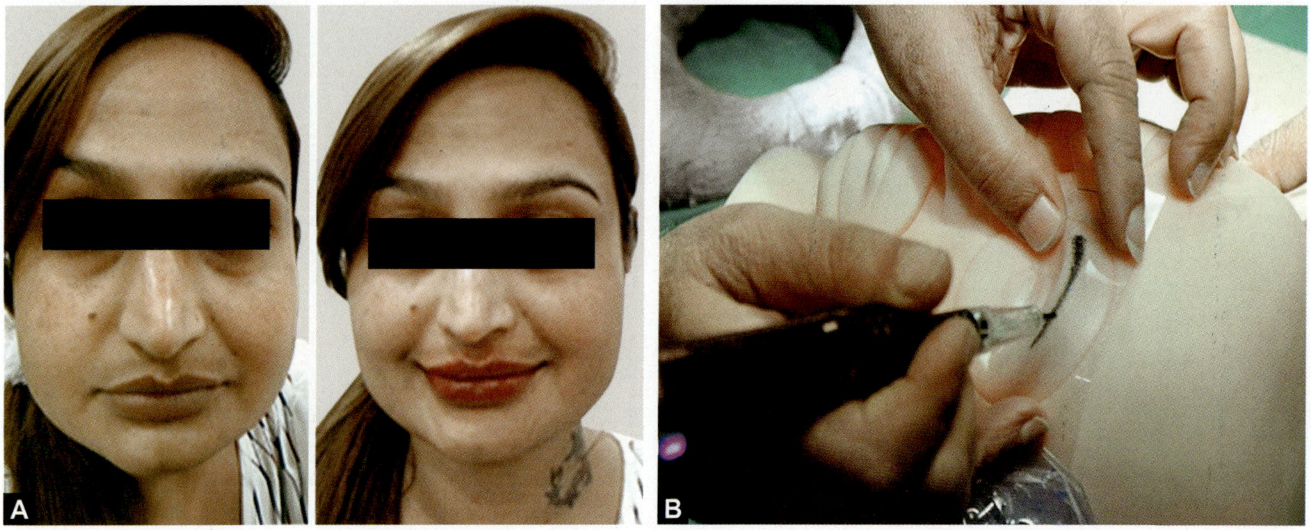

Figs. 52.7A and B: (A) Permanent make up for lips before and after; (B) Demonstration of micropigmentation of eyebrow on a mannequin.

After Procedure

There may be some redness, swelling and sometimes bruising lasting up to a few hours to few days. The color may appear darker and brighter than the healed and final result.

After the first week of peeling, the color will be lighter by 30%–50%. After 3–4 weeks, when the color becomes softer, lighter and even, a second sitting can be performed.

Postprocedure Care

A pressure dressing, along with prophylactic antibiotics and anti-inflammatory drugs, may be given postoperatively. Patient is advised to avoid contact with water for 3–4 days. The postprocedure crust and scab falls off in about 7 days. The patient can be reviewed after 4 weeks to assess, if any further corrective touch-up micropigmentation is required.

Adverse Effects

The immediate adverse effects—ecchymosis, crusting, and edema lasting for 2 to 3 days, reactivation of herpes infection, secondary bacterial infection, and contact allergy to pigments can be seen in the first week following the procedure. A number of infections have been known to be transmitted through the repeated use of the same needles from one patient to another without proper sterilization.

Other risks involved may be photosensitization allergy, mainly to cadmium sulfate, and blurring of pigment (color leaks from original site).

Existing Evidence

Recalcitrant lesions of vitiligo, especially over distal digits, lips (Figs. 52.8A and B), hands, wrists, axillae, elbows, perianal areas, lower legs, mucosae, and mucocutaneous junctions.

- Nevus depigmentosus (Figs. 52.9A to D)
- Postinflammatory hypopigmentation
- Idiopathic guttate hypomelanosis
- To camouflage FUT scar and hairless patches.
- Nipple-areola reconstruction (Fig. 52.10)
- Enhancement of eyebrows and eyelashes
- Esthetic improvements of scars and skin grafts (Figs. 52.11A and B).

Micropigmentation can be a good therapeutic method for FPHL. Unlike in MPB, in FPHL the overall hair density is reduced without the hairline retreating (Fig. 52.12).

The reduction in hair density is noticed when the scalp is seen through the hair, commonly referred to as a "see-through appearance."

In such cases, micropigmentation can decrease the "see-through appearance" and is a great help in camouflaging the intensity of the hair loss.

Performing micropigmentation alone or in addition to hair transplantation can bring about very good improvements.

Complications

The incidence of reported complications in micropigmentation is relatively rare in comparison with other cosmetic

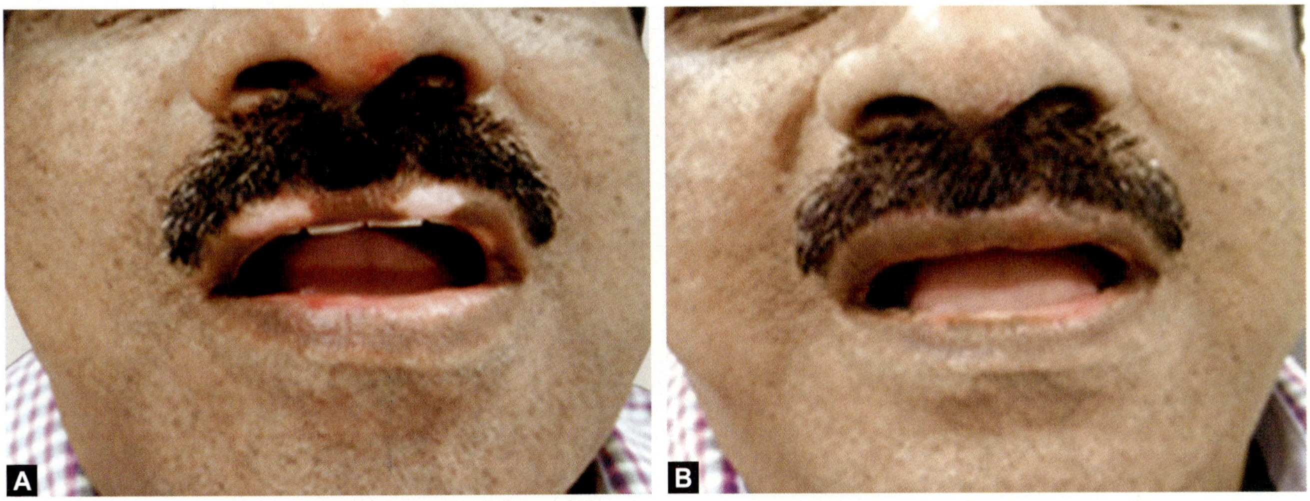

Figs. 52.8A and B: Recalcitrant lip vitiligo (A) Before (B) After micropigmentation.

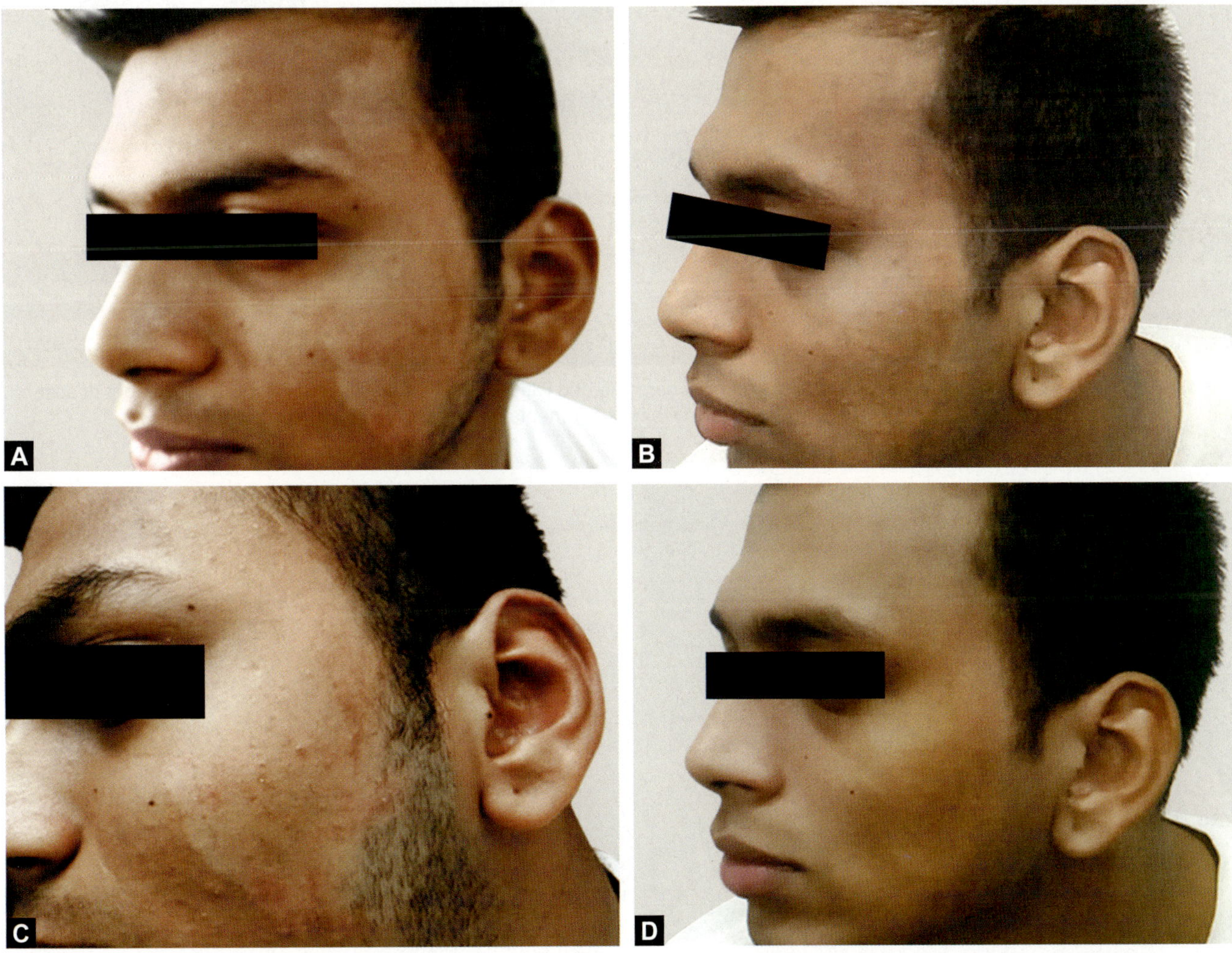

Figs. 52.9A to D: (A) Nevus depigmentosus; (B and C) Partial color match; (D) Satisfactory color match achieved with micropigmentation.

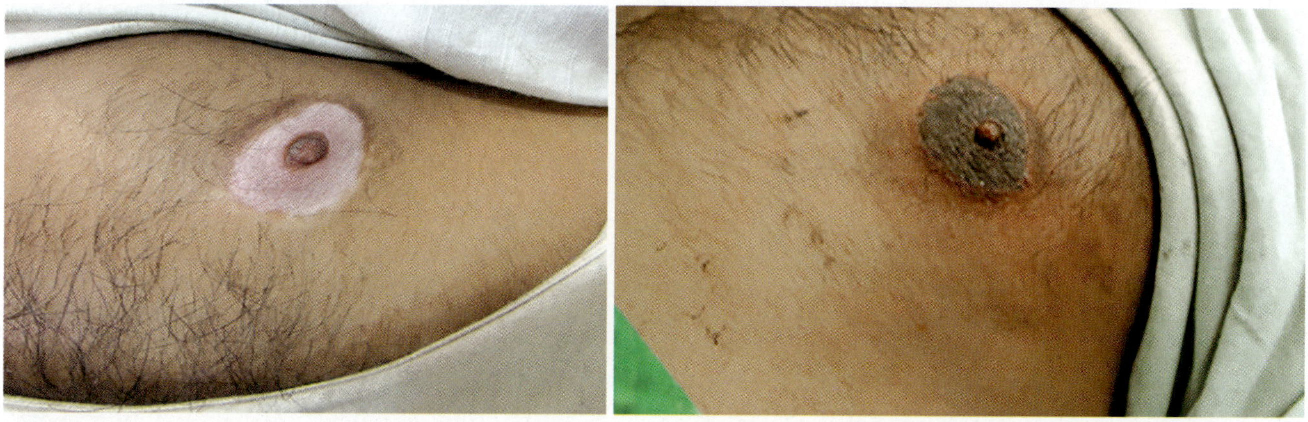

Fig. 52.10: Vitiligo of the areola-excellent result with micropigmentation.

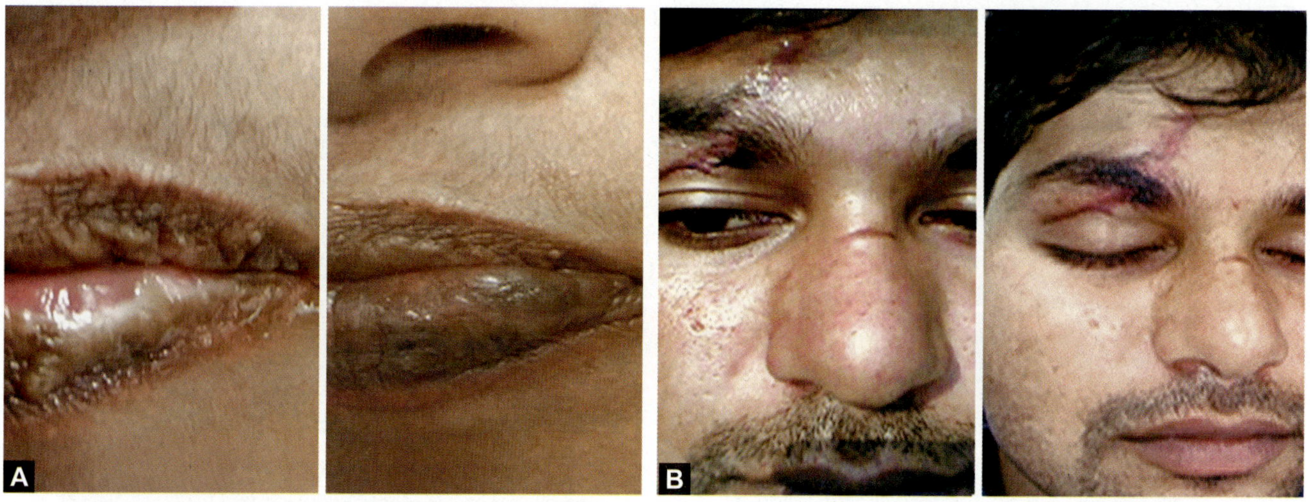

Figs. 52.11A and B: (A) Color mismatch following skin graft camouflaged with micropigmentation. (B) Partial improvement of scar on forehead with micropigmentation.

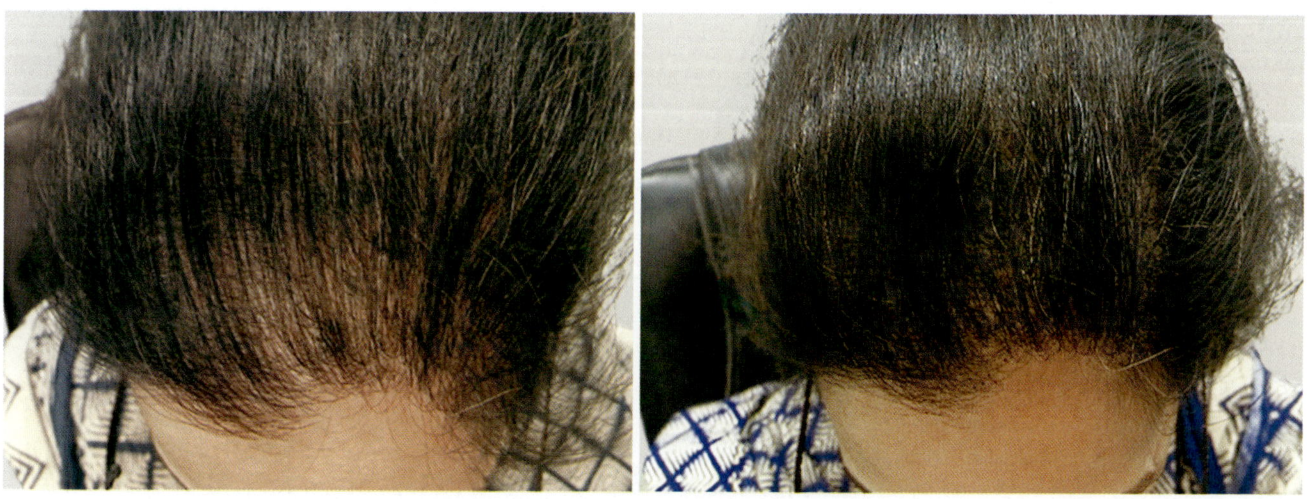

Fig. 52.12: FPHL before and after micropigmentation.
Courtesy: Dr Rachita Dhurat, Mumbai, Maharashtra, India

surgeries. The complications may occur when unsterile pigments are used or if the procedure is performed without sterile precautions. Bacterial or viral infection can occur at the site of procedure. Infections like mycobacterial or fungal can take months or years to develop.

Allergic reactions to the micropigmentation pigment can be seen but this is more common when mercury salt (red), cadmium (yellow), cobalt (blue) and dichromate (green)-based pigments are used. Also, allergic reactions can occur, if the pigment is contaminated by nickel sulfate.

Koebnerization can occur in skin diseases like vitiligo, lichen planus or psoriasis and the disease may exacerbate.[5]

Micropigmentation can cause granulomatous reactions which can be present either as sarcoidal granulomas or can also present as other granulomatous reactions like foreign body granulomas.[6]

Benign lesions like milia, epidermal cysts and seborrheic keratosis are other possible complications which may occur due to micropigmentation; and very rarely malignant lesions, such as malignant melanoma, basal cell carcinoma, squamous cell carcinoma, keratoacanthoma and dermatofibrosarcoma protuberans may be seen.[7] Black pigment containing benzopyrene can be carcinogenic.

REFERENCES

1. Singh AK, Karki D. Micropigmentation: tattooing for the treatment of lip vitiligo. J Plast Reconstr Aesthet Surg. 2010;63(6):988-91.
2. Traquina AC. Micropigmentation as an adjuvant in cosmetic surgery of the scalp. Dermatol Surg. 2001;27(2): 123-8.
3. Garg G, Thami GP. Micropigmentation: tattooing for medical purposes. Dermatol Surg. 2005;31(8 Pt 1):928-31.
4. DeCuyper C. Permanent makeup: indications and complications. Clin Dermatol. 2008;26(1):30-4.
5. Tiziano JP. Dermography: a complement to esthetic surgery. Ann Chir Plast Esthet. 1990;35(6):489-95.
6. Singh AK, Karki DJ. Micropigmentation: tattooing for the treatment of lip vitiligo. Plast Reconstr Aesthet Surg. 2010;63(6):988-91.
7. Halder RM, Pham HN, Breadon JY, et al. Micropigmentation for the treatment of vitiligo. J Dermatol Surg Oncol. 1989;15(10):1092-8.

Index

Page numbers followed by *b* refer to box, *f* refer to figure, *fc* refer to flowchart and *t* refer to table.

D

E

G

H

I

J

K

N

O

P

T